PSYCHIATRY
UPDATE

S0-EDQ-550

AMERICAN PSYCHIATRIC ASSOCIATION

Annual Review

— Vol. 6

| Bipolar Disorders |
| Neuroscience Techniques |
| Differential Therapeutics |
| Violence and the Violent Patient |
| Psychiatric Epidemiology |
| Psychopharmacology |

CONTINUING MEDICAL EDUCATION SUPPLEMENT

Editors

Robert E. Hales, M.D. and Allen J. Frances, M.D.

Associate Editors

Janet M. Anastasi, Lise Coty, M.D., and Arthur M. James, M.D.

APA Office of Education

Carolyn B. Robinowitz, M.D., Sara F. Carroll, M.S. and Jean M. Forrest

Contributors

The chapter authors of the *Annual Review: Volume 6* contributed questions for the development of this supplement.

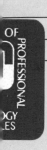

Continuing Education Credit—The American Psychiatric Association designates this continuing medical education activity for up to 24 credit hours in Category I of the Physician's Recognition Award of the American Medical Association and for the CME requirement of the APA.

CATEGORY I CME CREDIT

The American Psychiatric Association is accredited by the Accreditation Council for Continuing Medical Education (ACCME) to sponsor continuing medical education for physicians, and the use of *Annual Review, Volume 6* in conjunction with the completion and submission of this CME Supplement meets the criteria for continuing medical education, Category I credit.

A participant earns up to 24 Category I CME credit hours following the submission and subsequent scoring of the completed answer sheet. The completion of each of the six sections in the "Supplement" carries with it four Category I credits. Participants may complete as many or as few sections as they wish and earn their CME credits accordingly; i.e., one section = 4 CME credits; two sections = 8 credits; three sections = 12 credits; etc.

ALL INDIVIDUAL SCORES KEPT CONFIDENTIAL

GENERAL INSTRUCTIONS

1. Please enter your name, address, APA membership number (if applicable), and telephone number in the appropriate spaces on the answer sheet provided.
2. This booklet contains two types of questions. There are special directions for each type of question inside the booklet. Be sure that you understand the directions before attempting to answer any questions.
3. After you have decided upon the best answer for a question, blacken the circle containing the corresponding letter on the answer sheet. Use only #2 pencils (soft lead) and be sure that each mark is black and completely fills the answer space.
4. Only one choice should be marked for each question. If you change an answer, be sure that all previous marks are erased completely.
5. After you have completed the answer sheet, check it to make sure that the answers marked correspond to the answers you have chosen, that there is only one mark for each question, and that there are no extra marks on the answer sheet.
6. Mail the answer sheet to:

American Psychiatric Association
Office of Education
1400 K Street N.W.
Washington, D.C. 20005

SECTION ONE: BIPOLAR DISORDERS

1. A patient who has been treated with lithium for several years is noted to have breakthrough depressive episodes. His blood level, taken 12 hours after his last dose, is 1.2 mEq/L. Appropriate treatment responses include all of the following *EXCEPT*:

   A. Addition of a tricyclic antidepressant.
   B. Addition of thyroid hormone.
   C. Substitution with carbamazepine.
   D. Addition of a monoamine oxidase inhibitor.
   E. Addition of a neuroleptic drug.

2. In most epidemiological studies the incidence of suicide in the general population has been found to be greatest in:

   A. Late summer.
   B. Mid-fall.
   C. Mid-winter.
   D. Late spring.
   E. None of the above.

1

For each of the questions or incomplete statements below, **ONE** or **MORE** of the suggested answers or completions given is correct. On the answer sheet fill in the space containing

    A   if ONLY 1, 2, and 3 are correct,
    B   if ONLY 1 and 3 are correct,
    C   if ONLY 2 and 4 are correct,
    D   if ONLY 4 is correct,
    E   if ALL are correct.

**FOR EACH QUESTION FILL IN ONLY ONE SPACE
ON YOUR ANSWER SHEET**

Directions Summarized				
(A)	**(B)**	**(C)**	**(D)**	**(E)**
1,2,3	1,3	2,4	4	All are
only	only	only	only	correct

3.   Which of the following are correct about the lifetime incidence of bipolar disorder?

   1. It is approximately 1% for men.
   2. It is higher in people in lower socioeconomic classes.
   3. It is similar in men and women.
   4. It is equal to the lifetime incidence of unipolar depression.

4.   Which of the following are correct concerning mania?

   1. Organic causes of mania are more common than functional causes.
   2. Hypomania is usually diagnosed with high reliability.
   3. A diagnosis of bipolar disorder, manic requires the presence of psychotic symptoms.
   4. Functional mania is unlikely to occur for the first time after the age of 50.

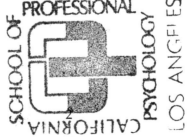

5. In general, the "gold standard" predictor(s) of a favorable treatment response in patients with bipolar disorder is/are:

   1. Neuroendocrine output and response.
   2. Calcium increase in the CSF.
   3. Increase of somatostatin in the CSF.
   4. Clinical criteria.

6. An increased frequency of cycles between mania and depression occurs as a long-term effect in patients treated with:

   1. Tricyclic antidepressants.
   2. Hypermetabolic doses of thyroid hormone.
   3. Monoamine oxidase inhibitors.
   4. Carbamazepine.

7. Acute mania may be effectively treated by administering:

   1. Lithium.
   2. Carbamazepine.
   3. Neuroleptic drugs.
   4. Electroconvulsive therapy.

8. Lithium holidays have been advocated for:

   1. Minimizing long-term side effects.
   2. Increasing compliance by having drug-free periods as a reward.
   3. Preparation for pregnancy.
   4. Stimulating the immune system.

9. Factors involved in a patient's ability to cope with suicidal thoughts include:

   1. A capacity to control behavior; the person can stand pain or impulsivity.
   2. A capacity to relate readily and in a meaningful way to someone else.
   3. A motivation for help and willingness to work actively on the problem.
   4. The variety of resources which facilitate the therapeutic process and the transition back to a stable life pattern.

10. Correct statements concerning how to develop a positive therapeutic alliance with bipolar patients include:

    1. The physician should over-estimate treatment results of a particular drug.
    2. The physician should not educate the patient about his/her illness.
    3. The physician should emphasize that the patient and not the physician will determine whether a successful treatment outcome occurs.
    4. The physician should explain that drug trials are experimental and that poor responses are not defeats.

11. Research suggests which of the following drug(s) to be sound treatment options for the refractory bipolar patient?

    1. Phenobarbital.
    2. Valproic acid.
    3. Phenytoin.
    4. Carbamazepine.

12. Increased carbamazepine levels and toxicity may be produced by:

    1. Erythromycin.
    2. Phenobarbital.
    3. Isoniazid.
    4. Primidone.

13. Side effects of carbamazepine include:

    1. Decreased white blood cell count.
    2. Hepatitis.
    3. Agranulocytosis.
    4. Hyperthyroidism.

14. Factors strongly associated with rapid cycling affective disorders include:

    1. Hypothyroidism.
    2. Women.
    3. Tricyclic antidepressants.
    4. Bipolar course.

15. Depressive symptoms most commonly found in seasonal affective disorder include:

    1. Insomnia.
    2. Weight gain.
    3. Agitation.
    4. Carbohydrate-craving.

16. The importance of sleep in the pathophysiology of affective illness is suggested by observations that:

    1. Short REM sleep latency is a specific diagnostic marker of depression.
    2. Total sleep deprivation is capable of inducing temporary improvement in depression.
    3. Selective REM sleep deprivation is capable of inducing improvement in depression.
    4. Most effective antidepressant drugs reduce sleep duration.

DIRECTIONS (Items 17-23):
Each of the questions or incomplete statements below is followed by suggested answers. Select the **ONE** that is **BEST** in each case and fill in the circle containing the corresponding letter on the answer sheet.

---

17. Which statement best describes research findings on the relationship of plasma haloperidol, butaperazine, and fluphenazine levels to clinical response?

   A. There is an inverted U-shaped relationship between plasma levels and clinical response such that non-responders usually have either very low plasma levels or very high levels and responders have intermediate plasma levels.
   B. There is no relationship between plasma levels and clinical response.
   C. There is an inverted U-shaped relationship between clinical response and plasma levels such that non-responders usually have intermediate plasma levels and responders have either very low plasma levels or very high levels.
   D. Many non-responders have low plasma levels and many responders have high levels.
   E. Many responders have low plasma levels and many non-responders high levels.

18. Based on combined data, the urinary excretion of MHPG in unipolar depressed patients is:

   A. Substantially below that of a control population.
   B. Approximately equal to age and sex-matched controls.
   C. Substantially above that of a control population.
   D. Approximately equal to bipolar, manic patients.
   E. None of the above.

7

19. Which statement(s) correctly reflect(s) recent research findings on the ability to use urinary MHPG levels to predict differential response to imipramine and amitriptyline?

A. In both unipolar and bipolar patients, there is no relationship between urinary MHPG levels and response to amitriptyline.
B. Normal or elevated urinary MHPG levels predict response to amitriptyline in bipolar patients.
C. Low urinary MHPG levels predict favorable response to imipramine in bipolar patients.
D. Low urinary MHPG predicts a favorable response of unipolar depressed patients to imipramine.
E. None of the above.

20. Which one of these findings is not associated with REM sleep?

A. Dreaming.
B. Loss of temperature regulation.
C. Rapid eye movements.
D. Continued normal muscle tone.
E. None of the above.

21. Which of the following sites are associated with NREM sleeping?

A. Basal forebrain.
B. Dorsal raphe nucleus.
C. Solitary tract nucleus of the medulla.
D. All of the above.
E. None of the above.

22. Which of the following is thought to be associated with circadian rhythmicity?

A. Suprachiasmatic nucleus.
B. Pontine reticular activating formation.
C. Occipital cortex.
D. Dorsal raphe nucleus.
E. Globus pallidus.

23. Which of the following medications is contraindicated in sleep apnea?

   A. Lithium.
   B. Sedative/hypnotics.
   C. Antidepressants.
   D. Methoxyprogesterone.
   E. Ritalin.

DIRECTIONS (Items 24-34):

For each of the questions or incomplete statements below, **ONE** or **MORE** of the suggested answers or completions given is correct. On the answer sheet fill in the space containing

A   if ONLY 1, 2, and 3 are correct,
B   if ONLY 1 and 3 are correct,
C   if ONLY 2 and 4 are correct,
D   if ONLY 4 is correct,
E   if ALL are correct.

**FOR EACH QUESTION FILL IN ONLY ONE SPACE
ON YOUR ANSWER SHEET**

		Directions Summarized		
(A)	**(B)**	**(C)**	**(D)**	**(E)**
1,2,3	**1,3**	**2,4**	**4**	**All are**
only	**only**	**only**	**only**	**correct**

24. Performance of the dexamethasone suppression test includes which of the following steps:

1. Administration of dexamethasone 1 mg p.o. at 11 p.m.
2. Blood sample the next day at 4 p.m.
3. Blood sample the next day at 8 a.m.
4. Administration of dexamethasone 1 mg p.o. the next day at 4 p.m.

25. Which of the following statements about the dexamethasone suppression test are true?

1. The test gives false-positive results in the face of severe illness of the heart, kidneys or liver, or pregnancy.
2. The test gives false-positives in patients taking dilantin, phenobarbital, or birth control pills and in chronic alcoholics.
3. Normal suppression is plasma cortisol less than 5 ug/dl at 8 a.m.
4. The test is affected by concurrent administration of tricyclic antidepressants.

26. Which of the following statements about psychiatric medication is/are true?

    1. Lithium carbonate may cause goiter, hypothyroidism, and hypercalcemia with hyperparathyroidism.
    2. The prolactin stimulating potencies of the phenothiazines correlate with their clinical effectiveness.
    3. Galactorrhea may be caused by reserpine, opiates, tricyclics, and phenothiazines.
    4. Neuroleptics may increase the risk for breast cancer in women.

27. Which of the following statements about psychiatric manifestations of endocrine disease is/are true?

    1. Patients with hyperthyroidism may display apathy or anxiety.
    2. The behavior of hypothyroid subjects may resemble mental retardation or depression.
    3. Cushing's syndrome may present with depressed mood, impaired concentration, and impaired memory.
    4. Hypoparathyroidism may be accompanied by nervousness and organic mental disorders.

28. The concept of neuromodulation of immunity is supported by:

    1. Receptors for neurotransmitters on lymphocytes.
    2. Stress effects on immunity.
    3. The influence of hypothalamic lesions on humoral and cell mediated immune responses.
    4. Direct innervation of lymphoid tissue.

11

29. Three dimensional functional brain imaging techniques include:

    1. Single Photon Emission Computed Tomography (SPECT).
    2. Xenon-133 regional cerebral blood flow (rCBF).
    3. Positron Emission Tomography (PET).
    4. Computerized EEG and evoked potential mapping.

30. "Organizing theories" in psychiatric research have focused interest in the following brain regions:

    1. Left hemisphere.
    2. Frontal lobes.
    3. Temporal lobes.
    4. Occipital lobes.

31. The following brain imaging techniques use radioactive isotopes:

    1. Positron Emission Tomography (PET).
    2. Magnetic Resonance Imaging (MRI).
    3. Single Photon Emission Computed Tomography (SPECT).
    4. Computerized EEG and evoked potential mapping.

32. The following techniques can provide measures of brain blood flow:

    1. Positron Emission Tomography (PET).
    2. Xenon-133 regional cerebral blood flow (rCBF).
    3. Single Photon Emission Computed Tomography (SPECT).
    4. Computerized EEG and evoked potential mapping.

33. Patients with clinically significant depression who are hospitalized, when compared to controls, have been shown to have:

    1. Increased lymphocyte responses to mitogen stimulation.
    2. Increased frequency of antinuclear antibodies.
    3. Increased total number of B cells.
    4. Decreased number of lymphocytes.

34. Research concerning the relationship between stress and humoral and cell-mediated immunity has shown that:

    1. Acute exposure to a stressor may suppress humoral immune responses.
    2. Acute exposure to a stressor may suppress cell-mediated immune responses.
    3. Extended exposure to a stressor may enhance humoral immune responses.
    4. Extended exposure to a stressor may enhance cell-mediated immune responses.

SECTION THREE: DIFFERENTIAL THERAPEUTICS

> **DIRECTIONS (Items 35-44):**
> Each of the questions or incomplete statements below is followed
> by suggested answers. Select the **ONE** that is **BEST** and fill in the
> circle containing the corresponding letter on the answer sheet.

35. The strongest indication for family/marital treatment is:

    A. A cooperative family.
    B. When the patient's chief complaint is an eating disorder.
    C. When the identified patient is a child.
    D. When the patient's chief complaint is a family/marital
       problem.
    E. To remove stigma from the identified patient.

36. The median length of outpatient psychotherapy in the United
    States, according to Taube and colleagues, is:

    A. 6 sessions.
    B. 16 sessions.
    C. 36 sessions.
    D. 50 sessions.
    E. 150 sessions.

37. There are convincing data supporting the special effectiveness of:

    A. The 50-minute hour.
    B. Twice a week vs once a week psychotherapy.
    C. The use of the couch in psychoanalysis.
    D. Continuous vs intermittent psychotherapy.
    E. None of the above.

38. The number of psychotherapy treatments currently found in the
    armamentarium of mental health professionals is:

    A. Less than 25.
    B. Approximately 50.
    C. Approximately 100.
    D. Approximately 200.
    E. Over 1000.

39. Which of the following statements is FALSE concerning the use of therapy manuals?

   A. The more faithfully the manual is followed, the more effective the treatment.
   B. Clinicians are frequently reluctant to apply therapy manuals.
   C. The reliability of manualized therapies has not yet been established.
   D. Manuals based on a number of different therapy approaches have been developed.
   E. The use of manuals is helpful in psychotherapy outcome research.

40. The disorder for which there is the most consistent evidence that a specific intervention is related to a specific outcome is:

   A. Generalized anxiety disorders.
   B. Major depressive disorder.
   C. Sexual dysfunctions.
   D. Simple phobias.
   E. Borderline personality.

41. Research suggests that the best predictor of psychotherapy efficacy is:

   A. Patient diagnosis.
   B. Patient and therapist matching.
   C. Therapist orientation.
   D. Personal characteristics of the patient.
   E. Therapist age.

42. The psychotherapy outcome literature has documented that:

   A. Various types of psychotherapy produce approximately equal effects.
   B. Behavior therapy is superior to psychodynamic therapy.
   C. Psychodynamic therapy is superior to behavior therapy.
   D. Cognitive modification is superior to interpersonal psychotherapy.
   E. Psychotherapy is ineffective.

43. Interest in differential therapeutics suggests that:

   A. All patients cannot benefit from a uniform treatment approach.
   B. There is a need for diversification in outpatient psychiatry services.
   C. There is a need for a network of referral practitioners.
   D. There is an administrative dilemma in centers that are experts in delivering just one or a few treatments.
   E. All of the above.

44. With regard to the frequency of outpatient psychotherapy, it has been shown that:

   A. Patients seen with greater frequency have greater therapeutic benefits.
   B. There is no such thing as a therapeutic relationship that is too intense.
   C. Patients seen with less frequency have fewer therapeutic benefits.
   D. Frequency should be based on an independent determination of the patient's assets and needs.
   E. Frequency should be rigidly set such that the patient always has "his time" predictably assigned.

For each of the questions or incomplete statements below, **ONE** or **MORE** of the suggested answers or completions given is correct. On the answer sheet fill in the space containing

> A if ONLY 1,2, and 3 are correct,
> B if ONLY 1 and 3 are correct,
> C if ONLY 2 and 4 are correct,
> D if ONLY 4 is correct,
> E if ALL are correct.

**FOR EACH QUESTION FILL IN ONLY ONE SPACE
ON YOUR ANSWER SHEET**

Directions Summarized				
(A)	**(B)**	**(C)**	**(D)**	**(E)**
1,2,3	1,3	2,4	4	All are
only	only	only	only	correct

45. Compared to inpatient hospitalization, partial hospital programs are:

    1. Less acceptable to patients and families.
    2. Underutilized.
    3. Less effective.
    4. Less expensive.

46. Research studies concerning day hospital treatment suggest that:

    1. Patients pay a greater direct cost for day treatment.
    2. Clinicians underutilize day treatment as an alternative to inpatient care.
    3. Acute care outpatient treatment may reduce the length of inpatient hospitalization.
    4. For many patients day treatment may produce more favorable outcomes than inpatient care.

47. Group treatments were developed, in part, because they:

    1. Were economical.
    2. Were an effective means of reducing resistances expressed in individual therapy.
    3. Provided adjunctive ego supports in the form of other patients.
    4. Provided a setting in which interactional forces could be examined.

48. In an outpatient psychiatry clinic with residents:

    1. Supervisor and trainee disagreements should be discussed with the service director.
    2. Trainees should be held responsible for their treatment decisions.
    3. Trainees should be exposed to multiple supervisors.
    4. It is best for a trainee to be exposed to only one supervisor.

This statement pertains to Questions 49 and 50.

OCCASIONALLY IN LONG-TERM PSYCHOTHERAPY THE PATIENT AND THERAPIST MAY STRUGGLE WITHOUT OPENLY ACCEPTING THAT A DEFINITIVE TERMINATION IS NOT LIKELY, THUS A STALEMATE SITUATION IS REACHED.

49. Stalemate situations pose which of the following potential dangers for the therapeutic relationship?

    1. The treatment ends in a default because of frustration and bitterness in both parties.
    2. The patient may acknowledge that psychotherapy has inherent limitations; thus, the problem will not be examined nor worked through.
    3. The patient may be erroneously seen as resisting treatment.
    4. The patient may become hopeless because the anticipated termination has not been achieved.

50. In a stalemate situation the therapist may consider:

    1. Changing the duration from long-term psychotherapy to continuous psychotherapy.
    2. Prescribing "treatment holidays" which can be weeks or months, then reassess the treatment.
    3. Making changes in the format, setting, or technique of the psychotherapy.
    4. Changing the duration from long-term psychotherapy to intermittent psychotherapy.

51. Effective treatment(s) of delusional depression are:

    1. Antidepressants alone.
    2. ECT.
    3. Neuroleptics alone.
    4. Antidepressants combined with neuroleptics.

52. Therapeutic approaches to patients with depression who do not respond to antidepressants include(s):

    1. Review diagnosis.
    2. Check compliance and dosage.
    3. Switch to another antidepressant.
    4. Use adjunctive medication.

SECTION FOUR: VIOLENCE AND THE VIOLENT PATIENT

DIRECTIONS (Items 53-61):
Each of the questions or incomplete statements below is followed
by suggested answers. Select the **ONE** that is **BEST** and fill in the
circle containing the corresponding letter on the answer sheet.

---

53. Which of the following is not true concerning patients who make
    homicidal threats?

    A. They are about as likely to commit suicide as to commit
       murder.
    B. The police can do nothing because it is not a crime to make
       threats.
    C. Threats to public figures should be treated like any other
       threat.
    D. A sizable proportion of those who subsequently murder, kill
       someone other than the person threatened.
    E. None of the above.

54. Which of the following statements about robbery is correct?

    A. Robbery rates are highest in the summer.
    B. Less than 10 percent of robberies result in incarceration of the
       offender.
    C. Higher income groups have the highest rate of robbery
       victimization.
    D. Police records of a patient's arrest history are an accurate
       guide to past criminal conduct.
    E. None of the above.

55. Which of the following statements about homicide is correct?

    A. Mentally disordered murderers are particularly likely to kill
       strangers.
    B. Homicide rates have increased continuously since 1970.
    C. A third or more of all homicides stem from trivial altercations
       and other arguments.
    D. Homicide is the leading cause of death among blacks aged
       20-34.
    E. None of the above.

56. All of the following are true EXCEPT:

A. Violence among epileptic patients during seizures is rare.
B. The surface EEG is an insensitive measure of limbic ictus.
C. Temporal lobe epilepsy is a frequent cause of violence in society.
D. Violent epileptic patients often have other concurrent conditions related to poor impulse control.
E. None of the above.

57. Evidence for a hormonal effect on violent behavior is WEAKEST for:

A. Androgens.
B. Hypoglycemia.
C. Corticosteroid excess.
D. Premenstrual syndrome.
E. None of the above.

58. Among patients admitted to psychiatric hospitals, those with the LEAST likelihood of violent behavior are those with:

A. Mania.
B. Schizophrenia.
C. Organic mental disorders.
D. Personality disorders.
E. None of the above.

59. A test which used alone may predict future assaultiveness by a patient is:

A. The Minnesota Multiphasic Personality Inventory (MMPI).
B. The Rorschach Psychodiagnostic Test.
C. The Thematic Apperception Test (TAT).
D. The Wechsler Adult Intelligence Test (WAIS).
E. None of the above.

60. Which of the following best describes the current status of psychiatric patients' right to refuse treatment?

   A. All patients have the right to refuse treatment unless found incompetent to do so.
   B. Definitions of the right and procedures to implement it vary widely across jurisdictions.
   C. The courts have held that the rights of voluntary and involuntary patients are identical when it comes to treatment refusal.
   D. The U.S. Supreme Court has never indicated whether it believes that psychiatric patients have a right to refuse treatment.
   E. None of the above.

61. Which of the following statements is correct?

   A. A patient who keeps a diary purporting to describe assassination plans can be assumed to be harmlessly documenting a vivid fantasy life.
   B. Because they have discharged all of their aggression outwardly, mass murderers are at unusually low risk of suicide.
   C. The majority of serial killers suffer from longstanding psychotic illnesses.
   D. No casualties resulted from the 35 terrorist bombings in the United States in 1983 and 1984.
   E. None of the above.

For each of the questions or incomplete statements below, **ONE** or
MORE of the suggested answers or completions given is correct. On the
answer sheet fill in the space containing

A   if ONLY 1, 2, and 3 are correct,
B   if ONLY 1 and 3 are correct,
C   if ONLY 2 and 4 are correct,
D   if ONLY 4 is correct,
E   if ALL are correct.

**FOR EACH QUESTION FILL IN ONLY ONE SPACE
ON YOUR ANSWER SHEET**

	Directions Summarized			
(A)	**(B)**	**(C)**	**(D)**	**(E)**
1,2,3	**1,3**	**2,4**	**4**	**All are**
only	**only**	**only**	**only**	**correct**

62. When interviewing an assaultive patient who has been brought to
the emergency room by police, one should:

1. Ask the law enforcement officer to leave the area so as not to
upset the patient.
2. Never forget that the patient is also a criminal, and thus
potentially dangerous.
3. Initially try to interview the patient alone in order to develop a
therapeutic relationship.
4. Make every effort to interview the officer before he departs.

63. With respect to violence, which of the following is/are true of
mental patients?

1. Violent behavior is an essential feature of antisocial personality
disorder, aggressive.
2. Violent behavior is an associated feature of organic mental
disorders.
3. Violent behavior is an infrequent feature of histrionic
personality disorders.
4. Violent behavior is an infrequent feature of mental retardation.

23

64. Relative contraindications to rapid tranquilization include:

    1. Overdose with alcohol or sedative-hypnotic drugs.
    2. Manic symptoms.
    3. Toxic-metabolic confusional states.
    4. Paranoid delusions.

65. Proper indications for seclusion and/or restraint include:

    1. Prevention of imminent harm to patient or others.
    2. Punishment for verbal abuse of staff.
    3. Prevention of serious damage to the physical environment.
    4. Social control of milieu when short of staff.

66. Standards of proper care and monitoring of a patient in seclusion/restraint include the following:

    1. Doctors visit twice daily, approximately 12 hours apart.
    2. Nursing "checks" every 15 minutes.
    3. Toileting every four hours.
    4. A written report to the director of the hospital within 4 hours of seclusion.

67. The difference between the earlier cases imposing liability in the event of patients' negligent release or escape and the more recent cases following the precedent of *Tarasoff* include which of the following:

    1. The older cases defined a narrower duty for psychiatrists.
    2. The *Tarasoff*-like decisions are less supportive of the need to take chances to encourage patients' rehabilitation.
    3. The older cases were more tolerant of errors in judgment that did not deviate from the standard of care.
    4. Psychiatrists were never previously held liable to third parties for their patients' violent acts.

68. The reasons why outpatient commitment is not used widely in the United States include which of the following explanations?

   1. Few states' statutes permit the option of outpatient commitment.
   2. Outpatient commitment is discouraged under the doctrine of the least restrictive alternative.
   3. The expense of outpatient commitment is greater than the cost of inpatient care.
   4. No effective enforcement mechanisms exist for outpatient commitment orders.

69. Rapid neuroleptization is most effective against the following symptoms in psychiatric patients:

   1. Excitement.
   2. Hostility.
   3. Assaultive behavior.
   4. Chronic thought disorder.

SECTION FIVE: PSYCHIATRIC EPIDEMIOLOGY

DIRECTIONS (Items 70-74):
Each of the questions or incomplete statements below is followed by suggested answers. Select the **ONE** that is **BEST** and fill in the circle containing the corresponding letter on the answer sheet.

---

70. The clinical and the epidemiologic approach to the study of diseases are:

    A. Incompatible.
    B. Merging.
    C. Identical.
    D. Developing in different directions.
    E. None of the above.

71. The risks to the fetus from maternal alcohol consumption during pregnancy are greatest during:

    A. The first trimester.
    B. The second trimester.
    C. The third trimester.
    D. All of the above.
    E. None of the above.

72. Types of symptoms generally experienced by disaster victims include the following:

    A. They display a single response pattern characterized by psychic numbing.
    B. Their mental health improves in the short term.
    C. They display a range of affective and somatic symptoms.
    D. Their mental health is unaffected.
    E. They exhibit symptoms almost always within one month of the disaster.

73. The personal risk factor most consistently associated with a negative response to disaster has been:

   A. Being female.
   B. Being elderly.
   C. History of a psychiatric disorder.
   D. Being black.
   E. Being poor.

74. Greater involvement with a disaster:

   A. Produces increased distress.
   B. Produces decreased distress.
   C. Is not as important as intrapsychic predisposition.
   D. Delays response.
   E. Usually results in chronicity.

DIRECTIONS (Items 75-87):

For each of the questions or incomplete statements below, **ONE** or **MORE** of the suggested answers or completions given is correct. On the answer sheet fill in the space containing

A if ONLY 1,2, and 3 are correct,
B if ONLY 1 and 3 are correct,
C if ONLY 2 and 4 are correct,
D if ONLY 4 is correct,
E if ALL are correct.

**FOR EACH QUESTION FILL IN ONLY ONE SPACE
ON YOUR ANSWER SHEET**

Directions Summarized				
(A)	**(B)**	**(C)**	**(D)**	**(E)**
1,2,3	**1,3**	**2,4**	**4**	**All are**
only	**only**	**only**	**only**	**correct**

75. Epidemiologic studies done in the U.S. during the late 1950s and 1960s:

1. Demonstrated high rates of psychiatric disorders.
2. Demonstrated high rates of mental impairment.
3. Used poor methodology in defining samples.
4. Had no reliable method of assigning diagnoses.

76. The major achievements in psychiatry of the last decade which have made possible psychiatric epidemiologic studies of clinical value include:

1. Specified diagnostic criteria.
2. Improved diagnostic reliability.
3. Standardized methods of assessing signs and symptoms.
4. Understanding the causes of the major psychiatric disorders.

77. New computer scored interviews can provide:

1. Lifetime diagnoses.
2. Symptom patterns.
3. Current diagnoses.
4. Age of onset.

78. Problems with epidemiologic studies based only on psychiatric record data from psychiatric facilities are:

    1. They omit cases treated by non-specialists.
    2. They provide no data on the frequency of untreated cases in the community.
    3. They may report diagnoses which were not made according to research standards.
    4. They do not provide demographic information about patients before they became sick.

79. Which of the following were among the objectives of the Epidemiological Catchment Area (ECA) study?

    1. To replicate the classic Hollingshead and Redlich study of Social Class and Mental Illness.
    2. To determine the prevalence and incidence rates of specific mental disorders as defined by DSM-III.
    3. To determine the rates of mental illness on a graded scale of impairment from mild to severe.
    4. To assess the use of mental health services in specialty mental health, general medical, and other human service settings.

80. The 6-month prevalence rates of mental disorders from the first three Epidemiological Catchment Area (ECA) sites were as follows:

    1. Overall rates ranged from 16–23% of the population.
    2. Schizophrenic disorders were found at 0.6 to 1.1% of the population.
    3. Affective disorders were found at rates of 4.6-6.5% of the population.
    4. Personality disorders were found at rates between 15 and 20%.

Directions Summarized

(A)	(B)	(C)	(D)	(E)
1,2,3	1,3	2,4	4	All are
only	only	only	only	correct

81. Evidence for the involvement of genetic factors in the etiology has been found for which of the following psychiatric disorders?

    1. Schizophrenia.
    2. Alcoholism.
    3. Bipolar depression.
    4. Antisocial personality disorder.

82. The risk of transmitting psychiatric disorders to children is greatest when parental illness is accompanied by:

    1. Marked marital discord.
    2. Serious distortion in parenting.
    3. Scapegoating of the child.
    4. Illness in the father rather than the mother.

83. The following conditions represent disorders which are currently considered preventable:

    1. Major affective disorder.
    2. Autism.
    3. Attention deficit disorder.
    4. Subacute sclerosing panencephalitis.

84. To establish a causal connection between risk factors for a disorder and the disorder itself:

    1. A statistically significant relationship between them must exist after the disorder is established.
    2. A causal mechanism must be understood.
    3. Laboratory demonstration is required.
    4. The risk factors must be shown to exist prior to onset of the disorder.

85. Goldberger's discovery of the nutritional basis of pellagra was based on:

    1. Measuring the niacin content of foods.
    2. Eliminating various infectious diseases as causes.
    3. Understanding the mechanism of vitamin deficiency.
    4. Manipulating the diet of institutional inmates.

86. Characteristics of a preventive trial include:

    1. Random allocation of experimental and control groups.
    2. "Blind" determination of outcome.
    3. Clear definition of risk factions.
    4. Prior demonstration that prevention is more cost-effective than treatment of the targeted condition.

87. Which of the following are clinical or public health uses of epidemiology?

    1. Completing a clinical picture.
    2. Assessing individual risks.
    3. Community diagnosis.
    4. Planning treatment programs.

SECTION SIX: PSYCHOPHARMACOLOGY: DRUG SIDE EFFECTS AND INTERACTIONS

DIRECTIONS (Items 88-97):
Each of the questions or incomplete statements below is followed by suggested answers. Select the **ONE** that is **BEST** and fill in the circle containing the corresponding letter on the answer sheet.

88. Which of the following conditions is LEAST likely to be adversely affected by bedtime use of a benzodiazepine?

    A. Asthma.
    B. Chronic bronchitis.
    C. Snoring.
    D. Sleep apnea.
    E. Substance abuse.

89. Which of the statements concerning benzodiazepine overdose is most true?

    A. Coma with associated hypotension and hypothermia is frequent.
    B. Recovery of consciousness usually requires more than 24 hours.
    C. Dialysis is a useful adjunctive treatment in benzodiazepine overdoses.
    D. Benzodiazepine overdose is much less lethal than barbiturate overdose.
    E. Fatalities with benzodiazepine overdose are common.

90. The only sedative antidepressant free of cardiotoxicity is:

    A. Trazodone.
    B. Doxepin.
    C. Maprotiline.
    D. Desipramine.
    E. None of the above.

91. The estimated prevalence of aplastic anemia due to carbamazepine treatment is approximately:

    A. 1:500
    B. 1:5000
    C. 1:50,000
    D. 1:500,000
    E. 1:1,000,000

92. In a patient with severe extrapyramidal symptoms with fever, vigorous treatment of which of the following signs or symptoms should be of immediate concern to the physician?

    A. Fever.
    B. Immobilizing rigidity.
    C. Fever with hypertension.
    D. Acute dystonia.
    E. Tremor.

93. Tardive dyskinesia is:

    A. Essentially irreversible.
    B. Likely to become worse if the dosage of neuroleptics is increased.
    C. Likely to improve eventually if neuroleptics are stopped.
    D. Likely to improve as soon as neuroleptics are stopped.
    E. Confined to patients over 60 years of age.

94. The cardiovascular effect of neuroleptics that leads to the most morbidity is:

    A. Hypotension.
    B. Arrhythmias.
    C. T-wave changes in the EKG.
    D. Decreased cardiac contractility.
    E. P-R interval prolongation in the EKG.

95. Concurrent use of a phenothiazine and a tricyclic antidepressant (TCA) is most likely to cause:

A. No change in the plasma level of either drug.
B. A significant increase in plasma levels of the TCA since both drugs use the same hepatic microsomal enzyme system.
C. A significant decrease in plasma levels of the TCA since both drugs use the same hepatic microsomal enzyme system.
D. A significant decrease in the plasma levels of both drugs.
E. A significant decrease in plasma levels of the phenothiazine since both drugs use the same hepatic microsomal enzyme system.

96. Cimetidine interacts pharmacokinetically with both benzodiazepines (bz) and tricyclic antidepressants (TCA). The outcome of this interaction is most likely to cause:

A. No change in plasma level of either bz or TC.
B. Increased plasma levels of bz, but not TCA.
C. Increased plasma levels of TCA, but not bz.
D. Increased plasma levels of both bz and TCA.
E. Decreased plasma levels of both bz and TCA.

97. Which of the following antidepressants is least likely to potentiate the effects of drugs with CNS depressant properties (i.e., alcohol, barbiturates, etc)?

A. Amitriptyline.
B. Maprotiline.
C. Nomifensine.
D. Trazodone.
E. Imipramine.

For each of the questions or incomplete statements below, **ONE** or
MORE of the suggested answers or completions given is correct. On the
answer sheet fill in the space containing

A   if ONLY 1, 2, and 3 are correct,
B   if ONLY 1 and 3 are correct,
C   if ONLY 2 and 4 are correct,
D   if ONLY 4 is correct,
E   if ALL are correct.

**FOR EACH QUESTION FILL IN ONLY ONE SPACE
ON YOUR ANSWER SHEET**

		Directions Summarized		
(A)	**(B)**	**(C)**	**(D)**	**(E)**
1,2,3	1,3	2,4	4	All are
only	only	only	only	correct

98. Side effects of the MAO inhibitors include:

   1. Supine hypotension.
   2. Carpal tunnel syndrome.
   3. Anorgasmia in females.
   4. Priapism in males.

99. Major side effects of the tricyclic compounds include:

   1. Premature ejaculation.
   2. Reduction in seizure threshold.
   3. Nocturnal enuresis.
   4. Anticholinergic effects.

100. Correct statement(s) about the side effects of lithium on
    reproduction include:

   1. It is common for men to experience reduced libido and erectile
      dysfunction.
   2. Mutagenesis has not been found.
   3. Breast feeding is encouraged since lithium is not present in
      breast milk.
   4. The fetus is exposed to lithium levels at least as high as those
      in the maternal blood.

101. To what extent were you satisfied with the continuing medical education learning experience provided by this program?

   A. Very satisfied.
   B.
   C.
   D.
   E. Not satisfied at all.

102. To what extent did the program meet your expectations?

   A. Exceeded my expectations.
   B.
   C. As expected.
   D.
   E. Less than expected.

103. Do you plan to subscribe to next year's Annual Review?

   A. Definitely yes.
   B. Probably yes.
   C. Undecided.
   D. Probably no.
   E. Definitely no.

104. The questions are:

   A. Very difficult.
   B. Difficult.
   C. About right in difficulty.
   D. Easy.
   E. Very easy.

AMERICAN PSYCHIATRIC ASSOCIATION - CME Supplement for Annual Review, Volume 6

APA Membership Number	TELEPHONE NUMBER

(Grid of bubbles numbered 0–9 for each digit column)

PLEASE READ INSTRUCTIONS
1. Use ONLY no. 2 pencil to fill in this form. DO NOT USE A PEN.
2. Erase errors completely and cleanly.
3. Fill appropriate circles with heavy black marks.
4. Mark only one circle for each answer.
5. Complete both sides of answer sheets.
6. Complete all requested information.
7. Make no stray marks.

1. Ⓐ Ⓑ Ⓒ Ⓓ Ⓔ
2. Ⓐ Ⓑ Ⓒ Ⓓ Ⓔ
3. Ⓐ Ⓑ Ⓒ Ⓓ Ⓔ
4. Ⓐ Ⓑ Ⓒ Ⓓ Ⓔ
5. Ⓐ Ⓑ Ⓒ Ⓓ Ⓔ
6. Ⓐ Ⓑ Ⓒ Ⓓ Ⓔ
7. Ⓐ Ⓑ Ⓒ Ⓓ Ⓔ
8. Ⓐ Ⓑ Ⓒ Ⓓ Ⓔ
9. Ⓐ Ⓑ Ⓒ Ⓓ Ⓔ
10. Ⓐ Ⓑ Ⓒ Ⓓ Ⓔ
11. Ⓐ Ⓑ Ⓒ Ⓓ Ⓔ
12. Ⓐ Ⓑ Ⓒ Ⓓ Ⓔ
13. Ⓐ Ⓑ Ⓒ Ⓓ Ⓔ
14. Ⓐ Ⓑ Ⓒ Ⓓ Ⓔ
15. Ⓐ Ⓑ Ⓒ Ⓓ Ⓔ

16. Ⓐ Ⓑ Ⓒ Ⓓ Ⓔ
17. Ⓐ Ⓑ Ⓒ Ⓓ Ⓔ
18. Ⓐ Ⓑ Ⓒ Ⓓ Ⓔ
19. Ⓐ Ⓑ Ⓒ Ⓓ Ⓔ
20. Ⓐ Ⓑ Ⓒ Ⓓ Ⓔ
21. Ⓐ Ⓑ Ⓒ Ⓓ Ⓔ
22. Ⓐ Ⓑ Ⓒ Ⓓ Ⓔ
23. Ⓐ Ⓑ Ⓒ Ⓓ Ⓔ
24. Ⓐ Ⓑ Ⓒ Ⓓ Ⓔ
25. Ⓐ Ⓑ Ⓒ Ⓓ Ⓔ
26. Ⓐ Ⓑ Ⓒ Ⓓ Ⓔ
27. Ⓐ Ⓑ Ⓒ Ⓓ Ⓔ
28. Ⓐ Ⓑ Ⓒ Ⓓ Ⓔ
29. Ⓐ Ⓑ Ⓒ Ⓓ Ⓔ
30. Ⓐ Ⓑ Ⓒ Ⓓ Ⓔ

31. Ⓐ Ⓑ Ⓒ Ⓓ Ⓔ
32. Ⓐ Ⓑ Ⓒ Ⓓ Ⓔ
33. Ⓐ Ⓑ Ⓒ Ⓓ Ⓔ
34. Ⓐ Ⓑ Ⓒ Ⓓ Ⓔ
35. Ⓐ Ⓑ Ⓒ Ⓓ Ⓔ
36. Ⓐ Ⓑ Ⓒ Ⓓ Ⓔ
37. Ⓐ Ⓑ Ⓒ Ⓓ Ⓔ
38. Ⓐ Ⓑ Ⓒ Ⓓ Ⓔ
39. Ⓐ Ⓑ Ⓒ Ⓓ Ⓔ
40. Ⓐ Ⓑ Ⓒ Ⓓ Ⓔ
41. Ⓐ Ⓑ Ⓒ Ⓓ Ⓔ
42. Ⓐ Ⓑ Ⓒ Ⓓ Ⓔ
43. Ⓐ Ⓑ Ⓒ Ⓓ Ⓔ
44. Ⓐ Ⓑ Ⓒ Ⓓ Ⓔ
45. Ⓐ Ⓑ Ⓒ Ⓓ Ⓔ

46. Ⓐ Ⓑ Ⓒ Ⓓ Ⓔ
47. Ⓐ Ⓑ Ⓒ Ⓓ Ⓔ
48. Ⓐ Ⓑ Ⓒ Ⓓ Ⓔ
49. Ⓐ Ⓑ Ⓒ Ⓓ Ⓔ
50. Ⓐ Ⓑ Ⓒ Ⓓ Ⓔ

(continued on back)

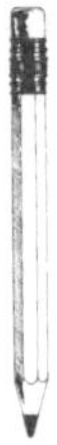

#2

PENCIL

ONLY

Name

Street Address

City | State | Zip Code

PLEASE READ INSTRUCTIONS

1. Use ONLY no. 2 pencil to fill in this form.
   DO NOT USE A PEN.
2. Erase errors completely and cleanly.
3. Fill appropriate circles with heavy black marks.
4. Mark only one circle for each answer.
5. Complete both sides of answer sheet.
6. Complete all requested information.
7. Make no stray marks.

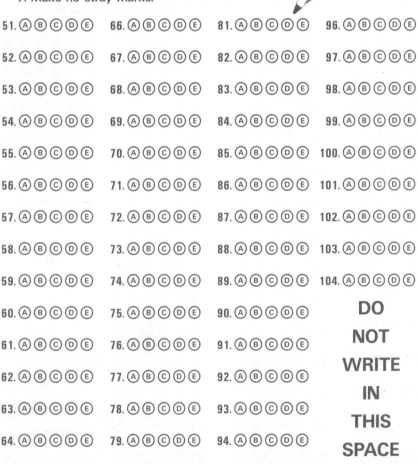

51. Ⓐ Ⓑ Ⓒ Ⓓ Ⓔ	66. Ⓐ Ⓑ Ⓒ Ⓓ Ⓔ	81. Ⓐ Ⓑ Ⓒ Ⓓ Ⓔ	96. Ⓐ Ⓑ Ⓒ Ⓓ Ⓔ
52. Ⓐ Ⓑ Ⓒ Ⓓ Ⓔ	67. Ⓐ Ⓑ Ⓒ Ⓓ Ⓔ	82. Ⓐ Ⓑ Ⓒ Ⓓ Ⓔ	97. Ⓐ Ⓑ Ⓒ Ⓓ Ⓔ
53. Ⓐ Ⓑ Ⓒ Ⓓ Ⓔ	68. Ⓐ Ⓑ Ⓒ Ⓓ Ⓔ	83. Ⓐ Ⓑ Ⓒ Ⓓ Ⓔ	98. Ⓐ Ⓑ Ⓒ Ⓓ Ⓔ
54. Ⓐ Ⓑ Ⓒ Ⓓ Ⓔ	69. Ⓐ Ⓑ Ⓒ Ⓓ Ⓔ	84. Ⓐ Ⓑ Ⓒ Ⓓ Ⓔ	99. Ⓐ Ⓑ Ⓒ Ⓓ Ⓔ
55. Ⓐ Ⓑ Ⓒ Ⓓ Ⓔ	70. Ⓐ Ⓑ Ⓒ Ⓓ Ⓔ	85. Ⓐ Ⓑ Ⓒ Ⓓ Ⓔ	100. Ⓐ Ⓑ Ⓒ Ⓓ Ⓔ
56. Ⓐ Ⓑ Ⓒ Ⓓ Ⓔ	71. Ⓐ Ⓑ Ⓒ Ⓓ Ⓔ	86. Ⓐ Ⓑ Ⓒ Ⓓ Ⓔ	101. Ⓐ Ⓑ Ⓒ Ⓓ Ⓔ
57. Ⓐ Ⓑ Ⓒ Ⓓ Ⓔ	72. Ⓐ Ⓑ Ⓒ Ⓓ Ⓔ	87. Ⓐ Ⓑ Ⓒ Ⓓ Ⓔ	102. Ⓐ Ⓑ Ⓒ Ⓓ Ⓔ
58. Ⓐ Ⓑ Ⓒ Ⓓ Ⓔ	73. Ⓐ Ⓑ Ⓒ Ⓓ Ⓔ	88. Ⓐ Ⓑ Ⓒ Ⓓ Ⓔ	103. Ⓐ Ⓑ Ⓒ Ⓓ Ⓔ
59. Ⓐ Ⓑ Ⓒ Ⓓ Ⓔ	74. Ⓐ Ⓑ Ⓒ Ⓓ Ⓔ	89. Ⓐ Ⓑ Ⓒ Ⓓ Ⓔ	104. Ⓐ Ⓑ Ⓒ Ⓓ Ⓔ
60. Ⓐ Ⓑ Ⓒ Ⓓ Ⓔ	75. Ⓐ Ⓑ Ⓒ Ⓓ Ⓔ	90. Ⓐ Ⓑ Ⓒ Ⓓ Ⓔ	DO
61. Ⓐ Ⓑ Ⓒ Ⓓ Ⓔ	76. Ⓐ Ⓑ Ⓒ Ⓓ Ⓔ	91. Ⓐ Ⓑ Ⓒ Ⓓ Ⓔ	NOT
62. Ⓐ Ⓑ Ⓒ Ⓓ Ⓔ	77. Ⓐ Ⓑ Ⓒ Ⓓ Ⓔ	92. Ⓐ Ⓑ Ⓒ Ⓓ Ⓔ	WRITE
63. Ⓐ Ⓑ Ⓒ Ⓓ Ⓔ	78. Ⓐ Ⓑ Ⓒ Ⓓ Ⓔ	93. Ⓐ Ⓑ Ⓒ Ⓓ Ⓔ	IN
64. Ⓐ Ⓑ Ⓒ Ⓓ Ⓔ	79. Ⓐ Ⓑ Ⓒ Ⓓ Ⓔ	94. Ⓐ Ⓑ Ⓒ Ⓓ Ⓔ	THIS
65. Ⓐ Ⓑ Ⓒ Ⓓ Ⓔ	80. Ⓐ Ⓑ Ⓒ Ⓓ Ⓔ	95. Ⓐ Ⓑ Ⓒ Ⓓ Ⓔ	SPACE

PSYCHIATRY
UPDATE

AMERICAN PSYCHIATRIC ASSOCIATION

Annual Review

Vol. 6

EDITED BY ROBERT E. HALES, M.D.
ALLEN J. FRANCES, M.D.

American Psychiatric
Press, Inc.

American Psychiatric Press, Inc.
1400 K Street, N.W.
Washington, DC
1987

American Psychiatric Press, Inc.

Typeset by VIP Systems, Alexandria, VA
Manufactured by Arcata Graphics, Fairfield, PA

Psychiatry Update: Volume 6
ISSN 0736-1866
ISBN 0-88048-243-5 (hardbound with CME Supplement)
ISBN 0-88048-242-7 (pbk.)

To Dianne and Julia, who are a constant source of joy and inspiration.

R.E.H.

To Craig and Bobby, in appreciation for all you have taught me.

Your Dad (A.J.F.)

PSYCHIATRY UPDATE: THE AMERICAN PSYCHIATRIC ASSOCIATION ANNUAL REVIEW, VOLUME 4 (1985)

Robert E. Hales, M.D., and Allen J. Frances, M.D., Editors

An Introduction to the World of Neurotransmitters and Neuroreceptors
Joseph T. Coyle, M.D., Section Editor

Neuropsychiatry
Stuart C. Yudofsky, M.D., Section Editor

Sleep Disorders
David J. Kupfer, M.D., Section Editor

Eating Disorders
Joel Yager, M.D., Section Editor

The Therapeutic Alliance and Treatment Outcome
John P. Docherty, M.D., Section Editor

PSYCHIATRY UPDATE: THE AMERICAN PSYCHIATRIC ASSOCIATION ANNUAL REVIEW, VOLUME 5 (1986)

Allen J. Frances, M.D., and Robert E. Hales, M.D., Editors

Schizophrenia
Nancy C. Andreasen, M.D., Ph.D., Section Editor

Drug Abuse and Drug Dependence
Robert B. Millman, M.D., Section Editor

Personality Disorders
Robert M.A. Hirschfeld, M.D., Section Editor

Adolescent Psychiatry
Carolyn B. Robinowitz, M.D., and Jeanne Spurlock, M.D., Section Editors

Psychiatric Contributions to Medical Care
David Spiegel, M.D., and W. Stewart Agras, M.D., Section Editors

Group Psychotherapy
Irvin D. Yalom, M.D., Section Editor

PSYCHIATRY UPDATE: THE AMERICAN PSYCHIATRIC ASSOCIATION ANNUAL REVIEW, VOLUME 6 (1987)

Robert E. Hales, M.D., and Allen J. Frances, M.D., Editors

Bipolar Disorders
Frederick K. Goodwin, M.D., and Kay Redfield Jamison, Ph.D., Section Editors

Neuroscience Techniques in Clinical Psychiatry
John M. Morihisa, M.D., and Solomon H. Snyder, M.D., Section Editors

Differential Therapeutics
John F. Clarkin, Ph.D., and Samuel W. Perry, M.D., Section Editors

Violence and the Violent Patient
Kenneth Tardiff, M.D., M.P.H., Section Editor

Psychiatric Epidemiology
Myrna M. Weissman, Ph.D., Section Editor

Psychopharmacology: Drug Side Effects and Interactions
Philip Berger, M.D., and Leo Hollister, M.D., Section Editors

AMERICAN PSYCHIATRIC PRESS REVIEW OF PSYCHIATRY, VOLUME 7 (1988)

Allen J. Frances, M.D., and Robert E. Hales, M.D., Editors

Panic Disorders
M. Katherine Shear, M.D., and David Barlow, Ph.D., Section Editors

Unipolar Depression
Martin B. Keller, M.D., Section Editor

Suicide
J. John Mann, M.D., and Michael Stanley, Ph.D., Section Editors

Electroconvulsive Therapy
Robert M. Rose, M.D., and Harold Pincus, M.D., Section Editors

Cognitive Therapy
A. John Rush, M.D., and Aaron T. Beck, M.D., Section Editors

CONTENTS

Section

V

Psychiatric Epidemiology

Introduction

As the President of the American Psychiatric Association, one of my more plea-
surable tasks is writing the introduction to this year's volume of the *Annual
Review*. Volume 6 represents the completion of the first three-year set of volumes
under the editorship of Drs. Robert E. Hales and Allen J. Frances. They have
done a marvelous job in selecting distinguished psychiatrists and psychologists
to serve as section editors and chapter authors for the series and in instituting
a number of constructive changes to improve the content and relevance for
practicing psychiatrists. The *Annual Review* provides the field with the state of
the art in selected topical areas and provides a degree of comprehensiveness,
scholarship, and readability not found in other publications. The book also
serves an important function in filling the gap between information presented
in our excellent psychiatric journals and material that appears in major textbooks.

I don't know how we got along without the *Annual Review* before 1982. By
presenting the latest scientific findings of immediate clinical relevance, the series
serves an important educational function. It is also of such high quality that I
find myself reading a chapter several times and acquiring new information after
each reading. The series is particularly helpful to psychiatric residents in reviewing in depth specific content areas and subjects.

The topics chosen for this year exemplify the excitement in advances occurring
in the field of psychiatry. Frederick Goodwin, M.D., and Kay Jamison, Ph.D.,
have assembled an outstanding team to discuss "Bipolar Disorders." Their panel
of experts, from the National Institute of Mental Health, the Massachusetts
General Hospital, and UCLA have presented a mini-volume on much of what
the clinician needs to know in treating patients with bipolar disorders, to include
biological findings and clinical approaches to patients who fail to respond to
traditional treatments. As with the other major psychiatric disorders, it became
clear to me after reading this section that treatment of patients with bipolar
disorders requires an integration of psychopharmacology with psychosocial
methods to achieve the most successful results. This section is one of the best
presentations on this topic that I have ever read. The authors should be congrat-
ulated for a job superbly done.

I am equally impressed by the fine job done by John Morihisa, M.D., and
Solomon Snyder, M.D., on the section entitled, "Neuroscience Techniques in
Clinical Psychiatry." How many of us wonder what tests we should order for
our patients and what is the clinical relevance of some of the newer test procedures? In addition, with newer research findings in psychoendocrinology,
psychoimmunology, and imaging techniques, psychiatrists may sometimes be
confused about how to translate the information being published in psychiatric
journals and to apply it in their clinical practice. Drs. Morihisa and Snyder have
selected highly qualified investigators who are conducting ongoing research in
these new neuroscience techniques, investigators who have emphasized the
current and future application of these techniques for clinicians. The authors
have summarized a wealth of material in a scholarly fashion.

The section entitled "Differential Therapeutics," edited by John Clarkin, Ph.D., and Samuel Perry, M.D., is a fine series of chapters for clinicians that will help to determine the mix of treatment approaches for selected patients. As you know, in 1984 and 1985 the section editors, together with Dr. Allen Frances, published two books that introduced us to the concept of differential therapeutics. This section updates material previously presented by including additional outside authors and by integrating the most recent research and clinical findings into their discussion of treatment strategies. This section discusses how the setting, format, and duration of treatment affect the choice and selection of treatment modalities. Important factors for clinicians to consider in deciding upon a particular psychotherapeutic intervention are highlighted in an elegantly prepared chapter. Psychopharmacologic issues and ways to integrate psychopharmacology with psychotherapy is presented in a well organized chapter. Finally, the clinical, teaching, research, and administrative issues that educators and clinicians should consider in integrating psychosocial and psychopharmacologic treatments is summarized comprehensively.

One of the most important topics for psychiatrists in clinical practice is "Violence and the Violent Patient." This section, edited by Dr. Kenneth Tardiff, one of the country's foremost experts in this area, presents much current information concerning violence and how to manage the violent patient. This section begins in a systematic way by discussing the patterns and determinants of violence. It then moves to the evaluation and emergency treatment of the violent patient. Because nearly one-half of all psychiatrists are involved in outpatient practice, a chapter is devoted to the management of the violent patient in an exclusively outpatient setting. Finally, forensic issues, vitally important in dealing with violent patients and, in particular, violent psychiatric patients, are summarized in a scholarly review. This section should be required reading for all residents, since the majority of violent acts against psychiatrists occur with our younger colleagues.

One of the most exciting fields of psychiatric research in the last decade concerns "Psychiatric Epidemiology." Who but Dr. Myrna Weissman should edit such a section? She has done a marvelous job and has put together, in my opinion, the best comprehensive review of this important topic that I have yet read. She begins by providing an overview of epidemiological principles and then discusses related issues as they pertain to the proper diagnosis of psychiatric patients. The Epidemiological Catchment Area (ECA) Study is comprehensively summarized. Other important topics that are discussed include genetic epidemiology, familial risk factors, and prevention. Finally, clinical applicability of epidemiologic methods to disaster research is nicely summarized.

The final section, edited by Leo Hollister, M.D., and Philip Berger, M.D., entitled, "Psychopharmacology: Drug Side Effects and Interactions," is a most comprehensive and clinically useful discussion of this important topic. Each of the chapter authors is a prominent investigator. Side effects for each of the major psychotropic medications are summarized: benzodiazepines, antidepressants, lithium and carbamazepine and neuroleptics. In addition, a comprehensive chapter summarizes the interaction of each of these psychoactive drugs with other medications prescribed in medical practice. Numerous tables are distributed throughout the chapters and serve as a ready source of reference for busy clinicians.

The *Annual Review*, and in particular Volume 6, is an important contribution to psychiatry and is an excellent update and reference for clinicians and residents. Based on current books' sales, it is estimated that one out of every three to four psychiatrists in the United States will have purchased each volume. As an educator, I'm grateful to the editors, Drs. Hales and Frances, to the section editors, and to all the authors for providing such an excellent, timely, and useful book. I predict that Volume 6 will be the most successful and widely acclaimed in the current series. I encourage colleagues to join me in reading and rereading the excellent chapters and sections.

Robert O. Pasnau, M.D.

Foreword to Volume 6

by Robert E. Hales, M.D., and Allen J. Frances, M.D.

When friends comment to us on our participation in the *Annual Review*, it is usually in a grateful and complimentary way, saying that they have enjoyed the books and have found them useful. But we can also often detect a sense of pity in their tone (as in, "How can you stand reading that stuff over and over?") and sometimes even a touch of contempt (as in, "Don't you guys have anything better to do?"). Indeed, editing is something of a mixed blessing. It promotes bad eyesight (one of us has taken to wearing reading glasses); ruins friendships (at least one of our former section editors and several former chapter authors seem to turn away when we meet on the street, and everyone with a future commitment tries to avoid us whenever possible); clogs one's files, haunts one's dreams, and, worst of all, distracts from our own work.

Nonetheless, we feel quite grateful for the opportunity to plan and assemble the last three volumes of the *Annual Review* series. The biggest personal return is also the most obvious—in reading and rereading and rereading the chapters, we have learned a great deal about psychiatry. If you take the time to read the *Annual Review* even once, you should develop a fairly comprehensive, timely, and in-depth acquaintance with the topics covered. The second greatest reward comes from our relationships with the sections editors and chapter authors. Beyond the inevitable nagging, it has been a rare privilege for us to work closely with some of the outstanding leaders in the field of psychiatry, and we will remain greatly in their debt.

The third reward is perhaps least obvious. It is great fun to plan the book and then watch it grow up from a glimmer of discussion to a fully realized product. It is a responsibility, but also a pleasure, to pick the topics and the section editors, and then to work with them in organizing a scheme of presentation and in selecting chapter authors. The process of revising and editing also appeals to a latent instinct for order that both of us share.

Well, what about the current volume—Why were the topics chosen and what do the sections cover?

Our first section is on "Bipolar Disorders," ably edited by Drs. Frederick K. Goodwin and Kay Redfield Jamison. Aside from the great clinical relevance of this topic, we were intrigued by the findings relating the rhythmicity that characterizes the course of bipolar disorders with the basic rhythms of nature, by the importance of treating these disorders with both pharmacologic and psychotherapeutic approaches, and, finally, by the development of new interventions for dealing with the treatment resistant patient.

We included the section on "Neuroscience Techniques in Clinical Psychiatry," edited by Drs. John M. Morihisa and Solomon H. Snyder, because we believe this is an appropriate time to take stock of the many recent advances in neuroscience technology that have enriched our profession—both to learn about their applications (and limitations) to current clinical practice and to prepare our readers for the future wave of new results that will be generated by them.

"Differential Therapeutics," edited by Drs. John F. Clarkin and Samuel W.

Perry, was selected as a topic, despite the fact that it is a special interest of one of us (AJF), because the other (REH) felt that it would be interesting and timely to summarize the available outcome data concerning the selection of psychiatric treatments and the tailoring of specific treatment settings, formats, orientations, durations, and medications to the specific needs of selected patients.

"Violence and the Violent Patient," edited by Dr. Kenneth Tardiff, was chosen because it is a major social problem and one in which psychiatric expertise (if not predictive power) has greatly expanded in recent years. It is also a topic that makes teachers, students, clinicians, and researchers nervous and therefore receives too little attention. The section on violence provides a wealth of practical material and should be of great value, particularly to residents and psychiatrists in full-time clinical practice.

"Psychiatric Epidemiology," edited by Dr. Myrna Weissman, has recently flourished into a vital and fascinating area of psychiatric research with major implications for clinical practice. The recently completed Epidemiological Catchment Area Study solved many of the major methodological problems in conducting epidemiological surveys in the community. It has produced a data base which suggests that our clinical populations represent only a highly selected sample of psychiatric disorders in the community. Psychiatric epidemiology has a great deal to say about how we conduct our clinical practices, how resources are allocated for public health initiatives, and ultimately what steps may be taken to prevent psychiatric illness, especially in high risk populations.

Our final section, "Psychopharmacology: Drug Side Effects and Interactions," edited by Drs. Leo Hollister and Philip Berger, is essential reading. It provides a remarkably scholarly and comprehensive overview of an area that is absolutely crucial in psychiatric practice, and does this in a way that encourages retention of a vast amount of information.

We don't have space to acknowledge all the people who helped us with the book, but we would like to acknowledge several people who were especially helpful. We first would like to thank our able Administrative Assistant, Ms. Sandy Landfried, who in addition to coordinating many administrative tasks related to the Annual Meeting, ensures that the *Annual Review* chapters are submitted and reviewed in a timely fashion. This book simply would not be published on schedule without her significant involvement. We also would like to thank our editor at the American Psychiatric Press (APPI), Ms. Eve Shapiro, for her careful and meticulous editing of every page of this year's *Annual Review* and the two previous volumes. She has earned our respect and admiration for a job well done. Ron McMillen, the General Manager of APPI, has been supportive of our suggestions about improving the series and has been remarkably creative in designing the book. Richard Farkas, as APPI Production Manager, has done a superb job in ensuring the fast turn-around time between receipt of manuscripts and actual publication. We would like to acknowledge the faithful service of Ms. Joanne Mas in the preparation of this manuscript. We would like to thank our Departmental Chairmen, Drs. Harry Holloway and Bob Michels, for their support and encouragement of our work. We are especially appreciative of our understanding wives, Dianne Hales and Vera Frances, who allowed us to spend so much free time on evenings, weekends, and holidays working on the book.

Finally, we thank our chapter authors and section editors for placing such a high priority on this volume. All of the contributors are busy, productive, and well-respected academicians. Their commitment to the education of their colleagues by preparing chapters or sections is greatly appreciated by us and, we hope, by you, as you begin to read and study the *American Psychiatric Association Annual Review: Volume 6.*

Contributors

Carol B. Allen, M.D.
Department of Psychiatry, Bronx Veterans Administration
Medical Center, New York, New York

Nancy C. Andreasen, M.D., Ph.D.
Professor of Psychiatry, University of Iowa College of Medicine,
Iowa City, Iowa

Paul S. Appelbaum, M.D.
A.F. Zeleznik Professor of Psychiatry; Director, Law and
Psychiatry Program, Department of Psychiatry, University of
Massachusetts Medical School, Worcester, Massachusetts

George U. Balis, M.D.
Professor of Psychiatry, University of Maryland School of
Medicine, Institute of Psychiatry and Human Behavior,
Baltimore, Maryland

Philip A. Berger, M.D.
Norris Professor of Psychiatry, Stanford University Medical
Center, Stanford, California

Larry E. Beutler, Ph.D.
Professor and Chief, Clinical Psychology, Department of
Psychiatry, University of Arizona Health Sciences Center,
Tucson, Arizona

Barry Blackwell, M.D.
Professor and Chairman, Department of Psychiatry, University
of Wisconsin Medical School (Milwaukee Clinical Campus),
Milwaukee, Wisconsin

David B. Bresnahan, M.D.
Assistant Professor of Psychiatry, University of Illinois College
of Medicine at Chicago; Research Fellow, Illinois State
Psychiatric Institute, Chicago, Illinois

Evelyn J. Bromet, Ph.D.
Associate Professor of Psychiatry and Epidemiology; Director,
Psychiatric Epidemiology Program, Department of Psychiatry,
University of Pittsburgh School of Medicine, Pittsburgh,
Pennsylvania

Jack D. Burke, Jr., M.D., M.P.H.
Deputy Director, Division of Clinical Research, National
Institute of Mental Health, Rockville, Maryland

John F. Clarkin, Ph.D.
Professor of Clinical Psychology in Psychiatry, Cornell
University Medical College, White Plains, New York

Marjorie Crago, Ph.D.
Research Assistant, Department of Psychiatry, University of
Arizona College of Medicine, Tucson, Arizona

John G. Csernansky, M.D.
Assistant Professor of Psychiatry, Stanford University School of
Medicine, Stanford, California; Medical Director, Schizophrenia
Biologic Research Center, Veterans Administration Medical
Center, Palo Alto, California

Bonnie M. Davis, M.D.
Professor of Psychiatry, Bronx Veterans Administration Medical
Center, New York, New York

John M. Davis, M.D.
Director of Research, Illinois State Psychiatric Institute; Gilman
Professor of Psychiatry, University of Illinois at Chicago
School of Medicine, Chicago, Illinois

Kenneth L. Davis, M.D.
Professor of Psychiatry and Pharmacology, Mount Sinai School
of Medicine, New York, New York; Chief, Psychiatry Service,
Veterans Administration Medical Center, Bronx, New York

Park Elliott Dietz, M.D., M.P.H., Ph.D.
Professor of Law; Professor of Behavioral Medicine and
Psychiatry; Medical Director, Institute of Law, Psychiatry and
Public Policy, University of Virginia Schools of Law and
Medicine, Charlottesville, Virginia

Felton Earls, M.D.
Blanche F. Ittleson Professor of Psychiatry (Child); Director,
William Greenleaf Eliot Division of Child Psychiatry,
Washington University School of Medicine, St. Louis, Missouri

Allen J. Frances, M.D.
Professor of Psychiatry, Cornell University Medical College,
New York, New York

Minna Fyer, M.D.
Lecturer of Psychiatry, Cornell University Medical College,
New York, New York

J. Christian Gillin, M.D.
Professor of Psychiatry, University of California, San Diego;
The San Diego Veterans Administration Medical Center,
San Diego, California

Frederick K. Goodwin, M.D.
Director, Intramural Research, National Institute of Mental
Health, Bethesda, Maryland

Alan I. Green, M.D.
Assistant Professor of Psychiatry, Harvard Medical School;
Associate Director of Psychopharmacology, Massachusetts
Mental Health Center, Boston, Massachusetts

John H. Greist, M.D.
Professor of Psychiatry, University of Wisconsin Medical
School, Madison, Wisconsin

Gretchen L. Haas, Ph.D.
Assistant Professor of Psychology in Psychiatry, Cornell
University Medical College, New York, New York

Robert E. Hales, M.D.
Associate Professor of Psychiatry, Uniformed Services
University of the Health Sciences, F. Edward Hébert School of
Medicine, Bethesda, Maryland; Director of Psychiatry
Residency Training, Walter Reed Army Medical Center; Clinical
Associate Professor of Psychiatry, Georgetown University
School of Medicine, Washington, D.C.

Leo E. Hollister, M.D.
Professor of Medicine, Psychiatry and Pharmacology, Stanford
University Medical Center; Senior Medical Investigator,
Veterans Administration Medical Center, Palo Alto, California

Kay Redfield Jamison, Ph.D.
Associate Professor; Director, UCLA Affective Disorders Clinic, Department of Psychiatry, UCLA School of Medicine, Los Angeles, California

George E. Jaskiw, M.D.
Clinical Fellow in Psychiatry, National Institute of Mental Health Intramural Research Program, St. Elizabeths Hospital, Washington, D.C.

James W. Jefferson, M.D.
Professor of Psychiatry, University of Wisconsin Medical School, Madison, Wisconsin

Martin B. Keller, M.D.
Associate Professor of Psychiatry, Harvard Medical School; Director of Clinical Research, Department of Psychiatry, Massachusetts General Hospital, Boston, Massachusetts

Steven E. Keller, Ph.D.
Research Associate Professor of Psychiatry, Mount Sinai School of Medicine, New York, New York

Howard Klar, M.D.
Assistant Professor of Psychiatry, Mount Sinai School of Medicine, New York, New York

Douglas F. Levinson, M.D.
Assistant Professor of Psychiatry; Director, Neuropsychiatric Unit, Medical College of Pennsylvania at Eastern Pennsylvania Psychiatric Institute, Philadelphia, Pennsylvania

John R. Lion, M.D.
Clinical Professor of Psychiatry, University of Maryland School of Medicine, Institute of Psychiatry and Human Behavior, Baltimore, Maryland

Irwin Lucki, Ph.D.
Assistant Professor of Psychology in Psychiatry, University of Pennsylvania School of Medicine, Philadelphia, Pennsylvania

Kathleen R. Merikangas, Ph.D.
Assistant Professor of Psychiatry and Epidemiology, Yale University School of Medicine; Depression Research Unit, New Haven, Connecticut

John M. Morihisa, M.D.
Professor and Chairman, Department of Psychiatry,
Georgetown University School of Medicine; Psychiatry Service,
Veterans Administration Medical Center, Washington, D.C.

Robert O. Pasnau, M.D.
Professor of Psychiatry, University of California, Los Angeles;
President, American Psychiatric Association, Washington, D.C.

Samuel W. Perry, M.D.
Associate Professor of Clinical Psychiatry, Cornell University
Medical College, New York, New York

Robert M. Post, M.D.
Chief, Biological Psychiatry Branch, National Institute of Mental
Health Intramural Research Program, Bethesda, Maryland

William Z. Potter, M.D., Ph.D.
Chief, Section on Clinical Pharmacology, Laboratory of Clinical
Science, National Institute of Mental Health Intramural
Research Program, Bethesda, Maryland

Mark H. Rapaport, M.D.
Chief Resident in Psychiatric Research, Department of
Psychiatry, University of California, San Diego; The San Diego
Veterans Administration Medical Center, San Diego, California

Darrel A. Regier, M.D., M.P.H.
Director, Division of Clinical Research, National Institute of
Mental Health, Rockville, Maryland

William H. Reid, M.D., M.P.H.
Medical Director, Colonial Hills Hospital, San Antonio, Texas

Karl Rickels, M.D.
Stuart and Emily B.H. Mudd Professor of Human Behavior;
Professor of Psychiatry, University of Pennsylvania School of
Medicine, Philadelphia, Pennsylvania

Lee N. Robins, Ph.D.
Professor of Sociology in Psychiatry, Department of Psychiatry,
Washington University School of Medicine, St. Louis, Missouri

Norman E. Rosenthal, M.D.
Chief, Unit on Outpatient Studies, Clinical Psychobiology
Branch, National Institute of Mental Health Intramural
Research Program, Bethesda, Maryland

Peter Roy-Byrne, M.D.
Associate Professor of Psychiatry, Washington University
School of Medicine, Seattle, Washington

Matthew V. Rudorfer, M.D.
Senior Staff Fellow, Section on Clinical Pharmacology,
Laboratory of Clinical Science, National Institute of Mental
Health Intramural Research Program, Bethesda, Maryland

Michael Rutter, C.B.E., M.D., F.R.C.P., F.R.C. Psych.
Honorary Director, MRC Child Psychiatry Unit, Institute of
Psychiatry, Denmark Hill, London, England

David A. Sack, M.D.
Chief, Clinical Research Unit, Clinical Psychobiology Branch,
National Institute of Mental Health Intramural Research
Program, Bethesda, Maryland

Carl Salzman, M.D.
Associate Professor of Psychiatry, Harvard Medical School;
Director, Psychopharmacology, Massachusetts Mental Health
Center, Boston, Massachusetts

Steven J. Schleifer, M.D.
Assistant Professor of Psychiatry, Mount Sinai School of
Medicine, New York, New York

Herbert C. Schulberg, Ph.D.
Professor of Psychiatry and Psychology; Director, Social and
Community Psychiatry Program, Department of Psychiatry,
Western Psychiatric Institute and Clinic, University of
Pittsburgh, Pittsburgh, Pennsylvania

Edward E. Schweizer, M.D.
Assistant Professor of Psychiatry, University of Pennsylvania
School of Medicine, Philadelphia, Pennsylvania

M. Katherine Shear, M.D.
Assistant Professor of Psychiatry, Cornell University Medical
College, New York, New York

Priyattam J. Shiromani, Ph.D.
Postgraduate Psychobiologist, Department of Psychiatry,
Veterans Administration Medical Center, University of
California, San Diego, California

George M. Simpson, M.D.
Professor of Psychiatry; Director, Clinical Psychopharmacology,
Medical College of Pennsylvania at Eastern Pennsylvania
Psychiatric Institute, Philadelphia, Pennsylvania

Solomon H. Snyder, M.D.
Department of Neuroscience, Johns Hopkins Medical School,
Baltimore, Maryland

Paul H. Soloff, M.D.
Associate Professor of Psychiatry, Western Psychiatric Institute
and Clinic, University of Pittsburgh School of Medicine,
Pittsburgh, Pennsylvania

Marvin Stein, M.D.
Esther and Joseph Klingenstein Professor and Chairman,
Department of Psychiatry, Mount Sinai School of Medicine,
New York, New York

Kenneth Tardiff, M.D., M.P.H.
Associate Dean for Student Affairs and Academic Programs,
Associate Professor of Psychiatry and of Public Health, Cornell
University Medical College, New York, New York

Thomas W. Uhde, M.D.
Chief, Unit on Anxiety and Affective Disorders, Biological
Psychiatry Branch, National Institute of Mental Health,
Bethesda, Maryland

Thomas A. Wehr, M.D.
Chief, Clinical Psychobiology Branch, National Institute of
Mental Health Intramural Research Program, Bethesda,
Maryland

Daniel R. Weinberger, M.D.
Chief, Clinical Neuropsychiatry and Neurobehavior Section, Neuropsychiatry Branch, National Institute of Mental Health Intramural Research Program, Washington, D.C.

Myrna M. Weissman, Ph.D.
Professor of Psychiatry and Epidemiology; Director, Depression Research Unit, Yale University School of Medicine, New Haven, Connecticut

Harvey A. Whiteford, M.B., B.S., M.R.A.N.Z.C.P.
Research Fellow, Department of Psychiatry and Behavioral Sciences, Stanford University School of Medicine, Stanford, California

I

Bipolar Disorders

I

Bipolar
Disorders

Contents

Section I

Bipolar Disorders

Foreword

by Frederick K. Goodwin, M.D., and Kay Redfield Jamison, Ph.D., Section Editors

More than five years ago the editors of this section began work on a comprehensive book about manic-depressive illness, the first to be written in more than 30 years. In our early planning (Goodwin and Jamison, in press), we were initially motivated, and then humbled, by the enormity of the accumulated scientific and clinical information about the affective illnesses. This rapidly expanding knowledge base was paralleled by a growing recognition of the public health significance of these disorders and the enormous economic and social impact derived from their successful treatment. We chose to focus on bipolar manic-depressive illness because it fit well into a disease model with its relatively clear syndromal boundaries and its remarkably consistent descriptions (over many decades and across numerous cultures) of symptoms, natural history, and familial patterns. We were also impressed that, unlike unipolar major depressive disorders, so little systematic and integrated review existed.

While taking note of modern contributions, we found it especially appropriate to pay special tribute to Professor Emil Kraepelin. Time and time again we "rediscovered" contemporary findings in the original writings of this remarkably astute and careful observer. He not only laid the groundwork for a systematic nosology and clinical description of manic-depressive illness, but he anticipated, either explicitly or implicitly, many recent theoretical developments. In psychiatry, he was the first to fully develop a disease model backed by extensive and carefully organized observations and descriptions; his synthesis has had a profound and lasting impact on the field. His contribution was truly original and revolutionary, not only because of the extensive clinical descriptions, however elegant, but also because his classification system was based on the validation of diagnoses by *independent* assessments of course, outcome, and family history. Given the current (and not inappropriate) concern over biological reductionism, it is important to note that Kraepelin's disease model included psychological factors, and he was one of the first to point out explicitly the importance of psychological stresses as precipitating factors for episodes. Further, by noting "slight colorings of mood which pass over without sharp boundary into the domain of personal predisposition," Kraepelin provided the basis for the recent development of spectrum concepts which focus on the relationship between aspects of manic-depressive illness and normal variance in mood, energy patterns, and behavior.

Bipolar illness remains fascinating because, far more than other psychiatric illnesses, it has been the central focus of psychobiological research for over two

The opinions expressed herein are those of the authors and do not reflect official policy of the NIMH.

decades. This has been true for several reasons. First, as noted by Dr. Keller (Chapter 1), the diagnostic criteria for bipolar disorder have enjoyed a consistently high rate of agreement among independent observers, even in the *DSM-II* era. Second, manic and depressive episodes tend to spontaneously remit. The opportunity to compare biological measures during the illness with the same measures in the recovered state permits longitudinal paradigms that can circumvent the problem of interindividual variability. Third, many manic-depressive patients experience regular recurrences of their episodes. This means that, in a research setting, the onset of a given phase can be predicted to some extent, allowing the investigator to schedule data collection at critical points. Fourth, the period of change from one phase to another (the switch) is often both rapid and profound, especially during the switch into mania. This switch period offers maximum opportunity to uncover behaviorally relevant biochemical changes. Finally, as noted by Dr. Potter and his colleagues (Chapter 2), there is an especially rich array of pharmacological–behavioral correlations that can be observed in manic-depressive illness. With two distinct, and in many respects opposite, illness phases to study, the study of drug–behavioral relationships is multiplied and enhanced. Of the drugs that precipitate mania, some are antidepressants, others are not; some of the drugs that diminish mania produce depression, while others either do not or are actually antidepressants. Thus, bipolar illness provides at least six distinct patterns of response to pharmacological agents: increase and decrease of mania, increase and decrease of depression, and increased or decreased frequency of episodes. Because the onset of an episode (especially mania or hypomania) is relatively easy to identify and measure, bipolar illness provides an excellent model for the study of the relations among stress, biological changes, and illness onset.

Not only does this illness play a central role in clinical psychobiology, but its role in basic neurobiology can easily be appreciated when one examines a number of papers published on the mechanism of action of mood altering drugs. Lithium is, of course, the most striking example. Prior to its establishment as an effective maintenance treatment for bipolar illness, there existed only a handful of studies into the effects of this ion on brain function. Over the last 20 years, the literature on the neurobiological effects of lithium has exploded and now exceeds one thousand papers per year. That lithium can treat the "opposite" states of mania and depression, and that it can prevent as well as treat both phases, continues to provide specific challenges for neurobiology.

From yet another perspective, bipolar illness is fascinating in that it provides rich opportunities for the study of fundamental human characteristics—elation, creativity, depression, impulsivity, psychosis, and the coexistence of opposites.

The opening chapter by Dr. Keller focuses on the fundamentals of manic-depressive illness: diagnosis, natural course, and epidemiology. To the task of integrating contemporary diagnostic systems with traditional concepts, Keller brings his intimate knowledge of the ongoing NIMH collaborative study of depression, with its extensive longitudinal clinical data from a large cohort of bipolar patients. The stability of diagnostic constructs of bipolar disorder over the years made the integration easier. In considering the distinction between bipolar and unipolar disorders, it is important to evaluate *cyclicity* as well as polarity. It is a reasonable hypothesis that the highly recurrent, cyclic forms of unipolar depression are closely related to bipolar illness, but the definitive studies have not yet been done. As Keller points out, most unipolar/bipolar comparisons involve considerably more heterogeneity in the unipolar than in the bipolar groups. Questions concerning the boundary between bipolar II and bipolar I and the existence of unipolar mania would be sharpened by the inclusion of Professor Jules Angst's subclassification system for bipolar disorders (1978). He divides bipolar patients into "MD," "Md," and "mD" groups, with "M" and "D" indicating a manic or depressive episode requiring hospitalization, while "m" and "d" designate episodes clearly different from normal, but not of sufficient severity to require hospitalization. Angst's "mD" group is analogous to bipolar II in the *DSM-III*, but the American system has no subcategory analogous to Angst's "Md" group. This is unfortunate since he has reported interesting differences among these subgroups: for instance, the ratio of females to males is substantially higher in the predominantly depressed subgroups (unipolar depression and "Dm"), while males are more frequent in the subgroups with full manic episodes ("MD" and "Md"). Almost certainly the reports of unipolar mania reflect predominantly patients with the "Md" form of bipolar illness.

Keller's review of "organic" causes of mania gives useful emphasis to what is an important clinical differential diagnosis as well as an avenue for potential new insights into neuroanatomical substrates for primary mania, an approach recently reviewed by Jeste and colleagues (manuscript in submission). Dr. Keller's descriptions of well intervals and personality factors in bipolar illness anticipate topics developed more fully in Dr. Jamison's chapter on psychotherapeutic issues.

One important aspect of epidemiology—seasonality—is included in the discussion of biological rhythms (Chapter 3), rather than in Chapter 1. Given space limitations, Keller's review of family history does not include development of the genetic models for bipolar disorder, which fortunately have been well reviewed elsewhere (Gershon, 1983).

In undertaking the review of an enormous, rapidly expanding body of knowledge, Dr. Potter and his colleagues judiciously chose to focus on biological findings in which bipolar/unipolar differences have been reported. In doing so, they note the difficulty in confronting a literature largely developed before the bipolar/unipolar distinction was commonplace. Starting from the classical concept of the "pharmacological bridge," Potter and colleagues focus on cyclicity—a fundamental aspect of bipolar illness not previously addressed in pharmacological modeling. While avoiding a premature integration of the diverse array of biological findings, the authors nevertheless point the way by emphasizing dysregulation rather than classical formulations based simply on deficits or excesses of monoamine neurotransmitters. Their focus on the importance of a biological marker for bipolarity is noteworthy and it anticipates the discussions of pharmacologically precipitated mania and cycle induction in Chapters 3 and 4.

Chapter 3, by Dr. Wehr and his colleagues, integrates clinical and research observations of sleep in bipolar disorder into the general framework of biological rhythms. Biological rhythm research represents one of the most exciting and fruitful new frontiers in the study of manic-depressive illness, and Wehr and his group have pioneered its development in this country. In tracing the origins of their focus on rhythm disturbances in bipolar disorder, the authors return to the focus on cyclicity introduced by Keller and give it additional emphasis, particularly with regard to possible neurobiological and pharmacological implications. Wehr and his colleagues were the first to report systematically the impact of tricyclic antidepressants on cycle frequency in bipolar patients, and their initial observations have now been widely replicated and represent a significant consideration for the practicing clinician. Of equal clinical significance is their focus on the critical role of sleep. Thus, manipulation of sleep not only provides a nonpharmacological alternative for the treatment of depression, but is also capable of precipitating mania. This latter observation leads to practical and sensible recommendations for clinicians; for example, that bipolar patients should avoid activities and substances with a high potential for sleep disruption, and that sleep assisting medications should be considered for short-term use in bipolar patients. The recent indentification by Wehr's group of seasonal affective disorder (a subtype of bipolar II disorder) has generated considerable interest, not only because of its biological implications, but also because it has formed the basis for the development of another nonpharmacological treatment (artificial light).

In Chapter 4, Drs. Goodwin and Roy-Byrne emphasize practical clinical applications, drawing not only from the research literature, but also from the authors' clinical experience and the responses of 40 experts in the field to a systematic questionnaire originally developed to provide material for the treatment chapters in *Manic-Depressive Illness*. Goodwin and Roy-Byrne deal with the treatment of breakthrough episodes in Chapter 4 rather than in Chapter 6 on treatment resistance, as breakthrough episodes are part of routine management.

Dr. Jamison's chapter on psychotherapeutic issues and suicide brings together two topics which are extremely important, but too frequently overlooked. The interaction of psychotherapy and drug therapy in bipolar disorders, although not as well explored as those in unipolar disorders, is an area of rich potential. It has been our clinical impression that the psychological component of the treatment of bipolar disorder is a major factor behind the wide variation in the reported success rates with prophylactic medications. In addition to Dr. Jamison's specific principles of psychotherapy with manic-depressive patients on maintenance medication, we would add the importance of clinicians having a solid knowledge of the illness—its phenomenology, biology, pharmacology, genetics, and psychology—in order to function effectively as psychotherapists. The central issue in the psychological management of bipolar patients is medication compliance, and recent studies show substantial enhancement of treatment outcome associated with adjunctive psychotherapy, no doubt reflecting the contribution of improved compliance.

Today, we are encountering a new wave of professional and public interest in the problem of suicide and, with it, much confusion about risk factors—a confusion which comes partly from obscuring the distinction between completed suicide and attempted suicide. Dr. Jamison's chapter reminds us that the single most important contributing factor to actual suicides is the presence of a major affective disorder. Among the major affective disorders, bipolar illness conveys the highest risk, with suicide as the cause of death in approximately 25 percent of bipolar patients in the pre-lithium era. A recent survey of several thousand patients being followed in four lithium clinics indicates that the suicide rate is strikingly less than would have been expected from the pre-lithium outcome data. Dr. Jamison emphasizes the important point that the most effective prevention of suicide lies in the competent management of the underlying affective illness.

Chapter 6, by Drs. Post and Uhde on treatment-resistant bipolar illness, opens by returning to fundamentals—the assessment of natural course. The authors build on Keller's chapter by emphasizing a practical methodology for charting the life course and illness as a precondition for quality treatment. Post and Uhde appropriately chose to focus on the anticonvulsants which, in our opinion, comprise one of the major contemporary developments in the treatment of bipolar illness. As developed by Post and his group, the use of anticonvulsants in bipolar illness represents a unique example in psychiatry of a practical treatment which developed from theoretical models; that is, kindling and sensitization. It is a pleasure to see the final chapter both open and close with a theoretical focus.

REFERENCES

Angst J: The course of affective disorders, II: typology of bipolar manic-depressive illness. Archiv for Psychiatrie und Nervenkrankheiten 226:65-73, 1978

Gershon ES: The genetics of affective disorders, in Psychiatry Update: The American Psychiatric Association Annual Review, vol. 3. Edited by Grinspoon L. Washington, DC, American Psychiatric Press, Inc., 1983

Goodwin FK, Jamison KR: Manic-Depressive Illness. New York, Oxford University Press (in press)

Chapter 1

Differential Diagnosis, Natural Course, and Epidemiology of Bipolar Disorders

by Martin B. Keller, M.D.

OVERVIEW

History and Theory

The evolution of the concept of bipolar disorder began with Kraepelin (1921), who included both unipolar and bipolar affective disorders in his definition of manic-depressive illness. Leonhard et al (1962) proposed the separation of patients with manic-depressive insanity into two groups: bipolar and monopolar. Patients termed bipolar had a history of depression and mania whereas those termed monopolar experienced only depressive or only manic/hypomanic episodes (Klerman et al, 1984). As the definition of bipolarity developed further, it became inclusive of manic or hypomanic patients with or without a history of depression. Following work by Perris (1966) and Winokur et al (1969), bipolar disorder became a widely accepted concept in psychiatry (Coryell et al, 1984).

A major theoretical question is whether unipolar and bipolar illnesses are variants of one disorder or are two distinct disorders (Klerman et al, 1984). There are familial/genetic, neurophysiological, biochemical, personality, and clinical correlates that validate bipolar illness as a separate diagnostic entity. However, there is not etiological evidence to support this distinction (Krauthammer and Klerman, 1978). The marked differential treatment response of unipolar and bipolar disorder warrants the distinction for clinical and research purposes, pending more conclusive data (Klerman et al, 1984).

Throughout this chapter, unless otherwise specified, mania and hypomania will refer to those conditions without any known organic etiology. A later section in this chapter will cover a detailed review of the differential diagnosis of organic etiologies of mania and hypomania.

CLASSIFICATION OF BIPOLAR DISORDERS

This section includes a description of existing and proposed categories of bipolar disorder. Bipolar I and bipolar II disorder will be discussed briefly here and in detail in each of the ensuing sections of this chapter. Bipolar III, cyclothymia, and unipolar mania will be covered almost exclusively in this section, since much less is known about these categories.

Klerman (1982) delineated six variations of elated mood to encompass the spectrum of manic states:

1. normal states: happiness, pleasure, joy
2. neurotic elations: cyclothymic personality, hypomanic personality
3. hypomania (nonpsychotic)
4. mania (nonpsychotic)
5. mania (psychotic): delusions or other manifestations of impaired reality testing
6. 'delirious' mania: severe overactivity, hostile attitude toward others, destruction of property, assaultiveness toward others, paranoid delusions (Klerman, 1982, pg. 448)

It is now widely recognized that more normal feelings of happiness, joy, and pleasure are rarely present during full blown manic or hypomanic syndromes.

Bipolar I

The *Diagnostic and Statistical Manual of Mental Disorders, Third Edition (DSM-III)* (1980) criteria for bipolar disorder require an episode of mania with or without a history of depression. The Research Diagnostic Criteria (RDC) diagnosis of bipolar I requires that at least one manic episode and depressive episode have occurred during the patient's lifetime.

The *DSM-III* and RDC for mania are identical, with the exception that the RDC includes impairment criteria (Spitzer et al, 1985). The diagnostic features of mania are presented in Table 1.

Bipolar II

There is increasing agreement about the value of distinguishing bipolar I from bipolar II disorder (Dunner and colleagues, unpublished paper; Perris, 1982). Patients with bipolar I disorder suffer from episodes of depression and mania, whereas those with bipolar II disorder have brief hypomanic episodes, and episodes of major depression (Perris, 1982). It is the presence of hypomanic episodes which differentiates patients with bipolar II disorder from patients with recurrent unipolar disorder.

Hypomania is a nonpsychotic elevated, expansive, or irritable mood. According to the RDC, for a definite hypomanic episode the expansive mood must persist for at least one week, while two days are required for a "probable" episode. Two of the descriptive criteria for mood in the manic disorder must be met if the mood is irritable rather than euphoric (Spitzer et al, 1985).

While RDC bipolar II patients would be classified as atypical bipolar disorder in the *DSM-III*, the revision of the *DSM-III*, *DSM-III-R*, has developed a new category for bipolar II classification. The *DSM-III-R* classifies bipolar II as "bipolar disorder not otherwise specified," which is also used to categorize chronic hypomania (Spitzer et al, 1985; *DSM-III-R*, in press).

There is evidence that although some bipolar II patients may eventually have a manic episode and thus meet criteria for bipolar I disorder (Akiskal et al, 1978; 1983b; Dunner, 1983), many will not. The next section of this chapter will include a more detailed discussion of bipolar II disorder and its relationship to bipolar I disorder and recurrent unipolar disorder.

Table 1. Diagnostic Features of Manic Episode*

Essential Features	Associated Features
A. Periods of elevated, elated, expansive, or irritable mood: This mood is predominant, although it may be interrupted by depressive mood	Lability of mood, often with rapid, brief shifts to anger or depression
	Increased sociability
B. Hospitalization—or duration of at least one week—with at least three of these symptoms, or four, if the mood is irritable:	Intrusive, demanding, tactless behavior
	Flamboyant dress; excessive makeup
1. Increased activity or restlessness	Giving away candy, belongings, money to strangers
2. Pressure of speech or increased talkativeness	Speech rapid, loud, often filled with jokes, puns, or rhymes
3. Flight of ideas	Occasionally, loosening of associations and incoherence, even to the point of disorientation and confusion, particularly when exhausted or on medication
4. Inflated self-esteem (grandiosity)	
5. Reduced sleep	
6. Distractibility (i.e., reacting to many, often irrelevant stimuli of the environment)	
7. High risk-taking and poor judgment (e.g., reckless driving, buying sprees, sexual indiscretions)	
C. No mood-incongruent delusions or hallucinations, and no bizarre behavior if the affective syndrome (A and B) is not present	
D. Not associated with schizophrenia, schizophreniform disorder, or paranoid disorder	
E. Not due to organic or toxic mental disorder	

*Adapted from American Psychiatric Association: Diagnostic and Statistical Manual of Mental Disorders, Third Edition. Washington, DC, American Psychiatric Association, 1980

Reprinted from Lehmann HE: Affective disorders: clinical features, in Comprehensive Textbook of Psychiatry IV, vol. 1. Edited by Kaplan HI, Sadock BJ. Baltimore, Williams & Wilkins, 1984. Copyright 1984 by Williams & Wilkins Co. Reprinted by permission

Bipolar III

It has been hypothesized that antidepressant medication may trigger the onset of manic symptoms (Dunner et al, 1976), and Klerman (1981) has suggested classifying these patients as bipolar III.

Bunney (1978) reviewed 80 reports which documented antidepressant induced changes in polarity from depression to mania. The majority of the 10 percent of the 3,923 patients with induced mania had a history of bipolar disorder (Klerman, 1981). However, the magnitude of the risk of this side effect of antidepressant drugs has not yet been established with precision. This is because it is difficult to disentangle the medication effect from the natural tendency of some patients to cycle to hypomania or mania, even in the absence of antidepressant medication (Keller et al, 1986, submitted for publication).

Unipolar Mania

A very small proportion of the population has only manic episodes (Boyd and Weissman, 1982). In a longitudinal study, Helgason (1979) found that only .1 percent of 5,395 persons had a manic episode without a history of depression. Hence, he uses the terms 'bipolar' and 'mania' to distinguish those who experience both mania and depression from unipolar manics. A more recent investigation provides some data that unipolar mania may be more common than was once thought. Nurnberger et al (1979) found that approximately one out of every six patients in an outpatient lithium clinic had mania as defined by the RDC, and no history of major depression.

It has been observed that the symptoms of unipolar and bipolar manic syndromes are identical. Additionally, the age of onset and sex ratios for both disorders are similar. Among first degree relatives of the two groups there are no consistent differences in the risk for affective illness (Pfohl et al, 1982).

In summary, patients who have manic episodes without depression do exist, but that does not necessarily mean that they constitute a distinct diagnostic group. It is expected that a number of 'unipolar manics' would be seen, given the varied distribution over the course of a person's life of the age at which manic and depressive episodes first become manifest. While the case for unipolar mania as a distinct entity should not be considered closed (Pfohl et al, 1982), the continued classification of unipolar mania and bipolar disorder under the same category in the *DSM-III-R* seems justified based on the data described above.

Cyclothymia

Historically, cyclothymia has been classified as a personality disorder in most diagnostic nomenclatures. The *DSM-III* grouped cyclothymia with other affective disorders, since its symptomatology resembles bipolar I and bipolar II disorder (Klerman et al, 1984).

The periods of elation in cyclothymia are short-lived and less severe than manic episodes. Because cyclothymics have self-control, they often present without exhibiting symptoms and may function well in interviews (Tyrer and Shopsin, 1982). Symptoms are usually muted, "e.g., loss of interest or pleasure, instead of feelings of hopelessness and depression; irritable or expansive mood, instead of manic euphoria" (Lehmann, 1985, p. 804). The longstanding nature of cyclothymia frequently causes substantial social and occupational impairment; however, due to the insidious onset and long duration, such patients may learn to adapt to their symptoms so that they have minimal disruption in functioning (Lehmann, 1985). In particular, during the elated periods, these people are often considered by themselves, family, and friends to be normal, outgoing, energetic individuals.

Cyclothymic disorder has been reported to most frequently begin in early adulthood, and appears to occur more often in women than men, in contrast to full-blown bipolar affective disorder which equally affects men and women. As with bipolar I and bipolar II, it is more common in families of patients who have a major affective disorder (Lehmann, 1985).

The cyclothymic temperament was considered by Kraepelin to be a "form-fruste" of manic depressive illness. Although data is limited, it has been observed that a high proportion of people who become manic have a premorbid cyclothymic personality. This view is widely accepted in European psychiatry and described in the writings of Kretschmer and Schneider.

Given the many clinical similarities between cyclothymia and bipolar I and bipolar II disorder, cyclothymia is often a difficult differential diagnosis for clinicians. Currently the evidence is insufficient to determine whether cyclothymia is an independent entity or a mild form of bipolar affective disorder.

CONTROVERSIES IN THE CLASSIFICATION OF BIPOLAR DISORDERS

Many nosologic questions regarding mania and hypomania require validation. Rather than cover all of these issues, this section will consist of an in-depth discussion of two major questions about classification: First, what is the relationship of bipolar II disorder to bipolar I disorder? Second, what is the relationship between bipolar I disorder and psychotic states, particularly schizoaffective disorder?

Are Bipolar I and Bipolar II Distinct Entities?

The issue is unresolved as to whether bipolar disorder and unipolar illness are separate disorders, or whether they form a continuum. Recent efforts to address this problem have included the applications of genetic models (Gershon, 1983; Reich, unpublished paper), but the answers are not yet established (Klerman et al, 1984). Related to this controversy is the relationship of bipolar II disorder to bipolar I disorder and to recurrent unipolar disorder.

Data have emerged recently on prior course, characteristics of the index episode, diagnostic stability, and familial aggregation of patients with bipolar II disorder, which support separating bipolar II disorder from patients with both bipolar I and those with recurrent unipolar disorder.

Less evidence supports the separation of patients with bipolar I and bipolar II disorder. Similarities among these groups include age of onset, increased tendency to cycle within episodes, and a similar proportion of relatives and family units who have had a manic or hypomanic episode. In contrast, patients with recurrent unipolar disorder have significantly lower rates of mania or hypomania in their relatives than patients with bipolar I or bipolar II disorder.

Despite the specific similarities described above, there are also differences of potential clinical and research importance between bipolar I and bipolar II patients (Endicott et al, 1985). Bipolar II patients and their relatives appear to be heterogeneous, including individuals at high risk to 'switch' to bipolar I disorder (Dunner et al, 1976; Akiskal et al, 1977, 1978, 1983b; Klerman, 1980). Although individuals may be manifesting a milder bipolar I disorder, evidence is accumulating that suggests some bipolar II patients may 'breed true' and not simply be a less severe type of bipolar I disorder (Endicott et al, 1985).

Until definitive data become available, the results described above, which identify similarities and differences for the three conditions in prior course, phenomenology, and familial rates of disorder, have led Coryell et al (1985) and others to recommend that at the present time bipolar II patients be categorized separately from both recurrent unipolar and bipolar I patients.

The Distinction Between Bipolar Illness and Schizoaffective Disorder

Patients who are manic and who have psychotic behavior often are found to have symptoms typical of schizophrenia, but there is considerable debate as to whether these states should be regarded as affective variants, schizophrenic variants, or as a separate diagnostic entity (Klerman, 1982).

The label schizoaffective was first used by Kasanin (1933) to refer to patients presenting with these symptoms. Before Kasanin, multiple terms had been created, including: 'schizophreniform psychosis,' 'cycloid psychosis,' 'atypical psychosis,' 'good prognosis schizophrenia,' 'reactive psychoses,' and 'atypical schizophrenic.'

These disorders were classified under the schizophrenias in the DSM-I and DSM-II. DSM-III (1980) allows these patients to be placed under the heading of 'psychoses not elsewhere classified' without specifying criteria, or to be classified as manics or major depressives with mood-incongruent psychotic features. In the DSM-III-R (in press), schizoaffective disorder is placed in the category of 'psychotic disorders not elsewhere classified.'

Clayton (1982) and others suggest that schizoaffective mania is best considered as a severe form of bipolar affective disorder, whereas schizoaffective depression is thought to represent a more diverse group of conditions. This section considers the relationship of bipolar disorder to schizoaffective mania separately from its relationship to schizoaffective depression.

Evidence has been accumulating over the past 10 years that schizoaffective manic patients resemble bipolar patients (Cadoret et al, 1974; Abrams et al, 1976; Brockington et al, 1980) in the following ways: an early age of onset, an acute onset of each episode, and similar sex ratios. Schizoaffective manics have also been found to have high rates of affectively ill relatives, particularly of the bipolar type (Van Eerdewegh, unpublished paper).

In contrast, schizoaffective depressives probably comprise a mixed group of patients, including: schizophrenics with depression; major depressives with psychotic features; and patients with primary conditions, such as obsessive-compulsive disorder and somatoform disorder, who develop a psychotic depression (Clayton, 1982). The data supporting this position will be summarized in the rest of this section.

An increase of schizophrenia has been reported in the families of schizoaffective depressed patients, when compared to families of patients with major depression and to families of patients with schizoaffective mania.

Greater similarities in course are reported between patients with schizoaffective mania and bipolar disorder than between schizoaffective depressed patients and those with bipolar disorder (Brockington et al, 1980; Clayton, 1982; Abrams and Taylor, 1976; Pope et al, 1980; Miller and Libman, 1979). In particular, Cadoret et al (1974) found a greater number of lifetime episodes in schizoaffective mania than in schizoaffective depression, which is consistent with the increased number of episodes in bipolar patients compared to unipolar patients.

Brockington et al (1980) found that past history, clinical features, and patterns of outcome were more variable in schizoaffective depressed patients than in schizoaffective manic patients. They also found that very few of the patients developed bipolar affective disorder, as some followed a typical unipolar depressive course and others appeared to be more typically schizophrenic (Clayton, 1982).

In conclusion, current knowledge suggests that it is important to look at schizoaffective patients in a dichotomous fashion, separating schizoaffective manic patients from schizoaffective depressed patients. This has prognostic value clinically and research utility.

DIAGNOSIS OF BIPOLAR DISORDERS

In this section I will discuss three aspects of the differential diagnosis of mania and hypomania: 1) organic conditions which have manic and hypomanic symptoms; 2) distinguishing between mania and hypomania and other nonorganic psychiatric disorders; and 3) the reliability of diagnosing mania and hypomania.

Functional Versus Organic Causes of Mania and Hypomania

Most manic episodes are phases of a nonorganic bipolar disorder. However, a significant number of manic episodes occur secondary to organic conditions in patients with or without a history of affective disorder (Klerman, 1982).

SPECIFIC ORGANIC CAUSES OF MANIA. Hendrie (1978) and Krauthammer and Klerman (1978) propose the division of organic causes of mania into two groups: 1) organic conditions that are associated with or gradually develop into an organic syndrome, and 2) organic conditions that induce mania that is phenomenologically indistinguishable from functional bipolar disorder (Lazare, 1979). Multiple sclerosis and drug withdrawal states are examples of the first group. The second group includes agents such as L-dopa and steroids. Table 2 is a comprehensive listing of organic causes of mania.

The concept of secondary mania is not recognized in the *DSM-III* (1980) or the RDC (Spitzer et al, 1985). However, the *DSM-III-R* (in press) acknowledges that organic factors may induce mania.

In the *DSM-III-R* secondary mania can be classified as a 'Non-Substance Induced Organic Mental Syndrome and Disorder,' or a 'Substance Use Disorder.' More specifically, mania that is secondary to a neurologic or metabolic condition can be classified as an 'Organic Affective Syndrome.' For mania that is drug related there are three categories under the 'Substance Use Disorder' heading for classification. The 'Psychoactive Substance Induced Organic Mental Disorder' category can be used for mania induced by a specific drug or alcohol, or for manic

Table 2. Organic Causes of Manic and Hypomanic Symptoms

Drug related
Steroids and ACTH*
Isoniazid*
Bromides*
L-dopa*
Antidepressants
Hallucinogens (marijuana, LSD, mescaline, psilocybin, STP, cocaine)
Sympathomimetic amines (dexedrine, methedrine, Preludin, Ritalin)
Disulfiram (Antabuse)
Alcohol
Barbiturates
Anticholinergics (Symmetrel, Pagitane, Akineton, Cogentin, Artane)
Anticonvulsants (Phenurone, Zarontin, Milontin)
Benzodiazepines

Neurologic conditions
Tumors (parasagittal meningioma, diencephalic glioma, suprasellar
    craniopharyngioma)*
Epilepsy
Infection (postviral encephalitis, influenza)*
General paresis
Multiple sclerosis
Huntington's disease
Postcerebrovascular accident
Right temporal lobectomy
Posttraumatic confusion
Postelectroconvulsive therapy
Deliriform organic brain disease

Metabolic conditions
Postoperative states*
Hemodialysis*
Hyperthyroidism
Postinfectious hypomania
Cushing's disease
Addison's disease

Other conditions
Postisolation syndrome

*Meets criteria of Krauthammer and Klerman (1978) for secondary mania

Reprinted from Lazare A: Manic behavior, in Outpatient Psychiatry: Diagnosis and Treatment. Edited by Lazare A. Baltimore, Williams & Wilkins, 1979. Copyright 1979 by Williams & Wilkins Co. Reprinted by permission states that are precipitated by substance withdrawal. For induction of mania from substances unspecified in the *DSM-III-R*, such as L-dopa, Cogentin, Artane, or unknown, the 'Other Drug or Unspecified Psychoactive Substance Induced Organic Mental Disorders' category can be used. The category, 'Other Drug or Unspecified Psychoactive Substance Affective Disorder,' indicates the occurrence of an affective episode in response to an unknown or unspecified substance. **CLINICAL APPROACH TO DIFFERENTIAL DIAGNOSIS.** The best approach for diagnosing an organic cause of manic behavior is knowledge of the disorders outlined in Table 2, and familiarity with the specific symptoms of these syndromes. Factors that should alert a clinician to a possible organic etiology include: no past history of clear-cut affective episodes, no family history of mania or depression, sudden onset in a well-functioning individual, and lack of treatment response. Other indications of an organic etiology are persistent confusion following improvement in manic symptoms, shifts from confusion to a clear sensorium, and exposure to any of the exogenous agents listed in Table 2 (Lazare, 1979).

Initial screening begins with a detailed history, especially inquiry about drug ingestion, medication, and recent infection. More extensive medical evaluation may be necessary, and this will usually involve a neurological examination, EEG, skull x-ray, and toxic screening (Krauthammer and Klerman, 1978).

Clinical treatment of secondary mania should focus on correcting the organic dysfunction, while also attending to the patient's psychological well-being. A trial of lithium carbonate or neuroleptic therapy is often indicated (Krauthammer and Klerman, 1978).

Differential Diagnosis from Nonorganic Psychiatric Syndromes

The differentiation of mania from non-organic psychiatric syndromes is of clinical importance. Four conditions to always consider include: schizophrenia, schizoaffective disorder, hysteria, and adolescent conduct disorder. Each of these disorders has features that may resemble those found in a manic syndrome.

As I have already mentioned, distinguishing schizoaffective mania from mania is difficult, and many people believe the two disorders are either on a continuum or represent one syndrome. For those who separate the disorders, the main symptom which separates schizoaffective psychosis from mania is the presence of mood-incongruent schizophrenic symptoms (Tyrer and Shopsin, 1982).

Thought disorder and characteristics of the patient's mood usually make it possible to distinguish schizophrenia from mania. For example, in schizophrenia, especially catatonia, there is rarely any elevation in mood (Tyrer and Shopsin, 1982).

Adolescent conduct disorder, especially in females, often presents with an irritable or expansive excitement. A history of delinquency should alert the clinician to a diagnosis of conduct disorder as opposed to mania, although such behavior may also be prodromal to a manic episode (Tyrer and Shopsin, 1982).

Hysterical neurosis, also termed conversion disorder in the *DSM-III*, should be distinguishable from mania, since when manic symptoms appear, they are rarely sustained (Tyrer and Shopsin, 1982).

Reliability of Diagnosing Mania and Hypomania

The reliability of diagnosing a past or current history of bipolar I disorder is very good, based on a series of interrater and test-retest reliability studies (Andreasen et al, 1981).

Table 3. SADS–L Test-Retest Study: Diagnostic Reliability*

SADS–L–RDC Lifetime Diagnoses	Base Rate, %	Intraclass R	
		Morning vs. Afternoon	Initial vs. Consensus
Bipolar 1	10	1.00	.88
Bipolar 2	6	.62	.06
Major depressive disorder	44	.87	.75
Primary	33	.70	.59
Secondary	6	.60	.51
Recurrent	15	.78	.21
Psychotic	9	.79	.24
Incapacitating	9	.19	.40
Alcoholism	25	.94	.72
Never mentally ill	33	.70	.63

*SADS–L indicates the Schedule for Affective Disorders and Schizophrenia–Lifetime Version; RDC, Research Diagnostic Criteria. $N = 50$

Reprinted from Andreasen NC, Grove WM, Shapiro RW: Reliability of lifetime diagnosis: a multicenter collaborative perspective. Arch Gen Psychiatry 38:400-405, 1981. Copyright 1981 by the American Medical Association. Reprinted by permission

However, bipolar II disorder is diagnosed with very poor reliability (Andreasen et al, 1981). The low reliability of diagnosing hypomania probably is a result of low rates of the disorder in the population, and the difficulty that patients and interviewers have in recalling and assessing mild symptoms that border on normality (Andreasen et al, 1981). Furthermore, since hypomanic episodes often coincide with periods of excellent productivity, and seldom lead to treatment intervention, it is plausible that these episodes may be ignored or forgotten (Endicott and colleagues, unpublished paper).

Data from Rice and colleagues (unpublished paper) suggest that although hypomania has low sensitivity, it has high specificity. This means that if a positive diagnosis at one of any number of separate interviews are used as a criteria, the chances of making a correct diagnosis are increased substantially. Since there is a high likelihood that a single interview will fail to elicit a past episode of hypomania, repeat assessments, along with a careful family history, are recommended when considering the diagnosis of hypomania.

In summary, the diagnosis of major depression or mania should present minimal problems for the well trained and experienced clinician, while the diagnosis of hypomania is considerably more difficult.

NATURAL COURSE

Bipolar patients have more episodes during their lifetime than unipolars, and this is not thought to be a consequence of an earlier age of first onset (Coryell and Winokur, 1982; Perris, 1982; Coryell et al, 1984).

The world literature on the natural course of manic-depressive illness has been comprehensively reviewed by Goodwin and Jamison (1984). Here we will focus on new information becoming available from naturalistic prospective longitudinal research protocols and from long-term randomized trials of maintenance treatment. There is substantially more information on bipolar I than bipolar II so most of the attention in this section will be on bipolar I patients.

Bipolar I

RECOVERY.   Coryell and Winokur's (1982) comparison of recovery rates in unipolar versus bipolar illness shows faster rates for unipolar illness in three reports (Bratfos and Haug, 1968; Shobe and Brion, 1971); Morrison et al, 1973) and for bipolar illness in three others (Hastings, 1958; Lundquist, 1945; Rao and Nammalvar, 1977). Recent findings from the NIMH Program on the Psychobiology of Depression show that the polarity of the episode at the time the patient seeks help significantly affects outcome (Keller et al, 1986, submitted for publication). For example, patients whose index episode was purely manic at entry recovered faster (median five weeks after entry) than patients whose index episode was purely depressed (median nine weeks after entry), whereas patients whose index episode was mixed or cycled between poles recovered much more slowly (median 14 weeks). Furthermore, bipolar patients who seek treatment for purely manic or purely depressed episodes are at high risk for cycling or becoming mixed prior to recovery (Keller et al, 1986, submitted for publication). Hence, the classification of bipolar disorders in the *DSM-III-R* based on the polarity of current episodes is of prognostic value.

Clinical factors identified as predictors of a slow recovery rate among bipolar patients include endogenous features, severity of depressive features, psychotic and secondary RDC subtypes of depression, alcoholism, psychomotor retardation, suicidal tendencies, anxiety, and a longer episode before entry into the study (Keller and colleagues, unpublished paper).

RELAPSE/RECURRENCE.   Zis and Goodwin (1979) reviewed a series of studies and documented high rates of relapse among bipolar patients. According to Zis and Goodwin (1979), one-third of Kraepelin's (1921) manic-depressive patients had a mixed or circular course. Chronicity or relapse was observed in almost all of the bipolar patients in Bratfos and Haug's (1968) follow-up study. Similarly, Rennie (1942) and Stendstedt (1952) found high rates of relapse, with 64 and 86 percent of bipolars having three or more episodes, respectively. Recurrence among Pollock's (1931) bipolar patients was less common, with 19 percent of subjects having three or more episodes. Nearly 60 percent of the bipolars in Perris' (1966) study had six or more episodes, and bipolar patients in Taschev's study (1974) averaged 4.7 episodes. Methodological limitations in these studies are discussed in detail by Zis and Goodwin (1979) and they conclude that further research on relapse is necessary in order to specify the lifetime rates of relapse and recurrence for bipolar disorders.

There is some evidence that patients with bipolar disorder have an increasing risk of experiencing a manic or depressive episode as they grow older, which may be a result of decreasing intervals between episodes as patients become older (Weissman and Boyd, 1985).

WELL INTERVALS. Although there is some evidence that the duration of the intervals between the episodes decreases with subsequent episodes (Coryell and Winokur, 1982), several investigations report that once a patient has had a certain number of episodes, the duration of the cycle (defined as the time from the beginning of one episode to the beginning of the next episode) becomes more stable and ultimately bottoms out at a cycle time of approximately six to nine months. This is thought to occur after the patient has had at least five episodes (Grof et al, 1974; Clayton, 1981; Coryell and Winokur, 1982; Angst et al, 1973; Lundquist, 1945). The phenomenon of changing cycle length over a person's lifetime is of great value in terms of prognosis and treatment planning, and is currently being studied intensively in several naturalistic prospective studies and long-term controlled treatment trials.

CHRONICITY. The precise risk of chronicity in bipolar disorder is unknown. This is partly true because lithium therapy has been so effective in shortening the course of episodes of mania (Clayton 1981). Coryell and Winokur (1982) report rates of chronicity in bipolar I disorder ranging from 15 to 53 percent based on their review of seven long-term follow-up studies. A limitation of these comparisons is that varying definitions of chronicity have been used in most of these studies.

Bipolar patients in the NIMH Program on the Psychobiology of Depression who presented with a purely depressed episode experienced rates of chronicity (22 percent) which were very close to those of non-bipolar patients (21 percent) entering the same study when they sought treatment with an episode of major depressive disorder. Mixed/cycling patients were found to be at high risk for chronic illness, with a 32 percent probability of remaining ill after one year, whereas patients presenting with only manic symptoms had a seven percent chronicity rate after one year (Keller et al, 1986, submitted for publication).

Bipolar II

There is considerably less known about the course of bipolar II disorder. In comparison with bipolar I patients, Coryell et al (1985) found that bipolar II subjects had shorter and less severe episodes.

In separate reports, Endicott and colleagues (unpublished paper) and Coryell et al (1985) found complicated histories of psychopathology among bipolar II patients. They observed a greater likelihood of schizotypal features and nonaffective disorders, such as obsessive compulsive disorder, alcoholism, drug abuse, antisocial personality and Briquet's disorder, in bipolar II patients compared to either bipolar I or unipolar patients. Furthermore, Endicott and colleagues (unpublished paper) found significantly higher rates of premenstrual dysphoria in bipolar II females (71 percent) compared to bipolar I (44 percent) and recurrent unipolar (42 percent) patients.

Bipolar II patients also exhibited psychopathology at an earlier age, were more often symptomatic on follow-up, and made more suicide attempts than bipolar I or unipolar patients (Coryell et al, 1985).

PERSONALITY FACTORS IN BIPOLAR DISORDERS

Although there are a limited number of empirical studies of the relation between personality traits and bipolar disorder (Hirschfeld and Klerman, 1979) there has been tremendous interest in the personality of patients with bipolar disorder since the writings of Kraepelin (1921). This section describes personality factors that have been observed in patients prior to their manifesting mania and depression, examines personality features that persist during symptom-free intervals, and explores those personality factors that may modify manic episodes.

"Premorbid" Personality Features

In 1921, Kraepelin noted that manic-depressive patients had pre-existing temperaments, from which he thought manic and depressive episodes developed. "Thus, depressive, manic, irritable (mixed), and cyclothymic (circular) personalities were considered the temperamental bases of respective full-blown forms of illness" (Akiskal et al, 1983a). Kretschmer (1936) extended the Kraepelinian concept, and concluded that bipolars had a cycloid personality that was predispositional to manic-depressive illness. Cohen and colleagues' (1954) clinical-dynamic approach focused on personality factors as precursors to manic-depressive disorder. They purported that in response to parental attitudes bipolar patients developed extroverted, ambitious, and hard-driven personalities that predisposed them to manic-depressive illness (Akiskal et al, 1983a). A more recent prospective study (Akiskal et al, 1977) has supported the Kraepelinian view of cyclothymia as a genetic predispositional personality that may develop into full-bloom manic-depressive episodes (Akiskal et al, 1983a). Perris' (1966) review of research on premorbid personalities of bipolars indicates that while studies such as Rowe and Daggett's (1954) find no deviations from normality, personality sensitivity and subclinical mood swings are commonly observed (Chodoff, 1972). In studies using personality scales and catamnestic data (Metcalfe, 1968; Perris, 1966; Coppen, 1966), neuroticism was found to be in the normal range when bipolar patients were asked to retrospectively rate their personality before their first manic or depressive episode (Chodoff, 1972).

Personality Features During Well Intervals

Bleuler (1924) described well-intervals between episodes of mania and depression that are marked by a return to the patient's premorbid cyclothymic and cycloid personality. With a return to the premorbid state, mild oscillations of mood may persist, as well as an optimistic or gloomy personality (Chodoff, 1972).

Hirschfeld and Klerman's (1979) assessment of personality characteristics of manic patients when the manic symptoms abated indicated relatively normal personality profiles among manics with deviations on obsessional state and obsessional traits. This finding contradicts Kendall and Discipio's (1970) assertion that obsessionality is a protector from mania, and rarely is a precursor to manic episodes in patients with bipolar disorder.

The Influence of Personality Factors on the Course of Bipolar Disorders

Studies of the relationship between personality factors and symptomatology in unipolar depression indicate that personality traits may modify affective episodes

(Lazare and Klerman, 1968; Akiskal et al, 1983a). However, there is much less known about how personality modifies the symptomatic expression of mania. While there are bipolar patients with premorbid personality features most closely resembling unipolar depressives ('melancholic type'), and those with hypomanic or manic features during their premorbid state ('manic type'), it is unclear how these features influence the frequency, severity, or duration of manic episodes (von Zerssen, 1982).

Of clinical relevance is the common observation that the personality style of bipolar patients often seems to lead to a resistance to treatment, therefore prolonging the duration of the manic episode (Akiskal et al, 1983a). Because of this, a high level of clinical skill is usually required for the optimal psychopharmacologic and psychotherapeutic treatment of patients with bipolar disorder.

EPIDEMIOLOGY

Several excellent studies on the epidemiology of psychiatric disorders in adults have recently been completed. As noted by Boyd and Weissman (1982, p. 100), these studies can generate new ideas about etiology, pathogenesis, treatment, and prevention and can provide insights to improve practice and planning for care by gathering data on: "1) rates (prevalence and incidence); 2) variations of these rates by person, time and place; and 3) identification of risk factors which increase the probability of developing the disorder."

Definition of Epidemiological Terminology

Standard definitions of several of the more commonly used epidemiological terms are as follows. 'Point prevalence' is that proportion of the population which has the disorder being studied at a given point in time. 'Morbid risk' is the individual's lifetime risk of having an episode of illness. 'Incidence' is the number of new cases of a disorder occurring in the population per unit of time (Boyd and Weissman, 1981, 1982).

LIFETIME RISK. The lifetime risk of bipolar disorder in the Epidemiologic Catchment Area (ECA) survey was found to be 0.9 to 1.1 percent for men and 0.6 to 1.3 percent for women, and these rates were quite comparable across New Haven, Baltimore, and St. Louis (Weissman and Boyd, 1985).

Separate reviews of the epidemiological literature found the lifetime risk of bipolar disorder to be approximately 1.0 percent, ranging from 0.6 to 0.9 percent in industrialized nations (Weissman and Boyd, 1985). Of interest is a much lower (and unexplained) lifetime rate of 0.2 percent from a study in New Zealand, which is inconsistent with the higher rates in other countries (Boyd and Weissman, 1982).

INCIDENCE. Boyd and Weissman (1985) recently reported that the annual incidence of bipolar disorder ranged from 0.009 to 0.020 percent for men and from 0.007 to 0.030 percent for women.

Demographic Variables

The onset of bipolar disorder is now thought to occur most commonly in late adolescence and the early 20s, contradicting previous observations of first episodes occurring between ages 24 to 32 (Boyd and Weissman, 1982; Weissman and

Boyd, 1985; Krauthammer and Klerman, 1979). As with unipolar depression, although the age of onset of the first episode may be young, the age of patients when they first seek treatment is often older.

Evidence exists for an increased rate of bipolar disorder in the upper socio-economic classes. It has been hypothesized that this "may be a consequence of the periods of hypomanic activity found in bipolar patients in which the individual can function at an increased level without significant impairment of judgment and thereby, achieve higher levels of success" (Cancro, 1985, p. 761). No evidence has been found to support a relation between prevalence and incidence of bipolar disorder and rural–urban status, marital status, religion, and race (Cancro, 1985). However, the low base rates for bipolar disorder would make it difficult to detect these associations if they did exist. Although one recent study suggests that life events may precipitate manic episodes (Cancro, 1985), this finding has not been replicated.

Frequency of Bipolar Disorders in Relatives of Bipolar Patients

Bipolar disorder is more familial than unipolar depression in all reported studies (Winokur, 1978; Clayton, 1981). Clayton's review of the literature reveals that approximately 50 percent of patients with bipolar disorder have at least one parent with an affective disorder, and approximately 50 percent of patients with bipolar disorder have a parent and a grandparent or a child with a bipolar disorder. Between 4 and 10 percent of bipolar patients were found to have a first degree relative with mania (Clayton, 1981), which is significantly greater than the rate of .6 to 1.0 percent found in the general population (Kidd and Weissman, 1978; Boyd and Weissman, 1982).

"Patients with bipolar disorder have high rates of relatives with either bipolar I or unipolar disorders, whereas patients with unipolar disorder generally show a high rate of unipolar but not bipolar illness in first degree relatives" (Weissman et al, 1984, p. 20; Gershon et al, 1982; Angst, 1979; Winokur et al, 1982).

SPECIFICITY OF BIPOLAR II DISORDER IN RELATIVES OF BIPOLAR II PATIENTS.   Bipolar II disorder is significantly more frequent among relatives of bipolar II patients than relatives of patients with unipolar or bipolar I illness (Coryell et al, 1984; Dunner et al, 1983; Gershon et al, 1982), whereas rates of bipolar II disorder are similar among relatives of nonbipolar and bipolar I patients (Coryell et al, 1984). There is also an increased rate of bipolar disorder in the biological relatives of patients with cyclothymia (Akiskal et al, 1977; Klein et al, 1985).

RATES OF BIPOLAR DISORDER IN THE OFFSPRING OF BIPOLAR PATIENTS.   Offspring of bipolar patients have significantly higher rates of the broad range of affective disorders, including bipolar II, cyclothmyia, and dysthymia than do the offspring of patients with nonaffective psychiatric disorders. In one study, 24 percent of the offspring of bipolar but none of the offspring of control subjects were diagnosed as cyclothymic (Klein, 1985). Akiskal and colleagues (1985) cite evidence of a 27 percent rate of bipolar spectrum disorders in chidren with one affected parent and significantly greater rates if both parents are ill.

BIPOLAR DISORDERS IN CHILDREN

High quality epidemiological studies of psychiatric disorders in children and adolescents are not yet available, and the existence of bipolar disorder in children has been disputed (Anthony and Scott, 1960; Tyrer and Shopsin, 1982). However, as early as 1921, Kraepelin noted that 0.4 percent of his manic-depressive patients had symptoms of sporadic mania prior to age 10.

Clinical Profile

Varied descriptions have been given of childhood mania (Davis, 1979; Weinberg and Brumback, 1976; Tyrer and Shopsin, 1982). Most often there is a definite mood change with exuberance and noisy hilarity, increased activity, high-flown ideas, and disturbed sleep. As in the adult, other symptoms may be prominent. Children tend, while in a manic state, to be physically aggressive, overactive and accident-prone, eat poorly, complain of abdominal pain, and have a short attention span (*British Medical Journal* 1:214–215, 1979). Another characteristic feature is low frustration tolerance, with explosive anger. Davis (1979) describes these features as affective storms, involving loss of emotional control without an adequate precipitant. Additional diagnostic features include a family history of affective illness, poor personal relationships, extroverted personality, and cyclothymia before the illness develops. Depression is commonly found in children with mania and is thought to appear even more commonly than in manic adults (Weinberg and Brumback, 1976; Tyrer and Shopsin, 1982).

Course

Bipolar disorder often begins in late childhood and adolescence with relatively minor oscillations in mood, most characteristically depressive in nature (Akiskal et al, 1985; Winokur et al, 1969). Some children do relatively well whereas others remain chronically ill, in spite of treatment, with persistent mood swings and poor psychosocial adjustment. It is generally believed that more "episode-free" time makes it possible for the youngster to progress with many of the developmental tasks of adolescence (Carlson, 1985).

Suicidal ideation and behavior is a risk in young people with bipolar affective disorder as it is in older people (Carlson, 1985) and must be watched for carefully.

Differential Diagnosis with Other Nonorganic Psychatric Disorders

CONDUCT DISORDER. Adolescents with bipolar disorder are often diagnosed as having conduct disorder "because the presentation may be mixed with antisocial disorder, temperamental patterns, or polydrug use" (Weissman and Boyd, 1985, p. 765). The high rates of hyperactivity, delinquent acts, and immature behavior found in the offspring of bipolar patients further serve to make this a difficult differential diagnosis (Greenhill and Shopsin, 1979; Tyrer and Shopsin, 1982).

ATTENTION DEFICIT DISORDER. Frequently children with bipolar disorder are initially diagnosed as having an attention deficit disorder, based on the presence of inattention, inpulsivity, and hyperactivity. When present, a thought disorder should exclude the diagnosis of attention deficit disorder and make the clinician consider schizophrenia, schizoaffective disorder, or mania.

CHILDHOOD SCHIZOPHRENIA. Early-onset psychosis may occur within the first two years of life and manifest itself with delayed language development, lack of response, or extreme hyperactivity and irritability (Chess and Hassibi, 1978), which may appear similar to a manic syndrome. The presence of bizzare thought content in older children should help to differentiate middle onset psychosis from mania. However, aggressive behavior, and preoccupation with injury, violence, and death may also mimic a manic syndrome (Potter, 1983).

BORDERLINE PERSONALITY DISORDER. At an early age, borderline personality disorder and manic depressive disorder often appear very similar, and borderline personality should be included in the differential diagnosis of early onset mania or hypomania (Potter, 1983).

Conclusion

"Bipolar disorder beginning in adolescence occurs with greater frequency than clinicians heretofore believed. Although there are a number of factors complicating recognition of the disorder, it is important . . . to identify and treat the disorder before the secondary complications of a disrupted life make treatment and adjustment more difficult" (Carlson, 1985, p. 386). It is strongly recommended that clinicians look for the early and subtle temperamental, as well as the more extreme psychotic features (Akiskal et al, 1985) that are indicative of bipolar illness among children.

SUMMARY

The distinction between unipolar and bipolar affective illness has been refined substantially since the writings of Kraepelin in 1921, and has been validated in recent years by the identification of genetic, biochemical, and clinical correlates that differentiate these conditions.

A more controversial diagnostic issue is whether to consider bipolar I and bipolar II as separate disorders. While the Research Diagnostic Criteria (RDC) differentiates bipolar I and bipolar II patients based on the presence of mania and hypomania, respectively, the *DSM-III* does not have a category for bipolar II. Recent research indicates that the two disorders are similar in regard to age of onset and circular course, but are distinguished by familial aggregation, psychiatric history, and suicidal tendencies. Hence, the *DSM-III-R* includes a new category, bipolar disorder not otherwise specified, for patients who have a history of depression and hypomania.

In comparison with bioplar I disorder, it appears that schizoaffective mania is more similar to mania than schizoaffective depression is to depression. Clayton's (1982) review indicates that schizoaffective depression is related to a wide spectrum of disorders, whereas schizoaffective mania resembles manic episodes of bipolar disorder in regard to age and severity of onset.

When considering the differential diagnosis of bipolar disorder, the clinician should search for organic causes of mania and hypomania, and be aware of the nonorganic psychiatric disorders which may present with these features. Krauthammer and Klerman (1978) have documented that exogenous agents and organic conditions can induce mania in patients with or without a history of mania, and clinicians should screen patients presenting with mania to determine the etiology of their illness. The *DSM-III-R* has the category, 'substance use disorders' for mania induced by drugs, and the 'organic mental syndromes and disorders (non-substance induced)' for mania secondary to medical illness. Examples of nonorganic psychiatric disorders that have features resembling mania and hypomania include: schizophrenia, schizoaffective disorder, hysteria, and adolescent conduct disorder.

The reliability of diagnosing mania and hypomania is an important consideration for the clinician. Research findings indicate that while the reliability for diagnosing mania is quite good, the diagnosis of hypomania has low reliability. Therefore, the clinician should be alerted by mild symptoms that border on normality for the detection of hypomania.

The natural course of bipolar I disorder is characterized by high rates of relapse and chronicity. Zis and Goodwin have reported high rates of relapse among bipolars, with 19 to 86 percent having three or more episodes. Coryell and Winokur's (1982) review of follow-up studies indicates that 15 to 53 percent of bipolar I patients were chronically ill.

The polarity of the episode is of prognostic importance when assessing the course of bipolar I disorder. The NIMH-Collaborative Study on the Psychobiology of Depression found that patients seeking treatment for pure manic episodes recovered more quickly than bipolars presenting with pure depressed and mixed/cycling episodes (Keller et al, 1986).

Although much less is known about the course of bipolar II disorder, Coryell and colleagues (1985) found that affective episodes were less severe and of shorter duration in patients with bipolar II disorder compared to those with bipolar I disorder.

The Kraepelinian concept of a cyclothymic pre-existing temperament for many patients who develop bipolar disorder has been supported by current research findings (Perris, 1966). Investigation of personality features that persist during well-intervals indicate that minor oscillations in mood may continue and thereby constitute a return to these patients' premorbid cyclothymic state. According to Hirschfeld and Klerman (1979), personality traits of bipolar patients do not deviate from normality, with the exception of obsessionality. Of much interest is the role of personality features in the course of bipolar disorder. However, there is a dearth of information related to how personality modifies the duration, frequency, or severity of manic episodes.

Epidemiologic studies indicate a lifetime risk of approximately one percent in men and women for bipolar disorder in the general population. Bipolar disorder is a familial illness with high rates of affective illness among parents, children, and other first and second degree relatives of bipolar patients. Akiskal and colleagues (1985) have also reported a 24 percent rate of cyclothymia in children of bipolar patients.

Although less common than in adults, bipolar disorder does exist in children. The age of onset of bipolar illness is earlier than once thought, often occurring during late childhood and early adolescence. Features of childhood mania, including an exuberant mood, increased activity, and short attention span, may appear similar to characteristics of nonorganic psychiatric illnesses such as conduct disorder, attention deficit disorder, and borderline personality disorder.

REFERENCES

Abrams R, Taylor MA: Mania and schizoaffective disorder, manic type: a comparison. Am J Psychiatry 133:1445-1447, 1976

Akiskal HS, Dijenderdjian AH, Rosenthal RH, et al: Cyclothymic disorder: validating criteria for inclusion in the bipolar affective group. Am J Psychiatry 134:1227-1233, 1977

Akiskal HS, Bitar AH, Puzantian VR, et al: The nosological status of neurotic depression: a prospective three or four year follow-up examination in light of the primary-secondary and unipolar-bipolar dichotomies. Arch Gen Psychiatry 35:756-766, 1978

Akiskal HS, Hirschfeld RMA, Yerevania BI: The relationship of personality to affective disorders: a critical review. Arch Gen Psychiatry 40:801-810, 1983a

Akiskal HS, Walker PW, Puzantian VR: Bipolar outcome in the course of depressive illness. Journal of Affective Disorders 5:115-128, 1983b

Akiskal HS, Downs J, Jordon P, et al: Affective disorders referred in children and younger siblings of manic-depressives: mode of onset and prospective course. Arch Gen Psychiatry 42:996-1003, 1985

American Psychiatric Association: Diagnostic and Statistical Manual of Mental Disorders, Third Edition (DSM-III). Washington, DC, American Psychiatric Association, 1980

American Psychiatric Association: Diagnostic and Statistical Manual of Mental Disorders, Third Edition (DSM-III-R). Washington, DC, American Psychiatric Association, in press

Andreasen NC, Grove WM, Shapiro RW: Reliability of lifetime diagnosis: a multicenter collaborative perspective. Arch Gen Psychiatry 38:400-405, 1981

Angst J: The reliability of morbidity risk figures, in Genetic Aspects of Affective Illness. Edited by Mendlewicz J, Shopsin B. New York, Spectrum Publications, 1979

Angst J, Baastrup P, Grot P, et al: The course of monopolar depression and bipolar psychosis. Psychiatria Neurologia Neurochirurgia 76:489-500, 1973

Anthony EJ, Scott P: Manic-depressive psychosis in childhood. Journal of Child Psychology and Psychiatry and Allied Disciplines 1:53-72, 1960

Bleuler EP: Lehrbuch der Psychiatrie. New York, Macmillan, 1924

Boyd JH, Weissman MM: Epidemiology of affective disorders: a reexamination and future directions. Arch Gen Psychiatry 38:1039-1046, 1981

Boyd JH, Weissman MM: Epidemiology, in Handbook of Affective Disorders. Edited by Paykel ES. New York, Guilford Press, 1982

Bratfos O, Haug JO: The course of manic depressive psychosis: a follow-up investigation of 215 patients. Acta Psychiatr Scand 44:89-112, 1968

Brockington IF, Wainwright S, Kendell RE: Manic patients with schizophrenic or paranoid symptoms. Psychological Medicine 10:665-675, 1980

Bunney WE: Psychopharmacology of the switch process in affective illness, in Psychopharmacology: A Generation Process. Edited by Lipton MA, Dimascio A, Killiam KF. New York, Raven, 1978

Cadoret RJ, Fowler RC, McCabe MS, et al: Evidence for heterogeneity in a group of good-prognosis schizophrenics. Compr Psychiatry 15:443, 1974

Cancro R: Overview of affective disorders, in Comprehensive Textbook of Psychiatry IV, vol 1. Edited by Kaplan HI, Sadock BJ. Baltimore, William & Wilkins, 1985

Carlson GA: Bipolar disorder in adolescence. Psychiatric Annals 15:379-386, 1985

Chess, S, Hassibi M: Principles and Practice of Child Psychiatry. New York, Plenum Press, 1978

Chodoff P: The depressive personality. Arch Gen Psychiatry 27:666-673, 1972

Clayton PJ: The epidemiology of bipolar affective disorder. Compr Psychiatry 22:31-43, 1981

Clayton PJ: Schizoaffective disorders. J Nerv Ment Dis 170:646-650, 1982

Cohen MS, Baker G, Cohen RA, et al: An intensive study of 12 cases of manic-depressive psychosis. Psychiatry 17:103-138, 1954

Coppen A: The Marke-Nyman Temperament Scale: an English translation. Br J Med Psychol 39:55-60, 1966

Coryell W, Winokur G: Course and outcome, in Handbook of Affective Disorders. Edited by Paykel ES. New York, Guilford Press, 1982

Coryell W, Endicott J, Reich T, et al: A family study of bipolar II disorder. Br J Psychiatry 145:49-54, 1984

Coryell W, Endicott J, Andreasen N, et al: Bipolar I, bipolar II, and nonbipolar major depression among the relatives of affectively ill probands. Am J Psychiatry 142:817-821, 1985

Davis RE: Manic-depressive variant syndrome of childhood: a preliminary report. Am J Psychiatry 136:702-706, 1979

Dunner DL: Subtypes of bipolar affective disorder with particular regard to bipolar II. Psychiatr Dev 1:75-86, 1983

Dunner DL, Fleiss JL, Fieve RR: The course of development of mania in patients with recurrent depression. Am J Psychiatry 133:905-908, 1976

Endicott J, Nee J, Andreasen N, et al: Bipolar II: combine or keep separate? J Affective Disord 8:17-28, 1985

Gershon ES: The genetics of affective disorders, in Psychiatry Update: The American Psychiatric Association Annual Review, vol II. Edited by Grinspoon L. Washington, DC, American Psychiatric Press Inc., 1983

Gershon ES, Hamovit J, Guroff JJ, et al: A family study of schizoaffective, bipolar I, bipolar II, unipolar, and normal controls. Arch Gen Psychiatry 39:1157-1167, 1982

Gershon ES, Nurnburger JI, Berrettini WH, et al: Affective disorders: genetics, in Comprehensive Textbook of Psychiatry IV, vol 1, fourth edition. Edited by Kaplan HI, Sadock BJ. Baltimore, Williams & Wilkins, 1985

Goodwin FK, Jamison KR: The natural course of recurrent affective illness, in Neurobiology of the Mood Disorders. Edited by Post RM, Ballenger JC. Baltimore, Williams & Wilkins, 1984

Greenhill LL, Shopsin B: Survey of mental disorders in the children of parents with affective disorder, in Genetic Aspects of Affective Illness. Edited by Mendelwicz J, Shopsin B. New York, SP Medical and Scientific Books, 1979

Grof P, Angst J, Haines T: The clinical course of depression: practical issues, in Classification and Prediction of Outcome and Depression. Edited by Angst J. New York, FK Schattauer Verlag, 1974

Hastings DW: Follow-up results in psychiatric illness. Am J Psychiatry 114:1057-1066, 1958

Helgason T: Epidemiological investigations concerning affective disorders, in Origin, Prevention and Treatment of Affective Disorders. Edited by Schoe M, Stromgren E. New York, Academic Press, 1979

Hendrie HC (Ed): The Psychiatric Clinics of North America: Symposium on Brain Disorders, Clinical and Diagnosis and Management, vol 1, number 1. Philadelphia, Saunders & Co., 1978

Hirschfeld RMA, Klerman GL: Personality attributes and affective disorders. Am J Psychiatry 136:67-70, 1979

Kasanin J: The acute schizoaffective psychoses. Am J Psychiatry 13:97-126, 1933

Keller MB, Lavori PW, Coryell W, et al: Differential outcome of episodes of illness in bipolar patients: pure manic, mixed/cycling and pure depressive. JAMA 256:3138-3142, 1986

Kendall RE, Discipio WJ: Obsessional symptoms and obsessional personality traits in patients with depressive illnesses. Psychol Med 1:65-72, 1970

Kidd KK, Weissman MM: Why we do not yet understand the genetics of affective disorders, in Depression: Biology and Psychodynamics and Treatment. Edited by Cole JO, Schatzberg AF, Frazier SH. New York, Plenum Press, 1978

Klein DN, Depue RA: Continued impairment in persons at risk for bipolar affective disorder: results of a 19-month follow-up study. J Abnorm Psychol 93:345-347, 1984

Klein DN, Depue RA, Slater JF: Cyclothmyia in the adolescent offspring of parents with bipolar affective disorder. J Abnorm Psychol 94:115-127, 1985

Klerman GL: Long-term outcomes of neurotic depressions, in Human Functioning in Longitudinal Perspective. Edited by Sells S, Crandall R, Strauss JS, et al. Baltimore, Williams & Wilkins, 1980

Klerman GL: The spectrum of mania. Comp Psychiatry 22:11-20, 1981

Klerman GL: Practical issues in the treatment of depression and mania, in Handbook of Affective Disorders. Edited by Paykel ES. New York, Guilford Press, 1982

Klerman GL, Hirschfeld RMA, Andreasen NC, et al: Major depression and related affective disorders. Presented at American Psychiatric Association Invitational Workshop: DSM-III: An Interim Appraisal. Washington, DC, Oct. 12–15, 1983. Published in Proceedings. Washington, DC, American Psychiatric Press, Inc., 1984

Kraepelin E: Manic-Depressive Insanity and Paranoia. Edinburgh, Livingstone, 1921

Krauthammer CD, Klerman GL: Secondary mania: manic syndromes associated with antecedent physical illness or drugs. Arch Gen Psychiatry 35:1333-1339, 1978

Kretschmer E: Psychique and Character. Translated by Miller E. London, Kegan Paul, Trench, Trubner, and Co, Ltd, 1936

Lazare A: Manic behavior, in Outpatient Psychiatry: Diagnosis and Treatment. Edited by Lazare A. Baltimore, Guilford Press, 1979

Lazare A, Klerman G: Hysteria and depression: the frequency and significance of hysterical personality features in hospitalized depressed women. Am J Psychiatry 124:48-56, 1968

Lehmann HE: Affective disorders: clinical features, in Comprehensive Textbook of Psychiatry IV, vol 1, fourth edition. Edited by Kaplan HI, Sadock BJ. Baltimore, Williams & Wilkins, 1985

Leonhard K, Korff I, Shulz H: Die temperamente in den familien der monopolaren und bipolaren phasischen psychosen. Psychiatry and Neurology 143:416, 1962

Lundquist G: Prognosis of course in manic depressive psychoses: a follow-up study of 319 first admissions. Act Psychiatr Neurol (Supplement 1) 35:1-96, 1945

Lundquist G: Manic states in affective disorders of childhood and adolescence. Br Med J 1:214-215, 1979

Metcalfe M: The personality of depressed patients, in Recent Developments in Affective Disorders. Edited by Coppen A, Walk A. London, Royal Medico-Psychological Association, 1968

Miller FT, Libman H: Lithium carbonate in the treatment of schizophrenia and schizoaffective disorder: review and hypothesis. Biol Psychiatr 14:705-710, 1979

Morrison J, Winokur G, Crowe R, et al: The Iowa 500, the first follow-up. Arch Gen Psychiatry 29:678-682, 1973

Myers JK, Weissman MM, Tischler GL, et al: Six-month prevalence of psychiatric disorders in three communities: 1980–1982. Arch Gen Psychiatry 41:959-967, 1984

Nurnberger J, Roose SP, Dunner DS, et al: Unipolar mania: a distinct clinical entity? Am J Psychiatry 136:1420-1423, 1979

Perris C: A study of bipolar (manic depressive) and unipolar recurrent depressive psychosis, I: genetic investigations. Acta Psychiatr Scand (Suppl) 194:15-44, 1966

Perris C: The distinction between bipolar and unipolar affective disorders, in Handbook of Affective Disorders. Edited by Paykel ES. New York, Guilford Press, 1982

Pfohl B, Vasquez N, Nasrallah H: Unipolar versus bipolar mania: a review of 247 patients. Br J Psychiatry 141:453-458, 1982

Pollock HM: Recurrence of attacks in manic-depressive psychoses. Am J Psychiatry 11:568-573, 1931

Pope HG, Lipinski JF, Cohen BM, et al: "Schizoaffective disorder": an invalid diagnosis? A comparison of schizoaffective disorder, schizophrenia, and affective disorder. Am J Pyschiatry 137:921-927, 1980

Potter RL: Manic-depressive variant syndrome of childhood. Clin Pediatr 22:496-499, 1983

Rao AV, Nammalvar N: The course and outcome of depressive illness: a follow-up study of 122 cases in Madurai, India. Br J Psychiatry 130:392-396, 1977

Rennie T: Prognosis in manic-depressive psychoses. Am J Psychiatry 98:801-814, 1942

Rowe CJ, Daggett BR: Prepsychotic personality traits in manic-depressive disease. J Nerv Ment Dis 119:412-420, 1954

Rowe CJ, Daggett BR: Prepsychotic personality traits in manic-depressive diseases. J Nerv Ment Dis 137:162-172, 1963

Shobe FO, Brion P: Long-term prognosis in manic depressive illness. Arch Gen Psychiatry 24:334-337, 1971

Spitzer RL, Endicott J, Robins E: Research Diagnostic Criteria (RDC) for a selected group of functional disorders, third edition. New York, New York State Psychiatric Institute, 1985

Stenstedt A: A study in manic-depressive psychosis. Acta Psychiatr Scand 79(suppl 1): 1-111, 1952

Taschev T: The course and prognosis of depression on the basis of 652 patients deceased, in Classification and Prediction of Outcome of Depression. Edited by Angst J. New York, FK Schattauer Verlag, 1974

Tyrer S, Shopsin B: Symptoms and assessment of mania, in Handbook of Affective Disorders. Edited by Paykel ES. New York, Guilford Press, 1982

von Zerssen D: Personality and affective disorders, in Handbook of Affective Disorders. Edited by Paykel ES. New York, Guilford Press, 1982

Weinberg WA, Brumback RA: Mania in children. Am J Dis Child 130:380-385, 1976

Weissman MM, Boyd JH: Affective disorders: epidemiology, in Comprehensive Textbook of Psychiatry IV, vol 1, fourth edition. Edited by Kaplan HI, Sadock BJ. Baltimore, Williams & Wilkins, 1985

Weissman MM, Gershon ES, Kidd KK, et al: Psychiatric disorders in the relatives of probands with affective disorders. Arch Gen Psychiatry 41:13-21, 1984

Winokur G: Mania and depression: family studies and genetics in relation to treatment, in Psychopharmacology: A Generation of Progress. Edited by Lipton MA, DiMascio A, Killam KF. New York, Raven, 1978

Winokur G, Clayton PJ, Reich T: Manic Depressive Illness. St. Louis, Missouri, CV Mosby, 1969

Winokur G, Tsuang MT, Crave RR: The Iowa 500: affective disorder in relatives of manic and depressive patients. Am J Psychiatry 139:200-212, 1982

Zis AP, Goodwin FK: Major affective disorder as a recurrent illness: a critical review. Arch Gen Psychiatry 36:835-839, 1979

Chapter 2

Biological Findings in Bipolar Disorders

by William Z. Potter, M.D., Ph.D., Matthew V. Rudorfer, M.D., and Frederick K. Goodwin, M.D.

Biological investigations of manic-depressive illness can only be understood in the context of the broader matrix of psychiatric syndromes that involve depressive symptoms. Ideally, we would like to know to what extent patients who suffer from both recurrent depression and hypomania or mania are biologically unique. If we limit ourselves to this question we would be restricted to the small number of studies that clearly distinguish bipolar patients and specifically compare them to other populations. Since biologic approaches and diagnostic criteria have been evolving concurrently, it would be premature to take such a restrictive approach. Important diagnostic issues, as well as our current knowledge of the natural course of manic-depressive illness, are discussed in Chapter 1. Because most biologic studies involving bipolar patients include direct reference or comparison to unipolar ones, it is particularly necessary to be clear about how we view this diagnostic distinction.

DIAGNOSTIC CAVEATS

Family history and twin data suggest that bipolar and unipolar patients may be able to be separated, in part, on a genetic basis. On the other hand, the genetic data do not support a view that unipolar and bipolar are entirely separate illnesses (Gershon et al, 1982). A continuum model may be most appropriate with bipolar as the more severe, and recurrent unipolar as the less severe form of the same illness. It would be useful to identify *recurrent* unipolar in any comparisons with bipolar patients. The relation between bipolar depression and depression in general (which often tends to be called unipolar simply on the basis of not being bipolar) is unclear. New data provide additional support for the concept that subtyping nonbipolar depression into unipolar endogenous using recurrence as a criterion (Newcastle scale) best identifies subjects with a familial and presumably more biological illness (Andreasen et al, 1986). Thus, for comparisons with bipolar patients, we attempt to limit unipolar patients to those who have major depressive illness with endogenous features. However, it must be recognized that the data base unavoidably includes some biologic studies performed on a clearly heterogeneous "unipolar" population.

Moreover, biological studies in most unipolar and bipolar patients have not been analyzed separately. In the many studies done before the bipolar/unipolar distinction, this is an unavoidable omission. Currently, however, many studies still fail to analyze data separately for bipolar and unipolar patients. And even

The opinions expressed herein are those of the authors and do not reflect official policy of the NIMH.

in reports which do provide results according to diagnostic subgrouping, the criteria for selection of the unipolar group are often not adequately described.

Thus, although our review of biological findings focuses primarily on bipolar illness, it necessarily includes extensive data on forms of unipolar illness. We do not view this only as a capitulation to the state of the literature; rather, it seems reasonable that bipolar and recurrent unipolar illness must be related and have at least some common pathophysiology.

TYPES OF BIOLOGICAL FINDINGS

Table 1 lists classes of replicated biological abnormalities in patients with major depressive illness and indicates whether those findings differentiate bipolar depressed from unipolar patients. Methodological issues bearing on the interpretation of these data are noted later in this chapter, when the individual categories are reviewed. The studies represented in this summary did not include a sufficient number to systematically evaluate the hypothesis that the more recurrent forms of unipolar illness may be biologically closer to bipolar illness. Instead, we limited ourselves to two dichotomies: depressed versus normal and bipolar versus unipolar. Unipolar/bipolar differences required a minimum of three positive studies which had to constitute the majority of qualified studies. Findings based on less than three studies are indicated with a question mark. Negative reports with a high probability of a Type II error (potential false negatives due to small sample size and/or large variance) have been excluded. For the purposes of the Table, a negative report would be expressed as no difference between groups and indicated with an " = " sign.

Inspection of the Table reveals that there are very few instances of replicated bipolar/unipolar differences. Possible differences based on one or two studies with as yet no replications are, as indicated above, not represented in the Table. Even those differences satisfying criteria to be included are not universally accepted as reflecting a true biologic bipolar/unipolar dichotomy. It is interesting that some of the most robust bipolar/unipolar differences emerge from earlier studies dealing with membrane function. These findings (RBC/plasma lithium ratio and 5HT uptake by platelets) involve a possible expression of genetic differences and have sometimes been claimed to be state independent. More recent data, however, raises questions about the state independence of these findings. The other bipolar/unipolar differences which emerge from several studies involve the function of the norepinephrine system during the depressed or (hypo) manic state (for example, urinary 3–methoxy–4–hydroxyphenylglycol (MHPG) and plasma norepinephrine).

RESEARCH FINDINGS VERSUS CLINICAL APPLICATIONS

Thus, we have biologic data supporting some pathophysiologic abnormalities in the illness and, to a lesser extent, some support for the unipolar/bipolar distinction. Why haven't these findings been developed to the point of practical diagnostic tests? It is becoming increasingly clear that the biologic systems which have been studied are vulnerable to multiple sources of dysregulation; in other words, it is exceedingly difficult to establish the specificity of any of the abnormalities summarized in Table I.

Table 1. Six Classes of Replicated Biologic Findings in Depression[1]

	Depressed versus Normal	Bipolar versus Unipolar
1. Electrolytes		
Calcium in CSF	↑	?
2. Membrane Transport		
RBC/Plasma lithium ratio	±	↑
5HT uptake by platelets	↓	↓
³H–Imipramine binding in platelets	↓	?↓
3. Peptides		
Somatostatin (CSF)	↓	=
4. Neuroendocrine Output and Response		
Cortisol (plasma, urine and CSF)	↑	=
Cortisol post-dexamethasone (DST)	↑	=
Growth hormone responses	↓	=
TSH to TRH	↓	=
5. Neurotransmitter Receptors		
Platelet α₂ receptors	↑	?
Platelet α₂ sensitivity	↓	?
Lymphocyte β–receptor sensitivity	↓	?
6. Neurotransmitters, Metabolites, and Related Enzymes		
HVA in CSF	↓	=
MHPG in CSF	=	?↓
NE in plasma	↑	↓
MHPG in urine	?↓	
Platelet MAO	*↓	?↓

*Only in bipolar versus control

" ↑ " = increased; " ↓ " = decreased; " ± " = data supporting both increased and decreased; "=" = no differences; "?" = insufficient data available to make any judgment; "?↑ or ↓" = trend toward increase or decrease, but data preliminary or questionable

[1] Some, but not all, of the references upon which this Table is based are discussed in the text. A complete bibliography is available on request from the authors.

The question of specificity, central to biological research, requires that we ask whether a given biological finding is specific to manic-depressive illness or may also be found in other major psychiatric illnesses. Related to this is the importance of evaluating other relevant parameters such as whether a biological "finding" is associated with the full syndrome of depression or mania, or with an individual symptom or symptom cluster. The distribution of the biological finding in the patient population is important; a non-normal distribution might suggest subgroups. Additionally, the distribution and variance in a comparison patient or normal population could shed light on the role of the biological factor in manic-depressive patients. These issues should be borne in mind as the individual biological findings are reviewed in greater detail.

THE PHARMACOLOGICAL BRIDGE

Classic Formulation

The stimulus for the study of particular systems in vivo was provided by the discovery of effective pharmacologic treatments for depression and mania. These treatments led to the formulation of the so-called pharmacological bridge between depressive illness and neurotransmitter systems in the brain. In brief, research in animals first focused on identifying those systems which were acutely influenced by antidepressants and, more recently, on those influenced by several weeks of treatment (that is, to parallel the time course of therapeutic effect).

The foundation for the pharmacological bridge was the observation that reserpine use was associated with an unexpected high incidence of depression; this antihypertensive was later shown to deplete amine neurotransmitters in animals. Rather than causing depression, it now appears that reserpine activates a preexisting vulnerability (Goodwin et al, 1972). It is not clear, however, whether a bipolar versus unipolar history confers a different degree of vulnerability to this drug, or whether continuously administered it could precipitate recurrent depressive or manic depressive illness. Methyldopa, now believed to act via stimulation of presynaptic receptors which inhibit norepinephrine release, can also precipitate depression (Whitlock and Evans, 1978). The peripheral and centrally active beta receptor antagonist, propranolol, may rarely precipitate depressive episodes in patients being treated for cardiovascular disease (Whitlock and Evans, 1978). Whether, like reserpine, this effect is confined to vulnerable individuals (as reflected in a past history or family history of affective illness) has not been studied.

Table 2 summarizes the major known drug–amine–behavioral associations relevant to manic-depressive illness. We will only briefly discuss this extensive literature since it has been well reviewed and critiqued elsewhere (Goodwin and Jamison, in press). The specific drug effects indicated in Table 2 are those generally reported as the acute effects in most animal species, although these effects are often complex and controversy remains concerning their specific mechanisms of action. First, it can be noted that drugs that are stimulants in normal individuals are not generally found to be therapeutic in patients suffering from major depressive illness (Goodwin and Sack, 1973). Conversely, those drugs that do have antidepressant activity are not stimulants in normals (Oswald et al, 1972). Amphetamine, a stimulant in normals, is generally conceded not to be an effective antidepressant agent. Cocaine, also a powerful stimulant in normals, is a potent inhibitor of catecholamine reuptake at the synapse, an effect similar to that of the tricyclic antidepressants. L–dopa, primarily a precursor of dopamine (DA), and secondarily of norepinephrine, acutely, at least, increases the output of both, but is not an effective antidepressant (Goodwin et al, 1970). Nevertheless, it does produce some activation, as evidenced by increased anger and psychosis ratings in some patients, and hypomanic episodes superimposed on depression in a high proportion of bipolar patients (Murphy et al, 1971).

It is well established that reserpine depletes a variety of catecholamines, a

Table 2. The Pharmacological Bridge: Drug-Neurotransmitter Relations and Behavioral Effects in Humans[1]

Drug	Acute Effects on the Functional Output of Neurotransmitters	Predisposed to Affective Illness	Depressed Patients	Manic Patients	Normals
MAOI	↑ (NE, DA)	Can precipitate mania	Antidepressant	Aggravates mania	?
Tricyclic antidepressants	↑ (NE, 5HT)	Can precipitate mania	Antidepressant	Aggravates mania	?
Amphetamine	↑ (NE, DA)	Can precipitate mania (?)	Poor antidepressant		Stimulant
Cocaine	↑ (NE, DA)	Can precipitate mania	Poor antidepressant		Stimulant
L-dopa	↑ (DA, ?NE)	Can precipitate hypomania	Activation—no antidepressant effect		No effect
Reserpine	↓ (NE, 5HT, DA)	Can precipitate depression	?	Partial antimanic	Can precipitate depression
Lithium	?	Does not precipitate depression	Antidepressant (some patients)	Antimanic	Mild sedation
Neuroleptics	↓ (DA)	?	?	Partial antimanic	Sedation
AMPT	↓ (DA, NE)	?	Does not reverse imipramine antidepressant effects	Antimanic	Sedation (?)
Piribedil	↑ (DA)	Can precipitate mania	? Antidepressant	?	?
Bromocriptine	↑ (DA)	Can precipitate mania		?	Euphorogenic
Physostigmine	↑ (AcH)	Can precipitate depression in euthymic bipolars	Worsens	Transiently antimanic	Transient depressive symptoms

"?" = insufficient data available to make any judgment

Abbreviations: MAOI = monoamine oxidase inhibitors; NE = norepinephrine; DA = dopamine; 5HT = serotonin; AMPT = alpha methylparatyrosine; AcH = acetylcholine

[1]Table adapted from Goodwin and Sack (1973)

fact to which we have already referred. Lithium's effects are less clear: earlier data were interpreted to indicate a drug induced decrease of functional amines (for references see Goodwin and Sack, 1973), although these findings have been subsequently questioned (see below). Neuroleptics, in contrast, have at least one clear effect: blockade of dopamine's actions on the D_2 subtype of dopamine receptors. Alphamethylparatyrosine (AMPT), next on the list in Table 2, is a relatively specific inhibitor of dopamine synthesis and, therefore, will deplete the amounts available for release. Piribedil and bromocriptine are both partial dopamine agonists that appear to sometimes induce mania; moreover, bromocriptine sometimes is euphorogenic.

An imbalance in the noradrenergic and cholinergic transmitter systems regulating affect—a relative predominance of noradrenergic over cholinergic tone associated with mania and the reverse with depression—gained currency as a specific hypothesis of biological mood disorders in the 1970s (Janowsky et al, 1972). Evidence for a pharmacological bridge to manic-depressive illness was provided by studies demonstrating the ability of intravenous physostigmine, a central cholinesterase inhibitor, to briefly, but dramatically, reduce symptoms in manic patients (Janowsky et al, 1973) and to precipitate depression in euthymic bipolar patients maintained on lithium (Oppenheim et al, 1979). However, the therapeutic activity of antidepressant and antimanic drugs does not consistently parallel effects on the cholinergic system, and a number of these agents, including MAOIs and various "second generation" antidepressants, lack any interaction with cholinergic receptors (Rudorfer et al, 1984). Thus, the noradrenergic/cholinergic balance theory has not led to reproducible direct biochemical studies in humans.

The most striking pharmacological bridge that can be built on the data in Table 2 does not lead directly to depression, but to the consistent findings that direct or indirect norepinephrine and dopamine agonists precipitate episodes of mania or hypomania in patients with underlying manic-depressive illness. This effect is usually observed as a switch from depression to mania or hypomania (since the compounds which produce it are given as antidepressants), although it can also occur from the euthymic state.

Many of the "classical" biochemical effects outlined in Table 2 are based on the ability of drugs to alter the so-called turnover of the neurotransmitter. This term refers to the combined rate of synthesis, release, and elimination of a particular substance. High turnover traditionally implies a higher level of function—low, the reverse—although we have learned that there are many exceptions to this rule. Table 2 characterizes the net action of a drug on an amine system, rather than dealing with the complexities of drug effects on different measures of these systems. The wide variety of drug effects that have been revealed by new receptor based and electrophysiological techniques primarily in animals is reviewed in *Psychiatry Update: The American Psychiatric Association Annual Review*, Volume 4 (Paul et al, 1985).

Where relevant data in humans or primates exist, they are consistent with the simple formulations outlined in Table 2. For instance, focusing for the moment on the classification of drugs as catecholamine agonists, the potent norepinephrine uptake inhibitors, imipramine and desipramine, increase plasma norepinephrine in depressed patients and normal volunteers (Lake et al, 1979; Ross et al, 1983; Veith et al, 1983) and increase norepinephrine in the cerebrospinal fluid (CSF) of monkeys (Lerner et al, 1980). Postmortem samples from patients treated with monoamine oxidase inhibitors (MAOIs) reveal elevated hypothalamic norepinephrine (Bevan-Jones et al, 1972), and L–dopa administration produces elevated metabolites of norepinephrine and dopamine in the CSF (Goodwin et al, 1970). Thus, there are now drug–amine relationships established directly in patients. They lend support to an association between a hyperadrenergic and/or hyperdopaminergic state and the onset of hypomania or mania. This interpretation is also consistent with longitudinal studies of norepinephrine and its metabolites in body fluids (to be reviewed later), which are generally low in bipolar depression and high in mania.

The Extended Bridge

There remain, however, even more striking pharmacologic findings going beyond effects on a single episode of depression or mania; that is, the effects of drugs on the long-term course of bipolar illness. As discussed in Chapters 3 and 4 of this volume, antidepressants in general, and tricyclics in particular, may increase the frequency of cycles and worsen long-term outcome. MAOIs can precipitate mania, apparently with about the same frequency as TCAs, and may be associated with an increased frequency of cycles. The data on cycle induction after MAOIs, as compared to TCAs, are relatively sparse, although it seems to occur. Whether through drugs or simply spontaneous recurrences, the phenomenon of increased frequency and/or worsening of cycles can be viewed as a type of kindling—a concept developed in detail in Chapter 6 of this volume.

Carbamazepine, an interesting drug with antikindling properties, is antimanic and may be partially antidepressant as well as anticycling. It does not precipitate manias or induce cycles. Another important treatment, electroconvulsive therapy (ECT), can apparently precipitate as well as terminate manias in bipolar patients, depending on the phase of illness in which it is administered. Systematic studies show termination of mania by ECT; even without such studies, switches from depression to mania are observed often enough to be accepted as real phenomena. Although not systematically studied, a review of treatment histories from patients with rapid cycles suggests that ECT can also increase as well as decrease cycle frequency. Finally, thyroid hormone, which has been used in modest doses as an adjunct to potentiate response to tricyclic antidepressants, may itself have anticycling properties when used in hypermetabolic doses (see Chapter 3 of this volume). It too, however, may initially potentiate or worsen manias. Again, the distinction between systematic and case studies needs to be kept in mind before using findings as a basis for broader generalizations.

These various clinical actions in bipolar patients are summarized in Table 3, along with potencies of the three most common treatments with multiple effects. Six fundamental categories of actions on the illness can be identified, four relating to effects on a given episode (precipitate or reverse depression, precipitate or reverse mania) and two relating to the long-term course of the illness (increase or decrease cycle frequency). Thus, tricyclic antidepressants can reverse depression (#1), precipitate mania (#3), and increase cycle frequency (#5) in at least a subgroup of bipolar patients. Monoamine oxidase inhibitors can reverse depression (#1), precipitate mania (#3), and in the case of the (experimental) MAO type A inhibitors, decrease cycle frequency (#6); although the nonspecific

Table 3. Drugs with Three Classes of Actions on Bipolar Illness[1]

Classes of Actions	Drug Types		
Single Episode (weeks to months)	**TCA**	**MAOI** (relative potency)	**Lithium**
1. Antidepressant	+ + +	+ + +	+ +
2. Precipitate depression	0	0	0
3. Precipitate mania	+ + +	+ + +	0
4. Antimanic	0	0	+ + +
Long-Term (years)			
5. Increase cycle frequency	+ +	0/ + *	0
6. Reduce cycle frequency	0	0/ + *	+ +

0 = no effect
+ = weak effect
+ + = moderate effect
+ + + = strong effect
*Action may be related to balance of MAO Type A versus B inhibition
[1]Table adapted from Goodwin and Jamison (in press)

MAOIs may, like TCAs, increase cycle frequency (#5). Lithium can reverse depression (#1), reverse mania (#4), and decrease cycle frequency (#6). Carbamazepine, less extensively evaluated biochemically than any of the above and therefore not included in Table 3, also may have three classes of action: It is partially antidepressant (#1), certainly antimanic (#4), and probably anticycling (#6).

In Table 3, an attempt has been made to roughly quantify the overall relative potency and/or range of effectiveness among compounds for each class of action. Keep in mind that this is an attempt to examine the question of whether there are any general patterns, and we must necessarily ignore individual differences, grey areas, and clinically important distinctions. For example, we have listed MAOIs and TCAs as having approximately equal antidepressant activity in bipolars. As elaborated in later chapters, this is a complex question, the answer to which may depend on such things as the severity of the depressive episode. At any rate, both TCAs and MAOIs seem more potent than lithium for most depressive episodes, and lithium seems more potent than carbamazepine. Lithium is firmly established as reducing cycle frequency, and carbamazepine appears to be capable of this as well; whether these two "stabilizers" really have their effects on different ranges of cycle frequency remains to be seen. TCAs and MAOIs appear to be equipotent in their ability to precipitate a manic episode, and lithium and carbamazepine may be equipotent in treating mania. Only TCAs are well established as increasing the frequency of cycles, although other agents, including nonspecific MAOIs (Kukopoulos et al, 1980), may have such effects as well.

Some of these issues involving patterns of response to treatment will be touched on in greater detail in later chapters. Here, what we wish to emphasize is the way in which pharmacologic treatments direct our attention to neurotransmitters (Table 2) as involved in the mechanism of antidepressant and antimanic drug actions. It is tempting to reason that dysregulation of these systems may also play some primary role in the pathophysiology of manic-depressive illness. The multiple functions of central neurotransmitter systems, however, makes it difficult to conceptualize, let alone demonstrate, true specificity of detected abnormalities. Even investigations of electrolytes (for example, magnesium or calcium) or membrane function (for example, red blood cell sodium-potassium ATPase) involve parameters with widespread functional implications. Thus far, attempts to find unique biochemical substances and/or permanent structural abnormalities in some specific brain area have not been fruitful. Instead, we have unusually low or high amounts of normal substances and/or responses to normal stimuli. We now return to a consideration of those biologic studies that can be directly or indirectly related to the hypotheses generated by various pharmacological bridges.

BIOLOGIC STUDIES IN DETAIL

Caveats in the Interpretation of Biologic Data

As will emerge from what follows, even those biologic findings meeting criteria for Table 1 do not reflect a true consensus, despite the fact of some replications. We have already discussed the problem of diagnostic specificity of patient populations. A closely related issue involves comparability of state of patients across studies even in those who truly have the same diagnosis. Are they studied at the same point of their recurrent illness? How long have they been drug free? It is now clear, for instance, that withdrawal from the high therapeutic doses of antidepressants currently employed produces biochemical changes which persist for at least three and up to six weeks following discontinuation. For more than a decade, the bulk of psychiatric patients available for biochemical studies have recently been or are on medication at the beginning of an investigation. None of the studies below specify a minimum withdrawal over three weeks and most involve only a one- to 2-week drug-free period. There are, however, a few studies in which a parameter is followed longitudinally over different states in one or two untreated subjects. From a research point of view such studies are particularly valuable, although they clearly must be generalized with caution, since investigated patients are those able and willing to tolerate prolonged periods without drugs and, therefore, may be atypical.

Many other factors such as age, sex, and body size, as well as assay validity— too often taken for granted—can contribute to the lack of consensus across studies. In general, however, it is our belief that unrecognized differences in diagnosis, assessment of severity of illness, and failure to allow for an adequate period free of medications are the major sources of variance.

Six Categories of Biologic Studies

With these points in mind, we will briefly review those biologic studies that are summarized in Table 1, along with others that do not meet the criteria of replication for inclusion in the Table. Following the review we will go into somewhat greater detail with regard to very recent studies which relate to unipolar/bipolar differences in functioning of norepinephrine systems. For a more comprehensive discussion of these six categories of biological studies in manic-depressive illness, see Goodwin and Jamison (in press).

The biologic parameters can be categorized into six classes:

1. electrolytes
2. membrane transport
3. peptides
4. neuroendocrine output and response
5. neurotransmitter receptors
6. neurotransmitters, their metabolites, and related enzymes

1. ELECTROLYTES: SODIUM, MAGNESIUM, AND CALCIUM. Although some of the earliest biochemical investigations of manic-depressive illness focused on electrolytes, very little has been done in the last 15 years. This may seem rather curious since if one were to be guided by the pharmacologic bridge strategy of studying parameters related to the action of drugs with wide and important ranges of effects, electrolytes should be of special interest in light of the action of lithium on various endogenous ions (see Emrich, 1982). The three electrolytes reported to be abnormal in some respect during depression and/or (hypo)mania are sodium, magnesium, and calcium. Interestingly, abnormalities in potassium are not found as a function of manic-depressive illness.

Although there were earlier reports of abnormalities in sodium concentration in plasma or CSF, these have not been replicated (Bech et al, 1978; Jimerson et al, 1979). In contrast to direct measures of concentration, use of radioactive sodium permits the study of sodium transfer from plasma to CSF; an early application of this technique revealed decreased sodium transfer in depressed patients as compared to controls (Coppen, 1960). This finding was replicated by another British investigator (Baker, 1971) who, however, showed the same deficit in a group of manic patients. A subsequent study (Carroll, 1972) was consistent with decreased sodium transport in both depressed and manic patients. Another group (Glen et al, 1968) had noted decreased salivary sodium transport in manic-depressive patients.

Using red blood cell (RBC) concentrations as a possible index of intracellular sodium in all body compartments, some groups initially found abnormal concentrations in unipolar and bipolar depressed or manic patients, but more recent studies have failed to replicate this finding (Frazer et al, 1983). The other major factors in understanding sodium concentrations are the membrane mechanisms responsible for sodium transport—we will return to these.

Despite the meager data, it is still attractive to consider the possibility that bipolar illness may involve some generalized abnormality (with a genetic basis?) producing altered regulation of some major electrolyte which might be corrected or compensated for by lithium.

Magnesium is of more recent interest because of the positive finding from the large-scale NIMH collaborative study of depression, that plasma magnesium is elevated in both depressed and manic patients compared to controls (Frazer et al, 1983). However, the ionized fraction (considered to represent the physiologically active form) was not different among the groups. Moreover, CSF studies reveal no subgroup differences or differences from controls in magnesium concentrations (reviewed by Mellerup and Rafaelsen, 1981; Jimerson et al, 1979). In the absence of any theoretical reason for incorporating abnormalities of magnesium, we are tempted to view the few findings that have emerged as not specific to the illness.

In contrast, there is something of a pharmacological bridge to the electrolyte calcium, an increase of which has been associated with depressive symptoms, while hypocalcemia is often accompanied by mood instability, irritability, and hyperactivity (for review see Katzman and Pappius, 1973). For methodologic reasons, direct studies of blood calcium are difficult to interpret. Measures of CSF calcium are less problematic and beginning with a report over 60 years ago (Weston and Howard, 1922), four of seven studies found significantly higher, while none found lower, concentrations in depressed patients versus controls. The unipolar/bipolar distinction, however, was not made in these studies. Within bipolars, CSF calcium has been studied longitudinally with some evidence for decreases following treatment of bipolar depression with ECT (Carman et al, 1977) or lithium (Jimerson et al, 1979); however, there is one study reporting no effect of ECT on CSF calcium. Finally, in a small group of unmedicated bipolar patients, CSF calcium was higher in depression than in mania. Overall, the studies support the notion of increased CSF calcium in bipolar depression. Whether this can be related to the neurotransmitter alterations discussed later remains to be seen. Nonetheless, it suggests that systematic studies of drugs affecting calcium balance and/or transport, for example, calcitonin and calcium channel blockers, may be of particular relevance for manic-depressive illness.

2. MEMBRANE AND TRANSPORT STUDIES: RBC/PLASMA LITHIUM RATIO, RBC NA-K ATPase, PLATELET 5HT UPTAKE, AND (^{3}H)-IMIPRA-MINE BINDING.

Rather than focus primarily on the absolute amount of a substance (for example, electrolytes, as discussed above) in various compartments, some investigators have studied membrane transport functions more directly. Alterations of enzyme dependent ion transfer systems in membranes could account for any abnormalities in concentrations. The major focus, however, has not been on transport of sodium or calcium, but on lithium. It was observed in patients that although lithium in the RBC is usually about 50–60 percent of that in plasma—the RBC/plasma lithium ratio—there was wide interindividual variability in the ratio which appeared to reflect both genetic and clinical response characteristics. The mechanisms underlying the ratio involve a sodium–lithium energy dependent countertransport system; thus there is a correlation between the activity of the RBC countertransport system measured in vitro in cells taken from patients, and the RBC lithium ratio observed in vivo when the patients are treated with lithium.

There are the usual methodological problems in actual studies of these parameters especially with regard to patient selection and, importantly, the length of periods on and off lithium. When data from 13 studies comparing the in vivo lithium ratio in treated unipolar and bipolar patients are pooled, however, a significantly higher ratio is found in bipolars (Goodwin and Jamison, in press). Consistent with this observation, three out of five studies show decreased activity of the RBC sodium–lithium countertransport system in bipolars as compared to normals; decreased transport out would be expected to result in higher RBC levels of lithium in bipolars. Again, however, interpretation is confounded by the apparent long-term inhibitory effects of lithium treatment on the system. Taken together, the data still suggest that some bipolar patients may have an abnormality in the membrane processes responsible for the movement of sodium into and lithium out of the cell.

It is logical next to consider the function of a major membrane enzyme, Na-K ATPase, responsible for maintenance of the critical physiologic ionic gradient which arises from sodium being pumped out of and potassium into the cell. One can directly assay this enzyme activity in RBCs from patients by measuring release of phosphate from ATP. The handful of reports on Na-K ATPase in depressed bipolars, unipolars, and controls so far yield inconsistent results. When, however, the depressed state is compared to recovered or manic states, Na-K ATPase does show a significant decrease; therefore, enzyme activity may at least be relatively low in depression versus euthymia or mania within individuals (reviewed in Nurnberger et al, 1982).

It has been speculated that circulating substances that change with mood might account for the change in Na-K ATPase activity. One possible candidate is the element vanadium, but initial positive results (Naylor et al, 1984) have not been replicated (Ali et al, 1985). The point to be emphasized is that the source of variation in the enzyme activity need not reflect any primary alteration at the membrane.

Although there have been a few studies on other specific membrane enzymes and functions in manic-depressive patients (for example, calcium ATPase), the only ones which have so far generated widespread interest are those on serotonin uptake in platelets. In some respects, the platelet is a reasonable model of events at serotonin nerve endings in the brain, especially with regard to providing a peripheral index of drug induced inhibition of serotonin uptake. Serotonin uptake is coupled to platelet Na-K ATPase and is reported to be reduced in many, but not all, studies of depressed patients, especially bipolars (Meltzer et al, 1981). A related finding in depression is of reduced tritiated (^{3}H)-imipramine binding to a site closely associated with the serotonin uptake site (reviewed in Paul et al, 1985). The majority of studies in this area reveal a modest decrease in ^{3}H-imipramine platelet binding; two studies suggest that this is restricted to bipolar patients or those with familial pure depressive disease (Wood et al, 1983; Lewis and McChesney, 1985). To date, however, there has been no comparison of Na-K ATPase, serotonin uptake, and ^{3}H-imipramine binding sites in the same subject. Interestingly, when serotonin uptake and ^{3}H-imipramine binding are measured simultaneously in the same platelets, they do not always correlate (Raisman et al, 1982).

Nonetheless, all of the above approaches taken together suggest that some variable factors, perhaps circulating in blood and most likely present in bipolar depression, reduce Na-K ATPase and related enzyme activities and/or binding sites on membranes, such that transport of selected ions and at least one neurotransmitter, serotonin, is decreased. This pattern suggests that we should continue to look for evidence of altered central serotonin output in CSF studies; as mentioned below, some groups continue to report lower levels of 5HIAA, the serotonin metabolite, in CSF from depressed patients.

3. PEPTIDES: ENDORPHINS AND SOMATOSTATIN. Peptidergic hormones, their precursors, and fragments are now known to be present in brain tissue, have nonrandom patterns of localization, and produce various effects when directly injected, at least in animals. Since such substances do not readily cross the blood–brain barrier, the only logical tissue available for clinical studies is CSF. Before considering CSF studies, however, clinical trials of substances related to endorphins should be mentioned. Endorphins are, of course, the class of endogenous peptides that act at the receptors which were identified as the site of action of administered opiates. Given the range of opiates' effects and the long history of their use, it seemed obvious that they might be important in manic-depressive illness. Too much endorphin might account for the euphoria of mania, too little, for depression. Although there have been reports of some antimanic effects with the opiate antagonist naloxone, as well as of antidepressant effects with opiates, the data are weak and inconsistent. Not surprisingly (considering the blood–brain barrier), intravenous administration of endorphins and enkephalins have not produced effects beyond the expected placebo ones when a new compound is administered by an enthusiastic investigator. It may still emerge that some component of the endorphin system is important for manic-depressive illness, a view strongly held by at least some European investigators (Emrich, 1982), but definitive abnormalities have not yet been demonstrated in actual attempts to measure endorphins in blood or CSF.

In fact, the strongest findings have emerged around peptides that are usually thought of as being concerned with physiologic functions far removed from mood. Although so far only six studies have been done, consistent decreases of the gut peptide somatostatin have been found in both unipolar and bipolar depression, as well as in bipolar depression as compared to euthymia or (hypo) mania. Somatostatin is widely distributed in the central nervous system (CNS), including cortical, limbic, and hypothalamic areas, where it exerts inhibitory control over the hypothalamic–pituitary–adrenal axis. It also alters appetite, pain, sleep, and motor activity functions, which are often abnormal or dysregulated in affective illness. Somatostatin not only modulates a variety of classic neurotransmitter substances (NE, 5HT, DA, GABA, AcH), but it coexists in neurons containing NE, AcH, or GABA, suggesting important regulatory functions in these systems (reviewed in Rubinow et al, 1983). A very recent study (Doran et al, 1986) suggests that CSF somatostatin is lower in patients who escape from dexamethasone suppression and hence those who are hypernoradrenergic (see below). It may emerge that decreased somatostatin, elevated corticotropin releasing factor (CRF), and exaggerated norepinephrine release to stress are closely related findings in depression. It is important to note, however, that these are not unique to bipolar depression and are at best equally abnormal in severe unipolar depression.

There are a few studies on CSF concentrations of each of a variety of centrally active peptides: vasopressin, oxytocin, calcitonin, substance P, cholecystokinin, thyrotropin releasing hormone (TRH), neurotensin, vasoactive intestinal peptide (VIP), and CRF—all of which can be argued to have a possible role in mediating at least some symptoms of depression. So far, it is unclear whether direct measures of these various peptides in CSF will reveal consistent data on the biology of bipolar depression. Implicit in the neuroendocrine studies that are discussed next, however, is the assumption that the regulation of many of these peptides must be altered in some specific sites if not the whole brain. CSF peptide concentrations need not necessarily reflect alterations at sites of interest; it will require many more years of investigation in which systems are characterized at multiple levels to explore the potential, if any, of such measures to biologically characterize bipolar illness.

4. NEUROENDOCRINE OUTPUT AND RESPONSE. It is now generally accepted that one or more measures that reflect function of the hypothalamic-pituitary-adrenal (HPA) axis are abnormal in the majority of depressed patients. Abnormalities appear to be state dependent and are not specific to depression. Table 4 expands on Table 1 and summarizes neuroendocrine measures related to HPA function which are most consistently noted to be abnormal in depression, with a focus on whether they appear to be able to discriminate unipolar

Table 4. Reported Neuroendocrine Abnormalities in Depression[1]

	Depressed versus Control	Bipolar(D) versus Unipolar	Bipolar (D) versus (Hypo)mania	(Hypo)Mania versus Control or Unipolar
Cortisol				
Resting—CSF	=, ↑	=	*	? ↑
—plasma	↑	=	↑	
—urine	↑	=	↑	? ↑
Post-Dexamethasone				
—plasma	↑	=	=, ↑	=, ↑
Post 5HTP—(plasma)	=, ↑			
ACTH response to CRF	↓	=		
Growth hormone				
response to clonidine, insulin, amphetamine,	↓	=, ↑		? ↓ (to insulin)
and L–dopa to CRF		? ↑		
Prolactin response				
to L–tryptophan	↓	=		
to TRH	↓	=		
TSH response to TRH	↓	? ↑		

" ↑ "—increased in most studies
" ↓ "—decreased in most studies
" = "—some studies show no difference
" =, ↑ or ↓ "—some studies show no difference, others show increase or decrease
"?, ↑ or ↓ "—preliminary studies showing increase or decrease

*Absence of symbol indicates studies not available

Abbreviations: (D) = depressed; CSF = cerebrospinal fluid; 5HTP = 5–hydroxytryptophan; ACTH = adrenocorticotropic hormone; CRF = corticotropin releasing factor; TRH = thyrotropin releasing hormone; TSH = thyroid stimulating hormone

[1]The bibliography forming the basis for this Table is available upon request from the authors.

from bipolar depression or, for that matter, either from mania. What emerges is that cortisol is elevated in plasma, urine, and probably CSF, as well as "escaping" from dexamethasone suppression in plasma both in unipolar and bipolar depressed patients, but less frequently in mania. Unipolar and bipolar patients also have an exaggerated cortisol response to ACTH, as well as a blunted ACTH response to CRF (not found in mania). The blunted ACTH response to exogenous CRF is interpreted to reflect hypersecretion of CRF in depressed patients, and the exaggerated cortisol response to ACTH may be secondary to adrenal hypertrophy (Gold et al, 1984). The point to be emphasized here, however, is that unipolar and bipolar depression are not distinguishable.

Another endocrine response, growth hormone (GH) release following clonidine, L–dopa, insulin induced hypoglycemia, amphetamine, or desipramine administration is blunted in approximately 90 percent of patients with depression, unipolar and bipolar. The blunting has not been clearly related to other neuroendocrine abnormalities; for instance, it is found in depressed patients who have both normal and elevated cortisol. One study reports a paradoxical stimulation of GH by CRF in bipolar depression—comparison data in unipolars is not available (Gold et al, 1984). In any event, it should be noted that the GH response to many stimuli may be mediated in part by hypothalamic $alpha_2$ receptors, which could be down-regulated secondary to a hyperadrenergic (and hypercortisolimic) state (see below). Any GH response to CRF would presumably be mediated through some other receptor(s).

Two other hormones, prolactin and thyroid-stimulating hormone (TSH), have been extensively studied, each from a different theoretical model. Prolactin release stimulated by serotonin agonists (direct and indirect) is a putative marker of CNS serotonergic function, although ACTH and cortisol release following the same compounds may emerge as better indices. In any event, initial studies indicate that prolactin response to serotonin agonists is blunted, but again both in unipolar and bipolar depression (Heninger et al, 1984; Siever et al, 1984).

As for TSH and the hypothalamic-pituitary-thyroid axis, findings on the therapeutic effects of thyroid, already discussed in the context of the pharmacological bridge, suggest that this might be a particularly relevant system. One should recall that modest doses of thyroid may potentiate responses to standard tricyclic antidepressants in either unipolar or bipolar depression, and that hypermetabolic doses of thyroid may interrupt rapid manic-depressive cycling. As reviewed in Chapter 3 of this volume, there is a very high incidence of hypothyroidism in rapid cycling bipolar patients, usually revealed by an exaggerated TSH response to TRH. It is not clear, however, that this TSH response can be used prospectively to distinguish a subgroup of rapid cyclers. The problem arises from the phenomena that some depressed patients (perhaps 30 percent) show a blunted TSH response to TRH (Loosen and Prange, 1982). There is some evidence suggesting that the blunted TSH response is confined primarily to unipolar depression, in which case an elevated one would indicate either hypothyroidism and/or bipolar depression. As further advances are made in studying the hypothalamic-pituitary-thyroid axis, they should be applied to the biological characterization of subtypes of depression with an aim toward refining these suggestive leads.

The present ability of neuroendocrine measures to specifically address the biology of *bipolar* illness is thus surprisingly limited. It is, nonetheless, obviously important that any inclusive formulation be able to explain the association of endocrine abnormalities with both bipolar and unipolar depression. In what follows we will briefly return to this issue.

5. NEUROTRANSMITTER RECEPTORS. Since chronic administration of all antidepressant and antimanic treatment can be shown to alter one or more neurotransmitter receptors in rodent brains, an obvious strategy is to measure such receptors in patients. Given that direct brain measures are not feasible, one must use peripheral sources of receptors. Some generalized abnormal membrane function might be equally reflected in most receptor populations, a concept which relates back to the previously discussed studies on electrolyte and membrane transport alterations in depression. Such an approach does not, however, appear to reflect the intent of direct studies on neurotransmitter receptors, usually in platelets and lymphocytes. Rather, the unusually labor intensive investigations (at least from the laboratory point of view) are so far directed at possible specific receptor defects, primarily of noradrenergic alpha$_2$ and beta receptors.

A recent discussion of the problems in the interpretation of altered alpha$_2$ receptor number and/or function on platelets (Kafka and Paul, 1986) concludes with the caveat that findings could be explained simply on the basis of elevated circulating catecholamines (see below). Were this so, then findings of increased alpha$_2$ agonist binding accompanied by desensitization (that is, reduced norepinephrine mediated inhibition of cAMP formation) in platelets from unipolar patients without significant findings in bipolars would be consistent with the unipolar/bipolar difference in norepinephrine output discussed below. On the other hand, no single study to date has obtained relevant platelet alpha$_2$ parameters and measures of norepinephrine output in both unipolar and bipolar depressed patients. Furthermore, there are no studies in unmedicated mania.

Interpretation of the very few studies of lymphocyte beta receptor number and function in depressed patients is difficult. Receptor number appears to be unchanged, whereas beta receptor mediated cyclic AMP response to isoproterenol is clearly blunted in unipolar depression (Pandey et al, 1979; Mann et al, 1985); there is not sufficient data on bipolars. Preliminary data on circulating norepinephrine and epinephrine do not appear to account for the variance observed in the sensitivity or affinity states of the beta receptors in depressed patients, although such a relationship can be observed in normal volunteers under controlled experimental conditions (Feldman et al, 1984). This apparent dissociation between transmitter and receptor could be interpreted as further evidence of dysregulation of the norepinephrine system in depression, although, to date, there is insufficient information on whether it will prove useful in clarifying the unipolar/bipolar dichotomy.

6. NEUROTRANSMITTERS AND THEIR METABOLITES. *CSF Studies.* At the outset it is worth emphasizing that of the three monoamine neurotransmitters most extensively evaluated in preclinical studies, two—serotonin and dopamine—have been studied in depressed patients almost exclusively in terms of concentrations of their receptive *metabolites*, 5–hydroxy–indoleacetic acid (5HIAA) and homovanillic acid (HVA) in CSF. Under carefully controlled conditions, the neurotransmitter metabolites will, in part, reflect relative differences in the output and metabolism of dopamine and serotonin in those brain regions which contribute the most to CSF concentrations. However, in humans, the relative contribution of different brain areas is not well understood. Moreover, it is not really possible to study the responsiveness of 5HT and dopamine neuronal systems using a single point measure of transmitter metabolite in CSF; at most, longer term changes can be reflected in CSF studies. Thus, CSF studies of HVA and 5HIAA in untreated depressed patients can identify some relative differences, but cannot directly address the source of any alteration, even to the extent of distinguishing changes of output from those of metabolism and/or elimination. When considering actual studies, it is also important to recognize that limitations of assay methodology make it difficult to feel confident about many earlier studies. The technique of performing two lumbar punctures within a few days of each other, before and after the administration of probenecid to block the active acid transport of 5HIAA and HVA out of the CSF, was an ingenious approach to obtaining an estimate of 5HT and DA function and release (that is, the amount of accumulation of 5HIAA and HVA between the period of probenecid administration and the lumbar tap). Such probenecid induced accumulations sometimes revealed group differences not observed in using so-called baseline measures (Goodwin et al, 1973).

The pertinent CSF literature through the late 1970s has been thoroughly reviewed elsewhere (Post et al, 1980). Overall, there is a trend for HVA to be lower in depressed patients (whether bipolar or unipolar) than in controls, with most studies involving the probenecid technique showing reduced HVA accumulation. HVA values in manic as compared to depressed patients or controls are nonsignificantly higher in most studies. Recent studies with relatively large sample sizes both from this country (Koslow et al, 1983) and Scandinavia (Ågren, 1980; Åsberg et al, 1984) provide additional evidence that HVA is reduced in depression, especially patients with melancholia (Åsberg, 1984), again without any evidence of unipolar/bipolar differences.

Earlier findings on 5HIAA in CSF are also in the direction of reductions in depressed patients, but with much less consistency, perhaps because of reliance on a fluorometric assay. There is also a trend in this data for bipolar patients to have lower 5HIAA than unipolars (reviewed in Goodwin and Jamison, in press). Probenecid induced accumulations of 5HIAA are consistently lower in depressed patients than in controls (Post et al, 1980). Interestingly, unlike the HVA pattern observed in comparison of mania with depression, 5HIAA concentrations are not different in the two states. In fact, 5HIAA may be reduced in mania as compared to controls to the same extent as observed in depression. More recent studies of baseline 5HIAA in CSF of unmedicated depressed patients are inconsistent: the NIMH Collaborative Study reports *increased* 5HIAA in depressed women (Koslow et al, 1983). In 83 patients with melancholia diagnosed and treated at the Karolinska Institute in Sweden, 5HIAA was modestly, but significantly, reduced (Åsberg et al, 1984). In the former study there was a trend for female bipolar patients to have lower 5HIAA than unipolars; in the latter study, there were no unipolar/bipolar differences in this measure.

The CSF norepinephrine metabolite, 3–methoxy–4–hydroxyphenylglycol (MHPG) in depressed patients is consistently reported as not different from controls, both in earlier and current studies, except for higher levels in postmenopausal women (Koslow et al, 1983). Within the depressed group, however, significant subgroup differences in MHPG do emerge, although not in the data from the NIMH collaborative study. One Scandinavian series, which did not include a control group, showed lower MHPG in CFS from bipolar I than from unipolar patients (Ågren and Potter, unpublished data). Similarly, we have observed that norepinephrine itself in CSF is lower in age- and sex-matched bipolar than unipolar patients (Rudorfer et al, 1983).

Earlier investigations had shown that CSF norepinephrine was higher during mania than depression (Post et al, 1978). In the NIMH collaborative study, MHPG in the CSF was higher in mania than in depressed unipolar or bipolar patients or in controls (Table 5).

Table 5. Cerebrospinal Fluid Studies of Neurotransmitters and/or Their Metabolites in Depression and Mania

Substance and Comparison**	HVA, 5HIAA, and MHPG		
	Review of World Literature (Post et al, 1980) 1969–1979 *n = 352 (120)	Karolinska Series (Åsberg et al, 1984) 1970–1980 n = 83 (0)	NIMH Collaborative Study (Koslow et al, 1983) 1975–1980 n = 92 (14)
HVA—D vs. C	↓	↓	↓
BP vs. UP	=	=	=
M vs. BP	? ↑	N/A	↑
5HIAA—D vs. C	? ↓	↓	=
BP vs. UP	=	=	=
M vs. BP	=	N/A	=
MHPG—D vs. C	=	=	=
BP vs. UP	?	?***	=
M vs. BP	? ↑	N/A	↑

	Norepinephrine	
	Radioenzymatic Method (Post et al, 1978) n = 20 (8)	HPLC–EC Method (Rudorfer et al, 1983) n = 21 (0)
NE—D vs. C	=	N/A
BP vs. UP	***	↓
M vs. D	↑	N/A

" ↑ " = increased; " ↓ " = decreased; "±" = data supporting both increased and decreased; "="—no differences; "?" = insufficient data available to make any judgement; "? ↑ or ↓ " = trend toward increase or decrease, but data preliminary or questionable; N/A means not applicable

*n = total population of depressed patients in whom HVA or 5HIAA was available; number in parentheses indicates size of manic sample

**D = depressed (unipolars + bipolars); C = control; BP = bipolar depressed (includes types I and II); UP = unipolar depressed; M = mania (includes hypomania)

***Insufficient depressed and BPs studied or specified; two BPI patients in Karolinska series

Taken together, the CSF studies of norepinephrine and its metabolite MHPG suggest that depression versus mania and unipolar versus bipolar depression are associated with differences in norepinephrine output. However, as will become clear from what follows, it is possible that the CSF findings reflect events occurring in the sympathetic nervous system as much as events occurring in the brain. But this distinction is rather artificial since there are intimate links between CNS function and peripheral sympathetic norepinephrine output. We therefore find it most useful to consider as many components of the norepinephrine system(s) as possible before making an interpretation.

Studies of norepinephrine and MHPG in Plasma. During the last decade there have been an increasing number of investigations of plasma norepinephrine and MHPG. Consistent with the fact that there is a significant correlation between MHPG in CSF and plasma, no differences emerge from comparison of depressed patients and controls. Too few bipolars and unipolars have been compared in the same studies to evaluate the possibility of bipolar/unipolar differences in plasma MHPG.

In contrast, plasma norepinephrine is consistently reported to be different from controls in groups of depressed patients, although there is considerable overlap. Interestingly, in the earliest study, plasma norepinephrine was found to be elevated during depression (Wyatt et al, 1971). Subsequent studies have shown that in a total group of depressives (Lake et al, 1982), in a clearly endogenous subgroup (Esler et al, 1982), and in patients with a positive dexamethasone suppression test (DST) (Barnes et al, 1983), plasma norepinephrine is elevated compared to controls or to depressed dexamethasone suppressors. Another study that did not include plasma norepinephrine found elevated MHPG in depressed patients who had a positive DST (Jimerson et al, 1983). Most of the patients in these studies had unipolar illness. Two recent NIMH studies have shown elevated standing norepinephrine in unipolar depressives; only one found that the supine level was elevated (Rudorfer et al, 1985; Roy et al, 1985). Moreover, in one of these studies, we found lower resting plasma norepinephrine in bipolars than in age- and sex-matched controls or unipolars. These findings are summarized in Table 6.

How can one reconcile the various studies? We have argued the point in detail elsewhere (Rudorfer et al, 1985) and will only summarize the conclusion here. First, depressed bipolar patients, on average, especially if maintained in a setting where stress is minimized, have a lower output of norepinephrine. We see evidence of this in a sufficient proportion of studies, whether of CSF, plasma, or urine (see below). Moreover, in mania, plasma and CSF norepinephrine are elevated in comparison to depression (reviewed in Potter et al, 1985a), although not necessarily in comparison to control values. Similar findings of elevations during mania are observed for CSF and urinary MHPG. Thus, the early notion (Schildkraut, 1965; Bunney and Davis, 1965) that bipolar depression is relatively hyponoradrenergic and mania a relatively hyperadrenergic state has stood the test of time.

Second, it is clear that unipolar and bipolar patients show an exaggerated functional norepinephrine increase after the physiologic "stress" of going from a lying to a standing position. Unipolar patients appear to be particularly sensitive to a variety of stresses, at least as regards plasma norepinephrine. Thus, establishing a "true" resting level, even in the supine position, can be proble-

Table 6. Plasma Norepinephrine Concentrations in Depression

Study	D versus C*	BP versus UP	High NE Associated with:
Wyatt et al (1971)	↑		
Lake et al (1982)	↑		
Esler et al (1982)	↑		Endogenicity
Veith et al (1983)	=, ↑		+DST
Roy et al (1985)	↑	? ↓	+DST
Rudorfer et al (1985)	=, ↑,**	↓	

" ↑ "—elevated in most studies; " ↓ "—lowered in most studies; "=, ↑ or ↓ "—some studies show no difference, others show increase or decrease; "?, ↑ or ↓ "—preliminary studies showing increase or decrease
*D = depressed; C = control; BP = bipolar depressed; UP = unipolar depressed
**Supine values same in depressed and controls; standing values elevated in depressed

matic without maintaining subjects at bed rest over night. This may explain some of the discrepancies in supine values among studies; in contrast, the "stressed" standing plasma norepinephrine is consistently elevated. These methodologic issues may also be relevant to discrepancies in measures of integrated norepinephrine output over time, such as 24-hour urinary excretion of MHPG. For instance, a unipolar patient who is stressed in various ways over an extended period of time would be expected to have a relatively high total norepinephrine output, whereas one who is only intermittently stressed could show elevated plasma norepinephrine at that time, but an integrated output within the normal range. These concepts may help to understand the conflicting data in urine, which will be reviewed next.

Urinary Studies of Norepinephrine and its Metabolites. Attempts to characterize output of the norepinephrine system in depressed patients have focused on measurements of MHPG in urine more than any other single parameter. Under appropriately controlled conditions, urinary MHPG does provide an accurate index of the total excretion of norepinephrine plus its metabolites (Linnoila et al, 1982). A detailed review of the literature on this measure through 1980 suggests that there is a modest reduction of urinary MHPG in depressed individuals compared to controls (Potter et al, 1985b); taking only those studies which separately consider unipolar and bipolar patients and have satisfactory methods, the MHPG reduction is accounted for exclusively by bipolars. Reduced urinary MHPG may be present only in bipolar I and not in bipolar II patients (Muscettola et al, 1984). In any event, MHPG is clearly not reduced in unipolar populations. If anything, there may be a subgroup of unipolar patients who have elevated MHPG as compared to controls (Schatzberg et al, 1982), and compared to bipolar subjects. However, urinary MHPG was no different in a relatively large group of mixed bipolar I and II depressives as compared to unipolars or controls, in whom urinary norepinephrine itself was higher in the unipolars than bipolars (Koslow et al, 1983). It is not clear whether the relative dissociation of urinary norepinephrine and MHPG in this latter multicenter study reflects a true phenomena or a methodological artifact, since there is a close association between urinary norepinephrine and MHPG when studied in a single center using a single assay methodology (Linnoila et al, 1982).

It is interesting to note that one group has been able to utilize urinary measures of norepinephrine and all of its metabolites to develop a discriminant function analysis, which correctly identified almost all bipolar versus unipolar patients in a subsequent group of patients studied in the same setting (Schildkraut et al, 1978). Unfortunately, such discriminant functions developed within a center are not generalizable as such, perhaps because of the lack of standardization of research procedures and assays. In any event, it may prove possible to distinguish unipolar from bipolar depressed subjects by using all norepinephrine related measures in urine rather than MHPG alone.

Summary of Bipolar/Unipolar Differences in Norepinephrine Systems. The common theme which emerges from the above is that when bipolar I is compared to unipolar depression, one or more possible indices of norepinephrine output are reduced. This finding also emerges from some studies in which a bipolar I versus II distinction is not made. The different types of evidence are summarized in Table 7. It is tempting to conclude that if we had consistent measures in CSF, plasma, and urine, we would be able to identify a depressed individual as unipolar or bipolar. On the other hand, the norepinephrine system is influenced by so many factors that, in practice, it may not be feasible to provide sufficient controls to develop a sensitive and specific diagnostic test that distinguishes most unipolars from bipolars. Nonetheless, if the data are valid, a test that specifically identifies a proportion of bipolar depressed subjects should be possible; this arises from the consideration that most exogenous variables will elevate rather than reduce norepinephrine output. Thus, in the absence of other organic disease that produces a reduction of sympathetic outflow (such as Shy-Drager syndrome), a depressed patient who 1) has substantially lower than average (for example, a 30 percent or greater reduction) urinary MHPG or norepineph-

Table 7. Summary of Noradrenergic Measures Reported to Distinguish Bipolar from Unipolar Depression

	Bipolar I*	Bipolar I and II
Measure		
CSF–NE	↓	↓
–MHPG	=, ↓	=
Plasma–NE		↓
Urine–NE		↓
–MHPG	↓	=

*direction in comparison to unipolar depression
" ↓ "—decreased in most studies
" = "—some studies show no difference
" =, ↓ "—some studies show no difference; others show decrease

rine as compared to age- and sex-matched controls or depressed patients taken as a whole, *and* who 2) has a similarly reduced supine plasma norepinephrine combined with an elevated fractional norepinephrine increase on standing, is likely to be suffering from bipolar depression. The specificity and predictive power of these parameters are currently undergoing evaluation.

Integration of Biologic and Treatment Response Findings

We turn now to the broader question of the implications that many biologic abnormalities are common both to bipolar and unipolar depression. So far, no underlying trait abnormality separating bipolar from unipolar depression has been convincingly demonstrated—at the moment the two most plausible candidates are increased RBC Li^+ ratio and decreased 5HT platelet uptake in bipolars (Table 1 and the section on membrane transport, above). We therefore believe it is prudent to operate under the assumption that all findings may be in some way "secondary" to the state of depression or mania. Since central nervous system noradrenergic projections have perhaps the widest range of targets that control other types of parameters documented to be abnormal in depression (for example, neuroendocrine), we feel that the most appropriate integration is in terms of norepinephrine function. It is clear from the data that norepinephrine output and/or response is altered in both unipolar and bipolar patients, and can be either high or low depending on the circumstances. What then are the likely consequences of such abnormalities?

To obtain a sense of the overall function of norepinephrine systems in intact organisms, we turn to preclinical studies. Electrophysiologists have developed a concept of norepinephrine in the CNS as a modulator of other signals, rather than as a primary signal transducer, which it seems to be in the sympathetic nervous system (SNS) (Woodward et al, 1979). At least in the cerebellum, norepinephrine released following locus coeruleus (LC) stimulation *decreases* the spontaneous firing of purkinje cells, thereby increasing the relative signal from exogenous stimuli (Woodward et al, 1979). In other words, norepinephrine increases the signal-to-noise ratio in this area of the brain, thereby increasing the sensitivity to stimuli. Thus, norepinephrine projections from the LC to other areas may amplify the overall functional role of norepinephrine by rendering various brain regions more responsive to a number of stimuli.

Another way to put the different roles of norepinephrine into perspective is to evaluate the consequences of disease related deficits in total norepinephrine output in man. Patients with idiopathic hypotension have greater than 70 percent reductions in circulating plasma norepinephrine (Polinsky et al, 1981), as well as markedly decreased total norepinephrine output (56 percent), presumably as a consequence of a reduction in postganglionic SNS neurons (Kopin et al, 1983). This example, however, pertains only to the SNS as far as is known and CNS production of norepinephrine is presumed to be intact. Only in animal studies do we see direct evidence of CNS consequences. Agents (including clonidine) in doses which deplete central norepinephrine plus its metabolites in rodents or primates by 50–90 percent reduce normal responses to a whole variety of stressors, both along physiological and behavioral axes (for relevant reviews see Porsolt, 1981; Hellhammer, 1983). In a general way this would be compatible with a major role of norepinephrine as an important modulator of other systems, as discussed above. Obviously following treatments such as reserpine, which are not selective for the CNS, animals' SNS functions will be altered as well, with resultant miosis, diarrhea, hypersalivation, lacrimation, gastric hypersecretion, and bradycardia (Garrattini and Jori, 1967). A reasonable interpretation of these findings by those working with animal models of depression is that a well-functioning norepinephrine system is protective; a deficient one predisposes to pathologic effects of whatever induced syndrome one is studying, whether stress (Katz and Baldrighi, 1982; Weiss et al, 1981), separation (Kraemer and McKinney, 1979), or learned helplessness (Weiss et al, 1976). It may well be that norepinephrine is far more related to these models than the models are to depression; the point, however, is that at least in animals, norepinephrine has an important modulatory role beyond the cardiovascular one.

In light of the above, it seems reasonable to speculate that, in man, norepinephrine may also play a protective role and be important in responding to various stresses, not only as a mediator of immediate SNS output, but also as a means of altering the "gain" of multiple systems in the central nervous system (that is, increasing or decreasing the signal-to-noise ratio). A deficient norepinephrine system would thus increase the susceptibility to depression and/or permit depression to become manifest.

And what effects do the treatments which have the widest range of effects on depressive illness (Table 4) have on norepinephrine systems? As shown in Table 8, the three most studied—TCAs, MAOIs, and lithium—produce a range of effects on norepinephrine as well as serotonergic (5HT) parameters. Consistent effects on dopamine are *not* apparent. With regard to the norepinephrine effects, we have suggested on the basis of our clinical studies that these antidepressant induced alterations of output or receptor response can be best understood as reflections of increased efficiency of the noradrenergic system—in other words, in the face of less norepinephrine, necessary endogenous functions are maintained or restored despite reduced response to exogenous agonists (Table 8) (see Potter et al, in press for a detailed discussion). On the basis of a review of previous literature, mostly in animals, Stone (1983) has also advanced the notion that antidepressants increase the efficiency of the noradrenergic system.

If treatments increase norepinephrine (and perhaps 5HT) efficiency, are the abnormalities interpretable as indicating reduced efficiency in the untreated state? We would argue that in depression, whatever the resting output, "excess" norepinephrine is released on standing (stress?) in untreated depressed patients in both absolute and proportional terms, and that this norepinephrine increase seems to be dissociated from cardiovascular function. This excess norepinephrine in search of a function may be in fact wasted and hence "inefficient." One could speculate that the association between elevated plasma norepinephrine and cortisol escape from dexamethasone suppression is another example of inefficiency, since the excess cortisol appears to serve no useful function. In depressed patients, we see direct evidence of inefficiency in the norepinephrine system, at least as regards SNS release following an orthostatic challenge. As far as we know, this inefficiency is not linked to the increased total norepinephrine turnover seen in unipolar patients. Thus, as noted above, even in bipolar patients in whom total norepinephrine turnover is decreased, as evidenced by both lower supine plasma norepinephrine and urinary MHPG or norepinephrine, there is an exaggerated increase of plasma norepinephrine on standing.

Table 8. Effects of TCAs, MAOIs, and Lithium on Neurotransmitter Systems in Animals and Humans

Chronic Biochemical Effects in Animals			
	TCAs	MAOIs	Lithium
NE uptake inhibition	↓↓↓	0	0–↑
5HT uptake inhibition	↓–↓↓↓	0	0
Monoamine oxidase inhibition	↓	↓↓↓	0

Chronic Effects on Receptor Density or Coupling to Cyclic AMP in Animals			
	TCAs	MAOIs	Lithium
Beta adrenergic	↓↓	↓↓	0–↓
Alpha 1	0–↑	0	0
Alpha 2	0–↓↓	↓↓	0–↓
$5HT_1$	0	↓↓	0–?↓
$5HT_2$	↓–↓↓	↓↓	0–↓
Dopamine–2	0	0–?	0–↓
GABA–B	↑↑	0–↑	?

Human Studies of Neurotransmitter Turnover			
	TCAs	MAOIs	Lithium
MHPG in urine or CSF	↓↓	↓↓	0–↓
"Sum" of metabolites in urine	↓↓	↓↓↓	0–↓
5HT via 5HIAA in CSF	↓↓	↓	0–?
Dopamine via HVA in CSF	0	↓–↓↓	0–?

Responses Related to Neurotransmitter Function in Humans			
Norepinephrine (NE)	TCAs	MAOIs	Lithium
Plasma NE increase on standing	↑↑	0	?
Heart rate	↑–↑↑	0–↓	0
Blood pressure response to clonidine	↓–↓↓	0–↓	?
Blood pressure response to phenylephrine	0–↓	↑↑↑	?
Growth hormone response to NE agonists	↑–↓	↓	?
Melatonin output	↑	↑	?

Serotonin (5HT)	TCAs	MAOIs	Lithium
Prolactin response to L–tryptophan	↑	?	↑
Prolactin response to TRH	?	?	?↑
Cortisol response to 5HTP	↓	↑	↑

Table adapted from Goodwin and Jamison (in press)

"0"—no effect

" ↓ "—slight decrease

" ↓ ↓ "—moderate decrease

" ↓ ↓ ↓ "—marked decrease

" ↑ "—slight increase

" ↑ ↑ "—moderate increase

" ↑ ↑ ↑ "—marked increase

"?"—data unavailable or unclear

Abbreviations: CSF = cerebrospinal fluid; HVA = homovanillic acid; MHPG = 3–methoxy–4–hydroxyphenylglycol; TRH = thyrotropin releasing hormone

We do not mean to exclude other neurotransmitter candidates from pivotal roles in the action of antidepressants or pathophysiology of depression. As emphasized elsewhere, the primary measure of 5HT, its metabolite 5HIAA in CSF, seems affected whenever central norepinephrine function is altered (Potter et al, 1985a). Urinary 5HT and 5HIAA are less consistently affected, but may come predominantly from irrelevant peripheral sources. The dopamine metabolites HVA and DOPAC in CSF, as well as dopamine itself, HVA, and DOPAC in urine, are not consistently altered by antidepressant treatments (Linnoila et al, 1983). Interestingly, two treatments with anticycling properties, lithium and an MAO Type A inhibitor, are those that affect dopamine, either in terms of products in urine or CSF. It is also of interest to recall that classically the most noradrenergic (and dopaminergic) drugs (Tables 2 and 8) are the ones that can precipitate mania and/or cycling (Table 4). This suggests that a low average norepinephrine output in bipolar depression may render patients subject to other than antidepressant effects. From a therapeutic point of view, it would be of great importance to establish whether this notion holds, since it would provide a rationale for identifying patients at risk for TCA or MAOI induced manias or cycles.

SUMMARY

Biologic findings in bipolar disorders have been reviewed in the context of findings in endogenous unipolar depression, as well as of the major biochemical effects of drugs used in the treatment of manic-depressive illness. A great number of studies implicating other substances, especially cholinergic ones, have not been included. Connections between the cholinergic and noradrenergic systems, particularly with regard to stress responses, are clearly widespread and likely to be involved in aspects of bipolar illness. To even begin to do justice to the range of studies of the cholinergic and other systems is beyond the scope of this chapter. Thus, we have opted to avoid lists of all known findings accompanied by passing reference to each relevant series of hypotheses. Rather, the concentration has been on those classes of findings that have been most often claimed to distinguish bipolar from unipolar depression. One major integrative approach has then been selected—to understand the extent to which norepinephrine function is altered in bipolar versus unipolar depression, and the extent to which effects on the norepinephrine system explain the action of drugs used in the treatment of these conditions.

We conclude by emphasizing the importance of continuing to pursue the interface between biologic findings and treatment. In general, looking for predictors of response has been frustrating and somewhat academic, since clinical criteria provide the "gold standard." Without a history of (hypo)mania, however, it is not possible to assess whether a depression is bipolar or unipolar. Thus, possible long-term adverse consequences of treating bipolar or "pseudo unipolar" depression with mania (or cycle) inducing drugs gives a sense of urgency to the search for a biologic test. In the foreseeable future, some combination of norepinephrine related measures appears most likely to be able to identify the bipolar population most at risk. It is hoped that simpler and more robust measures will emerge, but we should try to find a means of better utilizing the knowledge that we already have.

REFERENCES

Ågren H: Symptom patterns in unipolar and bipolar depression correlating with mono-amine metabolites in the cerebrospinal fluid, I: general patterns. Psychiatr Res 3:211-223, 1980

Ali SA, Peet M, Ward NI: Blood levels of vanadium, caesium, and other elements in depressive patients. J Affect Dis 9:187-191, 1985

Andreasen NC, Scheftner W, Reich T, et al: The validation of the concept of endogenous depression: a family study approach. Arch Gen Psychiatry 43:246-251, 1986

Åsberg M, Bertilsson L, Martensson B, et al: CSF monoamine metabolites in melancholia. Acta Psychiatr Scand 69:201-219, 1984

Baker EFW: Sodium transfer to cerebrospinal fluid in functional psychiatric illness. Canadian Psychiatric Association Journal 16:167-170, 1971

Barnes RF, Veith RC, Borson S, et al: High levels of plasma catecholamines in dexameth-asone-resistant depressed patients. Am J Psychiatry 140:1623-1625, 1983

Bech P, Kirkegaard C, Bock E, et al: Hormones, electrolytes, and cerebrospinal fluid proteins in manic-melancholic patients. Neuropsychobiology 4:99-122, 1978

Bevan-Jones AB, Pare CMB, Nicholson WJ, et al: Brain amine concentrations after mono-amine oxidase inhibitor administration. Br Med J 1:17-19, 1972

Bunney WE, Davis JM: Norephinephrine in depressive reactions: a review. Arch Gen Psychiatry 13:483-494, 1965

Carman JS, Post RM, Goodwin FK, et al: Calcium and electroconvulsive therapy of severe depressive illness. Biol Psychiatry 12:5-17, 1977

Carroll BJ: Sodium and potassium transfer to cerebrospinal fluid in severe depression, in Depressive Illness. Edited by Davies B. Springfield, Illinois, Charles C Thomas, 1972

Coppen A: Abnormality of the blood-cerebrospinal fluid barrier of patients suffering from a depressive illness. J Neurol Neurosurg Psychiatry 23:156-161, 1960

Cowen PJ, Geaney DP, Schachter M, et al: Desipramine treatment in normal subjects: effects on neuroendocrine responses to tryptophan and on platelet serotonin (5–HT)-related receptors. Arch Gen Psychiatry 43:61-67, 1986

Doran AR, Rubinow DR, Roy A, et al: CSF somatostatin and abnormal response to dexa-methasone administration in schizophrenic and depressed patients. Arch Gen Psychiatry 43:365-369, 1986

Emrich HM: A possible role of opioid substances in depression. Adv Biochem Psycho-pharmacol 32:77-84, 1982

Esler M, Turbott J, Schwarz R, et al: The peripheral kinetics of norepinephrine in depressive illness. Arch Gen Psychiatry 39:295-300, 1982

Feldman RD, Limbird LE, Nadeau J, et al: Leukocyte beta-receptor alterations in hypertensive subjects. J Clin Invest 73:648-653, 1984

Frazer A, Ramsey TA, Swann A, et al: Plasma and erythrocyte electrolytes in affective disorders. J Affective Disord 5:103-113, 1983

Garrattini D, Jori A: Interactions between imipramine-like drugs and reserpine on body temperature, in Antidepressant Drugs. Edited by Garrattini S, Dukes MNG. Amsterdam, Excerpta Media Foundation, 1967

Gershon ES, Hamovit J, Guroff J, et al: A family study of schizoaffective, bipolar I, bipolar II, unipolar, and normal controls. Arch Gen Psychiatry 39:1157-1167, 1982

Glen AIM, Ongley GC, Robinson K: Diminished membrane transport in manic-depressive psychosis and recurrent depression. Lancet 2:241, 1968

Gold PW, Chrousos G, Kellner C, et al: Psychiatric implications of basic and clinical studies with corticotropin-releasing factor. Am J Psychiatry 141: 619-627, 1984

Goodwin FK, Jamison KR: Manic-Depressive Illness. New York, Oxford University Press (in press)

Goodwin FK, Sack RL: Affective disorders: the catecholamine hypothesis revisited, in Frontiers in Catecholamine Research. Edited by Usdin E, Snyder S. New York, Pergamon Press, 1973

Goodwin FK, Brodie HKH, Murphy DL, et al: L–dopa, catecholamines and behavior: a clinical and biochemical study in depressed patients. Biol Psychiatry 2:341-366, 1970

Goodwin FK, Ebert MH, Bunney WE: Mental effects of reserpine in man: a review, in Psychiatric Complications of Medical Drugs. Edited by Shader RI. New York, Raven Press, 1972

Goodwin FK, Post RM, Dunner DL, et al: Cerebrospinal fluid amine metabolites in affective illness: the probenecid technique. Am J Psychiatry 130:73-79, 1973

Hellhammer D: Learned helplessness—an animal model revisited, in The Origins of Depression: Current Concepts and Approaches. Edited by Angst J. Berlin, Dahlem Karprenzen, Springer-Verlag, 1983

Heninger GR, Charney DS, Sternberg DE: Serotonergic function in depression: prolactin response to intravenous tryptophan in depressed patients and healthy subjects. Arch Gen Psychiatry 41:398-402, 1984

Janowsky DS, El-Yousef MK, Davis JM, et al: A cholinergic-adrenergic hypothesis of mania and depression. Lancet 2:632-635, 1972

Janowsky DS, El-Yousef MK, Davis JM, et al: Parasympathetic suppression of manic symptoms of physostigmine. Arch Gen Psychiatry 28:542-547, 1973

Jimerson DC, Post RM, Carman JS, et al: CSF calcium: clinical correlates in affective illness and schizophrenia. Biol Psychiatry 14:37-51, 1979

Jimerson DC, Insel TR, Reus VI, et al: Increased plasma MHPG in dexamethasone-resistant depressed patients. Arch Gen Psychiatry 40:173-176, 1983

Kafka MS, Paul SM: Platelet alpha$_2$-adrenergic receptors in depression. Arch Gen Psychiatry 43:91-95, 1986

Katz RJ, Baldrighi G: A further parametric study of imipramine in an animal model of depression. Pharmacol Biochem Behav 16:969-972, 1982

Katzman R, Pappius HM: Brain Electrolyte and Fluid Metabolism. Baltimore, Williams & Wilkins, 1973

Kopin IJ, Gordon EK, Jimerson DC, et al: Relation between plasma and cerebrospinal fluid levels of 3–methoxy–4–hydroxyphenylglycol. Science 219:73-75, 1983

Koslow SH, Maas JW, Bowden CL, et al: Cerebrospinal fluid and urinary biogenic amines and metabolites in depression and mania: a controlled, univariate analysis. Arch Gen Psychiatry 40:999-1010, 1983

Kraemer GW, McKinney WT: Interactions of pharmacological agents which alter biogenic amine metabolism and depression: an analysis of contributing factors within a primate model of depression. J Affect Dis 1:33-54, 1979

Kukopoulos A, Reginalde D, Laddomada P, et al: Course of the manic depressive cycle and changes caused by treatments. Pharmakopsychiatry Neuropsychopharmakology 13:156-167, 1980

Lake CR, Mikkelsen EJ, Rapoport JL, et al: Effect of imipramine on norepinephrine and blood pressure in enuretic boys. Clin Pharmacol Ther 26:647-653, 1979

Lake CR, Pickar D, Ziegler MG, et al: High plasma norepinephrine levels in patients with major affective disorder. Am J Psychiatry 139:1315-1318, 1982

Lerner P, Major LF, Ziegler M, et al: Central noradrenergic adaptation to long-term treatment with imipramine in rhesus monkeys. Brain Res 200:220-224, 1980

Lewis DA, McChesney C: Tritiated imipramine binding to platelets in manic subjects. J Affect Dis 9:207-211, 1985

Linnoila M, Karoum F, Potter WZ: High correlation of norepinephrine and its major metabolite excretion rates. Arch Gen Psychiatry 39:521-523, 1982

Linnoila M, Karoum F, Potter WZ: Effects of antidepressant treatments on dopamine turnover in depressed patients. Arch Gen Psychiatry 40:1015-1017, 1983

Loosen PT, Prange AJ Jr: Serum thyrotropin response to thyrotropin-releasing hormone in psychiatric patients. Am J Psychiatry 139:405-416, 1982

Mann JJ, Brown RP, Halper JP, et al: Reduced sensitivity of lymphocyte beta-adrenergic receptors in patients with endogenous depression and psychomotor agitation. N Engl J Med 313:715-720, 1985

Mellerup ET, Rafaelsen OJ: Electrolyte metabolism and manic-melancholic disorder, in The Handbook of Biological Psychiatry. Edited by van Praag HM, Rafaelson O, Lader M, et al. New York, Marcel Dekker, Inc., 1981

Meltzer HY, Arora RC, Baber R: Serotonin uptake in blood platelets of psychiatric patients. Arch Gen Psychiatry 38:1322-1326, 1981

Murphy DL, Brodie HKH, Goodwin FK, et al: Regular induction of hypomania by L–dopa in "bipolar" manic-depressive patients. Nature 229:135-136, 1971

Muscettola G, Potter WZ, Pickar D, et al: Urinary MHPG and major affective disorders: a replication and new findings. Arch Gen Psychiatry 41:337-342, 1984

Naylor GJ, Smith AHW, Bryce-Smith D, et al: Tissue vanadium levels in manic-depressive psychosis. Psychol Med 14:767-772, 1984

Nurnberger J Jr, Jimerson DC, Allen JR, et al: Red cell ouabain-sensitive Na^+-K^+-adenosine triphosphatase: a state marker in affective disorder inversely related to plasma cortisol. Biol Psychiatry 17:981-992, 1982

Oppenheim G, Ebstein RP, Belmaker RH: The effect of lithium on the physostigmine-induced behavioral syndrome and plasma GMP. J Psychiatr Res 15:133-138, 1979

Oswald I, Brezinova V, Dunleavy DLF: On the slowness of action of tricyclic antidepressant drugs. Br J Psychiatry 120:673-677, 1972

Pandey GN, Dysken MW, Garver PL, et al: Beta-adrenergic receptor function in affective illness. Am J Psychiatry 136:675-678, 1979

Paul SM, Janowsky A, Skolnick P: Monoaminergic neurotransmitters and antidepressant drugs, in Psychiatry Update: The American Psychiatric Association Annual Review, vol. 4. Edited by Hales RE, Frances AJ. Washington, DC, American Psychiatric Press, Inc., 1985

Polinsky RJ, Kopin IJ, Ebert MH, et al: Pharmacologic distinction of different orthostatic hypotension syndromes. Neurology 31:1-7, 1981

Porsolt RD: Behavioural despair, in Antidepressants: Neurochemical, Behavioural, and Clinical Perspectives. Edited by Enna SJ, Malick JB, Richelson E. New York, Raven Press, 1981

Post RM, Lake CR, Jimerson DC, et al: Cerebrospinal fluid norepinephrine in affective illness. Am J Psychiatry 135:907-912, 1978

Post RM, Ballenger JC, Goodwin FK: Cerebrospinal fluid studies of neurotransmitter function in manic and depressive illness, in The Neurobiology of Cerebrospinal Fluid, vol. I. Edited by Wood JH. New York, Plenum Press, 1980

Potter WZ, Ross RJ, Zavadil AP III: Norepinephrine in the affective disorders: classic biochemical approaches, in The Catecholamines in Psychiatric and Neurologic Disorders. Edited by Lake CR, Ziegler MG. Stoneham, MA, Butterworth, Inc., 1985a

Potter WZ, Scheinin M, Golden RN, et al: Selective antidepressants and cerebrospinal fluid: lack of specificity on norepinephrine and serotonin metabolites. Arch Gen Psychiatry 42:1171-1177, 1985b.

Potter WZ, Rudorfer MV, Linnoila M: New clinical studies support a role of norepinephrine in antidepressant action, in Perspectives in Psychopharmacology. Edited by Barchas J, Bunney WE. New York, Alan R. Liss, in press

Raisman R, Briley MS, Bouchami F, et al: ^{3}H-imipramine binding and serotonin uptake in platelets from untreated depressed patients and control volunteers. Psychopharmacology 77:332-335, 1982

Ross RJ, Zavadil AP III, Calil HM, et al: Effects of desmethylimipramine on plasma norepinephrine, pulse, and blood pressure. Clin Pharmacol Ther 33:429-437, 1983

Roy A, Pickar D, Linnoila M, et al: Plasma norepinephrine level in affective disorders: relationship to melancholia. Arch Gen Psychiatry 42:1181-1185, 1985

Rubinow DR, Gold PW, Post RM, et al: CSF somatostatin in affective illness. Arch Gen Psychiatry 40:409-412, 1983

Rudorfer MV, Lesieur P, Ross RJ, et al: Norepinephrine in depression: up or down? Paper presented at the 136th Annual Meeting of the American Psychiatric Association, New York, 1983

Rudorfer MV, Golden RN, Potter WZ: Second generation antidepressants. Psychiatr Clin North Am 7:519-534, 1984

Rudorfer MV, Ross RJ, Linnoila M, et al: Exaggerated orthostatic responsivity of plasma norepinephrine in depression. Arch Gen Psychiatry 42:1186-1192, 1985

Schatzberg AF, Orsulak PJ, Rosenbaum AH, et al: Toward a biochemical classification of depressive disorders, V: heterogeneity of unipolar depressions. Am J Psychiatry 139:471-474, 1982

Schildkraut JJ: The catecholamine hypothesis of affective disorders: a review of supporting evidence. Am J Psychiatry 122:509-522, 1965

Schildkraut JJ, Orsulak PJ, LaBrie RA, et al: Toward a biochemical classification of depressive disorders, II: application of multivariate discriminant function analysis to data on urinary catecholamines and metabolites. Arch Gen Psychiatry 35:1436-1439, 1978

Siever LJ, Murphy DL, Slater S, et al: Plasma prolactin changes following fenfluramine in depressed patients compared to controls: an evaluation of central serotonergic responsivity in depression. Life Sci 34:1029-1039, 1984

Stone EA: Problems with current catecholamine hypotheses of antidepressant agents: speculations leading to a new hypothesis. Behav Brain Sci 6:535-547, 1983

Veith RC, Raskind MA, Barnes RF, et al: Tricyclic antidepressants and supine, standing, and exercise plasma norepinephrine levels. Clin Pharmacol Ther 33:763-769, 1983

Weiss JM, Glazer HI, Pohorecky LA: Coping behavior and neurochemical changes: an alternative explanation for the original "learned helplessness" experiments, in Relevance of the Psychopathological Animal Model to the Human. New York, Plenum, 1976

Weiss JM, Goodman PA, Losito BG, et al: Behavioural depression produced by an uncontrollable stressor: relationship to norepinephrine, dopamine, and serotonin levels in various regions of rat brain. Brain Research Review 3:167-205, 1981

Weston PG, Howard MQ: The determination of sodium, potassium, calcium, and magnesium in the blood and spinal fluid of patients suffering from manic-depressive insanity. Arch Neurol Psychiatry 8:179-183, 1922

Whitlock FA, Evans LEJ: Drugs and depression. Drugs 15:53-71, 1978

Wood PL, Suranyi-Cadotte BE, Nair NPV, et al: Lack of association between ^{3}H-imipramine binding sites and uptake of serotonin in control, depressed and schizophrenic patients. Neuropharmacology 22:1211-1214, 1983

Woodward DJ, Moises HC, Waterhouse BD, et al: Modulatory actions of norepinephrine in the central nervous system. Fed Proc 38:2109-2116, 1979

Wyatt RJ, Portnoy B, Kupfer DJ, et al: Resting plasma catecholamine concentrations in patients with depression and anxiety. Arch Gen Psychiatry 24:65-70, 1971

Chapter 3

Sleep and Biological Rhythms in Bipolar Illness

by Thomas A. Wehr, M.D., David A. Sack, M.D., Norman E. Rosenthal, M.D., and Frederick K. Goodwin, M.D.

Many psychiatrists who have treated affective patients and followed the course of their illness have become interested the role of biological rhythms in the illness. Partly this is because the illness itself is a kind of biological rhythm. Episodes of mania and depression remit and relapse spontaneously, and recur in a quasi-periodic manner. Also, the occurrence and severity of affective symptoms sometimes seem to be strongly influenced by normal biological rhythms. For example, the classical feature of diurnal variation in mood in endogenous depression suggests that some daily physiological rhythm aggravates or mitigates the depressive process. The association of exacerbations of affective symptoms with phases of the menstrual cycle and seasons of the year has been repeatedly observed by physicians treating individual patients and by epidemiologists surveying populations of patients. In recent years experimental evidence has accumulated that shows that rhythms in the body, especially the daily sleep–wake cycle, may be centrally involved in the processes responsible for depression and mania. This evidence reveals that manipulation of daily and seasonal rhythms by means of nonpharmacological interventions (such as alterations of sleep–wake and light–dark cycles), as well as by means of pharmacological interventions, can alter the course of the illness. As this statement implies, experimental investigations of the role of biological rhythms in affective illness have begun to yield benefits for the treatment of patients. This chapter reviews recent developments in this area and emphasizes those that may be of practical use to the psychiatrist treating patients with affective disorders.

THE SLEEP–WAKE CYCLE IN BIPOLAR ILLNESS

Physiological aspects of sleep in depression have been studied extensively in the last 20 years. Physiological changes during sleep have been measured and characterized on the basis of polygraphic recordings of electroencephalogram (EEG), eye movements, and muscle tone through the night. Normally, sleep is a rhythmic process, with stages of rapid eye movement (REM) sleep alternating with non-REM sleep approximately every 90 minutes during the sleep period. Typically, slow-wave sleep (2–4 cycles per second) is most prominent during non-REM periods in the first part of the night. REM sleep typically begins about 90 minutes after sleep onset and is most prominent in the later part of the sleep period, in the hours before waking. These patterns in the occurrence of sleep stages arise from an oscillatory mechanism that generates the REM–non-REM

The opinions expressed herein are those of the authors and do not reflect official policy of the NIMH cycle during sleep, and from other processes that occur during the waking state as well. The amount of slow wave sleep, for example, is partly a function of the duration of prior wakefulness; the timing and amount of REM sleep is partly controlled by a circadian pacemaker that generates a circadian rhythm in REM sleep propensity. The REM circadian rhythm reaches its maximum at about dawn and its minimum in the late evening hours. The increasing amounts of REM sleep in the later part of the sleep period reflect the circadian rhythm in REM sleep propensity.

Sleep EEG Abnormalities in Bipolar Illness

Several abnormalities of polygraphically monitored sleep have been consistently reported in major depression (reviewed in Gillin et al, 1984). These include: 1) short REM sleep latency (time from sleep onset to REM sleep onset); 2) reduced slow-wave sleep; 3) increased frequency of rapid eye movements during REM sleep (increased REM density); 4) a shift in the temporal distribution of REM sleep so that more occurs in the early part of the night (shorter REM latency and longer first REM periods); 5) reduction of sleep, with longer sleep latency (time from lights out to sleep onset), intermittent awakening, early awakening, and, therefore, decreased sleep efficiency. Most, if not all of these changes appear to be rather nonspecific, inasmuch as they can each be found in a number of other psychiatric illnesses and in nonpsychiatric illnesses (Gillin et al, 1983). Furthermore, it has not been clearly established that a specific combination of these abnormalities is characteristic of depression. Thus, as Gillin (1983) has observed, the situation with sleep EEG findings in depression is rather similar to that of the dexamethasone suppression test. The findings appear to reflect abnormal functioning in sleep related processes, but lack diagnostic specificity.

In the few instances where the results of sleep studies of depression have been analyzed separately for bipolar patients, abnormalities similar to those described for unipolar depression have generally been found. However, these abnormalities are not invariably present. In some studies REM sleep latencies (Linkowsky et al, 1985; Sack et al, submitted for publication) or the temporal distribution of REM sleep during the night (Duncan et al, 1979) have been reported to be normal. REM sleep has been reported to be more fragmented in depressed bipolar patients compared with unipolar patients and normal individuals (Duncan et al, 1979). Insomnia is almost invariably associated with mania, and often occurs in depression. In bipolar patients, depression is also frequently associated with normal or increased sleep (hypersomnia) (Detre et al, 1972; Duncan et al, 1979; Garvey et al, 1984; Rosenthal et al, 1984). Since most sleep laboratories impose external constraints on patients' sleep schedules (for example, patients are awakened at 7 A.M.), sleep duration in hypersomnic patients is almost certainly underestimated. In a depressed bipolar patient who was permitted to sleep *ad libitum*, daily sleep periods reached 12 hours and encompassed as many as nine REM–non-REM cycles (Wehr et al, 1985b).

There is relatively little information about polygraphically monitored sleep in mania. Some findings in mania resemble those in depression. Of course, sleep is often reduced in mania. Furthermore, REM sleep latency has been reported to be short during mania (Mendels and Hawkins, 1971; Post et al, 1976; Gillin et al, 1977).

Longitudinal studies of sleep in rapid cycling manic-depressive patients have shown changes in REM sleep latency, sleep duration, first REM period duration, and slow-wave sleep that parallel clinical changes that occur during the courses of the mood cycles (Post et al, 1976; Wehr, 1977). In general, changes in REM sleep variables and slow-wave sleep that are reported to be characteristic of depression are more accentuated during the depressive phases of the manic-depressive cycles in rapid cycling patients, and in some cases sleep EEG changes appear to anticipate the switch into depression (Post et al, 1976; Wehr, 1977). When such patients switch from the depressed to the manic phase, they frequently exhibit alternate nights of total insomnia (Wehr et al, 1982). Similar 48-hour sleep–wake cycles sometimes occur in normal individuals whose circadian rhythms are free-running in special experimental conditions, where all external time cues have been eliminated (Wehr et al, 1982). Thus, 48-hour sleep–wake cycles in manic patients may depend on a process that is involved in normal sleep regulating mechanisms, but which ordinarily is expressed only in unusual experimental conditions.

Biological Rhythm Models of Depressive Sleep Abnormalities

Basic research in biological rhythms has led to the development of models of the processes thought to be responsible for the daily sleep–wake cycle and the intrasleep 90-minute REM–non-REM cycle. These models, in turn, have led to hypotheses about the origins of sleep abnormalities in depression and mania. Hobson and McCarley (1975) have developed a "reciprocal interaction" model to describe the intrasleep REM–non-REM cycle. The model was based on interactions between noradrenergic and cholinergic centers in the brainstem that could be measured with neurophysiological techniques. Certain aspects of depressive sleep, such as short REM sleep latencies, could be simulated by hypothesizing that the level of activity of the noradrenergic component of the system is abnormally low at sleep onset, causing the oscillatior to begin its cycle in an unusual phase (McCarley, 1982). After the moment of sleep onset the model functions according to its usual constraints but generates REM sleep patterns reminiscent of those seen in depression. A novel prediction of the model is that the frequency distribution of REM sleep latencies in depressive patients should be bimodal, with a cluster of sleep-onset REM episodes and REM episodes with normal latencies of onset (Beersma et al, 1984). This bimodal pattern has in fact been described by some investigators (Schultz et al, 1979). Thus, according to this model, the problem of depressive sleep is essentially a sleep-onset problem; the REM–non-REM oscillator starts in an abnormal state but functions normally thereafter. As indicated, the model implicates decreased noradrenergic function in depressive sleep abnormalities, a venerable if controversial proposition. In a later refinement, the sleep-onset level of activity of the noradrenergic component of the REM–non-REM oscillator is modulated by a circadian rhythm (McCarley, 1986). Thus, hypotheses about the involvement of this intrasleep oscillator might be compatible with hypotheses about the role of circadian rhythms in manic-depressive sleep disturbances.

There is general agreement that at least two types of processes appear to be responsible for the behavior of the daily sleep–wake cycle. The propensity to sleep or awaken is partly related to a homeostatic process corresponding to the intuitive idea that a person becomes increasingly drowsy the longer he or she remains awake, and less drowsy the longer he or she sleeps. The propensity to sleep or wake is also related to a circadian process. A biological clock in the brain makes a person more sleepy at certain times of day than at others, regardless of the duration of prior wakefulness. The amount of slow-wave sleep during sleep is mainly a function of the duration of prior wakefulness, and has been identified with the homeostatic process. In one model of depressive sleep (Borbely and Wirz-Justice, 1982), decreased sleep duration and decreased slow-wave sleep are attributed to a deficiency in the rate of increase of the sleep-inducing, homeostatic process during wakefulness (process S). In another model of depressive sleep, decreased sleep, short REM latency, and the abnormally early temporal distribution of REM sleep within the sleep period are attributed to a phase advance or early timing of the circadian rhythm controlling sleep propensity and REM sleep propensity (Papousek, 1975; Wehr and Wirz-Justice, 1982). The two hypotheses are not mutually exclusive, and there is some empirical evidence in support of each.

HOMEOSTATIC MECHANISMS. The amount of slow-wave sleep, which is reduced in depression, is postulated to reflect the level of process S in the model; S increases during wakefulness and is rapidly discharged during sleep in an exponential manner. In quantitative analyses of sleep EEG data, the level of S is equated with power in the EEG spectrum (~2 to 20 cycles per second). Kupfer and colleagues (1984) found the predicted low levels of delta sleep measured with an automated analyzer, and Borbely and colleagues (1984) found correspondingly low levels of power density of the EEG in patients. However, two recent studies (see van den Hoofdakker and Deersma, 1985; Mendelson et al, 1986) in which EEG spectral analysis was performed yielded the somewhat surprising finding of no difference in EEG power density between depressives and normal subjects, even when conventional manual scoring of EEG records showed slow-wave sleep reductions in the depressives. The latter findings imply that the amount of slow-wave activity in depressive sleep EEG recordings may be normal, but that slow-waves are dispersed and/or attenuated in such a way as to escape detection by manual scoring criteria.

The process S deficiency hypothesis provides a conceptual framework for the antidepressant effects of sleep deprivation (discussed below). Since S rises during wakefulness and falls during sleep, sleep deprivation is hypothesized to compensate for depressives' abnormally low rate of accumulation of S during wakefulness by extending the duration of their wakefulness.

CIRCADIAN RHYTHM MECHANISMS. According to the circadian rhythm phase advance hypothesis of depression (Papousek, 1975; Wehr and Goodwin, 1981), sleep reduction and altered temporal distribution of REM sleep arise from an advance in the phase position or timing of a pacemaker controlling circadian rhythms in sleep propensity and REM sleep propensity. This pacemaker is also considered to control circadian rhythms in cortisol secretion, core body temperature, and many other variables. In depressives, the timing of these circadian rhythms is hypothesized to be shifted abnormally early relative to the sleep schedule. An analogous situation can be established in normal subjects by shifting the timing of their sleep schedule later relative to the timing of their circadian rhythms, a situation equivalent to jet lag after westward flight. In this type of experiment, certain features of depressive sleep can be reproduced in normal subjects, including reduced sleep with early awakening, short REM sleep latency, and early temporal distribution of REM sleep (Weitzman et al, 1968). Long sleep latency, decreased slow-wave sleep, and increased REM density are not reproduced. Some normal subjects who have been evaluated by blind ratings during such experiments have become moderately depressed (Knowles et al, 1986). The phase advance hypothesis has been investigated in two ways: 1) circadian rhythms in cortisol, core body temperature, and other variables have been examined for evidence of an abnormally early phase position; 2) shifting depressive sleep period several hours earlier than usual, a manipulation designed to correct the putative abnormal phase-relationship between their sleep schedule and their circadian rhythms, has been investigated for its possible antidepressant effects.

Wehr and Goodwin (1981) reviewed nearly 20 published studies of circadian rhythms in depressed patients. An analysis of the results of these studies showed that the phase position of depressives' circadian rhythms was abnormally advanced one or more hours in many cases. As is often the case in clinical research, however, one's confidence in these findings is limited by methodological problems in the various studies (Wehr and Goodwin, 1981). Recently, additional studies have been published. Investigations of the cortisol circadian rhythm in depression show either a phase-advance (Linkowsky et al, 1985; Sherman and Pfohl, 1984) or no phase abnormality (von Zerssen et al, 1985). Recent cross-sectional (one-day) investigations of the temperature circadian rhythm in depression generally have not supported the phase-advance hypothesis (von Zerssen et al, 1985; Avery et al, 1982; van den Hoofdakker and Deersma, 1985), while longitudinal studies indicate that the phase is unstable (sometimes advanced, sometimes normal) (Pflug et al, 1976; Wehr and Goodwin, 1983a). In one extensive longitudinal study of manic-depressive cycles, shifts in the timing of REM sleep were correlated with shifts in the timing of the circadian temperature rhythms, as predicted by the phase-advance hypothesis (Wehr and Goodwin, 1983a). It is difficult to measure variation due to the circadian pacemaker isolated from other influences, such as meals, sleep schedules, activity, and so on, that distort the expression of the rhythm. These distorting, or masking factors, reduce one's confidence in the validity of descriptions of circadian rhythms measured in the usual clinical setting. A recent approach to the problem of masking has been to study patients on a constant routine, where they remain awake, at bedrest, and eat isocaloric meals every hour for 30 hours or so. In the first clinical study of this type, the phase position of the cortisol circadian rhythm was advanced in depressed patients relative to age- and sex-matched controls (Sack et al, manuscript submitted for publication). The melatonin circadian rhythm in these patients was normal. More such studies are needed to resolve the still conflicting evidence bearing on the question of whether the phase position of depressives' circadian rhythms is phase-advanced. The phase-advance hypothesis is compatible with the finding that tricyclic and monoamine oxidase inhibitor (MAOI) antidepressants delay the phase-position of circadian rhythms in experimental animals (Wehr and Wirz-Justice, 1982; Tamarkin et al, 1983; Duncan et al, 1986), and therefore might be expected to correct the putative abnormal phase-advance of depressives' circadian rhythms. The hypothesis is also compatible with the finding that manic-depressives are supersensitive to hypothalamic effects of light (Lewy et al, 1985a), an alteration that could cause their circadian rhythms to be abnormally phase-advanced (Wehr and Wirz-Justice, 1982).

Effects of sleep schedule shifts appear to support the phase advance hypothesis in some cases (Wehr et al, 1979; Sack et al, 1985; Souetre et al, 1985) but not others (van den Hoofdakker, personal communication), but have been evaluated mainly in uncontrolled studies. These experiments are discussed below.

EXPERIMENTAL ALTERATIONS OF THE SLEEP–WAKE CYCLE IN BIPOLAR ILLNESS

Effects of Experimental Alterations of Sleep on Mood

As noted above, dramatic changes in the timing and duration of sleep occur during mania and depression, and there is considerable experimental evidence that the changes in sleep that accompany clinical state changes in bipolar patients are not epiphenomena but rather play an important role in the pathophysiological process that is responsible for the clinical changes. This evidence can be simply summarized: sleep deprivation is capable of causing switches from depression to mania, and sleep (recovery sleep after sleep deprivation) is capable of causing switches from mania to depression. It is well established that total sleep deprivation (Pflug and Tolle, 1971), or partial sleep deprivation in the second half of the night (Schilgen and Tolle, 1980), is capable of inducing temporary remissions in depressed unipolar and bipolar patients. The responses of over one thousand patients to sleep deprivation have been investigated (reviewed in Gillin, 1983). Between 60 and 70 percent of patients respond with improvement in depression. Patients usually relapse back into depression after recovery sleep. There is some experimental evidence that the timing of sleep may have effects on mood. Shifting the timing of sleep five or six hours earlier than usual sometimes induces switches out of depression in unipolar and bipolar patients (Wehr et al, 1979; Sack et al, 1985). Antidepressant effects of this phase-advance treatment suggest that being awake or asleep in the later part of the night is a critical factor in patients' responses to sleep manipulations. This hypothesis gains further support from studies that indicate that partial sleep deprivation in the first half of the night is less effective than partial sleep deprivation in the second half of the night in improving patients' depressive symptoms (Goetze and Tolle, 1981).

Sleep Deprivation: Implications for Management of Depression

The usefulness of sleep deprivation therapy in the clinical management of depression has been limited by the fact that most patients relapse after recovery sleep. There have been several attempts to overcome this problem. Sleep deprivation has been combined with antidepressant drug therapy in hopes that the rapid antidepressant effects of the former could be sustained by the latter. Evidence concerning the efficacy of this approach is preliminary and partly contradictory. Elsenga and van den Hoofdakker (1983) found that antidepressant effects of clomipramine could be accelerated by repeated sleep deprivation treatments during the initial phase of treatment. However, they were unable to replicate this finding in a later study. Recently Baxter (1985) has reported that antidepressant effects of sleep deprivation can be sustained by the administration of lithium beginning on the day after the sleep deprivation night. Sack and colleagues (1985) reported that responses to antidepressant drugs could be potentiated by phase-advance of the sleep–wake cycle in an uncontrolled study. Another approach has been to try to find a way to administer sleep interventions on a chronic basis (after all, the therapeutic effects of electroconvulsive treatment (ECT) might not look promising if the treatment were only administered once). Repeated partial sleep deprivations in the later half of the night and phase advance of the sleep–wake cycle are more readily tolerated by patients than repeated total sleep deprivations, and are the focus of ongoing clinical studies. Some patients appear to respond to this type of treatment (Sack et al, unpublished data).

Sleep Deprivation: Implications for Management of Mania

There have been several reports that sleep deprivation is capable of inducing switches into mania in bipolar patients, but this phenomenon has been systematically investigated in only one study. Wehr et al (1982) found that a majority of depressed rapid cycling manic-depressives switched into hypomania or mania following one night's total sleep deprivation. In some cases patients switched back into depression after recovery sleep. In others mania persisted for days or weeks. Phase advance of the sleep–wake cycle has also been reported to induce switches from depression to hypomania or mania in a few bipolar patients (Wehr et al, 1979; Wehr et al, 1982; Wehr and Goodwin, 1983a, 1983b).

Considering that experimental evidence shows that bipolar patients can be made to switch into mania when they are deprived of sleep, it follows that any factor that is capable of depriving patients of sleep may be capable of precipitating mania through this mechanism. In this way, sleep reduction may serve as final common pathway for diverse factors that have been thought to induce mania (Wehr et al, paper submitted for publication). Sleep reduction is likely to occur during disruptions of routine due to travel, shift work, social events, and medical and other types of emergencies. Emotional reactions to persons or events, such as anxiety, fear, anger, infatuation, or bereavement can cause insomnia. Drugs, such as amphetamines, caffeine, and monoamine oxidase inhibitors, and withdrawal from drugs such as antidepressants, neuroleptics, and sedatives can cause insomnia. Each of these factors, which have been reported to induce mania, could act through a common mechanism involving sleep reduction.

Mania, itself, causes insomnia. Thus, the relationship between sleep loss and mania is bidirectional and self-reinforcing. Once set in motion by other factors, mania and sleep reduction could participate in a vicious cycle that might escalate out of control (as appears to happen in the clinical setting).

The sleep-reduction hypothesis of the switch into mania has obvious implications for treatment and prevention of mania. Patients at risk for mania could be counselled to avoid situations that are likely to cause disruptions in sleep routine. Psychological management of emotional crises that might be capable of disturbing sleep could be provided. Use of drugs known to interfere with sleep could be avoided. Care could be taken to avoid insomnia related to too rapid withdrawal of drugs, such as antidepressants. Sedatives might be used to control insomnia.

The Mechanism of Sleep Deprivation Therapy

One of the shortcomings of currently available antidepressant drugs is their slow onset of action. In contrast, patients can experience complete remissions in depressive symptoms within hours after beginning sleep deprivation. These rapid responses strongly suggest that the two- to four-week latency of antidepressant responses to drugs results from a peculiarity of the mechanism of action of the drugs rather than any inherent inertia of the depressive syndrome itself. Discovery of the mechanism of action of sleep deprivation could be expected to lead to the development of new, rapidly acting antidepressant drugs. Our understanding of the mechanism of action may depend on the development of a more specific intervention than total sleep deprivation, which, after all, involves many interventions (exposure to light, changes in posture, increased activity, social stimulation, and so on). Some progress has been made in this direction. Partial sleep deprivation in the later half of the night appears to be as effective as total sleep deprivation, and superior to partial sleep deprivation in the first half of the night (Schilgen and Tolle, 1980; Goetze and Tolle, 1981). Exposure to light at night is not a necessary condition for the response (Wehr et al, 1985a). Selective REM sleep deprivation, in one study, has been shown to have antidepressant effects (Vogel et al, 1980). Thus, sleep deprivation may act more specifically through REM sleep deprivation. In support of this hypothesis is the observation that partial sleep deprivation in the later half of the night (the effective treatment) reduces REM sleep, while partial sleep deprivation in the first half of the night (the less effective treatment) does not (Sack et al, paper submitted for publication). Also, in a recent study, patients who responded to total sleep deprivation and who were allowed to nap during the following day relapsed only if those naps contained REM sleep (Wiegand et al, 1985). Thus, processes that occur during REM sleep, that are interrupted by REM sleep deprivation, are good candidates for mechanisms of action of the sleep intervention treatments.

Sleep and sleep deprivation are known to have powerful effects on certain neuroendocrine systems. For example, sleep deprivation disinhibits cortisol (Weitzman et al, 1982) and thyrotropin stimulating hormone (TSH) secretion (Parker et al, 1976) and inhibits prolactin (Parker et al, 1974) and growth hormone secretion (Takahashi et al, 1968). TSH secretion normally increases at night (Parker et al, 1974), but is inhibited by sleep; sleep deprivation has a permissive effect on nocturnal TSH secretion. The nocturnal rise of TSH secretion and its responses to sleep deprivation is blunted in rapid cycling bipolar patients (Sack et al, manuscript submitted for publication); nevertheless, sleep deprivation restores nocturnal TSH secretion to levels observed during sleep in normal subjects (of course, sleep deprivation also restores their mood to normal or above-normal). Thus, effects of sleep deprivation on TSH may be involved in the mechanism of action of sleep intervention therapies. This, and other possibilities, can be investigated with pharmacological probes of these systems that might mimic or block the effects of sleep deprivation.

RAPID CYCLING AFFECTIVE DISORDER

Rapid cycling affective disorder is a form of bipolar illness that usually follows a circular course with alternating episodes of mania and depression. Furthermore, as the name implies, the frequency of recurrences is high, four or more per year, according to a traditional definition (Dunner and Fieve, 1974). Two processes seem to be involved in the rapid cycling: a cycling process, corresponding to the overall cycle of mania and depression and having a period of days, weeks or months; and a switch process, corresponding to the rapid transitions between mania and depression and spanning minutes or hours. Usually the switch from depression to mania is associated with marked changes in physiological and behavioral variables and is a more dramatic event than the switch from mania to depression (Bunney et al, 1972; Wehr, 1977).

Patients with rapid cycling affective disorder have played an important role in the history of psychiatry. Through longitudinal observations of such patients, the 19th-century French psychiatrists, Baillarger (1854) and Falret (1890), were able to determine that mania and depression were not separate illnesses, but were actually different manifestations of the same illness. In some such patients, the prophylactic efficacy of lithium carbonate was first demonstrated by Baastrup and Schou (1967). These observations were made possible by the frequent and somewhat predictable patterns of recurrence in such patients.

Rapid cycling patients appear to be uncommon; furthermore, they seem to respond poorly to the conventional treatments for bipolar illness (Dunner and Fieve, 1974; Wehr et al, submitted for publication). Thus, although they are infrequently encountered in clinical practice, they present special problems in management for the treating psychiatrist. In recent years, much new information has become available about risk factors associated with this disorder and approaches to its treatment.

In many respects the clinical picture in rapid cycling affective disorder is similar to that in other forms of bipolar illness. First of all, most if not all rapid cycling patients have a bipolar form of affective disorder (Kukopulos et al, 1983). Furthermore, the cross-sectional phenomenonology of mania and depression and the age of onset of illness are indistinguishable in rapid and nonrapid cycling bipolar patients (Dunner and Fieve, 1974). In addition, there is a high incidence of nonrapid cycling forms of unipolar and bipolar affective illness, and a low incidence of rapid cycling forms in first degree relatives of rapid cycling patients (Dunner and Fieve, 1974), suggesting that the two types of bipolar illness are genetically related. Although rapid cycling affective disorder appears to be phenotypically and genetically related to more common forms of bipolar illness, it is distinguished by 1) a predominance of women patients, 2) a high incidence of thyroid disease, and 3) poor response to standard treatments.

The Female Reproductive System and Rapid Cycling

Rapid cycling affective disorder appears to be much more common in women than in men (Dunner et al, 1977; Kukopulos et al, 1980; Hatotani et al, 1983; Alarcon 1985). An exception is the more rare form with 48-hour mood cycles, which is more common in men, begins at an older age, and often follows a unipolar course (Alarcon, 1985). Rapid manic-depressive cycles in women do not appear to be generated by menstrual cycle. This conclusion is supported by observations that rapid cycling may begin or persist after menopause in many cases and can persist during pregnancy. Furthermore, extensive longitudinal observations have shown that the two types of cycles are not precisely synchronized, but gradually go in and out of phase with one another, even in cases where they initially appeared to be synchronized. The rapid cycling process, however, may be influenced by events connected with the female reproductive system. Reports of individual cases suggest that the onset of rapid cycling and the rate of rapid cycling may be affected by hormones of the female reproductive system (Wehr et al, manuscript submitted for publication). There are some indications that rapid cycling can be induced by administration of estrogen

(Oppenheim, 1984) and suppressed by administration of progesterone (Hatotani et al, 1983).

Thyroid Dysfunction and Rapid Cycling

Thyroid disease occurs in association with rapid cycling affective disorder in 30 to 40 percent of cases, usually in the form of hypothyroidism after treatment with lithium. This association was first noted by Cho and colleagues (1979), who found that most cases of hypothyroidism in a lithium clinic had occurred in rapid cycling patients. Cowdry and colleagues (1983) reported similar findings, and found that more than 90 percent of rapid cycling patients on lithium had TSH levels that were higher than those of nonrapid cycling patients on lithium. In an investigation of 50 rapid cycling patients, Wehr and colleagues found the incidence of thyroid dysfunction requiring treatment to be over 40 percent.

What is the nature of the relationship between rapid cycling affective disorder and thyroid dysfunction? Two lines of evidence suggest that thyroid dysfunction may play a role in the pathophysiology of rapid cycling. In experimental animals, lesions of the thyroid are capable of inducing long-term cycles in which activation and inhibition of behavior alternate (Richter, 1965). Motor activity recordings from such animals resemble those obtained from rapid cycling manic-depressives. Hypermetabolic doses of thyroxine appear to be capable of interrupting rapid cycling in manic-depressives, according to reports by Gjessing (1976) and Stancer and Persad (1982); however, the beneficial effect of the treatment may be temporary (Sack et al, manuscript submitted for publication).

Diagnosis and treatment of thyroid disease in rapid cycling patients almost always occur some time after the onset of rapid cycling. Therefore, if rapid cycling is partly caused by thyroid dysfunction, it must involve a subclinical form of thyroid disease, as proposed by Extein and colleagues (1982), or a factor predisposing to thyroid disease. Sack and colleagues have reported that rapid cycling patients exhibit abnormal patterns of TSH secretion that are only detectable at night, not in the morning when such patients usually are tested. The normal nocturnal rise in TSH is absent in rapid cycling patients, and their secretion of TSH responds very weakly to sleep deprivation. This and other sensitive challenge tests may prove to be useful in the detection of subclinical forms of thyroid dysfunction in such patients.

Induction of Rapid Cycling by Antidepressants

Reversible rapid cycling can be induced by antidepressant drugs, especially tricyclics (Wehr and Goodwin, 1977, 1979; Siris et al, 1979; Lerer et al, 1980; Mattson and Seltzer, 1981; Oppenheim, 1984; Tondo et al, 1981; Ko et al, 1981). In certain cases it has been shown clearly that rapid cycling occurs during periods of drugs administration, and ceases when the drugs are withdrawn (Wehr and Goodwin, 1979). Rapid cycling in such cases does not require that the drugs be administered in a periodic or cyclical fashion. Drug induced rapid cycling can occur when the drug is administered at a fixed dose. Many patients begin rapid cycling while they are being treated with antidepressants (Tondo et al, 1981). In many cases the rapid cycling persists when antidepressants are withdrawn. In these cases antidepressants may have induced rapid cycling that subsequently became autonomous. This possibility needs to be considered because of the known capability of such drugs to induce reversible rapid cycling in other patients; however, it is difficult to prove and should be considered speculative.

The mechanism of antidepressant-induced rapid cycling may be fundamentally related to the mechanism of the usual antidepressant effect of these drugs. This idea is supported by the observation that depressive phases of drug induced rapid manic-depressive cycles are similar in duration to the intervals during which patients remain depressed after they begin treatment with these drugs (the latency of response). It is as though rapid cycling patients repeatedly go through the two- to four-week process that is required for the more conventional antidepressant response to these drugs. The possibility that antidepressants interact with an impaired thyroid axis to produce rapid cycling has implications for their mechanism of action in depression and could be explored in animal models involving thyroid lesions (Richter, 1965).

Treatment of Rapid Cycling Affective Disorder

In Baastrup and Schou's classical lithium studies (1967) it was apparent that some rapid cycling patients responded well to this drug. In a recent review of the treatment of over 50 such patients, Wehr and colleagues found rapid cycling ultimately ceased in 36 percent. Successful outcomes, defined as cessation of rapid cycling with rare or no affective recurrences, was associated most often with discontinuation of tricyclic antidepressants and treatment with lithium carbonate and/or low doses of monoamine oxidase inhibitors. In patients who continued to cycle during treatment, lithium and/or carbamazepine appears to attenuate the severity and shorten the duration of manic phases of the cycles, as reviewed by Post and colleagues in Chapter 6 of this volume. In evaluating published reports of treatments of such patients, it is important to remember that antidepressants may induce rapid cycling and that rapid cycling may cease when they are withdrawn. When a new treatment follows a period of tricyclic administration, it is never clear whether rapid cycling stopped because of the new treatment or because tricyclics were discontinued. Some data indicate that lithium is not capable of suppressing rapid cycles induced by concurrently administered tricyclics, but is quite effective when administered alone (Wehr and Goodwin, 1979). Thus, patients should not be considered to be lithium nonresponsive until they have been treated with lithium alone.

The foregoing observations have some clear implications for the treatment of rapid cycling affective disorder. Some patients may improve when tricyclic and other adjunctive medications are discontinued. In these cases treatment with lithium alone may be effective (sometimes it may be necessary for the patient to endure one or two manic or depressive episodes without adding adjunctive medications). Low doses of monoamine oxidase inhibitors alone or in combination with lithium may be necessary in cases where cycling stops when tricyclics are discontinued, but the patient becomes mired in depression. Because of the evidence linking hypothyroidism to rapid cycling and the evidence that hypermetabolic doses of thyroxine are capable of suppressing rapid cycling, physicians should be prepared to recognize and treat hypothyroidism in these patients, even in its earliest stage. Approaches to the treatment of rapid cycling and other treatment resistant patients are discussed in detail by Dr. Post and colleagues in Chapter 6.

SEASONALITY OF BIPOLAR ILLNESS

Seasonal aspects of affective disorder have been a part of clinical lore since ancient times. Seasonality of bipolar illness can be viewed from two perspectives: seasonal trends in the epidemiology of populations of patients and seasonal patterns in the course of illness in individual cases. Somewhat different pictures emerge from these two perspectives.

Seasonal Trends in the Epidemiology of Mania and Depression

Patients may become manic or depressed at any time of year, but the incidence of these types of episodes shows some seasonal variation (reviewed in Rosenthal et al, 1983). The most consistent finding is that attacks of mania are more frequent in the summer than at other times of year. In studies of the seasonal incidence of depression, results for bipolar patients usually are not reported separately from those for unipolar patients. These statistics indicate that the incidence of depression (or hospitalizations for depression, ECT treatments, or suicides) is relatively more common in the late spring. The pattern is similar, that is, related to season, not month, south of the equator. In the few studies that have examined bipolar depression separately no consistent pattern emerges.

In a review of the world's literature regarding the seasonal incidence of suicide, Aschoff (1981) made a number of interesting observations concerning environmental factors that might play a role in the increased risk of suicide at certain times of year. He found that the amplitude of seasonal variation was greatest in the least industrialized nations, and had declined as nations became more industrialized during the past 100 years. Thus, some aspect of industrialization (for example, artificial light, central heating, and so forth) may insulate patients from an environmental factor that augments or attenuates their risk for affective episodes. Aschoff also found a relationship between seasonality of suicide and latitude. Seasonal variation was greatest, not in the north, but in the temperate latitudes. Of various environmental variables, this pattern correlated best with seasonal variation in hours of clear sunshine (not day length per se). This observation, which implicates brightness and duration of light (rather than its timing) in the seasonal occurrence of depression, is similar to conclusions about the properties of phototherapy in seasonal affective disorder.

Seasonal Recurrences in Individual Cases: Seasonal Affective Disorder (SAD)

In the 19th century psychiatrists had the opportunity to observe the course of untreated bipolar affective disorder for long periods. Several of the leading psychiatrists of this era, including Esquirol (Baillarger, 1854), Griesinger (1882), Falret (1890), Baillarger (1854) and Kraepelin (1921), recorded cases in which the pattern of recurrences was seasonal, with fall–winter depression and spring–summer mania or hypomania. This pattern can also be observed in longitudinal data published by Baastrup and Schou, in their now classical lithium studies (1967) and, more recently, by Kukopulos and Reginaldi (1973). In recent years the syndrome of seasonal affective disorder (SAD) has been systematically investigated by Rosenthal and colleagues (1984), Lewy et al (1982), and Wirz-Justice et al (1985). Nearly 200 cases have been investigated. Patients are mostly women with bipolar II illness (hypomania and depression). As with other forms of bipolar illness, onset most often occurs in the second and third decades of life, and a number of cases in children have been reported. Depressions usually begin in November and are characterized by hypersomnia, anergia, carbohydrate craving and weight gain, symptoms that are considered "atypical" in depression but which commonly occur in bipolar patients. Other symptoms include the usual features of depressed mood, hopelessness, suicidal thoughts, decreased libido, and social withdrawal; the syndrome is generally associated with considerable functional impairment. In evaluating published studies of SAD it is important to keep in mind that the Hamilton Rating Scale for Depression underestimates the severity of this type of depression, since increased sleep and weight, and improvement in these symptoms after treatment, are scored negatively. Depressions usually end in March, and may be followed by hypomania, mania, or normal mood in the spring and summer. The seasonal pattern for mania is consistent with that observed in population studies discussed previously. Nonseasonal unipolar or bipolar affective disorder is found among first degree relatives in most cases, indicating that SAD is likely to be genetically related to the commoner forms of affective illness. The clinical features of the syndrome have proven to be quite consistent among the different populations studied at different centers.

Biological correlates of SAD have only recently been investigated. Sleep EEG recordings confirmed patients' reports of increased sleep in winter compared with summer (Rosenthal et al, 1984). In comparison with normal persons, SAD patients showed reductions in slow-wave sleep in winter, but none of the other features usually found in depression, such as reduced REM sleep latency or increased REM density. Dexamethasone suppression and TRH tests are normal in depressed SAD patients (Rosenthal et al, 1984; James et al, in press).

Melatonin and prolactin, hormones known to play important roles in animal seasonal rhythms, have been measured in SAD patients. Preliminary studies indicate that levels of both hormones are abnormally high at certain times of day but these potentially important findings need to be replicated.

Phototherapy of SAD

It is well established that many types of seasonal changes in animal behavior and physiology are triggered by seasonal changes in the timing and/or duration of daylight (Gwinner, 1981; Hoffman, 1981). Furthermore, artificial light can be used to control seasonal behaviors in animals, and this effect of light has been exploited in food production industries by bringing plants into bloom and animals into breeding out of season. Because of the central importance of light in the regulation of seasonal rhythms in biology, it was reasonable to consider whether changes in natural light might trigger clinical changes in SAD and whether artificial light might be used to treat winter depression in affected patients.

Numerous clinical trials at several centers, involving more than 100 patients, have established that phototherapy is an effective treatment for winter depression in SAD (Rosenthal et al, 1984; Rosenthal et al, 1985a; Lewy et al, 1986; Wirz-Justice et al, 1985; Terman et al, 1986). Approximately 80 percent of patients respond to the treatment with significant improvement. Based on the results of these studies, several generalizations can be made about the properties of effective phototherapy. To be effective, phototherapy requires light that is several times brighter than that which is ordinarily encountered in most indoor environments. In most studies, patients have been exposed to light emitted through a diffusing screen from eight four-foot fluorescent bulbs at a distance of three feet (2,500–3,000 lux). Originally, on the basis of animal models, it was hypothesized that light would be effective only if it were administered in such a way as to extend the apparent duration of the short winter day. The weight of experimental evidence, however, indicates that the time of day of light treatments is not critical. For example, light administered in the middle of the day appears to be more or less as effective as light administered at the extremes of the day (Wehr et al, in press). There are some indications that phototherapy in the morning is *relatively* more effective than phototherapy administered in the evening, however (Lewy et al, 1986; Terman et al, 1986). There is increasing evidence of a dose-response relationship in phototherapy (Terman et al, 1986). Effective treatment seems to require at least two hours of exposure per day, and four hours of treatment are more effective than two. Finally, the therapeutic effects of phototherapy appear to be mediated by the eyes and not the skin (Wehr et al, manuscript submitted for publication). There is no evidence to date concerning the wavelength of light that is effective.

The course of the response to phototherapy is relatively rapid (Rosenthal et al, 1985b). Patients sometimes experience slight improvement after one or two treatments and attain maximal benefit after four to seven days. Relapses after withdrawal of light are similarly rapid. The rapidity of patients' responses to the vicissitudes of their exposure to light has practical implications for their management. Patients sometimes notice a deterioration in mood after a series of overcast days, even in summertime. Furthermore, patients in whom maintenance phototherapy seems to lose its effectiveness often are found to have neglected their treatment schedules. In uncontrolled studies, phototherapy appears to have prophylactic efficacy against winter depression in SAD (Rosenthal et al, manuscript submitted for publication).

The mechanism of phototherapy is unknown. Two principal hypotheses have been advanced, but neither has received consistent support from the experimental evidence. Based on animal models, Rosenthal and colleagues (in press) hypothesized that the mechanism of action of phototherapy involved suppression of nocturnal pineal melatonin secretion by light. The following observations, however, go against this hypothesis: 1) administration of melatonin to remitted patients during light treatments reproduces some of the atypical symptoms of depression, such as fatigue, hypersomnia and hyperphagia, but fails to induce relapses with typical symptoms as reflected in the Hamilton Rating Scale for Depression; 2) administration of atenolol, a beta adrenergic antagonist that suppresses melatonin secretion, is relatively ineffective in the treatment of SAD (Rosenthal et al, in press); and 3) light administered in the middle of the day, which has little effect on the already low daytime levels of melatonin, is an effective treatment for SAD (Wehr et al, in press). Lewy and colleagues (1986) proposed that the mechanism of action of phototherapy involves its capacity, when administered in the morning, to advance the timing or phase of abnormally delayed circadian rhythms, and they have provided some supporting experimental evidence. Results of other investigators who found positive effects of light in the middle of the day or in the evening (Wehr et al, in press; Terman et al, 1986), however, are inconsistent with this hypothesis. Further progress toward identification of a mechanism of action of phototherapy may require additional basic research on the biological effects of light.

A major problem in the evaluation of the clinical trials of phototherapy is the difficulty of establishing blind treatment conditions. It is difficult to imagine how patients can be kept blind to a treatment that they literally must see in order for it to be effective. In this situation, one can never be certain that patients' responses are not engendered by their expectations of the procedure, especially in an environment where there has been so much publicity about the procedure. Of course, this problem is not unique to phototherapy; many patients involved in clinical trials of antidepressants are able to determine when they are receiving capsules containing active drugs because of their obvious side effects. There are several reasons to believe that patients' responses to phototherapy are not related to nonspecific aspects of the intervention (placebo responses). Patients fail to respond to sham treatments involving yellow light of ordinary intensity, even though they were told that we were interested in the effects of color on mood (Rosenthal et al, 1984). There is usually a latency of response and relapse relative to initiation and termination of treatment. Furthermore, patients do not appear to develop tolerance to the procedure, as often occurs with placebo. Finally, in a recent study, patients' expectations of benefit from phototherapy administered via the eyes and phototherapy administered via the skin were similar, but they responded only to the eye condition (Wehr et al, manuscript submitted for publication).

The responses of SAD patients to drugs have not been systematically investigated.

Relationship Between Phototherapy and Sleep Deprivation

In their rapid onset and rapid termination of action, sleep deprivation therapy and phototherapy are rather similar to one another, and, as has been previously mentioned, are rather different from antidepressant drugs. In some experiments the effects of sleep deprivation and phototherapy have been confounded. When patients are awakened for early morning light treatments, they are incidentally partially sleep deprived. When patients undergo sleep deprivation therapy they are incidentally exposed to light at times when they would ordinarily be asleep in the dark. Furthermore, some patients with SAD have been shown to respond to sleep deprivation (Wehr et al, 1985a).

In spite of their similarities, and their having been confounded in some experiments, a series of controlled experiments indicates that the two types of treatment are fundamentally separate and can operate independently. Patients respond to phototherapy without sleep deprivation (Rosenthal et al 1985a), and they respond to sleep deprivation without exposure to light (Wehr et al, 1985a).

SUMMARY

Investigation of the rhythmic behavior of bipolar illness, and of its modulation by daily and seasonal biological rhythms, has led to new hypotheses about the pathogenesis of mania and depression and to new kinds of treatments for those conditions. Experimental evidence indicates that changes in the sleep–wake cycle that occur spontaneously in the course of the illness are not epiphenomena, but probably play an important role in the processes responsible for switches into mania and depression. This experimental evidence also indicates that in some cases mania can be prevented and depression treated by appropriate manipulations of the sleep–wake cycle. Furthermore, viewing bipolar illness as a type of biological rhythm has led to the discovery that in some cases antidepressants are capable of drastically accelerating the frequency of that rhythm, leading to a continuous, circular, rapid cycling course of illness. Recognition of this frequency modulating effect of the drugs can lead to better management of patients who appear to be resistant to treatment. Antidepressants have also been shown to markedly slow the oscillations of the biological clock that drives daily rhythms, such as the sleep–wake cycle; this discovery may lead to better understanding of the mechanism of action and of the side effects of these drugs in patients treated for depression. Finally, application of basic research in seasonal biological rhythms to clinical investigations of a seasonal form of recurrent bipolar illness has led to an entirely new type of treatment for depression: phototherapy. These tangible results indicate that ongoing research on biological rhythms and bipolar illness is likely to produce new insights into the causes of bipolar illness, and fundamentally new approaches to its treatment.

REFERENCES

Alarcon RD: Rapid cycling affective disorders: a clinical review. Compr Psychiatry 26:522-540, 1985

Aschoff J: Annual rhythms in man, in Handbook of Behavioral Neurobiology. Edited by Aschoff J. New York, Plenum Press, 1981

Avery D, Wildschiodtz G, Rafaelsen O: REM latency and temperature in affective disorders before and after treatment. Biol Psychiatry 17:463-470, 1982

Baastrup PC, Schou M: Lithium as a prophylactic agent: its effect against recurrent depression and manic-depressive psychosis. Arch Gen Psychiatry 16:162-172, 1967

Baillarger: Note sur un genre de folie dont les acces sont caracterises par deux periodes regulieres, l'une de depression et l'autre d'excitation. Gazette Hebdomadaire de Medecine et de Chirurgie 132:263-265, 1854

Baxter LR: Can lithium carbonate prolong antidepressant effect of sleep deprivation? Arch Gen Psychiatry 42:635, 1985

Beersma DGM, Daan S, Van den Hoofdakker RH: Distribution of REM latencies and other sleep phenomena in depression as explained by a single ultradian rhythm disturbance. Sleep 7:126-136, 1984

Borbely AA, Wirz-Justice A: Sleep, sleep deprivation and depression—a hypothesis derived from a model of sleep regulation. Hum Neurobiol 1:205-210, 1982

Borbely AA, Tobler I, Loepfe M, et al: All-night spectral analysis of the sleep EEG in untreated depressives and normal controls. Psychiatry Res 12:27-33, 1984

Bunney WE Jr, Goodwin FK, Murphy DL, et al.: The "switch process" in manic-depressive illness, II: relationship to catecholamines, REM sleep and drugs. Arch Gen Psychiatry 27:304-309, 1972

Cho JT, Bone S, Dunner DL, et al: The effect of lithium treatment on thyroid function in patients with primary affective disorder. Am J Psychiatry 136:115-116, 1979

Cowdry R, Wehr TA, Zis AP, et al.: Thyroid abnormalities associated with rapid cycling bipolar illness. Arch Gen Psychiatry 40:414-420, 1983

Detre T, Himmelhoch J, Swartzburg M, et al.: Hypersomnia and manic-depressive disease. Am J Psychiatry 128:1303-1305, 1972

Duncan WC, Pettigrew MA, Gillin JC: REM architecture changes in bipolar and unipolar depression. Am J Psychiatry 136:1424-1427, 1979

Ducan WC, Tamarkin L, Wehr TA: Clorgyline increases the circadian period and the activity-rest ratio in Syrian hamsters. Abstracts of the Second Montreux Conference on Chronopharmacology, Montreux, Switzerland, March 10–13, 1986

Dunner DL, Fieve RR: Clinical factors in lithium prophylaxis failure. Arch Gen Psychiatry 30:229-233, 1974

Dunner DL, Patrick V, Fieve RR: Rapid cycling manic depressive patients. Compr Psychiatry 18:561-566, 1977

Elsenga S, van den Hoofdakker RH: Clinical effects of sleep deprivation and clomipramine in endogenous depression. J Psychiatr Res 17:361-374, 1983

Extein I, Pottash ALC, Gold MS: Does subclinical hypothyroidism predispose to tricyclic-induced rapid mood cycles? J Clin Psychiatry 43:290-291, 1982

Falret J: La folie circulaire ou folie a formes alternes, in Etudes Cliniques sur les Maladies Mentales et Nerveuses. Paris, Librairie J B Bailliere et Fils, 1890

Garvey MJ, Mungas D, Tollefson GD: Hypersomnia in major depressive disorders. J Affect Dis 6:283-286, 1984

Gillin JC: The sleep therapies of depression. Prog Neuropsychopharm and Biol Psych 7:351-364, 1983

Gillin JC, Mazure C, Post RM, et al: An EEG sleep study of a bipolar (manic-depressive) patient with a nocturnal switch process. Biol Psychiatry 12:711-718, 1977

Gillin JC, Sitaram N, Wehr TA, et al: Sleep and affective illness, in Neurobiology of Mood Disorders. Edited by Post RM, Ballenger JC. Baltimore, Williams & Wilkins, 1984

Gjessing RR: Thyroid and adrenal function, in Contributions to the Somatology of Periodic Catatonia. Edited by Gjessing L, Jenner FA. Oxford, Pergamon, 1976

Goetze U, Tolle R: Antidepressive wirkung des partiellen schlafentzuges wahrend der 1. halfte der nacht. Psychiatr Clin (Basel) 14:129-149, 1981

Griesinger W: Mental Pathology and Therapeutics, 2nd edition. New York, William Wood and Co, 1885

Gwinner E: Annual rhythms: perspective, in Handbook of Behavioral Neurobiology. Edited by Aschoff J. Plenum Press, New York 1981

Hatotani N, Kitayama I, Inoue K, et al: Psychoneuroendocrine studies of recurrent psychoses, in Neurobiology of Periodic Psychoses. Edited by Hatotani N, Nomura J. Tokyo, Igaku-shoin, 1983

Hellekson CJ, Rosenthal NE: Phototherapy of winter depression in Alaska. Philadelphia, Abstracts of the Fourth World Congress of Biological Psychiatry, 1983

Hobson JA, McCarley RW, Wyzinski PW: Sleep cycle oscillation reciprocal discharge by two brainstem neuronal groups. Science 189:55-58, 1975

Hoffman K: Photoperiodism in vertebrates, in Handbook of Behavioral Neurobiology. Edited by Aschoff J. Plenum Press, New York, 1981

James SP, Parry BL, Carpenter CJ, et al: Evening light treatment of seasonal affective disorder. Br J Psychiatry 147:424-428, 1985

James SP, Wehr TA, Sack DA, et al: The dexamethasone suppression test in seasonal affective disorder. Compr Psychiatry (in press)

Knowles JB, MacLean AW: A critical evaluation of two models of depression, in Biological Psychiatry, 1985, vol. 6. Edited by Shagass C, Josiassen RC, Wagner HB. New York, Elsevier, 1986

Ko GN, Leckman JF, Heninger GR: Induction of rapid mood cycling during L–dopa treatment in a bipolar patient. Am J Psychiatry 138:1624-1675, 1981

Kraepelin E: Manic-depressive Illness and Paranoia. Edited by Robertson GM, Livingstone E, Livingstone S. Translated by Barclay RM. Edinburgh, E & S Livingstone, 1921

Kukopulos A, Reginaldi D: Does lithium prevent depressions by suppressing manias? International Journal of Pharmacopsychiatry 8:152-158, 1973

Kukopulos A, Reginaldi D, Laddomada P, et al: Course of the manic-depressive cycle and changes caused by treatments. Pharmakapsychiatrie-Neuro-Psychopharmakologie 13:156-167, 1980

Kukopulos A, Caliari B, Tondo A, et al: Rapid cyclers, temperament, and antidepressants. Compr Psychiatry 24:249-258, 1983

Kupfer DJ, Ulrich RF, Coble PA, et al: Application of automated REM and slow wave sleep analysis, II: testing the assumptions of the two-process model of sleep regulation in normal and depressed subjects. Psychiatry Res 13:335-343, 1984

Lerer B, Birmacher B, Ebstein RP, et al: Forty-eight-hour depressive cycling induced by antidepressant. Br J Psychiatry 137:183-185, 1980

Lewy AJ, Kern HA, Rosenthal NE, et al: Bright artificial light treatment of a manic-depressive patient with a seasonal mood cycle. Am J Psychiatry 139:1496-1498, 1982

Lewy AJ, Nurnberger JI, Wehr TA, et al: Supersensitivity to light may be a trait marker for manic-depressive illness. Am J Psychiatry 142:725-727, 1985a

Lewy AJ, Sack RL, Miller LS, et al: Treatment of winter depression with light, in Biological Psychiatry 1985, vol. 6. Edited by Shagass C, Josiassen RC, Wagner HB. New York, Elsevier, 1986

Linkowsky P, Mendlewicz J, LeClercq R, et al: The 24-hour profile of adrenocorticotropin and cortisol in major depressive illness. J Clin Endocrinol Metab 61:429-438, 1985

Mattson A, Seltzer RL: MAOI-induced rapid cycling bipolar affective disorder in an adolescent. Am J Psychiatry 138:677-679, 1981

McCarley RW: REM sleep and depression: Common neurobiological control mechanisms. Am J Psychiatry 139:565-570, 1982

McCarley RW, Massaquoi SG: The REM sleep limit cycle model and depression, in Biological Psychiatry 1985, vol. 6. Edited by Shagass C, Josiassen RC, Wagner HB. New York, Elsevier, 1986

Mendelson WB, Martin JV, Wagner R, et al: Do depressed patients have decreased delta power in the sleep EEG? Abstracts of the American Association of Psychophysiological Studies of Sleep, 1986

Mendels J, Hawkins DR: Longitudinal sleep studies in hypomania. Arch Gen Psychiatry 25:274-277, 1971

Oppenheim G: A case of rapid mood cycling with estrogen: implications for therapy. J Clin Psychiatry 45:34-35, 1984

Papousek M: Chronobiologische aspekte der zyklothymie. Fortschritte der Neurologie Psychiatrie 43:381-440, 1975

Parker DC, Rossman LG, Vanderlan EF: Relation of sleep-entrained human prolactin release to REM–non-REM cycles. J Clin Endocrinol Metab 38:646-651, 1974

Parker DC, Pekary AE, Hershman JM: Effect of normal and reversed sleep-wake cycles upon nyctohemeral rhythmicity of plasma thyrotropin: evidence suggestive of an inhibitory influence in sleep. J Clin Endocrinol Metab 43:318-329, 1976

Pflug B, Tolle R: Disturbance of the 24-hour rhythm in endogenous depression and the treatment of endogenous depression by sleep deprivation. Int Pharmacopsychiatry 6:187-196, 1971

Pflug B, Erikson R, Johnsson A: Depression and daily temperature: a long-term study. Acta Psychiatr Scand 54:254-266, 1976

Post RM, Stoddard FJ, Gillin JC, et al: Slow and rapid alterations in motor activity, sleep and biochemistry in a cycling manic-depressive patient. Arch Gen Psychiatry 34:470-477, 1976

Richter CP: Biological Clocks in Medicine and Psychiatry. Springfield Ill, Charles C Thomas, 1965

Rosenthal NE, Sack DA, Wehr TA: Seasonal variation in affective disorders, in Biological Rhythms and Psychiatry. Edited by Wehr TA, Goodwin FK. Pacific Grove, California, Boxwood Press, 1983

Rosenthal NE, Sack DA, Gillin JC, et al: Seasonal affective disorder: a description of the syndrome and preliminary findings with light therapy. Arch Gen Psychiatry 41:72-80, 1984

Rosenthal NE, Sack DA, Carpenter CJ, et al: Antidepressant effects of light in seasonal affective disorder. Am J Psychiatry 142:163-170, 1985a

Rosenthal NE, Sack DA, James SP, et al: Seasonal affective disorder and phototherapy. Ann N Y Acad Sci 453:260-269, 1985b

Rosenthal NE, Sack DA, Jacobsen FM, et al: The role of melatonin in seasonal affective disorder. J Neural Transm (in press)

Rosenthal NE, Carpenter CJ, James SP, et al: Seasonal affective disorder in children and adolescents. Am J Psychiatry (in press)

Sack DA, Nurnburger J, Rosenthal NE, et al: The potentiation of antidepressant medications by phase-advance of the sleep–wake cycle. Am J Psychiatry 142:606-608, 1985

Schilgen B, Tolle R: Partial sleep deprivation as therapy for depression. Arch Gen Psychiatry 37:267-271, 1980

Schultz H, Lund R, Cording C, et al: Bimodal distribution of REM sleep latencies in depression. Biol Psychiatry 14:595-600, 1979

Sherman B, Pfohl B, Winokur G: Circadian analysis of plasma cortisol levels before and after dexamethasone administration in depressed patients. Arch Gen Psychiatry 41:271-275, 1984

Siris SG, Chertoff HR, Perel JM: Rapid cycling affective disorder during imipramine treatment: a case report. Am J Psychiatry 136:341-342, 1979

Souetre E, Salvati E, Pringuey D, et al: Sleep and mood of depressed patients are improved by a phase advance process. Proc Wrld Cong Biol Psychiatry, Philadelphia 1985 (in press)

Stancer HC, Persad E: Treatment of intractable rapid cycling manic-depressive disorder with levothyroxine. Arch Gen Psychiatry 39:311-312, 1982

Takahashi Y, Kipnis DM, Daughaday WH: Growth hormone secretion during sleep. J Clin Invest 47:2079-2090, 1968

Tamarkin L, Craig CJ, Garrick NA, et al: Effect of clorgyline (a MAO type A inhibitor) on locomotor activity in the Syrian hamster. Am J Physiol 245:R215-R221, 1983

Terman M, Quitkin FM, Terman JS: Bright light treatment of seasonal affective disorder. New Research Abstracts, 139th Annual Meeting of the American Psychiatric Association, 1986

Tondo L, Laddomada P, Serra G, et al: Rapid cyclers and antidepressants. Int Pharmacopsychiatry 16:119-123, 1981

van den Hoofdakker RH, Deersma GM: On the explanation of short REM latencies in depression. Psychiatry Res 16:155-163, 1985

Vogel GW, Vogel C, McAbee RS, et al: Improvement of depression by REM sleep deprivation. Arch Gen Psychiatry 37:247-253, 1980

von Zerssen D, Barthelmes H, Dirlich G, et al: Circadian rhythms in endogenous depression. Psychiatry Res 16:51-63, 1985

Wehr TA: Phase and biorhythm studies of affective illness in the switch process in manic-depressive psychosis. Ann Intern Med 87:321-324, 1977

Wehr TA, Goodwin FK: Tricyclics modulate the frequency of manic-depressive cycles. Chronobiology 4:161, 1977

Wehr TA, Goodwin FK: Rapid cycling in manic-depressives induced by tricyclic antidepressants. Arch Gen Psychiatry 36:555-559, 1979

Wehr TA, Goodwin FK: Biological rhythms and psychiatry, in American Handbook of Psychiatry, vol. 7, 2nd Edition. Edited by Arieti S, Brodie HKH. New York, Basic Books, 1981

Wehr TA, Goodwin FK: Biological rhythms and manic-depressive illness, in Biological Rhythms and Psychiatry. Edited by Wehr TA, Goodwin FK. Pacific Grove, California, Boxwood Press, 1983a

Wehr TA, Goodwin FK: Introduction, in Biological Rhythms and Psychiatry. Edited by Wehr TA, Goodwin FK. Pacific Grove, California, Boxwood Press, 1983b

Wehr TA, Wirz-Justice A: Circadian rhythm mechanisms in affective illness and in antidepressant drug action. Pharmacopsychiatry 15:31-39, 1982

Wehr TA, Wirz-Justice A, Duncan W, et al: Phase-advance of the circadian sleep–wake cycle as an antidepressant. Science 206:710-713, 1979

Wehr TA, Wirz-Justice A, Goodwin FK, et al: 48-hour sleep–wake cycles in manic-depressive illness: naturalistic observations and sleep deprivation experiments. Arch Gen Psychiatry 39:559-565, 1982

Wehr TA, Rosenthal NE, Sack DA, et al: Antidepressant effects of sleep deprivation in bright and dim light. Acta Psychiatr Scand 72:161-165, 1985a

Wehr TA, Sack DA, Duncan NE, et al: Sleep and circadian rhythms in affective patients isolated from external time cues. Psychiatry Res 15:327-339, 1985b

Wehr TA, Sack DA, Jacobsen F, et al: Timing of phototherapy and its effect on melatonin secretion are not critical for its antidepressant effect in seasonal affective disorder. Arch Gen Psychiatry (in press)

Weitzman ED, Goldmacher D, Kripke D, et al: Reversal of sleep–waking cycle: effect on sleep stage pattern and certain neuroendocrine rhythms. Transactions of the American Neurological Association 93:153-157, 1968

Weitzman ED, Czeisler CA, Zimmerman JC, et al: The sleep–wake pattern of cortisol and growth hormone secretion during non-entrained (free-running) conditions in man, in Circadian and Ultradian Variations of Pituitary Hormones in Man. Edited by Nijhoff M. Brussels, Elsevier, 1982

Wiegand M, Berger M, Zulley J, et al: The influence of daytime naps on the therapeutic effect of sleep deprivation, in Biological Psychiatry 1985, vol. 6. Edited by Shagass C, Josiassen RC, Wagner HB. New York, Elsevier, 1986

Wirz-Justice A, Bucheli Ch, Graw P, et al: The Swiss SAD study: incidence of seasonal depression and light therapy. Philadelphia, Abstracts of the Fourth World Congress of Biological Psychiatry, 1985

Chapter 4

Treatment of Bipolar Disorders

by Frederick K. Goodwin, M.D., and Peter Roy-Byrne, M.D.

The development of safe, effective pharmacologic treatment for bipolar affective disorder constitutes one of the major advances in modern psychiatry. While the use of pharmacotherapy to treat acute episodes of mania and depression has been lifesaving for many patients, the availability of effective pharmacological strategies for the prevention of future affective episodes is certainly one of the most powerful and important pharmacological developments in modern psychiatry. In this chapter, we will focus on the practical aspects of pharmacotherapy for the acute and prophylactic treatment of bipolar affective disorder. Because certain topics (that is, the treatment resistant patient, and nonpharmacologic treatments such as sleep deprivation and phototherapy) are extensively reviewed in other chapters of this section, we will only deal with them briefly, referring the reader to these other chapters for a more in-depth review.

In outlining important general principles of clinical care, it is obvious that their application will depend upon the specifics of the clinical situation—that is, the phase of the illness being treated, the severity of symptoms, the setting, and whether the nature of intervention is acute or maintenance treatment.

Pretreatment evaluation is the most important phase of treatment and should be as extensive as the clinical condition of the patient allows. If at all possible, the patient's spouse or close family member should participate in the evaluation and perhaps in follow-up treatment as well. For differential diagnosis (see Chapter 1 of this volume) as well as for effective treatment planning, a careful exploration of the past history is at least as important as full description of the presenting episode. Whenever possible, the onset, duration, and treatment response of all past episodes should be graphically recorded on a "life chart," along with important life events (Roy-Byrne et al, 1985). Data collection for past history can begin with a structured form filled out by the patient and/or family member.

A thorough medical evaluation serves two basic purposes. First, it provides information about possible vulnerabilities in those systems that can be adversely affected by drug treatment, especially the central nervous system, the kidneys, the thyroid, the liver, and the heart. Second, it provides baseline measures useful in the future should medical complications develop. An outline of pretreatment evaluations that would be adequate for all patients is not practical, but the ideal minimum evaluation can be described. In some situations, such as an acutely manic patient, it is occasionally necessary to initiate treatment with little or no medical data. Obviously, in these instances, the data (history, physical, lab studies) should be obtained as soon as possible after treatment is started. The medical history should include a careful review of systems, a full survey of current and past medications, and a family history of medical problems.

The use of large numbers of laboratory tests as a nonspecific screen for pathol-

The opinions expressed herein are those of the authors and do not reflect official policy of the NIMH.

ogy in a healthy patient is of questionable value. Lab tests should be tailored to the planned treatment. Thus, when lithium is being considered, more attention should be given to thyroid and renal function; when tricyclics or MAO inhibitors are to be used, the cardiovascular status should receive relatively more focus. Routine liver function studies and blood count (including platelets) are of special importance when neuroleptics or carbamazepine might be used.

It is also useful to obtain a baseline evaluation of potential "side effects," since many symptoms attributed to drug treatment may have existed previously; the patient's baseline weight should also be recorded. Generally, a brief physical exam including blood pressure and gross neurological exam should be completed, especially in acute situations where little or no medical history can be obtained. It is wise to obtain an electrocardiogram (EKG) in patients over 50, unless a recent one is available. If possible, the patient and/or a family member should start behavioral ratings several days prior to treatment, using one of the instruments available for this (Murphy et al, 1982).

CLINICAL MANAGEMENT OF ACUTE MANIA

Clinical Factors Influencing Drug Choices in Mania

SETTING. The decision to initiate treatment with lithium alone, neuroleptics alone, a lithium–neuroleptic combination, carbamazepine (alone or in combination with lithium), or electroconvulsive therapy (ECT) depends to some extent on the setting. The antimanic effects of lithium are more gradual in onset compared to the neuroleptics and ECT (and probably also carbamazepine) (Chapter 6, this volume). There are some settings where the "lithium lag" in therapeutic onset (7 to 12 days for moderate to severe mania) might be tolerable, such as in a well staffed inpatient research unit. In most settings, however, very rapid control of symptoms is a priority consideration, and in some situations (for example, an emergency room without a closed psychiatric unit for backup) rapid control is clearly a necessity.

SYMPTOMS. The nature and severity of manic symptoms are the most important factors influencing treatment choice. In general, mild manic symptoms (hypomania or Stage I mania) respond well to lithium alone. As the symptoms increase in severity, and particularly as they begin to be dominated by gross hyperactivity and psychotic features, the neuroleptics assume increasing importance. Both the research literature and clinical experience suggest that neuroleptics, and perhaps also carbamazepine, are superior to lithium in the *early* phase of treating severe mania; that is, the first week or two (Goodwin and Zis, 1979). In the later phases of treatment—beyond two weeks—lithium and carbamazepine are superior to neuroleptics. The superiority of lithium and carbamazepine at this later phase derives from their greater specificity (that is, calming the patient with a minimum of sedation and nonspecific "tranquilization"), and from their ability to decrease the likelihood of a post-mania depression. The question of the efficacy of carbamazepine alone compared to lithium or neuroleptics is discussed in Chapter 6 by Robert Post.

MEDICAL COMPLICATIONS AND/OR RELATIVE CONTRAINDICATIONS TO TREATMENT. In some instances, pre-existing medical conditions and/or concurrent medications influence the choice of drugs in the treatment of mania. Although we are concerned here with the short-term use of drugs for the treatment of acute mania, the medical factors discussed below are also relevant to discussions about long-term prophylactic treatment.

Because lithium can influence renal tubular function, the presence of renal functional impairment presents a relative contraindication to this treatment. In this situation, carbamazepine is the preferred alternative, although if the impairment is moderate and stable, lithium can still be used, but with caution. If it is used, the lithium blood level should be monitored carefully; the dose required to achieve a therapeutic level is generally lower (DePaulo et al, 1981; Ramsey and Cox, 1982; DePaulo and Correa, 1985).

Pre-existing cardiac disease can influence treatment decisions in mania. Lithium produces changes in the EKG (particularly T wave flattening) which are generally benign and reversible. Rare and scattered case reports indicate that, in the presence of certain kinds of pre-existing cardiac pathology and/or other drugs with cardiac effects, there is a slight risk of complications due to lithium, including conduction defects and aggravation of ventricular ectopic beats. In the case of myocardial infarction, although lithium might aggravate the increased irritability of an already compromised myocardium, it might be the preferred antimanic agent, since both alternate treatments and untreated mania may present more risk to the heart (that is, the hypotensive effects of neuroleptics on the one hand, or the impact of uncontrolled activity and uncertain compliance with medications on the other). Carbamazepine may provide a useful alternative to lithium or neuroleptics in this situation. For a comprehensive review of the cardiac effects of lithium, the reader is referred to the excellent review by Mitchell and MacKenzie (1982).

Neurological conditions that affect treatment decisions in mania include: epilepsy, parkinsonism, dementia, cerebellar disease, myasthenia gravis, and neuroleptic induced tardive dyskinesia. The risk of this latter complication increases with age, particularly in females; and patients with affective illness, compared to schizophrenics, may be at greater risk. Although both lithium and the neuroleptics can have activating effects on the EEG, neither is contraindicated in classic epilepsy. Nevertheless, the anticonvulsant carbamazepine is the obvious choice for treating patients in whom a seizure disorder and manic-depressive illness coexist. Because one of lithium's biochemical actions is to decrease dopamine synthesis, it can produce symptoms of parkinsonism (Kane et al, 1978; Lang, 1984), and probably can aggravate pre-existing Parkinson's disease and perhaps tardive dyskinesia. Since carbamazepine does not affect the dopamine system, it might be preferred in the management of mania in parkinsonian patients on L–dopa, or in manic patients with pre-existing tardive dyskinesia. In treating manic patients with pre-existing dementia or cerebellar disease, neuroleptics or carbamazepine may be preferable because lithium is more likely to intensify the underlying dysfunctions. However, some patients with dementia are more sensitive to the organic–confusional effects of neuroleptics (probably because of their more potent hypotensive effects) and anticonvulsants. The tendency for lithium to produce muscle weakness makes it unsuitable for use in patients with myasthenia gravis. Lithium has been successfully used to treat the pathological mood lability associated with multiple sclerosis, without aggravating the neurological disorder (Kemp et al, 1977).

There are other medical conditions that have potential interactions with the drugs used in the treatment of mania. For example, compromised liver function and porphyria could weigh against neuroleptics. Although transient mild elevations of liver enzymes are commonly seen during the early stages of carbamazepine treatment and need not necessitate drug discontinuation (Ramsay et al, 1983), more substantial liver function disturbance is a clear contraindication for carbamazepine treatment. Diabetes is not a contraindication to lithium treatment, but the disease should be monitored more closely as the drug is initiated. Thyroid disease can be aggravated by lithium, but is not generally an important consideration in the choice of drugs for the acute treatment of mania, since any lithium effects can be offset by the administration of thyroid hormone. Conditions in which electrolyte imbalance exists, such as severe diarrhea, make the use of lithium and perhaps also carbamazepine more problematic, and therefore neuroleptics might be favored. Any abnormality in the hematopoietic system may complicate the use of carbamazepine (Hart and Easton, 1982; Joffe et al, 1985).

PREGNANCY. The incidence of birth defects (principally cardiac) in babies born to mothers who were on lithium in the first trimester is significantly higher than normal (Kallen and Tandberg, 1983), and therefore, its use should be avoided during pregnancy, particularly during the first trimester. Milder manic episodes during pregnancy should probably be managed without drugs, but it is still prudent to treat more severe episodes, since the risk to the fetus from the manic hyperactivity is considerable. Carbamazepine, when administered alone, is not known to be associated with fetal abnormalities and, therefore, might be used in these circumstances. Robert Post discusses this further in Chapter 6. The question of discontinuing long-term maintenance lithium in anticipation of pregnancy will be discussed below.

CONCURRENT MEDICATIONS. The drug interactions that should be considered in relation to lithium, neuroleptics, and carbamazepine are specified in Chapter 6 of this volume and in the individual sections below. In addition, with regard to lithium, diuretics deserve special attention. "Loop" diuretics such as furosemide (Lasix) do not substantially alter lithium excretion and can be coadministered safely (Jefferson and Kalin, 1979; Safer and Coppen, 1983). The thiazide drugs, however, decrease tubular readsorption of sodium and indirectly increase lithium reabsorption and decrease excretion (Jefferson and Kalin, 1979). Therefore, with these drugs, lithium should be initiated at a low dose and increased very gradually with frequent monitoring of the blood level. Other medical drugs with potential lithium interactions include: the anti-inflammatory agents indomethacin and phenylbutazone, which can increase lithium levels (Reimann et al, 1983), and certain antibiotics with nephrotoxic potential. These interactions are discussed in detail by Jefferson and colleagues (1981). Carbamazepine drug interactions are discussed by Robert Post and Thomas Uhde in Chapter 6.

Determining Medication Dosage

NEUROLEPTICS. The treatment of acute mania with neuroleptics alone often can require larger doses than are routinely used in the treatment of schizophrenic psychosis. For example, in the various controlled studies, the chlorpromazine dose averaged over 1,000 mg. Similar high doses are reported for haloperidol use in mania. Unlike lithium, neuroleptic blood level determinations are not yet routinely available nor clinically meaningful. Clinical titration of dose involves consideration of age, sex, and weight, with higher doses required for males, younger patients, and heavier patients. With high dose neuroleptic treatment of mania it is important to continually reevaluate dosage requirements. Dosage should be reduced as soon as the manic symptoms begin to subside in order to minimize the possibility of neurotoxicity, extrapyramidal side effects, or post-mania depression (Kukopulos et al, 1980).

LITHIUM. The management of mania with lithium is best achieved by a dosage schedule that produces the highest plasma level consistent with acceptable side effects; the blood levels usually achieved in acute treatment are higher than is necessary or safe for maintenance treatment. In using lithium, it is important to be aware that the gap between therapeutic and toxic levels is narrow. Clinical factors that affect the dose/blood level relation are sex, age, weight (especially muscle mass), salt intake, amount of sweat, the individual's intrinsic renal clearance capacity for lithium, and, as noted previously, other medications (Lesar et al, 1985). A relatively higher dose/blood level ratio is associated with being younger, male, and heavier (especially muscle mass) and having dietary habits involving higher salt intake.

For the lithium management of mania, one of the most important factors affecting the dose/blood level relationship is the patient's clinical state. A given patient, when manic, will be in positive lithium balance; that is, the patient will retain lithium in body pools outside the plasma, probably largely in bone (Trautner et al, 1955; Hullin et al, 1968; Greenspan et al, 1968; Almy and Taylor, 1973). Thus, it will require more lithium to achieve a given blood level during mania than during euthymia or depression (Greenspan et al, 1968; Goodwin et al, 1969; Serry, 1969). What this means in practical terms is that when the mania begins to respond to lithium, a downward dosage adjustment is usually necessary in order to ensure that the patient does not slip into lithium toxicity. Obviously, blood levels should be monitored more frequently when the clinical state is changing. Some authors have suggested a test dose of lithium followed at 24 hours by a plasma level determination as a way of predicting dosage requirements (Cooper and Simpson, 1976; Champ et al, 1979; Fava et al, 1984; Perry et al, 1984). However, its practical value in the treatment of acute mania is limited by the fact that the kinetics of lithium are state dependent. In particular, changes in sleep and activity level have been shown to invalidate this technique (Perry et al, 1984).

There are substantial individual differences in the plasma level of lithium necessary for clinical response in mania as well as for toxicity, probably reflecting widespread interindividual differences in the ratio of intra- to extracellular lithium. Stokes and his colleagues (1976) have shown an association between increasing plasma levels of lithium (up to 1.4 mEq/1) and the percentage of manic patients showing a therapeutic response. Blood levels above 1.5 are not recommended, and for levels between 1.2 and 1.5, considerable care is required to avoid toxicity. In the great majority of cases, levels in the therapeutic range will be achieved at doses between 900 and 2,100 mg per day. In making decisions concerning the maximum lithium level for the treatment of a manic patient, the most important potential toxic effects to attend to are those involving the central nervous system (CNS). Severe mania can involve some delirium-like symptoms which may be difficult to distinguish from these neurotoxic effects.

Some authors have suggested a "loading dose" strategy for the treatment of mania with lithium, in order to achieve the maximum blood level quickly and to diminish the lag in therapeutic onset. However, the value of this is questionable, particularly in light of animal and human data indicating considerable delay in the entry of lithium from blood into brain even at high plasma levels. In a study of cerebrospinal fluid (CSF) lithium levels, there was an average 50 percent increase in CSF lithium from the first to the third week on a constant dose (Rey et al, 1979).

LITHIUM PLUS NEUROLEPTICS. Dosage considerations involve respect for the additive and, to some extent, synergistic effects of these two classes of drugs. Lithium has been shown to potentiate both the therapeutic (Biederman et al, 1979) and some neurotoxic effects of neuroleptics (Branchey et al, 1976; Spring, 1979). When used in combination with lithium, the dose of neuroleptic should be substantially lower than when given alone, while the lithium level should be kept below 1.2 mEq/1. Administered this way, lithium and neuroleptics can be combined safely and effectively (Baastrup et al, 1976; Abrams and Taylor, 1979).

ELECTROCONVULSIVE THERAPY (ECT). ECT remains today a treatment alternative that is used only occasionally for mania. Numerous clinical reports indicate that it is a rapidly effective antimanic treatment, but no prospective studies have been performed to determine its efficacy in comparison with standard drug treatments (Fink, 1979). However, a recent study does suggest that bilateral ECT is probably more effective than unilateral ECT for *manic* symptoms (Small et al, 1985). There are some situations in which ECT would seem to represent a reasonable alternative. Such instances would include patients who consistently refuse medication, those in whom there are medical contraindications to medication, and those who have proven unresponsive to medication. If ECT is going to be used, it is probably best that lithium not be administered simultaneously (or given in reduced doses), in light of reports of neurotoxic complications with this combination (Remick, 1978; Hoenig and Chaulk, 1977; Small et al, 1980; Mandel et al, 1980). The ECT treatment of breakthrough depressions in patients on maintenance lithium will be discussed later.

Suggested Outline of the Drug Treatment of Severe Mania

For the acute treatment of moderately severe to severe mania (Stages II or III), treatment can be initiated with neuroleptics (or carbamazepine); because it is believed to achieve motor control more rapidly, haloperidol is the preferred neuroleptic for many clinicians. One should give doses of 5 to 10 mg I.M. every 4 to 6 hours, with gradual replacement of oral doses up to 100 mg per day; for chlorpromazine, the dose would be 50 to 100 mg I.M. every 6 hours, replaced by oral doses up to 2,500 mg per day. After three to four days, or as soon as the acute hyperactive and psychotic symptoms begin to subside, the dose of neuroleptic can be reduced as lithium is added, initially in small doses of 300 to 600 mg per day. With careful monitoring of both clinical effects and side effects, the dose of neuroleptic is gradually decreased in conjunction with a gradual increase in the lithium dose. By the third week, most patients can be maintained on lithium alone, although with some it will be necessary to continue modest doses of neuroleptics for a longer time. For patients with substantial schizo-affective features, adjunctive neuroleptics may have to be maintained indefinitely.

As discussed extensively in Chapter 6, carbamazepine, initially reserved for lithium nonresponders, is now being given serious consideration as a first choice alternative to neuroleptics, as an adjunct to lithium in the treatment of mania. If additional studies continue to show that it is at least as effective as neuroleptics without the same potential for post-mania depression or cycle induction, carbamazepine may be preferable to neuroleptics. Also reviewed in Chapter 6 are other anticonvulsants with antimanic properties, such as the benzodiazepine clonazepam, and valproic acid. Additional reports and small scale studies have suggested a possible role for L–tryptophan (Chouinard et al, 1985), propranolol (Emrich et al, 1979), lecithin (Cohen et al, 1982), and clonidine (Jouvent et al, 1980) in the acute treatment of mania. Until more information is available, however, these agents cannot be recommended for routine use. Robert Post and Thomas Uhde discuss additional treatment alternatives for acute mania in Chapter 6.

Hospitalization

When the patient is exhibiting the fully developed picture of frank mania (psychotic mania, Stage III mania) there is usually no question that hospitalization is necessary. Under these circumstances, one must frequently resort to involuntary hospitalization. When the manic symptoms are still in the mild to moderate range, the question of whether and when to hospitalize can be a more difficult one. The support and collaboration of the family is extremely important here, not just to help get the patient hospitalized if necessary, but to provide the external controls (including medication compliance) if the patient is to stay out of the hospital. The basic question is this: Is the patient more likely to be disadvantaged by the potential stigma of hospitalization or by the social, occupational, or legal consequences of manic behavior? In assessing this, it is well to keep in mind that the "switch" from the milder to the more severe stages of mania can occur very rapidly and unexpectedly.

Since manic patients rarely see the need for or the wisdom of hospitalization, informed consent presents a dilemma. On the one hand, involuntary commitment is not only difficult and cumbersome for the clinician, but it increases the likelihood of stigmatization and can result in the patient losing other legal rights. On the other hand, to acquiesce to the patient's refusal is to court disaster. A humane alternative to this "no win" dilemma is to obtain *consent-in-advance*, as is now permitted in some jurisdictions under the new so-called odysseus principal. Under this arrangement, an individual who knows that he or she has manic depressive illness can, when in a well state, give fully informed consent to a *future* hospitalization as it is deemed necessary by the physician he or she chooses and by the family.

CLINICAL MANAGEMENT OF ACUTE BIPOLAR DEPRESSION

This section deals with the management of depression in a bipolar patient not already on lithium. Management of "breakthrough" depressions occurring during prophylactic treatment will be covered in the following section. Our discussion of general principles in the management of depression focuses on those issues most relevant to bipolar patients. For further discussion of overall management of depressive disorders in general, the reader is referred to the many useful reviews of this subject (Klein et al, 1980; Stern et al, 1980; Kupfer and Detre, 1978; Baldessarini, 1977; Goodwin, 1977).

Pretreatment Evaluation

In dealing with the acutely depressed (and perhaps suicidal) patient, the clinician faces an urgent and, at times, even an emergency situation. There is often great pressure to begin treatment immediately, perhaps before adequate information has been obtained. Adding to this difficulty is the fact that depressed patients may be too preoccupied by their symptoms or too confused or retarded to give a comprehensive history in the all-too-short time that many busy practitioners give them. It cannot be overemphasized that the time and care invested in the pretreatment evaluation is vital to the success of the therapeutic effort. Depressed patients will frequently underestimate prior hypomanic or manic symptoms, often recalling them simply as their well state, so that it is important to interview the spouse as well.

In exploring past history, it is important to know the age of onset of the first definable depressive (or manic/hypomanic) episode, and the general characteristics of each episode, including severity, duration, nature of symptoms, and patterns of recurrence, including seasonal patterns. Important to treatment decision is any information bearing on the nature of any response to prior exposure to psychotrophic drugs. Sometimes the only evidence for any latent bipolarity will be a brief hypomanic period following an earlier exposure to antidepressant drugs. As mentioned previously, graphic visualization of this information may facilitate evaluation and treatment. In addition, data on the family history of response to drug treatment are important, since there is evidence suggesting that response to lithium, tricyclic antidepressants, and monoamine oxidase inhibitors has a familial component (Pare, 1962).

General Indications for Drug Treatment

The decision to use drugs for acute treatment depends on an assessment of the overall severity of the depression, the nature of the symptoms, and the extent of functional impairment. As with depressions in general, pharmacological intervention is more likely to be indicated the greater the degree of functional impairment, the less reactivity to the environment, and the more the symptoms reflect physiological dysfunction (sleep, appetite, diurnal pattern, and so forth). The presence or absence of convincing psychosocial precipitants is irrelevant to the question of whether pharmacotherapy is indicated.

A Drug "Decision Tree" Approach

Lithium should be started first, absent contraindications or prior evidence of intolerance. For depressions of only moderate severity, it is well to allow three, four, or even five weeks to evaluate the antidepressant effects of lithium alone. Many will respond, and since most will subsequently be kept on lithium for prophylaxis, starting with a trial of lithium as an antidepressant means that some patients will be spared being on two drugs (lithium plus an antidepressant) unnecessarily. In this regard, we should recall that the risk of precipitating mania with antidepressants is considerable: the data reviewed elsewhere (Goodwin, 1981; Wehr and Goodwin, in press) indicate that, for many bipolar patients, manic reactions occur within the first few weeks; that is, within the time it takes to evaluate antidepressant effects. In Chapter 3 of this section Wehr and his colleagues review the convincing evidence that tricyclic antidepressants can be associated with the onset of rapid cycling in some bipolar patients. Thus, the reassuring notion that one can initiate antidepressant treatment with impunity in any bipolar patients, as long as the treatment is not maintained too far beyond a favorable response, is not supported by the data.

With more severe bipolar depressions, an adjunctive antidepressant (tricyclic, heterocyclic, or MAO inhibitor) may be needed at the outset. In such situations, treatment should be initiated with lithium and the antidepressant together. Among the tricyclics, one of the more activating, less sedating drugs may be preferable (desipramine, imipramine, nortriptyline) since psychomotor retardation is often prominent in bipolar depression; also this avoids the excessive sedation that can sometimes occur on the combination of an anxiolytic tricyclic (such as amitriptyline) and lithium. A wide variety of "second generation" heterocyclic antidepressants are now available. Which will, among these, in the long run, prove to be as good as or superior to the tricyclics as antidepressants remains to be seen. One of them (bupropion) has been suggested by some as especially useful in bipolar depression because of its effects on psychomotor retardation, and because it may carry a relatively lower risk of precipitating mania (Shopsin, 1983). Recent evidence (Quitkin et al, 1984) suggests that it is necessary to wait six weeks for a response rather than the traditional figure of three or four weeks, before declaring the patient a nonresponder.

USE OF MONOAMINE OXIDASE (MAO) INHIBITOR. Traditionally these drugs are often reserved for tricyclic nonresponders. However, today many experienced clinicians prefer to employ the MAOI–lithium combination before a tricyclic, especially when the depression is characterized by extreme anergy, hypersomnia, and excessive appetite (Himmelhoch et al, 1972; Kupfer and Detre, 1978). The differential efficacy of tricyclics and MAOIs in bipolar depression is a major unanswered question in psychopharmacology, and controlled studies are urgently needed. Clinical experience suggests that many lithium nonresponsive bipolar depressed patients will respond to the addition of an MAOI.

Some clinicians recommend the combination of a tricyclic and an MAOI when neither alone has produced a response. Although the question of whether such a combination is associated with any additional efficacy is not yet settled, the safety of this combination has now been convincingly established (Schuckit, et al, 1971; Spiker and Pugh, 1976; White and Simpson, 1980; Marley and Wozniak, 1983; Razani et al, 1983). The safety of this combination when given with lithium has not been studied systematically, but clinical experience suggests that they can be coadministered safely as long as attention is paid to potentially additive effects. In using TCA and MAOI combinations, it is important not to add the TCA to a patient already established on an MAOI. The two drugs should either be started simultaneously (at lower than usual doses for each used above), or the MAOI can be added to pre-existing tricyclics. One additional advantage of the combination derives from the ability of small doses of tricyclics (25–50 mg at bedtime) to diminish the sleep disruptions associated with the MAOIs. For more details on the proper use of these combinations, the reader is referred to the reviews cited above.

ELECTROCONVULSIVE THERAPY. ECT continues to have a place in the treatment of some cases of bipolar depression. In our view, it should be given consideration as the initial treatment if the patient is severely ill, especially if delusional and/or at high risk for suicide. Many clinicians often prefer to reserve ECT for patients who have failed to respond to drugs because of an inability to personally administer it, because of misconceptions about its risks and benefits, or because of actual legal barriers in some areas. However, reserving ECT only for drug failures ignores data on the poor response of delusional depressives to tricyclics in contrast to the remarkably high rate of response to ECT. It also ignores the evidence that repeated exposure to tricyclics may alter the long-term course of bipolar illness toward more frequent recurrence, whereas ECT does not seem to incur this risk.

Dosage, Blood Levels

When coadministering tricyclics or MAOIs with lithium, it is advisable to start with somewhat lower doses of the added drug since some of the side effects (for example, sedation) are additive. However, once initial accommodation to the drugs has occurred, doses should be increased until either response or unacceptable side effects ensue. Many treatment "failures" with tricyclics or MAOIs are simply due to inadequate dosage (Quitkin, 1985). Throughout the trial of the tricyclic or MAOI, the lithium level should be maintained between 0.6 and 1.0 mEq/1; that is, somewhat lower than recommended for lithium alone.

Tricyclic blood levels may be helpful, keeping in mind the evidence that the relationship to clinical response appears to be linear for imipramine and desipramine, whereas nortriptyline has a "therapeutic window." The current state of the art on TCA blood levels has been the subject of excellent reviews (Potter and Linnoila, 1984; Amsterdam et al, 1981; Van Brunt, 1983; APA Task Force Report, 1985).

The use of alternative and/or adjunctive agents to treat depression in bipolar patients will be discussed later in this chapter, under the heading, Treatment of Breakthrough Depressions.

Hospitalization

The majority of bipolar depressions can be managed on an outpatient basis. When is hospitalization advisable? There are no universal guidelines, but in considering each patient's individual situation it is important to evaluate the availability of the clinician and of support in the environment, the risk of suicide, and the social, economic, and occupational costs to the patient as a result of being hospitalized—or conversely, of being kept out of the hospital.

Duration of Treatment

Assuming that the patient has responded to pharmacological intervention, how long should the drug or drugs be continued? Here we are *not* addressing the question of maintenance treatment aimed at preventing *new* episodes in the future. The question here is continuation treatment: to prevent *relapse*, what is an adequate duration of treatment for a depressive episode in a bipolar patient? If the patient has responded to lithium alone and is tolerating it well, it should be continued for 9 to 12 months after remission, at which point the question of maintenance treatment can be considered, employing the criteria outlined below. If the patient responded to a combination of lithium and tricyclic or lithium and MAOI, it is probably advisable to gradually withdraw the tricyclic or MAOI after the patient has been in remission for one or two months. It should be noted that antidepressant withdrawal has been reported to precipitate mania in some patients (Nelson et al, 1983), so clinical state should be carefully monitored at this time. If for some reason treatment was started with tricyclic or MAOI alone, then lithium could be either added or substituted as soon as the patient is in remission. As stated before, we don't recommend this particular sequence because of the risk of drug induced mania.

MAINTENANCE (PROPHYLACTIC) TREATMENT OF MANIC-DEPRESSIVE ILLNESS

For the great majority of bipolar patients, the cornerstone of maintenance treatment will be lithium alone or in combination. However, the following general guidelines would apply to the use of alternate prophylactic drugs as well.

Selection of Patients for Maintenance Treatment

Patient selection involves balancing projected benefits against risks. Put simply, a decision to initiate maintenance medication is fundamentally an expectation that the treatment will do more good than harm. A decision to *continue* such treatment once it has begun is a different matter that involves continuous evaluation of many factors in the individual patient (side effects, impact on interepisode functioning, psychological reactions to lithium, and so forth); assessment of these factors requires many months of observation. Of course, when a drug such as lithium is initiated as a treatment for an episode, one already has weighed any potential medical complications and has some experience with the patient's ability to tolerate it. Generally, the effects of a drug should be observed for at least one year before a decision about long-term use is reached.

In the consideration of maintenance treatment, the fundamental question facing the clinician and the patient is: What is the likelihood of a relapse in the absence of prophylactic medication compared to that same likelihood in its presence? As reviewed by Keller in Chapter 1 of this volume, two fundamental conclusions about the natural course of bipolar illness are that it recurs and that the recurrences tend to become more frequent as the illness progresses. However, even though the majority of bipolar patients will *eventually* have recurrences frequent enough to justify prophylactic treatment, this does not mean that all patients should be placed on maintenance treatment after the first sign of the illness.

Efforts to develop criteria for patient selection have focused on the *frequency* of prior episodes and the *total number* of episodes. Obviously, in a patient whose history is similar to those selected for the prophylactic studies in the literature (multiple episodes with a frequency ranging from two per year to one every two years), the need for prophylaxis is clear, given the very high relapse rate on placebo in these studies, averaging 73 percent within the first year (Schou, 1978). What about the need for prophylaxis among patients with lower relapse rates? Based on naturalistic observation of 95 bipolar patients over many years,

Angst and Grof (1979) have concluded that a total of two or three previous episodes is the best minimum criterion for lithium prophylaxis. To require more than three episodes, or that these episodes occur within two or three years, excludes from treatment a substantial number of patients who would relapse during the first two years without it. Considering the relative safety of long-term lithium and the devastation that episodes of bipolar affective illness can bring, treating some patients during a period when they would not relapse anyway seems preferable to excluding from treatment many patients who would otherwise relapse quickly. For example, if the criterion of two episodes within two years had been applied, two-thirds of the patients excluded from lithium would have relapsed within two years. Another reason why a selection criterion based on frequency is not as reliable as one based on total number of episodes is the evidence that the natural course of the illness can be quite irregular, with episodes sometimes occurring in "bursts." Many experienced clinicians will initiate maintenance lithium after the first manic episode, even when there has not been a prior depressive episode.

As reviewed in Chapter 1, it is now well established that episodes of bipolar affective illness tend to occur closer together as the illness progresses, particularly through the first several episodes. There is some evidence that the latency between the first and second episodes may be related to age of onset. Zis and colleagues (1979) analyzed the longitudinal course of illness in 105 bipolar patients followed in three countries over many years, and found a correlation between the age of onset and the length of the first cycle; that is, the time between the first and second episode. Patients with an age of onset below 30 had a 20 percent chance of a relapse within two years after the first episode; those with an age of onset between 30 and 50 had a 50 percent chance, and late age of onset (50+) was associated with an 80 percent chance of a relapse within two years. These data are in agreement with those of Angst (1980), but not those of Dunner and colleagues (1979). The data are also consistent with an earlier observation by Schou of an often prolonged "latent period" between the first and second episode in patients who have their first episode early. This latent period may allow a lithium-free period during the prime childbearing years in the mid- to late 20s, an important advantage given the potential negative impact of lithium on the fetus in the first trimester.

There is some suggestion in the literature (Perris, 1966) that bipolar patients whose first episode is manic are more likely to experience a subsequent course in which mania predominates, compared with those patients whose illness starts with a depression. Since vulnerability to mania represents a more potent indication for lithium prophylaxis than does depression, a manic first episode might justify prophylaxis sooner. Also, the evidence that among bipolar patients the ratio of manic to depressive episodes is higher in males compared with females (Angst, 1978), provides some justification for considering prophylaxis earlier in males.

Other features of the illness to be considered in making decisions about prophylaxis include the severity of previous episodes and whether their onset was sudden or gradual. If the onset of the prior manic episode was sudden, then the indications for prophylaxis are stronger, since there may be no warning period of hypomania during which treatment could be started again.

There are, in addition, features of the individual patient that should affect decisions about prophylaxis. For example, how reliable is the patient likely to be in noting early signs and seeking early treatment? Is he or she likely to deny difficulty until it is too late? What is the status of the family and other support systems available to the patient? A concerned family member is especially important for the early detection of hypomania because many patients do not experience this state as a problem and would be unlikely to seek help for it on their own. Some clinicians recommend that physiological disruptions (such as physical illness and drug induced states), possibly contributing to the onset of the first manic episode, be taken into account in deciding about prophylaxis. This recommendation is based on the notion that such "secondary" manias (Krauthammer and Klerman, 1978) represent less inherent vulnerability, and therefore, less need for prophylaxis.

In summary, although there is no set of guidelines that can be uniformly applied to all patients, some general principles can be followed. For almost all bipolar patients, lithium maintenance is indicated after the second or third major episode. Prophylaxis should be considered earlier if the patient is male, if onset occurs after age 30, with the first episode manic, with sudden onset, with onset not precipitated by external factors, and in the face of a poor family and social support system.

Pretreatment Evaluation

As was discussed under acute treatment, this evaluation focuses on certain medical contraindications that occasionally mitigate against lithium maintenance. Most, if not all, of these contraindications are relative rather than absolute; they focus on the three systems prominent in our discussion of side effects: the kidney, the cardiovascular system, and the central nervous system. These relative contraindications, described earlier in the section on acute treatment of mania, may justify the use of alternative medications (see below).

Monitoring of Maintenance Lithium

THE APPROPRIATE LITHIUM LEVEL. The optimal level for maintenance treatment is generally between 0.6 and 1.2 mEq/1, somewhat lower than that recommended for the acute treatment of mania. In earlier studies of prophylaxis, blood levels were maintained near the high end of this range, but more recently a somewhat lower range has become the accepted norm; several studies indicate that a drop in prophylactic efficacy is unlikely to occur until blood levels fall below 0.6–0.7 mEq/1. However, these are group data; since individuals vary in their response at a given level, the best approach is to start with a blood level near the point where side effects become troublesome, and then very gradually bring it down to a level where side effects almost, but not completely, disappear, indicating the lower range of an effective dose.

The frequency of blood level monitoring varies with the clinical situation. For the first several weeks, levels need to be evaluated from every few days to every week in order to determine the dose/blood level ratio for that particular patient. As noted earlier, the clinical state of the patient, as well as a variety of other individual factors (sex, age, muscle mass, and diet), contribute to that ratio. Frequent monitoring in this early phase of treatment also helps establish compliance by emphasizing to the patient the importance of the blood level. Once the dose and blood level have been stabilized, most patients can be adequately managed by monitoring every four to eight weeks. Continuous monitoring remains important, not only because of the possibility of unexpected medical conditions that can alter the lithium level, but also because it has an important psychological impact: it is the major way in which the patient participates in the management of the illness, and it serves as a reminder both of the illness and of the importance of the medication.

FREQUENCY OF OTHER LABORATORY TESTS. Table 1 outlines a routine monitoring program for patients on lithium in the absence of clinical indications of developing problems; authorities differ on the extent of minimum monitoring, as indicated in the Table.

SPECIAL CIRCUMSTANCES. A variety of situations can affect the lithium level and it is important that both the clinician and the patient be aware of them. Probably the most common of these is the occurrence of medical illness. For example, even brief episodes of the flu, if severe enough to substantially reduce food (and therefore salt) intake and produce changes in fluid balance, can elevate the plasma lithium level beyond the safe range. Sometimes it can be difficult to distinguish the early signs of lithium toxicity from symptoms of the medical illness itself; if the illness persists for more than a few days, plasma lithium should be checked, and if accompanied by vomiting and/or diarrhea, plasma electrolytes should be measured.

Surgical procedures that involve general anesthesia require attention. Although there are no absolute contraindications to general anesthesia, it is generally advisable to reduce the lithium dose by one-half two to three days preceding the surgery, withholding it altogether for 24 hours before the procedure. Therapeutic lithium levels can be re-established as soon as fluid and electrolyte balance is normalized. Lithium has been found to potentiate analgesics in animals

Table 1. Pretreatment Evaluation for Lithium Maintenance (Healthy Individuals Under Age 45)

Minimum Recommendation:	BUN
	Creatinine
	T–4
	TSH
	Urinalysis including protein and microscopic exam
Additional tests recommended by some authorities:	
	24-hour urine volume
	Creatinine clearance
	Urine Osmolality
	T–3 resin uptake
	Complete blood count
	Electrolytes
	EKG
	Blood pressure

(Havdala et al, 1979) and patients on lithium have been noted to need less pain medication during post-operative recovery.

Alterations in diet can occasionally be a puzzling source of change in the lithium level. Most frequently encountered is the initiation of a crash diet without the physician's knowledge. The bulk of daily salt intake comes from food and severe dieting can cause sodium depletion, producing increased plasma lithium levels. Patients on diets should pay special attention to salt intake; more frequent plasma monitoring is also advisable.

Major *changes in physical activity* can be important; for example, when a program of strenuous exercise is started such as long distance running, care is required to maintain adequate hydration, replace lost electrolytes (especially sodium and potassium), and monitor lithium more closely. Strenuous physical activity in hot climates may increase the risk of lithium intoxication, principally because of selective loss of sodium and fluid in the sweat. However, a recent study showed that long distance runners may also lose lithium through the sweat, thereby lowering the lithium level (Jefferson et al, 1982). In these situations, it may be advisable to monitor lithium levels and adjust the dose accordingly.

In some patients on a constant dose, changes in the blood level can occur in association with major shifts in mood state. A shift into depression can be accompanied by an increase in plasma lithium, while a shift into hypomania can be associated with a decreased level. One final consideration is the impact of age on lithium level; renal lithium clearance gradually decreases with age, indicating that periodic downward dosage adjustment may be necessary in the course of long-term lithium administration.

MANAGEMENT OF LITHIUM SIDE EFFECTS. The first response to an unacceptable side effect is to decrease the dose; obviously any effect which is dose related should respond to such a maneuver, at least partially. However, one is often reluctant to lower the dose enough to abolish a side effect, particularly if prior experience suggests that the risk of relapse becomes unacceptably high. Fortunately, some side effects can be managed by supplemental treatment.

One of the most common side effects of lithium, fine tremor, is also one of the easiest to treat; and, if left untreated, it can contribute to poor compliance. Although reducing the blood level may help, the tremor often persists even at the minimum level needed for prophylaxis. Propranolol (10–40 mg per day) controls tremor very effectively and, at this modest dosage, is essentially without other effects including, probably, the drug induced depression that has been reported by some investigators. The onset and timing of propranolol's anti-tremor action is usually within 30 minutes, lasting for four to six hours.

Excessive polyuria, that is, lithium induced nephrogenic diabetes insipidus (NDI), can occasionally become so severe that either the patient or the clinician stops the drug. In the presence of a clearly demonstrated need for lithium, two alternate strategies are available. The addition of diuretics to the lithium regimen may be helpful; as noted earlier, for this indication, loop diuretics such as furosemide (Lasix) are safer than thiazides, although Himmelhoch et al (1977) offers guidelines for the combined use of lithium and thiazide diuretics. The second strategy is to substitute (completely or partially) carbamazepine for lithium, since the former does not antagonize the antidiuretic hormone. Carbamazepine will not reverse NDI in the presence of a continued high level, but it may substantially decrease the need for lithium.

The antithyroid effects of lithium can and should be treated with supplemental thyroid if there is laboratory as well as clinical evidence of hypothyroidism. Clinical manifestations may be limited to such nonspecific symptoms as lassitude, tiredness, and decreased cognitive functioning. The use of thyroid hormone as an experimental treatment for "breakthrough" depressions in the absence of chemical evidence of hypothyroidism is discussed below.

The most troublesome of the common side effects of lithium, and frequently associated with poor compliance, is weight gain. Here we are not referring to the small amounts of weight gain (under 10 pounds) experienced by most patients during the initiation of lithium therapy; much of this is probably due to fluid retention and can be expected to recede gradually. However, approximately 25 percent of patients will experience weight gain greater than 10 pounds. Women, especially those who have had prior difficulty controlling their weight, are particularly likely to experience lithium induced weight gain. It is central to compliance that weight gain be managed early and vigorously. First, restrict carbohydrates. Frequently, lithium treatments can produce a mild hypoglycemia-like pattern in which the patient will experience carbohydrate craving associated with low plasma glucose two to three hours after the ingestion of carbohydrates, especially sugar. Often, simply eliminating sugar-containing foods (for example, orange juice at breakfast) can alleviate the mid- or late-morning hunger which, of course, contributes to the weight problem. Lithium induced hypothyroidism may be associated with weight gain and, if present, this contributing factor can easily be corrected. Last, patients should not inadvertently increase their caloric intake by responding to lithium induced thirst with high caloric drinks.

TREATMENT OF LITHIUM TOXICITY. Prevention is the most important principle in the management of lithium toxicity. The most sensitive indicator of incipient lithium toxicity is the central nervous system. It is imperative that patients be alerted in advance to CNS symptoms, and each patient contact should include some assessment of CNS functioning. It can sometimes be difficult to distinguish between the agitation and restlessness of early intoxication and similar symptoms seen as part of mixed affective states. If the intoxication is so severe that lithium withdrawal is not sufficient, then the patient should be admitted to a hospital and cared for by a specialist well versed in the treatment of poisoning. A variety of methods have been used to treat lithium poisoning. First, general supportive measures, such as would be appropriate in any CNS poisoning, should be pursued vigorously. Obviously, kidney function should be preserved by maintaining blood pressure and by replacing fluids and salt. If kidney function falters, hemodialysis is necessary. Although the majority of patients who overdose on lithium, deliberately or accidentally, will recover, some die or are left with a persistent neurological or renal defect. Because of these severe complications, the possibility of lithium intoxication should never be taken lightly. Obviously, patients with pre-existing vulnerabilities, particularly in kidney function, require more careful monitoring.

Interaction of Lithium with Other Drugs

In general, there are surprisingly few problems associated with the use of lithium in combination with other drugs. Although several of the interactions have been discussed previously, we will outline them here briefly for the sake of completeness.

PSYCHOACTIVE DRUGS. Sedative hypnotics, as well as the benzodiazepines and other related minor tranquilizers, have no clinically significant interactions with lithium, although the CNS depressant effects can be additive. The most widely studied interaction is that with neuroleptic drugs, particularly haloperidol. A reasonable conclusion derived from these studies is that lithium and neuroleptics can be coadministered safely, as long as the clinician is aware of potential additive effects (sedation, extrapyramidal symptoms) and uses the lowest effective doses of both drugs. Lithium is quite compatible with tricyclic antidepressants, monoamine oxidase inhibitors, and carbamazepine, although some side effects may be additive. Theoretically, lithium plus a tricyclic could have additive effects on cardiac conduction in susceptible individuals, and it is probably unwise to use this combination in patients with pre-existing severe or unstable cardiac conduction defects.

NONPSYCHOACTIVE DRUGS. The interaction of lithium with diuretics has been discussed. The effects of certain drugs (such as quinidine) on cardiac conduction could, at least theoretically, be potentiated by lithium. There are some animal data which suggest that lithium potentiates digitalis toxicity by lowering intracellular potassium, but whether this occurs in humans is not clear. In conclusion, the combination of lithium with cardiac drugs, although not contraindicated, requires more careful monitoring, including periodic EKGs.

Any drug that alters renal function should be used cautiously in patients on lithium, especially if there is any history of kidney disease. There are two case reports of alpha-methyldopa (Aldomet) (O'Reagan, 1976; Byrd, 1977) and one report of a tetracycline antibiotic (McGennis, 1978) interfering with lithium clearance by the kidney. The interaction of lithium with anticonvulsants is discussed by Robert Post and Thomas Uhde in Chapter 6.

Although lithium does not generally interfere with alcohol induced highs, some patients report that they need more alcohol to produce the desired alteration in mood, and some inadvertently increase their consumption of alcoholic beverages in response to the lithium induced increase in thirst. Thus, these effects of lithium can indirectly cause alcohol related complications, such as cirrhosis, due to gradually increased alcohol consumption. On the other hand, an attenuation of alcohol seeking behavior is seen in some, particularly if the behavior has been strongly linked to extremes of mood. Lithium has been reported to interfere with cocaine and amphetamine induced highs.

Lithium may actually *decrease* the need for certain medications. For example, some forms of headache, as well as labile hypertension, respond to lithium, at least partially. The interaction of lithium with other drugs has been extensively reviewed by Himmelhoch and Neil (1980) and by Jefferson et al (1981).

Impact of Lithium on Other Functions

As we noted earlier, there are important effects of lithium in addition to its alteration of manic or depressive episodes; these other effects tend to be noticed predominantly during the interepisode periods. Commonly reported by patients on lithium is an apparent intensification of smaller cycles. For example, women may become aware of the mood changes accompanying the menstrual cycle; and other patients may become aware of subtle cycles of activity and energy, perhaps reflecting the attenuation of the major cycles of the illness, allowing these more subtle phenomena to manifest themselves.

Lithium has an effect on EEG monitored sleep: overall depth and length is increased, as is the duration of REM and its latency (Chernick et al, 1974). To what extent these changes represent alterations in the illness versus generalized effects of lithium per se is not clear, but clinically the effects of lithium on sleep are not striking; in most patients, a large dose at bedtime has a mild sedative effect. Occasionally, patients will report feeling activated following their nighttime dose of lithium, perhaps reflecting a high blood level.

Management of "Breakthrough" Manias and Depressions in Lithium Treated Patients

Since the management of breakthrough episodes fundamentally involves strategies very similar to those described earlier in the section on the acute treatment of mania and depression, we will review them here only briefly.

For *breakthrough symptoms of hypomania*, the first approach is generally an increase in the lithium dose while closely monitoring the blood level. If hypomanic symptoms persist after reaching a maximum tolerable lithium level, a neuroleptic or carbamazepine should be added, initially in small doses and preferably at bedtime. One alternative suggestion is to add L–tryptophan 1.5 to 3 gms (with 100–300 mg Vitamin B_6); although this has been reported as effective in some studies, not everyone agrees. Early detection of hypomania is most critical; often a decreased need for sleep is the first clue. In the face of a rapid onset of manic symptoms, a neuroleptic or carbamazepine should be added immediately without waiting to adjust the lithium level. If neuroleptics are used in this way, they should be tapered and discontinued soon after the symptoms are under control. A few bipolar patients, generally those with schizoaffective symptoms, will need continued management with neuroleptics. Even in these cases, the effort to get them off the drug or on lower doses should not be abandoned.

Breakthrough depressions of varying severity constitute one of the most important challenges in the management of bipolar patients on lithium. The first response to the appearance of depressive symptoms should include a reevaluation of the lithium level and thyroid function, as well as a reassessment of the patient's life situation with particular reference to real or perceived losses. The lithium level should be raised to at least 1.2 mEq/1 or higher, since some of breakthrough depressions will respond to increased lithium, usually within a week to 10 days.

As noted earlier, thyroid medication is clearly appropriate when there is chemical evidence of hypothyroidism. Is thyroid supplement ever appropriate as a treatment for breakthrough depression in the absence of clear evidence of hypothyroidism? Since chemical thyroid indices have a wide "normal range," it is not always clear whether a "normal" value is really optimal for a given patient. Frequently, one finds that the prelithium baseline values were also in the low normal range, so that there is no chemical indication of a lithium induced hypothyroidism. But, since affective illness itself may be associated with low thyroid function, the fact that baseline values were in the same range does not rule out supplemental thyroid. It is the authors' experience that rigid adherence to the "normal" range of thyroid indices would deny many patients the considerable benefit attendant to the use of small doses of supplemental thyroid medication. Doses should start at 25 micrograms of T_4 once a day (but not in the evening or night) and progress in increments of 25 micrograms with monitoring of blood thyroid indices.

If the response to thyroid optimization and increased lithium is not satisfactory, the clinician and patient must decide whether to add an antidepressant drug. If the depression is only moderately severe, it might be better to provide more psychological support and avoid antidepressants because of their potential for worsening the course of the illness (Wehr and Goodwin, in press). This conservative approach is especially worthwhile when the patient has been on lithium for only a year or two, since there is a tendency for the prophylactic efficacy of lithium to improve with time.

On the other hand, if the depression is severe enough to cause considerable suffering, and especially if normal functioning becomes significantly impaired, antidepressants are indicated. Tricyclics are still the most frequently used antidepressants in this situation, and among them, those with less sedative effect (such as imipramine, desmethylimipramine, or nortriptyline) are preferred, since breakthrough depressions in bipolar patients are frequently characterized by anergy and lassitude, while anxiety, sleep disturbance, and psychic pain are not as prominent. One of the "second generation" heterocyclic antidepressants may also be considered, especially if one is concerned about the greater likelihood of side effects with the "traditional" tricyclic drugs. On the other hand, the efficacy of these new drugs is generally not as well established, especially when the breakthrough depression is quite severe. Doses of the antidepressant should generally be somewhat lower than those used in the absence of lithium, since some side effects, such as tremor and sedation, can be additive. Because of the risk of precipitating mania/hypomania (even in the presence of lithium), these drugs should be gradually withdrawn shortly after the antidepressant response is achieved.

Recently, the use of monoamine oxidase inhibitors has undergone somewhat of a renaissance, and they are increasingly used as an alternative to tricyclic (or heterocyclic) antidepressants for the treatment of breakthrough depressions in patients on lithium. In fact, some authorities now recommend MAOIs as the treatment of choice in such cases. Studies on the administration of MAO inhibitors in combination with lithium have been reviewed elsewhere (Kupfer and Detre, 1978).

Several reports suggest a role for other pharmacologic agents (besides thyroid hormone) as adjunctive treatments in combination with tricyclic antidepressants. These include psychostimulants (Ayd and Zohar, 1985), reserpine (Ayd, 1985), and gonadal steroids (Klaiber et al, 1979; Vogel et al, 1985). Although technically contraindicated, psychostimulants have recently been successfully combined with MAOIs without serious side effects (Feigner et al, 1985). Two recently developed nonpharmacologic approaches also deserve mention. Partial sleep deprivation—that is, keeping the patient awake from 2 A.M. through 11 P.M.—has been found to produce antidepressant effects similar to an entire night's sleep deprivation, but has the advantage of being able to be administered repetitively. Some recent evidence (Sack et al, 1985; Baxter et al, 1985) suggests that this technique may potentiate and/or accelerate response to both tricyclic antidepressants and lithium. Finally, phototherapy (high intensity light) may provide a good antidepressant effect for breakthrough depressions, especially those occurring during the fall and winter, and is discussed in more detail by Wehr and colleagues in Chapter 3 of this volume.

Miscellaneous Issues in Lithium Maintenance

TIMING OF THE DOSE. A great deal has been written about the pharmacokinetics of lithium and the advantages and disadvantages of various preparations and schedules of administration. One question is whether "sustained release" preparations offer sufficient advantage to justify their increased cost. For the data supporting the various positions in this argument, we refer the reader to reviews (Amdisen, 1980; Grof, 1979). The higher peak of lithium obtained with a single daily dose of the standard preparation has been associated with a lesser incidence of renal side effects (Plenge and Rafaelson, 1982), presumably due to the "rest" given the kidneys during the trough in plasma lithium levels 18–24 hours after the single dose. One argument against the sustained release preparations, in addition to their higher cost, focuses on some reports of variability in absorption.

In general the fewer doses per day the better, primarily as a matter of convenience and therefore compliance; many patients find it difficult to remember to take a pill several times a day, especially when there are few, if any, symptoms to remind them of why they are taking it. Also, once-a-day dosing decreases the social embarrassment that can be associated with being on lithium. Taking the entire dose at bedtime means that the blood level decreases progressively during the day, a desirable occurrence if one considers side effects. There is extensive evidence that once-a-day administration provides as satisfactory a prophylactic result as divided doses do. In the authors' experience, the great majority of patients tolerate a single bedtime dose quite well, and with this regimen they will experience the peak levels while asleep; any side effects they do experience during the day will be concentrated in the early morning. There are patients, on the other hand, with exquisite sensitivity to the cognitive side effects of lithium, whose illness requires that they be maintained at relatively high levels; such patients will often do better on sustained release preparations since, given the high total dose needed for prophylaxis, peak levels in response to standard lithium preparations would not be tolerable.

PLASMA MONITORING. Plasma monitoring should be obtained as close as possible to 12 hours following the last doses of lithium; that is, the morning after a bedtime dose. In patients who take their entire dose at night, the 12-hour blood level will be approximately 15 percent higher than on a divided dose of the standard preparation. Patients who cross several time zones while on lithium must be careful to avoid confusion about the timing of the doses. Anecdotal evidence that "jet lag" can be associated with mood destabilization in some patients indicates that an adequate lithium level can be especially important. The approach that we follow is to "split the difference" between the old and the new time in planning the dosage schedule. It is also very important to scrupulously maintain adequate hydration during such travel, since transmeridial flying can induce shifts in fluid and electrolyte balance.

LITHIUM "HOLIDAYS." Lithium "holidays" have been advocated for some patients analogous to the recommendation of neuroleptic holidays (Ayd, 1981). The rationale is that holidays might minimize long-term side effects by giving the body's systems an opportunity to recover from sustained exposure to the drug. Ayd reports mixed results; some patients have sustained progressively longer holidays (to the point of withdrawal) without relapse, but others have relapsed relatively quickly. Although this is an interesting research technique that deserves further exploration, it cannot be recommended as a clinical practice at this point. In the first place, a brief holiday is really equivalent to lowering the lithium level; as we have noted earlier, there is good reason to use the lowest maintenance levels that preserve effective prophylaxis, but this can be accomplished best by gradual reduction in the daily dose, since this does not involve repeated sudden changes in plasma level. Another problem with lithium holidays is the potential for subtle encouragement of poor compliance. A patient who finds himself symptom free while off lithium, with the doctor's blessing, may mistakenly assume that he or she no longer needs the drug. Every experienced clinician knows that often when a patient is taken off lithium for a medical or surgical reason, it can be difficult to convince that patient to go back on it. If the clinician feels that the patient might be receiving more lithium than he or she really needs, the preferable approach is to gradually lower the daily dose. On the other hand, if one wishes to try a period without lithium, the safest approach is to gradually decrease the dose until it is fully withdrawn, rather than to gradually lengthen the drug-free periods.

The most common reason for an off-lithium period is preparation for pregnancy. In some patients, it may be feasible to select a "lower vulnerability" time of the year that can be used for the off-lithium period. Although for most manic-depressive patients pregnancy itself is a period of mood stability, it is important to resume lithium at least a few weeks before the birth is expected because of the high risk of postpartum mania and/or depression. Lithium levels should, of course, be lowered immediately before parturition, and be followed carefully during the immediate postpartum period until fluid and electrolyte balance is normalized again.

One interesting and related unstudied aspect of long-term lithium maintenance is the potential for some positive contributions to general health associated with the treatment. Many lithium treated patients note a decreased frequency of common colds and flu-like episodes—a phenomenon which, if real, may be traceable to certain stimulatory effects of the ion on the immune system. Anecdotal reports have also suggested a decrease in the expected incidence of myocardial infarction in males maintained on lithium. If true, this might be partially due to a general decrease in mood related stress.

SUMMARY

The first step in initiating treatment is a pretreatment evaluation, including a detailed assessment of past course of illness, a medical history focused according to the drug treatment under consideration, a baseline evaluation of side effects, and selection of a rating scale for baseline and subsequent mood evaluation. For acute mania, the choice of drug depends on the setting, symptoms, concurrent medical conditions, and drugs used. Mainstays of treatment for acute mania include lithium, neuroleptic drugs, carbamazepine, and ECT. In general, dose titration depends on the severity of mania, the rapidity of clinical response, and certain physical characteristics of the individual. Lithium levels change with clinical state, and the levels required to produce therapeutic and toxic effects vary individually. ECT is a rapid, effective antimanic agent that is probably underutilized. Carbamazepine may work as rapidly as neuroleptics and is now being given consideration as a first choice alternative to neuroleptic drugs as an adjunct to lithium. Hospitalization may be required depending on the situation, and because of the severity of mania, obtaining informed consent in advance for treatment and/or hospitalization is advisable. For acute depression, the pretreatment evaluation is similar, but must also include careful assessment of suicidality, as well as the presence or absence of past manic episodes and the family history of drug responsiveness, since there is some evidence that there is a genetic component to drug response.

The decision to initiate treatment usually depends on the overall severity of the condition, the particular symptoms, and the extent of functional impairment. Lithium should be started first and may, by itself, be an effective antidepressant, although more severe depressions may require adjunctive antidepressant treatments at the outset. There is also the risk of precipitating a mania with antidepressant treatment even if the patient is on lithium. Both tricyclic antidepressants and monamine oxidase inhibitors are effective antidepressants, and the latter class of drug, often reserved for tricyclic antidepressant nonresponders, may be especially effective in bipolar depression and is probably underutilized. Tricyclic and monoamine oxidase inhibitor antidepressants, given in combination, are also safe and potentially effective. Antidepressant treatment failures are commonly due to inadequate dosage or inadequate time on the drug. Again, ECT is probably underutilized in depression, and is especially effective in delusional depressions. Indications for hospitalization for acute bipolar depression are similar to those previously mentioned for acute mania, with the additional need to assure the safety of a suicidal patient. The duration of antidepressant treatment should be 9 to 12 months before treatment is tapered and discontinued.

The possibility of precipitating hypomanic reactions on tapering or discontinuation of antidepressants must also be kept in mind. Selection of the patient for maintenance treatment involves balancing projected risks and benefits of both future episodes of illness and taking a drug. Factors that need to be kept in mind in making this decision include the likelihood of relapse (increased with both age and with past number of episodes), the likelihood of a manic course (increased in males), the severity of illness, the onset of episodes (gradual versus sudden), and the adequacy of support systems for detecting early symptoms and bringing the patient into treatment.

The optimal lithium level needs to be individualized and ranges from 0.6 to 1.2 mEq/l. Plasma lithium level monitoring should be continuous (every 4 to 8 weeks) to ensure a patient's continued awareness of the illness and thereby facilitate compliance. Circumstances affecting the lithium level can include flu, anesthesia, alterations in diet, and alterations in both physical activity and mood state. The occurrence of side effects due to lithium can be managed, depending on the side effect, with dose reduction, adjunctive medications, and alteration of habits.

Lithium can interact with a wide variety of different drugs. Breakthrough manic episodes can be treated with the addition of neuroleptic drugs or carbamazepine to lithium, and perhaps even the addition of 1.5 to 3 grams of L–tryptophan. The occurrence of breakthrough depression should prompt evaluation of thyroid function and consideration of supplemental thyroid medication. Continued depression should prompt initiation of either tricyclic antidepressant or monoamine oxidase inhibitor drugs.

Finally, regarding the chronic use of lithium, there are no hard and fast rules concerning dosing regimen or type of preparation, with the clinician's choice depending on the individual's needs. Plasma monitoring should always occur about 12 hours after the last dose. Patients crossing several time zones while traveling need to split the difference in the time to maintain an adequate lithium level. Finally, the advocacy of lithium "holidays" by some investigators has not been systematically tested. Such "holidays" may pose a danger by encouraging noncompliance and precipitating a breakthrough manic or depressive episode.

REFERENCES

Abrams A, Taylor MA: EEG observations during combined lithium and neuroleptic treatment. Am J Psychiatry 136:336-337, 1979

Almy GL, Taylor MA: Lithium retention in mania. Arch Gen Psychiatry 29:232-234, 1973

Amdisen A: Lithium, in Applied Pharmacokinetics. Edited by Evans WE, Schentag JJ, Jusko WJ. San Francisco, Applied Therapeutics, Inc, 1980

American Psychiatric Association Task Force on the Use of Laboratory Tests in Psychiatry: Tricyclic antidepressants—blood level measurements and clinical outcome. Am J Psychiatry 142:155-162, 1985

Amsterdam J, Brunswick D, Mendels J: The clinical application of tricyclic antidepressant pharmacokinetics and plasma levels. Am J Psychiatry 137:653-662, 1981

Angst J: The course of affective disorders, II: typology of bipolar manic-depressive illness. Archiv Fur Psychiatrie und Nervenkrankheiten 226:65-74, 1978

Angst J, Grof P: Selection of patients with recurrent affective illness for a long term study: testing research criteria on prospective follow-up data, in Lithium: Controversies and Unresolved Issues. Edited by Cooper TB, Gershon S, Kline NS, et al. Amsterdam, Excerpta Medica, 1979

Angst J: Verlauf unipolar depressiver, bipolar manisch-depressiver und schizo-affectiver erkrankungen und psychosen ergebnisse einer prospektiven studie. Fortschr Neurol Psychiatr 48:3-30, 1980

Ayd FR Jr: Lithium holidays. International Drug Therapy Newsletter 16:17-19, 1981

Ayd FJ Jr: Reserpine therapy for tricyclic-resistant depression. International Drug Therapy Newsletter 20:17-18, 1985

Ayd FJ Jr, Zohar J: Psychostimulant (amphetamine or methylphenidate) therapy for chronic and treatment-resistant depression, in Treating Resistant Depression. Edited by Zohar J, Belmaker RH. New York, Spectrum Press (in press)

Baastrup PC, Hollnagel P, Sorensen R, et al: Adverse reactions in treatment with lithium carbonate and haloperidol. JAMA 236:2645-2646, 1976

Baldessarini RJ: Chemotherapy in Psychiatry. Cambridge, Harvard University Press, 1977

Baxter LR Jr: Can lithium carbonate prolong the antidepressant effect of sleep deprivation? Arch Gen Psychiatry 42:635, 1985

Biederman J, Lerner Y, Belmaker RH: Combination of lithium carbonate and haloperidol in schizo-affective disorder: a controlled study. Arch Gen Psychiatry 36:327-333, 1979

Brancher MH, Simpson GM: Cogwheel rigidity early in lithium treatments. Am J Psychiatry 134:211, 1977

Branchey MH, Charles J, Simpson GM: Extrapyramidal side effects in lithium maintenance therapy. Am J Psychiatry 133:444-445, 1976

Byrd GL: Lithium carbonate and methyldopa: apparent interaction in man. Clinical Toxicology 11:1-4, 1977

Champ SS, Pandey GN, Cooper RC, et al: Pharmacokinetics of lithium: predicting optimal dosage, in Lithium Controversies and Unresolved Issues. Edited by Cooper T, Gershon S, Kline NS, et al. Amsterdam, Excerpta Medica, 1979

Chernik DA, Cochrane C, Mendels J: Effects of lithium carbonate on sleep. J Psychiatry Res 10:133-146, 1974

Chouinard G, Young SN, Annable L: A controlled clinical trial of L–tryptophan in acute mania. Biol Psychiatry 20:546-557, 1985

Cohen BM, Lipinski JF, Altesman RI: Lecithin in the treatment of mania: double-blind, placebo-controlled trials. Am J Psychiatry 139:1162-1164, 1982

Cooper TB, Simpson GM: The 24-hour lithium level as a prognosticator of dosage requirements: a 2-year follow-up study. Am J Psychiatry 133:440-443, 1976

DePaulo JR Jr, Correa EI, Sapir DG: Renal glomerular function and long-term lithium therapy. Am J Psychiatry 138:324-327, 1981

DePaulo JR Jr, Correa EI: Renal effects of lithium. International Drug Therapy Newsletter 20:13, 1985

Dunner DL, Murphy D, Stallone F, et al: Episode frequency prior to lithium treatment in bipolar manic-depressive patients. Compr Psychiatry 20:511-515, 1979

Emrich HM, von Zerssen D, Moller HJ, et al: Action of propranolol in mania: comparison of effects of the d- and the l-stereoisomer. Pharmakopsychiatrie 12:295-304, 1979

Fava GA, Molnar G, Block B, et al: The lithium loading dose method in a clinical setting. Am J Psychiatry 141:812-813, 1984

Feighner JP, Herbstein J, Damlouji N: Combined MAOI, TCA, and direct stimulant therapy of treatment-resistant depression. J Clin Psychiatry 46:206-209, 1985

Fink M: Convulsive Therapy—Theory and Practice. New York, Raven Press, 1979

Goodwin FK: Drug treatment of affective disorders: general principles, in Psychopharmacology in the Practice of Medicine. Edited by Jarvik M. New York, Appelton Century Crofts, 1977

Goodwin FK: The impact of antidepressant treatment on the course of recurrent affective disorders, in Epidemiological Impact of Psychotropic Drugs. Edited by Tognoni G, Bellantuono C, Lader M. New York, Elsevier/North Holland Biomedical Press, 1981

Goodwin FK, Jamison KR: The natural course of recurrent affective illness, in Neurobiology of the Mood Disorders. Edited by Post RM, Ballenger JC. Baltimore, Williams & Wilkins, 1984

Goodwin FK, Zis AP: Lithium in mania: comparisons with neuroleptics and the issue of specificity, in Lithium: Controversies and Unresolved Issues. Edited by Cooper T, Gershon S, Kline NS, et al. Amsterdam, Excerpta Medica, 1979

Goodwin FK, Murphy DL, Bunney WE Jr: Lithium carbonate treatment in depression and mania: a longitudinal double-blind study. Arch Gen Psychiatry 21:486-496, 1969

Greenspan K, Green R, Durrell J: Retention and distribution patterns of lithium: a pharmacologic tool in studying the pathophysiology of manic-depressive psychosis. Am J Psychiatry 125:512-519, 1968

Grof P: Some practical aspects of lithium treatment: blood levels, dosage prediction, and slow-release preparations. Arch Gen Psychiatry 36:891-893, 1979

Grof P, MacCrimmon DJ, Smith EKM, et al: Long-term lithium treatment and the kidney. Can J Psychiatry 25:535-545, 1980

Hart RG, Easton JD: Carbamazepine and hematological monitoring. Ann Neurol 11:309-312, 1982

Havdala HS, Borison RL, Diamond BI: Potential hazards and applications of lithium in anesthesiology. Anesthesiology 50:534-537, 1979

Himmelhoch JM, Neil JF: Lithium therapy in combination with other forms of treatment, in Handbook of Lithium Therapy. Edited by Johnson FN. Lancaster, England, MTP Press, Ltd, 1980

Himmelhoch JM, Detre T, Kupfer DJ, et al: Treatment of previously intractable depressions with tranylcypromine and lithium. J Nerv Ment Dis 155:216, 1972

Himmelhoch JM, Forrest J, Neil JF, et al: Thiazide–lithium synergy in refractory mood swings. Am J Psychiatry 134:149-152, 1977

Hoenig J, Chaulk R: Delirium associated with lithium therapy and electroconvulsive therapy. Community Medical Association Journal 116:837-838, 1977

Hullin RP, McDonald R, McAnderson W, et al: Prophylactic lithium. Lancet 1:1155-1156, 1968

Jefferson JW, Kalin NH: Serum lithium levels and long-term diuretic use. JAMA 241:1134-1136, 1979

Jefferson JW, Greist JH, Baudhuin M: Lithium: interactions with other drugs. J Clin Psychopharmacol 1:124-134, 1981

Jefferson JW, Greist JH, Clagnaz PJ, et al: Effect of strenuous exercise on serum lithium levels in man. Am J Psychiatry 139:1593-1595, 1982

Joffe RT, Post RM, Roy-Byrne PP, et al: Hematological effects of carbamazepine in patients with affective illness. Am J Psychiatry 142:1196-1199, 1985

Jouvent R, Lecrubier Y, Peuch AJ, et al: Anti-manic effect of clonidine. Am J Psychiatry 137:1275-1276, 1980

Kallen B, Tandberg A: Lithium and pregnancy. Acta Psychiatr Scand 68:134-139, 1983

Kane J, Rifkin A, Quitkin F, et al: Extrapyramidal side effects with lithium treatment. Am J Psychiatry 135:851-853, 1978

Kemp K, Lion JR, Marpram G: Lithium in the treatment of a manic patient with multiple sclerosis: a case report. Diseases of the Nervous System 38:210-211, 1977

Klaiber EL, Broverman DM, Vogel W, et al: Estrogen therapy for severe persistent depression in women. Arch Gen Psychiatry 36:550-560, 1979

Klein DF, Gittelman R, Quitkin F, et al: Diagnosis and Drug Treatment of Psychiatric Disorders: Adults and Children. Baltimore, Williams & Wilkins, 1980

Krauthammer C, Klerman G: Secondary mania. Arch Gen Psychiatry 35:1333-1339, 1978

Kukopulos A, Reginaldi D, Laddomada P, et al: Course of the manic-depressive cycle and changes caused by treatment. Pharmakopsychiatrie Neuro-psychopharmakologie 13:156-167, 1980

Kupfer DJ, Detre TP: Tricyclic and monoamine oxidase inhibitor antidepressants: clinical use, in Handbook of Psychopharmacology, vol. 14. Edited by Iversen LL, Iversen SD, Snyder SH. New York, Plenum Press, 1978

Lang AE: Lithium and parkinsonism. Ann Neurol 15:214, 1984

Lesar TS, Tollefson G, Koch M: Relationship between patient variables and lithium dosage requirements. J Clin Psychiatry 46:133-136, 1985

Mandel MR, Madsen J, Miller AL, et al: Intoxication associated with lithium and ECT. Am J Psychiatry 137:1107-1109, 1980

Marley E, Wozniak KM: Clinical and experimental aspects of interactions between amine oxidase inhibitors and amine re-uptake inhibitors. Psychol Med 13:735-749, 1983

McGennis AJ: Lithium carbonate and tetracycline interaction. Br Med J 1:1183, 1978

Mitchell JE, Mackenzie TB: Cardiac effects of lithium therapy in man: a review. J Clin Psychiatry 43:47-51, 1982

Modell JG, Lenox RH, Weiner S: Inpatient clinical trial of lorazepam for the management of manic agitation. J Clin Psychopharmacol 5:109-113, 1985

Murphy DL, Pickar D, Alterman IS: Methods for the quantitative assessment of depressive and manic behavior, in The Behavior of Psychiatric Patients: Quantitative Techniques for Evaluation. Edited by Burdock EI, Sudilovsky A, Gershon S. New York, Marcel Dekker, Inc, 1982

Nelson JC, Schottenfeld RS, Conrad CD: Hypomania after desipramine withdrawal. Am J Psychiatry 140:624-625, 1983

O'Reagan JB: Adverse interaction of lithium carbonate and methyldopa. Can Med Assoc J 115:385-386, 1976

Pare CMB: Differentiation of two genetically specific types of depression by the response to antidepressants. Lancet 2:1340-1343, 1962

Perris C: A study of bipolar (manic-depressive) and unipolar recurrent depressive psychoses. Acta Psychiatr Scand (Suppl. 194) 42:9-184, 1966

Perry PJ, Prince RA, Alexander B, et al: Prediction of lithium maintenance doses using a single point prediction protocol. J Clin Psychopharmacol 3:13-17, 1983

Perry PJ, Alexander B, Prince RA, et al: Prospective evaluation of two lithium maintenance dose schedules. J Clin Psychopharmacol 4:242-246, 1984

Plenge P, Rafaelson OJ: Lithium treatment: does the kidney transfer one daily dose instead of two? Arch Psychiatr Scand 66:121-128, 1982

Potter WZ, Linnoila M: Tricyclic antidepressant concentrations, clinical and research implication, in Neurobiology of the Mood Disorders. Edited by Post RM, Ballenger JC. Baltimore, Williams & Wilkins, 1984

Quitkin FM: The importance of dosage in prescribing antidepressants. Br J Psychiatry 147:593-597, 1985

Quitkin FM, Rabkin JG, Ross D, et al: Duration of antidepressant drug treatment. Arch Gen Psychiatry 41:238-245, 1984

Ramsay RE, Wilder BJ, Berger JR, et al: A double-blind study comparing carbamazepine with phenytoin as initial seizure therapy in adults with epilepsy. Neurology 33:904-910, 1983

Ramsey TA, Cox M: Lithium and the kidney: a review. Am J Psychiatry 139:443-449, 1982

Razani J, White KL, White J, et al: The safety and efficacy of combined amitriptyline and tranylcypromine antidepressant treatment. Arch Gen Psychiatry 40:657-661, 1983

Reimann IW, Diener U, Frolich JC: Indomethacine but not aspirin increases plasma lithium ion levels. Arch Gen Psychiatry 40:283-286, 1983

Remick RA: Acute brain syndrome associated with ECT and lithium. Canadian Psychiatric Association Journal 23:129-130, 1978

Rey AC, Jimerson DC, Post RM: Lithium and electrolytes in cerebrospinal fluid of affectively ill patients during acute and chronic lithium treatment. Communications in Psychopharmacology 3:267-278, 1979

Roy-Byrne P, Post RM, Uhde TW, et al: The longitudinal course of recurrent affective illness: life chart data from research patients at the NIMH. Acta Psychiatr Scand (Suppl. 317) 71:1-34, 1985

Sack DA, Nurnberger J, Rosenthal NE, et al: Potentiation of antidepressant medications by phase advance of the sleep–wake cycle. Am J Psychiatry 142:606-608, 1985

Saffer D, Coppen A: Frusemide: a safe diuretic during lithium therapy? J Affective Disord 5:289-292, 1983

Schou M: Prophylactic lithium maintenance treatment in recurrent endogenous affective disorders, in Lithium: Its Role in Psychiatric Research and Treatment. Edited by Gershon S, Shopsin B. New York, Plenum Press, 1973

Schou M: Lithium for affective disorders: cost and benefit, in Mood Disorders: The World's Major Public Health Problem. Edited by Ayd F, Taylor I. Baltimore, Ayd Medical Communications, 1978

Schukit M, Robins E. Feignher J: Tricyclic antidepressants and monoamine oxidase inhibitors: combination therapy in the treatment of depression. Arch Gen Psychiatry 24:509-514, 1971

Serry M: The lithium excretion test: clinical application and interpretation. Aust NZ J Psychiatry 3:390-394, 1969

Shopsin B: Bupropion's prophylactic efficacy in bipolar affective illness. J Clin Psychiatry 44:163-169, 1983

Small JG, Kellams JJ, Milstein V, et al: Complications with electroconvulsive treatment combined with lithium. Biol Psychiatry 15:103-112, 1980

Small JG, Small IF, Milstein V, et al: Manic symptoms: an indication for bilateral ECT. Biol Psychiatry 20:125-134, 1985

Spiker DG, Pugh DD: Combining tricyclic and monoamine oxidase inhibitor antidepressants. Arch Gen Psychiatry 33:828-830, 1976

Spring GK: Neurotoxicity with combined use of lithium and thioridazine. J Clin Psychiatry 40:135-138, 1979

Stern SL, Rush J, Mendels J: Toward a rational pharmacotherapy of depression. Am J Psychiatry 137:545-552, 1980

Stokes PE, Koskis JH, Arcuni OJ: Relationship of lithium chloride dose to treatment response in mania. Arch Gen Psychiatry 33:1080-1084, 1976

Trautner EM, Morris R, Noack CH, et al: The excretion and retention of ingested lithium and its effect on the ionic balance of man. Med J Aust 2:280-291, 1955

Van Brunt N: The clinical utility of tricyclic antidepressant blood levels: a review of the literature. Therapeutic Drug Monitoring 5:1-10, 1983

Vogel W, Klaiber EL, Broverman DM: A comparison of the antidepressant effects of a synthetic androgen (mesterolone) and amitriptyline in depressed men. J Clin Psychiatry 46:6-8, 1985

Wehr TA, Goodwin FK: Can antidepressants precipitate mania and worsen the course of affective illness? Am J Psychiatry (in press)

White K, Simpson G: Combined MAOI–tricyclic antidepressant treatment: a reevaluation. Presented to the American College of Neuropsychopharmacology, 1980

Zis AP, Grof P, Goodwin, FK: The natural course of affective disorders: implications for lithium prophylaxis, in Lithium: Controversies and Unresolved Issues. Edited by Cooper TB, Gershon S, Kline NS, et al. Amsterdam, Excerpta Medica, 1979

Chapter 5

Psychotherapeutic Issues and Suicide Prevention in the Treatment of Bipolar Disorders

by Kay Redfield Jamison, Ph.D.

There is a growing tendency to recognize the importance of psychological issues and psychotherapeutic techniques in the effective and compassionate treatment of bipolar manic-depressive illness. Less frequently discussed, but crucial, is the prevention of suicide in bipolar patients. General psychological issues will be covered in the first section of this chapter and suicide prevention will be covered in the second. For a comprehensive review of these issues, see Goodwin and Jamison (in press).

GENERAL PSYCHOLOGICAL ISSUES

The Therapeutic Alliance in Drug Treatment

Earlier papers have dealt formally and extensively with the relationships between psychotherapy and drugs, especially lithium, in the management of bipolar patients (Goodwin, 1977; Jamison and Akiskal, 1983; Jamison and Goodwin, 1983a, 1983b). To restate a fundamental truth in psychopharmacology: for any drug to achieve its full therapeutic potential, it should be given in the context of a solid and positive doctor–patient relationship—that is, there must be a working therapeutic alliance. In most instances, this is best achieved by approaching the drug trial as an investigative undertaking, which depends on active collaboration between patient and clinician. It is well known that controlled double blind studies of antidepressant drugs consistently report success rates substantially below those reported in open trials (Klein and Davis, 1969). In part, these differences certainly reflect methodological bias. However, it is also likely that one of the reasons that drugs appear to work better in an open setting is that the positive and reinforcing effects of the therapeutic alliance are able to operate (Sheard, 1963).

The clinician is in the best position to help the manic-depressive patient when he or she is able to convey an attitude of serious concern for the individual's suffering, while communicating confidence in his or her own ability and expressing measured optimism about the *ultimate* outcome of the drug trials. It is exceedingly important not to overestimate treatment results with any particular drug. It is self-defeating since, if the first drug fails to work, the patient's trust is eroded and the physician feels defeated and discredited. These attitudes may, in turn, be subtly conveyed to the patient. When a trial of a given drug is viewed as an *experiment*, by doctor and patient alike, then even a poor response does not have to be experienced as a defeat, but rather as an important piece of new information not available previously that contributes substantially to the rational choice of subsequent drugs. It is helpful to make this explicit to the patient by pointing out that nonresponders to one class of drugs are more likely to be responders to an alternate class (Goodwin, 1977).

A good relationship between clinician and patient is particularly important in the *prophylactic* treatment of manic-depressive illness. Aside from the inherent course and severity of the illness, the single most important determinant of the success or failure in medication maintenance is the quality of the therapeutic alliance. When referring to the therapeutic alliance in prophylactic management, we do not mean formal psychotherapy in the traditional sense of a focus on psychodynamic conflicts (although dynamic psychotherapy is certainly appropriate for many patients on lithium), but rather refer to psychotherapy issues indispensable to long-term medication management. Thus, good prophylactic management includes sensitive teaching about the illness and its treatment. Second, it must be continuously emphasized that prophylactic management is a collaborative venture between the clinician and the patient, with each having an important and independent role. Finally, it is important that a family member be available whenever possible, particularly in dealing with acute phases of the illness. These issues are discussed more fully later in this section, and extensively in Goodwin and Jamison (in press).

COMMUNICATION OF INFORMATION. The explicit communication of information about the nature and treatment of manic-depressive illness is fundamental to responsible and effective medical care. Patients should be given written and verbal information about the natural history of their disease (especially its unrelentingly recurrent nature), its symptoms, relevant genetic information, and available treatments. Several aspects specific to medical care and to suicidality should be discussed with the patient and, where appropriate, the family. In addition to giving patients written material about their illness and medications prescribed, we have found it useful to emphasize, among others, these points:

- Manic-depressive illness is a serious, but treatable, illness.
- If left *untreated*, the risk of recurrence is high. Taking lithium and/or other medications as prescribed is imperative. Explaining to the patient and family that denial of recurrence is a very common phenomenon anticipates their feelings, and thereby lends credence to the clinician's recommendations.
- Lithium works as effectively in preventing depressions as it does manias, but there is usually more of a time delay in its effect in preventing depressions. It is important that the patient (and clinician) not be discouraged by this, nor assume that depressions are inevitable.
- Side-effects occur with most medications; many can be ameliorated, some cannot. Possible side-effects should be made explicit and information should be given about how transitory or permanent they are likely to be.
- Patients who are on antidepressant medications should be warned that the time course for a drug response may lead to a discrepancy between what their physician sees as improvement and what they themselves are experiencing. For example, the physician and family may see the patient as "improved" because he or she has more energy, sleep is better, and the patient's face and body are more animated. These changes generally occur earlier than improvements in mood and thinking, changes which are more likely to be important

to the patient. Predicting this discrepancy in perceptions can lessen some of the discouragement felt by patients. This is of concern because this stage in the patient's illness—that is, the beginning of recovery with increased energy—is a high risk time for suicide.

- As the patient's condition begins to improve, it is important to explain that this may be a particularly frustrating and difficult time because temporary setbacks are common; an explanation of this "saw tooth" pattern of recovery can be very reassuring.
- Patients should be informed that alcohol generally worsens depression, interferes with sleep, decreases judgment, and potentiates the side effects of other medications they may be taking.
- When depressed, patients should be advised to avoid significant social or personal changes and to obtain a leave of absence from school or work rather than quit.

MEDICATION MONITORING. Instructions about medications—dosages, timing, potential side effects, and dangerous adverse reactions, potentiation by alcohol and other drugs—should be explicit and, whenever possible, in writing. If it is feasible to involve another individual (family member or friend) in monitoring medications, it is often a good idea to do so. Confusion, subconscious suicidality, and ambivalence about taking medication make depressed patients particularly susceptible to errors in this area of their treatment. Plastic pill boxes with separate sections for each day of the week are helpful to many patients, particularly those taking more than one medication.

Active collaboration between physician and patient is extremely important during ongoing drug maintenance. For example, lithium levels often are coarsely, rather than finely, tuned. This is especially true when a patient is considerably improved clinically and the physician is reluctant to alter the lithium level that "seems to be working." Unfortunately, it is at precisely this point that fine tuning of lithium is most productive. Too low a maintenance dose can precipitate breakthrough depressions, manias, and hypomanias which not only threaten a stable existence but, in vulnerable bipolar patients, also increase the likelihood of suicide. Conversely, too high a dose can cause unnecessary side-effects, some of which can be debilitating, demoralizing, and influence compliance. Subtle changes in dosages and timing—often involving active collaboration, self-ratings, and self-titrations on the part of patients—can powerfully affect the patient's productivity, notions of control, and attitudes toward medication.

FOLLOW-UP CARE. The chronic, recurrent, and serious nature of manic-depressive illness makes follow-up care a necessary part of good treatment. Hankoff (1982) has emphasized the importance of specialty clinics in providing continuity of care, and comments that they have the advantage of carrying with them a certain prestige in the public eye. Because of their biological associations, they are also relatively free of the "stigmatization handicap of other psychiatric programs." Gitlin and Jamison (1984) have discussed other advantages of specialty clinics: they are equipped to make rigorous diagnoses, provide highly specialized and up-to-date treatment, and treat a large number of patients having similar types of problems. While it is true that affective disorders clinics can provide such services, most patients with manic-depressive illness are not treated by such facilities, nor is there any compelling reason why they should be. The important point is that continuity of care must be provided, and diagnostic and specialized treatment consultation should be obtained when necessary.

Psychotherapy

GENERAL PSYCHOTHERAPEUTIC ISSUES. The importance of psychotherapy and studies of its efficacy in treatment of manic-depressive patients are reviewed elsewhere (Jamison and Akiskal, 1983; Jamison and Goodwin, 1983a, 1983b). We covered at length in those chapters the general psychotherapeutic issues frequently arising during the treatment of bipolar patients and the essential role which psychotherapy can play in dealing with emotional turmoil, a reluctance to take long-term medications, or the establishment of psychological and interpersonal equilibrium. Here I will only reiterate and summarize briefly a few of the points made earlier. First and foremost, I again stress the importance of the clinician's thorough knowledge of manic-depressive illness: its natural history, psychobiology, diagnosis, and treatment. Such knowledge is critical to the competent and empathetic psychotherapy of manic-depressive patients. Specific psychotherapeutic issues which arise time and again in treating bipolar illness are discussed in detail in earlier papers (Jamison and Goodwin, 1983a, 1983b). Therefore, I list them here only as a reminder of concerns many patients have: 1) fears of recurrence; 2) denial of having a chronic and potentially life-threatening illness; 3) learning to discriminate normal from pathological moods; 4) effects of manic-depressive illness on relationships; 5) effects of the illness on normal developmental stages and tasks; and 6) genetic concerns.

We have also emphasized the clinical importance of understanding the positive aspects of manic-depressive illness (that is, the increased energy, drive, enthusiasm, mood, and so forth). An appreciation of possible advantageous features of the illness and a recognition of the potentially "addictive" qualities of hypomania increase the likelihood of attracting manic-depressive individuals into treatment, as well as maintaining them on lithium once a treatment program has begun (Jamison et al, 1980).

THERAPEUTIC STYLE AND COUNTERTRANSFERENCE. Psychotherapy with manic-depressive patients requires considerable flexibility in therapeutic style and an ability to maintain a "long lead" approach in order to maximize the patient's sense of control. The potential for power struggles with bipolar patients is virtually limitless; to the extent possible, such struggles, especially around lithium, should be minimized. However, at the same time, it is also critical to maintain a sensitivity to subtle mood and behavior changes which might be prodromal to an affective episode, or reflective of a problem in medication compliance. A collaborative approach to treatment—obtained through systematic patient education and the use of self-ratings of mood and behavior, limited patient titration of lithium dosages, and so forth—can minimize many clinical difficulties arising during the treatment of bipolar patients.

Countertransference issues can be problematic for several reasons: the contagious nature of moods; difficulties in distinguishing subtle fluctuations in mood states from characterological problems; misinterpretation of mild depressions as "resistance"; hypomania induced special sensitivity to vulnerabilities in the therapist; and problems deriving from certain appeals of the hypomanic state (for example, potential for envy, projective identification, collusion with lithium noncompliance, guilt or concern over depriving patients of a "special state," and so on).

Lithium Compliance

REASONS FOR NONCOMPLIANCE. We focus here on lithium compliance because it remains the principal agent used in the treatment of manic-depressive illness, and because it has been the subject of virtually all studies of compliance in manic-depressive illness. Noncompliance with lithium treatment is the major clinical problem encountered by most clinicians who treat manic-depressive patients. Research suggests that 25–50 percent of patients—for different reasons and varying periods of time—will stop their lithium against medical advice (Jamison et al, 1979). Among the major reasons for noncompliance are lithium side-effects, denial of a serious and recurrent illness, missing of hypomanic episodes, feeling well and therefore perceiving no need for ongoing medication, decreased productivity and creativity, depressive relapses, and being bothered by the idea of one's moods being controlled by medication. Additional factors include the delayed therapeutic action of lithium and delay in negative consequences following its cessation. Unfortunately, the reinforcement schedules operating with this drug involve pairing the start of treatment with unpleasant events (psychosis, depression, hospitalization, and relationship and job problems), while cessation of lithium is often accompanied by immediate positive experience, either because of the disappearance of side-effects or because of breakthrough hypomanias.

MANAGEMENT OF COMPLIANCE PROBLEMS. Although this discussion focuses on lithium, the general principles apply to other drugs that also might be used in long-term management. As with all medications, it is important not to oversell the efficacy of lithium nor unduly minimize its side-effects and potential negative impact on lifestyle and emotional intensity. Within these constraints, however, a generally positive and encouraging view of treatment outcome is both reasonable and useful. To the extent that possible side-effects are predicted and discussed in advance, the clinician's integrity is maintained and unnecessary concerns can be allayed. Whenever possible, side-effects should be treated aggressively, and patients should be educated about control they can exert (for example, in weight gain, the high caloric drinks consumed to quench lithium induced thirst). Complaints about diminished memory and other intellectual capacities should be taken seriously, even though the etiology of such symptoms is unclear. Lithium blood level monitoring on a regular basis is important not only for medical purposes, but also to impress upon the patient a certain mutual seriousness of purpose and collaboration. Regular inquiries into a patient's attitudes toward lithium and compliance demonstrate a recognition that these are potential problems or issues. Not uncommonly, such inquiries reveal early concerns and ambivalence, and occasional noncompliance, which has been undetected by serum lithium levels. Charting of moods and behaviors can underscore the pivotal role of lithium in mood stabilization, as well as reiterating the importance of genuine collaboration between physician and patient. Limited titration of lithium levels by a patient, under the close supervision of the clinician, can assist in the patient's sense of control over his or her own treatment.

The psychological issues and approaches outlined above are valid for all manic-depressive patients on maintenance medication. In addition, for individual patients, the clinician should evaluate the need for more formal and extensive psychotherapy—individual, group, or family.

EVALUATION AND MANAGEMENT OF SUICIDE

Prevention of suicide in bipolar manic-depressive patients is, of course, inextricably bound to the prevention of further affective episodes. Thus, suicide prevention is most powerfully accomplished through the effective treatment of the illness itself. Early and accurate diagnosis is critical, as suicide is more likely to occur in the initial phases of the disease (Johnson and Hunt, 1979; Ottosson, 1979; Weeke, 1979; Hankoff, 1982). This early suicide risk period has significant implications for clinical management, ranging from the timing of medication maintenance therapy to possible intensification of clinical help (for example, more frequent medication visits and psychotherapy) in the first months and years of the illness. The sophisticated and aggressive identification of bipolar patients, already at high risk for suicide, is important; so too is the identification of those bipolar patients at even higher risk because of personal or family history and clinical state.

Clinical Evaluation

Procedures for taking a thorough history and criteria needed for reliable diagnostic decisions and general information about suicide in manic-depressive illness are covered in Goodwin and Jamison (in press). In this section, I will emphasize those aspects of history and diagnosis which are relevant to the prediction and clinical management of suicidal behaviors in patients with manic-depressive illness. These include the assessment of personal and family history, the patient's present psychiatric status, interpersonal assets and liabilities, and treatment history.

FAMILY HISTORY.   Patients, and whenever possible their families, should be asked in detail about any history of *suicide, suicide attempts,* or *violence* in their first degree relatives.

PATIENT HISTORY.   *Diagnosis:* The diagnosis of bipolar manic-depressive illness carries with it a high risk for suicide. This fact is of basic importance; the rest of this section concerns itself with identification of subgroups of bipolar patients and clinical conditions that further increase the likelihood of suicide. Diagnostic studies indicate that within the general population of bipolar patients, there is some evidence of increased suicide risk in patients experiencing only hypomanic, rather than manic, episodes (Dunner et al, 1976; Stallone et al, 1980). However, this difference is neither sufficiently documented nor predictive to be of use in clinical practice at the present time.

History of suicide attempts or ideation: By history, many (19–24 percent) of those who actually commit suicide attempted it on at least one earlier occasion; conversely, 10 percent of those who attempt suicide go on to kill themselves within 10 years of the attempt. Barraclough et al (1974) concluded from their study of depressives who did and did not commit suicide, ". . . an important distinction between the two groups is the previous tendency of those who kill themselves to think of suicide more and to act on the thought" (p. 359). Robins et al (1959), in their postmortem analysis of 134 suicides, wrote:

. . . if we had found that suicide was an impulsive, unpremeditated act without rather well defined clinical limits, then the problem of its prevention would present insurmountable difficulties using presently available clinical criteria. The high rate of communication of suicidal ideas indicates that in the majority of instances it is a premeditated act of which the person gives ample warning.

Most clinicians acknowledge the importance of a history of attempted suicide in the determination of current or future suicide risk; the consistency of the research findings to this effect underscores the vital necessity for acquiring such a history, especially in bipolar patients. Less importance is generally attached to a history of suicidal *ideation*. Perhaps suicidal thinking is assumed to be more universal in depressed patients, and therefore, less predictive of suicide than it in fact is. Too, some clinicians may perceive a wider gap between thought and action than actually exists. Next to establishing the correct diagnosis, one of the most important things a clinician can do in ascertaining suicide risk is to take a thorough history of suicidal ideation, suicide attempts, and grossly morbid thought patterns. Major areas of inquiry for a patient with such a history are listed in Table 1.

Course of illness: Certain points in the course of an illness, and in the course of an individual episode, carry with them an increased risk for suicide. The items that should be covered in a thorough history are outlined in Table 2.

History of violence: It is difficult, but extremely important, to elicit from the patient an accurate history of violent feelings, thoughts, and behaviors. Many patients—particularly women—are reluctant to disclose thoughts and actions so at variance with socially accepted behaviors and traditional notions of femininity (and those who do reveal such histories often are diagnosed as borderline

Table 1. The Evaluation of Suicide Risk: Major Areas of Inquiry

---

Suicidal Ideation and Attempt
- how often suicidal
- longest time suicidal
- precipitating events
- correlates of suicidal ideation
- presence or absence of mixed states
- use of alcohol and other drugs to cope with feelings
- the most serious and potentially lethal thoughts and feelings
- suggestions from patient about what might be helpful if suicidal crisis recurs

Suicide Attempt
- feelings just prior to the attempt
- ability to communicate thoughts and feelings while suicidal
- degree of impulsivity vs. degree of planning
- length of time suicidal prior to attempt
- degree of cumulative stress and discouragement vs. acute exacerbation (or both)

Table 2. The Evaluation of Suicide Risk: Variables Related to the Course of Illness

Point in the *overall course of the illness* at which any past suicide attempts or severe suicidal ideation took place, especially:
- latency from onset of illness
- latency from onset of diagnosis and treatment

Point in the *sequence of episodes* at which attempts or ideation took place; i.e., did patient attempt suicide in a depressive episode preceding, or following, a manic episode?

Point in the *individual episode* at which patient appeared to be most vulnerable to suicidality. Was it:
- in the transition from manic to depressive, depressive to manic, manic or depressive to euthymic state?
- relatively soon after the beginning of a depressive episode or well into it? (The duration of past episodes, treated and untreated, is important here.)
- during the "recovery stage" of an episode? If so, did the patient perceive he or she was recovering, or was it the perception of the physician, family, and friends?

Point at which the patient, on the basis of past episodes (if any), might reasonably be expected to begin recovery, and to recover.

Point in menstrual cycle where the combination of that point and the affective episode might place patient in special jeopardy.

Other points where patient might be at increased risk for suicide; e.g., postpartum, annual, seasonal, time-of-day, or other patterns.

---

or hysteric). Many patients are not questioned in sufficient detail, and yet others—those from whom violent feelings and relationships are an integral part of their lifestyles—have no realistic, normative idea of what constitutes an abnormal level of violence or a sense that their lives or thoughts are unusual. The general areas that should be explored with the patient are outlined in Table 3.

Patients also should be asked about any cyclicity in their violent feelings and behaviors: Are there variations in these as a function of the menstrual cycle, do they have discernible diurnal or seasonal patterns, or are they particularly pronounced in a given mood state (for example, mixed states, depression, hypomania, or mania)?

Assets and liabilities: "Minimum pathology in a suicidal person bereft of strengths may be lethal, while severe pathology in a person with unusual strengths may constitute only a moderate risk" (Motto, 1975). The severity of manic-depressive illness and the associated biological factors underlying suicide account for most, but by no means all, of the variance in differentiating those who kill themselves

Table 3. The Evaluation of Suicide Risk: Violent and/or Impulsive Behavior

---

A history of:
- bad or violent temper
- frequent physical violence or fighting with others
- child, animal, or spouse abuse
- frequent provocation of violence in others
- frequent and pronounced irritability, or a "quick fuse"
- feeling "wired"; sense of pent up energy (usually dysphoric)
- frequent sense of wanting to put a fist through the wall or a pane of glass, to "lash out" physically (or actually doing so)
- frequent vitriolic scenes of verbal abuse ("Virginia Woolf" scenes)
- tempestuous relationships
- violent sexual behaviors (*not* induced to stimulate response, but from a sense of feeling overstimulated)
- impulsive behaviors such as throwing things, attempting to jump out of moving cars, bolting from restaurants, impetuousness in social situations
- impulsivity manifested by sociopathic behavior; e.g., shoplifting and frequent conflicts with authority figures

---

from those who do not. In addition, a wide range of personal assets and liabilities combine with the strength of the suicidal state to form a frighteningly delicate balance between the decision to live or die. To some extent, "assets" and "liabilities" become relative terms, for serious mood disorders, ironically, can cause certain characteristics which are strengths under normal circumstances (for example, independence, confidence, and self-determination) to become liabilities when an individual is depressed or suicidal. The existence of will, or the ability to cope well with life in general, become complicated concepts when put in the context of unnatural, superimposed, and highly pathological states. Suicide in otherwise normal, even extremely successful, people is not uncommon. This becomes even more important when one considers that manic-depressive illness is more common in the upper social classes and in those of high achievement. The inability to accept help, especially in men and in professional and otherwise accomplished individuals, has been described by many; Motto (1975) wrote:

> A person whose self-esteem rests on meeting high standards of performance, in a society which reveres rugged individualism, tends to avoid any situation that can be interpreted as reflecting weakness, dependence, or inability to cope with the stresses of living. Especially threatening is any suggestion of a "mental" disorder, with its implication of diminished control over one's behavior and intellectual functions. (p. 238)

Motto goes on to discuss several specific factors involved in the ability to survive suicidality, among them:

1. capacity to control behavior; that is, the person can stand the pain or impulse
2. capacity to relate readily and in a meaningful way to someone else . . . presence of family members and friends who are supportive
3. motivation for help and willingness to work actively on the problem
4. variety of resources which facilitate the therapeutic process and the transition back to a stable life pattern; for example, job skills, intelligence, physical health, communication skills, a capacity to trust, close ties to a church, or freedom from severe personality disturbance or addictive problems

To this list might be added financial resources (particularly important in gaining access to good medical treatment, covering financial excesses from manic episodes, and covering expenses during time lost from work); a strong marriage which is able to endure the disruptiveness of mania and the debilitation of depression; a willingness and ability to follow a prescribed treatment regimen; humor, and the kind of personality that, during normal times, will accumulate a backlog of good will. This backlog can be conceptualized as having a certain number of "jellybeans in the jar." Depression and mania deplete relationships enormously and there is little restocking during such states. The amount of support from others will be largely determined by the quality of predepression relationships. It is important that responsibilities and anxieties be distributed over a greater number, rather than a few, friends and family members.

Clearly, some types of depressions, or combinations of types of depressions with types of personalities, are less conducive to obtaining support than others. Hostile, paranoid, and irritable depressions are unlikely to bring out the same responses from others as do passive and sad depressions. This is especially true if an irritable depression is present in a somewhat nondescript and isolated person, and a less irritable depression occurs in a person who is normally outgoing and filled with *joie de vivre*. Unfortunately, those depressions, most dangerous in their own right, are also often the most alienating of affection and support.

CURRENT PSYCHIATRIC STATUS. Assessment of suicide risk is based both on history and clinical findings obtained during a psychiatric examination. The current severity of suicidal ideation and planning, as well as impulsivity, should be assessed; one of the most reliable and straightforward ways is to ask the patient directly whether or not he or she plans to commit suicide. If the patient denies immediate plans, the likelihood should be assessed of the patient's committing suicide within the next week, or the next month (on the assumption that he or she remains at the current level of distress). An attempt should be made to elicit any recent changes in mood, either for the better or worse. Severity of depression, marked hopelessness, and limited insight into the nature of the depression argue poorly for outcome (Paykel, 1979), and should be taken into account. Finally, specific symptoms and combinations of symptoms increase the probability of suicide and require close examination and monitoring: mixed states, psychomotor agitation, severe sleep disorders (or excessive concern about the quality and quantity of sleep), and delusions.

SUMMARY OF RISK FACTORS. Marie Asberg (personal communication, 1985) summarized what she sees as the primary suicide risk factors for bipolar patients:

1. patient's opinion (does the patient think he or she may commit suicide?)
2. previous suicide attempt, regardless of apparent intent and severity
3. low CSF 5–HIAA
4. apparent hostility (especially if expressed indirectly)
5. lack of social support and, even more, a lack of anyone (be it spouse, child, or pet) who is dependent on the patient
6. delusions and/or hallucinations

To this list of high risk variables I would add:

1. presence of mixed states, or history of same
2. family history of suicide
3. personal and/or family history of violence
4. short latency from onset of illness
5. poor lithium response or compliance
6. significant personal and interpersonal liabilities

Clinical Management

GENERAL ISSUES. Acutely suicidal patients, whether treated within a psychiatric hospital or as outpatients, require intensive care. This usually involves an increased time and psychological commitment on the part of the clinician; more vigorous or altered use of psychopharmacology and psychotherapy; and extensive involvement of family members and friends. If a suicidal crisis occurs while a patient is already under psychiatric care, there often is both an opportunity and impetus to reappraise previous working assumptions about diagnosis, psychiatric history, treatment response, and family and other relationships. Whatever the circumstances, certain clinical priorities remain clear. The first is, of course, to keep the patient alive. Relatedly, it is vital to develop a systematic plan for prophylaxis during future episodes of depression, mania, and suicidality. It is to these two points, primarily, that this clinical management section is addressed. Once the immediate danger of suicide is past, two other areas of concern bear mentioning. First, continued psychotherapeutic support is often extremely important after the immediate danger of suicide is past, and when the emotional repercussions of the patient's suicidal behavior become clearer to him or her and to those most immediately affected by it. Psychotherapy can be extremely important in helping the patient deal with the previously withheld anger and resentment of others, as well as in dealing with his or her own devastation. Second, it is essential to insure continuity of care for the basic psychiatric problem underlying the suicidal thoughts and behaviors.

General clinical management of acutely suicidal manic-depressives will be presented in this section; more specific psychotherapeutic and medical aspects will be presented in the next. The following recommendations are based on our clinical experience, as well as that of others.

Use of psychotherapy: Psychotherapy is usually required in treating the acutely suicidal bipolar patient, especially if the patient is not hospitalized. Suicidal patients, in general, need psychotherapy, but manic-depressive illness creates additional reasons for its use: changes in the illness create acute and dangerous perturbations in the patient's clinical state, best monitored by close contact with someone able to recognize and, it is hoped, ameliorate the situation.

Frequency of contact between clinician and patient: As a rule, suicidal patients should be seen and contacted more frequently than usually is the case. If financial or scheduling problems exist, attempts should be made to see the patient more often, but for a shorter period of time. Often it helps to establish a time each day, or every few days, for a brief telephone contact as well (Winokur et al, 1969; Motto, 1975). The patient's assessment of his or her own suicidality should be inquired about on a frequent and regular basis.

Availability of clinician: It should be absolutely clear to the patient how to reach the clinician in the event of an emergency or an acute exacerbation of suicidal thoughts and feelings. Directions for dealing with answering services, on-call systems, and coverage by other doctors should be explicit and in writing. Depressive confusional states and guilt or fear about overburdening and alienating doctors often prevent patients from indicating that they do not fully understand practical details about access. Even more important, most suicidal patients need frequent verbal assurance that they should contact the doctor if necessary. Putting this in writing on an appointment card (for example, "Please do not hesitate to call") is both concrete and reassuring. As with all suicidal patients, a clear understanding must be conveyed to the patient that he or she will call the clinician if in danger of losing control of feelings or actions, if acutely suicidal, or if feeling the need for immediate care.

Consultation with colleagues: Suicidal bipolar patients can present the clinician with exceedingly difficult problems, ranging from highly complicated and sophisticated diagnostic and psychopharmacological decisions, to problems of suicide management and countertransference (particularly in dealing with rage, frustration, and demands on time and emotional reserves). Consultation with specialists in the psychological and pharmacological treatment of affective illness can be helpful clinically, personally, and legally.

Involvement of family members and friends: The involvement of family members and friends can both minimize the need for hospitalization and maximize the family's and patient's sense of control over a potentially catastrophic situation. By participating during an acute risk period, families and patients can be actively involved in much of the decision-making (importantly, not all of it) and learn ways to avert future crises. The clinician can decrease the understandable sense of hopelessness and helplessness by providing information and reassurance to families, by giving them realistic expectations about likely difficulties in the acute and recovery phases, and by establishing clear contingency plans for serious problems that might arise. Families, similar to patients, should be given direct, and when possible, written information about the patient's illness, medications, suicide risk, and ways of contacting the clinician. A "suicide alert" system should be set up when necessary, and when it is particularly important to the patient to try and stay out of a hospital. This generally is best accomplished by a meeting including the patient, relevant members of the family, and a few close friends (if advisable). The purpose of the meeting should be to coordinate an effective and direct method of communication about particularly dangerous changes in the patient's mental condition and mood. The need for communication of this sort requires explication of the limits of confidentiality in situations involving potential suicide. The clinician should make it clear that the ultimate responsibility for assessing lethality and making decisions about hospitalization is his or hers alone; this avoids confusion about responsibility and lessens guilt about any subsequent misadventures that might occur. The clinician must maintain an ongoing surveillance of the system in order to assess the stress level within the family, friends, patients, and clinician, in order to determine if and when the patient needs inpatient care.

Hospitalization: The decision to admit a suicidal patient to a psychiatric hospital is often straightforward, obvious, and reassuring to all concerned. In many other instances—for example, when a patient equates hospitalization with failure and symbolic defeat, or where there exists a direct negative bearing on work or personal relationships—the assessment of costs and risks becomes far more complicated. The psychological, social, and clinical disadvantages to the patient must be weighed, not only against the risk of suicide, but also against the emotional stress to the family and the pragmatic and psychological limitations of the clinician if the patient remains out of the hospital. Even so, hospitalization, while clearly minimizing the risk of suicide, certainly does not eliminate it. Robins et al (1959) found that seven percent of the patients in their sample had committed suicide while in a psychiatric hospital; Weeke (1979) found that 27 percent of manic-depressive patients killed themselves while under hospital care, and that 50 percent of these were either on pass from a hospital or had absconded. Weeke, like Winokur et al (1969) and Roose et al (1983), emphasized the necessity for special suicide precautions as supplements to hospitalization. All emphasize that patients should be kept under close observation even after they appear substantially improved or recovered.

Motto (1975) recommends several specific ways to improve communication among staff members and the documentation of evidence, in order to prevent suicide:

1. There should be careful assessment of the degree of suicide risk. The risk should be explicit; for example, "low," "moderate," or "high."
2. There should be a statement of the measures to be taken to deal with the defined risk in clear, specific terms; for example, "visual contact with patient at least every 15 minutes," or "accompany at all times when off the ward." Do not use ambiguous terms such as "suicide observation" unless it refers to a specified set of procedures. If the orders change, be sure that it is indicated clearly in the record.
3. Assurance should be given that the measures indicated are carried out. This should be explicitly indicated in the nurse's notes and follow-up notes, as well as checked verbally with key ward personnel to assure that there are no misunderstandings.

Hawton and Catalan (1982) also emphasize the necessity for clear communication about clinical policies and specification of varying levels of observation. They note the importance of having a high staff to patient ratio, a reduced number of exits on the ward, an awareness that increased risk periods exist in the changeover of one nursing shift to another, and when a crisis on one part of the ward distracts staff attention from the suicidal patient. The same authors suggest that traditional methods of one-to-one, staff-to-patient suicide observation may be more harmful than helpful: "In addition, the resulting sense of confinement and intense observation may increase a patient's sense of hopelessness. It has even been suggested that such observation, especially if associated with low morale among staff, may actually increase the risk of suicide" (p. 112).

Psychological Aspects

> I remember sitting in your office a hundred times during those grim months and each time thinking: What on earth can he say that will make me feel better or keep me alive? Well, there never was anything you could say, that's the funny thing. It was all the stupid, desperately optimistic, condescending things you *didn't* say that kept me alive; all the compassion and warmth I felt from you that could not have been said; all the intelligence, competence, and time you put into it; and your granite belief that mine was a life worth living. You were terribly direct which was terribly important, and you were willing to admit the limits of your understanding and treatments and when you were wrong. Most difficult to put into words, but in many ways the essence of everything: You taught me that the road from suicide to life is cold and colder and colder still, but that—with steely effort, the grace of God, and an inevitable break in the weather—I could make it.
>
> —Patient with manic-depressive illness

The psychological treatment of suicidal bipolar patients is often emotionally draining, time consuming, and of critical importance. The suicidal manic-depressive patient has many problems which need psychological support of psychotherapy, reassurance, or general counseling of an informational nature. Ongoing professional assessment of suicide potential also is vital if the patient is to be treated as an outpatient. Often a suicidal depression will follow a manic episode, compounding the biological depression with many "precipitating" or "life" events—financial and employment chaos, marital problems, legal difficulties—which intensify the post-manic depression. These often need adjunctive management. Other psychological problems arise from the illness itself, such as frustration and hopelessness due to lithium's delayed antidepressant effect, and devastation at having been insane or severely lacking in judgment. This can result in a syndrome analogous to a traumatic neurosis and is particularly common after the first manic episode.

Several general psychotherapeutic issues arise in treating suicidal bipolar patients:

Therapeutic Style: Most clinicians agree that in-depth psychotherapy is contraindicated for most suicidal patients, especially manic-depressives (Winokur et al, 1969; Hankoff, 1982). Shneidman (1975) recommends a direct and active approach, as does the National Institute of Mental Health Task Force on Suicide, which suggests that the therapist maintain an "active relatedness" to the suicidal patient rather than a more "reflective approach." The therapist should be willing to take more initiative with poorly motivated patients than would be appropriate in other psychotherapeutic situations. Directness with suicidal patients is imperative for several reasons: the gravity of the situation, the patient's paralysis of will, and the fact that most suicidal bipolar patients are hyperalert and hypersensitive, and uncannily able to sense fear, cautiousness, and mincing of words in their therapists. Directness on the part of the clinician can help allay unnecessary anxiety and unwarranted fantasies, decrease a rather pervasive sense of negative omnipotence, and establish a basis for trust that can extend into other aspects of clinical care.

> Despite his status as an ally for life, the therapist must also have the capacity to hear out carefully and to tolerate the feelings of despair, desperation, anguish, rage, loneliness, emptiness, and meaninglessness articulated by the suicidal person. The patient needs to know that the therapist takes him seriously and understands. This understanding may require the therapist to explore the patient's darkest feelings of despair—a taxing empathetic task (Cassem, 1978, p. 595).

Reassurance: The liberal and intelligent use of reassurance is an integral part of the effective psychological care of suicidal manic-depressive patients. The extension of hope is not an unreasonable thing when dealing with a treatable and spontaneously remitting illness. Winokur and colleagues (1969) suggest frequent reassurance to patients and families that: a) manic-depressive illness *is* an illness; b) it is time limited; and c) that the clinician is familiar with this kind of problem. Suicidal patients need a great deal of reassurance, but because of depression, they are unlikely to acknowledge at the time they are depressed that the reassurance is helpful. More to the point, they are likely to reject the reassurance out-of-hand, and considerable skill is needed in order to reassure while still maintaining credibility. However, after the acute suicidal crisis is over, most patients spontaneously mention the importance of such reassurances.

Communication of Information: Explicit information about manic-depressive illness, its treatment, and suicide can be very helpful in reassuring patients and in minimizing feelings of hopelessness. Such information, discussed earlier in this chapter, should be written down, as well as communicated verbally. Among the first things to be clearly communicated should be the limits on confidentiality between the patient and the therapist when the patient is suicidal. This becomes of considerable concern when treating patients who are paranoid, irritable, and hostile, experiencing mixed states or rapidly fluctuating moods.

Countertransference: Feelings, thoughts, and actions engendered in a therapist by any patient are always important in the treatment process. However, when the patient is suicidal, it becomes essential that these feelings be examined. Such reactions often are a combination of the added stress, responsibilty, and time commitments involved in treating a suicidal patient, combined with the psycho-dynamics of the individual clinician. Problems can surface in different ways: overt or covert hostility toward the patient (for example, impatience, brusque-ness on the telephone), a tendency to avoid treating suicidal patients (thereby eliminating many bipolar patients from private practice), or more generally in the language used by clinicians, for example, suicidal "threat," or "successful" rather than "completed" suicide. Because manic-depressive illness is generally regarded as a biological disorder, psychoanalysts often refer suicidal bipolar patients to psychopharmacologists for treatment. These physicians may be well qualified to prescribe biological treatment, but not necessarily best suited to do the psychotherapy. Likewise, clinicians who are biologically oriented may overly rely on medication and slight the psychotherapy, while those who are primarily psychotherapists may de-emphasize the importance of psychopharmacology. Overidentification with patients, particularly successful ones, can result in increased psychological distress to the therapist and a corresponding risk of denial or overprotectiveness. The serious possibility of suicide reminds most therapists of their own vulnerabilities and limits.

SUMMARY

This chapter has emphasized the importance of psychological issues and active suicide prevention measures in the treatment of manic-depressive illness. General psychological issues discussed have included the therapeutic alliance in drug treatment, communication of care, psychotherapy, and lithium compliance. Discussion of the evaluation and management of suicidality in bipolar patients has focused on issues of detailed history taking, risk factors, course of illness, and current psychiatric status. Specific recommendations for clinical management have been presented.

REFERENCES

Barraclough B, Bunch J, Nelson B, et al: A hundred cases of suicide: clinical aspects. Br J Psychiatry 125:355-373, 1974

Cassem NH: Treating the person confronting death, in Harvard Guide to Modern Psychiatry. Edited by Nicholi AM. Cambridge, Harvard University Press, 1978

Dunner DL, Gershon ES, Goodwin FK: Hereditable factors in severity of affective illness. Biol Psychiatry 11:31-42, 1976

Gitlin MJ, Jamison KR: Lithium clinics: theory and practice. Hosp Comm Psychiatry 35:363-368, 1984

Goodwin FK: Drug treatment of affective disorders: general principles, in Psychopharmacology in the Practice of Medicine. Edited by Jarvik M. New York, Appleton-Century-Crofts, 1977

Goodwin FK, Jamison KR: Manic-Depressive Illness. New York, Oxford University Press, (in press)

Hankoff LD: Suicide and attempted suicide, in Handbook of Affective Disorders. Edited by Paykel ES. New York, Guilford Press, 1982

Hawton K, Catalan J: Attempted Suicide. New York, Oxford University Press, 1982

Jamison KR, Akiskal HS: Medication compliance in patients with manic-depressive illness. Psychiatr Clin North Am 6:175-192, 1983

Jamison KR, Goodwin FK: Psychotherapeutic treatment of manic-depressive patients on lithium, in The Interrelationship of Psychotherapy and Psychopharmacology. Edited by Greenhill M, Gralnick A. New York, MacMillan Co, 1983a

Jamison KR, Goodwin FK: Psychological issues in manic-depressive illness, in Psychiatry Update: The American Psychiatric Association Annual Review, vol. 2. Edited by Grinspoon L. Washington, DC, American Psychiatric Press, 1983b

Jamison KR, Gerner RH, Goodwin FK: Patient and physician attitudes toward lithium. Arch Gen Psychiatry 36:866-869, 1979

Jamison KR, Gerner RH, Hammen C, et al: Clouds and silver linings: positive experiences associated with the primary affective disorders. Am J Psychiatry 137:198-202, 1980

Johnson GF, Hunt G: Suicidal behavior in bipolar manic-depressive patients and their families. Compr Psychiatry 20:159-164, 1979

Klein DF, David JM: Diagnosis and Drug Treatment of Psychiatric Disorders. Baltimore, Williams & Wilkins, 1969

Motto JA: The recognition and management of the suicidal patient, in The Nature and Treatment of Depression. Edited by Flack FF, Draghi SC. New York, Wiley, 1975

Ottosson J: The suicidal patient—can the psychiatrist prevent his suicide?, in Origin,

Prevention and Treatment of Affective Disorders. Edited by Schou M, Stromgren E. London, Academic Press, 1979

Paykel ES: Management of acute depression, in Psychopharmacology of Affective Disorders. Edited by Paykel ES, Coppen A. New York, Oxford University Press, 1979

Robins E, Gassner S, Kayes J, et al: The communication of suicidal intent: a study of 134 consecutive cases of successful (completed) suicide. Am J Psychiatry 115:724-733, 1959

Roose SP, Glassman AH, Walsh BJ, et al: Depression, delusions and suicide. Am J Psychiatry 140:1159-1162, 1983

Shneidman ES: Suicide, in Comprehensive Textbook of Psychiatry II. Edited by Freedman AM, Kaplan HI, Sadock BJ. Baltimore, Williams & Wilkins, 1975

Sheard MH: Influence of doctor's attitude on patient's response to antidepressant medication. J Nerv Ment Dis 136:555-560, 1963

Stallone F, Dunner DL, Ahearn J. et al: Statistical predictions of suicide in depressives. Compr Psychiatry 21:381-387, 1980

Weeke A: Causes of death in manic-depressives, in Origin, Prevention and Treatment of Affective Disorders. Edited by Schou M, Stromgren E. London, Academic Press, 1979

Winokur G, Clayton P, Reich T: Manic-Depressive Illness. St. Louis, Mosby, 1969

Chapter 6

Clinical Approaches to Treatment-Resistant Bipolar Illness

by Robert M. Post, M.D., and Thomas W. Uhde, M.D.

Lithium carbonate is the mainstay treatment for the acute and long-term management of bipolar disorders. Its acute and long-term efficacy and relative lack of long-term side effects make lithium carbonate stand out as one of the major medical advances in this century in the treatment of severely ill patients with a chronic, debilitating disease. However, as has been noted elsewhere, not all patients tolerate or respond adequately to this treatment, and alternative therapies are necessary in some instances. Various estimates have suggested that some 20–40 percent of patients may not be adequately responsive to lithium, with the percentage of nonresponsive patients increasing in those with more rapidly cycling illness (Dunner et al, 1977; Prien, 1984, 1985; Himmelhoch, 1985; Secunda et al, 1985).

A series of alternative or adjunctive treatments have emerged that now appear to offer new clinical treatment options for the previously treatment-resistant bipolar patient. In this chapter we review the data supporting the clinical efficacy of the anticonvulsant compounds and related treatments for manic-depressive illness, and discuss the associated clinical and neurobiological implications. Treatment approaches for breakthrough episodes are reviewed by Drs. Goodwin and Roy-Byrne in Chapter 4, and the role of thyroid alterations in rapid cycling is reviewed by Dr. Wehr and his colleagues in Chapter 3.

GRAPHIC DEPICTION OF THE LIFE COURSE OF MANIC-DEPRESSIVE ILLNESS

In light of the recurrent nature of affective illness as summarized by Dr. Keller in Chapter 1 of this volume, an essential part of the evaluation and treatment strategy in approaching any bipolar patient and, especially, the treatment-resistant bipolar patient is the development of an accurate longitudinal assessment of the previous course of illness. Typical history taking based on casual inquiries about number of hospitalizations often grossly underestimates the frequency of previous episodes of mania and depression, and obscures their degree of treatment responsivity. We suggest that each individual patient and family members be requested to assess the previous course of illness in the most accurate way possible, and that the results be graphically plotted so that they can be clearly visualized by patient and physician. In this fashion, the previous course of illness, which is the best predictor of subsequent course of illness, can be most easily assessed. Moreover, the efficacy or partial efficacy of previous treatments can also be accurately delineated. Many patients present with a history of being

The opinions expressed herein are those of the authors and do not reflect official policy of the NIMH.

lithium-refractory or intolerant when, in fact, this estimate has not been based on systematic review. Careful inspection may reveal that the patient has had a substantial but partial response to lithium, or only had a brief bout of side effects which did not preclude the further use of this agent.

In a similar fashion, we strongly recommend the prospective use of a calendar for ongoing assessment of daily mood, sleep, and medication fluctuations, which can be performed in an unobstrusive way in a matter of seconds, by patients utilizing a 100 mm line for assessment of their mood ranging from worst ever (0) to best ever (100), with (50) being their "normal" self. If an individual patient has an especially prototypical symptom that fluctuates with mania and depression, such as energy level or difficulty concentrating, this might also be rated on another 100 mm line.

This systematic clinical approach to the patient serves a variety of purposes, many of which are not unlike daily measurement of glucose in the urine for the diabetic to assess degree of adequate control of diabetes mellitus with insulin. Not only can early warning signs of impending episodes be appropriately assessed and discussed by patient and physician, but the degree of efficacy of the current treatment regimen can be most accurately evaluated in this fashion. In addition, this approach emphasizes the seriousness of the illness, the necessity for medication compliance, the importance of a collaborative relationship with the physician, and the medical importance of the entire therapeutic process in the approach to this illness.

The retrospective life chart process has been described elsewhere (Squillace et al, 1984; Roy-Byrne et al, 1985; Post et al, in press) and will be only briefly outlined here. We suggest that three levels of severity of mania and depression be rated—*mild, moderate,* and *severe. Mild* would represent a subjective sense of depression that was clearly distinct from one's usual mood but did not lead to functional impairment. A *moderate* depressive episode would be one that would not only meet Research Diagnostic Criteria (RDC) and *Diagnostic and Statistical Manual of Mental Disorders, Third Edition (DSM-III)* criteria for major affective illness, but would also be associated with a substantial degree of functional impairment; that is, the patient would have difficulty in completing ongoing employment or social responsibilities but would still remain "on the job." The *severe* category would relate to a degree of functional incapacity indicating that the patient was no longer able to adequately keep up with social or occupational roles, and/or was incapacitated to the point of requiring hospitalization. Manic episodes would be related in similar fashion. In contrast to depressive episodes, where only moderate episodes would be counted in the quantitation of the total episodes, periods of even mild mania would be counted. This still represents a conservative approach, since hypomanic and manic episodes are often denied and underestimated by patients. Input from family members in this regard is invaluable. One should become familiar with which signs and symptoms are particularly characteristic of episodes of illness in a given individual, and which are likely to indicate the early warning signs of an episode.

Episodes of mania and depression with the three levels of severity should be plotted graphically above and below a euthymic line on a scale where at least one month is reflected per square. Medication and psychotherapy history should be appropriately coded above these episodes, and important environmental and psychosocial events can then be coded below this episode plot. This may aid in the systematic exploration of the role of psychosocial precipitants, potential anniversary events, vulnerable periods of the year, seasonal affective disturbances, and the like.

Once this life charting process has been initiated, we suggest that the patient receive a copy of it so that, in instances of transfer of medical care, this valuable aspect of the patient's medical record would be readily available without the undue delay that often occurs in the current era where regulations regarding confidentiality have, at times, impaired appropriate flow of medical information.

TREATMENT ALTERNATIVES: A FOCUS ON ANTICONVULSANTS

Carbamazepine

We focus on anticonvulsants as a class of agents in the treatment of bipolar illness because they have emerged as a leading clinical alternative to lithium. Of these agents, carbamazepine has been the most extensively studied, although, even with this drug, further clarification of its range of efficacy is required. Carbamazepine is a widely used drug in the treatment of trigeminal neuralgia and a variety of other related paroxysmal pain syndromes (Baker et al, 1985; Taylor et al, 1981; Fromm et al, 1984) and seizure disorders, particularly psychomotor epilepsy or complex partial seizures (Porter and Penry, 1978; Ramsay et al, 1983; Porter and Theodore, 1983; Callaghan et al, 1985). It is of interest that carbamazepine, which bears structural similarity to imipramine, was originally synthesized for its possible effects in depression. However, because it had atypical effects in a variety of animal models thought to relate to antidepressant efficacy, it was not considered further for this purpose, although its antinociceptive and anticonvulsant properties rapidly became established. Carbamazepine has been reported to have positive effects on mood and behavior in patients treated with it for their seizure disorder (Dalby, 1971, 1975) and to positively affect mood in a variety of other patient populations. These empirical data, taken in conjunction with the theoretical perspective that temporal lobe and limbic neural substrates are importantly involved in the regulation of emotional function, led us to an evaluation of carbamazepine in the treatment of primary affective disorders (Post et al, 1978, 1984a, 1985b, 1986a; Ballenger and Post, 1978, 1980).

Even at this current early stage in the study of carbamazepine, substantial evidence already exists for its acute and prophylactic efficacy in bipolar illness. Moreover, we will suggest that, with respect to carbamazepine, the clinical predictors of response, its side effects, and its possible mechanisms of action, each may differ from those of lithium carbonate.

ACUTE MANIA. Antimanic effects of carbamazepine have been documented in a series of double blind, controlled, and open studies (see detailed reviews and Tables in Post et al, 1985a; Post and Uhde, 1986). In most instances, the data from the open studies parallel those of the controlled trials, and indicate that carbamazepine has a magnitude and time course of efficacy equivalent to that of traditional antipsychotic or neuroleptic agents, which are thought to act by blockade of dopamine receptors. An example of this is shown in Figure 1, which illustrates the efficacy of carbamazepine in 19 acute manic patients; the

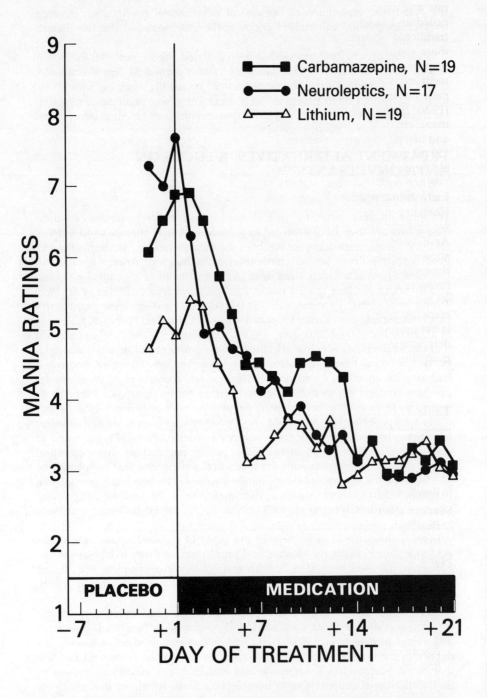

Figure 1. Time course of antimanic effects of carbamazepine compared to lithium and neuroleptics

rate and magnitude of response is closely parallel to that in 17 similarly diagnosed and rated patients on our clinical research unit who were treated with traditional neuroleptic agents such as chlorpromazine and thioridazine, or the more specific blocker of dopamine receptors, pimozide. The onset of clinical response to carbamazepine was often observed in the first several days of treatment and was evident in the ratings of nurses who were blind to which compounds patients might be treated with. Other studies, including those of Okuma et al (1979), Muller and Stoll (1984), and Grossi et al (1984) also report parallel antimanic effects of carbamazepine to other neuroleptics, including chlorpromazine and haloperidol when assessed under double blind conditions. Of 258 patients, 159 (62 percent) treated with carbamazepine had been reported to show moderate to marked improvement in mania.

When we divided our patient population into those who showed more clinically robust responses (improvement of two points or more on the Bunney-Hamburg manic rating scale) and those who showed less or no improvement, we observed several interesting correlates of clinical response to carbamazepine. As illustrated in Table 1, compared to nonresponders, the 12 patients who showed more robust responses to carbamazepine were more severly manic in the two days prior to the initiation of the carbamazepine trial, showed a trend for more manic dysphoria (increased ratings of depression during mania), and were more rapidly cycling in the year prior to NIH admission. The greater response to carbamazepine in those who were more severely manic at the outset is not a rating artifact or a reflection of regression to the mean, as most patients deteriorated following placebo substitution and again improved when carbamazepine was reinitiated on a double blind basis. Kishimoto and Okuma (1985)

Table 1. Predictors of Antimanic Response to Carbamazepine

	Non-responders (7)	Responders (12)	P
Severity of Mania			
Baseline mania ratings	3.4 ± .8	8.0 ± .4	.0001
Severity of Manic Dysphoria			
Baseline depression ratings (during manic episode)	4.5 ± .8	6.2 ± .5	.10
Rapid Cycling			
Episodes/years ill	1.2 ± .3	4.4 ± 1.7	.10
Episodes in year prior to NIMH admission	2.7 ± .9	7.0 ± 1.6	.03
Not:			
Age of onset first treatment	21.0 ± 1.9	21.0 ± 1.7	NS
Duration of illness (years)	15.0 ± 4.6	18.0 ± 3.3	NS

have similarly reported better response to carbamazepine in those who were more rapid cyclers.

Our data, taken with those of Okuma et al, are of particular interest in relationship to lithium carbonate. It has been well documented that patients with more severe and/or violent mania often require neuroleptic supplementation of lithium in the early phases of treatment. In addition, dysphoric mania has recently been associated with relatively poor antimanic response to lithium (Secunda et al, 1985). Finally, rapid cycling has been a predictor of relatively poor response to lithium (Dunner et al, 1976). Our carbamazepine responders were also over-represented in the group of patients without a family history of affective illness in first degree relatives. Thus, it would appear that several predictors of poor response to lithium tend to be associated with better response to carbamazepine.

ACUTE DEPRESSION. The acute antidepressant effects of carbamazepine have been less extensively studied than its acute antimanic effects. We have recently completed studying a series of 35 depressed patients in a double blind study utilizing a B–A–B design (Post et al, 1986a). We treated patients with an average dose of 971 mg/day achieving blood levels of 9.3 ± 1.9 µg/ml (range: 3–12.5 µg/ml). Twenty of these patients (57 percent) showed at least mild improvement while treated with carbamazepine, while 12 (34 percent) showed a more substantial improvement of two points or greater on the Bunney-Hamburg global depression scale. As illustrated in Figure 2, those who showed better response to carbamazepine were more severely depressed at the outset compared to those who did not respond. By the last week of treatment, those who improved were significantly better than the nonresponders in spite of their initially higher depression ratings. While improvement was statistically significant in the first week of treatment, it was not "clinically robust" until the second, third, and fourth weeks of treatment, consistent with the typical lag in onset of antidepressant effects reported with other antidepressant treatment modalities. Of the 12 substantial responders, nine would be considered to have shown a remission; they showed a mean rating of 3.0 on the 15–point Bunney-Hamburg scale.

In addition to initial severity of depression, other possible correlates of antidepressant response are summarized in Table 2. Responders had significantly more prior hospitalizations for mania compared with nonresponders, a finding that was not an artifact of response differences in unipolar and bipolar groups, as it persisted when bipolar patients were examined alone. Bipolar responders were also more rapid cyclers than the nonresponders (2.9 ± 3.0 episodes/years ill, compared with 1.0 ± 0.6 episodes/years ill, $p < .03$). All responders were less chronically ill prior to NIMH hospitalization as assessed by a lesser number of weeks ill with depression (137.7 ± 110) compared with nonresponders (237.6 ± 1.09, $p < .02$). Thus, it would appear that greater initial severity of depression, less chronicity of prior depression, and more discrete episodes of illness, which show a robust but transient response to sleep deprivation, tend to be associated with antidepressant response to carbamazepine. Many of these predictors are also associated with response to traditional antidepressants, and differential correlates of carbamazepine response remain to be elucidated.

PROPHYLAXIS. While we and Okuma have studied carbamazepine prophylaxis in a double blind, controlled fashion (Ballenger and Post, 1978, 1980; Post et al, 1983, 1984b; Okuma et al, 1981), most of the other clinical trials of carbamazepine for the long-term maintenance treatment of affective illness have been

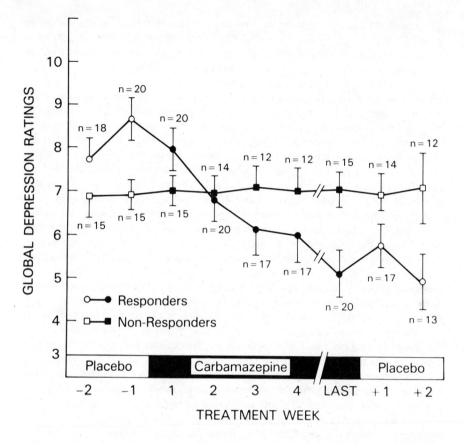

Figure 2. Antidepressant course in mild to moderate response to carbamazepine; these preliminary data require further clarification using other study designs.

Table 2. Possible Correlates of Antidepressant Response to Carbamazepine

Predictors	Non-Predictors
Initial severity of depression	Duration of illness
BP with history of manic episodes and hospitalization	Length of *episode* or *placebo* period
	Dose and blood level
Acute response to sleep deprivation	EEG abnormalities
Fewer psychosensory symptoms?	Family history of affective illness
Lower CSF HVA and c-GMP	CSF norepinephrine, somatostatin
Higher CSF opiate binding activity	Urinary free cortisol

uncontrolled clinical observations. Nonetheless, the two types of studies show parallel results, suggesting that some 65 percent of patients (161 of 248) may show substantial degrees of clinical improvement when carbamazepine is either used alone or added to previously ineffective treatment regimens.

In an initial series of nine good acute responders whom we have followed for an average 5.4 years in a mirror image design (we have compared an equal time on carbamazepine with that prior to drug administration), substantial improvement in the frequency, duration, and severity of both manic and depressive recurrences has been observed. While we have observed that the discontinuation of tricyclics can itself attenuate cycling frequency, as suggested by Wehr (1984), this did not appear to be a factor in our carbamazepine results, although it remains a factor to be evaluated in the bulk of the patients reported in the literature. As observed in Figures 3 and 4, many of our patients were extremely rapidly cycling with a high number of manic and/or depressive episodes in the years prior to institution of carbamazepine treatment, yet showed a substantial reduction in the frequency and duration of episodes in the time on carbamazepine. We employed maintenance doses of just under 1,000 mg/day, very similar to those used in the treatment of acute manic and depressive episodes, as described above. While most patients did not show complete absence of episodes, there was a marked reduction in morbidity in those patients who were severely ill, many of whom were ultra-rapid cyclers prior to carbamazepine treatment. The degree of efficacy in less severely ill patients, and in those not selected on the basis of initial positive acute response, requires further assessment. However, initial reports from Kishimoto and Okuma (1985) suggest that carbamazepine is as effective or more effective than lithium when each was administered alone for a minimum of one year's duration in an open study of bipolar patients.

It is important to note that many patients reported in the literature have been studied with the addition of carbamazepine to previously ineffective treatment regimens which have often included lithium carbonate. Thus, the long-term prophylactic efficacy of carbamazepine alone in comparison to lithium alone remains to be further elucidated. In addition, there is already clearcut evidence that there is a subgroup of patients who respond inadequately to either lithium or carbamazepine alone, but when the two agents are used in combination, show dramatic clinical benefit (Keisling, 1983; Moss and James, 1983; Lipinski and Pope, 1982; Fujiwara et al, 1984; Omura et al, 1984; Kishimoto et al, 1984). Thus, one might recommend the addition of carbamazepine to lithium carbonate in clinical treatment settings where there is some evidence of efficacy of lithium, even if it is inadequate. If the patient then shows remission of all symptoms, one might consider the withdrawal of lithium in order to assess whether carbamazepine is sufficient to "hold" the patient. However, it is clear that there is a subgroup of patients for whom the combination is required. Moreover, if prior episodes of illness have been severe and the potential consequence of a recurrence devastating enough, one might consider continuation of combination therapy if this proves clinically effective, even in the absence of unequivocal documentation of the need for both treatments. In our follow-up studies, we have observed relapses requiring hospitalization when doses of either lithium or carbamazepine have been reduced in some patients who require the combination.

DOSE AND BLOOD LEVELS OF CARBAMAZEPINE. We have not observed

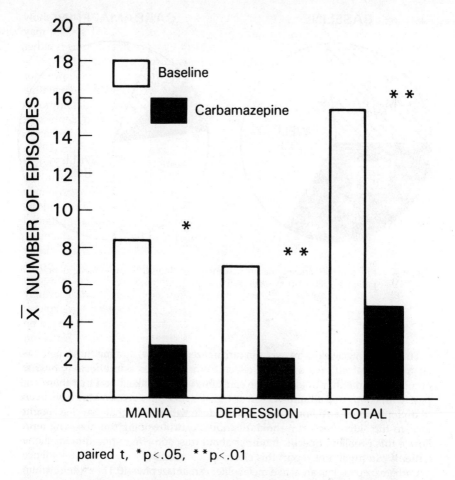

paired t, *p<.05, **p<.01

Figure 3. Reduction in manic and depressive episodes in nine patients followed on carbamazepine for an average of 2.7 years compared to 2.7 years baseline

clearcut relationships of carbamazepine blood levels to degree of acute clinical antidepressant or antimanic responses when the drug was administered in doses ranging from 400 to 2000 mg/day and generally achieving blood levels between 3–12 μg/ml. Individualization of dose of carbamazepine appears to be a most important part of the therapeutic regime, in order to minimize side effects. That is, there is a wide range of individual doses and blood levels that will be associated with side effects, and an average dose should not be employed in a casual manner. Some patients will have carbamazepine toxicity, including dizziness, ataxia, diplopia, dysarthria, on relatively low doses and blood levels of carbamazepine (as low as 5 μg/ml), while other patients will have none of these side effects on high doses and blood levels, even exceeding 12 μg/ml.

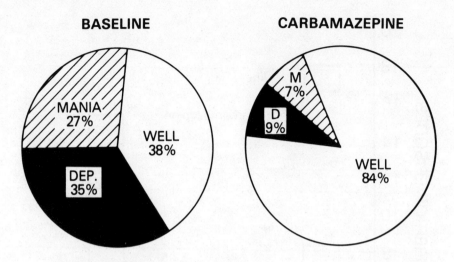

Figure 4. Effect of carbamazepine on percentage of time ill in nine manic depressive patients (follow-up average = 5.4 years)

Thus, we suggest slow increases in carbamazepine dose, titrating these increases against clinical efficacy and side effects. Where minor side effects appear to occur, one can either hold the dose constant, with the likelihood that these will pass with continued administration or transient dose reduction. Minor episodes of diplopia about two hours after a given dose will often signal that one is quite near to the side effects threshold; distributing or dropping the dose will ameliorate this problem. Specific inquiries about this side effect should be made, as patients often will not report this effect spontaneously.

Carbamazepine has an active metabolite, carbamazepine–10,11–epoxide, which itself is an anticonvulsant in animals, and is also effective in the treatment of trigeminal neuralgia in humans (Tomson and Bertilsson, 1984). Thus, there is some likelihood that levels of the epoxide contribute to the positive psychotropic effects of carbamazepine. Our initial studies suggested that the levels of the epoxide correlated better with the degree of clinical response to carbamazepine, although this has not continued in our larger series of depressed patients. The ratio of epoxide to carbamazepine might be associated with better degrees of antidepressant response; this remains to be further documented in a larger series of patients. The side effects profile of the epoxide appear to be parallel to, if not more benign than that of, carbamazepine (Tomson and Bertilsson, 1984, 1985; Patsalos et al, 1985a, 1985b).

Given the wide individual variability in dose and blood level associated with potential carbamazepine toxicity, it becomes important to become aware of pharmacological agents that might increase carbamazepine levels and induce carbamazepine toxicity if the patient is close to the side effects threshold. As summarized in Table 3, a variety of agents have been associated with increases in carbamazepine blood levels. The most important of these compounds are antibiotics

Table 3. Clinically Important Interactions Between Carbamazepine and Other Drugs*

Increased Carbamazepine Levels and Toxicity Produced by
  Erythromycin (and analogues)
  Triacetyloleandomycin
  Viloxazine
  Isoniazid
  Verapamil and diltiazem (not hifedipine)

Decreased Carbamazepine Levels Produced by
  Phenobarbital
  Phenytoin
  Primidone

Carbamazepine Decreases Effects of
  Haloperidol
  Clonazepam
  Phenytoin
  Valproate
  Ethosuximide
  Theophylline
  Dexamethasone
  Dicoumarol
  Warfarin
  Pregnancy tests

---

*See Post et al, 1985a, for references.

of the erythromycin and related category. These will markedly increase carbamazepine levels and may induce associated toxicity. The antitubercular drug isoniazid will also induce the same problem, although other monoamine oxidase inhibitors do not appear to share this proclivity. Propoxyphene (Darvon) and cimetidine (Tagamet) have been reported to produce relatively minor increases in carbamazepine levels.

SIDE EFFECTS. The side effects profile of carbamazepine appears to differ considerably from that observed with lithium carbonate, as summarized in Table 4. In particular, whereas patients on lithium sometimes report cognitive impairment, increased thirst, and urinary frequency, these are not routinely observed when patients are on carbamazepine. To the extent that these effects of lithium are related to its impairment of central and renal vasopressin function mediated by lithium's ability to inhibit the vasopressin stimulated adenylate cyclase activity, it is likely that carbamazepine would not be associated with these same properties. Carbamazepine appears to act in many ways opposite to that of lithium carbonate and may be a direct vasopressin agonist. Since lithium carbonate appears to act "below the receptor," the addition of carbamazepine to lithium treatment would not reverse lithium induced diabetes insipidus and, hypothetically, would not reverse lithium induced cognitive impairment. However, if these are problematic side effects of lithium, it is possible that carbamazepine

Table 4. Contrasting Side Effects Profiles

LITHIUM[a] (0.7–1.2 mEq/1)		CARBAMAZEPINE[b] (5–12 µg/ml)
Memory disturbances*		?
Thirst, polyuria	50–70%	— —
Tremor	30–50%	—
Weight gain*	10–30%	?
Diarrhea	10–20%	—
Hypothyroidism	5–10%	(essentially absent)
Psoriasis	1%	—
		Blood dyscrasias
		Hepatitis
		Dizziness/Ataxia
		Water intoxication

[a]Schou and Vestergaard, 1983
[b]Post, 1984a
*reasons for noncompliance (Jamison and Akiskal, 1983)

might provide an alternative treatment regimen. The substitution of carbamazepine in adequate lithium responders, however, should be considered with caution in light of observation by Paul Grof that good lithium responders may not respond adequately to carbamazepine, and the degree of overlap between response to these two agents remains to be further delineated.

In contrast to lithium carbonate, which increases the white count, carbamazepine consistently decreases the white count in most patients (Joffe et al, 1985). In most instances, white count does not drop below 3,000 white cells/cubic mm, and we have not had to discontinue carbamazepine in our series of 105 patients treated to date because of a low white count. The ability of lithium carbonate to stimulate white cell production will override the benign reductions in white count produced by carbamazepine (Brewerton, 1986). Thus, in patients with borderline low neutrophils (and other hematological indices in the normal range), one might consider the use of lithium for white cell stimulation, particularly if lithium supplementation was also indicated for clinical reasons.

However, there are reports of a more rare and idiosyncratic process developing during carbamazepine administration that has potentially serious side effects, that of agranulocytosis and aplastic anemia. There is currently great controversy as to the frequency and adequacy of hematological monitoring that should be employed in relationship to these potentially serious but extremely rare side effects. It is estimated that between 1 in 20,000 to 1 in 50,000 patients might be subject to aplastic anemia. In light of this vary rare problem and the likelihood that it might occur without warning, the utility of frequent blood counts has not been adequately elucidated in the literature. Recommendations in the neurology literature range from conservative taking blood counts weekly in the first several months and monthly thereafter to clinical experience in England (M. Trimble, personal communication), where white counts are rarely monitored, and patients are merely informed of the potential problem and told to report to their physician if any untoward side effects including fever, sore throat, rash, or petechiae should develop.

In contrast to lithium carbonate, which not only decreases thyroid indices but occasionally produces clinical hypothyroidism, and which requires supplementation with thyroid hormone (see Chapters 3 and 4 of this volume), carbamazepine is not associated with the onset of clinical hypothyroidism even though it lowers indices of circulating thyroid hormones. Of the many tens of thousands of epileptic patients treated with carbamazepine, only two patients have been reported to require thyroid supplementation. Thus, carbamazepine induces decreases in T_3 and T_4 without notable increases in thyroid stimulating hormone (TSH), as are observed during lithium. Moreover, those patients who responded best to carbamazepine had the largest drops in T_4 and free T_4, suggesting that the degree of hormone decrease is not only not clinically important, but potentially a correlate of degree of carbamazepine efficacy.

In patients treated with the combination of carbamazepine and lithium, the lithium effects such as increases in TSH predominate, and thyroid supplementation may be required. Thus, in each area of potential side effects from an interaction of carbamazepine with lithium (inhibition of vasopressin function, stimulation of white cells, and hypothyroidism manifested by increases in TSH), the lithium effect overrides that of carbamazepine.

Although the definitive studies remain to be conducted, preliminary inspection of available data does not suggest any major pharmacokinetic interaction between lithium and carbamazepine. While there are case reports of neurotoxicity during treatment with the combination (Chaudhry and Waters, 1983; Andrus, 1984; Shukla et al, 1984; Price and Zimmer, 1985), the symptoms reported can occur with normal blood levels of either agent alone. The vast majority of patients do not appear to experience important side effects during treatment with both drugs; and if neurotoxicity (sedation, ataxia, confusion, diplopia) should occur, it may respond to dose reduction, as is the case in the management of lithium and carbamazepine side effects when either drug is used alone. A generally benign side effects profile is also observed in an extensive series of patients (see review in Post and Uhde, 1986) during the combination of carbamazepine with neuroleptics, despite occasional case reports to the contrary (Stevens et al, 1979; Kanter et al, 1984; Yerevanian and Hodgman, 1985). We have observed one case of toxicity during haloperidol, lithium, carbamazepine combination; whether haloperidol (which is normally well tolerated in combination with carbamazepine [Klein et al, 1984]) is more likely to be involved than other neuroleptics remains to be explored. Carbamazepine will reduce haloperidol blood levels, however (Kidron et al, 1985; Jann et al, 1985). All of the combined toxicity reports should be reevaluated in light of the evidence reviewed above, that blood levels of carbamazepine, when used alone within the normal range (4–12 μg/ml), do not insure protection against side effects, that great variability in dose side effects thresholds occurs across individuals, and that a dose of carbamazepine not initially tolerated may subsequently be readministered without problems as chronic treatment proceeds and enzyme induction occurs. Thus, combination of carbamazepine with lithium or neuroleptics appears to be a clinically important strategy for the refractory patient, with no clearly demonstrated increased risk or differential presentation of side effects than that which can occur with each treatment alone.

We have observed 14 rashes in our first 105 patients exposed to carbamazepine and have discontinued treatment in these instances because of reports of exfoliative dermatitis and Stevens-Johnson syndrome in the literature. However, Vick (1983) indicates that steroid treatment with prednisone can suppress the rash in patients with otherwise uncomplicated reactions to carbamazepine. This should not be attemtped unless other treatment options are not readily available and other indications or more systemic reactions are absent (Hampton et al, 1985; De Swert et al, 1984).

Minor and transient elevations in liver enzymes are not uncommon during carbamazepine treatment and should be differentiated from the very rare and potentially fatal hepatitis that has either a toxic-hepatocellular or allergic-inflammatory picture on biopsy, and requires immediate drug discontinuation. In light of the rarity of this phenomenon, routine hepatic monitoring would not appear to be indicated.

While there is evidence that maintenance treatment with lithium during pregnancy may result in an increased incidence of congenital malformations, based on animal studies (Wray et al, 1982) and some clinical evidence, carbamazepine, among the anticonvulsants, has not been clearly linked to teratogenicity (Niebyl et al, 1979; Nakane et al, 1980; Friis, 1983; Butler, 1983)

Other aspects of carbamazepine side effects are reviewed in detail by J.H. Greist and J.W. Jefferson (see below).

Valproic Acid

Antimanic effects of an analogue of valproic acid (dipropyl acetamide) were first described by Lambert and colleagues in open clinical investigations (Lambert et al, 1975). These early observations have now been confirmed in double blind, placebo controlled observations (Emrich et al, 1984); (see Table 5). Emrich and colleagues observed improvement during double blind administration of valproic acid with deterioration on placebo substitution in four out of five patients. They then continued a series of inadequate responders to lithium carbonate on maintenance treatment with lithium in combination with valproic acid, and found substantial improvement in frequency of episodes. They employed doses up to 1,800 mg/day in the acute study, and similar doses during maintenance.

It appeared that valproate in combination with lithium was required for continued improvement since, in some instances, when lithium was discontinued, relapses occurred. Thus, it is unclear whether a subgroup of patients may respond to valproic acid alone, as in the case of carbamazepine, or whether, as it would appear in most instances, the use of valproate is required in conjunction with lithium carbonate. Puzynski and Klosiewicz reported that improvement was most notable in bipolar II patients, and sequentially less effective in bipolar I and schizoaffective patients. In patients with severe mania and mixed manic and paranoid psychoses, valproic acid treatment was not satisfactory, and additional therapy with neuroleptic drugs was required. These authors indicated that valproic acid was not as effective for depressive relapses and that, in several patients, the pattern of illness was changed from longer, more severe episodes to shorter, milder depressive episodes.

Table 5. Valproic Acid in Affective Illness

Study		Good or Excellent Response		
Lambert et al, 1984		**MDP**	**45/108**	**42%**
(valpromide)	(plus other	melancholia	8/38	21%
France	medications)	depression	12/47	26%
		mania	7/20	35%
		mixed	6/13	46%
		dysthymic schizophrenia	3/18	17%
Emrich et al, 1984		**M–D**	**7/11**	**66%**
Germany	(plus lithium)	affective schizoaffective		
		(acute mania)	(4/5)	(80%)
Puzynski and Klosiewicz, 1984		**M–D**	**8/10**	**80%**
Poland	(plus lithium and others)	BPII > BPI_D > SA		
Vencovsky et al, 1984		**M–D**	**?/38**	**—**
Czechoslovakia		(equal to lithium but less toxic)		
Brennan et al, 1984		**M–D**	**4/4**	**100%**
South Africa and U.S.A.	(plus lithium)	(acute mania)	(6/8)	(75%)
Prasad, 1984				
England		(acute mania)	(5/7)	(71%)

In studies of 38 manic-depressive patients, Vencovsky et al (1984) reported that valproic acid was of equal efficacy to lithium but less toxic. Brennan et al (1984) reported good prophylactic response to lithium in combination with valproic acid in four out of four patients, and acute antimanic response in six out of eight patients.

Our initial observations in several cases suggest that response to one anticonvulsant may not predict response to another. In particular, we observed a patient who was a clearcut responder to carbamazepine not responding to valproate (Post et al, 1984b); and in another patient, we observed a breakthrough mania during carbamazepine treatment, but successful long-term prophylaxis during valproic acid addition to previously ineffective lithium treatment (Post et al, unpublished, 1984). Thus, it would appear that in some refractory patients who were not responsive to lithium or carbamazepine alone or in combination, a clinical trial with valproate in combination with lithium might be indicated. While no or few side effects were reported in these series of psychiatric patients treated with valproic acid or its analogue, cases of severe and lethal hepatotoxicity have been reported in epileptics treated with valproic acid; thus, careful monitoring of liver function tests may be advisable during this treatment regimen.

Clonazepam

Chouinard et al (1983) reported that the anticonvulsant benzodiazepine, clonazepam, showed antimanic effects comparable to lithium carbonate in a double blind comparison. Supplemental neuroleptics were administered in both phases of the clinical trial and clonazepam was noted to be moderately sedative. Other authors have commented on the possible tolerance to its anticonvulsant effects, and one would wonder about the long-term efficacy of this compound for maintenance treatment. Data are not available on the prophylactic treatment of affective illness. Lechin and van der Dijs (1982) reported an increase in depressive problems in bipolar manic-depressive patients treated with clonazepam, however. Thus, the long-term efficacy of clonazepam would appear to require further study. Nonetheless, adjunctive treatment with this anticonvulsant benzodiazepine would appear to add another agent to the therapeutic armamentarium in the treatment of acute mania, particularly for **H.S.** medication, and in instances during inpatient hospitalizations when mild to moderate sedation would not be particularly problematic.

Phenytoin and Comparative Mechanisms of Action to Carbamazepine

While the uncontrolled observations of Kalinowsky and Putnam (1943) and Kubanek and Rowell (1946) suggested that phenytoin might have useful antimanic properties, Freyhan (1945) reported that five out of six of his patients were doubtful responders to treatment with this agent. However, he observed one manic-depressive patient with severe illness who responded on four occasions when phenytoin was administered and relapsed each time the drug was withdrawn. This sugests that at least some severely ill patients may be among those who respond to this anticonvulsant and that systematic controlled observations should be employed in the subsequent evaluation of its efficacy. Studies of the comparative efficacy of carbamazepine versus phenytoin in systematic, randomized, or crossover designs would not only be of clinical utility, but of some conceptual and heuristic value as well.

These clinical studies would help elucidate which potential mechanisms of action of carbamazepine and phenytoin might be important for their psychotropic activities, in contrast to their anticonvulsant effects. For example, both agents are potent in inhibiting binding of type 2 sodium channel receptors marked by ^{3}H–batachrotoxin–B–alpha–benzoate, and they also inhibit sodium fluxes preferentially under depolarizing and fast-firing conditions (Willow et al, 1985). Thus, this biochemical mechanism of action appears to be an excellent candidate for the anticonvulsant effects of these compounds and remains a putative mechanism for their psychotropic properties. However, if these two agents, which have approximately equal effects on sodium mechanisms and clinical anticonvulsant efficacy, are not of equal clinical efficacy in affective illness, it might suggest that other effects than those on sodium are important in affective illness.

Potential candidates might include a whole host of biochemical mechanisms, including carbamazepine's ability to increase plasma tryptophan, its ability to interact with adenosine receptors and "peripheral-type" benzodiazepine receptors, increase firing of the locus coeruleus, act as a vasopressin agonist, etc., as reviewed in detail elsewhere (Post el al, 1982, 1984a, 1985b). It is of interest that phenytoin and carbamazepine also have differential effects in amygdala versus cortical-kindled seizures, where carbamazepine is more effective than phenytoin in the amygdala-kindled variety (Racine, 1975; Albright and Burnham, 1980). Nonetheless, these two agents appear to have approximately equal clinical efficacy in the treatment of generalized and complex partial seizures. Therefore, systematic comparative studies of carbamazepine and phenytoin in affective illness would be invaluable in assessing their possible mechanisms of action.

Acetazolamide

Recently, Inoue et al (1984) reported that the anticonvulsant acetazolamide (Diamox), which is a carbonic anhydrase inhibitor, was effective in the treatment of some affectively ill patients who were unresponsive to either lithium or carbamazepine. In particular, patients who had affective illness in relationship to apparent endocrine disturbances, that is, either postpartum or perimenstrually related psychoses, were responsive to this agent. In addition, those who presented with "dreamy states" or confusional episodes were among those who were responsive. If these early data are confirmed in other patient populations, it would suggest that this anticonvulsant may become a treatment alternative for a symptomatically distinct subgroup of patients with severe and unresponsive affective disorders.

Alprazolam

Just as the early data would suggest that clonazepam has relatively "unimodal" effects in the treatment of mania, the early data would suggest that alprazolam has "unimodal" effects in the treatment of depression and may be relatively contraindicated in mania. Alprazolam is a triazolobenzodiazepine derivative, which is a potent anticonvulsant by virtue of its ability to displace compounds at the "central-type" benzodiazepine receptor. A series of systematic clinical trials suggest that it has important antidepressant effects in addition to its ability to reduce generalized anxiety and block panic attacks. However, several case reports suggest that treatment with alprazolam, like tricyclic and monoamine oxidase inhibitor antidepressant agents, may be associated with the induction of hypomanic and manic episodes (Arana et al, 1985; Strahan et al, 1985; Sack et al, unpublished manuscript, 1986).

Thus, preliminary data would suggest that alprazolam may be an alternative or an adjunctive treatment for the depressive phases of bipolar illness, but that extreme caution should be exercised in its use in patients who are likley to rapid-cycle or switch into serious manias. This warning would appear to be required for a series of tricyclic antidepressant compounds, as well as monoamine oxidase inhibitors (Wehr and Goodwin, 1979). However, preliminary data with a selective inhibitor of monoamine oxidase–A, clorgyline, suggests that some patients may have a decrease in rapidity of cycling when treated with this agent (Potter et al, 1982).

Progabide and Related GABA Agonists

Preliminary data suggest that progabide may have antidepressant properties equal to the tricyclic imipramine (Morselli et al, 1986) and one study suggests the possibility of acute antimanic efficacy as well (De Maio, 1984). While this drug is not currently available in the U.S., it is used in Europe as an anticonvulsant, and other analogues of this agent are currently undergoing clinical trials. These data suggest the possibility that an agent that acts as a direct GABA agonist may have some utility in the treatment of affectively ill patients, although maintenance studies have not yet been performed.

Electroconvulsive Therapy

Electroconvulsive therapy (ECT) is considered in this discussion of anticonvulsants because electroconvulsive seizures (ECS) in animals have been shown to be potently anticonvulsant to the development and manifestation of amygdala-kindled seizures (Post et al, 1984c). Moreover, data in humans suggest that ECT may also have clinically useful anticonvulsant effects in some seizure patients; it also increases the seizure and after-discharge thresholds in patients without seizure disorders (Sackheim et al, 1983).

Electroconvulsive therapy has long been noted to be useful in the treatment of acute mania (Fink, 1978), although recent studies by Small et al (1986) suggest that unilateral nondominant ECT may exacerbate mania in some patients, and that bilateral ECT is required for the successful treatment of acute mania. The efficacy of ECT in the treatment of acute depression is now unquestioned, and repeated studies have documented equal or better efficacy for ECT compared to a variety of other psychopharmacological treatment approaches in double blind comparison studies. What remains to be documented is whether periodic electroconvulsive treatment administered in a maintenance fashion would be successful for long-term prophylaxis of refractory patients with recurrent illness.

We have heard anecdotal reports of the efficacy of maintenance ECT for these refractory rapid cyclers, but also have observed one treatment failure. A 57-year-old patient with a history of several decades of rapid cycling (BP–II) initially responded dramatically to the first ECT treatment during a severe depressive episode, but rapidly develped a subsequent depressive episode despite prophylaxis with ECT in the interval. This latter episode was not responsive to the second complete course of ECT in another hospital, and the patient committed suicide shortly after leaving that institution. Thus, controlled clinical studies of ECT as a prophylactic treatment would appear indicated, in light of the lack of systematic data in the literature.

Calcium Channel Blockers

Verapamil and related calcium channel blockers have been reported, in a series of uncontrolled studies and case reports, to be effective in the treament of acute mania (Dubovsky et al, 1985). Only case reports exist regarding antidepressant prophylactic effects, and systematic controlled clinical trials are required in order to evaluate the early promising literature in regard to these agents. Verapamil is thought to only poorly cross the blood-brain barrier and, to our knowledge, has not been reported to be an effective anticonvulsant agent. It is also of interest that a variety of indirect lines of evidence suggest that carbamazepine may interact with calcium channels via its effects on adenosine receptors, "peripheral-type" benzodiazepine receptors, or a $GABA_b$ mechanism (Post et al, 1986b). Each one of these neurotransmitter receptor systems is thought to alter calcium fluxes, and it is possible that carbamazepine may likewise do so, although the preliminary evidence indicates that carbamazepine does not directly bind to the same calcium channels occupied by verapamil and nitrendipine.

Other Approaches

A series of other agents which do not possess anticonvulsant efficacy has also been employed in the treatment of acute mania and in the management of bipolar patients. These include neuroleptics, tryptophan supplementation of lithium carbonate (Beitman and Dunner, 1982), and the use of spironolactone in lithium refractory patients (Hendler, 1978). Other agents include 5–hydroxy-tryptamine (5HTP), clonidine, propranolol, buproprion, dopamine agonists, and sleep deprivation. The clinical utility of each of these approaches remains to be systematically explored. The importance of maintaining optimal thyroid function in the management of bipolar patients has already been emphasized by Drs. Goodwin and Roy-Byrne, and the special importance of thyroid function in rapid cycling has been reviewed by Dr. Wehr and his colleagues, in Chapters 3 and 4.

PHARMACOPROPHYLAXIS AS A FUNCTION OF COURSE OF ILLNESS

The longitudinal course of Parkinson's disease appears to be accompanied by differing degrees of biochemical pathology as a function of stage of illness, as well as a differential profile of pharmacotherapy. Early in Parkinson's disease, patients are exquisitely responsive to levodopa but, with progression of the illness, may require the addition of a direct dopamine agonist such as bromo-criptine. These agents are also likely to induce the rapid cycling motor phenom-ena observed in the "on-off" effect. A variety of treatments of this drug induced side effect have been recommended, but none has been unequivocally effective to date.

In a parallel fashion, it appears that different stages of the course of affective illness may require different pharmacotherapies. While controlled studies have not addressed this problem in a rigorous fashion, some of the available data for the differential response to lithium and carbamazepine reviewed above are, at least, not inconsistent with such a formulation.

It is noteworthy that the idea that a relatively unitary illness phenomenon is differentially responsive to pharmacotherapy as a function of stage of illness is most clearly documented experimentally within the amygdala kindling para-digm. As summarized in detail elsewhere (Weiss and Post, unpublished, 1986; Weiss et al, 1985; Post et al, in press), it is clear that agents effective in the early phases of kindling are not always effective in the late or spontaneous stages (such as diazepam), while some agents show the converse pattern (such as phenytoin) (Pinel, 1983). Moreover, we have observed that carbamazepine is unable to block the development of amygdala kindling in the rat, but is a highly effective anticonvulsant for completed kindled seizures. Conversely, carbamaze-pine is effective in blocking the early development of lidocaine kindled seizures, but is ineffective in blocking completed lidocaine seizures. These data strongly support the view that different stages of kindling processes are differentially pharmacologically responsive.

In a parallel fashion, in relation to affective illness, the preliminary data would suggest that psychotherapy and, perhaps, benzodiazepines, might be effective in the earliest phases of mild, stress related dysphorias. With more severe evolution of affective episodes, tricyclic antidepressants, monoamine oxidase inhibitors, or lithium carbonate may also be effective. However, with severe psychotic depressions, neuroleptics and other agents are sometimes required as supplements to tricyclics. In the latest stages of bipolar illness associated with severe manias, dysphoric manias, and rapid cycling illness, patients tend to be less responsive to lithium carbonate. In these instances, carbamazepine, valproic acid, and some of the related agents we have discussed in this chapter may then become more appropriate treatments, either as single agents or as adjuncts and in combination.

This conceptual schema is obviously highly preliminary and is presented for its heuristic value. As increasing numbers of patients are studied, it will be particularly valuable to attempt not only to subtype them in the traditional fashion, but also to relate their pharmaco-responsivity to their stage in the longitudinal course of their illness. In this fashion, data may be collected that could either support or refute this preliminary conceptualization of the evolution of pharmacotherapy as a function of course of illness in affective disorders. It is also possible that subgroups of affectively ill patients will be more clearly differentiated on the basis of other clinical and biological markers not directly related to course of illness.

The elucidation of these options should help clarify the sequence of pharmacological agents to be employed, so that the optimal agent can be applied earliest in the course of illness in order not only to decrease the substantial morbidity and mortality associated with affective disorders, but also, possibly, to inhibit the underlying sensitization process that might occur with the emergence of repeated episodes. Elsewhere, we have described the process in which each recurrence of affective illness appears to facilitate the occurrence of subsequent episodes (Post et al, 1986c). In fact, in more than 4,000 patients observed since the time of Kraepelin (1907), a pattern of decreasing well intervals has been observed as characteristic of the median course of affective illness. This natural tendency for the illness to speed up as a function of both patient age and number of affective episodes, which has been observed in both the prepharmacological and current psychopharmacological eras, may reflect a sensitization process that, in itself, merits direct attention and therapy. In addition to the previous numbers of episodes, severity of episodes, and duration of well interval, possible sensitization phenomena should be considered by the physician and patient when deciding when or whether to institute long-term maintenance treatment. Charting the life-course of illness will aid in this assessment, as well as the prospective evaluation of the effectiveness of subsequent treatment manipulations.

SUMMARY AND CONCLUSIONS

We have attempted to outline a series of treatment options, some of which might be employed sequentially or in combination in assessing the adequacy of pharmacoprophylaxis for the bipolar patient. As we have suggested, treatment may differ according to a variety of clinical and biological indicators, and possibly also as a function of course of illness. Nonetheless, it may be appropriate for several reasons to extend the list of current treatments that might be explored in the management of treatment-refractory bipolar patients. Physicians, patients, and their families should be aware that, in contrast to a decade ago when lithium was the only real treatment option, other agents are now available which have been more or less well studied, and which have some likelihood of being effective in the management of bipolar illness.

It would appear that the old approach of treating breakthrough manias with neuroleptics and breakthrough depressions with tricyclic antidepressants and monoamine oxidase inhibitors is not optimal for the bipolar patient. This type of treatment, particularly with antidepressant agents, has the liability of inducing manic episodes or increasing the frequency and severity of, if not inducing, rapid cycling bipolar illness. Periodic use of neuroleptics for breakthrough manias appears less likely to induce the next depression, although preliminary data from Kukopulos et al (1980) suggests that it, too, may be associated with an increasing severity of the next depressive episode. Moreover, the liability of neuroleptic treatment when employed chronically for inducing tardive dyskinesia may also be kept in mind, particularly in light of evidence suggesting that affectively ill patients may be particularly prone to the development of tardive dyskinesia.

While carbamazepine, valproic acid, and related anticonvulsant agents are not yet FDA approved for use in treating affective illness, the FDA does not object to such use on a physician-discretion basis. These agents are available as standard anticonvulsants, and the FDA acknowledges that their use for other indications may be appropriate, where available evidence supports this approach as a sound treatment (FDA Drug Bulletin, April 1982). It would appear that available data clearly do support this option for carbamazepine, and preliminary data with valproic acid from five centers in five different countries are also supportive of the use of this agent as a treatment option for refractory patients. Some of the other drugs reviewed are less well studied, but one or more may be effective in the otherwise refractory patient.

We early await continued delineation of possible clinical and biological markers of pharmacological response in bipolar patients, and documentation of the efficacy of a series of currently available treatments as well as the development of new treatment options.

REFERENCES

Albright PS, Burnham WM: Development of a new pharmacological seizure model: effects of anticonvulsants, on cortical- and amygdala-kindled seizures in the rat. Epilepsia 21:681-689, 1980

American Psychiatric Association: Diagnostic and Statistical Manual of Mental Disorders, Third Edition (DSM-III). Washington, DC, American Psychiatric Association, 1980

Andrus PF: Lithium and carbamazepine J Clin Psychiatry 45:525, 1984

Arana GW, Pearlman C, Shader RI: Alprazolam-induced mania: two clinical cases. Am J Psychiatry 142:368-369, 1985

Baker KA, Taylor JW, Lilly GE: Treatment of trigeminal neuralgia: use of baclofen in combination with carbamazepine. Clin Pharm 4:93-96, 1985

Ballenger JC, Post RM: Therapeutic effects of carbamazepine in affective illness: a preliminary report. Communications in Psychopharmacology 2:159-178, 1978

Ballenger JC, Post RM: Carbamazepine (Tegretol) in manic-depressive illness: a new treatment. Am J Psychiatry 137:782-790, 1980

Beitman B, Dunner D: L–tryptophan in the maintenance treatment of bipolar II manic-depressive illness. Am J Psychiatry 139:1498-1499, 1982

Brennan MJW, Sandyk R, Borsook D: Use of sodium-valproate in the management of affective disorders: basic and clinical aspects, in Anticonvulsants in Affective Disorders. Edited by Emrich HM, Okuma T, Muller AA. Amsterdam, Excerpta Medica, 1984

Brewerton TD: Lithium counteracts carbamazepine-induced leukopenia while increasing its therapeutic effect: a case report. Biol Psychiatry (in press)

Butler CD: Carbamazepine, seizure disorders, and pregnancy (letter). JAMA 250:3164, 1983

Callaghan N, Kenny RA, O'Neill B, et al: A prospective study between carbamazepine, phenytoin and sodium valproate as monotherapy in previously untreated and recently diagnosed patients with epilepsy. J Neurol Neurosurg Psychiatry 48:639-644, 1985

Chaudhry RP, Waters BGH: Lithium and carbamazepine interaction: possible neurotoxicity. J Clin Psychiatry 44:30-31, 1983

Chouinard G, Young SN, Annable L: Antimanic effect of clonazepam. Biol Psychiatry 18:451-466, 1983

Dalby MA: Antiepileptic and psychotropic effect of carbamazepine (Tegretol) in the treatment of psychomotor epilepsy. Epilepsia 12:325-334, 1971

Dalby MA: Behavioral effects of carbamazepine, in Complex Partial Seizures and Their Treatment: Advances in Neurology, Vol. 11. Edited by Penry JK, Daly DD. New York, Raven Press, 1975

De Maio D: Progabide in mania: preliminary observations. Proceedings of the IXth International Union of Pharmacology (IUPHAR) Congress, Paris, August 6–7, 1984

De Swert LF, Ceuppens JL, Teuwen D, et al: Acute interstitial pneumonitis and carbamazepine therapy. Acta Paediatr Scand 73:285-288, 1984

Dubovsky SL, Franks RD: Intracellular calcium in affective disorders: a review and an hypothesis. Biol Psychiatry 18:781-797, 1983

Dubovsky S, Franks R, Schrier D: Phenelzine-induced hypomania: effect of verapamil. Biol Psychiatry 20:1009-1014, 1985

Dunner DL, Fleiss JL, Fieve RR: Lithium carbonate prophylaxis failure. Br J Psychiatry 129:40-44, 1976

Dunner DL, Patrick V, Fieve RR: Rapid cycling manic-depressive patients. Compr Psychiatry 18:561-566, 1977

Emrich HM, Dose M, von Zerssen D: Action of sodium-valproate and of oxcarbazepine in patients with affective disorders, in Anticonvulsants in Affective Disorders. Edited by Emrich HM, Okuma T, Muller AA. Amsterdam, Excerpta Medica, 1984

Food and Drug Administration: Use of approved drugs for unlabeled indications. FDA Drug Bulletin 12:4-5, 1982

Fink M: Efficacy and safety of induced seizures (EST) in man. Compr Psychiatry 19:1-18, 1978

Freyhan FA: Effectiveness of diphenylhydantoin in management of nonepileptic psychomotor excitement states. Arch Neurol Psychiatry 53:370-374, 1945

Friis ML: Antiepileptic drugs and teratogenesis. Acta Neurol Scand Suppl 94:39-43, 1983

Fromm GH, Terrence CR, Maroon JC: Trigeminal neuralgia: current concepts regarding etiology and pathogenesis. Arch Neurol 41:1204-1207, 1984

Fujiwara Y, Ebara T, Fukuda K, et al: Prophylactic effect of the combination of lithium carbonate and carbamazepine on bipolar disorder. Folia Psychiatr Neurol Jpn 38:401, 1984

Grossi E, Sacchetti E, Vita A, et al: Carbamazepine vs. chlorpromazine in mania: a double-blind trial, in Anticonvulsants in Affective Disorders. Edited by Emrich HM, Okuma T, Muller AA. Amsterdam, Excerpta Medica, 1984

Hampton KK, Bramley PN, Feely M: Failure of prednisolone to suppress carbamazepine hypersensitivity. N Engl J Med 313:959, 1985

Hendler NH: Spironolactone prophylaxis in manic-depressive disease. J Nerv Ment Dis 166:517-520, 1978

Himmelhoch JM: Sources of lithium resistance in mixed mania. Abstracts of the Annual Meeting, American College of Neuropsychopharmacology Dec. 9–13, 1985

Inoue H, Hazama H, Hamazoe K, et al: Antipsychotic and prophylactic effects of acetazolamide (Diamox) on atypical psychosis. Folia Psychiatr Neurol Jpn 38:425-436, 1984

Jamison KR, Akiskal HS: Medication compliance in patients with bipolar disorder, in The Psychiatric Clinics of North America, vol 6. Edited by Akiskal HS. Philadelphia, W.B. Saunders, 1983

Jann MW, Ereshefsky L, Saklad SR, et al: Effects of carbamazepine on plasma haloperidol levels. J Clin Psychopharmacol 5:106-109, 1985

Joffe RT, Post RM, Roy-Byrne PP, et al: Hematological effects of carbamazepine in patients with affective illness. Am J Psychiatry 142:1196-1199, 1985

Kalinowsky L, Putnam T: Attempts at treatment of schizophrenia and other nonepileptic psychoses with Dilantin. Arch Neurol Psychiatry 49:414-423, 1943

Kanter GL, Yerevanian BI, Ciccone JR: Case report of a possible interaction between neuroleptics and carbamazepine. Am J Psychiatry 141:1101-1102, 1984

Keisling R: Carbamazepine and lithium carbonate in the treatment of refractory affective disorders. Arch Gen Psychiatry 40:223, 1983

Kidron R, Averbuch I, Klein E, et al: Carbamazepine-induced reduction of blood levels of haloperidol in chronic schizophrenia. Biol Psychiatry 20:199-228, 1985

Kishimoto A, Okuma T: Antimanic and prophylactic effects of carbamazepine in affective disorders. Abstracts of 4th World Congress of Biological Psychiatry, Philadelphia, Sept 8–13, 1985

Kishimoto A, Omura F, Umezawa Y, et al: Combined therapy with lithium and carbamazepine, in Abstracts of the 137th Annual Meeting of the American Psychiatric Association, NR22, Los Angeles, May 1984

Klein E, Bental E, Lerer B, et al: Carbamazepine and haloperidol in excited psychoses. Arch Gen Psychiatry 41:165-170, 1984

Kraepelin E: Clinical Psychiatry; a text book for students and physicians, abstracted and adapted from the seventh German edition of Kraepelin's Lehrbuch der Psychiatrie. Edited by Diefendorf R. New York/London, The MacMillan Company, 1907

Kubanek JL, Rowell RC: The use of Dilantin in the treatment of psychotic patients unresponsive to other treatment. Diseases of the Nervous System 7:47-50, 1946

Kukopulos A, Reginaldi D, Laddomada P, et al: Course of the manic-depressive cycle and changes caused by treatments. Pharmakopsychiatria 13:156-167, 1980

Lambert PA: Acute and prophylactic therapies of patients with affective disorders using valpromide (dipropylacetamide), in Anticonvulsants in Affective Disorders. Edited by Emrich HM, Okuma T, Muller AA. Amsterdam, Excerpta Medica, 1984

Lambert PA, Carraz G, Borselli S, et al: Le dipropylacetamide dans le traitement de la psychose maniaco-depressive. Encephale 1:25-31, 1975

Lechin F, van der Dijs B: Intestinal manometry as a guide to psychopharmacological therapy, in Clinical Pharmacology and Therapeutics. Edited by Velasco M. Amsterdam, Excerpta Medica, 1982

Lindhout D, Meinardi H: False-negative pregnancy test women taking carbamazepine (letter). Lancet 2:505, 1982

Lipinski JF, Pope HG Jr: Possible synergistic action between carbamazepine and lithium carbonate in the treatment of three acutely manic patients. Am J Psychiatry 139:948-949, 1982

Morselli PL, Fournier V, Macher, et al: Therapeutic action of progabide in depressive illness: a controlled clinical trial, in Laboratoires d'Etudes et de Recherches Synthélabo (L.E.R.S.) Monograph Series, vol 4: GABA and Mood Disorders. Edited by Bartholini G, Lloyd KG, Morselli PL. New York, Raven Press, 1986

Moss GR, James CR: Carbamazepine and lithium carbonate synergism in mania. Arch Gen Psychiatry 40:588-589, 1983

Muller AA, Stoll K-D: Carbamazepine and oxcarbazepine in the treatment of manic syndromes: studies in Germany, in Anticonvulsants in Affective Disorders. Edited by Emrich HM, Okuma T, Muller AA. Amsterdam, Excerpta Medica, 1984

Nakane Y, Okuma T, Takahashi R, et al: Multi-institutional study on the teratogenicity and fetal toxicity of antiepileptic drugs: a report of a collaborative study group in Japan. Epilepsia 21:663-680, 1980

Niebyl JR, Blake DA, Freeman M, et al: Carbamazepine levels in pregnancy and lactation. Obstet Gynecol 53:139-140, 1979

Okuma T, Inanaga K, Otsuki S, et al: Comparison of the antimanic efficacy of carbamazepine and chlorpromazine: a double-blind controlled study. Psychopharmacology 66:211-217, 1979

Okuma T, Inanaga K, Otsuki S, et al: A preliminary double-blind study of the efficacy of carbamazepine in prophylaxis of manic-depressive illness. Psychopharmacology 73:95-96, 1981

Omura F, Kishimoto A, Tsutsui T, et al: Combined therapy of lithium and carbamazepine in bipolar affective disorders. Folia Psychiatr Neurol Jpn 38:401, 1984

Patsalos PN, Stephenson TJ, Krishna S, et al: Side-effects induced by carbamazepine–10,11–epoxide. Lancet 2:496, 1985a; Lancet 2:1432, 1985b

Pinel JP: Effects of diazepam and diphenylhydantoin on elicited and spontaneous seizures in kindled rats: a double dissociation. Pharmacol Biochem Behav 18:61-63, 1983

Porter RJ, Penry JK: Efficacy and choice of antiepileptic drugs, in Advances in Epileptology, 1977: Psychology, Pharmacotherapy, and New Diagnostic Approaches. Edited by Meinardi H, Rowan AJ. Amsterdam, Swetz & Zeitlinger, 1978

Porter RJ, Theodore WH: Nonsedative regimens in the treatment of epilepsy. Arch Intern Med 143:945-947, 1983

Post RM, Uhde TW: Anticonvulsants in non-epileptic psychosis, in Aspects of Epilepsy in Psychiatry. Edited by Trimble MR, Bolwig TG. New York, John Wiley & Sons, 1986

Post RM, Ballenger JC, Reus VI, et al: Effects of carbamazepine in mania and depression. Scientific Proceedings of 131st Annual Meeting of the American Psychiatric Association, Atlanta, 1978

Post RM, Uhde TW, Ballenger JC, et al: Carbamazepine, temporal lobe epilepsy, and manic-depressive illness, in Advances in Biological Psychiatry, vol 8: Temporal Lobe Epilepsy, Mania, and Schizophrenia and the Limbic System. Edited by Koella WP, Trimble MR. Basel, S. Karger, 1982

Post RM, Uhde TW, Ballenger JC, et al: Prophylactic efficacy of carbamazepine in manic-depressive illness. Am J Psychiatry 140:1602-1604, 1983

Post RM, Ballenger JC, Uhde TW, et al: Efficacy of carbamazepine in manic-depressive illness: implications for underlying mechanisms, in Neurobiology of Mood Disorders. Edited by Post RM, Ballenger JC. Baltimore, Williams & Wilkins, 1984a

Post RM, Berrettini W, Uhde TW, et al: Selective response to the anticonvulsant carbamazepine in manic-depressive illness: a case study. J Clin Psychopharmacol 4:178-185, 1984b

Post RM, Putnam FW, Contel NR, et al: Electroconvulsive seizures inhibit amygdala kindling: implications for mechanisms of action in affective illness. Epilepsia 25:234-239, 1984c

Post RM, Uhde TW, Joffe RT, et al: Anticonvulsant drugs in psychiatric illness: new treatment alternatives and theoretical implications, in The Psychopharmacology of Epilepsy. Edited by Trimble MR. Chichester, England, John Wiley & Sons, 1985a

Post RM, Uhde TW, Rubinow DR, et al: Efficacy and mechanisms of action of carbamazepine in affective disorder, in Proceedings of the 4th World Congress of Biological Psychiatry, Philadelphia, Sept. 8–13, 1985. Amsterdam, Elsevier, 1985b

Post RM, Uhde TW, Roy-Byrne PP, et al: Antidepressant effects of carbamazepine. Am J Psychiatry 143:29-34, 1986a

Post RM, Uhde TW, Rubinow DR, et al: Carbamazepine in affective illness: implications for GABA mechanisms, in Laboratoires d'Etudes et de Recherches Synthélabo (L.E.R.S.), vol 4: GABA and Mood Disorders. Edited by Bartholini G, Lloyd KG, Morselli PL. New York, Raven Press, 1986b

Post RM, Rubinow DR, Ballenger JC: Conditioning and sensitization in the longitudinal course of affective illness. Br J Psychiatry 1986c

Potter WZ, Murphy DL, Wehr TA, et al: Clorgyline: a new treatment for refractory rapid cycling patients? Arch Gen Psychiatry 39:505-510, 1982

Prasad AJ: The role of sodium valproate as an antimanic agent. Pharmatherapeutica 4:6-8, 1984

Price WA, Zimmer B: Lithium-carbamazepine neurotoxicity in the elderly (letter). J Am Geriatr Soc 33:876-877, 1985

Prien RF: Five-center study clarifies use of lithium, imipramine for recurrent affective disorders. Hosp Community Psychiatry 35:1097-1098, 1984

Prien RF: Long-term maintenance drug treatment of mixed mania. Abstracts of the Annual Meeting, American College of Neuropsychopharmacology Dec 9–13, 1985

Puzynski S, Klosiewicz L: Valproic acid amide as a prophylactic agent in affective and schizoaffective disorders, in Anticonvulsants in Affective Disorders. Edited by Emrich HM, Okuma T, Muller AA. Amsterdam, Excerpta Medica, 1984

Racine RJ: Modification of seizure activity by electrical stimulation: motor seizures. Electroencephalogr Clin Neurophysiol 38:1-12, 1975

Ramsay RE, Wilder BJ, Berger JR, et al: A double blind study comparing carbamazepine with phenytoin as initial seizure therapy in adults. Neurology 33:904-910, 1983

Roy-Byrne PP, Post RM, Uhde TW, et al: The longitudinal course of recurrent affective illness: life chart data from research patients at the NIMH. Acta Psychiatr Scand Suppl 317, 71:5-34, 1985

Sackeim HA, Decina P, Malitz S, et al: Anticonvulsant and antidepressant properties of electroconvulsive therapy: a proposed mechanism of action. Biol Psychiatry 18:1301-1310, 1983

Schou M, Vestergaard P: Lithium treatment: problems and precautions, in Antidepressants. Edited by Burrows GD, Norman TR, Davies B. Amsterdam, Elsevier Biomedical Press, 1983

Secunda SK, Katz MM, Swann A, et al: Mania: diagnosis, state measurement and prediction of treatment response. J Affective Disord 8:113-121, 1985

Shukla S, Godwin CD, Long LEB, et al: Lithium–carbamazepine neurotoxicity and risk factors. Am J Psychiatry 141:1604-1606, 1984

Small JG, Milstein V, Klapper MH, et al: Electroconvulsive Therapy in the treatment of manic disorders. Ann NY Acad Sci 462:37-49, 1986

Squillace KM, Post RM, Savard R, et al: Life charting of the longitudinal course of affective illness, in Neurobiology of Mood Disorders. Edited by Post RM, Ballenger JC. Baltimore, Williams & Wilkins, 1984

Strahan A, Rosenthal J, Kaswan M, et al: Three case reports of acute paroxysmal excitement associated with alprazolam treatment. Am J Psychiatry 142:859-861, 1985

Stevens JR, Bigelow L, Denny D, et al: Telemetered EEG–EOG during psychotic behaviors of schizophrenia. Arch Gen Psychiatry 36:251-262, 1979

Taylor J, Brauer S, Espir M: Long-term treatment of trigeminal neuralgia with carbamazepine. Postgrad Med J 57:16-18, 1981

Tomson T, Bertilsson L: Potent therapeutic effect of carbamazepine–10,11–epoxide in trigeminal neuralgia. Arch Neurol 41:589-601, 1984

Tomson T, Bertilsson L: Side effects of carbamazepine: drug or metabolite? Lancet 2:1010, 1985

Vencovsky E, Soucek K, Kabes J: Prophylactic effect of dipropylacetamide in patients with bipolar affective disorder—short communication, in Anticonvulsants in Affective Disorders. Edited by Emrich HM, Okuma T, Muller AA. Amsterdam, Excerpta Medica, 1984

Vick NA: Suppression of carbamazepine-induced skin rash with prednisone. N Engl J Med 309:1193-1194, 1983

Wehr TA: Biological rhythms and manic-depressive illness, in Neurobiology of Mood Disorders. Edited by Post RM, Ballenger JC. Baltimore, Williams & Wilkins, 1984

Wehr TA, Goodwin FK: Rapid cycling in manic-depressives induced by tricyclic antidepressants. Arch Gen Psychiatry 36:555-559, 1979

Weiss SRB, Post RM, Patel J, et al: Differential mediation of the anticonvulsant effects of carbamazepine and diazepam. Life Sci 36:2413-2419, 1985

Willow M. Gonoi T, Catterall WA: Voltage clamp analyses of the inhibitory actions of diphenylhydantoin and carbamazepine on voltage-sensitive sodium channels in neuroblastoma cells. Mol Pharmacol 27:549-558, 1985

Wray SD, Hassell TM, Phillips C, et al: Preliminary study of the effects of carbamazepine on congenital orofacial defects in offspring of A/J mice. Epilepsia 23:101-110, 1982

Yerevanian BI, Hodgman CH: A haloperidol-carbamazepine interaction in a patient with rapid-cycling bipolar disorder (letter) Am J Psychiatry 142:785, 1985

Afterword

by Frederick K. Goodwin, M.D., and Kay Redfield Jamison, Ph.D.

We hope that the reader has found these chapters to be reasonably well balanced and integrated. Between an edited volume and an authored book there are inevitable tradeoffs. An edited volume exposes the reader to a variety of different perspectives and often at considerable depth. On the other hand, the level of integration and synthesis possible in a book authored by one or two individuals simply cannot be achieved in a collection of chapters which invariably have been conceived and written largely independently of one another.

However, most of the authors in this section work together in the same institution, thus making it easier for them to review and comment on each others' drafts as they were being prepared. This teamwork was particularly useful with respect to Chapters 2, 3, 4, and 6, where the potential overlap was significant.

We hope that by helping to update our colleagues on recent developments in bipolar disorders, their interest in our forthcoming comprehensive text/reference book on this topic will be enhanced.

The opinions expressed herein are those of the authors and do not reflect official policy of the NIMH.

II

Neuroscience Techniques in Clinical Psychiatry

Contents

Section II

Neuroscience Techniques in Clinical Psychiatry

Foreword

by John M. Morihisa, M.D., and Solomon H. Snyder, M.D.,
Section Editors

The rapid expansion of knowledge in the neurosciences has had a profound effect on the direction of psychiatric research as well as on the very way in which we view the nature of mental illness. In this section we attempt to provide a broad overview of those areas in which advances in the neurosciences have had a particularly dramatic impact in either clinical practice or in the ways in which we are investigating the underlying pathophysiology of psychiatric disorders.

We have divided this section into chapters on psychopharmacology, psychoendocrinology, psychoimmunology, sleep science, and structural and functional brain imaging. Each of these chapters could easily fill an entire volume with just the fundamental findings of the last decade. Nevertheless, we have tried to compile and discuss those neuroscience findings that appear to show the greatest promise or have had the greatest influence on the way in which we practice psychiatry. Furthermore, even as this volume goes to press, new findings are being reported that suggest different or new interpretations from those presented here. We are dealing with a dynamic process of evolution in the interactions between psychiatry and the neurosciences and any static view must endure certain limitations. Within these limitations we have endeavored to present an introduction to six of the major avenues of investigation that we feel represent areas of special interest in the neurosciences for psychiatric clinicians. It is our hope that this section will represent a starting point for a continuing examination of new findings in the brain sciences that will provide a useful context in which the reader can critically evaluate and choose among the ever growing cornucopia of information that this scientific discipline has generated.

Chapter 7

Psychopharmacology in Clinical Psychiatry

By John M. Davis, M.D., and David B. Bresnahan, M.D.

Pharmacology has radically altered the delivery of psychiatric services. It has had an equally profound effect on how psychiatrists speculate about and investigate the causes of mental illnesses and how they think about the applications of pharmacological treatment. In the 1940s, 1950s, and early 1960s, the dominant paradigm in psychiatry was the psychoanalytic one. To be sure, there were organically oriented psychiatrists in state hospitals providing custodial care, insulin coma, and electroconvulsive treatment, or screening plasma and urine of schizophrenics for the presence of abnormal compounds. The norepinephrine theory of affective disorders, as stated independently by Schildkraut in 1965, and Bunney and Davis in 1965, introduced a new paradigm to psychiatry: the neurotransmitter theory. Essentially the same paradigm was used for schizophrenia by Horn and Snyder (1971). This paradigm conceptualizes the biologic mechanism by which drugs may benefit a given disease and the biologic mechanism by which drugs may produce a given disease, and uses these mechanisms to formulate theories about the cause of that disease.

The norepinephrine theory of depression was based on the observation that there were three classes of antidepressant treatments at that time: the tricyclic antidepressants, the monoamine oxidase inhibitors (MAOIs), and electroconvulsive therapy (ECT). All three classes of treatment, in a functional sense, increased brain noradrenergic function. In addition, reserpine and alphamethyldopa, used in the treatment of hypertension, caused depression as a side effect. Both of these agents lower brain norepinephrine. It was suggested that depression was functionally caused by low brain norepinephrine and mania by high brain norepinephrine. Virtually the same evidence that supports the norepinephrine theory of depression can support a low serotonin theory of depression and a high serotonin theory of mania. The biogenic amine theory can be more precisely divided into two components: 1) that the common denominator by which the antidepressants help depression is their ability to potentiate norepinephrine (the mechanism of action by which the drug produces its therapeutic effect), and 2) that depression is caused by low norepinephrine in the brain and mania by high norepinephrine.

Horn and Snyder (1971) noted that a remarkable similarity existed between the structures of various antipsychotic compounds and the structure of dopamine, and postulated that the common denominator underlying the antipsychotic drugs was their ability to occupy the dopamine receptor and thus block dopaminergic transmission. Furthermore, Snyder (1972) noted that drugs which released dopamine, such as amphetamine, produced a paranoid psychosis, which was similar but not identical to schizophrenia.

We wish to gratefully acknowledge support for this work by the MacArthur Foundation.

There are two basic divisions of pharmacology: pharmacodynamics and pharmacokinetics. Pharmacodynamics studies the mechanism by which drugs produce their therapeutic or side effects. Pharmacokinetics studies the manner in which drugs are metabolized over time. The former studies what the drug does in the body; the latter studies how the drug is handled by the body. In this review we will focus upon both types of pharmacological theories. We will review the norepinephrine, serotonin, dopamine, and acetylcholine theories of disease, particularly those aspects which may be relevant to biochemical tests for depression. Specifically, can 3-methoxy 4-hydroxyphenylglycol (MHPG) be used as a test for depression or a test to predict the optimal type of antidepressant? We will then discuss how pharmacokinetics leads to a more rational psychopharmacology. In order to accomplish this, we will conduct a metanalysis or systematic review of the literature to ascertain what the current data indicate. Since this is a scholarly endeavor, the analytic techniques are necessarily complex, involving location of the relevant controlled studies and combining the data in a systematic fashion so that an unbiased conclusion can be drawn. We will follow these highly technical sections with general conclusions for the clinician.

THE TWO-DISEASE THEORY OF DEPRESSION

The norepinephrine theory suggests that depression is caused by low brain norepinephrine and mania is caused by high brain norepinephrine. Similarly, the serotinin theory suggests that depression is caused by low brain serotinin and mania by high brain serotonin. Maas and colleagues (1974) suggested that norepinephrine was metabolized in the brain to MHPG, but in the peripheral nervous system to vanillylmandelic acid (VMA). Maas and colleagues (1974), therefore, studied urinary MHPG in depressed patients and controls and found that although many depressed patients excreted normal MHPG, some excreted low MHPG. Similarly, Asberg and colleagues (1976) and Van Praag and colleagues (1973) used CSF 5-hydroxy indoleacetic acid (5HIAA) as a marker for brain serotonin and noted that a subgroup of depressed patients had low CSF 5HIAA. Maas and colleagues (1974) and Schildkraut (1973) suggested that a subgroup of depressed patients suffered from low norepinephrine depression, and this could be diagnosed by a measurement of low levels of urinary MHPG. Similarly, a subgroup of depressed patients had low serotonin depression, and this could be diagnosed by normal urinary MHPG. By implication, depressed patients with normal urinary MHPG were assumed to be in the low serotonin group with low CSF 5HIAA. It was further assumed that the tricyclic drugs benefit depression through their property of inhibiting norepinephrine or serotonin uptake. It was assumed that the parent tricyclics imipramine or amitriptyline were particularly potent in inhibiting serotonin uptake, but their desmethyl derivatives (nortriptyline or desipramine) were particularly potent in inhibiting the uptake of norepinephrine. Generally, the data for this assumption was based on acute test-tube experiments. Maas pointed out that in man, imipramine is substantially metabolized to desipramine, hence, it may be predominantly noradrenergic, and amitriptyline is only poorly metabolized to nortriptyline, hence, it may be a serotonergic drug.

We would assume that the tricyclic drugs block the reuptake of norepinephrine, therefore, making more norepinephrine available in the synaptic cleft, thus potentiating norepinephrine functionally. Since there is increased noradrenergic transmission, there is a down-regulation of the beta noradrenergic receptor sites. Down-regulation is a consequence of a decrease in the number of receptors. Through a feedback inhibitory mechanism, norepinephrine synthesis would decrease. We would further assume that there is also a compensatory decrease in norepinephrine synthesis. These are only partially compensating for the increase in noradrenergic transmission, so that norepinephrine is still potentiated, although to a lesser degree than it would have been had the compensatory mechanisms been absent.

One can list some of the assumptions in the two-disease MHPG theory as a test for predicting drug response. The assumptions are as follows: 1) MHPG is a marker for brain norepinephrine; 2) imipramine is extensively metabolized to desipramine, and amitriptyline is poorly metabolized to nortriptyline; 3) imipramine is a noradrenergic antidepressant and amitriptyline is a serotonergic antidepressant; 4) a subgroup of depressed patients have low MHPG; 5) low MHPG predicts response to imipramine or other so-called noradrenergic antidepressants; 6) normal MHPG predicts response to serotonergic antidepressants; 7) a subgroup of depressed patients have low 5-hydroxy indoleacetic acid (5HIAA). How well have these hypotheses held up to subsequent study?

MHPG As a Marker

Recently, it has been shown that MHPG can be converted to VMA. Hence, MHPG of central origin can be excreted as VMA. Finally, the theoretical components of the test have also been questioned. There is evidence to indicate that as little as 20 percent of MHPG in urine reflects brain activity.

The Specificity of Tricyclic Metabolism

Is imipramine heavily metabolized to desmethylimipramine and amitriptyline very poorly metabolized to nortriptyline? The answer is "yes" and "no." Generally, more imipramine is metabolized to desipramine than amitriptyline to nortriptyline. However, the difference is not that marked, and there are considerable individual differences. For example, the Depression Collaborative Study (Bowden et al, 1985; Hanin et al, 1985) found amitriptyline's plasma levels to be 142.1 ± 11.3 and CSF levels 9.3 ± 0.7, nortriptyline plasma levels 138.1 ± 11.3, CSF nortriptyline levels 12.6 ± 1.0, plasma imipramine levels 133.0 ± 14.2, and CSF imipramine levels 10.1 ± 1.0, plasma desipramine levels 170.9 ± 29.8, and CSF desimipramine levels, 21.1 ± 3.2. Other studies found comparable results. Although there is more desipramine present after imipramine than nortriptyline after amitriptyline, these differences are not marked.

Specificity of Tricyclic Action

Initially there was evidence that imipramine and other noradrenergic drugs affected norepinephrine in that they caused an expected decrease in urinary or CSF MHPG, and that the "serotonergic" drugs affected serotonin in that they produced the expected decrease in CSF 5HIAA. If imipramine was really noradrenergic and amitriptyline was serotonergic, then one would expect that in the majority of the patients treated with imipramine there would be a substantial decrease in urinary and CSF MHPG, and in the majority of the patients treated with amitriptyline there would be little change in MHPG but a marked reduction in 5HIAA. However, the Depression Collaborative Study (Bowden et al, 1985) did not find this. Rather, it found that both imipramine and amitriptyline decreased CSF and urinary MHPG and CSF 5HIAA to an equal extent. Insofar as these measures are indicative of a noradrenergic or serotonergic brain effect, we would have to conclude that in man, both imipramine and amitriptyline affect norepinephrine and serotonin equally. This evidence is contrary to the specificity hypothesis.

Is MHPG Really Low in Depression? (A Metanalysis)

We will review the literature on whether or not urinary MHPG is really low in depression, using what has become known as "metanalytic techniques." We previously (Davis, 1975) were the first to use such techniques for combining data from multiple studies on prevention of relapse. Such techniques are only valid when studies of a given design are analyzed and the design is reasonably adequate to the task. Subsequently, workers have misused the techniques in combining data from testimonials. Even the most complicated statistics do not alter the testimonial quality of uncontrolled studies. A number of controlled studies have investigated the 24-hour urinary excretion of MHPG, and we have combined the data from these. This can be a difficult problem since some workers will report a preliminary trial and then a subsequent trial, reporting both the additional subjects as well as those already reported. We only included patients in our review if we had positive evidence that a given patient was counted only once. As males excrete more MHPG than females, we separated the data so that male depressed patients are compared to male controls, and the same for females. When studies reported the number of subjects, the mean MHPG, and the standard deviation of the patients and controls, we were able to combine the data from the various studies (male and female results kept separate as if they were different studies), using the method of Hedges and Olkin (1985) (Table 1).

We also calculated the percentage increase that occurred in depressed patients in contrast to their sex-matched controls, weighing each study by the number of patients from the study. The percentage calculation is more intuitive than the D-plus index of Hedges and Olkin and is intended to give the reader a feel for the data. We find that the depressed patients excreted slightly more MHPG (0.5 percent) than the controls. As might be expected, if we pool the data statistically, there is no significant difference. We also did a test of homogeneity of findings: That is, do all studies in this set of data find the same results? The test for homogeneity in fact proved to be statistically insignificant here. When possible, since not all the studies divided the patients into unipolar versus bipolar, we evaluated the results in those studies which separated bipolar versus unipolar. Other investigators distinguish between unipolar, bipolar, and schizoaffective. Since Schildkraut hypothesized a diagnostic classification relevant to the MHPG hypothesis, we approximated, insofar as possible, the Schildkraut classification when we compared bipolar versus unipolar, and in weighing the number of patients in each study. Bipolars excreted 94 percent of the MHPG of unipolars, which we found to be statistically insignificant. The test for discrepancy of results between studies was clearly nonsignificant. We next compared unipolar patients against controls and found that unipolar patients excreted 10 percent more MHPG than the control patients. This is clearly contrary to the "low MHPG"

Table 1. Summary of MHPG in Unipolar and Bipolar Depression

Study	Sex	Number of Subjects		Mean MHPG		Percent MHPG depressed
		depressed	controls	depressed	controls	
Mass et al, 1974	M	20	48	1394	1694	83.27
	F	19	21	1155	1348	85.68
Schatzberg et al, 1982	M	38	13	2133	2021	105.54
	F	32	13	1691	1820	92.91
Beckman and Goodman, 1980	M	28	9	1810	1890	95.77
	F	38	18	1530	1830	83.61
Sharpless, 1977	M	10	6	2019	2105	95.91
	F	10	5	1357	1618	83.87
Hollister, 1981	M	30	17	2036	1888	107.84
Agren, 1983	M	27	8	3647	3481	104.77
	F	40	8	2910	2560	113.67
Taube et al, 1978	F	14	10	791	1029	76.87
Koslow et al, 1983	M	60	36	2273	2267	100.26
	F	54	36	1968	1660	118.55
Musscettola et al, 1984	M	10	7	1680	1440	116.67
	F	31	8	1500	1230	121.95

mean weighted percent = 100.5

(A)
Bipolars as a Percent of Controls

Schatzberg et al, 1982	70
	73
Beckman and Goodman, 1980	94
	80
Agren, 1983	109
	98
Koslow et al, 1983	120
	98
Musscettola et al, 1984	120
	78
Weighted mean	94

(B)
MHPG in Unipolars as Percent of Controls

Schatzberg et al, 1982	118
	102
Beckman and Goodman, 1980	100
	91
Agren, 1983	104
	119
Koslow et al, 1983	101
	100
Coppen et al, 1979	79
	108
Musscettola et al, 1984	142
	141
Weighted mean	110

Table 1. Summary of MHPG in Unipolar and Bipolar Depression (Continued)

(C) MHPG in Bipolars as a Percent of Unipolars	
Schatzberg et al, 1982	59
	72
Beckman and Goodman, 1980	94
	87
Edwards et al, 1980	92
Agren, 1983	105
	82
Koslow et al, 1983	97
	101
Musscettola et al, 1984	55
	68
Weighted mean	86

(D) Statistical Tests			
	dt (effect size)	Confidence Limits	Significance
Depressed patients versus controls	− .08	− .24 to .08	not significant
Bipolars versus controls	− .22	− .46 to .02	not significant
Unipolars versus controls	.54	.33 to .76	significant
Bipolars versus unipolars	− .34	− .50 to − .18	significant

This Table summarizes a metanalysis of the MHPG excretion in unipolar and bipolar patients in comparison to controls. When data were available, we compared male controls against male depressed patients, female controls against female depressed patients. In order to give the reader the feel for the data, we also calculated the percentage of MHPG excreted by depressed patients in comparison to the appropriate controls. However, the statistics computed were based on the original means, Ns, and standard deviations. Similarly, we compared bipolar patients to controls, unipolar patients to controls, and bipolar patients to unipolar patients, using the Hedges and Olkin technique again, but present percentages to give the reader the feel for the data. We have expressed in Tables 1A, 1B, 1C the percentage differences, and the Hedges/Olkin statistics are presented in 1D.

hypothesis. Indeed, based on this combined data, the unipolar depressed patients secreted statistically significantly more MHPG than controls. The effect sizes were not homogeneous ($p = .005$). Some studies show depressed patients excrete 40 percent more MHPG, others 20 percent, and still others no change or even a decrease. Part of the discrepancy in effect size between the studies is the degree to which depressed patients excrete more MHPG. This is indeed the case. But some studies find that bipolars excrete essentially similar MHPGs to unipolars, but most find that bipolars excrete less MHPG than unipolars. Overall, bipolars excrete 14 percent less MHPG than unipolars. And this is statistically significant, and some find that unipolars excrete more MHPG than bipolars.
CONCLUSION: MHPG IS NORMAL IN DEPRESSION. When we combine the data from all the studies, we find that MHPG is 105 percent of normals in

depressed patients. When separating bipolars from unipolars, the bipolar depressed patients' MHPG in comparison to normals is 94 percent and unipolar depressed patients' MHPG in comparison to normals is 110 percent. Because of the absence of statistically significant numbers, we would have to conclude that the MHPG in depressed patients is about the same as that in normals. MHPG may be slightly lower than normal in bipolars, slightly higher than normal in unipolars, and there may be a slight difference between bipolar depressed and unipolar depressed patients. Obviously, MHPG cannot be diagnostic for depression per se since we do not feel that MHPG can be used for the diagnosis of either bipolar or unipolar subtype and since these differences, even if real, are very modest. Hence, our conclusion is that MHPG is not diagnostically useful at this time.

Does Low MHPG Predict Response to Imipramine? (A Metanalysis)

The NIMH Collaborative Study (Maas, 1984) found that low MHPG predicted response to imipramine in bipolar but not unipolar patients. The initial positive study of Maas and his co-workers (1974) was based on mostly bipolar depressives and psychotic depressives. This suggests that the predictive power of MHPG should be re-examined in unipolars and bipolars separately. We systematically reviewed the literature, using data on unipolar or bipolar patients separately and recalculating the statistics from the raw data when possible. We corrected for sex or used MHPG/creatinine when this was possible. Where we could not separate patients into unipolar or bipolar types, we reported the results as mixed (unipolar and bipolar). We expressed the degree to which MHPG predicted clinical response as a correlation coefficient to have a common benchmark. There is really no adequate method to combine data from such disparate studies, but as an approximation we did calculate these correlations and then combined them, weighing each correlation by the number of subjects. Maas and colleagues (1974) in their original two studies, and Steinbook and colleagues (1979) did not separate unipolar and bipolar patients, and found low MHPG predicted a response to imipramine (Maas Study 1, $r = -.88$, $n = 11$; Study 2, $r = -.52$, $n = 12$; and Steinbook, $r = -.807$, $n = 7$). This yielded a combined correlation coefficient of $r = -.70$ in 35 subjects. Three studies on bipolars treated with imipramine found $r = -.38$, $n = 27$ (Maas et al, 1984); $r = -.67$, $n = 6$ (Hollister et al, 1980); and $r = .-48$, $n = 11$ (Musscettola et al, 1984). Combining the data, we found a pooled correlation of $-.44$ for 44 bipolar patients. The eight studies in unipolars on imipramine found correlations of $-.74$, $.34$, $-.22$, $-.42$, $-.49$, $.12$, $.13$ (Beckman et al, 1975; Hollister et al, 1980; Schatzberg et al, 1980b; Charney et al, 1981; Veith et al, 1983; and Janicak et al, 1986), yielding an average correlation of $-.17$ ($n = 162$).

Does Normal MHPG Predict Response to Amitriptyline?

Five studies on mixed patients found correlations of $.27$, $-.41$, $-.11$, 1.00, and $.32$ (Schildkraut, 1973; Steinbook et al, 1979; Gaertner et al, 1982; Sacchetti et al, 1979; Puzynski et al, 1984), the pooled correlation being $+.07$ for 82 subjects. The NIMH Collaborative Study results found low MHPG predicted response to amitriptyline in 11 bipolar patients $r = -.38$ (Maas et al, 1984), a result in the opposite direction from the hypothesis. Six studies of unipolars found correlations of 1.00, .16, −.27, .13, −.49 (Beckman et al, 1975; Coppen et al, 1979; Veith et al, 1983; Ward et al, 1983; Musscettola et al, 1984) and −.47 (our study) with a pooled correlation of +.01 for 86 subjects. The pooled data finds MHPG not to predict clinical response.

Conclusion on MHPG in Clinical Practice

In summary, evidence of distinct noradrenergic and serotonergically mediated depressions as well as the development of relatively specific antidepressants (that is, primarily noradrenergic or serotonergic) led researchers to look for methods to biochemically characterize depression and select antidepressants most likely to benefit each subtype. Foremost in this area has been examination of the norepinephrine metabolite MHPG in urine. Discovery of subpopulations of depressed patients with low urinary MHPG led to a classification scheme for depression based on MHPG levels, low MHPG being indicative of a noradrenergic depression most likely to respond to a noradrenergic agent (that is, desipramine). Conversely, normal or elevated MHPG was felt to indicate a serotonergic depression most likely to respond to a serotonergic agent. These predictions were based on a number of assumptions (that is, MHPG as a valid indicator of central nervous system (CNS) norepinephrine; neurotransmitter specificity of antidepressants, and so forth) which no longer appear to be valid. The predictive value of urinary MHPG has been unsubstantiated in a number of large studies, including the recent NIMH Collaborative Study and that of Janicak (1986). Because of some positive results from reliable laboratories and because the disparate result could be explained by methodologic artifacts, we feel it is premature to absolutely dismiss the MHPG hypothesis and regard the question as still open. However, a different standard should be applied when a test is used commercially. A routinely used clinical test must be a proven one that is clearly substantiated by the evidence. This is not the case with urinary MHPG.

Before leaving the question of urinary MHPG in clinical psychopharmacology, several practical problems should be highlighted. MHPG excretion decreases with previous tricylic treatment and may also vary significantly from day to day. In addition, there are differences in MHPG excretion patterns between males and females. Finally, the difficulty inherent in collecting adequate 24-hour urine specimens should not be underestimated. Even if MHPG's predictive value were clearly and unambiguously established, this could be a difficult test to administer in certain clinical populations (that is, psychotic depression, outpatient depressives). Given the evidence to date, we conclude that routine determination of urinary MHPG should not be employed clinically as a means of subtyping depression or selecting antidepressant treatment.

IS CSF 5HIAA LOW IN DEPRESSION?

There is an extensive literature indicating that CSF 5HIAA or CSF MHPG levels in depressives were higher, equal to, or lower than controls (see review of Koslow et al, 1983). But, most of the 25 or so studies of CSF MHPG, 5HIAA, or homovanillic acid (HVA) used, in whole or in part, neurological controls (since CNS or spinal cord diseases can influence CSF metabolite levels, any difference between neurological controls and depressed patients may reflect this). Many of these studies also used patients currently receiving psychotropic drugs, or who had less than a seven-day washout period. We will focus on a few studies that present baseline CSF metabolite values (not after probenecid), use healthy controls (not intermixed with neurological patients), and have a drug washout period of at least one week. This may not be long enough, but practical considerations make eight-week washout periods unfeasible. The Depression Collaborative Study (Koslow et al, 1983; Davis et al, 1983; and Berger et al, 1980) found 5HIAA values identical or slightly higher in depressives than normals. Traskman-Bendz and colleagues (1984) found a frequency histogram that in depressed patients CSF 5HIAA was bimodally distributed by visual inspection and that a subgroup of suicidal depressives had low CSF 5HIAA levels, while nonsuicidal patients were more similar to controls. We analyzed this data using our mixture-distribution paradigm and found 5HIAA to be bimodally distributed in depressed patients. We also reanalyzed Agren's (1983) data, finding a similar bimodal distribution. Furthermore, the results of the Asberg-Agren data are remarkably similar, finding most depressives have normal CSF 5HIAA levels, but there appears to be a distinct subgroup in each study characterized by these low CSF 5HIAA levels. Since low CSF 5HIAA is also characteristic of impulsive or violent patients, these low levels may be a characteristic of violence, impulsiveness, or some other variable pertinent to suicidal depression but not necessarily a core quality of all depressed patients. The Depression Collaborative Study was a very difficult protocol; hence, extremely disturbed and highly suicidal patients would not be likely to be referred to such a complicated study. This group did study severe chronic depressives, many of whom had suicidal ideation or had made previous suicidal attempts. The study of Asberg and colleagues (1976) was based on an unselected group of depressed patients, which included highly suicidal cases. Since there is consistent data from several large studies that there is a distinct subgroup with low 5HIAA, we find this convincing. Since this is a subgroup, it may be that certain studies have few such patients of this type included in their sample, and this may explain discrepancies in the data. None of the studies using normal controls found either a bimodal distribution or a subgroup of depressed patients to have uniformly low CSF MHPG (Koslow et al, 1983; Traskman-Bendz, 1984; Berger et al, 1980).

DOPAMINE IN DEPRESSION

Albeit some of the earlier studies used inadequate drug-free periods and neurological controls, there are a variety of studies which did find the dopamine metabolite, HVA, in depressed patients. Kasa et al (1982) found baseline CSF HVA to be 53 percent decreased in depression. Berger and colleagues (1980) found CSF HVA to be nearly equal, in that there was four percent less free HVA in depressed subjects in comparison to controls. Since we found CSF HVA to be decreased only in a subgroup of depressed patients, Berger's sample of 13 depressives may not have been large enough to ensure an adequate sample size in this low HVA subgroup. We have reanalyzed the published data of Traskman-Bendz (1984) and found that the healthy controls have a single Gaussian distribution with virtually identical peaks (ours peaks at 219 p moles/ml, Asberg's at 221 p moles/ml), and depressed patients have two peaks: one decreased (ours peaks at 125 p moles/ml, Asberg's at 109 p moles/ml) and one normal (ours peaks at 206 p moles/ml, Asberg's at 218 p moles/ml). Although most depressed patients have normal HVA, there is a clearly defined subgroup in a number of these studies that has low HVA. Note particularly a comparison between the NIMH Collaborative Study and the Asberg Study in which the peaks are almost exactly superimposed. Even though these studies are done in different countries, the estimate of the normal mean and the low mean agreed exactly in the second decimal place and only disagreed slightly in the third decimal place. Our reanalysis of Agren (1983) also indicated the presence of two HVA peaks similar to Asberg's and ours. This evidence taken in toto does suggest a subgroup of depressed patients who have decreased CSF HVA.

INCREASED PERIPHERAL CATECHOLAMINE EXCRETION IN A SUBGROUP OF DEPRESSED PATIENTS

Some years ago, the author (Davis), in collaboration with Bunney and Davis (1965) noted that a subgroup of depressed patients excreted markedly high levels of epinephrine and norepinephrine. Since epinephrine (E), norepinephrine (NE), metanephrine (MET), and normetanephrine (NMET) do not pass the blood-brain barrier, these compounds reflect only release from the peripheral autonomic nervous system. We made a very interesting observation about the excretion of the peripheral catecholamines in depressed patients. Davis and colleagues (1985) plotted the frequency histogram and found that while E and MET were distributed with the single Gaussian normal distribution in the healthy control population, E and MET were bimodally distributed in the depressed patients; one subgroup of depressed patients excreting normal levels and the others markedly high E and MET levels. Since E is metabolized to MET, we analyzed the joint distribution of E and MET with a two-dimensional frequency histogram. For the healthy control population, this study found a single normal distribution. In two dimensions in the depressed patient, we found a bimodal distribution on the joint excretion of epinephrine and metanephrine. Some depressed patient excreted essentially normal levels of E and MET. However, a subgroup of the depressed patients, consisting of slightly less than 50 percent, excreted markedly high levels of E and MET. This mixture of two Gaussian distribution analyses resulted in a much better fit of the data than a single Gaussian distribution (p less than .000001). We also did a four-dimensional analysis considering the excretion of E, MET, NE, and NM. The normal population essentially excreted normal levels of all these compounds. There were two subgroups in depressed patients, one excreting normal levels and one excreting high levels of all four compounds.

Several studies found depressed patients have high levels of plasma E or NE or both (Wyatt et al, 1971; Lake et al, 1982; Roy et al, 1985; Rudorfer et al, 1985). Esler and colleagues (1982) observed that depressed patients with an infusion of tritiated NE had elevated plasma NE spillover rates. This measures the rate of entry of NE to plasma from peripheral sympathetic nerves. Rosenblatt and colleagues (1969) also infused labeled NE, measuring the ratio of amines to oxidized metabolites (non-oxidized/oxidized ratio), and found that depressed patients excreted relatively more amine and less oxidized metabolites.

We suggest some depressives are releasing large amounts of catecholamines from the adrenal and sympathetic nervous system. Several studies found tyramine sensitivity decreased in depressives. Pandey and colleagues (1979) in our laboratory and Extein and colleagues (1979) noted that depressed patients' leukocytes were less (cAMP) responsive to isoproterenol, indicating beta receptor subsensitivity. The increased E and NE release may produce receptor subsensitivity in peripheral tissues, a so-called down regulation of vascular, platelet, and leukocyte adrenergic receptors, as well as produce other physiological changes that are seen in depression. Consistent data from several studies indicate CSF HVA is substantially reduced in depressives. This reduction is seen almost entirely in the high E + MET subgroup of depressed patients. This also suggests that HVA may be involved in some way with the peripheral noradrenergic activity. We note that dopamine agonists decrease peripheral noradrenergic secretion so that there may be a physiologic relationship of the low CSF HVA to the high E + MET in this subgroup.

Previous Drug Treatment as a Methodological Artifact

The same methodological problems plague virtually all biologic investigations into transmitter substance, their metabolites, and their synthetic or degradative enzymes. There is a possibility that previous drug treatment may alter platelet monoamine oxidase levels, autopsied brain dopamine binding sites, autopsied brain imipramine/desipramine binding sites, platelet imipramine sites, MHPG, or 5HIAA. It is even conceivable that there could be a rebound effect. This is an important distinction to make. One investigator could interpret a value drawn after discontinuing a drug as a rise above baseline, but, in reality, the value might not have completely returned to normal. Without having done studies to determine what normal is, any statement is purely speculative even though not necessarily labeled as such. Sometimes the existence of an artifact is only supported by rather limited data. To prove a methodological artifact, there must be some degree of rigorous proof. We should really look with some reasonable degree of skepticism at the methodology of studies which attempt to show that an artifact exists.

THE NOREPINEPHRINE HYPOTHESIS REVISITED

How has the norepinephrine hypothesis fared since it was first described 20 years ago? The original hypothesis suggested that depression may be a low norepinephrine state. In other words, it could be caused by either low brain norepinephrine or a decrease in synaptic transmission due to defective receptors and enhanced uptake systems. The latter possibility is important, since there may be a physiologic regulation of the reuptake process (Lee et al, 1983). The original hypothesis specifically made a functional statement and was not tied to norepinephrine levels. The attempt to estimate central norepinephrine levels by MHPG has failed to be proven. Research has not yet proved a norepinephrine defect in depressed patients. On the other hand, there is much new evidence to confirm the norepinephrine hypothesis, or at least to show that it is still a fruitful paradigm. A substantial number of new antidepressants have been discovered. The fact that many of these affect norepinephrine uptake should not be surprising since they were screened based on ability to affect norepinephrine uptake. The fact that these drugs proved efficacious is important. This inductive evidence suggests that the antidepressants may exert their antidepressant properties through their effect on norepinephrine. What is more important is the fact that these drugs did prove to be effective antidepressants. If the norepinephrine hypothesis was wrong, then it would have been expected that drugs screened to affect norepinephrine may not necessarily have been proved to be clinical antidepressants. Particularly important is the drug mianserin, which increases norepinephrine synthesis through a presynaptic mechanism. It represents a fourth class of antidepressants, where norepinephrine may be involved in the mechanism of action. Also of interest is the clinical antidepressant iprindole, which down-regulates norepinephrine. In our laboratory we have found that buproprion, in high doses, down-regulates norepinephrine receptors. The minor tranquilizer alprazolam (notwithstanding the difficulties in separating the antidepressant action secondary to its anxiolytic effect) clearly has therapeutic efficacy in outpatient depressions and may, indeed, be a true antidepressant, although further data on this is needed. In our laboratory, we found that alprazolam down-regulates beta adrenergic receptors. The fact that there are a substantial number of new treatments which benefit depression, and which affect norepinephrine, certainly suggests norepinephrine may be involved in the mechanism of action of antidepressant drugs.

THE SEROTONIN HYPOTHESIS REVISITED

Most of the new antidepressants affect norepinephrine and not necessarily serotonin. In addition, chlorimipramine is metabolized to desmethylchlorimipramine, which is a potent inhibitor of norepinephrine uptake. Zemelidine is metabolized to norzemelidine, which is also a potent uptake inhibitor of norepinephrine. Some of the other so-called specific serotonin drugs, such as trazodone, down-regulate beta-adrenergic receptors. So they may have a norepinephrine effect through a poorly characterized mechanism. Even so, there are some drugs which might possibly be specific serotonin potentiators. The existence of $5HD_2$ receptors and their down-regulation as a compensatory mechanism of chronic tricyclic treatment indicates that much the same evidence that supports the norepinephrine mechanism of action may also support a serotonergic mechanism of action for this family of drugs (Peroutka and Snyder, 1980). Furthermore, the noradrenergic and the serotonergic effects of tricyclics may be linked in some way.

Specific high affinity binding sites for imipramine have been demonstrated in human platelets which appear to be similar to those found in the human brain. Similar binding sites for tritiated desipramine are also present in the human brain. Imipramine and desipramine binding sites (receptors) are related functionally to presynaptic reuptake sites for serotonin and norepinephrine, respectively. A number of investigators have reported that the concentration of tritiated imipramine binding sites is decreased in depressed patients when compared with normal controls. Further, autopsied brain studies of depressed patients who have committed suicide and controls reveal a decrease in imipramine but not desipramine binding sites and an increase in 5HT sites in the depressed patients. The latter may be an up-regulation phenomenon of a post-synaptic receptor. In a broad sense, looking at the norepinephrine and serotonin hypothesis in the last 20 years, there is much new data that links these two transmitters to drugs which alter affective states. In revisiting these theories, the news is both good and bad. The bad news is that we cannot prove that one or another transmitter is actually involved in depression. The good news is that there is a substantial new body of evidence which links these transmitters to affective illness. In summary, the pharmacologic base of the norepinephrine hypothesis remains a viable paradigm. A number of avenues (that is, CSF 5HIAA) show potential promise and may someday be clinically useful tests, able to assist the clinician in evaluating and treating depressed patients. Trends indicate that in addition to CSF 5HIAA, CSF HVA and peripheral catecholamines may be useful in selecting subtypes of depressed patients. However, as with MHPG, there is lacking a convincing and consistent body of evidence supporting the usefulness of any of these neuropharmacologic tests. Their use in clinical practice is, therefore, not recommended at this time.

THE CHOLINERGIC HYPOTHESIS

While not as extensively studied at this point, there is also good evidence that the cholinergic system may play a role in affective illness. Changes in the cholinergic system (as produced by physostigmine) can influence affective states. Increased acetylcholine has been shown to transiently benefit mania (Davis et al, 1978). This has also been shown to affect cortisol and sleep patterns in a similar way to what is seen in depression. There is also evidence that physostigmine, presumably through a central action on increasing brain acetylcholine, increases the adrenal release of epinephrine, and we note that some depressed patients do have increased release of peripheral catecholamines.

ANTIDEPRESSANT PLASMA LEVELS

Since patients on the same dose have large interindividual differences in the tricyclic plasma level, can the lack of response be attributed to a difference in these plasma levels (Table 3; Figures 1, 2, 3)? We have summarized in this Table the empirical evidence on plasma levels, combining the data from different studies given in tables or graphs to see if the results are consistent. Some investigators presented the number of patients above or below a certain cut-off point, and we combined this data as best we could. When investigators reported data from several different weeks, we averaged those plasma levels to obtain a mean plasma level and related this to a mean clinical response.

Asberg and colleagues (1971) found that five patients failed to respond to plasma nortriptyline below 50 nl/gl. No other study had patients beneath the therapeutic window. The precise location of the "low window" derives principally from data on these five patients. Asberg further reported that patients who had plasma levels that exceeded 140 ng/ml tended to display an unfavorable clinical response. This seems not to be due to CNS toxicity (Figure 1). This paradoxical property of nortriptyline was confirmed in that two studies reported that poor responses occurred with plasma levels above 175 ng/ml and 200 ng/ml, respectively. The latter found that of 16 patients with high plasma levels who had had their clinical doses reduced, 12 improved within approximately one week. Kragh-Sorensen and colleagues (1976) adjusted doses to either above 180 ng/ml or below 150 ng/ml and reported that a disproportionately large number of subjects in the first group showed a poor clinical response. In a second phase, a subgroup selected at random from those with high plasma levels (180 + ng/ml) had their doses lowered to the therapeutic range. Five out of five patients improved. The six patients whose doses were not reduced had a poor response. The upper end of the therapeutic window varies substantially from study to study. Indeed, the 140 ng/ml upper limit, so widely quoted in secondary sources, is actually well within the range of the therapeutic window reported by most of the studies reviewed (Figure 1). Some review articles give the upper limit of the nortriptyline therapeutic window at 140 ng/ml, yet inspection of Figure 1 shows many responders have nortriptyline levels above 140 ng/ml.

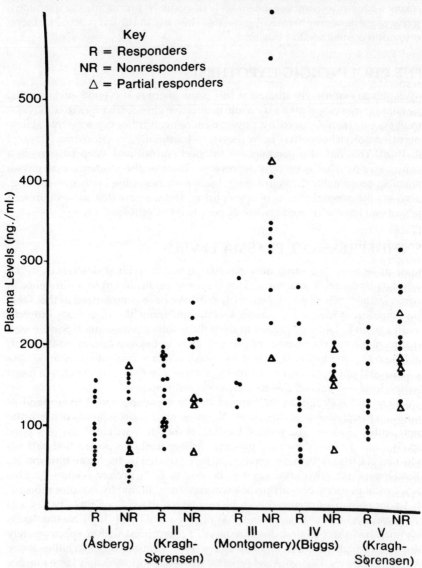

Figure 1. Nortriptyline plasma levels versus response

Data from two protriptyline studies are presented in Figure 2 (Davis et al, 1984). One study found several nonresponders with high plasma levels and two nonresponders with low levels. The results of the other study were below those of the first one. It is impossible to state the location of the therapeutic window limits for protriptyline because of the difference in absolute plasma levels. Protriptyline has an unusually long half-life, and therefore some patients may not necessarily have been at steady-state in the first two weeks. Fluorometric methods may be less specific than mass spectroscopic methods, but that is not the explanation for the discrepant finding here. Rickels and his co-workers (1983) found that four out of five nonresponders had plasma levels below 100 ng/ml[420].

When we tabulated the findings from an additional 10 amitriptyline studies and Rickel's results (Davis and colleagues' 1984 review) (Table 2), we found more good responders had levels above 100 ng/ml and more moderate or poor responders had levels below 100 ng/ml. Total amitriptyline plus nortriptyline plasma levels and final Hamilton scores were available in 10 studies, and hence were evaluated using a cubic regression model (Figure 3) but found no inverted U-shaped relationship between plasma levels and clinical response ($r^2 = 0.006$) (Davis et al, 1984). Responders had roughly the same plasma levels as the nonresponders, with no obvious upper end of the therapeutic window. When plasma levels fall below 100 ng/ml, the relative number of nonresponders increased, but most nonresponders had levels well above 100 ng/ml.

Summation of the data on desipramine indicates that the percent of response is low when plasma levels are below 115 ng/ml (Table 3). Imipramine studies (Table 3) find poor clinical responses with low plasma levels (under 180 ng/ml or under 240 ng/ml). These studies failed to find an upper end of the therapeutic window with a loss of efficacy at high plasma levels but did find toxicity at very high plasma levels. Of patients with plasma levels below 180 ng/ml, the response rate was 30 percent (which, parenthetically, is the placebo response rate). For patients with plasma levels above 240 ng/ml, 70 percent responded. These findings illustrate a somewhat indeterminate therapeutic range of 180–250 ng/ml.

All too often, authors place absolute limits on the upper and lower limits of the therapeutic window as if these were firmly established. It is incorrect to say, using an example where the therapeutic window is 100 ng/ml to 200 ng/ml, that a patient with 99 ng/ml would be below and surely a nonresponder, and a patient with 201 ng/ml would be above the window and equally sure a nonresponder. We see, from inspection of Figures 1 and 2, that such an absolute interpretation is not supported by the data. Most nonresponders are within the therapeutic window. We believe that the best way to interpret plasma levels is not through arbitrarily selected number values defining the upper or lower end but by the clinician placing a given plasma level in the context of the experimental data. When patients are at steady-state, a given plasma level should be considered an absolute number as it represents the physical presence of a substance in plasma, just as plasma Li or plasma sodium is a constant. Some of the variability observed can be explained by different authors measuring tricyclic levels on different occasions following the start of drug treatment. Some patients do not reach steady-state until three weeks or more. For example, Asberg and colleagues (1971) measured tricyclic levels during the first two weeks, while Kraugh-Sorensen (1976) made his determinations at the fourth week. Plasma

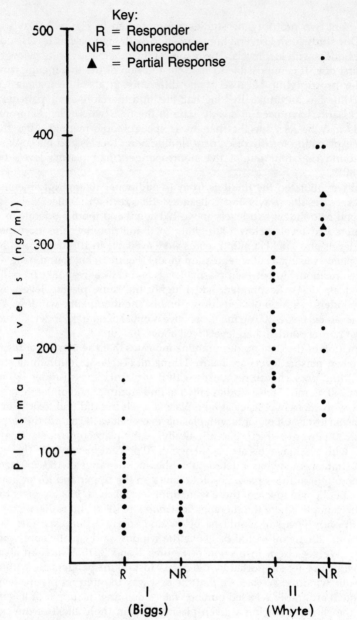

Figure 2. Protriptyline plasma levels versus response

levels should be proportionate to dose and hence, at steady-state, a given dose change should produce a given plasma level. Although the most fundamental information for dose adjustment are side effects and clinical response, plasma levels provide useful data earlier in time than side effects or response data.

No blanket statement can be made about the clinical usefulness of plasma

Table 2. Plasma Amitriptyline Levels

| | Plasma Level | |
Clinical Results	Low (less than 100 ng/ml)	High (greater than 100 ng/ml)
Good	12 (4%)	110 (40%)
Moderate–Poor	35 (13%)	120 (43%)
TOTAL	47 (17%)	230 (83%) (100%)

We combined the data from 11 controlled studies of amitriptyline clinical response and plasma levels and reported data on 277 patients, and found that for a low level of total amitriptyline (amitriptyline plus nortriptyline less than 100 ng/ml) only 1 out of 4 patients responded, but when the plasma levels were greater than this, about 1 out of 2 responded. Most nonresponders had plasma levels in the same range as the responders, however.

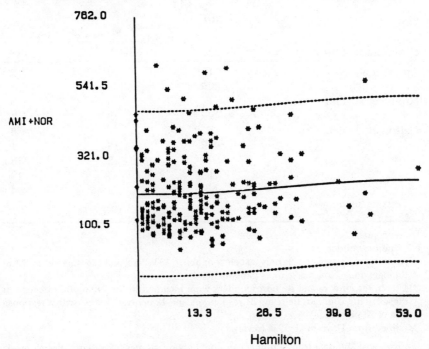

Amitriptyline vs Clinical Response (Hamilton scores)
Cubic Regression Model

Figure 3. Amitriptyline versus clinical response

Table 3. Plasma Levels versus Clinical Response Patients Treated with Desipramine and Imipramine**

		(A) Plasma Levels (ng/ml)		
Imipramine Study		0–180	180–240	+240
Glassman et al, 1977[+]	R	8	22*	
	NR	21	8*	
Matuzas et al, 1982[+]	R	1	1	0
	NR	6	2	0
Matuzas et al, 1983[+]	R	5	1	2
	NR	5	2	1
Reisbey et al, 1977[+]	R	11	4	18
	NR	23	5	5
Oliver-Martin et al, 1975[+]	R	0	2	4
	NR	3	1	4
Simpson[+]	R	8	3	7
	NR	6	1	2
Total	R	33	11	53***
	NR	64	11	20
Percent Response		34%	50%	73%

		(B) Plasma level ng/ml	
Desipramine Study		0–115	115+
Amin. et al, 1978[+]	R	0	2
	NR	1	2
Hrdina et al, 1981	R	0	3
	NR	3	1
Nelson et al, 1982	R	3	8
	NR	18	1
Total		0–115	115
	R	3	13
	NR	22	4
Percent Response		12%	76%

R = responder
NR = nonresponder
  *Author gave plasma levels only as below or above 180 (Perel and Glassman et al, 1978)
 **Endogenous + Nonendogenous patients
***The 22 responders and 8 nonresponders were included in the 240 ng/ml category. If these are not counted, there are 31 responders and 12 nonresponders, with a response rate of 72 percent.
[+]Modified from Davis et al, 1984 (review)

We reviewed the data from a number of double blind studies, classifying plasma levels as being below a cut-off point or within a given range, or above a cut off point and listing the number of patients who responded or did not respond.

levels of antidepressants. Since the shape of the plasma level clinical response curves and the adequacy of the data varies with different drugs, each one needs to be discussed separately. For many drugs, the available data is inadequate or contradictory, and we would not recommend use of plasma levels except to check for clinical extremes. For example, with two contradictory studies, as is the case with protriptyline, not enough data is available to meaningfully find a therapeutic range. There is also a poor correlation between amitriptyline plasma levels and clinical response. However, protriptyline or amitriptyline levels might be useful as a semi-quantitative measurement of compliance or in cases of overdose or toxic dose situations, to help define the magnitude of drug load and to monitor recovery. In general, we feel that the most reliable guide to dosing with antidepressants is clinical assessment of therapeutic effects and side effects. The inappropriate or excessive use of plasma levels can lead to a deterioration in the quality of care if doses are adjusted to plasma levels, ignoring important clinical variables.

Three drugs exist for which there are enough reliable data to warrant the use of plasma levels in clinical practice. These are: nortriptyline, imipramine, and possibly desipramine. We would emphasize, though, that with these agents, the data are not so overwhelming that plasma levels ought to be used routinely, but that their use should be considered elective. A number of clinical situations exist in which plasma levels for these agents may be clinically helpful. The first situation would be in the patient who is on an adequate dose of medication and in whom there is a poor clinical response. A low plasma level in such a patient might indicate that the dose should be increased. An extremely high level might indicate that nonresponse is not due to an inadequate level and suggest a change to another agent. A plasma level of imipramine between 180 ng/ml and 240 ng/ml is in a somewhat indeterminate range. For this, we would suggest a very modest increase in dose. It is important to remember that the correlation between plasma level and clinical efficacy is not tightly defined. Plasma levels are most useful when they are extreme. Desipramine has not been extensively investigated, but the available data suggest that if levels are clearly in excess of 115 ng/ml the dose is probably adequate, and if they are clearly below 115 ng/ml the dose is probably inadequate. For nortriptyline, the situation is more complicated in that there may be a failure to respond associated with high plasma levels. Clearly, for nortriptyline, if the plasma level is below 50 ng/ml, one would increase the dose. If the plasma level is between 50 and 120 and the patient is nonresponding, one might consider increasing the dose, particularly if it is in the low side of this range. Depending on the number of weeks of treatment, if the plasma level is clearly above 180 or so, one might consider decreasing the dose. A plasma level between 120 and 180 is difficult to interpret. Another example would be a patient with significant side effects on a relatively low dose. A high level in such a patient might identify a slow metabolizer who could be managed on a much lower dose of antidepressant.

If the patient has serious side effects, plasma levels may be helpful as follows: Certain subjective complaints of side effects can represent symptoms of depression rather than a true pharmacologic effect. Observing such subjective complaints in the face of low plasma levels and failure to respond clinically suggests that these are symptoms of depression and are not related to drug treatment. Some might say that normal plasma levels in a responding patient are not helpful and, therefore, are not indicated. Until the plasma level assay is done, however, one doesn't know that the plasma levels are normal. When a patient is having a reasonable clinical response with an extremely low plasma level, it may suggest that the patient is having a placebo response. If the patient's plasma level is normal, this information might be potentially useful in a future episode, since one knows the plasma level at which the patient has responded. In interpreting this, however, the clinician should remember the 30 percent base rate response of depression to placebo. For the responding patient, plasma levels are most useful if they are found to be unexpectedly high, but there may be some usefulness of knowing the levels are normal or low. Having a baseline plasma level drawn when the patient is in the hospital (when compliance is most assured) is also useful when one is using plasma levels as a monitor of compliance. Plasma levels early in treatment may be an aid to dose adjustment.

To conclude, use of antidepressant plasma levels can be clinically helpful but should be considered elective. If the patient is able to afford the assay and if a reliable laboratory is available, use of plasma levels for nortriptyline, imipramine, and, possibly, desipramine can be of modest clinical value.

BIOLOGICAL MECHANISM OF ACTION OF ANTIPSYCHOTICS

Despite the fact that we do not know the biological cause of schizophrenia, we do know the mechanisms by which the antipsychotic drugs benefit psychosis (that being their antidopaminergic effects). A wide variety of drugs benefit schizophrenia: the phenothiazine derivatives, the thioxanthene derivatives, the butyrophenonines, the indoles, the dibenzoxazepines, reserpine, and several experimental antipsychotic agents. Virtually all of these drugs cause parkinsonian side effects. Since Parkinson's disease is a dopamine deficiency state, we would assume that these parkinsonian side effects are caused by a dopaminergic mechanism. Reserpine and tetrabenazine lower brain dopamine levels and have antipsychotic activity. The other antipsychotic drugs block central dopamine receptors. Hence, the common denominator underlying most drugs that benefit schizophrenia is the action of central dopamine receptor blockade. Horn and Snyder in 1971 reviewed evidence based on x-ray crystallographic data, which indicated that chlorpromazine had a molecular configuration similar to that of dopamine (this structural similarity accounts for the ability of these drugs to block dopaminergic receptors). Furthermore, the potency of dopamine binding measured directly in the test tube correlates exactly to the potency of the agents in treating schizophrenics (Creese et al, 1976). Clinical potency and dopamine binding both correlate with pharmacological evidence of dopamine receptor blocking properties. Also, a double blind study found that the isomer of fluphenazine that blocks dopamine receptors is a potent antipsychotic in humans, but the isomer that does not block dopamine receptors is ineffective.

Clozapine is at least equally effective as the current antipsychotics. It has been argued that it blocks dopamine receptors with some degree of specificity for the mesolimbic dopaminergic system, but this is not firmly established. It does not produce extrapyramidal side effects. Insofar as it blocks dopamine receptors, its antipsychotic activity is consistent with the antidopaminergic mechanism. If we block dopamine synthesis with alpha-methyl-p-tyrosine, we can then reduce the amount of antipsychotic agent necessary for a beneficial effect in schizophrenia. The observation that alpha-methyl-p-tyrosine reduces the required antipsychotic dose of neuroleptics is evidence that the drugs produce their antipsychotic action by means of an interaction with a catecholamine (Walinder et al, 1976). We have found apomorphine, at a dose that stimulates presynaptic receptors, to reduce dopamine synthesis and, in preliminary single-dose studies, to have antipsychotic activity (Tamminga et al, 1978).

If decreasing dopaminergic activity benefits schizophrenia, increasing dopaminergic activity produces or aggravates schizophrenia. The psychomotor stimulants, such as amphetamine and methylphenidate, are potent releasers of dopamine. Magnesium pemoline can produce a paranoid psychosis when taken in higher amounts. It is well known that large doses of amphetamine can cause paranoid schizophrenia-like symptoms. A single large injection of amphetamine can produce a paranoid psychosis within hours in nonpsychotic amphetamine abusers. The duration of an amphetamine paranoid psychosis parallels the stay of amphetamine in the body. Cocaine blocks the reuptake of dopamine. The paranoid-suspiciousness syndrome (associated with cocaine use) disappears with a time course of approximately an hour or two after the last cocaine ingestion. This corresponds to our findings about cocaine's half-life in the body.

Janowsky and colleagues (1973) reported that small intravenous doses (such as 0.5 mg per kg) of methylphenidate can produce a marked worsening of an active schizophrenic episode in patients with florid symptomatic schizophrenic illness. It does not produce psychotic symptoms in normal patients, or in schizophrenic patients who are in either spontaneous or antipsychotic drug induced remission. The phenomenon of substantially worsening a preexisting psychosis may be a different one from that of amphetamine producing a typical paranoid psychosis in the nonschizophrenic subjects. In the former case, a patient's psychosis worsens both qualitatively and quantitatively in direction of his preexisting illness. Thus, catatonic and hebephrenic schizophrenics become more catatonic and hebephrenic. In the order of potency, methylphenidate is more potent than D-amphetamine, which itself is more potent than L-amphetamine. Methylphenidate releases central intraneuronal stores of dopamine from the reserpine-sensitive pool. Van Kammen also observed similar results. Angrist and colleagues (1984) investigated remitted schizophrenic patients when new maintenance antipsychotic drugs were discontinued. A temporary psychotic episode following an ingestion of these psychomotor stimulants predicted which patients would relapse in the forthcoming months. This observation is roughly consistent with our observation that psychomotor stimulants did not produce psychotic symptoms in patients with good solid remissions, but did so in those with active disease.

DOPA converted to dopamine can produce a psychosis in parkinsonian patients. Neurologists use a wide variety of agents which directly stimulate dopaminergic receptors to treat parkinsonian patients. The drugs do produce psychosis as a side effect in parkinsonian patients. Although amantadine has anticholinergic properties, it is also possibly a dopaminergic drug. It can produce a psychosis in parkinsonian patients or in schizophrenics who receive it for drug induced parkinsonian side effects.

Since there are many dopamine versus acetylcholine antagonistic systems in the brain, we examined whether increasing brain acetylcholine by physostigmine could block the psychosis-activating properties of methylphenidate (Janowsky et al, 1973). When physostigmine was administered before methylphenidate, we found it prevented the psychosis from worsening. If methylphenidate was administered and the psychosis worsened, an intravenous injection of physostigmine could bring the patient back to baseline within a minute or two. Physostigmine did produce an anergic syndrome, but it did not benefit the underlying psychotic illness per se. The observation that physostigmine does not reduce schizophrenia suggests that the underlying schizophrenic process is not as easily amenable to the effects of altering the cholinergic tone as is the worsening of the psychosis produced by methylphenidate.

The increase in dopamine activity by a variety of mechanisms seems to be a common denominator for a wide variety of drugs which cause paranoia, hallucinations, and so on. It suggests a mechanistic relationship, involving dopamine, between the antidopaminergic agents benefitting psychosis and dopaminergic agents producing paranoid symptoms or worsening psychoses. The dopamine theory of schizophrenia (Horn and Snyder, 1971), which suggests that certain schizophrenics have either high dopamine levels or supersensitive dopamine receptors, is still a viable theory.

THE ANTIPSYCHOTIC DOSE-RESPONSE RELATIONSHIP

We reviewed studies which randomly assigned subjects to different fixed doses in order to construct a dose-response curve from the pooled data. These studies investigated: A) newly admitted psychiatric patients with acute symptoms, using a fixed dose for several weeks; B) acutely ill patients in a psychotic break, using a fixed dose for a few hours or, at most, a day; or C) continued treatment studies of chronic schizophrenics (see Table 4).

We required an evaluation of superiority, a statistically significant difference on the total score or Global Improvement Score, or an overwhelming number of individual item scores. We constructed a dose-response curve on the basis of this data. The results of these studies are conservative because they are all relatively small, and may miss a group of patients who "need" higher doses. In other words, for an empirical study to show a higher dose to be better than a lower dose, there must be a sufficient number of nonresponding patients in both groups to produce a statistically reliable difference. These paired comparisons of fixed doses are used in defining the dose-response curve. Those patients receiving 300 mg (chlorpromazine equivalents) or less per day lie on the linear portion of the curve. Those receiving 500 mg per day or greater appear to lie on the plateau portion of the curve.

Antipsychotic Plasma Levels

There are relatively few controlled fixed-dose investigations of plasma levels of antipsychotic drugs and clinical efficacy. Flexible dose studies are worthless in making conclusions about plasma levels and efficacy since plasma levels reflect dose, and the flexible dose is determined by the clinician's reaction to the patient's clinical state. In a therapeutic blood level trial, it is necessary to study patients who have florid illness and thus are capable of showing a substantial degree of therapeutic improvement. We also distinguish rate of improvement from the

Table 4. High Dose versus Low Dose Chlorpromazine Data

Dose (Chlorpromazine Equivalents)	Number of Studies Where H Better Than L	Number of Studies Where H = L
1000 mg +	0	8
500–1000 mg	0	9
301–500 mg	0	1
0–300 mg	11	5

H = High dose
L = Low dose

We reviewed all the double blind studies for patients who were randomly assigned to two-dosage levels. We classified a study finding the relatively higher dose better than the lower dose, if there was statisticaly unequivocal evidence that proved the higher was more effective. When there was an occasional rating scale which found superiority but no consistent pattern of superiority, we classified the study as showing the two doses were equal. Occasionally, there was a study which found the lower dose more effective than the higher and vice-versa in terms of such questionably significant trends. The Table classifies the doses used in these studies after conversion to chlorpromazine equivalence by the lower dose of the pair.

maximum improvement possible. The former might be related to blood level, the latter to the underlying prognosis of the patient.

This problem was first investigated by Curry and colleagues (1970) who noted that there were marked individual differences in plasma levels among patients on comparable doses. Patients with a very low level of chlorpromazine failed to show either side effects or good clinical response. A few patients with a high chlorpromazine plasma level failed to respond, and for these, when the dose was lowered and plasma levels fell, clinical response improved. These findings suggest an inverted U relationship between plasma level and clinical response. Lader (1976) extended the first controlled study of Curry to include more floridly ill new patients, using a low dose (300 mg) and found a correlation of -0.32 between clinical efficacy and plasma levels (p less than 0.04 level, one-tailed). Wode-Helgodt and co-workers (1978) randomly assigned patients to fixed doses of 200, 400, or 600 mgs chlorpromazine, finding nonresponders to have slightly low chlorpromazine plasma levels during the first week or so. These studies using low doses are relevant only to the low end. Many metabolites of chlorpromazine are active. If a chemical assay measures only the unchanged chlorpromazine, and if the clinical effects are produced primarily by active metabolites, the unchanged drug may not be the appropriate compound to measure.

Van Putten and colleagues (1985), using one week's treatment data, Potkin and colleagues (1985), Mavroidis et al (1985), Davis (unpublished data), Bowers and colleagues (1985), and Smith et al (1985) have found an inverted U-shaped relationship between haloperidol levels and clinical response. The results of all these studies were consistent, showing an inverted U-shaped relationship with roughly the same therapeutic window and response with a lower end of 3–5 ng/ml and upper limit of 20 ng/ml. Dysken and co-workers (1981) have studied plasma fluphenazine levels and found an inverted U-shaped relationship between fluphenazine and clinical response. Most nonresponders have either very low fluphenazine levels or very high fluphenazine levels. Most antipsychotic drugs are bound to the plasma protein, but it is the plasma "free" drug that is in equilibrium with tissue levels. If the mechanisms involved in drug distribution across the red blood cell membrane mimic those governing the passage of drugs through the blood-brain barrier into brain tissue, then RBC drug levels may give additional information beyond that given by total plasma levels. We administered a constant dose of butaperazine to floridly ill schizophrenic patients, measuring plasma and RBC levels (Casper et al, 1980). The RBC levels versus response were best characterized by an inverted U-shaped curve, with poor responders having very low or very high plasma levels. An inverted U-shaped window has been found for haloperidol, butaperazine, and fluphenazine. All the data look similar in that the therapeutic window is not well defined, and there is a substantial amount of scatter. Although these results achieve some degree of statistical significance, they are not highly significant. The relationship of plasma/RBC levels and clinical response is only an approximate one with many values that do not fit. The results agree that there is only a modest effect of the inverted U-relationship. We feel that there are two consistent findings in the data so far: a) the hint of an inverted U-relationship, and b) evidence that this relationship is weak. The latter conclusion is as important as the former.

Conclusions About Usefulness of Antipsychotic Plasma Levels

We feel that the use of antipsychotic plasma levels is premature at this time. Some of the drugs have never been examined in an adequate study. Other drugs have been studied in only a limited fashion. Therefore, we do not feel enough data is available for them to be used clinically. The possible exception to this is haloperidol. The therapeutic range of haloperidol is somewhere between 5 ng/ml to 20 ng/ml; however, there is a good deal of scatter in the data. We think it is premature to recommend it now as an elective test, although it is getting close. We feel there is enough data so that individual differences in metabolism may be one of the reasons why different patients receive different doses. The theoretical knowledge might be of interest to the clinician as one of the reasons why he or she should adjust dose on a clinical basis.

CONCLUSION

In this chapter we have reviewed aspects of the neurotransmitter theories of depression and schizophrenia. In particular, we have focused on aspects of these theories that may be relevant to biochemical tests for the diagnosis and treatment of depression. We have also focused on the pharmacokinetics of antidepressant and antipsychotic medications, highlighting when and how plasma levels of these drugs can be used in clinical practice. From this discussion, the reader should conclude that it is vitally important to view laboratory tests from a critical perspective, just as one would critically view a new drug. As with the introduction of a new drug, there is often a surge of positive reports accompanying the introduction of a new laboratory test. However, new laboratory tests should not be accepted uncritically and prematurely. The uncritical physician may interpret laboratory test data using assumptions which are derived from largely unproven, and sometimes inaccurate, information. For example, some commercial laboratories advertise a normal range of therapeutic plasma levels for a drug without valid data for such a range. Obviously, the quality of care can suffer if we inappropriately make clinical decisions based on laboratory test results, especially when commonsense interpretations of clinical data are abandoned. In all cases, the clinician should treat the patient, not the laboratory test result. Although one should interpret laboratory test results cautiously, this caution should not be so excessive as to preclude the appropriate use of laboratory data. For example, even though the therapeutic window for a particular drug may not be precisely delineated, the clinician can appropriately use approximate plasma ranges by viewing them in the context of relevant clinical data. For instance, in a patient showing a good therapeutic effect, who experiences significant side effects and who has a plasma level three times the upper range value, the clinician should decrease the dose. If the patient has a plasma level two to three times lower than the minimum range value and is receiving no therapeutic benefit and is experiencing no side effects, the clinician should probably increase the dose.

It is impossible to complete controlled studies for every potential clinical situation. Most clinical decisions must be based on interpolation from basic pharmacological or pathophysiological findings and from pivotal controlled clinical studies, as well as from the physician's clinical experience and common sense. Laboratory tests do not provide clinically helpful information on all patients. To demand that controlled studies prove every possible application of laboratory tests is asking more than "science" can realistically deliver. In other words, it is possible to be excessively critical as well as excessively uncritical of laboratory tests.

As adjunctive tools, laboratory tests can help clinicians make safer and more effective diagnostic, treatment, and management decisions. In the future we may be able to predict the specific drug a particular patient will need from receptor function tests, or specific dosage requirements from test dose plasma studies. It is our belief that psychiatric science will eventually develop a wide variety of useful tests which will increase the quality of clinical practice.

REFERENCES

Agren H.: Depressive symptom patterns and urinary MHPG excretion. Psychiatry Res 6:185-196, 1982

Agren H: Depression and altered neurotransmission—states, traits, and interactions, in The Origins of Depression: Current Concepts and Approaches. Edited by Angst, J. New York, Springer-Verlag, 1983

Amin M, Cooper R, Khalid R, et al: A comparison of desipramine and amitriptyline plasma levels and therapeutic response. Psychopharmacol Bull 14:45-46, 1978

Angrist B, VanKammen DP: CNS stimulants as tools in the study of schizophrenia. Trends in Neuroscience 8:388-390, 1984

Asberg M, Cromholm B, Sjoquist F, et al: Relationship between plasma levels and therapeutic effect of nortriptyline. Br Med J 3:331, 1971

Asberg M, Thoren P, Traskman L, et al: Serotonin depression—a biochemical subgroup within the affective disorders? Science 191:478-480, 1976

Beckman H, Goodwin F: Antidepressant response to tricyclics and urinary MHPG in unipolar patients. Arch Gen Psychiatry 32:17-21, 1975

Beckman H, Goodwin FK: Antidepressant response to tricyclics and urinary MHPG in unipolar patients. Arch Gen Psychiatry 32:17-21, 1975.

Beckman H, Goodwin FK: Urinary MHPG in subgroups of depressed patients and normal controls. Neuropsychobiology 6:91-100, 1980

Berger PA, Faull KF, Kilkowski J, et al: CSF monoamine metabolites in depression and schizophrenia. Am J Psychiatry 137:174-180, 1980

Bowden CL, Koslow SH, Hanin I, et al: Effects of amitriptyline and imipramine on brain amine neurotransmitter metabolites in cerebrospinal fluid. Clin Pharmacol Ther 37:316-324, 1985

Bowers MB, Swigar ME, Jatlow MD, et al: Correlates of early haloperidol response using a uniform test dose—treatment dose protocol. Presented at the Annual Meeting of the American College of Neuropsychopharmacology, City? December 9–13, 1985

Bunney WE Jr, Davis JM: Norepinephrine in depressive reactions. Arch Gen Psychiatry 13:483-494, 1965

Bunney WE Jr, Davis JM, Weil-Malherbe H, et al: Biochemical changes in psychotic depression. Arch Gen Psychiatry 16:448-460, 1967

Casper RC, Garver DL, Dekirmenjian H, et al: Phenothiazine levels in plasma and red blood cells. Arch Gen Psychiatry 37:301-307, 1980

Charney DS, Heninger GR, Sterberg DE, et al: Plasma MHPG in depression: effects of acute and chronic desipramine treatment. Psychiatry Res 5:217-229, 1981

Cobbins DM, Requin-Blow B, Williams LR, et al: Urinary MHPG levels and tricyclic antidepressant drug selection. Arch Gen Psychiatry 36:1237-1264, 1967

Coppen A, Rama Rao VA, Ruthven CRJ, et al: Urinary 4-hydroxy-3-methoxyphenylglycol is not a predictor for clinical response to amitriptyline in depressive illness. Psychopharmacology 64:95-97, 1979

Creese K, Burt DR, Snyder SH: Dopamine receptor binding predicts clinical and pharmacological potencies of antischizophrenic drugs. Science 192:481-483, 1976

Curry SH, Marshall JHL, Davis JM, et al: Chlorpromazine plasma levels and effects. Arch Gen Psychiatry 22:289-296, 1970

Davis JM: Overview: maintenance therapy in psychiatry, I: schizophrenia. Am J Psychiatry 132:1237-1245, 1975

Davis JM, Gibbons RD, Maas JW, et al: Amine excretion in depressives and controls. American Psychiatric Association Syllabus and Scientific Proceedings, 136th Annual Meeting 48:127, New York, 1983

Davis JM, Javaid JI, Matuzas W: Plasma concentration monitoring of antipsychotic and tricyclic antidepressant treatment, in Handbook of Psychiatric Diagnostic Procedures. Edited by Hall RCW, Beresford TP. New York, Spectrum Publications, 1984

Davis JM, Javaid JI, Janicak PG, et al: Antipsychotics: plasma levels and clinical response, in Antipsychotic Drugs. Edited by Burrows G, Norman T, Davies B. New York, Elsevier/North Holland, 1985

Davis KL, Berger PA, Hollister LE, et al: Physostigmine in mania. Arch Gen Psychiatry 35:119-122, 1978

Dysken MW, Javaid JI, Chang SS, et al: Fluphenazine pharmacokinetics and therapeutic response. Psychopharmacology 73:205-210, 1981

Edwards DE, Spiker D, Neil J, et al: MHPG excretion in depression. Psychiatry Res 2:295-305, 1980

Esler M, Turbott J, Schwarz R, et al: The peripheral kinetics of norepinephrine in depressive illness. Arch Gen Psychiatry 39:295-300, 1982

Extein J, Tallman J, Smith CC, et al: Changes in lymphocyte beta-adrenergic receptors in depression and mania. Psychiatry Res 1:191-197, 1979

Gaertner H, Kreuter F, Scharek G, et al: Do urinary MHPG and plasma drug levels correlate with response to amitriptyline therapy? Psychopharmacology 76:236-239, 1982

Glassman AH, Perel JM, Shostak M: Clinical implications of imipramine plasma levels for depressive illness. Arch Gen Psychiatry 34:197-204, 1977

Hanin I, Koslow SH, Kocsis JH, et al: Cerebrospinal fluid levels of amitriptyline, nortriptyline, imipramine and demethyl-imipramine—relationship to plasma levels and treatment outcome. J Affective Disord 9:69-78, 1985

Hedges L, Olkin I: Statistical Methods for Meta-Analysis. New York, Academic Press, 1985

Hollister L: Excretion of 3-methoxy-4-hydroxy-phenylglycol in depressed and geriatric patients and normal persons. International Pharmacopsychiatry 16:138-143, 1981

Hollister L, Davis K, Berger P: Subtypes of depression based on excretion of MHPG and response to nortriptyline. Arch Gen Psychiatry 37:1107-1110, 1980

Horn AS, Snyder SH: Chlorpromazine and Dopamine: Conformational similarities that correlate with the antischizophrenic activity of phenothiazine drugs. Proceedings of the Academy of Science 65:2325, 1971

Hrdina P, Lapierre Y: Clinical response, plasma levels, and pharmacokinetics of desipramine in depressed patients. Progress in Neuropsychopharmacology 4:591-600, 1981

Janicak PG, Davis JM, Chan C, et al: Urinary MHPG as a predictor of response to treatment (in press)

Janowsky DS, El-Yousef MK, Davis JM: Provocation of schizophrenic symptoms by intravenous administration of methylphenidate. Arch Gen Psychiatry 28:185-191, 1973

Kasa K, Otsuki S, Yamamoto M, et al: Cerebrospinal fluid—aminobutyric acid and homovanillic acid in depressive disorders. Biol Psychiatry 17:877-883, 1982

Koslow SH, Maas J, Bowden C, et al: Cerebrospinal fluid and urinary biogenic amines and metabolites in depression and mania: a controlled univariate analysis. Arch Gen Psychiatry 40:999-1010, 1983

Kragh-Sorensen P, Eggert-Hansen C, Baastrup PC, et al: Self-inhibiting action of nortriptyline antidepressive effect at high plasma levels. Psychopharmacologia 45:305-312, 1976

Lader M: Monitoring plasma concentrations of neuroleptics. Pharmacopsychiatry 9:170-177, 1976

Lake CR, Pickar D, Ziegler MG, et al: High plasma norepinephrine levels in patients with major affective disorders. Am J Psychiatry 139:1315-1318, 1982

Lee CM, Javitch JA, Snyder A: Recognition sites for norepinephrine uptake: regulation by neurotransmitter. Science 220:626-629, 1983

Maas J, Dekirmenjian H, Fawcett J: MHPG excretion by patients with affective disorders. International Pharmacopsychiatry 9:14-26, 1974

Maas JW, Koslow SH, Katz MM, et al: Pretreatment neurotransmitter metabolite levels and response to tricyclic antidepressant drug response. Am J Psychiatry 141:10:1159-1171, 1984

Matuzas W, Javaid JI, Glass R, et al: Plasma concentrations of imipramine and clinical response among depressed outpatients. J Clin Psychopharmacol 2:140-142, 1982

Matuzas W, Javaid J, Uhlenhuth EH, et al: Plasma and red blood cell concentrations of imipramine and clinical response among depressed outpatients. Paper presented at the 136th Annual Meeting of the American Psychiatric Association, New York, May 1983.

Mavoroidis ML, Kanter DR, Hirschowitz J, et al: Therapeutic blood levels of fluphenazine: plasma or rbc determinations? Psychopharmacol Bull 20:168-170, 1985

Musscettola G, Potter WZ, Pickar D, et al: Urinary MHPG and major affective disorders: a replication and new findings. Arch Gen Psychiatry 41:337-342, 1984

Nelson JC, Jatlow P, Quinlan P, et al: Desipramine plasma concentration and antidepressant response. Arch Gen Psychiatry 39:1419-1422, 1982

Oliver-Martin R, Marzin D, Buschenschutz E, et al: Concentrations plasmatiques de l'imipramine et de la desmethylimipramine et effect an antidepresseur au cours d'un traitement controle. Psychopharmacology 41:187-195, 1975

Pandey GN, Dysken MW, Garver DL: Beta-adrenergic receptor function in affective illness. Am J Psychiatry 136:675-678, 1979

Pandey GN, Davis JM: Treatment with antidepressants, sensitivity of beta-receptors and affective illness, in Neuroreceptors: Basic and Clinical Aspects. Edited by Usdin E, Bunney Jr, WE, Davis JM. New York, John Wiley & Sons, 1981

Perel J, Stiller R, Glassman AH: Studies on plasma levels/effects relationships in imipramine therapy. Communications in Psychopharmacology 2:429-439, 1978

Peroutka S, Snyder SH: Long-term antidepressant treatment decreases spiroperidol labelled serotonin receptor binding. Science 210:88-90, 1980

Potkin SG, Shen YC, Pardes H: Does a therapeutic window for plasma haloperidol exist: preliminary Chinese data. Psychopharmacol Bull 21:59-61, 1985

Puzynski S, Rode A, Bedzinski A, et al: Failure to correlate urinary MHPG with clinical response to amitriptyline. Acta Psychiatr Scand 69:117-120, 1984

Reisby N, Gram LF, Bech P: Imipramine: Clinical effects and pharmacokinetic variability. Psychopharmacology 54:263-272, 1977

Rickels K, Weise C, Case G, et al. Tricyclic plasma levels in depressed outpatients treated with amitriptyline. Psychopharmacology 80:14-18, 1983

Rosenblatt S, Chanley JD, Leighton W: The investigation of adrenergic metabolism with $7H^3$-norepinephrine in psychiatric disorder–I and II. J Psychiatr Res 6:307-333, 1969

Roy A, Pickar D, Linnoila M, et al: Plasma norepinephrine level in affective disorders—relationship to melancholia. Arch Gen Psychiatry 42:1181-1192, 1985

Rudorfer MV, Ross RJ, Linnoila M, et al: Exaggerated orthostatic responsivity of plasma norepinephrine in depression. Arch Gen Psychiatry 42:1186, 1985

Sacchetti E, Allaria E, Negri F, et al: 3-methoxy-4-hydroxyphenylglycol and primary depression: clinical and pharmacological considerations. Biol Psychiatry 14:3:473-484, 1979

Schatzberg A, Orsulak P, Rosenbaum A, et al: Catecholamine measures for diagnosis and treatment of patients with depressive disorders. J Clin Psychiatry 41:12:35-39, 1980a

Schatzberg A, Orsulak P, Rosenbaum A, et al: Toward a biochemical classification of depressive disorders, IV: pretreatment urinary MHPG levels as predictors of antidepressant response to imipramine. Community Psychopharmacology 4:441-445, 1980b

Schatzberg A, Orsulak R, Rosenbaum A: Toward a biochemical classification of depressive disorders: heterogeneity of unipolar depression. Am J Psychiatry 139:471-475, 1982

Schildkraut JJ: The catecholamine hypothesis of affective disorders: a review of supporting evidence. Am J Psychiatry 122:509-522, 1965

Schildkraut JJ: Norepinephrine metabolites as biochemical criteria for classifying depressive disorders and predicting responses to treatment: preliminary findings. Am J Psychiatry 130:6, 695-699, 1973

Sharpless NS: Determination of 3-methoxy-4-hydroxy phenylglycol in urine and the effect of diet on its excretion. Res Commun Chem Pathol Pharmacol 18:257-273, 1977

Simpson G, White KL, Boyd JL, et al: Relationship between plasma antidepressant levels and clinical outcome for inpatients receiving imipramine. Am J Psychiatry 139:358-360, 1982

Smith RC, Baumgartner R, Shvartsburd A, et al: Red cell and plasma haloperidol and response in acutely ill schizophrenics: comparison of GLC and RRA. Psychopharmacol Bull 21:57-59, 1985

Snyder SH: Catecholamines in the brain as mediators of amphetamine psychosis. Arch Gen Psychiatry 27:743-747, 1972

Spiker DC, Edwards D, Hanin I, et al: Urinary MHPG and clinical response to amitriptyline in depressed patients. Am J Psychiatry 137:1183-1187, 1980

Steinbook R, Jacobson A, Weiss B, et al: Amoxapine, imipramine, and placebo: a double-blind study with pretherapy urinary 3-methoxy-4-hydroxyphenylglycol levels. Current Therapeutic Research 26:5:490-496, 1979

Tamminga CA, Schaffer MH, Smith RC: Schizophrenic symptoms improve with apomorphine. Science 200:567-568, 1978

Taube SL, Kirstein LS, Sweeney DR, et al: Urinary 3-methoxy-4-hydroxyphenylclycol and psychiatric diagnosis. Am J Psychiatry 135:78-82, 1978

Traskman-Bendz L, Asberg M, Bertilsson L, et al: CSF monoamine metabolites of depressed patients during illness and after recovery. Acta Psychiatr Scand 69:333-342, 1984

Van Praag NM, Korf J, Schut D: Cerebral monoamines and depression: an investigation with the probenecid technique. Arch Gen Psychiatry 28:827-831, 1973

Van Putten T, Marder SR, May PRA, et al: Is a plasma level of haloperidol clinically useful? Psychopharmacol Bull 21:61-64, 1985

Veith RC, Bielski RJ, Bloom V, et al: Urinary MHPG excretion and treatment with desipramine or amitriptyline: predictors of response, effect of treatment, and methodological hazards. J Clin Psychopharmacol 3:18-27, 1983

Walinder J, Skott A, Carlsson A, et al: Potentiation by metyrosine of thioridazine effects in chronic schizophrenics. Arch Gen Psychiatry 33:501-505, 1976

Ward NG, Bloom V, Fawcett JA, et al: Urinary 3-methoxy-4-hydroxyphenylethylene glycol in the prediction of pain and depression relief with doxepin: preliminary findings. J Nerv Ment Dis 171:55-58, 1983

Wode-Helgodt B, Borg S, Fyro B, et al: Clinical effects and drug concentrations in plasma and cerebrospinal fluid in psychotic patients treated with fixed doses of chlorpromazine. Acta Psychiatr Scand 58:149-173, 1978

Wyatt RJ, Portnoy B, Kupfer DJ, et al: Resting plasma catecholamine concentrations in patients with depression and anxiety. Arch Gen Psychiatry 24:65-70, 1971

Chapter 8

Psychoendocrinology in Clinical Psychiatry

by Carol B. Allen, M.D., Bonnie M. Davis, M.D., and Kenneth L. Davis, M.D.

Advances in basic neurobiology and neuroendocrinology have yielded avenues for psychiatric research. Similarly, as research methods in neuroendocrinology have improved, major alterations in endocrine gland activity have been documented in psychiatric illnesses. This chapter will present the major endocrine abnormalities found in affective disorders and schizophrenia, and discuss how these phenomena have been employed in the diagnosis, management, and treatment of psychiatric illness. The relationship of these findings to current research regarding hypotheses of pathophysiology of psychiatric disorder will be reviewed. Endocrine effects of psychiatric medications and endocrine abnormalities in substance abuse and aging will be discussed. In order for the clinician to be aware of the various endocrine disorders that present with prominent psychiatric manifestations, a discussion of these illnesses and their manifestations is included.

ENDOCRINE ABNORMALITIES IN AFFECTIVE DISORDER

Depression

Neuroendocrine abnormalities in patients with affective disorders might be expected because of the presence of signs and symptoms under hypothalamic regulation, such as disturbed appetite, sleep, sexual drive, diurnal mood regulation, and other autonomic functions. Furthermore, those biogenic amines hypothesized to be functionally abnormal in depressive disease (catecholamines, serotonin) are found in high concentrations in the hypothalamus, which regulates secretory activity of the anterior pituitary. Thus, the study of neuroendocrine abnormalities in various affective disorders may help to clarify the abnormalities of neurotransmitters in these disorders.

DEXAMETHASONE SUPPRESSION TEST. Patients with severe depressive illness frequently manifest several hormonal abnormalities. The best documented of these abnormalities is the hypersecretion of cortisol, with resistance to suppression by dexamethasone. In addition, patients with depression may exhibit loss of the normal diurnal variation in cortisol secretion. The dexamethasone suppression test (DST) was introduced by Liddle in 1960 to study Cushing's syndrome, a group of disorders characterized by hypercortisolism and frequently accompanied by behavioral manifestations, including depression. Abnormalities of the DST have been found in a host of disorders, including many behavioral disturbances with hypercortisolemia. Use of the DST has been extended to be part of the diagnostic evaluation of depression.

Dexamethasone, a potent synthetic glucocorticoid with a long serum half-life, taken at 11 P.M., suppresses the nocturnal secretion of adrenocorticotropin hormone (ACTH) by the pituitary gland and continues to suppress ACTH secretion throughout the following day. The suppression of ACTH thereby prevents cortisol secretion from the adrenal glands. The standard DST is performed by administering dexamethasone 1 mg orally at 11 P.M. Blood samples for assay of plasma cortisol are then drawn the following day at 8 A.M., 4 P.M., and 11 P.M. A normal response is suppression of plasma cortisol to less than 5 ug/dl as measured by radioimmunoassay. Failure to suppress to less than 5 ug/dl is considered an abnormal response, or a positive test. This procedure may be modified in outpatients by obtaining only a 4 P.M. sample; however, this results in a greater than 20 percent loss in sensitivity in the diagnosis of depressive illness.

Several factors may interfere with results obtained with the DST. In order for the DST to be reliable in the diagnosis of depression, each of these variables must be ruled out. False positive results can be obtained in patients with an altered pituitary-adrenal axis (such as cortisol-secreting adrenal tumors or ACTH-secreting pituitary or lung tumors (Cushing's syndrome), or in those with increased cortisol demands and altered resistance to dexamethasone. This occurs with acute hospitalization, severe illnesses of the heart, kidneys, or liver, pregnancy, hypertension, and uncontrolled diabetes mellitus. Estrogen administration, dilantin (accelerated metabolism by hepatic microsomal enzymes and biliary excretion), phenobarbital, primidone, alcoholism, and obesity either increase the dose of dexamethasone required for adrenal suppression or alter metabolic rate and subsequent duration of effect of dexamethasone. Other drugs that can cause a false positive test are tegretol, meprobamate, glutethimide, and methyprylon (Carroll, 1982, 1983).

Indomethacin, a prostaglandin inhibitor, is believed to inhibit corticotropin-releasing factor (CRF) and ACTH release. Its administration to depressed patients has been shown to cause false negative results. Indomethacin may act by altering the suppressibility of the hypothalamic-pituitary-adrenal (HPA) axis at a central site, since prostaglandin inhibitors can suppress the HPA axis when administered intrahypothalamically, an effect reversible by injection of prostaglandins (Mathe et al, 1982). The DST appears to be unaffected by most of the commonly used psychotropic medications, including tricyclic antidepressants, neuroleptics, and low dose benzodiazepines.

Interpretation of the DST is also affected by age. The decreased sensitivity and specificity of the DST, which have been reported in depressed children and adolescents, may reflect less well defined criteria for childhood as compared to adult depression. In addition, the optimal dose of dexamethasone for children has not yet been established (Carroll, 1983; Targum and Capodanno, 1983). Advanced age does not appear to affect the diurnal variations of cortisol or the DST (Raskin et al, 1982; Tourigny-Rivard et al, 1981); however, cortisol secretion in depressed patients increases with age (Asnis et al, 1981a). Research to clarify age as a parameter affecting the DST in normal individuals and depressed patients has yielded equivocal results. Recent data indicate a positive effect of age on basal cortisol levels and no significant effect of age on DST nonsuppressibility. It has been postulated that age-related degenerative changes in the locus coeruleus may occur in humans, paralleling that seen in animals, and that this decline in noradrenergic stimuli might induce an increase in basal cortisol secretion (Cohen et al, 1985).

Other illnesses that are known to affect the DST include nondepressed bulimic patients who are within 15 percent of their ideal body weight, anorexia nervosa, and primary obsessive-compulsive disorder (Hudson et al, 1982; Gerner and Gwirtsman, 1981). The DST is not useful in differentiating dementia from cognitive dysfunction secondary to depression. A 50 percent false positive rate has been reported in advanced primary degenerative disease (Spar and Gerner, 1982; Raskin et al, 1982).

Although the DST cannot guide the clinical selection of therapy, an abnormal DST may be a significant predictor of a good response to somatic treatment. An abnormal DST precedes the onset of depressive episodes and normalization heralds clinical recovery. A persistently positive DST despite clinical improvement is predictive of rapid relapse. Thus, the DST may help in timing the safe withdrawal of antidepressant therapy (Brown and Shuey, 1980; Carroll, 1982). Depressed patients with a positive DST are at a higher risk for serious suicide attempts than those with a negative DST. Therefore, monitoring the DST may help to decrease the possible mortality associated with depression (Carroll, 1983; Targum et al, 1983b).

Not all diagnostic categories of depression have abnormal dexamethasone suppressibility. The syndrome of depression, according to Research Diagnostic Criteria (RDC), can be subdivided into primary and secondary categories and further subtyped as endogenous or nonendogenous. This primary–secondary dichotomy is supported by the DST. Approximately 50 percent of primary depression patients had a positive DST. The rate of nonsuppression in secondary depression approaches that of normal control subjects. It is not established whether the DST will serve as a validating criterion of endogenous versus nonendogenous subtypes (Coryell et al, 1982; Brown and Shuey, 1980).

In summary, the DST may be useful in the diagnosis and management of depressive disorders; however, the DST is a nonspecific test. An abnormal DST is to be expected in several psychiatric and medical conditions, all of which must be ruled out before the diagnosis of primary depressive illness can be established.

THYROTROPIN-RELEASING HORMONE TEST. TSH releasing hormone (TRH) is a three-amino acid hypothalamic hormone which stimulates synthesis and release of thyrotropin (TSH) and prolactin from the anterior pituitary gland. TSH stimulates secretion of L-thyroxine (T_4) and triiodothyronine (T_3) from the thyroid gland. The TRH test is used in the diagnosis of thyroid, nonthyroidal, and psychiatric disease (depressive illness). The test is performed by giving an intravenous bolus injection over 30 seconds of synthetic TRH. The usual dose is 400 mcg, although doses from 200–600 mcg have been used. Serum samples for TSH assay are obtained immediately prior to the injection and at various intervals after the injection, depending upon which illness is suspected. To diagnose hyperthyroidism, one 20-minute or 30-minute post-injection sample is sufficient. In cases of suspected pituitary hypothyroidism, samples are obtained at 30, 60, 90, and 120 minutes after the injection. In suspected depression, a specimen is obtained at 30 minutes. A normal response to TRH is characterized by a rapid rise in TSH of 5–30 uU/ml (average = 15) above baseline within 20–30 minutes with a return to baseline over 2–3 hrs.

Table 1. Medical Conditions Associated with False Positive Dexamethasone Suppression Test

Cushing's syndrome

Cardiac, renal disease

Pregnancy

Estrogens

Dilantin, phenobarbital, tegretol

Alcoholism

Obesity

Dementia

When this procedure is applied to patients with depressive illness, the hormonal response is sometimes abnormal. The maximum TSH response is decreased (blunted) in those with unipolar or bipolar depression, mania or mixed manic-depressive illness, whereas normal responses are obtained in those patients with reactive or neurotic depression or reactive paranoid psychosis. These changes in TSH response do not appear to be due to altered thyroid function (T_3 or T_4) or thyroid hormone binding globulins (Kirkegaard et al, 1978). Furthermore, the altered TSH response has been correlated with the severity of depression and may remain blunted after clinical recovery (Asnis et al, 1981b). Those patients who fail to return to a normal TSH response are at increased risk of relapse. On the average, the incidence of blunted TSH response to TRH in depressive illness is approximately 25 percent.

The TSH response to TRH is partially under negative feedback control of circulating thyroid hormones and can be blunted by hypercortisolism. However, no correlation has been found between basal thyroid hormone levels and TSH responsiveness in depression. Furthermore, many depressives exhibit blunted TSH responsiveness after recovery, when cortisol secretion is known to be normalized (Loosen et al, 1977a). Blunting of TSH response to TRH is not specific for depressive illness. It has also been reported in alcoholism, anorexia nervosa, and other psychiatric illnesses. In normal subjects, TRH infusion does not stimulate a growth hormone response; however, such a response has been found in depressives. Prolactin response to TRH in depression has been found to be both increased and decreased.

Numerous nonpsychiatric factors can affect the TSH response to TRH. Of particular note is the fact that responsiveness to TRH declines in elderly men. Responsiveness is also decreased by pharmacological doses of glucocorticoids and in patients receiving exogenous thyroid hormone, growth hormone, levodopa, dopamine, and bromocriptine. Responses are augmented by metoclopramide or domperidone, dopaminergic antagonists. Other factors that decrease the TSH response include hypercortisolism, hyperthyroidism, lithium therapy, amphetamines, and estrogens. Most tricyclic antidepressants do not alter the test.

Depressed patients who have blunted TSH-responsiveness may also have lower excretion of methoxy-hydroxyphenyl glycol (MHPG), a major metabolite of norepinephrine (NE) of central nervous system origin. This finding is consistent with the assumption that a deficit in NE, which may stimulate TRH secretion, could be the core abnormality in depressed patients (Jimerson et al, 1983).

GROWTH HORMONE. Interest in growth hormone (GH) responsiveness in depression developed from evidence implicating biogenic amines in GH release and regulation (Martin, 1973; Chambers and Brown, 1976). Growth hormone is an eight amino-acid peptide whose release from the anterior pituitary gland is controlled by both growth hormone releasing hormone (GRH) and growth hormone release inhibiting factor (somatostatin). Both of these hormones have been characterized and synthesized. Stimuli to GH secretion presumably exert their effects by altering the secretion of these two substances.

The normal mean concentration of GH in plasma is 2–4 ng/ml in young adults and 5–8 ng/ml in children and adolescents. GH levels are affected by many factors, especially obesity, nutritional status, smoking, eating, sleep, and estrogen levels. For example, obese subjects have decreased GH secretion during sleep and decreased GH secretion in response to provocative stimuli. GH concentration has a reciprocal relationship with plasma glucose: a rise in plasma glucose suppresses GH secretion and a fall in glucose stimulates GH release. GH secretory spikes occur three to four hours after meals and about one hour after the onset of deep sleep.

Extrahypothalamic neural input, hypothalamic influences, metabolic fuels, hormones, and neurotransmitters all affect GH secretion. Physical exercise, stress, acute hypoglycemia, and the amino acids arginine and leucine have all been used to stimulate GH secretion. Central alpha-adrenergic agonists (for example, clonidine) also stimulate GH secretion. Growth hormone appears to have a negative feedback effect on its own secretion; however, it is not known whether this is a direct effect, or one which is mediated through somatomedins, the growth hormone effectors. Glucocorticoid excess suppresses GH, whereas estrogens increase basal GH secretion and enhance the GH response to provocative stimuli while simultaneously inhibiting somatomedin generation.

A normal response of GH to insulin induced hypoglycemia is a rise of at least 5 ng/ml. However, GH response to insulin induced hypoglycemia is diminished in major endogenous depression (Carroll, 1978). Responses of GH to other physiologic and pharmacologic stimuli in depression are less well established. In general, it appears that the response to L-dopa and apomorphine (dopaminergic agents) are normal. Several neurotransmitters mediate input to neurons involved in GH regulation. Alpha-adrenergic stimulation increases GH secretion and beta-adrenergic stimulation decreases GH secretion, both norepinephrine effects. Dopamine increases GH secretion in normal individuals. Acetylcholine (ACh) is believed to increase GH secretion because administration of a cholinergic antagonist, methscopolamine, diminishes the GH sleep spike. The serotonin antagonists cyproheptadine and methysergide blunt GH response to exercise and hypoglycemia; methysergide also augments the sleep spike of GH. These observations suggest that serotonin stimulates the GH response to hypoglycemia and exercise, but suppresses the response to sleep. No firm conclusions have emerged from studies of GH in patients with major depression.

INSULIN RESISTANCE. A mild insulin resistance has been observed in several studies of depressed patients. The normal response to an insulin tolerance test (ITT) is a decrease in blood glucose below 50 mg/dl, and at least a 50 percent drop below the baseline glucose level. A relatively smaller percentage of drop in blood glucose has been found during the intravenous insulin tolerance test (ITT) in depression than after recovery in response to the same dose of insulin (0.1 ug/kg). This occurs despite a normal baseline glucose level. This change in glucose cannot be accounted for by the growth hormone response to hypoglycemia. This response may be accounted for by the cortisol hypersecretion seen in depression (Sachar et al, 1980).

SUMMARY.   The neuroendocrine abnormalities mentioned presumably reflect underlying regulatory defects in the central nervous system. Current hypotheses of the etiology of depression are primarily concerned with the neurotransmitters norepinephrine, serotonin, dopamine, and acetylcholine. An abnormal DST is consistent with the catecholamine hypothesis of depression. The tonic inhibitory effect of NE on ACTH secretion may be decreased in depression if there is indeed a central defect of NE. Serotonin is believed to contribute to maintenance of the diurnal pattern of corticosteroid release, suggesting altered serotonergic function in depression. The blunted TSH response to TRH may be consistent with the biogenic amine hypothesis since NE and serotonin modulate thyroid function, in addition to stimulating GH release.

Diagnostic and research investigations of depressive illness involve a wide variety of techniques. The neuroendocrine parameters discussed here indicate that it may become possible to develop a clinically meaningful blood test for depressive illness. The DST is a safe, simple procedure which identifies approximately 50 percent of patients with major depression. The TRH test and GH stimulation tests identify smaller percentages of the same population. The theoretical implications of these tests await a better understanding of the neural regulation of hormonal release.

Anorexia Nervosa

The major features of anorexia nervosa are an intense fear of becoming fat, major weight loss, absence of an organic illness causing weight loss, and absence of primary psychiatric illness leading to loss of interest in eating. In addition to several major nonendocrine laboratory abnormalities (anemia, leukopenia, hypoalbuminemia, hypercholesterolemia), there are several endocrine abnormalites present in anorexia nervosa; however, there is no primary dysfunction of either the pituitary, the gonads, thyroid, or adrenal glands. Most changes appear to be secondary to the starvation and loss of body fat rather than reflecting a primary hypothalamic dysfunction.

Amenorrhea is a nearly constant feature of anorexia nervosa. One-half of subjects develop secondary amenorrhea with the onset of dieting, one-fifth cease menstruating before the onset of overt disease, and the remaining subjects develop amenorrhea after attaining marked weight loss (Schwabe et al, 1981). The primary defect appears to be localized to the hypothalamus and operates by impaired release of gonadotropin-releasing hormone (GnRH). Baseline gonadotropin values (luteinizing hormone, LH; follicle stimulating hormone, FSH) are decreased and diurnal secretory patterns regress to pubertal (nocturnal LH surge) or prepubertal (lack of surges) patterns (Boyar and Katz, 1977; Pirke et al, 1979). Men with anorexia nervosa have the same abnormalities in hypothalamic-pituitary-gonadal function as seen in females, and have low testosterone levels (McNab and Hawton, 1981). The mechanism of failure of GnRH release is unknown. Abnormalities in norepinephrine and dopamine metabolism in the central nervous system have been postulated (Schwabe et al, 1981). The low estrogen levels and lack of ovulation in anorexia nervosa are due to gonadotropin deficiency. These abnormalities may revert to normal with weight gain to 80 percent ideal body weight; however, superimposed psychological factors may prevent restoration of normal neuroendocrine function. The abnormal pituitary response to GnRH also returns to normal with restoration of body weight or GnRH administration (Beumont and Abraham, 1981).

Basal growth hormone values have been found to be elevated in one-third of patients, but the GH response to provocative stimuli is often impaired (Vigersky, 1977). Prolactin levels are usually normal (Isaacs et al, 1980; Skrabanek et al, 1981), but may have a paradoxical rise following GnRH administration. Basal TSH values are normal (Moshang and Utiger, 1977) and patients may have sick euthyroidism with either low T_3, elevated T_4, and elevated reverse T_3 (rT_3) or low T_4, low T_3, and elevated rT_3 with a blunted or delayed and prolonged TSH response to TRH (Casper and Frohman, 1982). These thyroidal abnormalities also reverse with weight gain.

Mean plasma cortisol levels measured over 24 hours are found to be high normal or elevated with flattening of the circadian curve possibly due to decreased cortisol metabolism or increased production (Walsh et al, 1981). Failure of cortisol suppression by dexamethasone may be due to either concomitant depression or is intrinsic to the primary condition.

Arginine vasopressin (ADH), normally released by the posterior pituitary in response to increased plasma osmolality and decreased circulating blood volume, is not released normally in response to an osmotic stimulus. In addition, its action in the kidney may be impaired. Levels of ADH in the cerebrospinal fluid are elevated (Gold et al, 1983). With successful treatment of anorexia nervosa all of these abnormalities of the various hypothalamic-pituitary-end organ axes have been shown to revert to normal.

Psychogenic Amenorrhea

Psychogenic amenorrhea is also referred to as "functional" or idiopathic amenorrhea. This form of secondary amenorrhea occurs in the absence of pregnancy without the presence of demonstrable abnormalities of brain, pituitary, or ovary. It may occur with minor degrees of psychic stress or with gross psychopathology. For example, psychogenic amenorrhea is associated with leaving home to attend school, life crises, bereavement, and the onset of psychiatric disorders such as acute depression or schizophrenia.

Basal levels of pituitary hormones are normal, and estrogen and progesterone levels are appropriate for the early follicular phase of the menstrual cycle. There appears to be a deficient feedback response of estrogen on LH which may be due to abnormal GnRH secretion. Some patients have demonstrated enhanced LH release after treatment with metoclopramide (a dopamine antagonist) or naloxone (an opioid antagonist). This suggests that the underlying abnormality may be related to excessive opioid or dopamine activity following the stressful event.

A possible variant of psychogenic amenorrhea, exercise amenorrhea, may be due to loss of body fat. This syndrome is seen in women who undergo intense physical training such as in competitive running and ballet dancing. These patients are always below ideal body weight and have low fat stores (Bates and Whitworth, 1984). If the training is begun prepubertally, sexual maturation may be delayed.

Premenstrual Tension Syndrome

The study of premenstrual tension syndrome (PMS) has been hampered by the lack of a common, generally agreed-upon definition of PMS and the lack of consensus concerning the hormonal onset of the premenstrual phase. Nonetheless, PMS can be defined as the presence of one or more psychological plus one or more physical symptoms. PMS is believed to affect as many as five percent of women. The psychological symptoms include depression, anxiety, increased fatigability, and easy crying. Physical symptoms include weight gain, breast tenderness, and swelling of the legs and abdomen. When stringent diagnostic criteria are applied, a percentage of women with PMS are at increased risk of developing psychiatric problems, especially affective disorders such as depression (Halbreich et al, 1973).

The etiology of PMS is not known. The most widely accepted hypothesis regarding its etiology involves the relationship between estrogen and progesterone during the premenstrual phase of the cycle. PMS has been attributed to 1) estrogen excess; 2) estrogen/progesterone imbalance due to relative progesterone deficiency; and 3) hyperprolactinemia. Prolactin levels have been reported to be higher during all phases of the cycle in women with PMS compared to asymptomatic controls. Many forms of treatment have been utilized, including diuretics, progestogens, nonsteroidal anti-inflammatory agents, and bromocriptine (Sommer, 1978; Tonks, 1975). None has been established as effective by rigorous double blind controlled studies.

Psychotic episodes which appear cyclic and are associated with the premenstrual phase have been described (Endo et al, 1978). These patients tend to be young (age of onset 13–23 years). This premenstrual psychosis in adolescents and young women differs from the previously described disorder in age of onset, severity and quality of symptoms, time course, and occasional dramatic response to treatment. It may represent a disorder distinct from PMS as commonly discussed in the literature.

ENDOCRINE ABNORMALITIES IN SCHIZOPHRENIA

The prevailing biochemical theory of schizophrenia is based on the concept of functional hyperactivity of central dopamine neuronal systems, particularly those that originate in the midbrain tegmental area and project to the limbic and cortical areas of the forebrain (Haracz, 1982). This concept is supported by the data which shows that essentially all drugs effective in treating active schizophrenic symptoms interfere with dopamine activity. The inability to directly measure activity of the mesolimbic and mesocortical dopamine systems, which are believed to be associated with psychosis, has led to the development of model dopamine systems that can be evaluated in schizophrenic subjects.

Growth Hormone and Prolactin

Growth Hormone (GH) and prolactin (PRL) are both one-chain somatomammotropin peptide hormones that are believed to have evolved by gene duplication. Prolactin, a 198-amino acid peptide hormone produced primarily within the lactrotrophe cell of the anterior pituitary gland, is also located in other brain areas, placenta, and neoplastic tissues. PRL release is stimulated by TRH, serotonin, acetylcholine, and opiates and inhibited by dopamine. Under normal conditions, therefore, the lactotrophe may be subjected to positive stimulation by these substances. Dopamine receptor agonists (for example, apomorphine, bromocriptine) suppress the release of PRL and, when administered chronically, possibly the synthesis of PRL. Normal serum levels of PRL are less than 25 ng/ml. Levels rise during sleep, usually between 3:00 A.M. and 5:00 A.M., provided that a prior slow-wave sleep stage has occurred. Levels may be higher during the luteal phase of the menstrual cycle and they are elevated 10–20 times during pregnancy.

The TRH test, previously described, is a pharmacologic stimulus to PRL release. Metoclopramide is used to assess PRL release, while apomorphine hydrochloride and bromocriptine suppress lactotrophic activity. The results of testing with these agents can be altered by concurrent administration of a variety of pharmacologic agents known to influence PRL release by causing hyperprolactinemia (Table 2). Hyperprolactinemia is also found in the presence of hypothalamic-pituitary disease (pituitary adenomas, craniopharyngiomas), hypothyroidism, polycystic ovary syndrome, and chronic renal failure. Although generally accepted that basal PRL secretion is normal both in acute and chronic schizophrenia, the severity of illness in drug-free chronic schizophrenic patients has been shown to correlate inversely with serum PRL concentrations. This finding suggests a relationship between the degree of dopaminergic activity and psychotic symptomatology in certain patients (Meltzer et al, 1974; Johnstone et al, 1977). In addition, all currently marketed antipsychotic drugs acutely increase PRL concentrations.

PRL response to neuroleptics has also been correlated with responses to treatment (Meltzer, 1980). The increase in serum PRL and clinical response was negatively correlated in females. This finding suggests that patients with the greatest increase in dopaminergic activity at the pituitary levels are the subgroup of schizophrenics for whom dopamine is a relevant factor etiologically. As such, these patients tend to be more responsive to neuroleptics.

Table 2.   Drug Induced Hyperprolactinemia

Psychotropics	Phenothiazines
	Butyrophenones
	Thioxanthenes
Antihypertensives	Reserpine
	Alpha-methyldopa
H_2-receptor blockers	Cimetidine
Opiates	Morphine
	Methadone
Antiemetics	Metoclopramide
Estrogens	Oral contraceptives

Growth hormone (GH) is regulated in part by neurotransmitters and peptides hypothesized to be abnormal in schizophrenia (see discussion under the section dealing with affective disorders). Obesity and age are nonpsychiatric factors that significantly influence GH levels. Interest in dopamine-mediated GH secretion has increased due to studies suggesting that the GH response is more closely associated with antipsychotic response to neuroleptics than that of dopamine-mediated prolactin secretion (Lal et al, 1982). For example, clozapine blocks apormorphine-induced GH release, but has little effect on PRL release. Furthermore, dopamine receptors mediating GH release are located centrally in the limbic system, while those mediating PRL release are located in the pituitary.

Apomorphine hydrochloride, a direct dopamine-receptor agonist, has been used to study the functional state of dopamine receptors involved in the release of PRL and GH. Apomorphine suppresses PRL release by a direct inhibitory action on dopamine receptors on the lactotrophes. The stimulation of GH release is believed to be mediated by way of dopamine receptors in the hypothalamus. Apomorphine induced GH response has been correlated with psychosis ratings and negative symptoms scale scores (Meltzer et al, 1984).

Schizophrenic subjects have other known alterations in hypothalamic-pituitary function, such as GH release in response to TRH and GnRH. Furthermore, basal LH and FSH levels are reduced with a reduced response to GnRH administration (Ferrier et al, 1983).

Endogenous Opiate System

The endogenous opioid system is believed to have an important role in mediating behavior. This is based upon observations of the marked behavioral effects of exogenous opiates and the distribution of opioid ligands and receptors in CNS sites thought to be involved in emotions and behavior (Simantov, 1981). There is increasing evidence that opioid peptides presynaptically modulate the release of classical neurotransmitters such as dopamine from nerve terminals. The modulatory effects of opioids on dopamine neuronal transmission have been convincingly demonstrated. Furthermore, opiate receptors have been shown to be located on dopamine neuronal elements. There are several lines of evidence to suggest a functional coupling of dopaminergic and opiate systems. Opiates, in general, increase the synthesis, release, reuptake, and metabolism of dopamine (DA). They have also been shown to increase pituitary prolactin release either by direct action or by an indirect DA antagonism. Dopamine agonists inhibit the release of pituitary beta-endorphin. In addition, lesions of the striatonigral DA pathway enhance the endogenous enkephalin content in the striatium.

An etiological role for endorphins in schizophrenia was suggested by behavioral experiments involving their injection into rodents. These investigations showed that beta-endorphins were capable of eliciting a long-lasting naloxone-reversible cataleptic syndrome. This syndrome was characterized by generalized muscular rigidity, absence of spontaneous movement, and maintenance of awkward postures, a state similar to that seen in schizophrenia. Therefore, a possible disturbance in availability of endorphins was proposed as an etiologic mechanism.

It is suggested that an imbalance of opiate-dopamine interactions might be involved in the pathogenesis of schizophrenia. Opioid agonists alter DA release, reuptake, and metabolism in the striatum and substantia nigra. In reverse, chronic neuroleptic treatment enhances the synthesis and release of pituitary beta-endorphin. Measurements of endorphin levels in chronic schizophrenics reveal elevated beta-endorphin levels, which gradually fall with neuroleptic treatment.

The endogenous opioid system has been studied clinically, predominantly by administering the opiate antagonist, naloxone, the rationale being that if a given symptomatology is related to excessive endogenous opioid activity, then blockade by naloxone should cause improvement. This approach is limited, however, by the greater affinity of endogenous opioids for receptors than that of exogenous agonists or antagonists. Naloxone has dose dependent behavioral and physiologic effects in normals. Low dose naloxone (0.3 mg/kg) has few effects, whereas high dose naloxone stimulates irritability, anxiety, sadness, and confusion. Data concerning the clinical effects of naloxone on schizophrenia are conflicting. While cessation of auditory hallucinations has been reported, other studies have reported either no clear effects or accentuation of negative symptoms of schizophrenia.

In general, most clinical studies of opioids in schizophrenia have been of the effect of opioids on psychotic symptoms. Additional studies of the effects on dopaminergic functions, such as PRL release, DA metabolites, and potentiation of opioid effects by neuroleptics, will extend knowledge of the role of DA and endogenous opioids in the pathogenesis of schizophrenia.

ENDOCRINE EFFECTS OF PSYCHIATRIC MEDICATIONS

Neuroleptics

All major classes of antipsychotic drugs commonly used (phenothiazines, butyrophenones, thioxanthines, dibenzoxazepines, and indolic compounds) stimulate prolactin (PRL) secretion. Neuroleptics inhibit dopamine transmission across neuronal synapses, apparently by blockade of dopamine receptors in the striatal, mesolimbic, and cortical regions (Bacopoulos et al, 1979). Dopamine receptors on pituitary lactotrophes (PRL-secreting cells) are also blocked by neuroleptics, thereby removing the tonic inhibitory influence of dopamine from the tuberoinfundibular tract (Gruen et al, 1978).

The PRL-stimulating potencies of neuroleptics correlate with their clinical effectiveness and their binding affinities to dopamine receptors (Langer et al, 1977). The PRL response increases with the dose of the neuroleptic, generally reaching a maximum at the equivalent of chlorpromazine 500–700 mg a day.

Not surprisingly, patients on neuroleptics may develop galactorrhea. Galactorrhea has also been associated with administration of reserpine, tricyclic antidepressants, and opiates. Women have higher PRL responses than do men, probably due to estrogen potentiation of lactotroph secretion. Elevated PRL levels have been linked to mammary tumors in rodents. However, epidemiologic studies of breast cancer in women treated with neuroleptics concluded that neuroleptics do not increase the risk for breast cancer in women despite their ability to cause hyperprolactinemia (Schyve et al, 1978).

PRL stimulation is the major hormonal effect of neuroleptics. GH and LH secretion and thyroid function are unchanged following neuroleptic administration. The ACTH response to stress is diminished, however basal and circadian

ACTH rhythms are not affected. Both men and women on neuroleptics can experience sexual dysfunction: menstrual dysfunction, diminished libido, erectile, ejaculatory, and orgasmic dysfunction. The mechanism of these changes is unclear, and may relate to dopamine receptor blockade, alpha-adrenergic blockade and anticholinergic activity, altered GnRH secretion, gonadotroph responsivity, or peripheral effects (Mitchell and Popkin, 1983). There is controversy concerning the effect of chronic neuroleptic therapy on serum testosterone levels. They have been reported as normal or low normal with increases after discontinuation of therapy.

Lithium

Lithium carbonate, used mainly in the treatment of manic-depressive disorders or recurrent depression, is known to cause alterations in the function of the thyroid and parathyroid glands. Lithium is concentrated within the thyroid gland and reaches a concentration four times that of serum. It inhibits the action of TSH on the thyroid, inhibits the uptake of iodine, impairs the conversion of iodotyrosines to iodothyronines (therefore the synthesis of T_3 and T_4), and interferes with the release of thyroid hormone. After a month of therapy, the blood levels of circulating thyroid hormones decrease in up to one-half of patients. These effects of lithium may result in the development of euthyroid goiter or frank hypothyroidism with or without the presence of a goiter. These clinical abnormalities have a prevalence of up to 15 percent (Lazarus and Bennie, 1972; Lindstedt et al, 1977). Patients who develop hypothyroidism may have circulating thyroid autoantibodies (antimicrosomal and antithyroglobulin), suggesting the coexistence of autoimmune thyroiditis. Clinical hypothyroidism developing as a result of lithium therapy responds to treatment with L-thyroxine.

Lithium therapy is rarely associated with the development of hyperthyroidism and may be a chance occurrence. Those patients who develop hyperthyroidism after withdrawal of lithium therapy may be manifesting rebound thyrotoxicosis following removal of the inhibition of thyroid function by lithium.

Lithium has been reported to raise serum calcium, to lower serum phosphate, and to increase urinary excretion of calcium. Serum calcium concentrations correlate with the serum lithium concentration (Davis et al, 1981). In fact, lithium can produce a drug-dependent reversible biochemical hyperparathyroidism. The complications of primary hyperparathyroidism, namely nephrolithiasis and osteitis fibrosa, are not known to occur with long-term lithium treatment. Furthermore, lithium has no effect on the serum calcium levels of patients with known primary hyperparathyroidism. Since chronic lithium administration has been associated with renal morphologic and functional pathology, early renal failure is a potential cause of PTH elevation during lithium therapy. Physiological causes of PTH elevation that may occur during lithium treatment include functional hypocalcemia (lithium has been shown to antagonize certain calcium-dependent processes) and renal impairment (Davis et al, 1981).

T_3 in Psychiatric Disease

Thyroid extract was first used to treat psychiatric disease by Kraepelin, with schizophrenics. Since that time many studies have been performed, but thyroid hormone has not been found efficacious in treating psychoses, with few exceptions. The rationale for using thyroid hormone in the treatment of depression is the observation that the affective state is similar in hypothyroidism and in depression. T_3 used daily in small doses potentiates the therapeutic efficacy of tricyclic antidepressant drugs in depressed women. The therapeutic dose of T_3 is 25 ug. The mechanism of this potentiation is unknown. The evidence in favor of this potentiation was the finding that administration of thyroid hormones to rats increased cyclic AMP levels in adipose tissue and also increased the toxicity of the tricyclic antidepressants. There is also clinical evidence that the level of thyroid activity is directly correlated with the level of adrenergic activity. Therefore, if some forms of depression are in fact due to decreased levels of catecholamines in the brain, one could conceivably enhance the sensitivity of the brain's catecholamine receptors by giving thyroid hormone and improving catecholamine-mediated neurotransmission.

One hypothesis suggests that T_3 sensitizes brain receptors to norepinephrine, thus facilitating the noradrenergic action of the antidepressant drugs. A second hypothesis postulates that T_3 reduces the protein binding ability of the drugs, thereby enhancing their antidepressant effect.

Several studies have been conducted using TSH and TRH in the treatment of both depression and schizophrenia. Unfortunately, they have yielded conflicting results and data has been difficult to compare. The use of thyroid hormone in the treatment of depression is still of questionable clinical value.

SUBSTANCE ABUSE

Chronic narcotic use is predominantly associated with alterations in gonadal function. Exogenous opiate administration reduces gonadotropin levels by way of a primary suppressive effect on hypothalamic LHRH-secreting cells. The decrease in luteinizing hormone (LH) secretion leads to a subsequent decrease in testosterone secretion in men (Mendelson et al, 1975). Naloxone administration has been shown to induce rises in serum LH levels associated with an increased frequency of LH secretory episodes. It thus seems likely that opioid peptides have a role in modulation of the hypothalamic control of LH secretion through variations in a tonic inhibitory influence (Moult et al, 1981).

Benzodiazepines interfere with the cortisol response to stress. This is a central phenomenon, not mediated by direct action of the pituitary. Benzodiazepines are also a stimulus for growth hormone secretion. This effect may be mediated by effects on dopaminergic transmission or by way of the benzodiazepines-gamma-aminobutyric acid receptor complex. As with narcotics and LHRH, tolerance develops to the GH-releasing effects (Shur et al, 1983).

Cocaine and other central stimulants increase dopaminergic and noradrenergic activity. Acute administration causes a decrease in serum PRL and an increase in GH. Chronic cocaine administration in animals causes a beta-adrenergic, alpha-adrenergic, and dopaminergic receptor supersensitivity and increased norepinephrine and dopamine turnover. There is evidence that cocaine may alter the thyroid axis. Cocaine activates central dopamine and norepinephrine systems by blocking neurotransmitter re-uptake (Ross and Renyi, 1966). Since these neurotransmitter systems are involved in TRH regulation, it is possible that cocaine abuse leads to thyroid axis disruption by way of chronic stimulation. In fact, the TSH response to TRH is blunted in cocaine abusers despite normal baseline T_4, T_3, and TSH levels. Chronic TRH release by cocaine could result in desensitized pituitary TRH receptors. Cocaine may also exert direct or indirect effects on T_4 receptors. Another central stimulant, d-amphetamine, produces elevated T_4 and TSH levels in monkeys and elevated T_4 levels in humans (Morley et al, 1980).

Neuroendocrine abnormalities have been found in 80 percent of chronic cocaine abusers immediately after cessation of use. GH levels are increased, PRL levels decreased, and dexamethasone suppression tests are abnormal despite normal basal cortisol values. These abnormalities have reverted to normal after more than four weeks of abstinence. These findings must be interpreted with caution, however, due to uncontrolled variables such as differences in purity of cocaine and street adulterants, routes of administration, and other substances abused among the study populations (Gawin and Kleber, 1985).

Alcohol ingestion causes a rapid decrease in serum testosterone. The lack of feedback inhibition causes a compensatory rise in plasma LH. Alcohol withdrawal is accompanied by elevated cortisol secretion, and blunting of the TRH test (Mendelson et al, 1978).

Chronic alcoholics in acute withdrawal have a hormonal profile suggesting thyroid activation and increased central dopaminergic activity. This is evidenced by elevated baseline levels of growth hormone, low levels of prolactin, and a blunted TSH response to TRH. GH and PRL abnormalities resolve in the remission state (Loosen et al, 1979). Chronic alcoholic patients have been found to have profound disturbances in the hypothalamic-pituitary-thyroid axis: 1) the "euthyroid sick syndrome" with low T_3 and high reverse T_3; 2) an increased binding capacity for thyroid hormone; and 3) blunted TSH response to TRH. The factors responsible for the blunted TSH response, which is not correlated with basal levels of T_4, T_3 or reverse T_3, are unknown.

A pseudo-Cushing's syndrome has been described in subjects with chronic alcoholism. These patients have elevated levels of plasma cortisol which normalizes spontaneously with abstinence. During the period of hypercortisolism they display an insufficient suppression by dexamethasone and absent diurnal variation in plasma cortisol. Although these findings revert to normal in parallel with normalization of liver function tests, the absence of a similar syndrome in patients with nonalcoholic liver disease excludes a straightforward relationship between cortisol and liver function tests.

ENDOCRINOLOGY OF AGING

Established normal values for laboratory tests may require modification when the patient is 65 years of age or older. For example, elderly subjects display delayed peak levels of glucose and delayed insulin response during a standard glucose tolerance test. Basal plasma levels of glucocorticoids appear to remain constant throughout life; however, diurnal patterns can be altered by chronic disorders such as heart disease, diabetes, and chronic brain syndromes. The circulating half-life of cortisol has been shown to be 40 percent longer for elderly subjects than in the young, and secretion rates have been shown to decrease 30 percent over the adult life span. There appears to be a decreased ability of the adrenal cortex to respond to ACTH. Urinary 17-ketosteroid excretion, one measure of androgen status, decreases with advancing age.

Thyroid hormone concentrations exhibit small changes with aging. While mean T_4 concentrations do not change significantly with age, T_3 concentrations are significantly lowered in older men. Mean thyroxine binding globulin concentrations are unchanged, but T_3 resin uptake declines slightly. The free T_4 index and free T_3 index have also been found to be significantly reduced in older men. An increase in TSH has been found, but TSH responses to TRH do not differ significantly with aging. These findings suggest that there is an age-related decrease in thyrotropic function (Harman et al, 1984).

Although endocrine diseases tend to occur in young women, thyroid hyper- or hypo-functioning often occurs in elderly individuals with Graves' disease, toxic multinodular goiter, prior radioiodine treatment of hyperthyroidism, or long-standing Hashimoto's disease. Apathetic hyperthyroidism is seen in elderly persons who typically have apathy or depression and weight loss, with or without an increase in appetite.

A study of plasma growth hormone during sleep in young and aged men found that the level of integrated plasma GH in aged men is significantly lower than in young men during the first three hours of sleep. A significant reduction is also found for the peak GH value. Compared with young men, nighttime peaks of GH were smaller or absent and were distributed more evenly across the night. The 24-hour GH levels are unaltered by age (Prinz et al, 1983).

The luteinizing-hormone-releasing hormone (LHRH) and TRH content in the hypothalamus of postmenopausal women has been studied. The hypothalamic content of TRH does not change significantly with age. In contrast, content of LHRH is lower in women who have been ovariectomized and in postmenopausal women. These findings suggest that the reduction in hypothalamic LHRH is a consequence of ovarian failure and not of aging (Parker and Porter, 1984).

Normal serum testosterone levels are 350 to 1,000 ng/dl regardless of age, with a small decrease in testicular volume normally occurring with age. Low levels of testosterone have been associated with physical illness and stress. Loss of libido in males age 50–70 is most likely attributable to nonhormonal factors such as poor health, marital factors, or psychologic conflicts. Serum testosterone levels do not decline with age in healthy men; therefore all borderline and low values need further evaluation. Regardless of age, elevated levels of luteinizing hormone (LH) and follicle-stimulating hormone (FSH) with low testosterone suggest primary testicular failure. Although the maximum response to LHRH is similar for all ages, the percent of baseline attained declines with age, and LH response may be delayed. There is very little evidence for a male menopause such as that seen in females.

PSYCHIATRIC ABNORMALITIES IN ENDOCRINE DISEASE

Endocrine hormones and the secretory products of their target tissues exert their effects on the brain both directly and indirectly. For example, gonadal and adrenal steroids act on target areas of the brain as well as on other body tissues. The effects of thyroid hormone deficiency during prenatal and postnatal development are striking. Changes in blood levels of calcium, glucose, thyroid, and steroid hormones can elicit marked behavioral changes.

In adults, failure of the pituitary or any of its target glands invariably gives rise to behavioral disturbances. Patients with hypopituitarism frequently become dependent, apathetic, drowsy, depressed, and fatigued. The mental effects range from confusion to frank psychosis. These symptoms may be seen in pituitary dysfunction of any etiology. Whether these behavioral changes are due to adrenocortical, thyroid, or gonadal failure is not clear.

Thyroid disease

A high proportion of patients with hypothyroidism exhibit evidence of mental disturbance. The effects of thyroid hormone deficiency on behavior can mimic mental retardation, schizophrenia, or depressive syndrome. Adult onset hypothyroidism is characterized by lethargy, apathy, psychomotor retardation, depression, confusion, cognitive impairment, and psychoses ("myxdema madness"). In severe hypothyroidism patients may have a frank psychosis with paranoid delusions, hallucinations, excitement, or mania. Although these psychiatric symptoms clear with appropriate treatment, residual intellectual deficit may persist. In cretinism, the degree of mental defect is proportional to the length of time prior to initiation of therapy.

Thyroid hormone may regulate sensitivity of brain catecholamine receptors (Prange et al, 1970), and a functional noradrenergic deficit caused by receptor insensitivity induced by thyroid hormone deficiency may account for the depressive phenomena of hypothyroidism as well as the disturbances in memory and attention. The mental effects of hyperthyroidism are anxiety, restlessness, fatigue, emotional lability, irritability, tremor, sleep disturbance, and difficulty with interpersonal relationships. In the elderly, apathy, withdrawal, depression, and weight loss may also occur, mimicking malignancy (apathetic hyperthyroidism). Severely hyperthyroid patients may actually develop perceptual disturbances including visual hallucinations. Thus, routine assessment of thyroid function is essential in psychiatric patients, especially those requiring hospitalization. Elevations of serum T_4, free T_4 index, and T_3 occur in up to 20 percent of short-term psychiatric admissions. Increase in thyroid function values are found in patients taking amphetamines or phencyclidine, and in patients with (paranoid) schizophrenia. In general, the elevated values tend to normalize during the first two weeks after psychiatric admission. It has been proposed that the elevations in thyroid function values may be due to an increase in phenylethylamine, an endogenous amphetamine-like compound, found in schizophrenic subjects. The mechanism of these abnormalities, however, remains to be elucidated (Morley et al, 1983; Spratt et al, 1982).

Cushing's Syndrome and Addison's Disease

Symptoms of Cushing's syndrome include depressed mood, decreased libido, insomnia, impaired concentration, impaired memory, fatigue, and diminished energy. Although the milder symptoms are difficult to separate from normal reactions to fatigue and physical disfigurement, the severe forms may be associated with delusions and suicidal tendencies, reportedly as high as 10 percent. Mild forms of mania are also seen: typically, talkativeness, overactivity, irritability, decreased sleep, and impulsiveness. In severe states, elation, grandiosity, and delusions occur. Schizophrenia-like symptoms are also seen, but are rare. Treatment with exogenous corticosteroids is also associated with the psychological and psychiatric disturbances as seen in Cushing's syndrome. Although depression is more common than mania with endogenous Cushing's syndrome, the reverse appears to occur in so-called "steroid psychosis." It was once thought that the mental effects of steroid therapy were related to the patient's premorbid personality, but evidence suggests that patients with prior mental illness are not at a greater risk of steroid-induced psychoses.

The common psychiatric manifestations of adrenal insufficiency include apathy, fatigue, somnolence, anorexia, nightmares, depression, poverty of thought, and a general negativism. In acute Addison's disease, a typical organic psychosis develops, with memory deficit, clouding of consciousness, and even stupor or loss of consciousness. There is also an increased sensitivity to taste, smell, and hearing despite an impaired ability to discriminate sensory input. The mechanism of action of glucocorticoids in Addison's disease is not completely understood, but it is known that when glucocorticoids are deficient the latency of neural transmission at central nervous system synapses is prolonged. This would be particularly marked in multisynaptic systems such as the reticular activating system, and in brain areas with a high affinity for glucocorticoids, such as the hippocampus and septum. Adequate steroid replacement therapy reverses the symptoms. One must be aware that the reappearance of psychiatric disturbances may indicate the need for temporary increase in replacement therapy dosage.

Other Endocrine Diseases

Parathyroid gland hyperfunction may first present with depression, lethargy, apathy, confusion, coma, or organic psychoses. In some patients, headache is a prominent feature. These abnormalities are related to the hypercalcemia that develops, rather than the level of parathyroid hormone. The EEG may show slowing and other nonspecific abnormalities that are reversible following treatment.

One-third of patients with longstanding untreated hypoparathyroidism suffer intellectual deterioration, nervousness, and organic mental syndromes including psychoses. After treatment a residual deficit often persists. Hypoparathyroidism due to surgery is associated with organic mental syndromes but intellectual deficit is rare, probably due to the rapidity of onset, recognition, and treatment.

Acute onset of hypoglycemia usually presents with adrenergic symptoms mimicking anxiety or panic disorders. Patients may experience anxiety, tremor, palpitations, sweating, and dizziness. Chronic hypoglycemia develops due to overtreatment of diabetes (especially with overuse of oral sulfonylurea drugs), extensive liver disease in advanced cancers, Addison's disease, or insulinoma. The symptoms of cerebral cortical dysfunction are most prominent and include headaches, faintness, confusion, restlessness, irritability, somnolence, and visual disturbances.

SUMMARY

This chapter has outlined the current interfaces between the disciplines of psychiatry and endocrinology—the study of psychoendocrinology—relying extensively on advances in basic mechanisms to understand clinical phenomena. Until recently the major endocrine tool in the investigation and diagnosis of psychiatric disease was the dexamethasone suppression test in depressive illness. Administration and interpretation of the DST is complicated by a host of factors that influence cortisol and cortisol suppression such as age, concurrent illness, and medications. Now, however, other tests of hypothalamic-pituitary-target gland responsiveness have been utilized in research protocols to obtain evidence in support of current neurotransmitter hypotheses of the pathophysiology of psychiatric illness; for example, measurements of growth hormone and prolactin and their responses to pharmacologic manipulations have given support to the dopamine hyperactivity theory of schizophrenia. This hypothesis has been modified by recent studies of effects of endogenous opioids on dopaminergic activity.

Psychiatric medications have several endocrine effects. Hyperprolactinemia and galactorrhea are caused by neuroleptics; hypothyroidism and hyperthyroidism are caused by lithium.

Neuroendocrine changes due to various substances of abuse are many. Study of the mechanisms involved are still in their infancy. Further study of neuroendocrine parameters in all psychiatric disease will hopefully lead to new therapeutic modalities in the treatment of psychiatric illness.

REFERENCES

Asnis GM, Sachar EJ, Halbreich U, et al: Cortisol secretion in relation to age in major depression. Psychosom Med 43:235-242, 1981a

Asnis GM, Sachar EJ, Halbreich U, et al: Endocrine responses to thyrotropin-releasing hormone in major depressive disorders. Psychiatry Res 5:205-215, 1981b

Bacopoulos NC, Spokes EG, Bird ED, et al: Antipsychotic drug action in schizophrenic patients: effect on cortical dopamine metabolism after long-term treatment. Science 25:1405-1407, 1979

Bates GW, Whitworth NS: Effects of body weight on female reproductive function, in The Hypothalamus. Edited by Givens JR. Chicago, Year Book, 1984

Beumont PJV, Abraham SF: Continuous infusion of luteinizing hormone releasing hormone (LHRH) in patients with anorexia nervosa. Psychol Med 11:477-484, 1981

Beumont PJV, Abraham SF, Turtle J: Paradoxical prolactin response to gonadotropin-releasing hormone during weight gain in patients with anorexia nervosa. J Clin Endocrinol Metab 51:1283-1285, 1980

Boyar RM, Katz J: Twenty-four-hour gonadotropin secretory patterns in anorexia nervosa, in Anorexia Nervosa. Edited by Vigersky RA. New York, Raven Press, 1977

Brown WA, Shuey I: Response to dexamethasone and subtypes of depression. Arch Gen Psychiatry 37:747-751, 1980

Carroll BJ: Neuroendocrine dysfunction in psychiatric disorders, in Psychopharmacology: A Generation of Progress. Edited by Lipton MA, DiMascio A, Killam KF. New York, Raven Press, 1978

Carroll BJ: Clinical applications of the dexamethasone suppression test for endogenous depression. Pharmacopsychiatry 15:19-24, 1982

Carroll BJ: Biological markers and treatment response. J Clin Psychiatry 44:30-40, 1983

Carroll BJ, Feinberg M, Greden J, et al: A specific laboratory test for the diagnosis of melancholia. Arch Gen Psychiatry 38:15-22, 1981

Caspar RC, Frohman LA: Delayed TSH release in anorexia nervosa following injection of thyrotropin-releasing hormone (TRH). Psychoneuroendocrinology 7:59-68, 1982

Chambers JW, Brown GM: Neurotransmitter regulation of growth hormone and ACTH in the rhesus monkey: effects of biogenic amines. Endocrinology 98:420-428, 1976

Cohen LS, Davis BM, Mathé AA, et al: Influence of age on the dexamethasone suppression test for depression. Geriatric Medicine Today 4:54-61, 1985

Coryell W, Gaffner G, Burkhardt P: DSM-III melancholia and the primary secondary distinction: a comparison of concurrent validity by means of the dexamethasone suppression test. Am J Psychiatry 139:120-122, 1982

Creese I, Burt DR, Snyder SA: Dopamine receptor binding predicts clinical and pharmacological potencies of anti-schizophrenic drugs. Science 192:481-483, 1976

Dackis CA, Estroff TW, Sweeney DR, et al: Specificity of the TRH test for major depression in patients with serious cocaine abuse. Am J Psychiatry 142:1097-1099, 1985

Davis BM, Pfefferbaum A, Krutzik S, et al: Lithium's effect on parathyroid hormone. Am J Psychiatry 138:489-492, 1981

Endo M, Daiguji M, Asano Y, et al: Periodic psychosis recurring in association with menstrual cycle. J Clin Psychiatry 39:456-466, 1978

Ferrier IN, Johnstone EC, Crow TJ, et al: Anterior pituitary hormone secretion in chronic schizophrenics. Arch Gen Psychiatry 40:755-761, 1983

Frank SS, Jacobs HS, Martin N, et al: Hyperprolactinemia and impotence. Clin Endocrinol 8:277-287, 1978

Gambert SR, Tsitouras PD, Duthie EH: Interpretation of laboratory results in the elderly, 2: a clinician's guide to endocrine tests. Postgrad Med 72:251-256, 1982

Gawin FH, Kleber HD: Neuroendocrine findings in chronic cocaine abusers: a preliminary report. Br J Psychiatry 147:569-573, 1985

Gerner GH, Gwirstman ME: Abnormalities of the dexamethasone suppression test and urinary MHPG in anorexia nervosa. Am J Psychiatry 138:650-653, 1981

Gold PW, Kaye W, Robertson GL, et al: Abnormalities in plasma and cerebrospinal-fluid arginine vasopressin in patients with anorexia nervosa. N Engl J Med 308:1117-1123, 1983

Goodwin FK, Post RM, Dunner DL, et al: Cerebrospinal fluid amine metabolites in affective illness: the probenecid technique. Am J Psychiatry 130:73-79, 1973

Greenwald BS, Mohs RC, Davis KL: Neurotransmitter deficits in Alzheimer's disease: criteria for significance. J Am Geriatr Soc 31:310-316, 1983

Gruen PH: Endocrine changes in psychiatric diseases. Med Clin North Am 62:285, 1978

Gruen PH, Sachar EJ, Langer G, et al: Prolactin response to neuroleptics in normal and schizophrenic subjects. Arch Gen Psychiatry 35:108-116, 1978

Halbreich U, Endicott J, Nee J: Premenstrual depressive changes. Arch Gen Psychiatry 40:535-542, 1973

Haracz JL: The dopamine hypothesis: an overview of studies with schizophrenic patients. Schizophr Bull 8:438-469, 1982

Harman SM, Tsitouras PD: Reproduction hormones in aging men, I: measurement of sex steroids, basal luteinizing hormone, and Leydig cell response to human chorionic gonadotropin. J Clin Endocrinol Metab 51:35-40, 1980

Harman SM, Wehmann RE, Blackman MR: Pituitary-thyroid hormone economy in healthy aging men: basal indices of thyroid function and thyrotropin responses to constant infusions of thyrotropin relasing hormone. J Clin Endocrinol Metab 58:320-326, 1984

Hudson JS, Laffer PS, Pope HG: Bulimia related to affective disorder by family history and response to dexamethasone suppression test. Am J Psychiatry 139:685-687, 1982

Isaacs AJ, Leslie RDG, Gomez J, et al: The effect of weight gain on gonadotrophins and prolactin in anorexia nervosa. Acta Endocrinol 94:145-150, 1980

Jimerson DC, Insel TR, Revus VI, et al: Increased plasma MHPG in dexamethasone-resistant depressed patients. Arch Gen Psychiatry 40:173-176, 1983

Johnstone E, Crow TJ, Mashiter K: Anterior pituitary hormone secretion in chronic schizophrenia—an approach to neurohumoral mechanisms. Psychol Med 7:223-228, 1977

Kirkegaard C, Bjorum N, Cohn D, et al: Thyrotropin-releasing hormone (TRH) stimulation test in manic-depressive illness. Arch Gen Psychiatry 35:1017-1021, 1978

Kolodny RC, Kahn CB, Goldstein HH, et al: Sexual dysfunction in diabetic men. Diabetes 23:306-309, 1974

Lal S, Nair NP, Iskandar HI, et al: Drug-induced growth hormone and prolactin responses in schizophrenia research. Prog Neuropsychopharmacol Biol Psychiatry 6:631-637, 1982

Langer G, Sachar EJ, Gruen PH, et al: Human prolactin responses to neuroleptic drugs correlate with antischizophrenic potency. Nature 266:639-640, 1977

Lazarus JH, Bennie EH: Effect of lithium on thyroid function in man. Acta Endocrinol 70:266-272, 1972

Lindstedt G, Nilsson L, Walinder J, et al: On the prevalence, diagnosis and management of lithium-induced hypothyroidism in psychiatric patients. Br J Psychiatry 130:452-458, 1977

Loosen PJ, Prange AJ, Wilson IC: Influence of cortisol on TRH-induced TSH response in depression. Am J Psychiatry 135:244, 1977a

Loosen PH, Prange AJ Jr, Wilson IC, et al: Thyroid stimulation hormone response after thyrotropin releasing hormone in depressed schizophrenic and normal women. Psycho-neuroendocrinology 2:137-148, 1977b

Loosen PT, Prange AJ Jr, Wilson ID: TRH (protirelin) in depressed alcoholic men: behavioral changes and endocrine responses. Arch Gen Psychiatry 36:540-547, 1979

Loosen PJ, Wilson IC, Dew BW, et al: Thyrotropin-releasing hormone (TRH) in abstinent alcoholic men. Am J Psychiatry 140:1145-1149, 1983

Martin JB: Neural regulation of growth hormone secretion. N Engl J Med 288:1384-1393, 1973

Mathé AA: False normal dexamethasone suppression test and indomethacin. Lancet 2:714, 1982

Mattsson B: Addison's disease and psychoses. Acta Psychiatr Scand (Suppl) 255:203-210, 1974

McNab D, Hawton K: Disturbances of sex hormones in anorexia nervosa in the male. Postgrad Med 57:254-256, 1981

Meltzer HY: Effect of psychotropic drugs on neuroendocrine function. Psychiatr Clin North Am 3:277-298, 1980

Meltzer HY, Sachar EJ, Frantz AG: Serum prolactin levels in unmedicated schizophrenic patients. Arch Gen Psychiatry 31:564-569, 1974

Meltzer HY, Goode DJ, Fang VS: The effect of psychotropic drugs on endocrine function, I: neuroleptics, precursors and agonists, in Psychopharmacology: A Generation of Progress. Edited by Lipton MA, Mascio AD, Killam KF. New York, Raven Press, 1978

Meltzer HY, Kolakowska T, Fang VS, et al: Growth hormone and prolactin response to apomorphine in schizophrenia and the major affective disorders: relation to duration of illness and depressive symptoms. Arch Gen Psychiatry 41:512-519, 1984

Mendelson JE, Meyer RE, Ellingboe J, et al: Effects of heroin and methadone on plasma cortisol and testosterone. J Pharmacol Exp Ther 195:296-302, 1975

Mendelson JH, Mello NK, Ellingboe J: Effect of alcohol on pituitary-gonadal hormones, sexual function, and aggression in human males, in Psychopharmacology: A Generation of Progress. Edited by Lipton MA, DiMascio A, Killam KF. New York, Raven Press, 1978

Mitchell J, Popkin M: The pathophysiology of sexual dysfunction associated with anti-psychotic drug therapy in males: a review. Arch Sex Behav 12:173-183, 1983

Morley JE, Shafer RB, Ellson MK, et al: Amphetamine induced hyperthyroxinemia. Ann Intern Med 93:707-709, 1980

Morley JE, Slay MF, Ellson MK, et al: The interpretation of thyroid function tests in hospitalized patients. JAMA 249:2377-2379, 1983

Moshang T Jr, Utiger RD: Low triiodothyronine euthyroidisms in anorexia nervosa, in Anorexia Nervosa. Edited by Vigersky RA. New York, Raven Press, 1977

Moult PJA, Grossman A, Evans JM, et al: Effect of naloxone pulsatile gonadotropin release in normal subjects. Clin Endocrinol 14:321-324, 1981

Parker CR Jr, Porter JC: Luteinizing hormone-releasing hormone and thyrotropin-releasing hormone in the hypothalamus of women: effects of age and reproductive status. J Clin Endocrinol Metab 58:488-491, 1984

Peterson P: Psychiatric disorders in primary hyperparathyroidism. J Clin Endocrinol Metab 28:1491-1495, 1968

Pirke KM, Fichter MM, Lund R, et al: Twenty-four hour sleep-wake pattern of plasma LH in patients with anorexia nervosa. Acta Endocrinol 92:193-204, 1979

Prange A, Meek J, Lipton MJ: Catecholamines: diminished rate of synthesis in rat brain and heart after thyroxine pretreatment. Life Sci 9:901-907, 1970

Prinz PN, Weitzman EP, Cunningham GR, et al: Plasma growth hormone during sleep in young and aged men. J Gerontol 38:519-524, 1983

Randrup A, Munkvad I, Fog R, et al: Mania, depression and brain dopamine, in Current Developments in Psychopharmacology, vol. 2. Edited by Essman WB, Valzelli L. New York, Spectrum Publishers, 1975

Raskin M, Raskin E, Rivard MF, et al: Dexamethasone suppression test and cortisol circadian rhythm in primary degenerative dementia. Am J Psychiatry 139:1468-1471, 1982

Reid RL, Yen SSC: Premenstrual syndrome. Am J Obstet Gynecol 139:85-104, 1981

Rose RM: Psychoneuroendocrinology, in Textbook of Endocrinology, seventh edition. Edited by Wilson JD, Foster DW. Philadelphia, W.B. Saunders, 1985

Ross SB, Renyi AL: Uptake of some tritiated sympathomimetic amines by mouse brain cortex slices in vitro. Acta Pharmacol Toxicol 24:297-309, 1966

Sachar EJ: Neuroendocrine responses to psychotropic drugs, in Psychopharmacology: A Generation of Progress. Edited by Lipton MA, DiMascio A, Killam KF. New York, Raven Press, 1978

Sachar EJ, Asnis G, Halbreich U, et al: Recent studies in the neuroendocrinology of major depressive disorders. Psychiatr Clin North Am 3:313-326, 1980

Schmauss C, Emrich HM: Dopamine and the action of opiates: a reevaluation of the dopamine hypothesis of schizophrenia. Biol Psychiatry 20:1211-1231, 1985

Schwabe AD, Lippe BM, Chang RJ, et al: Anorexia nervosa. Ann Intern Med 94:371-381, 1981

Schyve PM, Smithline F, Meltzer F: Neuroleptic-induced prolactin elevation and breast cancer. Arch Gen Psychiatry 35:1291-1301, 1978

Shur E, Petursson H, Checkley S, et al: Long term benzodiazepine administration blunts growth hormone response to diazepam. Arch Gen Psychiatry 40:1105-1108, 1983

Simantov R: Localization and modulation of enkephalins, endorphins and opiate receptors in the CNS and the pituitary gland, in The Role of Endorphins in Neuropsychiatry: Modern Problems of Pharmacopsychiatry. Edited by Emrich HM. Basel, S. Karger, 1981

Skrabanek P, Devlin J, McDonald D, et al: Plasma prolactin and gonadotrophins in anorexia nervosa and amenorrhea due to weight loss. Acta Endocrinol 97:433-435, 1981

Sommer B: Stress and menstrual distress. J Human Stress 4:5-10, 1978

Spar JE, Gerner R: Does the dexamethasone suppression test distinguish dementia from depression? Am J Psychiatry 139:238-240, 1982

Spratt DI, Pont A, Miller MB, et al: Hyperthyroxinemia in patients with acute psychiatric disorders. Am J Med 73:41-48, 1982

Starkman MN, Schteingart ED, Schork MA: Depressed mood and other psychiatric manifestations of Cushing's syndrome: relationship to hormone levels. Psychosom Med 43:3-18, 1981

Stokes PE, Stoll PM, Koslow SH, et al: Pretreatment DST and hypothalamic-pituitary adreno-cortical function in depressed patients and comparison groups: a multicenter study. Arch Gen Psychiatry 41:257-267, 1984

Targum SD, Capodanno AE: The dexamethasone suppression test in adolescent psychiatric inpatients. Am J Psychiatry 140:589-591, 1983

Targum SD, Rosen L, Capodanno AE: The dexamethasone suppression test in suicidal patients with unipolar depression. Am J Psychiatry 140:877-879, 1983

Tonks CM: Premenstrual tension. Br J Psychol 9:399-408, 1975

Tourigny-Rivard MF, Raskind M, Rivard D: The dexamethasone suppression test in an elderly population. Biol Psychiatry 16:1177-1184, 1981

Vigersky RA, Loriaux DL: Anorexia nervosa as a model of hypothalamic dysfunction, in Anorexia Nervosa. Edited by Vigersky RA. New York, Raven Press, 1977

Walsh BT, Katz JL, Levin J, et al: The production rate of cortisol declines during recovery from anorexia nervosa. J Clin Endocrinol Metab 53:203-205, 1981

Chapter 9

Psychoimmunology in Clinical Psychiatry

by Marvin Stein, M.D., Steven J. Schleifer, M.D., and Steven E. Keller, Ph.D.

The central nervous system (CNS) and the immune system are major integrative networks involved in biologic adaptation. Interaction between the CNS and immune system has been considered since the turn of the century, when the brain was thought to be the organ initiating the anaphylactic reaction. A series of studies conducted between 1910 and 1920 demonstrated, however, that the characteristic signs of anaphylaxis could occur in decerebrate guinea pigs and dogs. These and other observations led to discouragement in studying the influence of the nervous system on the immune system. With the development of immunobiology over the past several decades, an impressive amount of knowledge on the cellular and molecular aspects of immune processes has evolved. Until recently the immune system was considered a self-regulatory network of cells and cell products which functions to maintain immunological homeostasis.

With the explosion in knowledge and techniques in the neurosciences, consideration of the integrative capacity of the CNS on a variety of biological processes has stimulated a renewed interest in the role of the CNS in relation to immune function. Converging knowledge from a variety of areas utilizing findings and techniques derived from the neurosciences and immunology provides evidence of reciprocal interactions between the CNS and immune system. These include the effect of lesions of the hypothalamus and other areas of the brain on immune responses; the presence of receptors on lymphocytes for hormones and neurotransmitters; the influence of hormones, neurotransmitters, and peptides on immune function; the effect of immune responses on hypothalamic activity; and neuroanatomical and neurochemical evidence of direct innervation of lymphoid tissue.

An association between the CNS and immune processes is further suggested by a series of studies concerned with behavioral conditioning of immune responses. A variety of stressors in animals and humans alter immunity and the effects appear to be mediated by neuroendocrine, neurotransmitter, and neurosecretory systems. The demonstration that behavioral states and perturbations of the CNS are associated with immune function suggests that alterations in immunity may be found in patients with major psychiatric disorders.

Each of the above considerations of brain and behavior and immune function will be reviewed in this chapter, including the mechanisms by which the effects of brain and behavior on the immune system are mediated. A brief overview of the immune system will be presented to provide a general understanding of

This research was supported in part by a grant from the National Institute of Mental Health (MH39651) and by the Chernow Foundation.

the various components of the immune system and of the methods utilized to measure and evaluate immune function.

IMMUNE SYSTEM

The immune system is responsible for the maintenance of the integrity of the organism in relation to foreign substances such as bacteria, viruses, and neoplasia. The immune system can be divided into two major aspects: cell-mediated immunity and humoral immunity. The basic cellular unit of both cell-mediated and humoral immunity is the lymphocyte; however, there are differences in the lymphocytes in each immune component. The T lymphocyte is primarily involved in cell-mediated immunity, and the B lymphocyte is primarily involved in humoral immunity. Both T and B lymphocytes derive from pluripotent stem cells in the bone marrow, with T cell maturation in the thymus. Several subsets of T lymphocytes have been described and include helper T cells, suppressor T cells, and cytotoxic T lymphocytes. In addition to T and B lymphocytes, a number of other cell types are involved in immune processes and include monocytes, macrophages, mast cells, and neutrophils.

In the development of an immunologic response, antigens—substances recognized as foreign—attach to lymphocytes. Each lymphocyte is committed to recognize a specific target antigen which binds to its cell-surface receptor and, thereby, stimulates the cell. B and T lymphocytes initially contain the same genetic information as every other cell in the body. Each commits itself to develop a specific receptor by genetically programmed rearrangement of the DNA sequence which encodes the receptor structure. The end result is an immune system of extensive diversity such that in humans and other animals, B and T lymphocytes can recognize 10 million different antigenic structures. When an antigen binds to the surface of a specific lymphocyte, a process of cell division and differentiation occurs which results in a permanent increase in the number of circulating lymphocytes with its particular antigen-binding specificity. This clonal expansion results in a more rapid and extensive secondary reaction upon reexposure to the antigen. A subset of the lymphocytes involved in the proliferative response are committed to terminal differentiation as effector cells. The immune system, thus, provides wide diversity accompanied by exquisite specificity.

In humoral immunity, sensitized B lymphocytes, following activation by signals from marcrophages and T helper cells, proliferate and differentiate into plasma cells, which synthesize antigen-specific antibodies. Antibodies are immunoglobulins (Ig) and include five major classes: IgG, IgM, IgA, IgE, and IgD. The immunoglobulins IgM and IgG are produced in response to a wide variety of antigens, with the production of relatively small amounts of IgM soon after antigenic stimulation, followed by large amounts of IgG. IgA is involved in the protection of external surfaces of the body and is found in mucous secretions of the gut and respiratory tract, and in colostrum and milk. IgE is the reaginic antibody that binds to mast cells and, when a specific antigen combines with IgE, the mast cells release the mediators of immediate hypersensitivity. These mediators include histamine, kinins, and slow reacting substance of anaphylaxis (leukotrienes).

The primary protective function of humoral immunity is against infections by encapsulated bacteria (for example, pneumococci, streptococci). At times, however, the response can be pathologic, such as in anaphylaxis, in asthma, and, occasionally, in response to the organism's own tissues, in an autoimmune disorder such as systemic lupus erythematosus.

In contrast to the B cell, whose role is primarily secretory, the T cell itself participates in the cell-mediated immune response. T lymphocytes passing through the tissues are sensitized to a specific antigen peripherally and then progress to a local lymph node where they enter the free areas of the cortex follicles. The T cells proliferate and are transformed into larger lymphoblasts. After several days, the T lymphocytes become immunologically active. Effector T lymphocytes mediate delayed-type hypersensitivity such as occurs in chemical contact sensitivity or in the tuberculin reaction. T cells are also involved in cytotoxicity reactions and cytotoxic lymphocytes, also known as T killer cells, are a subset of effector cells in cell mediated immunity. They recognize, bind, and lyse target cells bearing the inducing foreign antigen. In addition, T cells release lymphokines such as macrophage migration inhibitory factor (MIF), chemotactic factors, cytotoxic factors, and interferon that are involved in the destruction of antigen. Cell-mediated immune responses include protection against viral, fungal, and intracellular bacterial infection; transplantation reactions; and immune surveillance against neoplasia.

It is now recognized that the classic division of the immune system into cellular and humoral immunity is oversimplified. The immune system consists of highly fine-tuned and self-regulatory processes with T-to-T and T-to-B lymphocyte interdependence and interactions. Subsets of the T cell population, T helper and T suppressor cells, have important regulatory functions that serve to control the initiation and termination of both T and B cell effector responses. A shift in the number or function of these cell types may result in either impaired or exaggerated immune responses with consequent pathological effects.

Furthermore, it has been demonstrated that exposure to antigen is not sufficient to stimulate T cell division. Macrophages or other accessory cells are required for T cell activation and produce a lymphocyte activating factor, known as interleukin-1 (IL-1). IL-1 does not directly stimulate T cell division but induces helper T cells to produce a T cell growth factor, interleukin-2 (IL-2), and to express cell-surface receptors for IL-2. The IL-2 lymphokine then stimulates T cells to proliferate. It appears that regulation of B cell proliferation and differentiation is similar to that of T cells. A B cell growth factor produced by T cells and IL-1 appear to be required to evoke the division of activated B cells. Specific differentiation factors are then required to elicit specific antibody production. The immune system thus operates by means of highly specific responses which incorporate an amplifying component involving a complex interplay of nonspecific chemical signals for growth and differentiation. These regulatory functions may have both protective and pathologic effects on the organism.

In addition to T and B lymphocytes, a subpopulation of lymphocytes that spontaneously recognize and selectively kill some virally infected cells and cancer cells has recently been described. These cells are known as natural killer (NK) cells since they mediate a cytotoxic reaction without the need for prior sensitization.

A variety of techniques and assays are available which permit detailed evaluation and investigation of the immune system in relation to brain and behavior. Cells of the immune system can be identified by surface markers with antigenic properties. The unique surface markers for the various cell types can be detected in vitro by specific monoclonal antibodies and the number of specific cells thereby enumerated (Diamond et al, 1981). Monoclonal antibodies are available to assess the total number of T and B lymphocytes as well as T helper and T suppressor cells. Cell markers have recently become available for NK cells. The quantitation of cell types provides information about the composition of lymphocyte subpopulations in the peripheral blood but does not provide information about lymphocyte function and other aspects of the immune response, including immunoregulatory processes.

A range of functional measures are available which can be employed in the study of brain and behavior and immunity. The in vivo measurement of an antibody response to a specific antigen provides evidence of the ability to acquire specific immunity. This procedure involves exposure to a novel antigen and measurement of specific antibody production. As an experimental paradigm in humans, immunization is limited by its invasiveness, and it also cannot be utilized in longitudinal studies since a second immunization will alter the pattern of antibody response compared with that of the primary immunization. In view of these limitations, many studies investigating immunity in behavioral states have used in vitro assays of immune function.

Lymphocyte stimulation is an in vitro technique which is commonly used to assess the in vivo function and interaction of lymphocytes participating in the immune response (Keller et al, 1981a). In the procedure, sensitized lymphocytes involved in the immune response are cultured and activated with specific antigens, or nonsensitized cells are activated with nonspecific stimulants, known as mitogens. A number of plant lectins and other substances have been utilized as mitogens. Phytohemagglutinin (PHA) and concanavalin A (ConA) are predominantly T cell mitogens, and pokeweed mitogen (PWM) stimulates primarily T-dependent B lymphocytes.

When lymphocytes are stimulated, there is an increase in DNA synthesis which eventually results in cell division and proliferation. The measurement of DNA synthesis is made by labeling stimulated cultures with a radioactive nucleotide precursor which is incorporated into newly synthesized DNA. The determination of the amount of precursor incorporated provides a measure of DNA synthesis and is employed as the standard measure of lymphocyte responsiveness.

B cell function may be assessed by the determination in plasma of immunoglobulin (Ig) secreted by differentiated B lymphocytes or plasma cells. Each of the Ig classes may be readily assessed in plasma utilizing a simple precipitation reaction. Ig levels provide a global index of B cell function but do not provide information at a cellular level or about immunoregulatory mechanisms involved in B cell function. PWM-induced differentiation of human B cells in vitro can be employed to assay cellular immunoregulatory mechanisms and, in particular, the functional effects of T helper and suppressor cells on PWM activated B cell differentiation (Chrest et al, 1983).

In addition to evaluating cellular immunoregulatory mechanisms, it is now possible to assess interleukins and their receptors utilizing lymphocyte stimulation techniques (Gillis et al, 1978; Hunig et al, 1983). The availability of procedures to assess immunoregulatory processes at a cellular and chemical level provides a means to further understand brain and behavior in relation to immune function.

Natural killer cell activity is assayed in vitro by the insertion of ^{51}Cr into specific established tumor cell lines and evaluating the lysis of the tumor cells by the release of the radioisotope following the addition of NK cells (Herberman and Ortaldo, 1981).

Many of the measures described above are influenced by day-to-day variations, diurnal rhythms, sex, age, and a range of nonimmunological factors such as medication effects. Special attention and controls for confounding variables must, therefore, be carefully considered in studies of brain, behavior, and immunity. These considerations will be noted in the review of the various paradigms described in this chapter.

CENTRAL NERVOUS SYSTEM MODULATION OF IMMUNITY

Effects of the Hypothalamus on Humoral Immunity

Some of the earliest reports linking the central nervous and immune systems utilized the investigation of the effect of destructive lesions of specific areas of the brain on immune function. Systematic investigation of the relationship between the brain and immune function was initiated in a series of studies concerned with the effects of lesions on lethal anaphylaxis. Anaphylaxis is a humoral immune response related to severe allergic and asthmatic reactions in humans. In experimental models of anaphylaxis, animals are sensitized to an antigen that induces a specific antibody, usually IgE or IgG, which attaches to cells such as mast cells in the lung. On reexposure to the antigen, an immune reaction between the antigen and tissue-fixed antibody occurs. This reaction results in the release of a variety of chemical mediators from the mast cell which, in guinea pigs and in humans, induce bronchiolar obstruction, resulting in dyspnea, wheezing, asphyxiation, and death.

In 1958, Freedman and Fenichel reported that bilateral midbrain lesions in the guinea pig inhibited anaphylactic death. Following that report, attention was directed primarily to the effect of lesions of the hypothalamus on anaphylaxis. The hypothalamus is involved in the regulation of endocrine and neurotransmitter processes, and both of these systems participate in the modulation of humoral and cell-mediated immunity. Szentivanyi and Filipp (1958) were among the first to study the role of the hypothalamus in anaphylaxis. They demonstrated that lethal anaphylactic shock in the guinea pig and rabbit could be prevented by bilateral focal lesions in the tuberal region of the hypothalamus. In our initial studies we found that anterior but not posterior hypothalamic lesions inhibited the development of lethal anaphylaxis in the rat (Luparello et al, 1964). Similarly, we found that there was significant protection against lethal anaphylaxis in guinea pigs with electrolytic lesions in the anterior hypothalamus using either picryl chloride (Macris et al, 1970) or ovalbumin (Schiavi et al, 1975) as the sensitizing antigen. Median and posterior hypothalamic lesions had no significant effect on lethal anaphylaxis (Macris et al, 1970).

The effects of hypothalamic lesions on anaphylaxis could be explained both by antigen specific and nonspecific changes in the immune system, as well as by changes in tissue factors and target organ responsivity (Stein et al, 1981). Studies investigating the influence of hypothalamic lesions on antibody levels have been inconclusive (Stein et al, 1981). The variability in the reported effects of hypothalamic lesions on antibody levels may be due to the heterogeneity of the study designs. Hypothalamic lesions may affect some components of humoral immunity and only under certain conditions of sensitization and challenge. Studies have utilized different animal species, a wide range of sensitizing and test doses, variable time schedules, and different antigens. In some cases, different types of immune responses have been involved. For example, in our laboratory, anterior hypothalamic lesions in guinea pigs suppressed antibody titers to picryl chloride (Macris et al, 1970) but not to ovalbumin (Schiavi et al, 1975). These antigens differ in the lymphocytes involved in the antibody response. Antibody production to the hapten picryl chloride is dependent upon recognition by T lymphocytes which may be particularly sensitive to CNS effects, while ovalbumin sensitization appears to be T-cell independent.

Several other immune components in addition to antibody production may be involved in the effects of hypothalamic lesions on the anaphylactic reaction. The lesions may interfere with antibody binding to host tissues, or they may alter the content and release of histamine and other mediator substances. Hypothalamic lesions may also diminish the responsivity of the lung, the target organ in guinea pig anaphylaxis, to the pharmacologic agents liberated by the antigen-antibody reaction (Schiavi et al, 1966). The modification of the target organ response may be related to changes in the autonomic nervous system which is associated with anterior hypothalamic function.

In an effort to clarify some of the mechanisms which may be involved in the protective effect of anterior hypothalamic lesions, we investigated the effect of the placement of lesions following and prior to sensitization (Keller et al, 1982). Anterior hypothalamic lesions placed in guinea pigs presensitization but not postsensitization provided protection against lethal anaphylaxis. These findings suggest that the hypothalamic effect appears to be related to immune components of the analphylactic reaction. While the hypothalamus may also influence the target organ, that is, the lung, the effects are not sufficient to inhibit anaphylaxis.

Effects of the Hypothalamus on Cell Mediated Immunity

Brain lesions have also been shown to have an effect on cell-mediated immunity. In 1970, our laboratory (Macris et al, 1970) reported that anterior hypothalamic lesions in the guinea pig suppressed the delayed cutaneous hypersensitivity response to picryl chloride and to tuberculin. Median and posterior hypothalamic lesions did not alter the response. We have also found that hypothalamic lesions in the guinea pig alter in vitro lymphocyte function (Keller et al, 1980). As in our studies of humoral immunity, bilateral electrolytic lesions were placed in the anterior hypothalamus one week prior to sensitization with tuberculin. The animals with hypothalamic lesions had significantly smaller cutaneous tuberculin reactions than nonoperated or sham-operated controls. Anterior hypothalamic lesions suppressed in vitro lymphocyte stimulation by the antigen PPD and by the mitogen PHA in whole blood cultures, demonstrating that the hypothalamus can directly influence lymphocyte function. In contrast, the lesions did not alter the response of isolated lymphocytes to the antigen or to the mitogen and no differences were found in the number of lymphocytes or in B or T cell numbers among the various groups.

These findings suggest that the lesions do not impair the primary acquisition of immunity to an antigen, but rather modify the efferent limb of the cell-mediated immune system. In addition, the absence of an effect in cultures of lymphocytes isolated from other blood components suggests that the modulating effect of anterior hypothalamic lesions may be related to humoral factors or to changes in accessory cells such as macrophages, monocytes, erythrocytes, and platelets.

Cross and co-workers (Cross et al, 1980; Cross et al, 1982) have demonstrated short term effects of brain lesions on cell-mediated immune function in the rat. Animals with bilateral anterior hypothalamic lesions had lower spleen and lymphocyte numbers than controls four days following the placement of lesions, but did not differ from controls at 14 days following the procedure. The response of spleen cells to the mitogen ConA was suppressed four days after hypothalamic lesioning but not at 7 or 14 days after lesion placement. In contrast, lesions in the amygdaloid complex or hippocampus were found to increase mitogen responses. Roszman and coworkers (1982), in an effort to explain the immunologic mechanisms by which brain lesions alter immunity, investigated the role of splenic macrophage suppressor function following anterior hypothalamic lesions. Although no increase in the number of splenic macrophages occurred following the placement of lesions, macrophages from anterior hypothalamic lesioned animals had more suppressor activity than those from control rats. It thus appears that anterior hypothalamic lesions may produce qualitative changes in macrophages and, thereby, influence lymphocyte function.

Anterior hypothalamic lesions in rats also result in decreased splenic natural killer activity which returns to normal activity by 14 days following lesion placement (Cross et al, 1984). The effect of hypothalamic lesions on NK activity was not related to cytotoxic macrophages nor was the altered NK function due to macrophage suppression. Different mechanisms therefore appear to be involved in the effect of CNS perturbations on various aspects of the immune system.

MEDIATORS OF CENTRAL NERVOUS SYSTEM EFFECTS ON IMMUNE FUNCTION

Neuroendocrine and Neurotransmitter Regulation

The hypothalamus is at the interface between the brain and a range of critical regulatory peripheral mechanisms that may alter the immune response. It is rich in neurotransmitters and neurohormones and is involved in the integration of endocrine secretion, autonomic processes, and behavior. A number of studies have examined some of the mechanisms whereby the hypothalamus may alter immune, and, in particular, lymphocyte activity. There is considerable evidence that changes in endocrine activity may be related, at least in part, to the effect of hypothalamic lesions on immune function (Stein et al, 1981).

In an effort to determine whether neuroimmunomodulation is mediated solely by the neuroendocrine system, Cross and colleagues (1982) investigated lymphocyte function in brain lesioned animals prior to and following hypophysectomy. The suppression of splenic mitogenic lymphocyte stimulation in anterior hypothalamic lesioned rats was abolished by hypophysectomy, as was the increase in splenic cell reactivity following hippocampal and amygdaloid lesions. However, hypophysectomy did not alter the suppression of thymocyte mitogenic responses following hypothalamic lesions. It is of note that hypophysectomy decreased NK activity in both intact and hypothalamic lesioned animals (Cross et al, 1984). Taken together, these findings suggest that some alterations in immunity following lesions of the brain involve an intact endocrine system and that multiple mechanisms appear to be involved in the CNS modulation of immune function.

There is considerable experimental evidence in support of the concept that neurotransmitters are involved in the modulation of immune function (Hall and Goldstein, 1985). The demonstration of receptors for neurotransmitters on the surface membranes of lymphocytes (Williams et al, 1976; Hohlfield et al, 1984) are in keeping with the possibility that neurotransmitters play a major role in the regulation of immunity. It has been shown that pharmacologic manipulation of norepinephrine in postganglionic sympathetic nerve fibers innervating lymphoid tissue results in alterations in immune function (Felten et al, 1985). It has also been demonstrated that serotonin has enhancing and inhibitory effects on immunity (Jackson et al, 1984).

Most of the research concerned with neurotransmitter regulation of immune function has involved peripheral or systemic manipulation of lymphoid tissues and has not investigated the effect of central neurotransmitter processes on immune reactivity. Recently, Cross and colleagues (1986) have shown that humoral immune responsiveness is impaired by the injection of 6-hydroxydopamine (6-OHDA) into the cisterna magna. 6-OHDA significantly reduced norepinephrine in the hypothalamus, midbrain, and pons-medulla. The treatment with 6-OHDA decreased the primary antibody response to sheep red blood cells and also impaired the development of immunological memory. If 6-OHDA was administered prior to immunization, it did not have an effect on the antibody response. These findings suggest that norepinephrine may play a role in the modulation of the afferent limb of the immune response and provide further evidence for CNS influences on immune function.

Direct Noradrenergic Innervation of Lymphoid Tissue

Considerable evidence has accumulated demonstrating direct autonomic innervation of parenchymal lymphoid tissue in the spleen, lymph nodes, thymus, appendix, and bone marrow (Felten et al, 1985; Bulloch and Pomerantz, 1984). Noradrenergic fibers innervate both the vasculature and parenchyma in lymphoid organs. This structural link between the nervous and immune systems provides another possible route for the neuromodulation of immunity. The effect may be related to catecholamine neurotransmitters altering blood flow and regulating humoral factors entering lymphoid tissue. Direct interaction on lymphocytes is also possible in view of the availability of noradrenergic and peptide receptors on the cell-surface of lymphocytes and could, thus, have a direct effect on lymphocyte function. Further in vitro and in vivo studies are required to investigate the effects of neurotransmitters on lymphoid tissue; however, the demonstration of direct sympathetic innervation of lymphoid tissue supports the concept of CNS modulation of immunity.

CONDITIONING OF IMMUNE PROCESSES

An association between the CNS and immune processes is further suggested by a series of studies concerned with behavioral conditioning of immune responses. This research is of considerable importance in that it considers a behavioral effect involving higher cortical function. Studies from Eastern Europe over the past 50 years based on Pavlovian concepts have attempted to condition a variety of immune responses with variable results (Ader, 1981). Ader and co-workers (Ader and Cohen, 1975) pursued the investigation of conditioning effects on the immune system and demonstrated that antibody responses can be suppressed by conditioned stimuli that had been paired previously with a pharmacologic immunosuppressant. The paradigm employed used taste aversion learning, a passive avoidance paradigm in which saccharin (the conditioned stimulus) was paired with cyclophosphamide, an immunosuppressive agent (the unconditioned stimulus). Three days after the conditioning procedure, which can be accomplished by a single pairing of the conditioned stimulus and unconditioned stimulus, the animals were immunized with sheep red blood cells (SRBC) and then exposed to the CS, US, or placebo. Six days later, hemagglutinating antibodies to SRBC were measured and were found to be significantly lower in the conditioned animals than in controls, although not as low as in animals injected with cyclophosphamide. These findings have been replicated by Rogers and co-workers (Rogers et al, 1976) and by Wayner and colleagues (Wayner et al, 1978).

Since the humoral immune response to SRBC involves T-helper cell function, Ader and co-workers undertook a study to determine whether B-cell function is subject to conditioning effects independent of effects on T cells (Cohen et al, 1979). Using the saccharin/cyclophosphamide conditioning paradigm, they found that the antibody response to the T-cell-independent antigen TNP-LPS was attenuated by exposure to the conditioned stimulus, although the findings were less consistent than those obtained with SRBC in rats. Since Wayner and associates (1978) found no significant conditioning effect in rats on the response to Brucella, a T-cell-independent antigen, further investigation of conditioning effects on the B cell is required.

Two other models of immune responsivity have also been found to be subject to conditioning effects. The graft versus host response, a function of cellular immunity, was found to be lower in conditioned rats than in controls (Bovbjerg et al, 1982). This response was assessed by measuring the size of draining lymph nodes after injection of splenic leukocytes from donor rats. Ader and Cohen (1982) also have reported conditioning effects in relation to cyclophosphamide induced suppression of autoimmune glomerulonephritis in mice, an animal model of systemic lupus erythematosus. Both proteinuria and mortality were significantly reduced by conditioning.

Smith and McDaniel (1983) reported an experiment suggesting that cell-mediated immune responses in humans may be subject to conditioning effects. Subjects were skin tested with tuberculin monthly, with antigen placed on one arm and saline on the other. At the sixth trial, however, the placement of tuberculin and saline was reversed without the knowledge of the subject or of the nurse who applied the antigen. A markedly diminished or absent delayed cutaneous response was found for the tuberculin placed on the arm where saline was expected. When the subjects were then informed of the identity of the test substances and the tuberculin again applied to the "saline" arm, a brisk response comparable to that of the first five trials was obtained. These findings may represent conditioning effects in which the skin testing protocol was the conditioned stimulus and the tuberculin response the unconditioned stimulus. Alternatively, as suggested by the investigators, the effects may have been related to the subjects' cognitive state of expectation unrelated to conditioning effects per se. Black and associates (1963), for example, reported inhibition of the tuberculin reaction by hypnotic suggestion. According to either hypothesis, the data demonstrate an association between higher cortical function and an immune response.

STRESS AND IMMUNE FUNCTION

Stress and Humoral and Cell-Mediated Responses

A variety of stressors have been found to alter humoral and cell-mediated immunity. These studies have been described in detail elsewhere (Stein et al, 1985b) and only a brief review will be presented to highlight some of the experimental issues involved in this area of investigation. Early studies of stress and humoral immunity indicated that avoidance learning stress decreases the susceptibility of mice to passive anaphylaxis (Rasmussen et al, 1959) and that the production of specific antibody was suppressed in a variety of species by distressing environmental stimuli such as noise, light, movement, or housing condition (Petrovskii, 1961; Hill et al, 1967; Vessey, 1964). Both primary and secondary antibody responses were suppressed by the stressors (Solomon, 1969). In contrast, exposure to other stressors such as repeated low voltage electric shock enhanced antibody responses (Solomon, 1969; Hirata-Hibi, 1967).

A number of studies have tended to support the observation that while acute exposure to a stressor may suppress humoral immune responses, repeated exposure may result in an enhanced immunologic response. For example, restraint or crowding, presented in a single session of varying lengths, induced suppression of antibody responses; but after three days of repeated presentation of the stimulus, the response returned to prestress levels (Gisler, 1974). Exposure of mice to sound stress for up to 20 days suppressed the response of splenic lymphocytes to the B cell mitogen lipopolysaccharide (LPS), but more extended exposure resulted in an enhanced response (Monjan and Collector, 1977). The complexity of stress effects on humoral immunity are further highlighted by a study which found differing effects on antibody responses for different stressors in rats depending upon the sex of the animal (Joasoo and McKenzie, 1976). These studies suggest that the effect of stress on the humoral immune system is related to the nature and intensity of the stimulus as well as to biological and social characteristics of the organism.

Stress has also been found to alter cell mediated immune processes. Monjan and Collector (1977) studied the effect of sound stress on the response of murine splenic lymphocytes to ConA. Parallel to their findings with the B cell mitogen LPS, they found suppression of the response following short-term exposure to the stressor and enhancement with extended exposure. Reite and co-workers (1981) have studied separation experiences in primates and found decreased T cell mitogen responses following peer separation for two weeks in pigtailed monkeys raised together from early infancy. Mitogen responses returned to baseline within several weeks of reunion. Studies from our laboratory (Keller et al, 1981b) have demonstrated a relationship between the intensity of an acute stressor and the degree of suppression of T lymphocyte function in rats. A graded series of stressors, applied over 18 hours, including restraint in an apparatus, low level electric tail shock, and high level shock, produced a progressively greater suppression of both the number of circulating lymphocytes and of PHA stimulation of peripheral blood lymphocytes.

Laudenslager and co-workers (1983) found that PHA and ConA stimulation of lymphocytes were suppressed in rats exposed to inescapable, uncontrollable electric tail shock for 80 minutes followed by several minutes of tail shock 24 hours later. However, animals receiving the same total amount of shock, using a yoked paradigm, but able to terminate the stressor, did not have decreased lymphocyte activity compared with nonstressed controls. These findings are consistent with hypotheses suggesting that the ability to cope with a stressor protects against its noxious effects.

Bereavement and Lymphocyte Function

Conjugal bereavement is among the most potentially stressful of commonly occurring life events and has been associated with increased medical mortality (Helsing et al, 1981). A link between bereavement and altered immunity was suggested by the report of Bartrop and co-workers (1977) who found that a group of bereaved individuals had decreased lymphocyte function compared with controls.

We have investigated the effect of bereavement on immunity in a prospective longitudinal study of spouses of women with advanced breast carcinoma (Schleifer et al, 1983). Lymphocyte stimulation was measured in 15 men before and after the death of their wives. Lymphocyte stimulation responses to the mitogens PHA, ConA, and PWM were significantly lower during the first two months postbereavement compared with prebereavement responses. The number of peripheral blood lymphocytes and the percentage and absolute number of T and B cells during the prebereavement period were not significantly different from the postbereavement period. Follow-up during the remainder of the postbereavement year revealed that lymphocyte stimulation responses had returned to prebereavement levels for the majority but not all of the subjects. Moreover, prebereavement mitogen responses did not differ from those of age- and sex-matched controls. These findings demonstrate that suppression of mitogen induced lymphocyte stimulation is a direct consequence of the bereavement event, and that a preexisting suppressed immune state does not account for the depressed lymphocyte responses in the bereaved. Furthermore, the long-term stress of the spouse's illness does not appear to result in a habituation of lymphocyte stress responses following bereavement. The long-term stress may, in fact, have sensitized the subject to the effects of bereavement.

The effects of bereavement on lymphocyte function in our sample, however, were not homogenous. A small subset of subjects did not have lowered mitogen responses at one to two months postbereavement, but tended to have decreased levels when restudied during the latter half of the postbereavement year. It is of note that these subjects were younger than the majority of the sample who had lowered responses immediately following the death of a spouse and a return to prebereavement levels after a number of months. The variability in altered mitogen responsivity is further reflected in the patterns of response to the three mitogens among individual subjects. Some subjects had a greater than 50 percent pre- to postbereavement decrease for PHA, ConA, and PWM, whereas others had an approximately 20 percent decrease in response to PHA, 35 percent decrease to ConA, and more than 50 percent decrease to PWM. It may well be that these patterns of response are specific for each individual. Further systematic investigation of the variability in immune changes associated with bereavement is required, including consideration of age, biologic predisposition, personality, and change in life-style and behavior related to bereavement, as well as consideration of the stability of the measures employed.

It is important to emphasize that the immune findings associated with bereavement do not adequately explain the epidemiologic findings of increased morbidity and mortality following bereavement. It remains to be determined whether stress induced immune changes such as decreased mitogen responses are related to the onset or course of physical illness following life stress (Schleifer et al, 1984b).

The processes linking the experience of bereavement with effects on lymphocyte activity are complex and require further investigation. Changes in nutrition, activity, exercise levels, sleep, and drug use, which are often found in the widowed, could influence lymphocyte function (Schleifer et al, 1983). Our subjects, however, did not report major or persistent changes in diet or activity levels or changes in the use of medication, alcohol, tobacco, or other drugs, and no significant changes in weight were noted. Further study is required to determine whether subtle changes on these variables are related to the effects of bereavement on lymphocyte function.

The effects of death of spouse on lymphocyte function could result from centrally mediated stress effects. Stressful life experiences may be related to changes in CNS activity associated with psychological states such as depression. Bereaved subjects have been characteristically described as manifesting depressed mood (Clayton et al, 1972; Parkes, 1972) and a subgroup of bereaved individuals has been reported to have symptom patterns consistent with the presence of a major depressive disorder (Clayton et al, 1972). There is now evidence, as described in another section of this chapter, for similar alterations in lymphocyte function in patients with depressive disorders.

Mediation of Stress Effects on Immune Function

A variety of biological factors may be involved in mediating the association among the brain, behavioral states, and the immune system. The endocrine system is highly responsive to both life experiences and psychological state, and has a significant although complicated effect on immune processes. The most widely studied hormones are those of the hypothalamic-pituitary-adrenal (HPA) axis. A wide range of stressful experiences are capable of inducing the release of corticosteroids (Rose, 1984) and corticosteroids have extensive and complex effects on the immune system. Of particular interest is the demonstration that glucocorticosteroids can suppress mitogen induced lymphocyte stimulation (Cupps and Fauci, 1982) and induce a redistribution of T cells and of T-helper cells from the circulating pool to the bone marrow (Claman, 1972; Cupps et al, 1984). Several reports have demonstrated that the recirculating lymphocyte traffic in humans is sensitive to endogenous corticosteroids and varies in relation to endogenous cortisol levels (Thomson et al, 1980; Abo et al, 1981) as does the response to PHA stimulation (Abo et al, 1981; Tavadia et al, 1975).

Secretion of corticosteroids has long been considered to be the mechanism of stress induced modulation of immunity and related disease processes (Riley, 1981; Selye, 1976). The regulation of immune function in response to stress, however, may not be limited to corticosteroids. As previously noted, we have shown in rats that unpredictable, unavoidable electric tail shock suppressed immune function as measured by the number of circulating lymphocytes and PHA stimulation (Keller et al, 1981b). In an effort to determine whether the adrenal is required for stress induced suppression of lymphocyte function in the rat, we investigated the effect of stressors in adrenalectomized animals (Keller et al, 1983). Four groups of rats were studied, including nonoperated, adrenalectomized, sham adrenalectomized, and adrenalectomized animals with a corticosterone pellet. Four behavioral conditions, identical to those used in our previous study, were used: home-cage control, apparatus control, low-shock, and high-shock animals. There was a progressive increase in corticosterone with increasing stress in both of the groups with adrenals; no corticosterone was detected in the adrenalectomized group; and the concentration of corticosterone in the adrenalectomized group that received the corticosterone pellets was constant. A progressive stress induced lymphopenia was found in the nonoperated and sham-operated groups, but no stress related changes in lymphocyte number were found in the adrenalectomized groups. In contrast, adrenalectomy did not prevent the stress induced suppression of lymphocyte stimulation by PHA, demonstrating that stress related adrenal secretion of corticosteroids and catecholamines is not required for the stress induced suppression of lymphocyte stimulation in the rat.

Our findings of adrenal dependent stress induced lymphopenia but of adrenal independent effects on lymphocyte stimulation indicate that stress induced modulation of immunity is a complex phenomenon involving several, if not multiple, mechanisms. Changes in the levels of thyroid hormones, growth hormones, and sex steroids have been associated with exposure to stressors (Rose, 1984), and each of these hormonal systems has been reported to modulate immune function (Fabris, 1973; Grossman, 1985; Snow, 1985). An immunoregulatory role has also been suggested for a variety of stress related peptides such as B-endorphin (Gilman et al, 1982; Shavit et al, 1984).

Neuroendocrine- and neurotransmitter-mediated CNS effects on immune function may result, in part, from changes in lymphocyte receptors. As described in the next section, major depressive disorder has been associated with altered lymphocyte function as well as HPA-axis dysregulation. Lowy and co-workers (1984) have investigated the in vitro effects of corticosteroids on lymphocyte cultures from depressed patients with varying levels of HPA dysregulation. They found that mitogen induced lymphocyte stimulation in dexamethasone suppression test (DST) positive subjects was less sensitive to corticosteroid induced suppression in vitro than were mitogen responses in DST negative subjects. The findings were consistent with down-regulation of corticosteroid receptors in DST positive subjects that resulted in decreased lymphocyte sensitivity to corticosteroids. The findings are also of interest in showing parallel responses for corticosteroid receptors in neuronal and immune tissues. This, and related observations in other receptor systems—for example, beta-adrenergic (Mann et al, 1985)—are of both theoretical and practical importance in the understanding of neural and immune functions and their interaction. For example, functional lymphocyte assays may be useful as test systems for investigating receptor activity relevant to neural processes in general. The specific findings concerned with receptor down-regulation in depression may also provide a model for the differential effects of acute and chronic stress on lymphocyte function.

IMMUNE–CENTRAL NERVOUS SYSTEM FEEDBACK

Recently, a series of observations has suggested that the relationship of the CNS and the neuroendocrine system with the immune system is not unidirectional, and that immune processes can modulate CNS function and neuroendocrine activity. In 1975, Besedovsky and co-workers found that rats with a primary immune response to sheep red blood cells had increased levels of corticosterone and decreased levels of thyroxine in temporal relationship with the development of the antibody response. These findings suggest that the primary immune response can influence the neuroendocrine system, perhaps by means of effects on the CNS. In further studies, Besedovsky and co-workers found an increase in the firing rate of neurons in the ventromedial nucleus of the hypothalamus during the course of an immune response in rats (Besedovsky and Sorkin, 1977) as well as altered hypothalamic noradrenergic activity (Besedovsky et al, 1983) concurrent with the immunization process. Others (Dafny et al, 1985) have shown that alpha interferon (IFN) applied microiontophoretically into the rat brain increased the firing of neurons of the cortex and hippocampus in a dose related manner, while in the ventromedial hypothalamus low doses of interferon tended to suppress firing while high doses enhanced the firing rate. In contrast, IFN did not alter the activity of thalamic neurons, and gamma IFN had no effect on any of the neuronal systems. These results suggest the presence of a feedback loop between specific components of the immune response and specific structures in the CNS. Besedovsky and co-workers (1985) recently demonstrated a possible mechanism of immune-neuroendocrine feedback. They found that mitogen-stimulated lymphocytes produce a factor which increases glucocorticoid levels by pituitary processes.

Another area of research has suggested that the immune system may also influence neuroendocrine activity by mechanisms not involving the classical hypothalamic-pituitary axis. Blalock and co-workers reported that lymphocytes can secrete an ACTH-like substance following viral infection (Smith et al, 1982). Hypophysectomized mice infected with Newcastle disease virus had increased corticosterone and IFN production. Furthermore, splenic cells from infected animals showed positive immunofluorescence with antibodies to ACTH, suggesting that the lymphocytes were secreting an ACTH-like substance along with the lymphokine, IFN. The viral induced increase in corticosterone but not IFN was blocked by dexamethasone.

It has also recently been shown, utilizing molecular cloning techniques, that mitogen activation of T-helper cells of mice induces the preproenkephalin gene in T cells (Zurawski et al, 1986). The production of a peptide neurotransmitter from activated T cells may provide a means by which T cells may be involved in the modulation of the CNS. Furthermore, the neurohypophyseal peptides, oxytocin and neurophysin, have been identified in human thymus, providing additional support for the notion of integrated neuroendocrine functions and immune processes (Geenen et al, 1986). These findings, taken together, suggest a regulatory feedback system involving the CNS, the neuroendocrine system, and the immune system.

IMMUNITY AND PSYCHIATRIC DISORDERS

The demonstration that the CNS and behavioral states can modulate immune function suggests that immune alterations might be found in patients with major psychiatric disorders, and that immune processes may be involved in the etiology and course of psychiatric illness. As early as 1930, Damashek (1930) noted abnormal leukocytes in the peripheral blood of patients with psychiatric disorders.

Depression and Altered Immunity

Several studies have assessed immunity in clinically depressed individuals. The frequency of antinuclear antibodies, which may reflect auto-immune processes, has been reported to be increased in patients with depression (von Brauchitsch, 1972; Deberdt et al, 1976; Johnstone and Whaley, 1975; Shopsin et al, 1973). More recently, investigators have begun to evaluate general measures of lymphocyte function in depression. Cappel and colleagues (1978) reported that lymphocyte stimulation responses to PHA were lower in a group of psychotically depressed patients during the acute phase of their illness than following clinical remission. PHA responses in the depressed group did not differ, however, from those of control subjects at either time, making interpretation of the findings difficult. Kronfol and co-workers (1983) reported that melancholic patients had lower lymphocyte responses to PHA, ConA, and PWM than groups of non-melancholic psychiatric patients and normal controls.

We have studied immune function in drug free hospitalized depressed patients (Schleifer et al, 1984a). The hospitalized patients were found to have a significantly decreased total number of lymphocytes and of T and B cells and decreased lymphocyte responses to the mitogens PHA, ConA, and PWM compared with age- and sex-matched controls. The findings demonstrated that the functional activity of the lymphocyte, as well as the number of circulating immunocompetent cells, are decreased in individuals hospitalized with major depressive disorder.

In order to determine whether altered immunity is associated specifically with depression and not related to hospital effects or nonspecifically to other psychiatric disorders, we investigated lymphocyte function in ambulatory patients with major depressive disorder and in patients hospitalized with schizophrenic disorders (Schleifer et al, 1985b). Lymphocyte stimulation responses were similar for the depressed outpatients and controls, suggesting that our findings of suppressed lymphocyte responses in hospitalized depressives may be related to hospitalization or to severity of the depression. A group of hospitalized schizophrenic patients was, therefore, studied, and we found no differences between the hospitalized schizophrenics and their controls on any of the lymphocyte measures. It is possible, however, that schizophrenic inpatients may have atypical responses to hospitalization. The effect of hospitalization on lymphocyte function was, therefore, also studied in a group of otherwise healthy patients admitted for elective herniorrhaphy, and no significant differences were found between the herniorrhaphy patients and matched controls (Schleifer et al, 1985b).

The decreased mitogen responses in hospitalized but not in ambulatory depressed patients suggests that altered immunity in depression may be related to the severity of depressive symptomatology. The hospitalized patients in our study were also older than the ambulatory depressives, and the sex distribution of the groups differed. Variables such as age and sex have been shown to be related to severity and other clinical aspects of depression, as well as to a range of biological changes associated with major depressive disorder.

In order to clarify further the association between depression and altered immunity, we recently investigated the effects of age, sex, and severity of depression on immune function in a not previously studied sample of 61 patients with major depressive disorder, unipolar subtype, compared with matched controls (Schleifer et al, 1985a). Analysis of partial variance, a special case of hierarchical multiple regression/correlation analysis, was used to analyze the effects of age, sex, severity, and hospitalization on the immune measures. This analysis also permitted statistical control for day-to-day variability in the lymphocyte assays.

We found that differences in mitogen responses between depressed patients and controls were related to age and severity of depression but not to sex or hospitalization. Controls had significant increases in lymphocyte responses to ConA, PHA, and PWM with advancing age. In contrast, patients with major depressive disorder had a significant negative correlation (ConA) or no significant relationship (PHA and PWM) between age and mitogen stimulation responses. These differential age related lymphocyte responses of controls and depressed patients were significantly different for all of the mitogens studied. We also found a significant positive correlation between the number of T-helper lymphocytes and age for controls, but no age effect on T-helper cells for the depressed patients. The relationship between the number of T-helper cells and age was significantly different for controls and depressed patients. In contrast, no age effects on T-suppressor cells were found. The differential effect of age on mitogen stimulation responses in depressed patients and controls may therefore be related to the alterations in immunoregulatory T lymphocyte subpopulations.

The age related changes in lymphocyte function in depression may be due to common underlying or interacting neurobiologic mechanisms, such as central noradrenergic processes associated with aging and depression, which may result in age-related dysregulation of immune function in major depressive disorder. Dysregulation of neurobiological and immune processes in depression may be due to genetic vulnerability in either or both biological systems, and to the effect of environmental stimuli. It must be determined whether age related alterations in immunity are specific for the state of depression or whether they persist into remission and may be trait markers.

Altered immunity appears to be a component of the complex psychobiology of affective disorders. Further studies of immunity in major depressive disorder may help to elucidate the pathophysiology of depressive states manifested in patterns of dysregulation of neuroendocrine, neurotransmitter, and immune systems.

Schizophrenia and Altered Immunity

The possibility that schizophrenia is associated with altered immunity has stimulated considerable interest for a number of years. The morphology of peripheral blood lymphocytes has been reported to be abnormal among patients with schizophrenia. Fessel and co-workers (Fessel and Hirata-Hibi, 1963; Fessel et al, 1965) showed an increased prevalence of abnormal leukocytes in both acute and chronic schizophrenic patients as well as in the family members of patients with chronic schizophrenia. These changes were found to be independent of neuroleptic medication.

With the development of immunologic techniques, a series of studies have investigated lymphocyte numbers and function in patients with schizophrenia. Suppressed mitogen responses have been reported in schizophrenic patients who were not drug free (Babayan et al, 1976; Vartanian et al, 1978); however, neuroleptics have been shown to suppress mitogen responses (Baker et al, 1977; Ferguson et al, 1978). A variety of inconsistently demonstrated changes have been reported in the percentage or numbers of T and B cells among schizophrenic patients (Vartanian et al, 1978; Coffey et al, 1983; DeLisi et al, 1982; Nyland et al, 1980; Zarrabi et al, 1979). Much of this variation may also have been related to the use of neuroleptics in the large majority of patients studied or to the lack of healthy age- and sex-matched controls. As previously noted, we have found no differences between hospitalized drug free patients with schizophrenia and age- and sex-matched controls in the mitogen stimulation responses or total numbers of lymphocytes (Schleifer et al, 1985b), suggesting that altered lymphocyte function or numbers are not intrinsic to schizophrenia.

A number of investigators have considered aspects of humoral immune function in schizophrenia, and the possibility has been raised that schizophrenia is an autoimmune disorder of the CNS. Amkraut and associates (1973) compared drug free acute schizophrenics with normal controls and found increased levels of IgM, IgA, and IgG in the patients. In addition, the schizophrenic patients with lower IgA and IgM levels showed significantly greater clinical improvement during the course of hospitalization. Other investigators have also reported increased immunoglobulin levels in schizophrenic patients (Strahilivetz and Davis, 1970), but some studies have shown decreased levels of IgM (Bock et al, 1970) or IgA (Domino et al, 1975), and others found no difference between schizophrenic and control groups (Bishop et al, 1966). A variety of factors could account for these discrepancies, including differences among the various study samples with regard to clinical characteristics, chronicity of illness, intercurrent illness, and pharmacologic treatment. For example, Fontana and co-workers (1980) found that medicated hospitalized schizophrenic patients had higher IgM and IgG levels when compared with blood donor controls but not when compared with hospitalized medical patients. It should also be noted that Ig levels are relatively nonspecific measures of immunity and subject to factors that alter serum proteins in general. More specific measures of B-cell function are now available to investigate humoral immunity in schizophrenia.

The hypothesis has been advanced that abnormal proteins and autoimmune antibodies contribute to the pathogenesis of schizophrenia (Heath et al, 1957; Knight, 1982). Heath and colleagues (1957) reported the presence of an abnormal Ig in the serum of patients with schizophrenia that was found to react with various regions of the brain. Using fluorescent antibody techniques, Heath and Krupp (1967) demonstrated antibodies bound to specific brain areas in 12 of 14 schizophrenic patients and in none of a control group. Baron and associates (1977) reported similar findings, indicating that schizophrenic patients tend to have higher levels of a serum globulin with a high affinity for the septal region of human brain, and Bergen and co-workers (1980) partially replicated Heath's reports of the ability of injected IgG fractions from schizophrenic patients to alter brain function in monkeys (Heath et al, 1967). Other groups, however, have been unable to replicate Heath's initial findings (Siegal et al, 1959).

Kuritzky and co-workers (1976) presented other data supporting the presence of auto-immunity directed against the CNS in some patients with schizophrenia. They reported an increased cell-mediated immune response to human myelin basic protein in chronic but not acute schizophrenia. Other Soviet workers (Vartanian et al, 1978; Luriya et al, 1974) have found that the sera of patients with schizophrenia contained antibodies against thymic antigens located on thymocytes and on T lymphocytes. Watanabe and co-workers (1982) reported similar findings and provided some evidence that neuroleptic medication was not solely responsible for these effects. In contrast to these studies, a number of authors have been unable to demonstrate excessive auto-immune related proteins, antibrain antibodies, or other auto-antibodies in schizophrenia (Fontana et al, 1980; Logan and Deodhar, 1970; Boehme et al, 1973; Mellsop et al, 1978).

In summary, although a number of investigators have found evidence suggestive of altered immunity and of autoimmunity in patients with schizophrenia, the specific findings have been difficult to replicate. Whether immune abnormalities are involved in the pathogenesis of some or all types of schizophrenia, or whether such changes are related to factors such as chronic institutionalization or neuroleptic treatment, remains to be determined.

Other Psychiatric Disorders and Immune Function

Little is known about immune function in patients with other psychiatric disorders, although there have been reports concerning immunity in Alzheimer's disease (Cohen and Eisdorfer, 1980) and Down's syndrome (Wisniewski et al, 1979), which will not be reviewed here. One study of autistic children (Weizman et al, 1982) found evidence of cell-mediated immune function directed against human myelin basic protein in 11 of 17 autistic children, but in none of a group of controls that included patients diagnosed with childhood schizophrenia. Although most of the autistic and control patients were not drug free, the investigators presented evidence suggesting that the observed effects were not due to medication. Further studies are required to elucidate these findings.

CONCLUSION

This chapter has reviewed knowledge and techniques derived from the neurosciences and immunobiology which further our understanding of the relationship between brain and behavior and immunity. An extensive network of CNS processes are involved in the modulation of the immune system in response to psychological phenomena which, in turn, may alter the development, onset, and course of a range of illnesses. The investigation of specific alterations in the immune system of patients suffering with psychiatric disorders and their behavioral and neurobiological correlates may provide a biologic basis for the identification of risk factors and for the ultimate development of intervention strategies.

The clinical application at this time of laboratory measures of immunity to psychiatric disorders for diagnostic purposes is premature. Clinically meaningful measures of the immune system in relation to disorders of immunity are usually at such variance with normal measures that reference values are not required. This, however, is not the case for the laboratory measurement of immunity in psychiatric disorders in which biologically and statistically significant alterations of immunity have been found, but extreme values have not been observed. Reference values for a variety of measures of immunity have not been established for psychiatric illnesses and may vary with determinations made in different laboratory settings as well as in psychiatric patients treated with psychopharmacologic agents or suffering with concomitant medical illnesses. Furthermore, laboratory values for different ages and for men and women must be developed in view of age- and sex-related alterations in immunity reported in psychiatric disorders.

Immune dysfunction in psychiatric illnesses may be associated with an isolated perturbation of the immune system such as of a lymphocyte subpopulation, e.g. T-helper cells, or may be related to multiple changes in immune function which interact to yield complex alterations in immune processes. As pointed out in this chapter, further research is required to identify appropriate immune measures related to specific psychiatric disorders and multiple measures of immunity may be required. This would include measurement of the numbers of lymphocyte subpopulations as well as specific measures of lymphocyte function and other indices of immunity.

Major psychiatric syndromes, such as affective disorders and schizophrenia, appear to be etiologically heterogeneous. Measures of immunity may be useful in the future in the identification of etiologically homogeneous subgroups.

New approaches utilizing cellular and molecular techniques derived from advances in immunobiology, genetics, and the neurosciences will further clarify the reciprocal interaction between the CNS and immune system and may provide fundamental knowledge about the impact of hereditary and environmental influences in psychiatric disorders. The application of cellular and molecular techniques to the investigation of CNS and immune processes will also help provide basic knowledge in immunobiology and neurobiology.

REFERENCES

Abo T, Kawate T, Ito K, et al: Studies on the bioperiodicity of the immune response, I: circadian rhythms of human T, B, and K cell traffic in the peripheral blood. J Immunol 126:1360-1363, 1981

Ader R: A historical account of conditioned immunobiologic responses, in Psychoneuroimmunology. Edited by Ader R. New York, Academic Press, 1981

Ader R, Cohen N: Behaviorally conditioned immunosuppression. Psychosom Med 37:333-340, 1975

Ader R, Cohen N: Behaviorally conditioned immunosuppression and murine systemic lupus erythematosus. Science 215:1534-1536, 1982

Amkraut AA, Solomon GF, Allansmith M, et al: Immunoglobulins and improvement in acute schizophrenic reactions. Arch Gen Psychiatry 28:673-677, 1973

Babayan NG, Sekoyan RV, Prilipko LL: Effect of blood serum from schizophrenics and healthy donors on DNA synthesis in lymphocytes. Exp Biol Med 81:527, 1976

Baker AG, Santalo R, Blumenstein J: Effect of psychotropic agents upon the blastogenic response of human T lymphocytes. Biol Psychiatry 12:159-168, 1977

Baron M, Stern M, Anavi R, et al: Tissue-binding factor in schizophrenic sera: a clinical and genetic study. Biol Psychiatry 12:199-219, 1977

Bartrop RW, Lazarus L, Luckherst E, et al: Depressed lymphocyte function after bereavement. Lancet 1:834-836, 1977

Bergen JR, Grinspoon L, Pyle HM, et al: Immunologic studies in schizophrenic and control subjects. Biol Psychiatry 15:369-379, 1980

Besedovsky H, Sorkin E: Network of immune-neuroendocrine interactions. Clin Exp Immunol 27:1-12, 1977

Besedovsky H, Sorkin E, Keller M, et al: Changes in blood hormone levels during the immune response. Proc Soc Exp Biol Med 150:466, 1975

Besedovsky H, del Ray A, Sorkin E, et al: The immune response evokes changes in brain noradrenergic neurons. Science 221:564-566, 1983

Besedovsky H, del Ray A, Sorkin E, et al: Lymphoid cells produce an immunoregulatory glucocorticoid increasing factor (GIF) acting through the pituitary gland. Clin Exp Immunol 59:622-628, 1985

Bishop MP, Hollister LE, Gallant BM, et al: Ultracentrifugal serum proteins in schizophrenia. Arch Gen Psychiatry 15:337-340, 1966

Black S, Humphrey JH, Niven JS: Inhibition of Mantoux reaction by direct suggestion under hypnosis. Br Med J 1:1649-1652, 1963

Bock E, Weeke B, Rafaelsen OJ: Immunoglobulins in schizophrenic patients. Lancet 2:523, 1970

Boehme DM, Cattrell JC, Dohan FC, et al: Fluorescent antibody studies of immunoglobulin binding by brain tissues. Arch Gen Psychiatry 28:202, 1973

Bovbjerg D, Ader R, Cohen N: Behaviorally conditioned suppression of a graft-versus-host response. Proc Natl Acad Sci USA 79:583-585, 1982

Bulloch K, Moore RY: Autonomic nervous system innervation of thymic-related lymphoid tissue in wild-type and nude mice. J Comp Neurol 228:57, 1984

Bulloch K, Pomerantz W: Autonomic nervous system innervation of thymic-related lymphoid tissue in wild-type and nude mice. J Comp Neurol 228:57, 1984

Cappel R, Gregoire F, Thiry L, et al: Antibody and cell mediated immunity to herpes simplex virus in psychotic depression. J Clin Psychiatry 39:266-268, 1978

Chrest FJ, Nagel JE, Pyle RS, et al: Human B cell function in responder and non-responder individuals, II: the role of T helper cells in promoting the PWM-induced B cell production of immunoprotein. Clin Exp Immunol 53:465-472, 1983

Claman HN: Corticosteroids and lymphoid cells. N Engl J Med 287:388-397, 1972

Clayton PJ, Halikes JA, Maurice WL: The depression of widowhood. Br J Psychiatry 120:71-78, 1972

Coffey CE, Sullivan JL, Rice JR: T lymphocytes in schizophrenia. Biol Psychiatry 18:113-119, 1983

Cohen D, Eisdorfer C: Serum immunoglobulins and cognitive status in the elderly: a population study. Br J Psychiatry 136:33-39, 1980

Cohen N, Ader R, Green N, et al: Conditioned suppression of a thymus independent antibody response. Psychosom Med 41:487-491, 1979

Cross RJ, Markesbery WR, Brooks WH, et al: Hypothalamic-immune interactions: the acute effect of anterior hypothalamic lesions on the immune response. Brain Res 196:79-87, 1980

Cross RJ, Brooks WH, Roszman TL, et al: Hypothalamic-immune interactions. Effect of hypophysectomy on neuroimmunomodulation. J Neurol Sci 53:557-566, 1982

Cross RJ, Markesbery WR, Brooks WH, et al: Hypothalamic-immune interactions. Neuromodulation of natural killer activity by lesioning of the anterior hypothalamus. Immunology 51:399-405, 1984

Cross RJ, Jackson JC, Brooks WH, et al: Neuroimmunomodulation: impairment of humoral immune responsiveness by 6-hydroxydopamine treatment. Immunology 57:145-152, 1986

Cupps TR, Fauci AS: Corticosteroid-mediated immunoregulation in man. Immunol Rev 65:134-155, 1982

Cupps TR, Edgar LC, Thomas CA, et al: Multiple mechanisms of B cell immunoregulation in man after administration of in vivo corticosteroids. J Immunol 132:170-175, 1984

Dafny N, Prieto-Gomez B, Reyes-Vazquez C: Does the immune system communicate with the central nervous system? Interferon modifies central nervous activity. J Neuroimmunol 9:1-12, 1985

Damashek W: The white blood cells in dementia praecox and dementia paralytica. Archives of Neurology and Psychiatry 24:855, 1930

Deberdt R, Van Hooren J, Biesbrouck M, et al: Antinuclear factor-positive mental depression: a single disease entity. Biol Psychiatry 11:69-74, 1976

DeLisi LE, Goodman S, Neckers LM, et al: An analysis of lymphocyte subpopulations in schizophrenic patients. Biol Psychiatry 17:1003-1009, 1982

Diamond B, Yelton D, Scharff MD: Monoclonal antibodies: a new technology for producing serologic reagents. N Engl J Med 304:1344, 1981

Domino EF, Krause RR, Thiessen MM, et al: Blood protein fraction comparisons of normal and schizophrenic patients. Arch Gen Psychiatry 32:717-721, 1975

Fabris N: Immunodepression in thyroid deprived animals. Clin Exp Immunol 15:601-611, 1973

Fauci AS, Dale DC: The effect of hydrocortisone on the kinetics of normal human lymphocytes. Blood 46:235-243, 1975

Felten DL, Felten SY, Carlson SL, et al: Noradrenergic and peptidergic innervation of lymphoid tissue. J Immunol 135:755s-765s, 1985

Ferguson RM, Schmidtke JR, Simmons RL: Effects of psychoactive drugs on in vitro lymphocyte activation, in Neurochemical and Immunologic Components in Schizophrenia. Edited by Bergsma D, Goldstein AL. New York, Alan R. Liss, 1978

Fessel WJ, Hirata-Hibi M: Abnormal leukocytes in schizophrenia. Arch Gen Psychiatry 9:91-103, 1963

Fessel WJ, Hirata-Hibi M, Shapiro IM: Genetic and stress factors affecting the abnormal lymphocyte in schizophrenia. J Psychiatr Res 3:275-283, 1965

Fontana A, Storck U, Angst J, et al: An immunological basis of schizophrenia and affective disorders? Neuropsychobiology 6:284-289, 1980

Freedman DX, Fenichel G: Effect of midbrain lesion on experimental allergy. Archives of Neurology and Psychiatry 79:164-169, 1958

Geenen V, Segros JJ, Franchimont P, et al: The neuroendocrine thymus: coexistence of oxytocin and neurophysin in the human thymus. Science 232:508-511, 1986

Gilman SC, Schwartz JM, Milner RJ, et al: β–endorphin enhances lymphocyte proliferative responses. Proc Natl Acad Sci USA 79:4226, 1982

Gillis S, Ferm MM, Ou W, et al: T cell growth factor: parameters of production and a quantitative microassay for activity. J Immunol 120:2027-2032, 1978

Gisler RH: Stress and the hormonal regulation of the immune response in mice. Psychother Psychosom 23:197-208, 1974

Gold WM: Cholinergic pharmacology in asthma, in Asthma Physiology, Immuno-Pharmacology and Treatment. Edited by Austen KF, Lichtenstein LM. New York, Academic Press, 1973

Grossman CJ: Interactions between the gonadal steroids and the immune system. Science 227:257-261, 1985

Hall NR, Goldstein AL: Neurotransmitters and host defense, in Neural Modulation of Immunity. Edited by Guillemin R, Cohn M, Melnechuk T. New York, Raven Press, 1985

Heath RG, Krupp IM: Schizophrenia as an immunologic disorder, I: Demonstration of antibrain globulins by fluorescent antibody techniques. Arch Gen Psychiatry 16:1-9, 1967

Heath RG, Martens S, Leach BE, et al: Effects on behavior in humans with the administration of taraxein. Am J Psychiatry 114:14-24, 1957

Heath RG, Krupp IM, Byers L. Schizophrenia as an immunologic disorder, II: effect of serum protein fractions on brain function. Arch Gen Psychiatry 16:10-23, 1967

Helsing KJ, Szklo M, Comstock GW: Factors associated with mortality after widowhood. Am J Public Health 71:802-808, 1981

Hendrie HC, Paraskevas F, Varsamis J: Gamma globulin levels in psychiatric patients. Canadian Psychiatric Association Journal 17:93-97, 1972

Herberman RB, Ortaldo JR: Natural killer cells: their role in defenses against disease. Science 214:24-30, 1981

Hill CW, Greer WE, Felsenfeld O: Psychological stress, early response to foreign protein, and blood cortisol in vervets. Psychosom Med 29:279-283, 1967

Hirata-Hibi M: Plasma cell reaction and thymic germinal centers after a chronic form of electric stress. Journal of the Reticuloendothelial Society 4:370-389, 1967

Hirata-Hibi M, Higashi S, Takehiko T, et al: Stimulated lymphocytes in schizophrenia. Arch Gen Psychiatry 39:82-87, 1982

Hohlfield R, Toyka KV, Heininger K, et al: Autoimmune T lymphocytes specific for acetylcholine receptors. Nature 310:244, 1984

Hunig T, Loos M, Schimpl A: The role of accessory cells in polyclonal T cell activation, I: both induction of interleukin 2 production and of interleukin 2 responsiveness by concanavalin A are accessory cell dependent. Eur J Immunol 13:1-6, 1983

Ikemi Y, Nakagawa S: Psychosomatic study of so-called allergic disorders. Japanese Journal of Medical Progress 50:451, 1963

Jackson JC, Cross RJ, Walker RF, et al: Neuroimmunomodulation: influence of serotonin on the immune response. Immunology 54:505, 1984

Joasoo A, McKenzie JM: Stress and the immune response in rats. Int Arch Allergy Appl Immunol 50:659-663, 1976

Johnstone EC, Whaley K: Antinuclear antibodies in psychiatric illness: Their relationship to diagnosis and drug treatment. Br Med J 2:724-725, 1975

Keller SE, Stein M, Camerino MS, et al: Suppression of lymphocyte stimulation by anterior hypothalamic lesions in the guinea pig. Cell Immunol 52:334-340, 1980

Keller SE, Schleifer SJ, Sherman J, et al: Comparison of a simplified whole blood and isolated lymphocyte stimulation technique. Immunological Communications 10:417-431, 1981a

Keller S, Weiss J, Schleifer S, et al: Suppression of immunity by stress: effect of a graded series of stressors on lymphocyte stimulation in the rat. Science 213:1397-1400, 1981b

Keller SE, Shapiro R, Schleifer SJ, et al: Hypothalamic influences on anaphylaxis. Psychosom Med 44:302, 1982

Keller SE, Weiss JM, Schleifer SJ, et al: Stress-induced suppression of immunity in adrenalectomized rats. Science 221:1301-1304, 1983

Knight JG: Dopamine-receptor-stimulating autoantibodies: a possible cause of schizophrenia. Lancet 2:1073-1075, 1982

Kronfol Z, Silva Jr J, Greden J, et al: Impaired lymphocyte function in depressive illness. Life Sci 33:241-247, 1983

Kuritzky A, Livni E, Munitz H, et al: Cell-mediated immunity to human myelin basic protein in schizophrenic patients. J Neurol Sci 30:369, 1976

Laudenslager ML, Ryan SM, Drugan SM, et al: Coping and immunosuppression: inescapable but not escapable shock suppresses lymphocyte proliferation. Science 221:568-570, 1983

Lazarus SC: Neurohumoral mechanisms in asthma, in Neuroregulation of Autonomic, Endocrine and Immune Systems. Edited by Frederickson RCA, Hendrie HC, Hingtgen JN, et al. Boston, M. Nijhoff, 1985

Logan DG, Deodhar SD: Schizophrenia, an immunologic disorder. JAMA 212:1703, 1970

Lowy MT, Reder AT, Antel JP, et al: Glucocorticoid resistance in depression: the dexamethasone suppression test and lymphocyte sensitivity to dexamethasone. Am J Psychiatry 141:1365-1370, 1984

Luparello TJ, Stein M, Park CD: Effect of hypothalamic lesions on rat anaphylaxis. Am J Physiol 207:911-914, 1964

Luriya EA, Domashneva IV: Antithymus antibodies in the blood serum of schizophrenics. Bulletin of Experimental Biology and Medicine 77:418, 1974

Macris NT, Schiavi RC, Camerino MS, et al: Effect of hypothalamic lesions on immune processes in the guinea pig. Am J Physiol 219:1205-1209, 1970

Mann JJ, Brown RP, Halper JP, et al: Reduced sensitivity of lymphocyte beta-adrenergic receptors in patients with endogenous depression and psychomotor agitation. N Engl J Med 313:715-720, 1985

Mellsop G, Whittingham S, Ungar B: Schizophrenia and autoimmune serological reactions. Arch Gen Psychiatry 28:194, 1978

Monjan AA, Collector MI: Stress-induced modulation of the immune response. Science 196:307-308, 1977

Nyland H, Ness A, Lunde H: Lymphocyte subpopulations in peripheral blood from schizophrenic patients. Acta Psychiatr Scand 61:313-318, 1980

Parkes CM: Bereavement: Studies of Grief in Adult Life. New York, International Universities Press, 1972

Petrovskii IN: Problems of nervous control in immunity reactions, II: the influence of experimental neuroses on immunity reactions. Zhurnal Mikrobiologii, Epidemiologii I Immunobiologii 32:63-69, 1961

Rasmussen AF Jr, Marsh JT, Brill NQ: Increased susceptibility to herpes simplex in mice subjected to avoidance-learning stress or restraint. Proc Soc Exp Biol Med 96:183-189, 1957

Rasmussen AF Jr, Spencer ET, Marsh JT: Decrease in susceptibility of mice to passive anaphylaxis following avoidance-learning stress. Proc Soc Exp Biol Med 100:878-879, 1959

Reite M, Harbeck R, Hoffman A: Altered cellular immune response following peer separation. Life Sci 29:1133-1135, 1981

Riley V: Psychoneuroendocrine influences on immunocompetence and neoplasia. Science 212:1100-1109, 1981

Rogers MP, Reich P, Strom TB, et al: Behaviorally conditioned immunosuppression: replication of a recent study. Psychosom Med 38:447-452, 1976

Rose RM: Overview of endocrinology of stress, in Neuroendocrinology and Psychiatric Disorder. Edited by Brown GM, Koslow SH, Reichlin S. New York, Raven Press, 1984

Roszman TL, Cross RJ, Brooks WH, et al: Hypothalamic-immune interactions, II: the effect of hypothalamic lesions on the ability of adherent spleen cells to limit lymphocyte blastogenesis. Immunology 45:737-742, 1982

Schiavi RC, Adams J, Stein M: Effect of hypothalamic lesions on histamine toxicity in the guinea pig. Am J Physiol 211:1269-1273, 1966

Schiavi RC, Macris NT, Camerino MS, et al: Effect of hypothalamic lesions on immediate hypersensitivity. Am J Physiology 228:596-601, 1975

Schleifer SJ, Keller SE, Camerino M, et al: Suppression of lymphocyte stimulation following bereavement. JAMA 250:374-377, 1983

Schleifer SJ, Keller SE, Meyerson AT, et al: Lymphocyte function in major depressive disorder. Arch Gen Psychiatry 41:484-486, 1984a

Schleifer SJ, Keller SE, Stein M: Brain, behaviour and the immune system (letter). Nature 310:456, 1984b

Schleifer SJ, Keller SE, Cohen J, et al: (abstract) Depression and immunity: role of age, sex, and severity. Paper presented at the Society for Neuroscience Annual Meeting, Dallas, Texas, October 23, 1985a

Schleifer SJ, Keller SE, Siris SG, et al: Depression and immunity: lymphocyte function in ambulatory depressed, hospitalized schizophrenic, and herniorrhaphy patients. Arch Gen Psychiatry 42:129-133, 1985b

Selye H: Stress in Health and Disease. Boston, Butterworth's, 1976

Shavit Y, Lewis JW, Terman GW, et al: Opioid peptides mediate the suppressive effect of stress on natural killer cell cytotoxicity. Science 223:188-190, 1984

Shopsin B, Sathananthan GL, Chan TL, et al: Antinuclear factor in psychiatric patients. Biol Psychiatry 7:81-86, 1973

Siegal M, Niswander CD, Sachs E Jr., et al: Taraxein, fact or artifact? Am J Psychiatry 115:819, 1959

Smith EM, Meyer WJ, Blalock JE: Virus-induced corticosterone in hypophysectomized mice: a possible lymphoid adrenal axis. Science 218:1311, 1982

Smith RG, McDaniel SM: Psychologically mediated effect on the delayed hypersensitivity reaction to tuberculin in humans. Psychosom Med 45:65-70, 1983

Snow EC: Insulin and growth hormone function as minor growth factors that potentiate lymphocyte activation. J Immunol 135:776s-778s, 1985

Solomon GF: Stress and antibody response in rats. International Archives of Allergy 35:97-104, 1969

Stein M, Keller S, Schleifer S: The hypothalamus and the immune response, in Brain, Behavior, and Bodily Disease. Edited by Weiner H, Hofer MA, Stunkard AJ. New York, Raven Press, 1981

Stein M, Keller SE, Schleifer SJ: Stress and immunomodulation: the role of depression and neuroendocrine function. J Immunol 35:827s-833s, 1985a

Stein M, Schleifer SJ, Keller SE: Immune disorders, in Comprehensive Textbook of Psychiatry IV. Edited by Kaplan HI, Freedman AM, Sadock BJ. Baltimore, Williams and Wilkins, 1985b

Strahilivitz M, Davis SD: Increased IgA in schizophrenic patients. Lancet 2:370, 1970

Szentivanyi A, Filipp G: Anaphylaxis and the nervous system, part II. Ann Allergy 16:143-151, 1958

Szentivanyi A, Szekely J: Anaphylaxis and the nervous system, part IV. Ann Allergy 16:389-392, 1958

Tavadia HB, Fleming KA, Hume RD, et al: Circadian rhythmicity of human plasma cortisol and PHA-induced lymphocyte transformation. Clin Exp Immunol 22:190, 1975

Thomson SP, McMahon LJ, Nugent CA: Endogenous cortisol: a regulator of the number of lymphocytes in peripheral blood. Clin Immunol Immunopathol 17:506, 1980

Vartanian ME, Kolyaskina GI, Lozovsky DV, et al: Aspects of humoral and cellular immunity in schizophrenia, in Neurochemical and Immunologic Components in Schizophrenia. Edited by Bergsma D, Goldstein AL. New York, Alan R. Liss, 1978

Vessey SH: Effects of grouping on levels of circulating antibodies in mice. Proc Soc Biol Med 115:252-255, 1964

von Brauchitsch H: Antinuclear factor in psychiatric disorders. Am J Psychiatry 128:102-104, 1972

Watanabe M, Funahashi T, Suzuki T, et al: Antithymic antibodies in schizophrenic sera. Biol Psychiatry 17:699-710, 1982

Wayner EA, Flannery GR, Singer G: The effects of taste aversion conditioning on the primary antibody response to sheep red blood cells and Brucella abortus in the albino rat. Physiol Behav 21:995-1000, 1978

Weizman A, Weizman R, Szekely GA, et al: Abnormal immune response to brain tissue antigen in the syndrome of autism. Am J Psychiatry 139:1462-1465, 1982

Williams LT, Synderman R, Lefkowitz RJ: Identification of B-adrenergic receptors on human lymphocytes by (^{3}H)-alprenolol binding. J Clin Invest 57:149-155, 1976

Wisniewski K, Cobill JM, Wilcox CB, et al: T lymphocytes in patients with Down's Syndrome. Biol Psychiatry 14:463-471, 1979

Zarrabi MH, Zucker S, Miller F, et al: Immunologic and coagulation disorders in chlorpromazine-treated patients. Ann Intern Med 91 194-199, 1979

Zurawski G, Benedik M, Kamb BJ, et al: Activation of mouse T-helper cells induces abundant preproenkephalin mRNA synthesis. Science 232:772-775, 1986

Chapter 10

The Neurobiology of Sleep: Basic Concepts and Clinical Implications

by Priyattam J. Shiromani, Ph.D., Mark H. Rapaport, M.D., and J. Christian Gillin, M.D.

Sleep and dreaming: What are their functions? How do they come about? What is their clinical significance? These unanswered questions have stirred the imagination since ancient times and continue to do so. The modern scientific attempt to answer these questions began just over 30 years ago with the discovery that sleep consists of two phases, rapid eye movement (REM) sleep and non-rapid eye movement (NREM) sleep. This observation has not diminished the mystery of sleep: Now we must explain the physiology and psychology of two states during sleep. On a psychological level, the discovery of REM sleep was particularly exciting. Awakenings during this state of sleep yielded dream recall about 80 percent of the time. During NREM sleep it was about 10 percent.

On a physiological level, the disparity between the two states stimulated other questions about the function and origin of sleep. Sleep had usually been conceived of as a time of energy conservation and quietude. REM sleep is, however, an internally aroused sleep state, characterized by autonomic variability, increased cerebral blood flow and metabolism, and EEG activation. The behavioral manifestations of the psychological and physiological activation of REM sleep are blocked by a peripheral muscle atonia. For these reasons REM sleep has often been called paradoxical sleep. In contrast, NREM sleep conforms more closely to the conventional notion that sleep is a time of psychological and physiological "rest." It has often been called orthodox sleep.

In the past 15 to 20 years, knowledge of clinical sleep disorders has exploded. Neither the diagnostic nosology of sleep disorders nor the number of patients involved had previously been appreciated. A new clinical subspecialty, clinical sleep disorders medicine, has arisen. A formal working nosology has been in use for more than five years. Clinical sleep disorders centers have been established throughout the country to provide specialized evaluation of patients with sleep disorders, to train and teach clinicians, and to conduct research. Much has been learned in recent years to aid general practitioners and psychiatrists in the office evaluation and treatment of sleep–wake disorders.

Changes in the sleep–wake cycle are integrally related to a number of psychiatric disorders, particularly depression and mania. Characteristic abnormalities of sleep have been described which appear to be relatively specific for certain clinical psychiatric disorders.

The sleep research laboratory is now part of many clinical research programs in psychiatry. All-night EEG, eye movements, and submental muscle tone are recorded on a polygraph for visual scoring of sleep stages. Important measures include: 1) sleep latency, the time to fall asleep; 2) REM latency, time from sleep onset to the first REM period; 3) REM density, a measure of the amount of eye movement activity per minute of REM sleep; 4) total sleep time; 5) amount and percentage of total sleep time spent in each of the stages of sleep; 6) sleep efficiency, percent of time in bed spent asleep; and 7) early morning awakening. In more specialized studies, respiration, blood oxygen saturation, heart rate, abnormal movements of the limbs, penile tumescence, or daytime sleepiness can be objectively measured. The sleep laboratory also permits detailed collection of dream reports, which can be readily obtained by awakening the subject during a REM period. The sleep laboratory remains largely a research tool in psychiatry, except in the evaluation of patients with specific sleep disorders.

Much has also been learned about the basic physiology of sleep and wakefulness. This knowledge provides a basis for interpreting the sleep abnormalities observed in clinical disorders. This chapter attempts to provide a background on basic sleep research principles arising out of human and animal sleep research laboratories, and to review clinical sleep disorders, especially from the perspective of the sleep laboratory.

NEUROBIOLOGY OF SLEEP

Early researchers believed that sleep was a passive phenomenon resulting from a cessation of afferent activity (Moruzzi, 1972). Such a view prevailed until the classic study by Moruzzi and Magoun (1949), which showed that electrical stimulation of the reticular formation produced arousal. This study indicated that the reticular formation, instead of the sensory impulses, was responsible for arousal. As already mentioned, another landmark in sleep research was the discovery of rapid eye movement (REM) sleep (Aserinsky and Kleitman, 1953).

The Characteristic Features of Non-REM and REM Sleep

Non-REM sleep normally precedes REM sleep (see Table 1). It is defined by EEG criteria: sleep spindles (12–14 cps waves), K–complexes, and delta waves (large voltage slow waves). In humans there are at least four stages (stages 1–4) of non-REM sleep. REM sleep is composed of tonic (occurring throughout the REM sleep episode) and phasic (occurring only sporadically during REM sleep) events (see Figure 1). The major tonic events include cortical desynchronization, loss of muscle tone in antigravity musculature, and theta activity in the dorsal hippocampus. The phasic events include monophasic waves in pons, lateral geniculate nucleus and occipital cortex (ponto-geniculo-occipital or PGO waves), and rapid eye movements (see Figure 1).

The Neuronal Mechanisms Responsible for Non-REM Sleep

Three sites have been thought to generate non-REM sleep (see Figure 2). One of the hypnogenic sites is the basal forebrain area. Lesions of the pre-optic basal forebrain area produced insomnia in rats (Nauta, 1946) and cats (McGinty and Sterman, 1968; Szymusiak and McGinty, 1985). Electrical stimulation of this region produces both EEG and behavioral signs of sleep (Sterman and Clemente, 1962), and Szymusiak and McGinty (1986) have found that neurons in the basal forebrain discharge selectively during non-REM sleep. In humans, it is possible, but unproven, that neuropathology in the basal forebrain contributes to the sleep disturbances commonly found in patients with Alzheimer's disease.

The second site is the serotonin-containing dorsal raphe nucleus, which at

Table 1. Physiological Characteristics of Non-REM and REM Sleep

	Non-REM	REM
EEG	Spindles, K-complexes, delta waves	Low voltage, fast "sawtooth" waves
EOG	Quiescent or slow movements	Bursts of rapid eye movements
EMG	Partially relax	Atonia
Blood pressure	Low	Variable
Heart rate	Slow	Variable
Cardiac output	Decreased	Decreased
Cerebral blood flow	Low, heterogeneous	Increased
Brain temperature	Decreased	Increased
Respiratory rate	Decreased	Increased
Minute ventilation	Decreased	Variable
Intercostal muscles	Partial relaxation	Atonia
Genioglossus and upper airway muscle	Partial relaxation	Atonia or hypotonic
Ventilatory response to CO_2	Intact	Partially impaired
Pulmonary stretch receptor	Intact	Partially intact
Genitals	Infrequent tumescence	Tumescence

one time was postulated to be the prime site for non-REM sleep. The original hypothesis was based on results from acute studies of lesions of the raphe and of pharmacological depletion of brain serotonin. Both procedures decreased total sleep (Jouvet, 1972). Chronic studies and other techniques have led to a reexamination of the original hypothesis, and it is no longer widely accepted that serotonin or the raphe nuclei are necessary for sleep. Nevertheless, elevation of serotonin by administration of its biosynthetic precursor, tryptophan, increases non-REM sleep in man and decreases the latency to sleep onset (Wyatt, 1972; Hartman, 1977).

The third postulated somnogenic area is located in the solitary tract nucleus of the medulla. Stimulation of this area produces EEG synchrony which outlasts the stimulation (Magnes et al, 1961), and lesions of the solitary tract nucleus considerably enhance and prolong the phasic arousal produced by reticular stimulation (Bonvallet and Allen, 1963). Application of serotonin (one of the neurotransmitters implicated in sleep onset) into the solitary tract nucleus induces non-REM sleep (Key and Mehta, 1977), and cells in this nucleus increase discharge rate during non-REM sleep (Eguchi and Satoh, 1979).

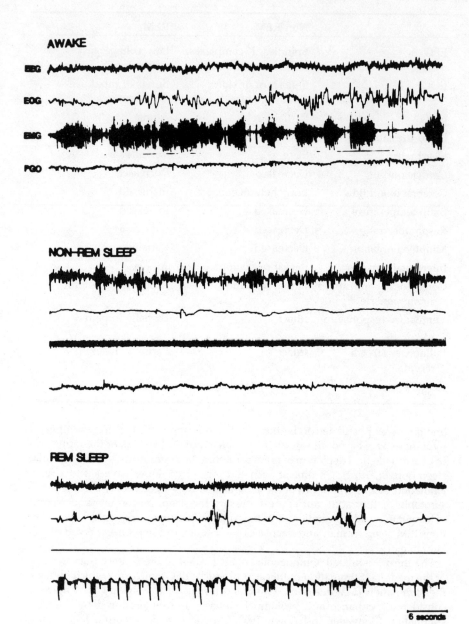

AWAKE

EEG

EOG

EMG

PGO

NON-REM SLEEP

REM SLEEP

6 seconds

Figure 1. Electrophysiological characteristics of the sleep–wake pattern in the cat

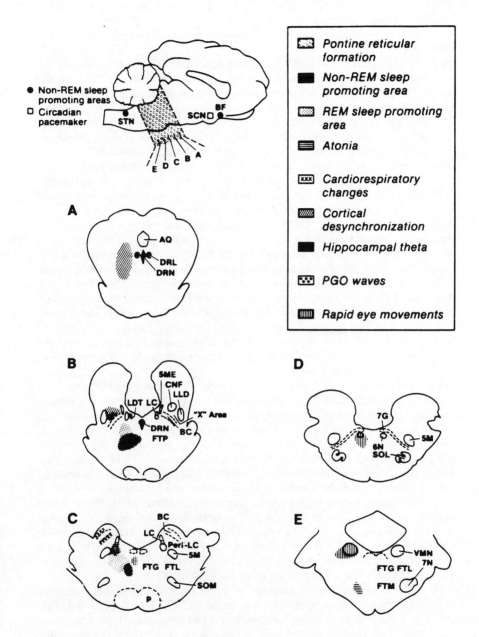

Figure 2. Localization of non-REM and REM sleep promoting areas in the brain

Cholinergic Mechanisms and REM Sleep

A diffuse network of cholinoceptive neurons in the pontine reticular formation (PRF) (perhaps less than 25 percent of PRF cells) primes, initiates, and maintains the consolidated state of REM sleep (see Figure 2). In addition, cholinergic neurons are intimately involved in the various tonic and phasic components of REM sleep.

ACETYLCHOLINE AND CORTICAL DESYNCHRONIZATION. The cholinergic system plays an important role in cortical desynchronization. Systemically administered atropine readily produces slow high amplitude waves, even during behavioral waking. Local infusion of cholinergic agonists, such as carbachol, bethanachol, or oxotremorine, into the reticular formation increases cortical desynchronization (Baghdoyan et al, 1984a, 1984b; George et al, 1964; Shiromani and McGinty, 1983). Intense behavioral and EEG arousal is noted with carbachol injections into the mesencephalic RF (Baghdoyan et al, 1984a; Baxter, 1969; Shiromani et al, 1986). Single unit studies have shown that mesencephalic RF cells increase discharge during waking and REM sleep compared with slow wave sleep (for review see Steriade et al, 1980).

ACETYLCHOLINE AND ATONIA. Much evidence supports the hypothesis that the cataplectic episodes of narcoleptic humans and dogs are related to the muscle atonia of normal REM sleep. The inhibition of antigravity musculature is hypothesized to result from activation of a discrete group of *non-monoaminergic* cells located ventrally in the locus coeruleus complex (Sakai, 1980) (see Figure 2). These peri-locus coeruleus neurons may exert an excitatory influence on magnocellular neurons located in the medullary RF (Sakai, 1980). The magnocellular neurons correspond to the medullary inhibitory center of Magoun and Rhines (1949) and are postulated to induce a generalized inhibition of spinal motor-neurons by exciting spinal inhibitory inter-neurons (Morales and Chase, 1978; Pompeiano, 1976, 1980).

Electrical stimulation of the medullary RF, especially the magnocellular nucleus, elicits generalized inhibition of spinal motor-neurons (Sakai, 1980), while bilateral electrical ablation of the peri-locus coeruleus and medial locus coeruleus abolishes the atonia during REM sleep (Henley and Morrison, 1974). Moreover, neuronal activity within the peri-locus coeruleus and the magnocellular nucleus is high during periods of atonia in REM sleep (Kanomori et al, 1980; Sakai, 1980). The dorso-lateral pontine tegmentum, which contains the peri-locus coeruleus, exhibits intense metabolic activity, as determined by the 2-deoxyglucose method, during concussion induced behavioral suppression (Hayes et al, 1984). It has been suggested that a common mechanism underlies the atonia of REM sleep and the behavioral suppression which follows concussion (Hayes et al, 1984; Katayama et al, 1984). Studies utilizing the horseradish peroxidase technique have shown connections between the peri-locus coeruleus, the magnocellular nucleus, and the spinal cord (Sakai et al, 1978, 1979).

The cholinergic system is implicated in atonia because infusion of carbachol into the pontine tegmentum readily induces cataplexy in cats (Baghdoyan et al, 1984a, b; Katayama et al, 1984; Shiromani and McGinty, 1983, 1986; Shiromani et al, 1986; Van Dongen et al, 1978). In narcoleptic dogs, systemically administered cholinomimetics increase the incidence of cataplectic episodes while muscarinic receptor blockers delay these episodes; nicotinic agents have no effect

(Baker and Dement, 1984; Delashaw et al, 1979). Moreover, in narcoleptic dogs, increased muscarinic receptor binding is found in several pontine sites (Baker and Dement, 1984).

ACETYLCHOLINE AND HIPPOCAMPAL THETA ACTIVITY. Regular 4–12 Hz waves can be obtained from the dorsal hippocampus during waking, REM sleep, and surgical anesthesia (Vanderwolf et al, 1978; Winson, 1972). This waveform, termed theta activity, can be further divided into two categories, depending upon the behavior of the animal and response to atropine (Vanderwolf and Robinson, 1981). The first type of theta (4–7 Hz) occurs during alert total immobility, inter-twitch intervals of REM sleep, and anesthesia (urethane, ether). It also occurs when the animal exhibits what has been termed Type II behavior, such as face-washing, shivering, chattering the teeth, and tremor. This type of theta is abolished by antimuscarinic drugs such as atropine, and stimulated by physostigmine. The second type of theta (7–12 Hz) occurs when the animal exhibits Type I behaviors such as walking, running, rearing, shifting of posture, and head movement. It also occurs during REM sleep-related phasic twitches and it is not abolished by antimuscarinic drugs. This type of theta is disrupted by anesthetics (ether, urethane) and morphine.

The system responsible for atropine-sensitive theta may be identical to the ascending cholinergic reticular system of Shute and Lewis (Vanderwolf and Robinson, 1981). Stimulation of the pontine reticular formation in rat (Klemm, 1972; Robinson and Vanderwolf, 1978) and cat (Macadar et al, 1974) triggers theta. Recently Vertes (1980) has confirmed these observations. In addition, some pontine reticular formation cells discharge maximally during theta (Vertes, 1979).

ACETYLCHOLINE AND RAPID EYE MOVEMENTS. The vestibular nuclei may be necessary for the rapid eye movements during REM sleep (Morrison and Pompeiano, 1966). For example, phasic changes in firing rates of vestibular neurons occur during REM sleep in intact cats (Bizzi et al, 1964), in the decerebrate preparation (Thoden et al, 1972a, 1972b), and in acute decerebrate animals treated with acetylcholine potentiating agents such as physostigmine (Thoden et al, 1972a, 1972b). Furthermore, Mergner and Pompeiano (1977) have shown that increased discharge rates of medial vestibular neurons and abducens motor-neurons precede activity in the lateral rectus muscle by 11–15 msec. Moreover, vestibular lesions abolish bursts of rapid eye movements but do not interfere with isolated, slow eye movements or with REM sleep per se. The excitation in vestibular and abducens motor-neurons may be generated by nuclei located within the para-median reticular formation (Cohen and Henn, 1972; Henn and Cohen, 1975).

ACETYLCHOLINE AND PGO WAVES. Ponto-geniculo-occipital (PGO) waves are slow monophasic waves which occur either singly or in clusters of three to four just prior to and during REM sleep (see Figure 1). These waves can be recorded from the pons, lateral geniculate nucleus, and occipital cortex. These areas are directly related to the visual system.

The neurons responsible for PGO waves are hypothesized to be located in and around the brachium conjunctivum (this area is called the "X" area), the rostral part of the lateral parabrachial nucleus which is just caudal to the "X" area, and the rostral part of the locus coeruleus (for review see Sakai, 1980) (see Figure 2). The PGO executive neurons appear to be cholinergic or at least cholinoceptive in nature. Atropine significantly reduces PGO bursts (Jacobs et al, 1972), while physostigmine triggers PGO bursts in collicular or pontine transected cats (Magherini et al, 1971). Microinfusions of carbachol in the dorsolateral pontine tegmentum have been shown to induce PGO activity selectively (Baghdoyan et al, 1984a; Shiromani and McGinty, 1983). A vestibular component also appears to be involved because carbachol microinfusion into the vestibular region evokes PGO waves tightly coupled to stereotyped eye movements (Shiromani, personal observations.)

The PGO mechanism is not exclusively under cholinergic control; noradrenergic and serotonergic inputs from the locus coeruleus and dorsal raphe nucleus are hypothesized to inhibit the cholinergic PGO executive neurons (Sakai, 1980; 1984; McGinty and Harper, 1976).

Acetylcholine and the Generation of the REM Sleep State

While discrete nuclei within the reticular formation may be responsible for generating the major tonic and phasic components of REM sleep, we suggest that a pontine reticular formation cholinoceptive mechanism primes the consolidated REM sleep state. Transection (Jouvet, 1972; Siegel et al, 1983, 1984) and electrical lesion studies (Jouvet, 1972) have made it clear that the machinery needed for REM sleep generation resides within the pontine reticular formation.

Jouvet initially postulated that brainstem cholinergic mechanisms played an important role in the generation of REM sleep (Jouvet, 1972). Increased acetylcholine is found during REM sleep in cortex (Celesia and Jasper, 1966; Jasper and Tessier, 1971) and striatum (Gadea-Ciria et al, 1973) of normal cats and in ventricular perfusates of conscious dogs (Haranath and Venkatakrisha-Bhatt, 1973). In normal humans (Sitaram et al, 1976, 1977, 1978a, 1978b; Sitaram and Gillin, 1980), intravenous infusions of physostigmine or arecoline during non-REM decrease the latency to REM sleep, although infusions during or immediately after REM sleep produce arousal. In addition, an orally active muscarinic agonist, RS-86, shortens REM latency in normal volunteers (Spiegel, 1984). In cats and rats (Baghdoyan et al, 1984a, 1984b; George et al, 1964; Hobson et al, 1983; Shiromani, 1983; Shiromani and McGinty, 1983, 1986; Shiromani et al, 1986), administration of cholinergic agonists, for example, carbachol, directly into the pontine reticular formation readily evokes elements of REM sleep (atonia, PGO waves, rapid eye movements), or complete REM sleep which may be unusually long. Infusions into midbrain or medullary sites fail to induce REM sleep (Baghdoyan et al, 1984b; Shiromani et al, 1986) while local infusion of scopolamine blocks the cholinomimetic induced REM sleep (Shiromani and McGinty, 1983). Shiromani and McGinty (1985, 1986) have shown that carbachol induced REM sleep occurs in conjunction with an increase in pontine neuronal activity. In our own investigation of the role of the pontine reticular formation in the regulation of REM sleep we have found that cholinoceptive neurons are responsible for REM sleep generation, but the identity of the cholinergic input remains unknown (Shiromani et al, 1986).

Sleep and Breathing

In the sleep apnea syndrome and in some cases the sudden infant death syndrome (SIDS) respiratory failure apparently occurs during sleep. Therefore, an understanding of the influence of sleep on breathing may provide clues about a variety of diseases and their pathophysiology.

Breathing is controlled by two separate but functionally integrated systems (Phillipson, 1978; Sullivan, 1980). One system is called the metabolic or automatic control system and its command center is located in the medulla and pons. This system is responsible for acid-base and blood-gas homeostasis. It provides an automatic neural drive to the respiratory pump by integrating input from central (CO_2 and pH sensitive) and peripheral (O_2 sensitive) chemoreceptors, and lung and chest wall mechanoreceptors. The other system is called the behavioral or voluntary control system. It resides within cortical and forebrain structures and allows the respiratory muscles to be used for nonrespiratory purposes, such as speech.

Both systems control breathing in wakefulness. During active waking the voluntary system is dominant, while during quiet wakefulness the automatic system exerts more control over breathing. It is clear that wakefulness provides a powerful drive to the respiratory pump since prolonged apneas occur only during sleep. In fact, patients with defective chemoreceptors or damage to the tract carrying the impulses from the pontine-medullary automatic metabolic system fail to breathe only during sleep. This condition is called Ondine's curse.

Throughout non-REM sleep, breathing is regular and it is controlled entirely by the automatic system. In REM sleep the picture is more complicated. The voluntary system is dominant during phasic REM sleep, while the automatic system is dominant in the quiet REM sleep periods. Therefore, in this aspect, the control of breathing during REM sleep is similar to that of waking. In contrast, however, respiratory drive is less sensitive to pCO_2 in REM sleep than wakefulness.

Breathing, heart rate, and blood pressure during REM sleep are irregular, a reflection of the phasic events of REM sleep. This is in sharp contrast to the regular sinusoidal pattern seen during non-REM sleep. Autonomic variability during REM sleep could be dangerous, especially to individuals with hypertension or respiratory and cardiovascular insufficiencies. Indeed, many cardiovascular deaths peak during the nocturnal hours.

In the case of sleep apneas it is important to point out that there are two types of apneas: obstructive and central. In the former, there is a cessation of airflow at the level of the nostrils and mouth in spite of persistent diaphragmatic respiratory effort. In central apnea airflow is absent in the mouth and nostrils and there is no respiratory effort. Most patients have both types of apneas (Guilleminault and Dement, 1978). The mechanism responsible for the apneas is unknown, but in the case of the obstructive apnea, it has been demonstrated that diminution of muscle tone in the oropharynx during sleep and REM sleep is a contributing factor. Typically, patients with obstructive sleep apnea snore loudly, which results from constricted upper airway passage. Guilleminault and Dement (1978) have provided a list of conditions associated with sleep apnea syndromes and some of these include enlarged tonsils, adenoids, micrognathia, obesity, and short necks.

Approximately 90 percent of all apneic episodes occur during non-REM sleep stages 1 and 2; apneas in deep non-REM sleep are rare. Because of the apneic episodes during the initial sleep stages, the subjects are deprived of stages 3 and 4. Therefore, the apneic episodes cause a sleep deprivation and fragmentation and the subject complains of hypersomnolence.

A critical element in treating apneas is to warn the patient against the use of sedatives or bedtime alcohol. Both of these have been shown to increase the incidence of apneas. Moreover, it is essential that reflexive mechanisms responsible for arousal not be compromised.

Temperature Regulation in Sleep

Temperature control is partially lost during REM sleep but not during non-REM sleep (see Parmeggiani, 1980). For example, during non-REM sleep, sweating occurs to lower body temperature when ambient temperature is high. Conversely, in low ambient temperature, shivering occurs during non-REM sleep. However, during REM sleep, sweating or shivering does not occur in response to altered ambient temperature. Additionally, hypothalamic cooling during non-REM sleep increases oxygen consumption and metabolic heat production. This response is lost during REM sleep. In cats, hypothalamic cooling elicits tachypnea during non-REM, but not in REM sleep.

Sleep and Chronobiology

The 24-hour sleep-wake cycle is but one example of a circadian rhythm. Other examples include body temperature, adrenocorticotropin hormone (ACTH) and cortisol, thyroid-stimulating hormone (TSH), and some mood and performance rhythms.

A modern, laboratory based approach to studying rhythms is the temporal isolation apartment. Subjects can live for extended periods of time in these environments without knowledge of clock-time, the natural light-dark cycle, or the usual social cues that time behavior. They need not be socially isolated. The subject is allowed to choose his or her own bedtime and wake-up time, meal time, and rest–activity times without reference to to any external Zeitgeber ("time-giver").

Several interesting changes typically occur when humans live in these circumstances. First, average duration of the sleep–wake cycle usually lengthens from the normal 24 hours to 24.5 to 25.0 hours. Thus, the subject goes to bed about 30–60 minutes later each "night" and arises 30–60 minutes later each "morning." In some cases, however, subjects may self-select markedly longer sleep–wake cycles; for example, 36-hour cycles with 24 hours of activity and 12 hours of rest. Both the long and the short changes occur without subjective awareness.

Second, REM latency typically shortens in free-running conditions. This probably reflects a change in the phase relationships between the onset of sleep and the rhythm of core body temperature. Indeed, not only REM latency but the duration of sleep appears to be a function of when sleep occurs in relation to the body temperature curve (Czeisler et al, 1980). REM sleep is inversely related to the body temperature (Czeisler et al, 1980). In addition, if sleep onset occurs soon after the circadian peak of body temperature, then the sleep periods tend to be long. On the other hand, sleep tends to be short when it begins near the temperature trough.

The biological clocks or oscillators are normally entrained to the external environment by the light-dark cycle and by social cues. In animals it has been demonstrated that pulses of light can either delay or advance certain rhythms, depending upon when the light is given with respect to the phase of the underlying oscillator. For example, light administered just before the rest period under free-running conditions will delay rest not only on that day but on subsequent days; conversely, light administered near the end of the rest period will advance the rest period on subsequent days. This phenomena is called the phase response curve.

Light also suppresses melatonin, a hormone normally released by the pineal gland during the dark phase of the 24-hour day. The amount of melatonin secreted varies with the seasonal photoperiod and has been implicated in seasonal breeding patterns in hamsters and sheep. Its function in man is largely unknown.

Chronobiology has important implications for the sleep disorders associated with affective illness, phase delay syndrome, jet lag, and shift work. For example, the short REM latency of depression has been interpreted as a "phase advance" of the circadian oscillator controlling REM sleep, similar to that seen in normal subjects living under free-running conditions (Kripke, 1983). Phase delay syndrome is a sleep disorder found in extreme "night owls," who go to bed late and arise late; that is, they are phase delayed with respect to the external environment. The problems of jet lag and shift work reflect a combination of sleep deprivation and desynchronization between internal clocks and the demands of the external environment.

Since light entrains the circadian oscillators, phase shifts rhythms in animals, and suppresses melatonin at night, it may have clinical utility in some clinical disorders. Perhaps the best demonstrated use of light in psychiatry is for seasonal affective disorders, a condition in which patients become depressed during the fall and winter months and hypomanic during the spring and summer (Rosenthal et al, 1984). Light may also have mild antidepressant effects in nonseasonal depression (Kripke, 1984). It may also be useful in treating patients with jet lag, shift work sleep problems, or other abnormalities of circadian phase.

The suprachiasmatic nucleus (SCN) of the hypothalamus is a pacemaker of the mammalian circadian system. For example, lesions of the SCN disrupt circadian rhythmicity in a number of systems, including the sleep–wake cycle (Moore and Eichler, 1972; Stephan and Zucker, 1972). After these lesions, for example, sleep and wakefulness occur in short bursts which are evenly distributed over the 24 hours. Inouye and Kawamura (1979) have found persistence of circadian rhythmicity, as demonstrated by neuronal activity, in a hypothalamic island containing the SCN. Their study also showed loss of circadian organization in structures outside of the SCN island. These studies demonstrate that the SCN is a potent autonomous circadian oscillator.

Although SCN lesions abolish the circadian sleep-wake cycle, they do not prevent the compensatory increase in total sleep time which typically follows sleep deprivation (Ibuka and Kawamura, 1975). These observations suggest that sleep is controlled by at least two processes: a circadian process which determines the propensity for sleep over the 24-hour period, and a homeostatic process (the longer wakefulness lasts, the greater the likelihood of sleep) (Borbely and Wirz-Justice, 1982). The "best sleep" occurs, therefore, when the subject has been awake for the optimal amount of time and goes to sleep at the "right" time of the circadian clock.

Endocrine Rhythms During Sleep

A number of endocrine hormones follow circadian patterns that are closely associated with the sleep–wake cycle (Parker et al, 1980). Takahashi et al (1968) were the first to find that growth hormone was secreted generally during non-REM sleep (stages 3 and 4). Infants under three months do not show a sleep-related increase in growth hormone, while during prepuberty growth hormone is secreted almost entirely during sleep. In puberty growth hormone shows the highest secretions during sleep but peaks are also seen during wakefulness. Sleep related release of growth hormone declines with age. If sleep is advanced or delayed, growth hormone release shifts to the new sleep period.

Prolactin secretion is also stimulated by sleep, with secretion commencing 30–90 minutes after sleep onset and reaching a peak in the early morning hours. Thyrotropin, on the other hand, is inhibited by sleep onset. Thyrotropin reaches peak levels every evening with a gradual decline occurring during sleep. If sleep is prevented then the thyrotropin levels continue to increase. Cortisol and ACTH secretion appear to also be regulated by a combination of circadian and sleep related influences. The circadian rhythm of cortisol and ACTH persist during sleep deprivation, but sleep onset has a modest inhibitory effect on these hormones.

Luteinizing hormone has a sleep related secretion pattern that changes with maturation. In early puberty, luteinizing hormone secretion increases during sleep; if the sleep-wake cycle is reversed, luteinizing hormone release will also be reversed to match the sleep phase (Boyar et al, 1972).

CLINICAL SLEEP DISORDERS AND IMPLICATIONS

The first half of this chapter focused on the neurobiology of sleep and emphasized the neuronal mechanisms involved in non-REM and REM sleep generation. The second half of this chapter attempts to link the basic neurobiology of sleep with current clinical research and practice. A brief description of the nosology of sleep disorders is followed by a section outlining the current function of a sleep laboratory in clinical psychiatry, and then some examples of how principles derived from basic neurobiological research can be applied to current clinical research questions.

The Nosology of Sleep

Although the physiological basis of many sleep disorders is not known at this time, considerable progress has been made in the recent past in classifying sleep disorders. Four major types of sleep disorder have been described:

1. *The Disorders of Initiating and Maintaining Sleep (DIMS)*, or the insomnias. Insomnia is, by definition, a subjective dissatisfaction with the amount or quality of sleep. It can result from a variety of causes, some trivial and some more serious. Transient insomnia is common in normal, healthy people undergoing acute stress. Chronic insomnia may be associated with psychiatric disorders such as depression or dysthymia, with alcoholism and drug abuse or misuse, with medical conditions, or pain syndromes, with sleep apnea or sleep related respiratory impairment, with abnormal movements during sleep such as nocturnal myoclonus, and with other conditions.

2. *The Disorders of Excessive Daytime Sleepiness (DOES)*. These disorders are characterized by inappropriate sleep without obvious reason and should be distinguished from fatigue. The two major causes are sleep apnea and narcolepsy, but it may be found occasionally in patients with "sleep-drunkenness" and Klein-Levine syndrome.
3. *The Disorders of the Sleep-Wake Cycle*. These include the sleep complaints associated with jet-lag, shift work, delayed sleep syndrome, and the non-24-hour-day syndrome.
4. *The Parasomnias*, or abnormal behaviors during sleep. These include bed-wetting, sleep-walking, pavor nocturnus, nocturnal epilepsy, nocturnal asthma, and other conditions.

These disorders are described in detail elsewhere (ASDC, 1979). In general, however, clinicians should be prepared to consider the differential diagnosis of the sleep complaint, to have an understanding of the characteristic signs and symptoms of each type of disorder, and to be prepared to refer patients to a sleep disorders specialist or other appropriate physician as needed.

Indications for Referral to a Sleep Laboratory

The primary care physician can quickly and easily perform a preliminary screening evaluation of patients who complain of sleep disorders. This office evaluation, as outlined in Table 2, allows the physician to categorize and make at least a tentative diagnosis of a patient's sleep problem. Patients who are thought to have problems with excessive daytime sleepiness, nocturnal epilepsy, intractable chronic insomnia that has been refractory to preliminary pharmacological and nonpharmacological therapies (sleep hygiene maneuvers, sleep period restriction, behavioral therapies, etc.), and male impotence should be referred to a qualified sleep disorders center for evaluation. Physicians should also consider getting a sleep disorders consultation on patients whose sleeping problems may be compromising their physical condition (such as patients with heart failure and suspected sleep apnea) and for patients whose diagnosis remains uncertain after the preliminary office evaluation.

The evaluation of a patient at a sleep disorders center usually includes a complete history, physical examination, screening blood and urine analysis and toxicology, a mental status examination, optional psychological testing, polysomnography recording (with EEGs, EOGs, EMGs) and, where appropriate, a monitoring for central and peripheral sleep apnea and peripheral muscle movements. Certain patients, particularly those with complaints of disorders of excessive daytime sleepiness, may require special daytime sleep evaluations such as the Multiple Sleep Latency Test (MSLT). In this test, the subject is given four or five different opportunities to nap during the day, for example at 10:00, 12:00, 2:00, 4:00, and 6:00. The time to fall asleep is measured polygraphically. If the subject fails to sleep within 20 minutes, the session is discontinued until the next test time. Patients with clinical excessive sleepiness will typically fall asleep within an average of five minutes or less. Normal subjects usually do not fall asleep within the first 15 minutes of the session.

Table 3 summarizes the sleep laboratory findings commonly seen with the major ASDC sleep disorders. As is illustrated by Table 3, a sleep laboratory

Table 2. Office Evaluation of the Patient with a Sleep Disorder

1. Nature, history, and duration of the complaint
2. Past history of sleep and its disorders
3. Medical history, physical examination, and laboratory tests, as indicated. Look for evidence of upper airway compromise, such as deviation of nasal system; enlargement of tonsils, adenoids, or tongue; a short, stubby neck; retrogathia; "bird-like" faces; malocclusion; obesity; impotence; head injury
4. Past and present psychiatric symptoms, diagnoses, and treatments
5. Use of prescription and nonprescription medications, sleeping pills, stimulants, nose-drops, analgesics, antihistamines, coffee, alcohol, "recreational drugs," smoking, nonpharmacological treatments, and so on
6. Detailed description of sleep habits, locations, sleeping partners, timing of sleep, napping, sleep latency, sleep duration, awakenings during sleep, bedtime and wake-up rituals, use of alarm clocks or other wake-up aids, sleeping environment, subjective satisfaction with sleep, attitudes and feelings about sleep, mental activity and concerns while in bed, expectations about sleep, bedtime rituals, exposure to light and dark
7. Evidence of unusual behavior or symptoms associated with sleep: snoring, shortness of breath, gasping, apnea, paroxysmal nocturnal dyspnea, orthopnea, enuresis, sleep-walking, night wandering, nocturnal falls, nightmares, night terrors, thrashing about and unusual movements during sleep, falling out of bed, restless legs, leg jerks, leg cramps, morning headaches, difficulty awakening, sleep paralysis, hypnogogic hallucinations, dreams, nightmares
8. Timing of sleep and wakefulness: When does patient go to bed and get up? Does patient nap either voluntarily or involuntarily? Tendencies to be "owl" or "lark"
9. Evidence of waking abnormalities possibly related to sleep–wakefulness: excessive daytime sleepiness, "dozing," fatigue, cataplexy
10. Social and occupational history, habits, exercise, diet
11. Family history of medical and psychiatric conditions, sleep patterns, excessive daytime sleepiness, sleep disorders
12. Sleep–wake diary for two weeks: bedtimes, wake-up times, sleep latency, sleep duration, number and duration of awakenings, early morning awakening, naps, involuntary sleepiness during the day, use of sleeping pills, alcohol, coffee, medications
13. Interview with bed-partner
14. Tape-recording of nocturnal respiratory sounds

consultation can provide a tremendous amount of useful information and can be a very important diagnostic tool for the referring psychiatrist.

Clinical Applications of Neurobiology

Important advances in the understanding and treatment of a variety of clinical disorders have developed through the application of neurobiological principles to these problems. Current clinical research in sleep disorders is very exciting because the field has just reached a point where basic neurobiological concepts, sleep laboratory technology, and clinical research techniques can come together to examine specific sleep problems.

SLEEP CHRONOBIOLOGY. The application of basic chronobiological principles to clinical research is currently yielding a tremendous wealth of new information. These principles, outlined earlier in this chapter, are being used to examine questions about the nature and function of sleep, depression, insominia, shift work problems, and jet lag. A particularly exciting aspect of these studies is that many of them involve treatment paradigms as part of the experiment. Preliminary studies using nonpharmacological interventions such as sleep restriction and light therapy have been shown to be beneficial for patients with insomnia and seasonal depression (Saskin et al, 1984; Rosenthal et al, 1985, Kripke et al, 1983). Saskin and colleagues (1984) have used the technique of sleep restriction to treat persistent psychophysiological insomnia. Lingjaerde and colleagues (1985) have demonstrated that patients who suffer from insomnia during the "dark period" in northern Norway can get at least some subjective relief of their symptoms with light therapy. Light therapy has also proven to be useful for the treatment of both seasonal and nonseasonal affective disorder (Rosenthal et al, 1985; Kripke et al, 1983).

Application of chronobiological principles to shift work and jet lag has not only added to our theoretical understanding of these problems but has also allowed us to develop pragmatic strategies to help individuals suffering from these syndromes. For example, shift workers can manipulate their rotations so that they phase-delay their schedule changes from days to evenings to nights and back to days in order to minimize fatigue and increase productivity and morale (Czeisler et al, 1983; Winget et al, 1984). Passengers on long transmeridian flights should expect that they will have more difficulty adjusting to time changes while traveling in an eastern direction because they must phase-advance their circadian rhythms (Winget et al, 1984). Thus, they can take this factor in account as they plan their itinerary and hopefully ease into more stressful activities.

NEUROBIOLOGY OF SLEEP DISTURBANCE IN DEPRESSION. Two important themes have emerged from sleep research in depression. First, most patients with moderate to severe depression show a state related constellation of changes in sleep architecture, such as short REM latency, elevated REM density, increased duration and REM density of the first REM period, and loss of stage 3 and 4 sleep (Gillin et al, 1979). Second, some sleep manipulations may ameliorate depression. The "sleep therapies" of depression include selective REM deprivation, partial and total sleep deprivation, and, possibly, phase advance of bedtime (Gillin, 1983; McCarley, 1982).

Several theoretical interpretations of the sleep disturbance of depression have been proposed (Gillin and Borbely, 1985). First, the sleep architecture changes may reflect an increase in cholinergic to aminergic neurotransmission in critical central synapses. As reviewed earlier, cholinergic synapses apparently trigger the onset of REM sleep. This interpretation is also consistent with the cholinergic-aminergic hypothesis of affective disordes proposed by Janowsky et al (1972).

Second, it has been hypothesized that a phase advance of the strong oscillator controlling the circadian appearance of REM sleep may be present in depression.

Table 3. Sleep Laboratory Findings in Major ASDC Disorders

ASDC[1] Disorders	Polysomnographic Findings	Apnea/EMG/Other
DIMS[2]		
Transient psycho-physiological DIMS	Decreased total sleep time Increased sleep latency	Associated with specific stressor and resolved within three weeks
Persistent psycho-physiological DIMS	Essentially normal total sleep time with possibly a slightly increased sleep latency	Patients perceive that they sleep less than they do. Patients sleep better in unfamiliar settings. Patients complain that their sleep is not refreshing
Depression A. major depression	Decreased total sleep time Decreased REM latency Decreased stages 3 and 4 Changes in REM architecture Early morning awakening	Patient with symptom complex seen in unipolar depression: decreased energy, decreased appetite, dysphoria, concentration problems
B. bipolar affective disorder, depressed	Increased total sleep time	Hyperphagia Hypersomnia Dysphoria
Anxiety	Increased sleep latency decreased total sleep	
Psychosis or mania	Increased sleep latency decreased total sleep	Acute psychotic or manic symptoms
CNS depressants A. tolerance	Decreased stages 3 and 4 sleep Decreased *REM* Increased stages 1 and 2 sleep Fragmentation of REM and NREM periods 14–18 Hz pseudospindles	
B. withdrawal	Decreased total sleep Increased REM density Increased awakenings	Nightmares, nausea cramping
CNS stimulants A. tolerance	Increased sleep latency Decreased total sleep Decreased stages 3 and 4 sleep Decreased REM	Anxiety, irrationality, paranoid thinking

Table 3. Sleep Laboratory Findings in Major ASDC Disorders (Continued)

ASDC[1] Disorders	Polysomnographic Findings	Apnea/EMG/Other
B. withdrawal	Increased total sleep time Decreased sleep latency	Daytime sleepiness Depressed mood
Alcohol		
A. tolerance	Decreased REM sleep Increased awakenings second half of the night	
B. acute withdrawal	Increased sleep onset Increased REM sleep	May have increased motor activity during sleep Irritability
C. chronic changes	Increased stage 1 sleep Decreased stage 4 sleep Increased wakefulness	
Childhood-Onset DIMS (See persistent psychophysiological DIMS)		Onset during childhood
Repeated REM sleep interruptions	Awakenings beginning with first REM and recurring in almost every subsequent REM period	Multiple awakenings during dreaming
Atypical polysomnographic features	1. Alpha waves superimposed on NREM EEG slow waves 2. Alpha intrusions	Patient complains of sleeping poorly. EMG bursts
DOES[3]		
Sleep apnea	Multiple partial arousals Decreased stages 3 and 4 sleep Increased stages 1 and 2 sleep	At least 30 apneic events lasting 10 seconds each. Complaints of unrefreshing sleep, snoring, daytime fatigue, headaches, nightsweats, or choking

		Central apnea
		  Cessation of airflow secondary to termination of the respiratory effort
		Obstructive apnea
		  Cessation of airflow, despite respiratory efforts secondary to obstruction, complete or partial
		Mixed apnea
		  Occurrence of central apnea followed by obstructive apnea; abnormal Multiple Sleep Latency Test

Table 3. Sleep Laboratory Findings in Major ASDC Disorders (Continued)

ASDC[1] Disorders	Polysomnographic Findings	Apnea/EMG/Other
Noctural myoclonus	Decreased stages 3 and 4 sleep Increased stages 1 and 2 sleep	Repetitive anterior tibial contractions lasting .5–10 seconds and occurring in at least 3 groupings lasting minutes to hours, with each group containing at least 30 leg contractions; complaints of no sleep or unrefreshed sleep; problems with "tearing-up" the bed while asleep; daytime fatigue
Restless leg syndrome (See findings for nocturnal myoclonus)		(See findings for nocturnal myoclonus) Irresistible urge to move legs when sitting or lying down; association with motor neuron disease
Narcolepsy	Sleep-onset REM periods (within 10 minutes of sleep onset) Decreased sleep latency	Peripheral EMG activity during sleep onset; sleep-onset REM periods during Multiple Sleep Latency Test *Tetrad of Narcolepsy* excessive daytime sleepiness; cataplexy; sleep paralysis; hypnagogic hallucinations
Idiopathic CNS hypersomnolence	Normal EEG findings	Very short sleep latencies on the Multiple Sleep Latency Test
Sleep drunkenness	Increased amounts of stages 3 and 4 sleep	Initially very short sleep latencies on Multiple Sleep Latency Test which increase to normal as the day progresses
Parasomnias Somnambulism (sleepwalking)	Complex behaviors initiated during stages 3 and 4 sleep followed by EEG flattening and nonreactive EEG alpha activity	Multiple complex motor activities, usually during the first ⅓ of the night

Table 3. Sleep Laboratory Findings in Major ASDC Disorders (Continued)

ASDC[1] Disorders	Polysomnographic Findings	Apnea/EMG/Other
Pavor nocturnus incubus (night terrors)	Arousal from Stages 3 and 4 sleep with high delta waves which progress to an alpha pattern with the sleep terror attack	Usually occurs during the first $\frac{1}{3}$ of the night and is associated with perseverative motor activity; other findings include increases in heart rate and respiration, and confusion and agitation for 5–10 minutes after waking from an attack
Sleep-related enuresis	May occur in any sleep stage	Children may be confused, disoriented, and hard to arouse after an episode
Dream anxiety states (nightmares)	Patient awakens from REM sleep	Patient is oriented and can recall dream and may have some anxiety and autonomic arousal
Sleep-related epileptic seizures	Seizure activity while patient is asleep	Tonic–clonic activity may be seen on peripheral EMG; seizures usually occur during first 2 hours of sleep, or between 4–6 AM
Sleep-related bruxism	May occur in all stages of sleep but primarily in stage 2 and transition stages	Rhythmic masseter muscle activity and increased peripheral body movement
Familial sleep paralysis	Occurs at sleep–wake transitions	Decreased EMG tone Dominant trait bound to the x chromosome
Impaired penile tumescence	Reduced REM sleep erections	Decreased amount and/or frequency of penile tumescence
Sleep-related vascular headaches	Onset of headache associated with REM periods or post-REM periods	Vascular headaches which begin while asleep

[1]ASDC = Association of Sleep Disorders Centers classification committee (1979)
[2]DIMS = Disorders of initiating and maintaining sleep
[3]DOES = Disorders of excessive daytime sleepiness

The depressed patient going to bed at 11 PM has sleep architecture similar to the normal subject going to bed at 11 AM.

Third, Borbely and Wirz-Justice (1982) have proposed that the wakefulness-dependent, homeostatic processes promoting sleep are deficient in patients with depression. This accounts for the loss of stage 3 and 4 sleep and the clinical response to sleep deprivation. It is assumed that the homeostatic process promoting stage 3 and 4 sleep exerts an inhibitory effect on REM sleep, thus accounting for short REM latency in depression.

Future research will be needed to determine a) the diagnostic significance of short REM latency and other abnormalities in depression; b) the physiological mechanisms responsible for these sleep changes; and c) the clinical and theoretical significance of the sleep therapies.

NARCOLEPSY. Basic sleep research has contributed significantly to our understanding of narcolepsy. This disease is characterized by excessive daytime sleepiness, sleep attacks, cataplexy, and hypnagogic hallucinations. Patients also frequently have sleep onset REM sleep periods. Some of the narcoleptic symptoms, such as cataplexy and hypnagogic hallucinations, are components of REM sleep which irresistibly encroach on wakefulness. Moreover, considering that narcoleptic patients frequently have sleep onset REM sleep periods, it would suggest that in narcolepsy there is a dysfunction of neuronal mechanisms responsible for REM sleep. Previously, we indicated that cholinergic mechanisms played an important role in REM sleep generation. Therefore, it is possible that in narcolepsy a hyperactive central cholinergic system is responsible for the inappropriate intrusions of REM sleep into waking episodes.

FUTURE OF SLEEP RESEARCH IN PSYCHIATRY

The value of EEG sleep studies in psychiatry has been most evident in depression. Short REM latency is probably the best established biological marker in psychiatry at this time. Although it is probably not specific for depression, short REM latency is also probably not just a nonspecific correlate of anxiety, distress, or psychosis. Although it has been reported in obsessive-compulsive disorder (Insel et al, 1982), it has not been found in most studies of anxiety disorder or schizophrenia. Considerable future research will be required to determine a) the diagnostic significance of short REM latency and other sleep abnormalities in depression; b) the physiological mechanisms responsible for these sleep changes; and c) the clinical and theoretical significance of the so-called sleep therapies (REM deprivation, total and partial sleep deprivation, and altered phase position of sleep), which have been reported to have antidepressant effects.

Another direction for the future will be the psychiatrist's contribution to sleep disorders medicine. In particular, the nature, etiology, and treatment of many forms of chronic insomina remain challenging, unresolved problems. Psychiatric and psychological factors probably are involved for many of these patients, but surprisingly little systematic research by psychiatrists with a knowledge of sleep has been directed toward solving these problems.

Other major clinical problems that need to be explored include sleep and aging, particularly in reference to Alzheimer's disease, and sleep and alcoholism. In both of these disorders, sleep problems are common and extremely difficult to treat.

Finally, clinical progress must be accompanied by basic scientific progress. Although much has been learned in the past 30 years about sleep, most of the fundamental questions remain unanswered: What is sleep for? How does sleep happen? What clinical significance does sleep have?

REFERENCES

Aserinsky E, Kleitman N: Regularly occurring periods of eye motility and concomitant phenomena during sleep. Science 118:273-274, 1953

Association of Sleep Disorders Centers Classification Committee: Diagnostic classification of sleep and arousal disorders, first edition. Sleep 2:1-137, 1979

Baghdoyan HA, Monaco AP, Rodrigo-Angula ML, et al: Microinjection of neostigmine into the pontine reticular formation of cats enhances desynchronized sleep signs. J Pharmacol Exp Ther 312:173-180, 1984a

Baghdoyan HA, Rodrigo-Angula ML, McCarley RW, et al: Site-specific enhancement and suppression of desynchronized sleep signs following cholinergic stimulation of three brainstem sites. Brain Res 306:39-52, 1984b

Baker TL, Dement WC: Canine narcolepsy-cataplexy syndrome: evidence for an inherited monoaminergic-cholinergic imbalance, in Brain Mechanisms of Sleep. Edited by McGinty D, Morrison A, Drucker-Colin RR, et al. New York, Raven Press, 1984

Baxter BL: Induction of both emotional behavior and a novel form of REM sleep by chemical stimulation applied to cat mesencephalon. Exp Neuro 23:220-30, 1969

Bizzi E, Pompeiano O, Somogyi I: Spontaneous activity of single vestibular neurons of unrestrained cats during sleep and wakefulness. Arch Ital Biol 102:308-320, 1964

Bonvallet M, Allen MB: Prolonged spontaneous and evoked reticular activation following discrete bulbar lesions. Electroencephalogr Clin Neurophysiol 15: 969-988, 1963

Borbely AA, Wirz-Justice A: A two process model of sleep regulation, II: implications for depression. Human Neurobiology 1:205-210, 1982

Boyar R, Finkelstein J, Roffwarg H, et al: Synchronization of augmented luteinizing hormone secretion with sleep during puberty. N Engl J Med 287:582-586, 1972

Celesia GG, Jasper HH: Acetylcholine released from cerebral cortex in relation to state of activation. Neurology 16:1053-1064, 1966

Cohen B, Henn V: Unit activity in the pontine reticular formation associated with eye movements. Brain Res 46:403-410, 1972

Czeisler CA, Weitsmaan ED, Moore-Ede WC, et al: Human sleep: its duration and organization depend on its circadian phase. Science 210:1264-1267, 1980

Czeisler CA, Moore-Ede MC, Coleman RM: Resetting circadian clocks in man: application to sleep disorders medicine and occupational health, in Sleep/Wake Disorder: Natural History, Epidemiology and Long-Term Evaluation. Edited by Guilleminault C, Lugaresi E. New York, Raven Press, 1983

Delashaw JB, Foutz AS, Guilleminault C, et al: Cholinergic mechanisms and cataplexy in dogs. Exp Neurol 66:745-757, 1979

Eguchi K, Satoh T: Characterization of the neurons in the region of solitary tract nucleus during sleep. Physiol Behav 24:99-102, 1980

Gadea-Ciria M, Stadler H, Lloyd KG, et al: Acetylcholine release within the cat striatum during the sleep–wakefulness cycle. Nature 243:518-519, 1973

George R, Haslett WL, Jenden DJ: A cholinergic mechanism in the brainstem reticular formation: induction of paradoxical sleep. Int J Neuropharmacol 3:541-552, 1964

Gillin JC: Sleep studies in affective illness: diagnostic therapeutic and pathophysiological implications. Psychiatric Annals 13:367-384, 1983

Gillin JC, Borbely A: Sleep: a neurobiological window on affective disorders. Trends in Neuroscience 8:537-542, 1985

Gillin JC, Duncan WC, Pettigrew K, et al: Successful separation of depressed, normal, and insomniac subjects by EEG sleep data. Arch Gen Psychiatry 36:85-90, 1979

Guilleminault C, Dement WC: Sleep apnea syndromes and related sleep disorders, in Sleep Disorders, Diagnosis and Treatment. Edited by Williams RL, Karacan I. New York, John Wiley & Sons, 1978

Haranath PS, Venkatakrishna-Bhatt H: Release of acetylcholine from perfused cerebral ventricles in unanesthetized dogs during waking and sleep. Jpn J. Physiol 23:241-250, 1973

Hartman E: L-tryptophan as an hypnotic agent. Waking and 334 Sleeping, 1:155-161, 1977

Hayes RL, Pechura CM, Katayama Y, et al: Activation of pontine cholinergic sites implicated in unconsciousness following cerebral concussion in the cat. Science 223:301-303, 1984

Henley K, Morrison AD: A re-evaluation of the effects of lesions of the pontine tegmentum and locus coeruleus on phenomena of paradoxical sleep in the cat. Acta Neurobiol Exp 34:215-232, 1974

Henn V, Cohen B: Activity in eye muscle motorneurons and brainstem units during eye movements, in Basic Mechanisms of Ocular Motility and their Clinical Implications. Edited by Lennestrand C, Back-y-Rita P. Oxford, Pergamon Press, 1975

Hobson JA, Goldberg M, Vivaldi E, et al: Enhancement of desynchronized sleep signs after pontine microinjections of the muscarinic agonist bethanechol. Brain Res 275:127-136, 1983

Ibuka N, Kawamura H: Loss of circadian rhythm in sleep–wakefulness cycle in the rat by suprachiasmatic nucleus lesions. Brain Res 96:76-81, 1975

Inouye ST, Kawamura H: Persistence of circadian rhythmicity in a mammalian hypothalamic "island" containing the suprachiasmatic nucleus. Proc Nat Acad Sci 76:5962-5966, 1979

Insel TR, Gillin JC, Moore AM, et al: The sleep of obsessive-compulsive disorder patients. Arch Gen Psychiatry 39:1371-1377, 1982

Jacobs BL, Henriksen SJ, Dement WC: Neurochemical bases of the PGO wave. Brain Res 48:406-411, 1972

Janowsky DC, El-Yousef MK, Dans JM: A cholinergic-adrenergic hypothesis of mania and depression. Lancet 2:632-635, 1972

Jasper HH, Tessier J: Acetylcholine liberation from cerebral cortex during paradoxical (REM) sleep. Science 172:601-602, 1971

Jouvet M: The role of monoamines and acetylcholine-containing neurons in the regulation of the sleep-waking cycle. Ergebnisse der Physiologie 64:166-308, 1972

Kanamori N, Sakai K, Jouvet M: Neuronal activity specific to paradoxical sleep in the ventromedial medullary reticular formation of restrained cats. Brain Res 189:251-255, 1980

Katayama Y, DeWitt DS, Becker DP, et al: Behavioral evidence for a cholinoceptive pontine inhibitory area: descending control of spinal motor output and sensory input. Brain Res 296:241-262, 1984

Key BJ, Mehta VH: Change in electrocortical activity induced by the perfusion of 5-hydroxytryptamine into the nucleus of the solitary nucleus. J Neuropharmacol 16:99-106, 1977

Klemm WR: Effects of electrical stimulation of brainstem reticular formation on hippocampal theta rhythm and muscle activity in unanesthetized cervical and midbrain-transected rats. Brain Res 41:331-344, 1972

Kripke DF: Phase advance theories for affective illnesses, in Circadian Rhythms in Psychiatry: Basic and Clinical Studies. Edited by Goodwin F, Wehr T. Pacific Grove, PA, Boxwood Press, 1983

Kripke DF: Critical interval hypotheses for depression. Chronobiology International 1:73-80, 1984

Kripke DF, Risch SC, Janowsky DJ: Bright white light alleviates depression. Psychiatry Res 10:105-112, 1983

Lingjaerde O, Bratlid T, Hansen T: Insomnia during the "dark period" in northern Norway. Acta Psychiatr Scand 71:506-512, 1985

Macadar AW, Chalupa LM, Lindsley DB: Differentiation of brainstem loci which affect hippocampal and neocortical electrical activity. Exp Neurol 43:499-514, 1974

Magherini PC, Pompeiano O, Thoden U: The neurochemical basis of REM sleep: a cholinergic mechanism responsible for rhythmic activation of the vestibulo-occulomotor system. Brain Res 35:565-569, 1971

Magnes J, Moruzzi G, Pompeiano O: Synchronization of the EEG produced by low-frequency electrical stimulation of the region of the solitary tract. Arch Ital Biol 99:33-67, 1961

Magoun HW, Rhines R: An inhibitory mechanism in the bulbar reticular formation. J Neurophysiol 9:165-171, 1949

McCarley RW: REM sleep and depression: common neurobiologial control mechanisms. Am J Psychiatry 139:569-570, 1982

McGinty DJ, Harper RM: Dorsal raphe neurons: depression of firing during sleep in cats. Brain Res 101:569-575, 1976

McGinty DJ, Sterman MB: Sleep suppression after basal forebrain lesions in the cat. Science 160:1253-1255, 1968

Mergner T, Pompeiano O: Neurons in the vestibular nuclei related to saccadic eye movements in the decerebrate cat, in Control of Gaze by Brainstem Neurons. Edited by Baker R, Bertholz A. Amsterdam, Elsevier/North-Holland, 1977

Moore RY , Eichler VB: Loss of a circadian adrenal corticosterone rhythm following suprachiasmatic lesions in the rat. Brain Res 42:201-206, 1972

Morales FR, Chase MK: Intracellular recording of lumbar motorneuron membrane potential during sleep and wakefulness. Exp Neurol 62:821-827, 1978

Morrison AR, Pompeiano O: Vestibular influences during sleep, IV: Functional relations between vestibular nuclei and lateral geniculate nucleus during desynchronized sleep. Arch Ital Biol 104:425-458, 1966

Moruzzi G: The sleep–waking cycle. Ergebnisse der Physiologie 64:1-162, 1972

Moruzzi G, Magoun HW: Brain stem reticular formation and activation of the EEG. Electroencephalogr Clin Neurophsiol 1:455-473, 1949

Nauta WJ: Hypothalamic regulation of sleep in rats: an experimental study. J Neurophysiol 9:285-316, 1946

Parker DC, Rossman L, Kripke DF, et al: Endocrine rhythms across sleep–wake cycles in normal young men under basal state conditions, in Physiology in Sleep. Edited by Orem J, Barnes CD. New York, Academic Press, 1980

Parmeggiani PL: Temperature regulation during sleep: a study in homeostasis, in Physiology in Sleep. Edited by Orem J, Barnes CD. New York, Academic Press, 1980

Phillipson EA: Control of breathing during sleep. Am Rev Respir Dis 118:909-939, 1978

Pompeiano O: Mechanisms responsible for spinal inhibition during desynchronized sleep: experimental study, in Narcolepsy. Edited by Guilleminault C, Dement WC, Passouant P. New York, Spectrum Publication, 1976

Pompeiano O: Cholinergic activation of reticular and vestibular mechanisms controlling posture and eye movements, in The Reticular Formation Revisited. Edited by Hobson AJ, Brazier M. New York, Raven Press, 1980

Robinson TT, Vanderwolf CH: Electrical stimulation of the brainstem in freely moving rats, II: effects of hippocampal and neocortical electrical activity and relations to behavior. Exp Neurol 61:485-515, 1978

Rosenthal NE, Sack DA, Gillin JC, et al. Seasonal affective disorder. Arch Gen Psychiatry 41:72-80, 1984

Rosenthal NE, Sack DA, Carpenter CJ, et al: Antidepressant effects of light in seasonal affective disorder. Am J Psychiatry 142:163-170, 1985

Sakai K: Some anatomical and physiological properties of ponto-mesencephalic-tegmental neurons with special reference to the PGO waves and postural atonia during paradoxical sleep in the cat, in The Reticular Formation Revisited. Edited by Hobson JA, Brazier MR. New York, Raven Press, 1980

Sakai K: Anatomical and physiological basis of paradoxical sleep, in Brain Mechanisms of Sleep. Edited by McGinty D, Morrison A, Drucker-Colin RR, et al. New York, Spectrum, 1984

Sakai K, Touret M, Salvert D, et al: Afferents to the cat locus coeruleus as visualized by the horseradish peroxidase technique, in Interactions Between Putative Neurotransmitters in the Brain. Edited by Garattini S, Pujol JP, Samanin R. New York, Raven Press, 1978

Sakai K, Sastre JP, Slavert D, et al: Tegmento–reticular projections with special reference to the muscular atonia during paradoxical sleep: an HRP study. Brain Res 176:233-254, 1979

Saskin P, Spielman AS, Jelinn MA: sleep restriction therapy for insomnia: six month follow-up. Sleep Res 13:163, 1984

Shiromani P: Long-term cholinergic stimulation of pontine nuclei. Effects on paradoxical sleep and memory. Ph.D. Thesis: The City University of New York, 1983

Shiromani P, McGinty DJ: Pontine sites for cholinergic PGO waves and atonia: Localization and blockade with scopolamine. Soc Neurosci Abstr 9(2):1203, 1983

Shiromani P, McGinty DJ: Pontine cholinergic mechanisms in the regulation of REM sleep, in Proceedings of the 23rd International Congress of Psychology. Edited by McGaugh J. Amsterdam, Elsevier Press, 1985

Shiromani P, McGinty DJ: Pontine neuronal response to local cholinergic infusion: relation to REM sleep. Brain Res 386:20-31, 1986

Shiromani PJ, Siegel J, Tomaszewski K, et al: Alterations in blood pressure and REM sleep following pontine carbachol microinfusion. Exp Neurol 91:285-292, 1986

Siegel JM, Nienhuis R, Tomaszewski KS: Rostral brainstem contributes to medullary inhibition of muscletone. Brain Res 268:344-348, 1983

Siegel JM, Nienhuis R, Tomaszewski KS: REM sleep signs rostral to chronic transections at the pontomedullary junction. Neurosci Lett 45:241-246, 1984

Sitaram N, Gillin JC: Development and use of pharmacological probes of the CNS in man: evidence for cholinergic abnormality in primary affective illness. Biol Psychiatry 15:925-955, 1980

Sitaram N, Wyatt RJ, Dawson S, et al: REM sleep induction by physostigmine infusion during sleep in normal volunteers. Science 191:1281-1283, 1976

Sitaram N, Mendelson WB, Wyatt RJ, et al: Time dependent induction of REM sleep and arousal by physostigmine infusion during normal human sleep. Brain Res 122:565-567, 1977

Sitaram N, Moore AM, Gillin JC: Experimental acceleration and slowing of REM ultradian rhythm by cholinergic agonist and antagonist. Nature 274:490-492, 1978a

Sitaram N, Moore AM, Gillin JC: Induction and resetting of REM sleep rhythm in normal man by arecoline: blockade by scopolamine. Sleep 1:83-90, 1978b

Spiegel R: Effects of RS-86, an orally active cholinergic agonist, on sleep in man. Psychiatry Res 11:1-13, 1984

Stephan FK, Zucker I: Circadian rhythms in drinking and locomotor activity of rats are eliminated by hypothalamic lesions. Proc Nat Acad Sci 69:1583-1586, 1972

Steriade M, Ropert N, Kitsikis A, et al: Ascending activating neuronal networks in midbrain reticular core and related rostral systems, in The Reticular Formation Revisited. Edited by Hobson JA, Brazier MB. New York, Raven Press, 1980

Sterman MB, Clemente C: Forebrain inhibitory mechanisms: sleep patterns induced by basal forebrain stimulation in the behaving cat. Exp Neurol 6:103-117, 1962

Sullivan CE: Breathing in sleep, in Physiology in Sleep. Edited by Orem J, Barnes CD. New York, Academic Press, 1980

Szymusiak R, McGinty DJ: Sleep-suppression after kainic acid-induced lesions of the basal forebrain in cats. Sleep Res 14:2, 1985

Szymusiak R, McGinty DJ: Sleep-related neuronal discharge in the basal forebrain of cats. Brain Res 370:82-92, 1986

Takahashi Y, Kipnis DM, Daughaday WH: Growth hormone secretions during sleep. J Clin Invest 417:2079-2090, 1968

Thoden U, Magherini PC, Pompeiano O: Cholinergic activation of vestibular neurons leading to rapid eye movements in the mesencephalic cat. Biological Ophthalmology 82:99-108, 1972a

Thoden U, Magherini PC, Pompeiano O: Cholinergic mechanisms related to REM sleep, II: effects of an anticholinesterase on the discharge of central vestibular neurons in the decerebrate cat. Arch Ital Biol 110:260-283, 1972b

Vanderwolf CH, Robinson TE: Reticulo-cortical activity and behavior: a critique of the arousal theory and a new synthesis. Behavior and Brain Sciences 4:459-514, 1981

Vanderwolf CH, Kramis R, Robinson TE: Hippocampal electrical activity during waking behavior and sleep: analysis using centrally acting drugs, in CIBA Foundation Symposium: Functions of the Septo-Hippocampal System. Edited by Elliott K, Whelan J. Amsterdam, Elsevier, 1978

Van Dongen PA, Broekamp LE, Coola AR: Atonia after carbachol microinjections near the locus coeruleus in cats. Pharmacol Biochem Behav 8:527-532, 1978

Vertes RP: Brainstem gigantocellular neurons: patterns of activity during behavior and sleep in the freely moving rat. J Neurophysiol 42:224-228, 1979

Vertes RP: Brainstem activation of the hippocampus: a role for the magnocellular reticular formation and the MLF. Electroencephalogr Clin Neurophysiol 50:48-58, 1980

Winget CM, DeReschia CW, Markley CL: A review of human physiological and performance changes associated with dysynchronosis of biological rhythms. Aviat Space Environ Med 55:1685-1696, 1984

Winson J: Interspecies differences in the occurrence of theta. Behavioral Biology 7:479-487, 1972

Wyatt RJ: The serotonin-catecholamine dream bicycle: a clinical study. Biol Psychiatry 5:33-63, 1972

Chapter 11

X-Ray Computed Tomography and Magnetic Resonance Imaging in Psychiatry

by George E. Jaskiw, M.D., Nancy C. Andreasen, M.D., Ph.D., and Daniel R. Weinberger, M.D.

Modern psychiatry was born approximately 100 years ago during the mid- to late-19th century. It was fathered by the general field of medicine, and neurology was its dizygotic twin. Both psychiatry and neurology were interested in the brain and the mind, and in how aberrations of either could lead to abnormalities in speech, emotional expression, motoric behavior, and cognitive function. The discipline that we now call neuroscience was then simply called "brain science," and it was clear that psychiatrists were brain scientists and that their major goals were to identify the neural substrates of mental illness and pharmacologic methods for healing them. In this milieu Kraepelin built one of the strongest departments of psychiatry. Under his leadership, Nissl, Brodmann, and Alzheimer were actively engaged in searching for various types of structural abnormalities in patients suffering from mental illness. Alzheimer was perhaps the most successful, in that he was able to identify a disease with its own specific neuropathology. But two other new diseases discovered by Kraepelin's department, dementia praecox and manic-depressive illness, were also extensively studied, although with somewhat less success.

Some time during the 20th century psychiatry and neurology developed an amnestic disorder which caused these facts to be forgotten. Instead, the notion of seeking for the causes of mental illness in brain structure seemed ludicrous and oversimplified. Evidence that had accumulated concerning neuropathological causes of schizophrenia and manic-depressive illness was conflicting rather than incisively convincing. As radiologic techniques developed, a few pneumoencephalographers attempted to look for abnormalities in anatomical structure in the brains of patients suffering from schizophrenia and perhaps observed some, but these studies were difficult to interpret because of the lack of appropriate controls (Storey, 1966). By 1960 or 1970, most psychiatrists were saying "we study the mind, while neurologists study the brain." Neither psychiatrists nor neurologists had much interest in asking whether structural brain abnormalities might occur in mental illness. When people did think about the causes of mental illness in terms of brain function, they assumed that they must be chemical or electrical.

The seminal work of Norman Geschwind had an important effect on refocusing our interest in the importance of brain structure (Geschwind and Levitsky, 1968). His imaginative studies of the asymmetry of the planum temporale reaffirmed the fact that brain function could be rooted in anatomy as well as chemistry and that in fact the two are intimately interrelated. Geschwind's work demonstrated that the primacy of human language function in the left hemisphere has a clear and consistently observed anatomic substrate that can be visualized in the neuroanatomy lab: the planum temporale is substantially larger on the left side, presumably because it has a much larger concentration of neurons dedicated to language perception and processing and because there is no corresponding language center on the right. Geschwind's discovery permitted a paradigm shift in our perceptions about what is interesting and permissible to research. Once again, one could with self-respect attempt to understand brain function through studying brain structure. One might be accused of being an "endophrenologist," but at least not a phrenologist.

Thus, when brain imaging techniques became available during the 1970s and 1980s, they fell on fallow soil. The relevance of dynamic techniques such as PET or regional blood flow was immediately evident, but the importance of structural techniques such as computerized tomography (CT) and nuclear magnetic resonance imaging (NMRI) was also obvious to many. The past few years of work in brain imaging have been productive and exciting, and the future years are likely to be even more so. While other chapters will review work done with the various dynamic techniques, this chapter will focus on the contributions of structural techniques.

COMPUTERIZED TOMOGRAPHY STUDIES

The modern search for brain abnormalities began in earnest shortly after the turn of this century. Investigations of brain structure, previously confined to gross and microscopic examination of post-mortem tissue, entered a new phase with the development of pneumoencephalography (PEG). Air could be injected into the lumbar space and the patient so positioned that the air migrated to the cerebrum and provided sufficient contrast on x-ray to allow delineation of air-fluid/tissue boundaries. An in vivo image of the inner and outer contours of the brain was thus produced. While promising, the application of the new technique to psychiatric research foundered on several methodological obstacles. Despite the nosological advances of Kraepelin and Bleuler, delineation of discrete psychiatric populations remained problematic. The latter, coupled with the difficulty of performing a potentially painful procedure on sufficient numbers of controls to establish normal standards, contributed to often inconsistent findings. Since no reproducible physical 'lesion' could be demonstrated in major psychiatric illnesses, they were held to be 'functional' rather than 'organic.' A combination of tautological reasoning and unfortunate terminology led to a premature, general discreditation of structural brain studies in psychiatry; the latter was in keeping with the prevailing skepticism of biological approaches to mental illness.

Discoveries through the 1950s of pharmacologic agents that could improve symptoms of mental illness marked the renaissance of neuroscience in psychiatry. The early research emphasis, however, was on a search for chemical imbalances that were thought to reflect pathophysiology at a microcellular level, a pathophysiology that was not expected to be reflected in structural changes. This unfortunate dichotomization of structure and function, often assumed but poorly substantiated, continued to limit psychiatry's neuroscientific field of study.

The road out of this quandary was paved by a dramatic technological advance in clinical radiology. The latter had been confined to interpreting *two*-dimensional images made with the x-ray source, the subject, and the detector aligned and fixed for the duration of each exposure. Spatial relationships were estimated by making exposures from different angles (for example, PA and lateral views of the chest), which the trained clinician would mentally combine to derive a three-dimensional image in the mind's eye. The advent of sophisticated computers capable of solving many simultaneous equations allowed information from multiple exposures made of a subject from different angles to be displayed in a single reconstructed image reflecting a cross-section or 'slice' of the subject. The development of computerized axial tomography (CT or CAT) in the early 1970s revolutionized the clinical investigation of brain disease. The new technique provided detailed, undistorted in-vivo images of gross cerebral structure, and was relatively noninvasive, painless, and quick; as such it was ideally suited for the study of psychiatric and control populations. Its utility in research as well as clinical practice was perceived swiftly.

Changes of comparable importance had been taking place in psychiatry. By the early 1970s standards were established that allowed greater consensual definition of psychiatric populations. Diagnostic schedules, rating scales, emphasis on 'blind' ratings, insistence on controls, and emphasis on possible placebo effects were products of the demand for increased scientific rigor in psychiatric research. These methodological advances, as much as the technological breakthrough of CT scanning, launched the brain imaging era in clinical neuroscience.

In 1976, Johnstone and colleagues reported that a small group of elderly, chronic schizophrenic patients had significantly larger lateral ventricles than a sex- and age-matched control group (Johnstone et al, 1976). Since that time, over 100 articles based on some 40 CT scan investigations have been published about schizophrenia alone. Some of the findings are more robust than others. To review this information, we will first delineate the general areas of investigation; second, we will consider possible sources of variance in the data; and third, we will assess the contributions of CT findings to the understanding of psychiatric illness.

Positive CT findings in psychiatric populations fall into six categories: lateral ventricular enlargement, third ventricular enlargement, cerebellar atrophy, widening of cortical fissures/sulci, reversed cerebral asymmetries, and brain density abnormalities. Inconsistencies in the results of studies appear to be traceable to differences in CT methodology, patient selection, and control group selection. The most robust CT research finding in psychiatry so far is enlargement of the lateral ventricles in schizophrenia, and these concerns are best discussed in relation to it.

Lateral Ventricular Enlargement

In their comprehensive review, Shelton and Weinberger (1986) note that of CT studies assessing lateral ventricular size in schizophrenic patients, about 75 percent demonstrated significant enlargement compared to a control group. Figure 1 is taken from one such study (Weinberger et al, 1979a), and illustrates the distribution for the VBR (ventricular–brain ratio), one index of lateral ventricular size. Several points should be noted. The ranges of values for the patient and control groups overlap. There are many patients with a VBR in the control group range. However, there are few controls with VBRs in the upper range of the schizophrenic group. The impression is that the distribution of the VBRs of the patient group is elongated and shifted upwards compared to the control group. While most radiologists will not classify a CT scan "read" off a viewing box as definitely abnormal until the VBR exceeds approximately 25 percent, even the high VBRs in the patient group in Figure 1 do not exceed a value of 20 percent. In other words, in the routine subjective evaluation of CT scans, individual patients with schizophrenia in Figure 1 would not be firmly separated from the control group on the basis of a difference in lateral ventricular size. To phrase it another way, enlargement of the ventricles in schizophrenia is detected as a quantitative *group* effect. Discussion of significant differences is confined to the *mean* ventricular size. It will be detected consistently only in appropriate groups of patients when quantitative techniques are employed.

These features render the results of CT studies particularly sensitive to variance, whether due to measurement techniques, patient selection, or control group selection. CT machines *per se* can differ in the images they produce. In addition, by changing a given CT scan's imaging parameters, the operator can modify the resulting image (Jernigan et al, 1979; Zatz and Alvarez, 1977; McCullough, 1977). Both machine and operator variance can be reduced within

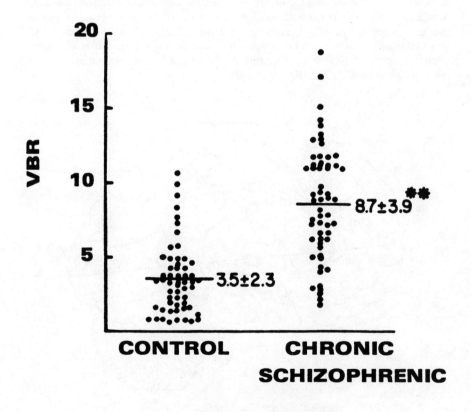

Figure 1. Distribution of ventricular brain ratio (from Weinberger et al, 1979a)

studies by employing the same operator and CT scanner for all patients and controls.

The use of different techniques to quantify ventricular enlargement can generate measurement variance. The simplest techniques are linear; they rely on a single measure or a ratio of measures, usually of the distance between corresponding points on each lateral ventricle (Evans, 1942; Hansson et al, 1975; Huckman et al, 1975), determined on the CT scan slice, where the latter are most prominent (see Figures 2, 3a, and 3b). The sensitivity of the linear techniques has been called into question (Huckman et al, 1975). The latter may account for the inconsistent CT findings when such measures are used (Shelton and Weinberger, 1986). The commonly employed VBR (ventricular–brain ratio) measures the area of the lateral ventricles relative to the area of the brain, on the CT scan slice where the area of lateral ventricles is maximal. Area can be determined manually by tracing the boundaries of brain parenchyma and ventricles, either with an engineering instrument called a planimeter (Synek and Reuben, 1976), or with a computer linked cursor (Andreasen et al, 1982b). VBR can also be determined densitometrically by programming a computer to read certain radiodensities on a CT image as corresponding to tissue, others as fluid, and summing their contributions (Jernigan et al, 1982). In general, empirical studies suggest that area measures are more sensitive than linear ones and correlate well with ventricular volume (Penn et al, 1978; Jernigan et al, 1979). Ventricular size has also been quantified by densitometric estimation of total ventricular volume (TVV) (Reveley, 1985).

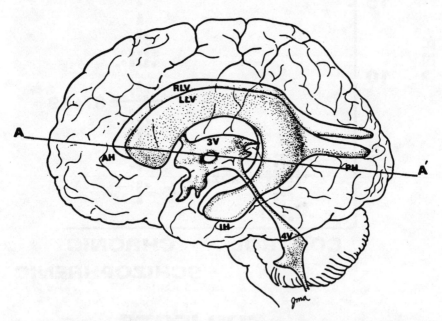

Figure 2. Schematic representation of cerebral ventricular system. CT images correspond to brain sections cut along planes at a 15-degree angle to the orbitomeatal line. Line A–A' marks one such plane.

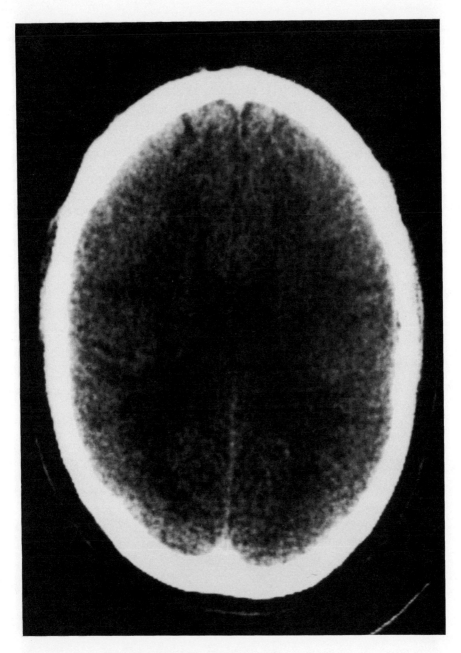

Figure 3a. CT scan with ventricular–brain ratio = 3.1

There is little question that different methods of measurement give different absolute values for certain indices. Jernigan and colleagues noted that two independent groups using the same set of scans differed twofold in their absolute

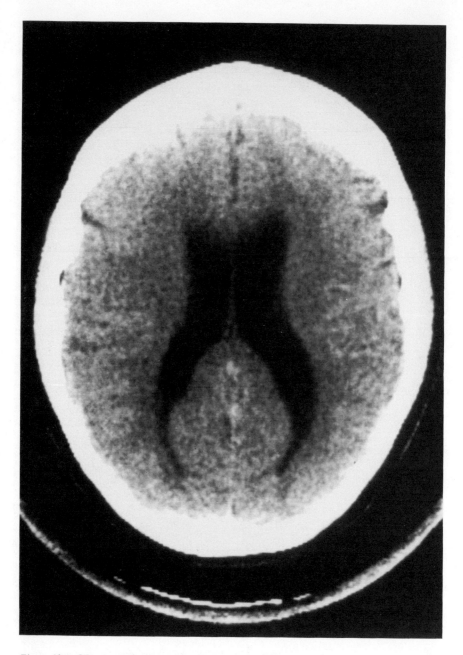

Figure 3b.   CT scan with ventricular–brain ratio = 11.6

estimation of mean VBR (Jernigan et al, 1982). Their study may have exaggerated this problem, however, because the two groups acknowledged using different modifications of the VBR method. While Reveley reported that several quantitative methods were able to separate the mean lateral ventricular size of a given group of schizophrenic patients from that of controls at the same level of significance (Reveley, 1985), a volumetric technique was most sensitive. In support of this, Raz and colleagues have found that a volumetric technique demonstrated significant lateral ventricular enlargement in a group of patients, where manual planimetric techniques had earlier shown no difference (manuscript in submission). Thus, a more sensitive measure of ventricular volume may have converted a false-negative study into a positive one. In general, while all methods are approximations of relative ventricular volume, their insensitivity militates for their *under*estimating subtle differences between patient and control groups.

The latter bias applies to control group selection as well. Controls should be at least age- and sex-matched with the patient group. Table 1 lists some of the conditions which have been associated with atrophic changes on CT scan. Yet some investigators have used for controls CT scans in radiology files, of migraine patients, patients undergoing chemotherapy for malignancy, and patients from general medical wards and clinics. Even if exclusionary criteria such as absence of positive signs on a routine neurological exam and lack of gross pathology on head CT scan are added, the use of such 'medical' controls may be a potential source of type I error, that is, failing to find a difference that exists. Dennert and Andreasen raised the opposite possibility that use of such radiology file 'normals' may, by excluding all patients with mildly enlarged ventricles, lower the mean VBR of the control group (Dennert and Andreasen, 1983). On the

Table 1. Conditions Associated with Signs of General Atrophy on CT Scan[1]

Neurological	Medical
Epilepsy	Nutritional deficiencies
Migraine	Cushing's disease
Parkinsons's disease	Systemic steroids
Huntington's disease	Intoxications:
Wilson's disease	alcohol
Post-encephalitic states	solvent
Multiple sclerosis	heavy metal
Alzheimer's disease	Radiation exposure
Multi-infarct dementia	Malignancy
Head injury	Cytotoxic drugs
Systemic lupus erythematosus	Birth complications
	Dialysis
Other	
Normal aging	Psychiatric
	Schizophrenia
	Affective disorders
	Anorexia nervosa
	Obsessive compulsive disorder

[1]Adapted from Shelton and Weinberger (1986)

other hand, Shelton and Weinberger note that of studies using medical or neurological controls, only four of eight (50 percent) showed a difference in lateral ventricular size between a group of schizophrenic patients and controls, whereas seven of eight (88 percent) studies relying on normal volunteers were positive (Shelton and Weinberger, 1986). In a group of schizophrenic patients studied by Doran and colleagues, significant lateral ventricular enlargement was demonstrated with respect to normal volunteers but not with respect to medical controls (Doran et al, 1985). Ideally true normals should be used for controls when possible.

Since measurement techniques and control selection both bias against detection of subtle differences in mean ventricular size, it is all the more remarkable that about 75 percent of all studies do find such differences between controls and patients with schizophrenia. The number rises to over 90 percent when studies using relatively insensitive indices of lateral ventricular size, non-rigorously diagnosed patient groups, or medical/neurological controls are excluded. As has been mentioned, lateral ventricular enlargement is consistently detected by comparing *mean* measures of ventricular volume of patient and control groups. Investigators have tried, in addition, to establish standards by which an *individual* measure of ventricular size could be classified as abnormal. Weinberger and colleagues suggested that 2 SD above the mean of a normal group marks a cutoff point above which a given VBR could be considered enlarged, and using manual planimetric techniques found the cutoff in their original study to correspond to a VBR value around 8.3 percent (Weinberger et al, 1979a). Studies based on different controls found cutoff points ranging from 5.8 percent (Barron et al, 1976) to 10.6 percent (Andreasen et al, 1982b). As Andreasen and associates have commented, depending on which of these cutoff points are used, the prevalence of lateral ventricular enlargement in a given patient population with schizophrenia may range from 6 to 62 percent (Andreasen et al, 1982b). Given that significant intergroup differences in measurement of VBR have been demonstrated, such cutoff points should never be used to guide clinical decisions, while their use in research must be viewed with caution. Whatever the cutoff point used, however, in most rigorous studies there are significantly fewer normal controls than patients with VBRs above the cutoff point. While it is not uncommon for a patient with schizophrenia to have a VBR in the "normal" range, it is highly unusual for a normal control to have a VBR greater than two standard deviations above the mean for the group. The latter bears directly on discussion of the implications of brain imaging findings.

Several controlled studies have failed to demonstrate significant lateral ventricular enlargement in schizophrenic patients. The negative results may be due to the patient sample used, a third source of variance. The latter results when a population is not homogeneous as far as the prevalence or degree of some measured variable is concerned, but is treated as homogeneous for sample selection purposes. There have been many subtypes proposed for the schizophrenic syndrome, some based on symptoms, others on illness course, treatment response, or family history. If the prevalence or degree of lateral ventricular enlargement is distributed unevenly, or segregates with certain clinical features, then depending on patient selection a difference may or may not be found between a patient group and a control population. Indeed in their original population, Johnstone and colleagues found (Johnstone et al, 1976), and in a followup study confirmed (Johnstone et al, 1978), that the degree of lateral ventricular enlargement correlated positively with some measures of cognitive impairment. The preponderance of subsequent studies support such a relationship (Donnelly et al, 1980; Golden et al, 1980a, 1980c, 1982; Andreasen et al, 1982a; Pandurangi et al, 1986). Johnstone and colleagues also reported that "negative symptoms" were more likely to occur in those patients with larger ventricles and cognitive deficits (Johnstone et al, 1976), thus linking a neuroanatomic finding with deficits on psychological testing and with clinical features. While many associations between CT findings, clinical symptoms, and other variables have been reported, most of the correlations are less robust than those linking lateral ventricular enlargement and cognitive impairment. The exception is the general trend for lateral ventricular enlargement to correlate positively with other measures associated with greater dysfunction (see Table 2). These include poor premorbid social adjustment (Williams et al, 1985; Weinberger et al, 1980b; Andreasen et al, 1982c; DeLisi et al, 1983) and poor outcome (Weinberger et al, 1980b; Andreasen et al, 1982c; DeLisi et al, 1983; Luchins and

Table 2. Some Reported Associations with Lateral Ventricular Enlargement in Patients with Schizophrenia

Associations	Studies
Neuropsychological impairment	Donnelly et al, 1980
	Golden et al, 1980a, 1980c, 1981, 1982
Poor premorbid adjustment	Williams et al, 1985
	Weinberger et al, 1980b
	Andreasen et al, 1982c
	DeLisi et al, 1983
Poor outcome	DeLisi et al, 1983
	Andreasen et al, 1982c
	Pearlson et al, 1985
	Kolakowska et al, 1985
More suicide	Levy et al, 1984
	Nasrallah et al, 1984
Poor neuroleptic response	Luchins et al, 1983b, 1984
	Weinberger et al, 1980a
	Schulz et al, 1983
More neuroleptic induced EPS	Luchins et al, 1983a, 1983b
More tardive dyskinesia	Albus et al, 1985
Less positive symptoms	Luchins et al, 1984
	Andreasen et al, 1982c
	Weinberger et al, 1980a
More negative symptoms	Williams et al, 1985
	Pearlson et al, 1985
	Andreasen et al, 1982a
	Kleinman et al, 1984

Meltzer, 1986; Pearlson et al, 1984a, 1985). Indeed, in a recent study where chronically hospitalized schizophrenic patients were *matched* for *age* and *illness duration* with acutely admitted patients, the chronic group had significantly greater lateral ventricular enlargement and spent a significantly greater percentage of time in hospital than the acute group (Luchins and Meltzer, 1986). Careful, controlled studies may not detect mean lateral ventricular enlargement in groups of patients selected from the "healthier" end of the spectrum, either because such patients as a group do not have it, or because current measurement techniques are too crude to detect very subtle differences. In the negative study by Benes and colleagues (1982), patients in a private psychiatric hospital were evaluated. Whether the latter biased the study is unclear. A subsequent study in the same hospital did find larger ventricles in another group of schizophrenic patients (Woods and Wolf, 1983). The negative results of Jernigan and colleagues (1982) are more problematic. It is possible that the exclusion of patients with abnormal neurological examinations and neuropsychological profiles may have reduced the fraction of more chronic patients.

It is close to an established fact that at least a subgroup of patients with schizophrenia have lateral ventricular enlargement compared to normal controls. Evidence also supports the contention that this finding cannot be explained by treatment. Most investigators find no relationship between degree of lateral ventricular enlargement and electroconvulsive therapy (ECT), total length of institutionalization, or cumulative neuroleptic dose (Shelton and Weinberger, 1986). More conclusively, ventricular enlargement has been reported in outpatients after little or no treatment (Weinberger et al, 1982; Schulz et al, 1984; Nyback et al, 1982). Age does appear to correlate positively with lateral ventricular size in the normal population, but the overwhelming majority of studies do not support such a relationship in patients with schizophrenia. If anything, the findings that mean ventricular size is increased early in the course of illness (Weinberger et al, 1982; Schulz et al, 1984; Nyback et al, 1982) and does not correlate with illness duration, suggest little if any progression of the process once the illness has manifested itself. The latter is supported by a preliminary study of a small group of schizophrenic patients, in which no significant change in mean VBR was found three years after the initial CT evaluation (Nasrallah et al, 1986).

Less conclusive results have emerged from studies of patients with unipolar, bipolar, or schizoaffective illness. Some investigators have found a degree of lateral ventricular enlargement comparable to that seen in schizophrenic patients (Pearlson et al, 1985; Luchins and Meltzer, 1983; Standish-Barry et al, 1982; Johnstone et al, 1981; Scott et al, 1983; Rieder et al, 1983); others have failed to do so. Differences in methodology, control population, and patient samples may account for much of the variance between studies. Several tentative conclusions may be reached, however. It seems that at least some groups of affectively ill patients cannot be separated on the basis of mean lateral ventricular size from patients with schizophrenia; both groups have significant enlargement compared to controls. As in schizophrenia, those among the affectively ill patients with the largest lateral ventricles appear to have a more severe or chronic form of the illness (Pearlson et al, 1985; Scott et al, 1983; Rieder et al, 1983; Targum et al, 1983; Jacoby et al, 1981; Luchins and Meltzer, 1983; Pearlson et al, 1984b). Unlike the schizophrenic process, age and duration of illness may have a significant effect on ventricular size in affective illness, suggesting that the causes of the CT findings in these psychiatric disorders may be different.

Third Ventricular Enlargement

Of the dozen studies in patients with schizophrenia, approximately 80 percent have found significant third ventricular enlargement compared to controls. Interestingly, as other reviewers have noted (Shelton and Weinberger, 1986), this high percentage of positive studies persists even in the subgroup of 10 studies that employed medical or neurological controls. Moreover, in one of these studies the group of patients with schizophrenia had significantly larger third ventricles but not lateral ventricles than a group of medical controls, several of whom also had some ventricular dilatation, perhaps secondary to medical illness (Boronow et al, 1985). These observations have led some investigators to suggest that third ventricular enlargement may be a more specific finding (Shelton and Weinberger, 1986) in schizophrenia.

The relationship between other variables and third ventricular enlargement is more complicated. While two studies demonstrated an age effect (Schulz et al, 1983; Nyback et al, 1982), three failed to do so (Boronow et al, 1985; Moriguchi, 1981; Shelton et al, 1985). A correlation of ventricular enlargement with illness duration and number of hospitalizations was found in four studies (Nyback et al, 1982; Gattaz et al, 1981; Shelton et al, 1985; Tanaka et al, 1981) but not seen in two (Moriguchi et al, 1984; Boronow et al, 1985). Findings have also been mixed as to the correlation of third ventricular enlargement with lateral ventricular enlargement. They have been found both together and independently. It has been proposed that patients with enlargement of both lateral and third ventricles comprise the most chronic subgroup of patients. Given the limited number of studies, it can be concluded that enlargement of the third ventricle does occur in patients with schizophrenia, but the relationship of this finding to other variables needs to be investigated further.

Cortical Surface Fissures/Sulci

Cortical fissures and sulci separate adjacent lobes and gyri of the brain, respectively. In several of the conditions listed in Table 1, fissures and sulci have been observed to become wider, deeper, and more prominent on CT scan. As was the case for lateral ventricles, several methods have been developed to quantify subtle changes in these surface markings. The simplest involves measuring the width of fissures and sulci. Investigators have differed in their selection. A second but also technically simple method involves visually assessing the prominence of cortical surface markings on CT scans and ranking them, either in relation to one another or according to some predetermined atrophy scale. In the densitometric method, a cutoff pixel density is assigned, and a computer program reads and sums all the areas below the cutoff density as fluid space and everything above the cutoff as tissue.

In a series of CT scan studies in schizophrenia reviewed previously (Shelton and Weinberger, 1986), 16 of 22 (73 percent) concluded that the patient sample had significantly increased surface markings compared to controls. When only studies using normal controls were considered, seven of eight (89 percent) were positive. The positive study of Doran and colleagues (1985) suggests that the use of medical controls can lead to a false-negative result. Taken together, the evidence strongly suggests that at least in some populations, increased cortical surface markings are associated with schizophrenia.

While the degree of enlargement of surface markings does seem to increase with age in normal individuals (Jacoby and Levy, 1980a) and in some with Alzheimer's disease (Fox et al, 1975; Jacoby and Levy 1980b), most studies find no such age effect in patients with schizophrenia (Schulz et al, 1984; Moriguchi, 1981; Weinberger et al, 1979b; Nasrallah et al, 1983). Several studies have found no correlation between widening of surface markings and illness duration (Weinberger et al, 1979b; Nasrallah et al, 1983). Overall, the number of reported attempts to correlate surface markings with cumulative medication dose, history of institutionalization, and ECT has been small. Further studies are needed. The same can be said of reports that degree of atrophy correlates with clinical features such as severity of illness, neuroleptic response, presence of positive versus negative symptoms. Two studies have suggested that patients with increased surface markings are more likely to manifest impairments on neuropsychological assessment (Weinberger et al, 1979b; Nasrallah et al, 1983).

Recent developments in the investigation of cortical markings suggest that the underlying pathology may be localizable. Several groups have reported selective widening of surface markings in the frontal cortex, with little or no widening of such markings in parieto-occipital areas (Boronow et al, 1985; Dewan et al, 1983; Pandurangi et al, 1984; Takahashi et al, 1981). Oxenstierna and colleagues (1984) reported that of their 10 patients with positive findings, four had significant widening of surface markings confined to the dorsolateral prefrontal cortex. The latter is an area where differences between controls and patients with schizophrenia have been demonstrated in electroencephalogram (EEG) (Morihisa and McAnulty, 1985) and cerebral blood flow studies (Weinberger et al, 1986; Berman et al, 1986). Shelton and colleagues found similar results in a large population of young patients compared to normal controls (Shelton and Weinberger, 1986). Corroborating data have recently been reported by Doran and colleagues (1985). Available evidence suggests, then, that widening of cortical surface markings is not only a robust group finding in patients with schizophrenia, but may have some localizing value.

There have been a few studies reporting increased cortical surface markings in affectively ill patients, but possible confounding factors (for example, alcohol use) have not been adequately evaluated. No study so far has demonstrated selective changes in the prefrontal region of this population.

Cerebellar Changes

Nestled in the posterior fossa, the cerebellum is relatively more difficult to assess by CT scan than the cerebrum. Measures of cerebellar CT changes have included visual assessments of atrophy, determination of fourth ventricular dimensions, and densitometric evaluation. The comparative sensitivity of these various approaches awaits clarification. Differences in measures, in control population, and in sample selection make comparisons between the limited studies difficult. The reported prevalence of cerebellar atrophy has ranged from 0 to 50 percent. Most studies cluster in the range of 5 to 17 percent (Shelton and Weinberger, 1986), seemingly higher than the 1 percent reported in large studies of general CT evaluated patients. In agreement with neuropathologic studies (Weinberger et al, 1980c; Luchins et al, 1981), most atrophy is seen around the area of the vermis. In at least one study of schizophreniform patients, vermian atrophy was not observed (Coffman et al, 1981).

It is known that cerebellar atrophy can result from drugs and some of the conditions listed in Table 1. Until confounding variables such as illness duration, cumulative neuroleptic dose, and others are evaluated, the finding of cerebellar changes in patients with schizophrenia is difficult to interpret.

Cerebral Asymmetry

Neuropathological and CT scan data suggest that most right handed individuals have subtle but significant right–left asymmetries of cerebral lobes; the right frontal is larger than the left frontal lobe, while the left occipital is larger than the right occipital lobe (Luchins et al, 1981). A small number of right handed individuals have reversed cerebral asymmetry; that is, larger left frontal and right occipital lobes. Cerebral asymmetry has been linked to the lateralization of cerebral functions. Language and handedness are probably the two most intensively studied lateralized skills, and indeed increased frequency of reversed asymmetry has been reported in disorders such as dyslexia (Hier et al, 1978b) and autism (Hier et al, 1978a), where development of language and motor dominance is often atypical. Asymmetry may be quantified by measuring the width of the frontal and occipital lobes on single CT cuts where they are most prominent, or by averaging their widths over several slices.

Of some 10 studies on patients with schizophrenia, only four reported increased frequency of reversed cerebral asymmetry (Shelton and Weinberger, 1986). Given that comparative sensitivities of measurement techniques are unknown, that most studies did not use normal controls, and that patients differed with respect to age and length of hospitalization, it is difficult to draw a firm conclusion. However, it is clear that some authors employed relatively sensitive measures, adequate sample and control groups, and failed to find significant cerebral asymmetry in schizophrenic patients (Andreasen et al, 1982). The status of cerebral asymmetry as a finding in schizophrenic patients is still unclear.

Brain Density

A CT scan maps radiodensity, expressed as x-ray attenuation values, which are in turn related to tissue density. A computer can be programmed to sum up the attenuation values of pixels in a specified area of the image and provide an estimate of the relative density of the corresponding tissue. In research studies, some investigators have sampled every "nth" pixel in a given area of a CT scan slice; others have summed all the pixel attenuation values within a specified area of a lobe or within an entire lobe on a given slice. Since attenuation values depend very much on machine type and x-ray energy and are particularly liable to distortion by bone, there has been considerable controversy about this technique in general. In particular, some of the earlier studies (Golden et al, 1980b; Lyon et al, 1981; Golden et al, 1981) assessed attenuation values over areas without differentiating tissue from ventricles, sulci and fissures, and were open to the charge that their measurements reflected the volumes of fluid filled spaces, rather than parenchymal densities.

Of early studies on patients with schizophrenia, one (Golden et al, 1980b) reported general decrease in tissue density at all levels, while two (Lyon et al, 1981; Golden et al, 1981) reported decreased density only in the left anterior frontal lobe. Later studies, performed with some of the earlier criticisms in mind, produced inconclusive findings. Largen and colleagues (1983) reported a trend for *increased* density in the right hemisphere of patients, but later found that this was not upheld by a conservative statistical analysis (Largen et al, 1984). Kanba reported *decreased* density bilaterally in frontal and occipital areas of patients (Kanba et al, 1984). The findings of Coffman and colleagues (1984) suggest a relative *decreased* density of the left cerebral hemisphere, while Dewan and associates (1983) found periventricular *increased* density, but no cortical differences between patients and controls. Given the few studies, their methodological limitations, and their differences, the disparate findings are not surprising. It is of concern that increases and decreases in density are hardly of equivalent meaning, yet both have been reported in schizophrenic patients.

To help resolve some of the contradictory findings Jacobson and colleagues undertook a systematic study of artefacts in densitometric studies (Jacobson et al, 1985). Density values appeared to be quite sensitive to the "beam hardening effect" resulting from the selective absorption of the lower energy X-rays by bone. In practical terms, skull size may have a highly significant effect on attenuation values for brain tissue. In addition, the algorithm which allows the reconstruction of a CT image from attenuation values may overcorrect for differences in skull shape, resulting in large hypodensity artefacts on the scan. The authors also found that attenuation values corresponding to a given tissue density tended to drift upwards over time; that is, the scanning system may be unstable over time, especially in the early years of use. The artefacts studied could give rise to changes in densitometric values, on the same order of magnitude as reported significant differences between patients and controls.

A recent study which considered many of these problems reported increased density in most cortical areas in those schizophrenics with enlarged lateral ventricles (Dewan et al, 1986). Further careful controlled studies and refinements in technique may establish whether and in what areas brain density differences between psychiatric patients and controls exist.

Summary

The CT scan is an instrument that provides in-vivo information about gross brain structure. Its use as a research tool for studying groups of psychiatric patients has led to a number of reported findings and associations, some better established than others. Disparate conclusions may be accounted for by differences in methodology, sample selection, and choice of control group. As a group, schizophrenic patients have enlargement of the lateral and third ventricles and of some cortical surface markings. The latter may be especially prominent in the frontal cortex. The findings are group phenomena, not in the sense that all of them invariably coexist, but in that their prevalence and degree are consistently different in patient and control groups. Such findings are subtle and would not be recognized on routine evaluation of a CT scan, but require special measurement techniques and appropriate control groups for detection. The degree of enlargement of the lateral ventricles and cortical surface markings appears to correlate with some indices of illness severity or dysfunction, but this too is a group phenomenon. In a given patient with suspected schizophrenia, the presence or absence of such CT findings is of no diagnostic or prognostic value. Cerebellar atrophy, cerebral asymmetry, and differences in brain density have also been studied in patients with schizophrenia, but findings have so far been inconclusive.

Some groups of patients with affective illness also appear to have enlargement of the lateral ventricles. The latter may be associated with a chronic course and poor prognosis. The independence of these findings from treatment artifact is unclear.

MAGNETIC RESONANCE IMAGING STUDIES

The application of nuclear magnetic resonance imaging (MRI) to psychiatry is in its infancy, or at least in its early childhood. This imaging modality has only been available since the mid-1980s. It has already become clear that MRI has many advantages that may lead to its eventually supplanting CT. The visual reconstruction of the human brain obtained with MRI is so clear that the pictures resemble slices of preserved brain. Excellent gray-white resolution is obtained. Further, unlike CT, MRI gives good visualization in the sagittal and coronal planes, in addition to the transverse plane. In a neuroanatomy lab, one can only slice the brain in one plane, but MRI permits a complete three-dimensional reconstruction. Further, it permits anatomical studies that bypass many of the problems inherent in postmortem studies, such as the examination of patients relatively late in life (making it difficult to disentangle the effects of the aging process, end-stage disease processes, preservation artifacts, and so on). Further, these anatomical studies can be done in human beings who can be simultaneously interviewed about the symptoms that they are experiencing. The procedure is essentially risk-free and does not require the use of ionizing radiation, thereby permitting repeated scans. Contraindications are relatively few and include primarily the presence of pacemakers and some types of aneurysm clips.

Figure 4 indicates the quality of image that can be obtained with MRI. It is a midsagittal cut. As the figure indicates, one can identify major sulci, such as the central sulcus that separates the frontal from the parietal lobes. The cingulate gyrus is well defined, as are the corpus callosum, the thalamus, the fornix, and other major brain structures.

Principles of Magnetic Resonance Imaging

Unlike CT, which relies on the attenuation of x-rays passing through tissues to generate an image, magnetic resonance imaging is relatively complicated and depends on a number of different parameters (Young, 1984; Bloch, 1946; Purcell et al, 1946; Pickett, 1982; Lauterbur, 1973; Fullerton, 1982; Axel et al, 1984; Ellis and Meiere, 1985; DeMyer et al, 1985). Table 3 summarizes the basic principles involved in nuclear magnetic resonance imaging. The images are produced when tissue is placed in a strong magnetic field, which is used to concentrate the inherent electromagnetic force contained in electrically charged particles found in the nuclei of atoms. In the human body, by far the most common of these is the hydrogen proton, which has a single positive charge. As the hydrogen proton spins, it generates a magnetic moment which makes it equivalent to a tiny magnet. When people speak of nuclear magnetic resonance imaging, the word *nuclear* refers to these particles found in the nuclei of atoms.

The technique is referred to as magnetic resonance imaging because magnets of large field strength (currently usually in the range of .5 to 1.5 Tesla) can be

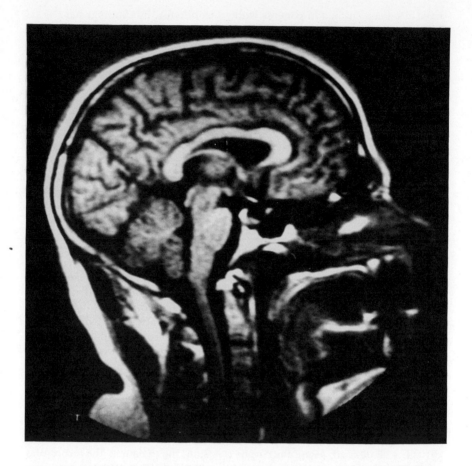

Figure 4. MRI midsagittal

used to concentrate this inherent EMF. In their natural state, the hydrogen protons are aligned randomly with respect to one another. When they are placed in the environment of a strong external magnetic field, however, they align parallel or antiparallel to that field. This concentrates the inherent magnetic moment and makes it strong enough to measure.

Because they spin, the protons also have a tendency to wobble (or precess, in technical language) when placed within a strong external field. This behavior is analogous to a spinning top in the earth's magnetic field. When a top spins, the spin is not uniform, but rather wobbles in response to the external forces generated by the earth's magnetic field. Different charged particles have varying rates of precession which are specific and are referred to as the Larmor frequency. If a radio signal is broadcast to them at their specific frequency, their energy state can be increased ("excited"). Thereafter, the gradual reduction ("decay") in excitation can be observed and measured. The broadcasting phase within magnetic resonance imaging occurs after the excitation phase during which the

Table 3. Principles of NMR Imaging

Nuclear	Based on the inherent magnetic moment associated with the nuclei of atoms (e.g., the hydrogen proton in water),
Magnetic	which is concentrated through the use of a magnetic field to align the nuclei in one plane, thereby creating a nonrandom magnetization that is strong enough to measure.
Resonance	These protons have their own specific spin and wobble (precession), which can be excited by a radio signal broadcast at their specific frequency (the Larmor frequency) by a radiofrequency transmitter; the gradual decay in this resonance can then be measured by a radiofrequency receiver.
Imaging	The radiofrequency signals can then be converted via computer to shades of gray, white, and black corresponding to the strength of the signal and used to make images or pictures.

Table 4. Components of the NMR Signal

Proton Density—An index of the number of protons present in the tissue

T1—An exponential growth constant that reflects the return of magnetization within the nuclei to the resting state in the z axis (also called longitudinal relaxation time, spin lattice relaxation)

T2—An exponential decay constant that reflects loss of signal strength as dephasing of the spin occurs

protons are stimulated. As their energy state declines, its decay can be measured by a radiofrequency receiver.

These radiofrequency signals transmitted back by the brain can then be assigned various shades of gray, white, or black, depending on the intensity of the signal. If only a single static magnet were used, this signal would come from the entire head. In actual practice in magnetic resonance imaging, gradient magnets are used in order to divide the brain into slices. In each slice a grid is imposed in order to produce tiny blocks or volume elements (voxels). These voxels are then changed to picture elements (pixels), which can be fused to make images or pictures.

The MR signal is based on more complicated phenomena than is the CT signal. Unlike CT, which is only based on x-ray attenuation through tissue, the MR signal has three major components. These are summarized in Table 4. The components of the MR signal include proton density, T1 relaxation time, and T2 relaxation time. For a more detailed defintion of these components, the reader is referred to a number of reviews of MR technology. In brief, proton density is an index of the number of hydrogen protons present in a tissue sample. Since the signal:noise ratio is poor, proton density alone is a poor index of tissue type or tissue pathology. T1 and T2 relaxation times are better indicators. Both of these are rate constants that represent different aspects of the decay of the MR signal over time. T1 is an exponential constant that reflects the return of the protons to their original net magnetization prior to excitation; it is defined as the time for them to return to 63 percent of their original net level. T2 is an exponential decay constant that represents the dephasing of spin as the protons relax after excitation.*

T1 and T2 are very sensitive discriminators of gray versus white matter in normal versus abnormal tissue. In general, gray matter relaxes more slowly than white matter and abnormal tissue more slowly than normal tissue. Pathological processes tend to lengthen both T1 and T2. Figure 5 shows actual measured T2 for gray matter, white matter, cerebrospinal fluid (CSF), and abnormal tissue (Pfefferbaum et al, 1985).

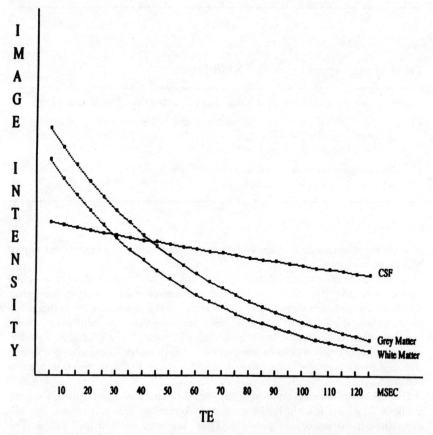

Figure 5. Actual measured T2 for gray matter, white matter, CSF, and abnormal tissue (Pfefferbaum et al, 1985)

As Figure 5 indicates, the time at which relaxation is sampled can significantly affect the type of image obtained. T1 and T2 are specific characteristics of tissue, but their relative contribution to the NMR signal is variable and depends on the timing of the excitation pulses from the radio transmitter and the timing of the measurements. Some pulse sequences elicit a stronger T1 component, while others are more heavily weighted by the T2 component. In general, in interpreting NMR images, one can use the following information as a guideline: increased signal intensity causes increased brightness in the image. Factors that increase signal intensity (and therefore brightness) include increased proton density, decreased T1, and increased T2. Pathological processes tend to lengthen T1 and T2. Gray and white matter can be bright or dark depending on the type of pulse sequence employed. When images have a strong T1 weighting, white matter tends to be relatively brighter than gray matter, while T2 weighted images make gray matter appear brighter than white matter and CSF brightest of all.

Approaches to Research Using MRI

CT research has the option of selecting between measures of tissue structure such as the VBR, and indices of x-ray attenuation ("density numbers"), although most of the work done to date has been anatomical and structural. As the above discussion indicates, the number and type of parameters available for research with MRI are much greater.

Because of the substantially improved gray-white resolution and the capacity to image in many different planes, the range of structural studies that can be done is substantially increased. With MRI one can examine the structure and shape of the corpus callosum, the size of the amygdala or hippocampus, the size of the frontal lobes, left versus right temporal lobe asymmetry, and so on.

Further, since T1 and T2 relaxation times reflect actual tissue characteristics, it is also possible to measure them directly in order to obtain indices of tissue pathology. When the structural information obtained through improved gray-white resolution is combined with measurement of T1 or T2, one has at least the potentiality for indirectly assessing pathology in specific structural regions of interest such as the basal ganglia, the amygdala, or frontal white matter tracts.

Studies Conducted to Date

ANATOMICAL STUDIES.   At present the largest anatomical study has been conducted at the University of Iowa College of Medicine (Andreasen et al, 1986; Nasrallah et al, 1986). Thirty-eight patients suffering from schizophrenia were compared with 49 normal controls. Structures that could be seen on the midline sagittal cut were measured. Figure 6 shows schematically the structures than can be identified and measured on this cut. Scans were enlarged using an overhead projector, then measured using a planimeter. A calibration line coded on each scan permitted calculation of actual brain area in square centimeters.

The patients consisted of consecutively admitted patients diagnosed as having schizophrenia by *The Diagnostic and Statistical Manual of Mental Disorders, Third Edition (DSM-III)*. They were evaluated clinically with the Comprehensive Assessment of Symptoms and History (CASH) which includes scales for assessing both positive and negative symptoms (Andreasen, 1984). The control subjects were healthy volunteers recruited from among hospital personnel.

TRACING OF MRI SAGITTAL SECTION

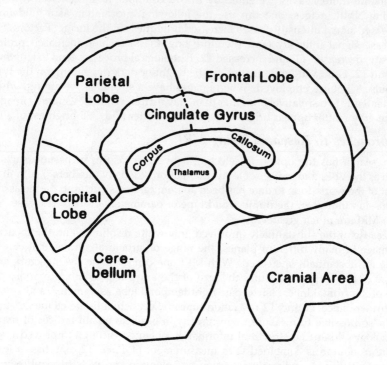

Figure 6. Midsagittal schematic

One set of analyses emphasized evaluation of frontal lobe size, based on the working hypothesis that frontal lobe abnormalities might be found in patients suffering from schizophrenia (Andreasen et al, 1986). A variety of studies in both animals and man have indicated that lesions in the prefrontal cortex lead to impairment in a wide range of cognitive functions (Fuster, 1980; Damasio, 1979; Luria, 1980; Nauta, 1971). Symptoms associated with frontal lobe injury include decreased spontaneity and fluency of speech, decreased volition and drive, a decrease in voluntary motor behavior, difficulty in focusing attention, and abnormalities in affect (especially apathy, indifference, and shallowness). Many of the symptoms of schizophrenia, particularly the negative symptoms, are strikingly similar to the symptoms associated with frontal lobe injury. Further studies using many other types of brain imaging modalities, such as positron emission tomography (PET), brain electrical activity mapping (BEAM), and regional cerebral blood flow (RCBF) have also provided some partial confirmation for the hypofrontality hypothesis (Ingvar and Franzen, 1974; Mathew et al., 1982;

Andreasen, 1986; Weinberger et al, 1986; Morihisa and Weinberger, 1986; Buchsbaum et al, 1985; Morihisa and McAnulty, 1985).

The Iowa study (Andreasen et al, 1986) does suggest that patients suffering from schizophrenia may have some type of structural abnormality in the frontal lobes. The schizophrenics as a group were found to have significantly smaller frontal lobes than did the control subjects. Because of sex differences in brain size, the findings for men and women were analyzed separately. The differences between male patients and controls were most striking. Figure 7 shows box-

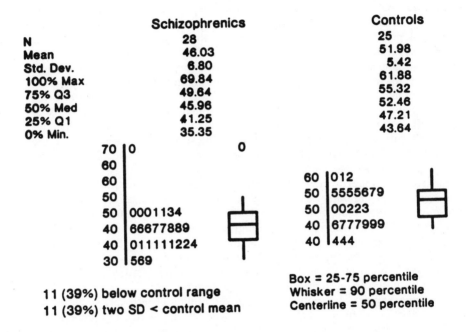

	Schizophrenics	Controls
N	28	25
Mean	46.03	51.98
Std. Dev.	6.80	5.42
100% Max	69.84	61.88
75% Q3	49.64	55.32
50% Med	45.96	52.46
25% Q1	41.25	47.21
0% Min.	35.35	43.64

Schizophrenics:
```
70 |0                    0
60 |
60 |
50 |
50 |0001134
40 |66677889
40 |011111224
30 |569
```

11 (39%) below control range
11 (39%) two SD < control mean

Controls:
```
60 |012
50 |5555679
50 |00223
40 |6777999
40 |444
```

Box = 25-75 percentile
Whisker = 90 percentile
Centerline = 50 percentile

Std. Dev. = Standard Deviation; 100% max = maximum value; 75% Q3 = 75th percentile; 50% median = median or 50th percentile; 25% Q1 = 25th percentile; 0% min = minimum value.

The numbers in the stem leaf diagrams represent brain area in square centimeters. The two digit numbers to the left of the line indicate the value in tens, while each of the numbers to the right represents the second digit; i.e., 30|569 represents values of 35, 36, and 39. Each of the numbers to the right of the line portrays a specific value for a specific subject in the study. These plots portray the distributional characteristics of all the raw data collected in the study.

Figure 7. Box-whisker plot of midsagittal frontal size (males only)

whisker plots of frontal lobe area in square centimeters for schizophrenic males versus control males. The differences between these two groups are highly significant ($p < .001$). Eleven patients (39 percent) were below the control mean in frontal size.

In the Iowa study, cerebral size and skull size were also measured. The patients also differed from controls in these two measures. Data for male patients are portrayed in Figures 8 and 9. Schizophrenic patients were also found to be significantly smaller in both brain and skull size. Seven patients (25 percent) were below the control range in cranial size, while six (21 percent) were more than two standard deviations away from the control mean. Five (18 percent) were outside the control range in cranial size, while five (18 percent) were more than two standard deviations below the control mean.

These findings could be explained by a variety of confounding variables. One obvious possibility is that the differences could be due simply to differences in body size, since one would expect cranial and brain size to be correlated with sex, height, and weight. The patient and control groups did not differ significantly in height or weight. Nevertheless, multiple regression was used to partial out the effects of sex, height, and weight. In the normal controls, cranial, cerebral, and frontal lobe size were found to be highly correlated with sex, height, and weight, with sex and height serving as the strongest predictors. When the regression equation developed for the normals was applied to the schizophrenics and the residuals calculated, most of the residuals were negative, indicating that schizophrenics do indeed have small cranial, cerebral, and frontal size when sex and height are statistically controlled. Thus it seems unlikely that the results are due to a sampling artifact related to body size. Many of the patients with negative residuals were female. Although as analysis of variance suggested that sex effect might explain part of the variance in the cranial, cerebral, and frontal findings, the regression data suggest that females may also have disproportionately small brain measures. A definitive answer as to whether there is a sex effect in these variables must await a larger sample.

Another important issue was whether the finding of relatively small frontal lobes was a specific regional finding, or whether it was due to a generalized decrease in cerebral size. Analysis of covariance was used in order to determine the relative influence of cranial and cerebral size on frontal lobe size. Even when frontal lobe size was "statistically corrected" for head and brain size, the small frontal lobe size remained highly significant. Consequently, the Iowa study suggests that schizophrenics may indeed have a specific structural abnormality in the frontal lobe.

Clinical phenomenology was examined in relation to these three brain measures. No association was observed among any of the measures and various positive symptoms (delusions, hallucinations, positive formal thought disorder, and bizarre behavior). On the other hand, negative symptoms (alogia, affective blunting, avolition, apathy, and attentional impairment) were associated with both decreased cerebral size and decreased cranial size. The *a priori* prediction of a relationship between negative symptoms and decreased frontal size was not confirmed, however.

These findings suggest that patients suffering from schizophrenia may have some type of early developmental abnormality that led to impaired capacity of

	Schizophrenics	Controls
N	28	25
Mean	86.47	96.31
Std. Dev.	11.38	9.38
100% Max	120.30	111.72
75% Q3	94.74	105.77
50% Med	85.85	94.73
25% Q1	78.16	88.65
0% Min.	67.20	79.35

```
120 |0                    0
110 |
110 |
100 |
100 |1
 90 |5555569
 90 |4
 80 |556789
 80 |014
 70 |567899
 70 |4
 60 |78
```

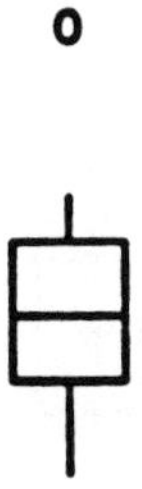

```
110 |12
100 |66799
100 |24
 90 |5666
 90 |00124
 80 |557889
 80 |
 70 |9
```

7 (25%) below control range
6 (21%) two SD < control mean

Box = 25-75 percentile
Whisker = 90 percentile
Centerline = 50 percentile

Std. Dev. = Standard Deviation; 100% max = maximum value; 75% Q3 = 75th percentile; 50% median = median or 50th percentile; 25% Q1 = 25th percentile; 0% min = minimum value.

The numbers in the stem leaf diagrams represent brain area in square centimeters. The two-digit numbers to the left of the line indicate the value in tens, while each of the numbers to the right represents the second digit; i.e., 60|78 represents values of 67 and 68. Each of the numbers to the right of the line portrays a specific value for a specific subject in the study. These plots portray the distributional characteristics of all the raw data collected in the study.

Figure 8. Box-whisker plot of midsagittal cerebral size (males only)

the brain to grow, particularly in the frontal region, thereby causing a correspondingly small cranial area. This could be due to a variety of factors, such as genetics, maternal nutrition, maternal alcohol consumption, difficulty during delivery, or environmental influences (for example, nutrition, parental nurture and stimulation, infection, and so on) during the first two years of life. The findings suggest that investigators must look to early developmental phenomena to explain at least part of the variance in the typology of schizophrenia.

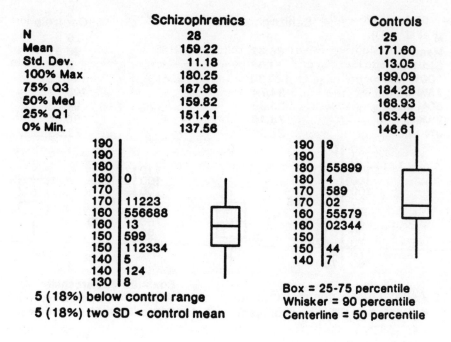

	Schizophrenics	Controls
N	28	25
Mean	159.22	171.60
Std. Dev.	11.18	13.05
100% Max	180.25	199.09
75% Q3	167.96	184.28
50% Med	159.82	168.93
25% Q1	151.41	163.48
0% Min.	137.56	146.61

```
190 |                          190 |9
190 |                          190 |
180 |                          180 |55899
180 |0                         180 |4
170 |                          170 |589
170 |11223                     170 |02
160 |556688                    160 |55579
160 |13                        160 |02344
150 |599                       150 |
150 |112334                    150 |44
140 |5                         140 |7
140 |124
130 |8
```

5 (18%) below control range

5 (18%) two SD < control mean

Box = 25-75 percentile

Whisker = 90 percentile

Centerline = 50 percentile

Std. Dev. = Standard Deviation; 100% max = maximum value; 75% Q3 = 75th percentile; 50% median = median or 50th percentile; 25% Q1 = 25th percentile; 0% min = minimum value.

The numbers in the stem leaf diagrams represent brain area in square centimeters. The two-digit numbers to the left of the line indicate the value in tens, while each of the numbers to the right represents the second digit; i.e., 130|8 represents a value of 138. Each of the numbers to the right of the line portrays a specific value for a specific subject in the study. These plots portray the distributional characteristics of all the raw data collected in this study.

Figure 9. Box-whisker plot of midsagittal cranial size (males only)

This sample was also examined in order to determine whether abnormalities in morphology of the corpus callosum could be observed (Nasrallah et al, 1986). Investigators interested in possible imbalances in hemispheric asymmetry in schizophrenia have long wondered whether interhemispheric communication might be impaired through defective callosal transfer. A variety of neurophysiologic studies have suggested some impairment in interhemispheric communication in schizophrenia (Gur et al, 1982; Diamond et al, 1980). A few anatomic studies have also suggested that schizophrenics and controls may differ in callosal thickness (Rosenthal and Bigelow, 1972; Beaumont and Diamond, 1973; Bigelow et al, 1983).

In the study by Nasrallah and colleagues (1986) the corpus callosum was divided into four quartiles. When the schizophrenics as a group were compared with the control subjects, the schizophrenics were found to have a significantly larger callosal area and thicker anterior and midcallosal thickness, thereby confirming previous postmortem findings of a thicker corpus callosum in a mixed schizophrenic sample.

Nevertheless, callosal thickness also has important confounders. Some reports have suggested that males and females may differ in callosal morphology, with females having a more bulbous callosum anteriorly (DeLacoste-Utamsing, 1982). When this sample was stratified by sex, it was found that most of the increase in callosal thickness in the schizophrenics was contributed by the female subjects. Male schizophrenics do not differ from controls in any of the callosal dimensions (except callosal length, which is greater in controls), but females continue to have significantly larger anterior and midcallosal dimensions.

Increased thickness in the corpus callosum is usually considered to represent a generalized increase in interhemispheric fibers, which might imply decreased hemispheric differentiation and less lateralization in cognitive task performance. If this is the case, then females suffering from schizophrenia might be hypothesized to have a lesser degree of functional hemispheric asymmetry than do normal females, while this functional abnormality would be less common in schizophrenic males.

The midsagittal cut also permits careful examination of cerebellar structure. Some earlier CT studies have reported an association between cerebellar atrophy and schizophrenia. Cerebellar size was also examined in the Iowa NMR study, and no differences were observed between schizophrenic patients and controls.

STUDIES OF T1 AND T2 RELAXATION. An alternate and highly promising technique for searching for brain abnormalities in the major mental illnesses is to use the actual raw data employed to reconstruct the NMR images: that is, proton density and T1 and T2 relaxation times. Operationally speaking, only T1 and T2 relaxation times can be well measured, and a number of investigators have begun to determine whether patients with major mental illnesses have different T1 and T2 relaxation times in various brain regions of interest.

Since T1 and T2 represent specific tissue parameters and in some sense reflect tissue *behavior*, they are potentially a more sensitive index of brain dysfunction, particularly regional brain dysfunction. Nevertheless, T1 and T2 are tricky to measure and require careful selection of pulse sequences. Since the actual measurement of T1 and T2 requires the calculation of their value extrapolating from several points on a curve (as displayed in Figure 5), at least two to three different pulse sequences must be used (for example, TE = 40, 80, and 160 in order to calculate T2). Further, the calculation of the actual value will become increasingly more precise if a greater number of different pulse sequences are used, since this will permit a more precise estimation of the relaxation decay curve. Yet increasing the number of pulse sequences increases the time of scanning. Consequently, investigators who choose to stress the evaluation of T1 and T2 may have to sacrifice in another area—for example, improved gray-white resolution on structural studies, a smaller number of cuts, or focus on a particular plane such as the coronal plane.

Further, although the study of calculated T1 and T2 appears theoretically promising, the methodological difficulties may be so great that the yield may not in fact be very high. For example, to date radiologists have found it difficult to distinguish between cancerous tissue and normal tissue using T1 and T2 relaxation times. Assuming that the abnormalities in major mental illnesses may be even more subtle, one might expect that they might be even more difficult to detect with these tissue parameters.

Nevertheless, some preliminary findings have been reported, although the sample sizes are relatively small and the results are necessarily to be interpreted with caution.

Besson and colleagues, working in Aberdeen, have examined T1 relaxation time in a group of 23 patients suffering from schizophrenia who were compared to 15 normal controls (Besson et al, 1984). They used a "region of interest" method in order to measure T1 values in specific brain regions. These included the genu and splenium of the corpus callosum, the thalamus (sagittal sections), temporal white matter (coronal sections), the inferior border of the temporal lobes, and left and right frontal, parietal, and occipital white matter (transverse cuts).

Their primary findings were an increase in T1 in the basal ganglia in some patients. There was some correlation between increased T1 and severity of tardive dyskinesia as measured by the Abnormal Involuntary Movement Scale (AIMS). Patients with prominent negative symptoms also tended to have increased T1 in the left basal ganglia.

The only other area to show statistically significant changes was the left frontal white matter. No large group differences were found when schizophrenic patients and controls were compared, but patients with prominent positive symptoms had a reduced T1 in the left frontal white matter. No relationship with negative symptoms was noted.

Since increased T1 is probably associated with tissue pathology, the finding of an association between increased T1 in the basal ganglia and tardive dyskinesia is particularly interesting. The findings concerning the relationship between positive symptoms and reduced T1 in the left frontal white matter are more difficult to interpret.

Fujimoto and colleagues (1984) have also examined T1 relaxation time in patients suffering from schizophrenia. They have studied 46 patients with schizophrenia compared to 20 normal controls. They also observed a decreased T1 in frontal white matter, and the findings are particularly strong on the left side. T1 was increased in the putamen as well, but no correlation with tardive dyskinesia was done, nor was there any attempt to relate observed abnormalities to positive and negative symptoms. Thus this work appears to confirm to some of the findings reported by the Besson group.

Rangel-Guerra and colleagues (1982) also examined T1 relaxation time in patients suffering from affective disorder. They studied 20 bipolar patients before and after treatment with lithium carbonate and compared their T1 values to 18 normal controls. They observed that 17 out of 20 patients had pre-lithium values higher than the controls, but that T1 values dropped to normal levels after lithium treatment. This study may suggest some abnormality in hydrogen proton behavior in patients suffering from bipolar affective disorder that normalized through lithium therapy.

Although it is outside the range of brain imaging per se, a study conducted by Rosenthal and colleagues (1986) has extended the work of Rangel-Guerra by examining the behavior of blood cells of patients suffering from affective disorder before and after lithium treatment using NMR spectroscopy. Their findings are in a similar direction to those reported by Rangel-Guerra, with T1 elevation prior to treatment and normalization after treatment.

Other investigators have sought for evidence of regional tissue abnormality using NMR, particularly in the periventricular region, which is of interest because of reports of periventricular gliosis by Stevens (1982). Studies that have used visual inspection alone have been negative (Andreasen, unpublished data; Crow, personal communication), but increasingly sophisticated techniques have been developed by the Stanford group using computerized maps of T1 and T2 (Pfefferbaum et al, 1985). These have been useful in identifying areas of periventricular lucency in patients suffering from dementia, and they offer potential for identifying similar areas in patients with schizophrenia, if they exist.

Clinical Use of CAT and MRI

While the CAT and MRI research findings discussed should not guide treatment decisions in psychiatry, both technologies are powerful tools for detecting clinically relevant structural brain changes. A number of conditions that affect central nervous system (CNS) structure can initially produce exclusively psychiatric symptoms (Weinberger, 1984). Until the 1970s the clinician who suspected such a condition had limited options. Relatively noninvasive approaches such as skull x-ray, brain scan, electroencephalogram (EEG), or neuropsychological testing were of low sensitivity. Cerebral angiography and pneumoencephalography were more sensitive, but their invasive nature precluded their use in most psychiatric patients unless definite neurological signs were present. Since the majority of structural CNS diseases eventually lead to neurologic impairment, all too often the clinician who suspected such a condition had to adopt a "wait and see" approach.

Today the CAT scanner provides the clinician with a relatively noninvasive, painless, and quick technique for producing detailed, undistorted images of gross cerebral brain structure. While CAT is familiar and widely available, a clear consensus on its indications in clinical psychiatry has been noticeably slow in emerging. Most psychiatric patients are referred for CAT to "rule out" structural lesions. The majority of patients with actual structural CNS pathology present with a *constellation* of psychiatric, neurological, and medical signs and symptoms that suggest the underlying condition. The utility of the CAT scan in this group is undisputed. However, the latter constitute but a small fraction of all psychiatric patients referred for CAT scan. While structural CNS lesions that initially produce only psychiatric symptoms are quite rare, such lesions can mimic virtually *any* psychiatric disorder. The *potential* number of psychiatric patients that may have a structural CNS lesion without concomitant gross medical/neurological signs and symptoms by far exceeds the *actual* number of such patients. In other words, the large majority of psychiatric patients without gross neurologic or medical impairment have relatively unremarkable CAT scans. Given the "low yield" of CAT scanning large numbers of unselected psychiatric patients, recommendations for its use have been shaped by cost–benefit discussions.

Since the brain is relatively radiation insensitive and the usual CAT scan radiation dose slightly exceeds that of a conventional x-ray skull series, the average adult faces no significant danger from a regular head CAT scan. However, if multiple scans are done in a short period, total radiation dose should be considered. Of patients who undergo contrast scans, few experience serious reactions to the contrast medium. As has been pointed out, the real cost of CAT scanning is the monetary one, anywhere from $150–$600, depending on the type of scan and where it is performed (Weinberger, 1984). Benefits are more difficult to quantify, though several investigators have attempted to evaluate the clinical utility of CAT scanning in psychiatric populations.

In a retrospective study of 123 consecutive psychiatric patients referred to rule out a CNS disorder, Larson and colleagues (1981) reported that in only four cases did the CAT findings affect the course of treatment. Since all of the latter had abnormal neurological exams, the authors suggested that CAT scans be administered only to patients with neurological signs. The ostensible yield of three percent is misleadingly low, however. Of all 123 patients, 35 percent had atrophy and 10 percent had focal lesions in the CNS. In those with focal lesions, the CAT scan was either diagnostic or led to definitive treatment in one-half of the cases. In addition, the authors did not consider that a negative scan, with its attendant reduction in uncertainty, had a value per se.

A different retrospective study of 135 psychiatric patients, referred for CAT scan to rule out "organic brain disease," reported that about 25 percent had abnormal scans when atrophy was included, but only three patients had focal findings (Tsai and Tsuang, 1981). When CAT results were compared to mental status evaluation, neurological examination, neuropsychological testing, and EEG it was found that even in the group with two abnormal clinical tests, the overall yield of abnormal scans was in the 25 percent range. The authors suggested that psychiatric patients below the age of 40 with no history of head injury and normal mental status and neurological examinations could be safely excluded from CAT scan screening.

Evans (1982) examined the case notes of 100 patients referred for CAT scan by community psychiatrists. Sixty-six patients were found to have cerebral atrophy, eight had specific lesions, while the scans of the rest were read as normal. The author commented that overall clincal outcome was not significantly affected even when specific lesions were detected. The disturbingly large fraction of abnormal but ostensibly clinically irrelevant scans may, in part, be accounted for by the high percentage of demented patients in the sample. Moreover, no value is assigned to the narrowing of differential diagnosis produced by CAT. In contrast, reviewers of 99 consecutive general hospital psychiatric consultations which led to referral for CAT scan concluded that the information obtained facilitated clinical decision-making in 25 percent of cases, even though in one-half of these the scans were negative (Holt et al, 1982). The reassurance provided by a negative scan was judged important to further clinical management.

Roberts and Lishman (1984) reviewed 323 records of hospitalized as well as outpatients referred for CAT scan by their psychiatrists to rule out structural abnormality. Scans were read as definitely abnormal in 29 percent of cases and equivocally abnormal in 26 percent. In the majority of cases atrophy and/or ventricular dilatation was the only abnormality. The authors judged that in 12 percent of cases the information from CAT scan had significant clinical impact.

A retrospective study covering 4,600 psychiatric admissions over 2½ years in a VA setting (where psychiatrists had unlimited access to CAT scanning) found that only 3.6 percent of all patients were scanned (Beresford et al, 1986). About one-third of the scans were read as abnormal. While 10 percent of scans had focal CAT findings, it is unclear how clinically relevant the latter were. CAT scan results contributed to a change of diagnosis in about 18 percent of all cases, though the number of definitive diagnoses was lower. Positive associations were reported between frequency of CAT findings and both abnormal neurologic and mental status examinations.

Overall, the prevalence of structural CNS disease other than diffuse atrophy appears to be 2 to 10 percent in preselected hospitalized psychiatric populations. The variance may, in part, be due to the considerable differences in patient selection criteria. Accordingly, interstudy comparisons and generalizations must be viewed with caution. There is no evidence to suggest that as a group, psychiatrists have been indiscriminately referring patients for CAT. Most studies do confirm what clinicians already know: that selecting patients with clinical evidence of CNS impairment increases the percentage of abnormal scans. While patients with structural CNS lesions who present with exclusively psychiatric symptoms are few, the cost of missing a potentially remediable condition is great. This consideration led Weinberger (1984) to propose selection criteria that encompass a relatively large group of patients (see Table 5). Since no set of guidelines can anticipate every situation, the clinician must apply or dispense with them as the situation requires.

Indications for clinical use of MRI are best presented in light of its differences and similarities with CAT. As has been discussed earlier, the CAT scan image is based on differential attenuation of x-rays. Calcified areas such as bone not only absorb more x-rays, but distort those that are transmitted. Areas where bony margins are very thick or irregular are difficult to visualize on CAT scan, due to dark streaking in the image (Hounsfield artifact). The posterior fossa, the brainstem, and the temporal and apical areas of the brain are particularly susceptible to this artifact. Since MRI records no significant signal from bone, it visualizes all areas except bone equally well. Though bone *marrow* is well visualized and the location of surrounding bone is evident, MRI is inferior to CAT in detecting calcium deposits in a lesion, for example in a meningioma (Edelman and Brady, 1985).

CAT is limited to images along a transverse plane (see Figure 2), while MRI

Table 5. Indications for CT Scan of Psychiatric Patients[1]

---

1. Confusion and/or dementia of unknown cause
2. First episode of a psychotic disorder of unknown etiology
3. Movement disorder of uncertain etiology
4. Anorexia nervosa
5. Prolonged catatonia
6. First episode of a major affective disorder or personality change after age 50

---

[1]Adapted from Weinberger, 1985

produces images along transverse as well as coronal and sagittal planes. Structures that run in certain planes may be better visualized by cuts along those planes. The longitudinal orientation of brainstem structures, for instance, make MRI sagittal images particularly informative in the area. CAT images depend on a physical property of tissue, its propensity to attenuate x-rays. The MRI technique exploits biochemical differences between neighboring tissues. It offers a high degree of resolution based on subtle differences in cellular environment irrespective of radiodensity. The latter becomes important in early stages of CNS demyelinating diseases such as multiple sclerosis. While CAT scanning can detect the larger foci of demyelination and inflammation in many parts of the CNS, MRI is far superior both in the scope of its imaging area and in its sensitivity to small plaques. Preliminary studies suggest that MRI will replace CAT scanning as the technique of choice for investigation of CNS white matter disease. In contrast, since many tumors and their perifocal edema have similar properties on MRI, CAT scan may be superior in discriminating such lesions from the surrounding edema (Huk and Gademann, 1984). Similarly, the CAT scan is better at distinguishing old from new CNS hemorrhage (Baker et al, 1985).

CAT requires exposure to ionizing radiation for up to 20 minutes. MRI depends on powerful magnetic fields applied to a patient for 20 minutes. Everything else being equal, MRI may be preferred for those patients requiring serial scans, to minimize total radiation dose. On the other hand, MRI is more sensitive to motion artifact and is therefore less useful in the very ill or the uncooperative. The MRI is contraindicated in patients with steel surgical clips, plates, cannulae, pacemakers, and so forth, that can be displaced by a magnetic field.

MRI is the more sensitive screening procedure. Its resolution for visualizing brain structure far surpasses that of CAT. It is also the procedure of choice for detecting pathology in the posterior fossa as well as several other areas, and for demyelinating disease. At the present time MRI is somewhat more costly and may be more time consuming than CAT imaging. Its use may be precluded in the agitated. Clinical, practical, and economic considerations will affect the clinician's choice between the two imaging techniques.

Current shortcomings of MRI are likely to be solved by technological advances. More powerful magnets and improved software can reduce scanning time, while economies of scale may lower operating cost. Since MRI is based on biochemical tissue differences, its future potential to detect subtle intracellular alterations is great. Accordingly, any conclusions about relative merits of and comparisons between CAT and MRI (see Tables 6 and 7) are short-lived.

Implications of Research Findings from Structural Brain Imaging

Imaging studies of cerebral structure have demonstrated that some psychiatric disorders are associated with anatomical pathology of the brain. In the case of schizophrenia, the data implicates a neuropathological condition of reduced tissue mass as defined by enlarged ventricles and prefrontal sulci, and reduced frontal lobe mass. The nature of this neuropathological condition, its etiology, primary location in the brain, and relationship to the pathogenesis of schizophrenia are the critical questions to emerge from this research. While definitive evidence is not available at present, tentative answers are suggested.

Lateral ventricular enlargement seen in patients with schizophrenia is not due

Table 6. Comparison of CAT and MRI

	CAT	MRI
Ionizing radiation	yes	no
Basis of soft tissue contrast	radiodensity	biochemistry
Typical scanning time	10–20 min.	20–60 min.
Imaging plane	transverse	transverse sagittal coronal
Image streaking due to bone artifact	in certain areas (especially posterior fossa)	no
Potential hazard with ferromagnetic objects	yes	no
Approximate cost of a scan (1986)	$150–$600	$500–$800

Table 7. Indications for Which One Imaging Technique Is Relatively Superior

CAT	MRI
Intracranial calcifications	Demyelinating disease
Tumor margins	Pathology of
Old versus new hemorrhage	posterior fossa
Agitated patient, limited time	apical areas
	temporal lobes
Contrast enhancement needed	brainstem
	spinal cord
	definition of brain structure

to abnormal CSF kinetics or dynamics (Pandurangi et al, 1984; Weinberger and Wyatt, 1982). In all likelihood, enlargement of the fluid-filled spaces occurs secondary to primary atrophy or dysplasia of brain parenchyma. Along with third ventricular enlargement, lateral ventricular enlargement is often referred to as a sign of central brain atrophy. It is tempting to infer that dilatation of the lateral ventricles occurs secondary to atrophy of the brain structures forming its boundaries, particularly since many of them have been implicated in recent, quantitative neuropathological studies (Stevens, 1982; Weinberger et al, 1983). However, lateral ventricular enlargement may be associated variously with atrophy of periventricular structures selectively, with generalized atrophy, and even with atrophy of distant cerebral areas. Similarly, no particular pathophysiologic process is implicated as underlying the findings. The gross anatomic findings of brain imaging simply indicate a reduction of tissue volume and imply reduction in brain mass; but whether the process is inflammatory, dysplastic, ischemic, and so on cannot be deduced from gross structural data. Future MRI studies may enable us to better localize the site or sites of primary neuropathology.

As was mentioned, most investigators find no correlation between the degree of lateral ventricular enlargement and patient age or duration of illness. This, along with the finding of lateral ventricular enlargement in recently diagnosed patients, suggests that structural changes and, by inference, the processes leading to them, have occurred either before the illness became manifest, or very early during its course. There is no strong evidence to suggest that lateral ventricular enlargement is a progressive phenomenon in patients with schizophrenia.

Most CT studies in schizophrenia report a distribution of ventricular size values that can be best described as unimodal, as opposed to bimodal or polymodal. This suggests that in schizophrenia lateral ventricular enlargement exists along a spectrum, and is not an all-or-nothing phenomenon. Whether lateral ventricular enlargement is a result of many different processes, or conversely the result of one process which may progress to different degrees in different individuals, is a matter for speculation.

Weinberger and colleagues (1981) found, in a study of families with affected individuals, a high degree of genetic control of lateral ventricular size among the normal members. The latter was confirmed in a careful, controlled CT study of identical twin pairs, at least one member of whom had schizophrenia (Reveley et al, 1982). In addition, Reveley and associates found that in twins discordant for schizophrenia, the affected twins as a group had significantly larger lateral ventricles than their nonschizophrenic co-twins (Reveley et al, 1982). However, in both studies there was also a nonsignificant trend for the nonschizophrenic siblings to have an increased VBR compared to normal controls. The speculation was that some pathologic process may have occurred in the intrauterine or perinatal period. Later studies suggested a negative correlation between lateral ventricular size and family history of psychiatric illness in the monozygotic probands with schizophrenia (Reveley et al, 1983a, 1983b). The inference drawn was that those probands with a lesser degree of genetic loading for the illness had to suffer an additional insult, which led to lateral ventricular enlargement and schizophrenia. The latter results and inference, however, are tentative and have not been supported by at least one subsequent study (DeLisi et al, 1985). Several familial investigations discount the likelihood that dilatation of lateral ventricles is a coincidental familial trait (Weinberger et al, 1981; Reveley et al, 1983a). One study suggests that the magnitude of the mean VBR increase correlates positively with the degree to which a physiologic measure is abnormal (Morihisa and McAnulty, 1985). That lateral ventricular enlargement is incidental to associated pathophysiology is possible but improbable.

The foregoing discussions are to different extents germane to the other brain CT findings presented. In patients with schizophrenia, the recent finding of selective prefrontal pathology is a particularly exciting one. It has not been reported so far in other groups of psychiatric patients, but then no one until now has extensively investigated such groups with the finding in mind. In at least one study, prefrontal atrophy was a significant finding though measures of generalized atrophy were not. Complementary results from NMR studies provide evidence that the underlying process is an early developmental one.

This is consistent with assumptions that the cause of ventricular enlargement also involves early developmental events (Weinberger, 1985). Moreover, evidence from cerebral blood flow and electrophysiologic studies in schizophrenia implicate the prefrontal cortex (Morihisa and McAnulty, 1985; Weinberger et al, 1986; Berman et al, 1986), providing a potential link to pathophysiology.

In conclusion, this chapter has summarized some of the developments that have hastened the integration of structural brain imaging into a neuroscience of psychiatry. Technological advances such as high-speed computers fostered the development of CT and MRI imaging. Increased nosological consensus in psychiatry, as well as demand for greater rigor in experimental design, made possible exploitation of the new technology. In this context, a conceptual revolution in neuroscience has occurred. The dissociation of pathophysiology from structural pathology and the subsequent exclusion of the latter from studies of so-called functional psychiatric disorders has ended. Converging evidence suggests that in major psychiatric disorders, structural and functional pathology are not only both present; they may be related. That structural brain studies are the legitimate domain of psychiatric inquiry is now beyond question. Structural imaging investigations of the brain, in concert with physiologic ones, offer valuable clues to the development of a neuroscientific basis for understanding mental illness.

REFERENCES

Albus M, Dieter N, Muller-Spahn F, et al: Tardive dyskinesia: relationship to computer tomographic, endocrine and psychopathological variables. Biol Psychiatry 20:1082-1089, 1985

Andreasen NC: Comprehensive Assessment of Symptoms and History (CASH). Iowa City, The University of Iowa, 1984

Andreasen NC (Ed): Can Schizophrenia Be Localized in the Brain? Washington, DC, American Psychiatric Press, Inc., 1986

Andreasen NC, Olsen SA, Dennert JW, et al: Ventricular enlargement in schizophrenia: relationship to positive and negative symptoms. Am J Psychiatry 139:297-302, 1982a

Andreasen NC, Smith MR, Jacoby CG: Ventricular enlargement in schizophrenia: definition and prevalence. Am J Psychiatry 139:292-296, 1982b

Andreasen NC, Olsen SA: Negative V positive schizophrenia: definition and validation. Arch Gen Psychiatry 39:789-794, 1982c

Andreasen NC, Dennert JW, Olsen SA, et al: Hemispheric asymmetries and schizophrenia. Am J Psychiatry 139:427-430, 1982d

Andreasen NC, Nasrallah HA, Dunn V, et al: Structural abnormalities in the frontal system in schizophrenia. Arch Gen Psychiatry 43:136-144, 1986

Axel L, Margulis AR, Meaney TF: Glossary of NMR terms. Magnetic Reasonance in Medicine 1:414-433, 1984

Baker HL Jr, Berquist TH, Kispert DB, et al: Magnetic resonance imaging in a routine clinical setting. Mayo Clin Proc 60:75-90, 1985

Barron SA, Jacobs L, Kinkel WR: Changes in size of normal lateral ventricles during aging determined by computerized tomography. Neurology 26:1011-1013, 1976

Benes F, Sunderland P, Jones BD, et al: Normal ventricles in young schizophrenics. Br J Psychiatry 141:90-93, 1982

Beaumont JG, Diamond SJ: Brain disconnection in schizophrenia. Br J Psychiatry 123:661-662, 1973

Beresford TP, Blow FC, Hall RCW, et al: CT scanning in psychiatric inpatients: clinical yield. Psychosomatics 27:105-112, 1986

Berman KF, Zec RF, Weinberger DR: Physiological dysfunction of the dorsolateral prefrontal cortex in schizophrenia, 2: role of neuroleptic treatment, attention and mental effort. Arch Gen Psychiatry 43:126-135, 1986

Besson JAO, Corrigan FM, Foreman EL, et al: T1 changes in schizophrenic disorders measured by proton NMR. Abstracts, Society for Magnetic Reasonance Imaging, 1984

Bigelow LB, Nasrallah HA, Rauscher FP: Corpus callosum thickness in chronic schizophrenia. Br J Psychiatry 142:284 287, 1983

Bloch F: Nuclear Induction. Physics Review 70:8, 1946

Boronow J, Pickar D, Ninan PT, et al: Atrophy limited to the third ventricle in chronic schizophrenic patients. Arch Gen Psychiatry 42:266-271, 1985

Buchsbaum MS, DeLisi LE, Holcomb HH, et al: Anterio-posterior gradients in cerebral glucose use in schizophrenia and affective disorder. Arch Gen Psychiatry 41:1159-1166, 1985

Coffman JA, Mefferd J, Golden CJ, et al: Cerebellar atrophy in chronic schizophrenia. Lancet 1:666, 1981

Coffman JA, Andreasen NC, Nasrallah HA: Left hemispheric deficits in chronic schizophrenia. Biol Psychiatry 19:1237-1247, 1984

Damasio A: The frontal lobes, in Clinical Neuropsychology. Edited by Heilman KM, Valenstein E. New York, Oxford University Press, 1979

De Lacoste-Utamsing C, Holloway RL: Sexual dimorphism in the human corpus callosum. Science 216: 1431, 1982

DeLisi LE, Schwartz CC, Tragum SD, et al: Ventricular brain enlargement and outcome of acute schizophreniform disorder. Psychiatry Res 9:169-171, 1983

DeLisi LE, Goldin LR, Hamovit JR, et al: Cerebral ventricular enlargement as a possible genetic marker for schizophrenia. Psychopharmacol Bull 21:365-367, 1985

DeMyer MK, Hendric HC, Gilmor RL, et al: Magnetic resonance imaging in psychiatry. Psychiatric Annals 15:262-267, 1985

Dennert JW, Andreasen NC: CT scanning and schizophrenia: a review. Psychiatric Developments 1:105-121, 1983

Dewan MJ, Pandurangi AK, Lee SH, et al: A comprehensive study of chronic schizophrenic patients. Acta Psychiatr Scand 73:152-160, 1986

Diamond SJ, Scammel RR, Price I, et al: Some failures of intermanual and cross-lateral transfer in chronic schizophrenia. J Abnorm Psychol 89:505-509, 1980

Donnelly EF, Weinberger DR, Waldman IW, et al: Cognitive impairment associated with morphological brain abnormalities on computed tomography in chronic schizophrenic patients. J Nerv Ment Dis 168:305-308, 1980

Doran AR, Pickar D, Boronow J, et al: CT scans in schizophrenic patients; medical and normal controls: replication and new findings. Abstracts of Panels and Posters Presented at the Annual Meeting of the American College of Neuropsychopharmacology, Maui, Hawaii, December 1985

Edelman RR, Brady TJ: Clinical applications of magnetic resonance imaging. Med Instrum 19:257-260, 1985

Ellis JH, Meiere FT: NMR Physics for Physicians. Indiana Medicine 78:20-28, 1985

Evans WA: An encephalographic ratio for estimating ventricular enlargement and cerebral atrophy. Archives of Neurology and Psychiatry 47:931-937, 1942

Evans WJR: Cranial computerized tomography in clinical psychiatry: 100 consecutive cases. Compr Psychiatry 23:445-450, 1982

Fox JH, Topel JL, Huckman MS: The use of computer tomography in senile dementia. J Neurol Neurosurg Psychiatry 38:948-953, 1975

Fujimoto T, Yokoyama Y, Fujimoto A, et al: Spin-lattice relaxation time measurement in schizophrenic disorders: abstracts. Society for Mag Reson Imaging, 1984

Fullerton GD: Basic concepts for nuclear magnetic resonance imaging. Magn Reson Imaging 1:39-55, 1982

Fuster JM: The Prefrontal Cortex. New York, Raven Press, 1980

Gattaz WF, Kasper S, Kohlmeyer K, et al: Die kraniale computertomographie in der schizophrenieforschung. Fortschrift Psychiatrie und Neurologie 49:286-291, 1981

Geschwind N, Levitsky W: Human brain: left-right asymmetries in temporal speech region. Science 151:186-187, 1968

Golden CJ, Moses JA, Zelazowski R, et al: Cerebral ventricular size and neuropsychological impairment in young chronic schizophrenics. Arch Gen Psychiatry 37:619-623, 1980a

Golden CJ, Graber B, Moses JA, et al: Differentiation of chronic schizophrenics with and without ventricular enlargement by the Luria-Nebraska Neuropsychological Battery. Int J Neurosci 11:131-138, 1980b

Golden CJ, Graber B, Coffman J, et al: Brain density deficits in chronic schizophrenia. Psychiatry Res 3:179-184, 1980c

Golden CJ, Graber B, Coffman J, et al: Structural brain deficits in schizophrenia. Am J Psychiatry 38:1014-1017, 1981

Golden CJ, MacInnes WD, Ariel RN, et al: Cross validation of the ability of the Luria-Nebraska neuropsychological battery to differentiate chronic schizophrenics with and without ventricular enlargement. J Consult Clin Psychol 50:87-95, 1982

Gur RC, Gur RE, Obrist WD, et al: Sex and handedness differences in cerebral blood flow during rest and cognitive activity. Science 217:659-661, 1982

Hansson J, Levander B, Lillequist B: Size of the intracerebral ventricles as measured with computer tomography, encephalography and echoventriculography. Acta Radiol [Suppl] (Stockh) 346:98-106, 1975

Hier DB, LeMay M, Rosenberger PB: Autism associated with reversed cerebral asymmetry. Neurology 28:348-349, 1978a

Hier DB, LeMay M, Rosenberger PB, et al: Developmental dyslexia: evidence for a subgroup with reversal of cerebral asymmetry. Arch Neurol 35:90-92, 1978b

Holt RE, Rawat SR, Beresford TP, et al: Computerized tomography of the brain and the psychiatric consultation. Psychosomatics 23:1007-1019, 1982

Huckman M, Fox J, Topel J: The validity of criteria for the evaluation of cerebral atrophy by computed tomography. Radiology 116:85-92, 1975

Huk WJ, Gademann G: Magnetic resonance imaging (MRI): method and early clinical experiences in diseases of the central nervous system. Neurosurg Rev 7:180-259, 1984

Ingvar DH, Franzen G: Abnormalities of cerebral blood flow distribution in patients with chronic schizophrenia. Acta Psychiatr Scand 15:425-462, 1974

Jacoby RJ, Levy R: Computed tomography in the elderly, 1: the normal population. Br J Psychiatry 136:249-255, 1980a

Jacoby RJ, Levy R: Computerized tomography in the elderly, 2: senile dementia diagnosis and functional impairment. Br J Psychiatry 146:256-269, 1980b

Jacoby RJ, Levy R, Bird M: Computed tomography and the outcome of affective disorder: a followup of elderly patients. Br J Psychiatry 139:288-292, 1981

Jernigan TL, Zatz LM, Naeser MA: Semiautomated method for quantifying information from CT scanner. Radiology 132:463-466, 1979

Jernigan TL, Zatz LM, Moses JA, et al: Computed tomography in schizophrenics and normal volunteers. Arch Gen Psychiatry 39:765-770, 1982

Johnstone EC, Crow TJ, Frith CD, et al: Cerebral ventricular size and cognitive impairment in chronic schizophrenia. Lancet 2:924-926, 1976

Johnstone EC, Crow TJ, Frith CD, et al: The dementia of dementia praecox. Acta Psychiatr Scand 57:305-324, 1978

Johnstone EC, Owens DGC, Crow TJ, et al: A CT study of 188 patients with schizophrenia, affective psychosis and neurotic illness, in Biological Psychiatry 1981. Edited by Perris C, Struwe G, Jansson B. Amsterdam, Elsevier, 1981

Kanba S, Shima S, Tsukuma D, et al: Brain CT density in chronic schizophrenia. Biol Psychiatry 19:273-274, 1984

Kleinman JE, Karson CN, Weinberger DR, et al: Eye-blinking and cerebral ventricular size in chronic schizophrenic patients. Am J Psychiatry 141:1430-1432, 1984

Kolakowska T, Williams AO, Ardern M, et al: Schizophrenia with good and poor outcome, I: early clinical features, response to neuroleptics and signs of organic dysfunction. Br J Psychiatry 146:229-235, 1985

Largen JW, Calderon M, Smith RC: Asymmetries in the density of white and gray matter in the brains of schizophrenic patients. Am J Psychiatry 140:1060-1062, 1983

Largen JW Jr, Smith RC, Calderon M, et al: Abnormalities of brain structure and density in schizophrenia. Biol Psychiatry 19:991-1013, 1984

Larson EB, Mack LA, Watts B, et al: Computed tomography in patients with psychiatric illness: advantage of a "rule in" approach. Ann Intern Med 95:360-364, 1981

Lauterbur PC: Image formation by induced local interactions: examples employing nuclear magnetic resonance. Nature, 1983.

Levy AB, Kurtz N, Kling AS: Associations between cerebral ventricular enlargement and suicide attempts in chronic schizophrenia. J Psychiatry 141:438-439, 1984

Luchins DJ, Meltzer HY: Ventricular size and psychosis in affective disorder. Biol Psychiatry 18:1197-1198, 1983

Luchins DJ, Meltzer HY: A comparison of CT findings in acute and chronic ward schizophrenics. Psychiatry Research 17:7-14, 1986.

Luchins DJ, Morihisa JM, Weinberger DR, et al: Cerebral asymmetry and cerebellar atrophy in schizophrenia: a controlled postmortem study. Am J Psychiatry 138:1501-1503, 1981

Luchins DJ, Jackman H, Meltzer HY: Lateral ventricular size and drug induced parkinsonism. Psychiatry Res 9:9-16, 1983a

Luchins DJ, Lewine RJ, Meltzer HY: Lateral ventricular size in the psychoses: relation to psychopathology and therapeutic and adverse response to medication. Psychopharmacol Bull 19:518-522, 1983b

Luchins DJ, Levine RJ, Meltzer H: Lateral ventricular size: psychopathology and medication response in the psychoses. Biol Psychiatry 19:29-44, 1984

Luria AR: Higher Cortical Functions in Man. New York, Basic Books, 1980

Lyon K, Wilson J, Golden CJ, et al: Effects of long term neuroleptic use on brain density. Psychiatry Res 5:33-37, 1981

Mathew RJ, Duncan GC, Weinman ML, et al: Regional cerebral blood flow in schizophrenia. Arch Gen Psychiatry 39:1121-1124, 1982

McCullough EC: Factors affecting the use of quantitative information from CT scanner. Radiology 124:99-107, 1977

Meltzer HY, Tong C, Luchins DJ: Serum dopamine-beta-hydroxylase activity and lateral ventricular size in affective disorders and schizophrenia. Biol Psychiatry 19:1396-1402, 1984

Moriguchi I: A study of schizophrenic brains by computerized tomographic scans. Folia Psychiatr Neurol Jpn 35:55-72, 1981

Morihisa JM, McAnulty GB: Structure and function: brain electrical activity mapping and computerized tomography in schizophrenia. Biol Psychiatry 20:3-19, 1985

Morihisa JM, Weinberger DR: Is schizophrenia a frontal lobe disease? an organizing theory of relevant anatomy and physiology, in Can Schizophrenia be Localized in the Brain? Edited by Andreasen NC. Washington, American Psychiatric Press, Inc., 1986

Nasrallah HA, Kuperman S, Jacoby CG, et al: Clinical correlates of sulcal widening in chronic schizophrenia. Psychiatry Res 10:237-242, 1983

Nasrallah HA, McCalley-Whitters M, Chapman S: Cerebral ventricular enlargement and suicide in schizophrenia and mania. Am J Psychiatry 141:919, 1984

Nasrallah HA, Olson SC, McCalley-Whitters M, et al: Cerebral ventricular enlargement in schizophrenia: a preliminary followup study. Arch Gen Psychiatry 43:157-159, 1986

Nasrallah HA, Andreasen NC, Coffman JA: A controlled magnetic resonance imaging study of corpus callosum thickness in schizophrenia. Biol Psychiatry 21:274-282, 1986

Nauta WJH: The problem of the frontal lobe: a reinterpretation. J Psychiatr Res 8:167-187, 1971

Nyback H, Wiesel F-A, Berggren B-M, et al: Computerised tomography of the brain in patients with acute psychosis and in healthy volunteers. Acta Psychiatr Scand 65:403-414, 1982

Oxenstierna G, Bergstrand G, Bjerkenstedt L, et al: Evidence of disturbed CSF circulation and brain atrophy in cases of schizophrenic psychosis. Br J Psychiatry 144:654-661, 1984

Pandurangi AK, Dewan MJ, Lee SH, et al: The ventricular system in chronic schizophrenic patients: a controlled computerized tomographic study. Br J Psychiatry 144:172-176, 1984

Pandurangi AK, Dewan MJ, Boucher M, et al: A comprehensive study of chronic schizophrenic patients. Acta Psychiatr Scand 73:161-171, 1986

Pearlson GD, Garbacz DJ, Breakey WR, et al: Lateral ventricular enlargement associated with persistent unemployment and negative symptoms in both schizophrenia and bipolar disorder. Psychiatry Res 12:1-9, 1984a

Pearlson GD, Garbacz DJ, Tompkins RH, et al: Clinical correlates of lateral ventricular enlargement in bipolar affective disorder. Am J Psychiatry 141:253-256, 1984b

Pearlson GD, Garbacz DJ, Moberg PJ, et al: Symptomatic familial, perinatal and social correlates of computerized axial tomography (CAT) changes in schizophrenics and bipolars. J Nerv Ment Dis 173:42-50, 1985

Penn RD, Belanger MG, Yasnoff WA: Ventricular volume in man computed from CAT scans. Ann Neurol 3:216-223, 1978

Pfefferbaum A, Zatz LM, Jernigan TL, et al: A quantitative approach to the analysis of CT and NMR brain scans. Abstracts of Panels and Posters Presented at the Annual Meeting of the American College of Neuropharmacology, City? December 1985

Pickett IL: NMR imaging in medicine. Scientific American 46:78-88, 1982

Purcell EM, Taurry HC, Pound RV: Resonance absorptions by nuclear-magnetic moments in a solid. Physics Review 59:37, 1946

Rangel-Guerra RA, Perez-Payan H, Todd LE, et al: Nuclear magnetic resonance in bipolar affective disorders. Magn Reson Imaging 1:229-239, 1982

Raz S, Raz N, Weinberger DR, et al: Morphological brain abnormalities in schizophrenia determined by computerized tomography: a reassessment based on volumetric quantification. Psychiatry Res (in press)

Reveley AM, Clifford CA, Reveley MA, et al: Cerebral ventricular size in twins discordant for schizophrenia. Lancet 1:540-541, 1982

Reveley AM, Reveley MA, Murray RM: Cerebral ventricular enlargement in non-genetic schizophrenia: a controlled twin study. Br J Psychiatry 144:89-93, 1983a

Reveley AM, Reveley MA, Murray RM: Enlargement of cerebral ventricles in schizophrenics is confined to those without known genetic predisposition. Lancet 2:525, 1983b

Reveley MA: CT scans in schizophrenia. Br J Psychiatry 146:367-371, 1985

Rieder RO, Donnelly EF, Herdt JR, et al: Sulcal prominence in young chronic schizophrenic patients: CT scan findings associated with impairment on neuropsychological tests. Psychiatry Res 1:1-8, 1979

Rieder RO, Mann LS, Weinberger DR, et al: Computed tomographic scans in patients with schizophrenia, schizoaffective and bipolar affective disorder. Arch Gen Psychiatry 40:735-739, 1983

Roberts JKA, Lishman WA: The use of the C.A.T. head scanner in clinical psychiatry. Br J Psychiatry 145:152-158, 1984

Rosenthal R, Bigelow LB: Quantitative brain measures in chronic schizophrenia. Br J Psychiatry 121:259-264, 1972

Rosenthal J, Strauss A, Minkoff L, et al: Identifying lithium responsive bipolar depressed patients using nuclear magnetic resonance. Am J Psychiatry 143:779-780, 1986

Schulz SC, Sinicrope P, Kishore P, et al: Treatment response and ventricular enlargement in young schizophrenic patients. Psychopharmacol Bull 19:510-512, 1983

Schulz SC, Keller MM, Kishore PR, et al: Ventricular enlargement in teenage patients with schizophrenia spectrum disorder. Am J Psychiatry 140:1592-1595, 1984

Scott MZ, Golden CJ, Ruedrich SL, et al: Ventricular enlargement in major depression. Psychiatry Res 8:91-93, 1983

Shelton RC, Weinberger DR: X-ray computerized tomography studies in schizophrenia: a review and synthesis, in The Neurology of Schizophrenia. Edited by Nasrallah H. Weinberger DR. Amsterdam, Elsevier, 1986

Shelton RC, Doran AJ, Pickar D, et al: Cerebral structural pathology in schizophrenia: a new cohort. World Congress of Biological Psychiatry, Philadelphia, 1985

Standish-Barry HMS, Bouras N, Bridges PK, et al: Pneumoencephalographic and computerized axial tomography scan changes in affective disorder. Br J Psychiatry 141:614-617, 1982

Stevens J: Neuropathology of schizophrenia. Arch Gen Psychiatry 39:1131-1139, 1982

Storey PB: Lumbar air encephalography in chronic schizophrenia: a controlled experiment. Br J Psychiatry 112:135-144, 1966

Synek V, Reuben JR: The ventricular-brain ratio using planimetric measurements of EMI scans. Br J Radiol 49:233-237, 1976

Takahashi R, Inaba Y, Inanga K, et al: CT scanning and the investigation of schizophrenia, in Biological Psychiatry 1981. Edited by Perris C, Struwe G, Jansson B. Amsterdam, Elsevier, 1981

Tanaka Y, Hazama H, Kawahara R, et al: Computerized tomography of the brain in schizophrenic patients. Acta Psychiatr Scand 63:191-197, 1981

Targum DS, Rosen LN, DeLisi LE, et al: Cerebral ventricular size and major depressive disorder: association with delusional symptoms. Biol Psychiatry 18:329-336, 1983

Tsai L, Tsuang MT: How can we avoid unnecessary CT scanning for psychiatric patients? J Clin Psychiatry 42:452-454, 1981

Weinberger DR: Brain disease and psychiatric illness: when should a psychiatrist order a CAT scan? Am J Psychiatry 141:1521-1527, 1984

Weinberger DR: Clinical-neuropathological correlations in schizophrenia; theoretical implications, in Controversies in Schizophrenia. Edited by Alpert M. New York, Guilford Press, 1985

Weinberger DR, Wyatt RJ: Brain morphology in schizophrenia: in vivo studies, in Schizophrenia as a Brain Disease. Edited by Henn FA, Nasrallah H. New York, Oxford University Press, 1982

Weinberger, DR, Torrey EF, Neophytides AN, et al: Lateral cerebral ventricular enlargement in chronic schizophrenia. Arch Gen Psychiatry 36:735-739, 1979a

Weinberger DR, Torrey EF, Neophytides An, et al: Structural abnormalities of the cerebral cortex of chronic schizophrenic patients. Arch Gen Psychiatry 36:935-939, 1979b

Weinberger DR, Kleinman JE, Luchins DJ, et al: Cerebellar pathology in schizophrenia: a controlled post-mortem study. Am J Psychiatry 137:359-361, 1980c

Weinberger DR, Cannon-Spoor E, Potkin SG, et al: Poor premorbid adjustment and CT scan abnormalities in chronic schizophrenia. Am J Psychiatry 137:1410-1423, 1980b

Weinberger Dr. Bigelow LB, Kleinman JE, et al: Cerebral ventricular enlargement in chronic schizophrenia, an association with poor response to therapy. Arch Gen Psychiatry 37:11-13, 1980a

Weinberger DR, DeLisi LE, Neophytides AN, et al: Familial aspects of CT scan abnormalities in chronic schizophrenic patients. Psychiatry Res 4:65-71, 1981

Weinberger DR, DeLisi LE, Perman GP, et al: Computer tomography in schizophreniform and other acute psychiatric disorders. Arch Gen Psychiatry 39:778-783, 1982

Weinberger DR, Wagner RL, Wyatt RJ: Neuropathological studies of schizophrenia: a selective review. Schizophr Bull 9:193-212, 1983

Weinberger DR, Berman KF, Zec RF: Physiological dysfunction of the dorsolateral prefrontal cortex in schizophrenia, 1: regional cerebral blood flow evidence. Arch Gen Psychiatry 43:114-124, 1986

Williams AO, Reveley MA, Kolakowska T, et al: Schizophrenia with good and poor outcome, II: cerebral ventricular size and its clinical significance. Br J Psychiatry 146:239-246, 1985

Woods BT, Wolf J: A reconsideration of the relation of ventricular enlargement to duration of illness in schizophrenia. Am J Psychiatry 140:1564-1570, 1983

Young SW: Nuclear Magnetic Resonance Imaging: Basic Principles. New York, Raven Press, 1984

Zatz LM, Alvarez RE: An inaccuracy in computed tomography: the energy dependence of CT values. Radiology 124:91-97, 1977

Chapter 12

Functional Brain Imaging Techniques

by John M. Morihisa, M.D.

One of the latest results of the evolution of the neurosciences is our ability to investigate brain function in the living human brain. This approach includes regional cerebral blood flow (rCBF), computerized EEG and evoked potential mapping, single photon emission computed tomography (SPECT), positron emission tomography (PET), and the potential application of magnetic resonance imaging (MRI) to functional brain imaging.

The neurosciences have given birth to these new approaches, not only in terms of the development and refinement of the applied mathematical and biophysical principles on which they are based, but also in terms of providing a mentor to help guide our application of these powerful new techniques. Indeed, much as a parent nurtures and shapes the direction of children, so too have the neurosciences provided a source of innovation and scientific direction as well as a structural framework of understanding. The neurosciences help tell us when we have digressed from the path of knowledge and how we may find our way back. In the heart of this new and expanding field of psychiatric research lies the promise that the child may yet be father to the man, as our psychiatric research findings may themselves provide the basis and direction for further neuroscience investigations.

FUNCTIONAL BRAIN IMAGING TECHNIQUES IN CLINICAL PSYCHIATRY

The purpose of this section is to discuss the various functional brain imaging techniques in terms of their potential clinical utility and their expanding relationship with the neurosciences. A comprehensive review of all the research reports and a detailed discussion of the principles underlying these approaches is beyond the scope of this chapter and is available elsewhere (Phelps et al, 1982; Morihisa, 1984; Andreasen, in press). Instead we will highlight the most promising and cohesive areas of research in an attempt to focus upon the most likely areas in which there may soon be some clinical application for this field of psychiatric research. With this aim we have chosen research findings that contribute to some of the organizing theories of brain dysfunction in the psychiatric disorders. The aim of this section is to serve as an introduction to a body of work that is growing and changing with each day. Indeed, a comprehensive discussion of all findings in the field would best be communicated in the form of a monthly newsletter. This section will attempt to provide the reader with the framework to begin what we hope will be a continuing interest and study of this dynamically evolving area of knowledge. Finally, this chapter will also attempt to suggest some of the areas in which there is a growing interaction between psychiatric research using functional brain imaging and the neurosciences.

POSITRON EMISSION TOMOGRAPHY (PET)

Positron emission tomography uses radionuclides to image brain function in vivo. Most studies, thus far, have created three-dimensional maps of brain metabolism. This technique uses positron-emitting isotopes to map brain function. The positrons interact with electrons in the brain resulting in their annihilation and the coincident generation of gamma rays. The coincident gamma radiation is quantified by arrays of detectors that relay this information to a computer. The computer, in turn, can apply standard computerized tomographic reconstruction algorithms to this data in order to create a three-dimensional representation of regionally specific brain functions.

This technique is dependent upon two general assumptions that are supported by basic science research. First, based upon neuroscience findings, it is assumed that there is a close relationship between the rate of regional glucose metabolism and the amount of functional activity in that brain region (Sokoloff, 1981, 1982). Second, that there is a body of neurophysiological evidence that brain metabolism is based almost exclusively on glucose as a substrate, and therefore measures of glucose utilization reflect regional brain energy production (Sokoloff 1981, 1982).

Briefly stated, in position emission tomography the subject is injected with a positron emitting isotope made by an accelerator such as a cyclotron. In addition, the relatively short half-life of positron emitting isotopes generally requires relatively easy access to this accelerator. The particular physiological characteristics of the isotope chosen will determine which aspects of brain function will be measured. The most commonly used isotope in psychiatric research has been FDG (F-18, fluorodeoxyglucose) which provides an estimate of the regional cerebral metabolism of glucose (Greenberg et al, 1981). The annihilation coincidence radiation from such positron emitting isotopes is measured by a ring of detectors positioned around the head of the subject. This data is used by a computer to reconstruct in three dimensions the regional use of glucose throughout the subject's brain. This data can then be presented in the form of color maps that can depict regions of varying degrees of glucose utilization according to a predetermined color code. For example, most color codes use white and reds for the greatest degree of glucose utilization.

Although the algorithms for image reconstruction are relatively standard, the actual statistical analysis of the data underlying these images is complex and a variety of techniques have been applied. Each of these approaches has a different set of strengths and limitations. Moreover, it is important to note that important basic science questions have been raised about some of the fundamental assumptions of PET scanning, ranging from the fact that the brain uses energy for a variety of purposes, many of which are maintenance (membrane repairs) as opposed to the actual energy used for thought, to fundamental questions concerning the mathematical translation of PET scan data to graphic representations of regional brain metabolism. Although these considerations of application and theory are far beyond the scope of his review, they represent an area of active investigation (Perlmutter et al, 1986; Phelps et al, 1984) and provocative discussion that will have important ramifications for PET research. Indeed, any possibility of clinical applications in the future will depend upon the resolution of such basic science concerns and the further refinement of techniques for measuring and statistically analyzing this data.

PSYCHIATRIC RESEARCH EMPLOYING PET

Positron emission tomography has the capability to study a number of functional aspects of the brain. Neurotransmitter precursors, drugs (for example, benzodiazepine antagonist) (Persson et al, 1985), amino acids, and glucose can be labeled with carbon-11 (C-11) or fluorine-18 (F-18). In this manner, PET can study glucose metabolism with F-18-2-deoxyglucose (FDG), and dopaminergic receptors (Figure 1) with C-11-chlorpromazine (Comar et al, 1979) or 3-N-(C11)methylspiperone (Wagner et al, 1983). Even brain blood flow can be measured in three dimensions using krypton-77, 13-NH-3, or oxygen-15-labeled water (Phelps, 1982).

A number of the earliest PET studies to investigate psychiatric populations used the isotope F-18-2-deoxyglucose (FDG) to measure regional brain metabolism in patients with schizophrenia. These initial studies focused upon differences in the anterior/posterior gradient of cortical metabolic rates for schizophrenic patients compared to controls. In studies from two separate groups utilizing FDG (Buchsbaum et al, 1982; Farkas et al, 1984) there were reports of decreased anterior/posterior ratios of glucose utilization in patients with schizophrenia. In addition, a group using 11-C-glucose also reported findings consistent with this abnormality of the anterior/posterior distribution of brain metabolism (Widen et al, 1984).

These initial findings provoked excitement, in part, because of a proposed congruence with the classical findings of Ingvar and Franzen (1974a, 1974b) who reported hypofrontality of regional cerebral blood flow in 31 schizophrenic patients compared to 10 neurologically normal male alcoholics. This apparent fit of functional brain imaging findings set the tone for further research and has shaped the focus of recent investigations.

There have been three basic limitations to this seemingly auspicious beginning: first, the original study by Ingvar and colleagues used a relatively small number of patients (as have subsequent functional studies) and had several methodological limitations (Berman et al, 1984). Second, the decreased ratio findings in at least one group were contributed more by higher absolute posterior values than a hypofrontality per se. Third, this interpretation focused only upon one of a group of findings and did not include the other findings that did not fit. In addition, some studies have failed altogether to find abnormalities in the frontal lobes.

The first problem has been partially addressed by the recent work of Weinberger and colleagues, who have extended the use of rCBF in the investigation of schizophrenia in a manner that has improved upon the research paradigm and has refined our focus to a specific component of the frontal lobes, the dorsolateral prefrontal cortex.

The second problem has been addressed by Wolkin and colleagues (1985) using FDG and PET methodology. This group has reported lower absolute metabolic activity in schizophrenic patients compared to normal controls in frontal and temporal regions. Thus, a direct finding is now described that specifically implicates the frontal lobes. However, in this study (Wolkin et al, 1985) the

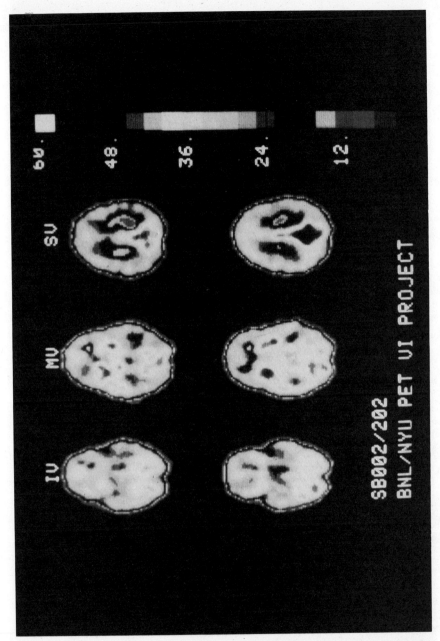

Figure 1. These are positron emission tomographic (PET) scan images using FDG (Fluorodeoxyglucose), of a 28-year-old patient with chronic paranoid schizophrenia; one month off of neuroleptics (top row) and after six weeks of thiothixene 100 mg/day. IV, MV, and SV denote horizontal slices approximately 30, 50, and 70 mm above the canthomeatal plane. Provided by Dr. Adam Wolkin and Dr. Alfred Wolf, New York University and Brookhaven National Laboratory PET Project.

temporal lobes are also implicated and this will require further elaboration of the theoretical model to address the possible meaning of this finding.

The third problem, however, has been exacerbated by a number of rCBF studies that failed to find any frontal abnormalities in schizophrenic patients (Mathew, 1982; Gur, 1984). Thus, despite the refinements provided by Weinberger's group there remains nothing close to a consensus concerning rCBF findings in this disorder.

Even more significantly, Sheppard and colleagues (1983), using oxygen-15 PET, studied 12 patients with schizophrenia (6 of whom had never received psychiatric mediations) compared to 12 controls and found no evidence of abnormalities of the anteroposterior metabolic gradient in schizophrenia. In this study, Sheppard and colleagues (1983) suggested that an abnormality of laterality might distinguish patients with schizophrenia from controls. In a study using FDG, Jernigan and colleagues (1985) studied six patients with chronic schizophrenia compared to six controls during performance of an auditory vigilance task and examined the utility of three separate techniques for measuring relative regional FDG distribution. This study did not confirm abnormalities of the anteroposterior metabolic gradient and their report concluded that this finding may be present to a variable degree in schizophrenia, and also that similar findings may be caused by a variety of other conditions.

In an attempt to extend our understanding of these findings, one group has investigated possible clinical correlations and assessed the effect of psychotherapeutic medications on this finding of abnormal frontal to posterior pattern of brain metabolic activity (DeLisi et al, 1985a, 1985b). This group (DeLisi et al, 1985a) used positron emission tomography with FDG to study 21 patients with chronic schizophrenia and compared them to an equal number of age- and sex-matched controls. In this study, 8 out of 21 patients demonstrated an abnormal reversal of the anteroposterior gradient of brain glucose utilization compared to 1 out of 21 control subjects. However, no statistically significant clinical correlates of this finding were delineated, and its possible relevance to psychopathology remains undetermined. The authors suggest that the lack of association between clinical symptoms and decreased anteroposterior metabolic gradients is consistent with this abnormality of glucose utilization representing a trait rather than a state variable. Thus, abnormal anteroposterior metabolic gradients might reflect a vulnerability to certain mental disorders rather than being tied directly to the clinical state of the patient. This interpretation, however, is based upon the failure to correlate clinical states with our findings, and thus the data does not address the most crucial question of whether the data is related at all to the disease process. Nevertheless, the interpretation is reasonable and theoretically compelling, but it would be prudent to tag it as circumstantial evidence until more direct correlations may be drawn from our investigations. Furthermore, in a logical application of combined brain imaging techniques, a structural measure (cerebral atrophy as delineated by CT scan) failed to demonstrate a correlation with this abnormal pattern of brain glucose utilization (DeLisi et al, 1985a). Thus, the important research step linking this hypothetical functional abnormality to structural pathology was not demonstrated.

Conversely, a PET study by Kling and colleagues (1986) using FDG, reported that a group of six patients with chronic schizophrenia and six patients with chronic depression were not significantly different from a group of 12 normal controls. In addition, although Kling and colleagues reported a tendency for lower global metabolism in patients with structural pathology (enlarged ventricles and widened sylvian fissures), a statistically significant correlation was not obtained. Thus, a fundamental relationship between structural pathology and functional pathology remains to be achieved.

In an attempt to investigate the effect of medications on regional brain metabolism, DeLisi and colleagues (1985b) used the isotope FDG in a PET study examining changes in glucose utilization in nine chronic schizophrenic patients, both on and off neuroleptic medications. No changes in the anteroposterior gradient following pharmacotherapy achieved significance. However, there was a significant increase in brain glucose utilization for total brain cortex, temporal cortex, as well as the basal ganglia. As is the case for most studies, the authors of this investigation correctly point out that their data may have been contaminated by artifactual effects of long-term medication. Nevertheless, their findings are consistent with a PET study by Brodie and colleagues (1984), who reported a 25 percent increase in mean glucose rates in six patients with chronic schizophrenia following neuroleptic treatment. However, these findings are the reverse of those found by Nilsson and colleagues (1977) using regional cerebral blood flow to assess the effect of haloperidol in 11 patients. Very significantly, these findings generally disagree with the basic science work of McCulloch and colleagues (1982), who found a significant decrease in rat brain glucose utilization after the administration of the neuroleptic haloperidol. It should be noted, however, that in the McCulloch study the nucleus accumbens and the pars compacta demonstrated an increase in glucose metabolism. Further, it is possible that the acute effects of neuroleptics may be different from the chronic effects, and there are some basic science findings to support this hypothesis (White and Wang, 1983). Interpretation of these studies is also limited by the use of different neuroleptics, which may have different effects on brain glucose utilization.

The study by DeLisi and colleagues (1985b) failed to demonstrate any significant difference in caudate glucose utilization between drug-free subjects with schizophrenia and normal control subjects; and when taken with the differences, demonstrated in these identical patients and controls following medication, we have specific evidence that neuroleptic medication affects central dopaminergic systems. Moreover, these findings do not provide any support for the classical hypothesis of a basic abnormality of brain dopamine systems in schizophrenia. However, the authors point out that one important limitation in the use of the FDG isotope for PET imaging is that this approach is not selective, and instead measures the activity of multiple systems for brain neurotransmission. Thus, this study should not be interpreted as a refutation of the dopamine hypothesis of schizophrenia. This emphasizes the need for studies employing ligands that are specific for a single type of receptor, as has been used to label dopamine receptors (Wagner et al, 1983; Garnett et al, 1983; Baron et al, 1985; Farde et al, 1986). This selectivity may provide more specific and clearly relevant information concerning the metabolic abnormalities associated with schizophrenia. Another general caveat exists in the interpretation of PET scan studies, and that is the fact that energy is utilized by the brain for a variety of purposes besides thought and affect (both normal and pathophysiologic), such as maintenance of cell structure and storage and transport of cellular components. Indeed, as we have learned from our neuroscience investigations of the brain, utilization of energy may be paradoxical and difficult to interpret.

Wolkin and colleagues (1985), using FDG, studied 10 chronic schizophrenic patients before and after somatic treatment compared to eight normal controls. In this PET study the untreated schizophrenic patients demonstrated lower absolute metabolic activity compared to controls in frontal and temporal regions, as well as a trend toward relative hyperactivity in the area of the basal ganglia. Following treatment, glucose utilization normalized toward the metabolic values of the control group. The exceptoin to this normalization was the frontal region. The authors emphasized that the persistence of abnormality in the frontal region supports the hypothesis of a loci of abnormal brain function in the frontal lobes. This first PET report of an absolute reduction of glucose metabolism in the frontal region is very significant to an organizing theory of frontal lobe dysfunction. All previous PET studies have reported an abnormality of the metabolic gradient from front to back, and thus did not give as compelling a specific localization of dysfunction. However, the finding of significantly lower metabolic activity in the temporal regions is the reverse of findings of a study by DeLisi and colleagues (submitted for publication), which reported increased glucose utilization in the temporal lobe regions of drug-free patients with schizophrenia. Thus, although certain clinically meaningful regions (for example, the frontal lobes) repeatedly appear in the reports of PET research, the body of findings remain inconsistent and at times contradictory. The disparity in our findings may reflect not only different technical and statistical approaches as well as different patient populations and test paradigms, but also the great heterogeneity of clinical presentation that is apparent in schizophrenia and other psychoses. Nevertheless, it is clear that the complexity and lack of consistency that characterize these findings represent some of the most significant challenges to deriving clinical applications from this research.

One of the first studies of patients with affective disorders used FDG to investigate regional brain metabolism (Buchsbaum, et al, 1984). The major finding of this study was to introduce yet another, complicating variable into our hypothesized "equation" of brain metabolism in mental illness. This study reported the finding of abnormal anteroposterior metabolic gradients in patients with affective disorders, as well as patients with schizophrenia and suggested, therefore, that the abnormality of anteroposterior metabolism joins the growing number of biological assessments that lack clear diagnostic specificity. It remains to be seen whether the findings of absolute decrease in metabolism in frontal regions reported by Wolkin and colleagues will also be found in patients with affective disorders. Finally, the study by Bushsbaum and colleagues (1984) did not find significant differences in left–right hemispheric nor whole brain metabolism in patients compared to controls. This is contrary to a number of PET and rCBF investigations that have focused attention on abnormalities of metabolic asymmetry (left–right hemispheric distribution), as well as global metabolic differences comparing measures of total brain activity.

Baxter and colleagues (1985) used the FDG isotope to PET scan 11 patients with unipolar depression, 5 patients with bipolar depression, 5 patients with mania, 3 patients with bipolar mixed states, and 9 normal controls. The major finding of this study was a whole brain reduction of glucose metabolism in bipolar and mixed patients compared to normal controls, unipolar depressed patients, and patients with mania. In an investigation of the abnormalities of anteroposterior metabolic gradient reported by other groups, Baxter and colleagues examined a related measure of frontal-occipital ratio of glucose utilization. They were unable to find statistically significant evidence of this type of abnormality in any of their diagnostic groups. In addition, patients with unipolar depression demonstrated a statistically significant decrease in the ratio of metabolism in the caudate nucleus to hemispheric metabolism compared to the normal controls and bipolar depression patients. This finding may provide preliminary evidence implicating the dopamine system in the pathophysiology of some affective disorders. This hypothesis could be further investigated by PET studies utilizing dopamine receptor specific ligands such as 3-N-(11C) methylspiperone (Wagner et al, 1983) to assess potential receptor changes associated with this suggestion of hypometabolism in the head of the caudate in unipolar depression.

A PET study (Rumsey, et al 1985) has been reported using FDG to study 10 men with a history of infantile autism compared to 15 normal controls. This group reported statistically significant elevations of glucose metabolism in diverse brain regions in the autism goup versus the control group. No regions of hypometabolism were identified in the autistic group and no characteristic pattern of abnormal increased metabolism could be delineated. As is the case with a number of psychiatric disorders there is evidence that autism may be a heterogeneous disorder, and this hypothesis would be consistent with the diverse distribution of abnormal glucose metabolism reported in this study.

A number of these studies used research paradigms studying a resting alert state. However, there are many difficulties associated with achieving "stable and reproducible 'resting'" state in the human brain (Mazziota et al, 1982). Strategies that utilize cognitive activation tests can enhance the experimental control over state variables as well as provide a more focused window on brain function (Gur, 1984; Morihisa, 1986b). A recent study by Cohen and colleagues (submitted for publication) uses the CPT (Continual Performance Task) to assess schizophrenic patients compared to normal control subjects. Such specific cognitive activation procedures represent an important strategy to refine our use of the positron emission tomography.

Although one of our basic strategies is to develop hypothetical equations that take into account the numerous variables and can explain the patterns of metabolism we delineate, there are dangers in this approach. Unfortunately, these equations take on a life of their own and threaten to outlive their usefulness. We must be quick to develop new equations and remain skeptical, with a constant demand for recertification of their utility as new findings emerge and our understanding of brain function grows.

Thus, positron emission tomography provides a probe of the topographic distribution of normal brain function as well as a window on regional metabolic abnormalities in psychiatric disorders. The cost of the PET scanner as well as the general requirement of a cyclotron will limit the widespread use of this powerful new brain imaging approach in psychiatric research. Moreover, important concerns about the basic science principles (Perlmutter et al, 1986) on which the PET scan is based as well as disagreement concerning the interpretation of this data (Reivich et al, 1985; Jernigan et al, 1985) must be resolved before the PET scan can fulfill its potential as a research tool. Despite a number of provocative findings, the clinical utility of this technique in the practice of psychiatry remains to be delineated. However, it continues to be a promising research tool that may eventually provide certain limited and specific clinical uses in the near future.

COMPUTERIZED EEG AND EVOKED POTENTIAL MAPPING OF BRAIN FUNCTION

The attempt to derive information about brain function from the patterns of electrical activity detected on the cortical surface is venerable by brain imaging historical standards (Berger, 1929). Indeed, the computer enhancement of this field constitutes a second generation of this research approach. The field of electrophysiological approaches to psychiatric illnesses has already experienced a cycle of excitement and ethusiastic expectation followed by disappointment and disillusionment when this approach failed to delineate the underlying pathophysiology of mental disorders during the middle of this century. This has represented both an advantage and a disadvantage to this approach. The advantage has been a talented body of senior researchers who have, over decades, developed and refined our understanding of the electrophysiological aspects of human brain function. The disadvantage has been unrealistic expectations of increased information comparable to the PET scan and a related misunderstanding of the significant limits to this particular brain imaging approach. In this section we will review some of the recent studies using computer imaging techniques to deal with the massive amounts of information derived from multiple lead recording of brain electrical activity. In the context of listing some of the limitations of this approach, we will address the present lack of clear clinical applications of this technique.

A number of mapping strategies have been applied over the last three decades to assist in the examination of electrophysiologic data. Building upon the work of pioneers such as Petsche (1976), Walter and Shipton (1951), Lehman (1971), Lemieux et al (1984), Itil et al (1972) and many others, Duffy and colleagues (1979) developed a system of EEG and evoked potential mapping called brain electrical activity mapping. This approach uses standard EEG amplifiers to record data from the skull surface, which is then subjected to a Fast Fourier Transform analysis, which breaks the EEG data into its component frequencies (that is, delta, theta, alpha, and beta). This data is then topographically displayed in the form of color maps. This technique was first sytematically applied to a psychiatric population in 1983 (Morihisa et al) in a study of 11 drug-free patients with chronic schizophrenia, 14 patients on a standard dose of haloperidol, and 11 normal control subjects. The major finding of this study was increased delta activity over the entire cortical surface of schizophrenic patients compared to controls. This finding of increased delta was less prominent in the medicated group of patients and therefore does not appear to represent an acute drug effect. A recent study from this same laboratory (Karson, Coppola, Morihisa, et al, submitted for publication) has replicated this finding of generally increased delta in schizophrenia in a new patient population (n = 11 versus n = 11) using a new EEG imaging system (Coppola et al, 1982), but also demonstrates the danger of contamination of delta by eye movements that are not detected and removed prior to analysis. For this reason topographic localizations of delta in schizophrenia should not be made unless the study utilizes an on-line electrooculogram that is subjected to the same spectral analysis program as the cortical data. Only in this manner can artifact-free data be secured and misleading topographic localizations of delta be avoided. Given this caveat, the findings of increased delta in schizophrenia should be interpreted as evidence for brain abnormalities in schizophrenia, but also as evidence that clear topographic localization of delta over specific brain regions are yet to be clearly demonstrated. A more comprehensive discussion of the process of deriving color maps from electrophysiologic data, as well as the strengths and limitations of this approach, is beyond the scope of this discussion and is available elsewhere (Morihisa, in press).

The use of evoked potentials has allowed some computerized topographic localization of brain abnormalities in psychiatric disorders and provides one of the only windows on brain function that can explore phenomena that occur in intervals measured in milliseconds. The work of Shagass and colleagues (1979, 1980), Roth (1977), Buchsbaum (1977) and many others in investigating abnormalities of evoked potentials or event related potentials has been fundamental in the development of techniques to examine this stimulus related brain electrical activity. In the classical evoked potential a stimulus (for example, light flash, auditory tone or click, somatosensory stimulation [Guenther and Breitling, 1985], pattern reversal or sometimes more complicated stimuli [Morstyn et al, 1983]) is presented multiple times to a subject. The brain electrical activity is recorded and averaged in order to remove the background EEG and delineate the characteristic electrical response to the specific stimulus. This data can be mapped in the form of different gray scales or colors with different shades or colors corresponding to different voltage ranges. One such mapping technique was developed by Coppola and colleagues (1982) and uses 28 different electrode sites to collect data, and displays this information on graphic representations of the left or right hemisphere (Figure 2). This technique has been particularly useful in the investigation of seizure disorders and medication effects. However, there has been limited demonstrated clinical utility of this computerized mapping technique in the major psychoses despite recent promising research findings (Buchsbaum et al, in press; Morstyn et al, 1983; Guenther and Breitling, 1985).

One of the most promising uses of brain imaging technology has been in the combined use of complementary methodologies that can measure and compare a variety of information concerning brain pathology. One such study (Morihisa and McAnulty, 1985) combined a structural (computed tomography/CT scan) and a functional (computerized evoked potential mapping) brain imaging technique to investigate patients with schizophrenia. This study suggests that, in schizophrenia, definable gross anatomic pathology may be associated with regionally specific electrophysiological differences (Figure 3).

Among brain imaging approaches, computerized mapping of EEG and evoked potentials have the greatest obstacles to overcome in the long hard journey to clinical application. Although the equipment and software are relatively inexpensive and becoming increasingly available, there are major limitations to this approach. First, in general the data collection is limited to recordings from the cortical surface (Morihisa, in press). The relationship between what can be detected at the skull surface and what is taking place electrophysiologically under the cortical surface is complex and remains largely undefined. Indeed, the very nature of the neural generators of this brain electrical activity is poorly under-

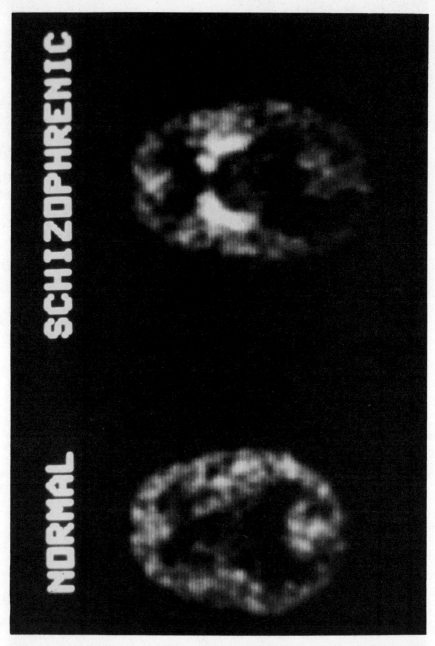

Figure 2. An investigation of dopamine receptor function is achieved in this PET image demonstrating the concentration of C-11-N-Methylspiperone in the caudate nucleus and putamen of a normal control and a patient with schizophrenia. In this PET image of the distribution of this compound, partial receptor blockade has been achieved by prior administration of a standard dose of haloperidol. This data provides evidence of abnormalities in dopamine receptor activity in schizophrenia. Provided by Dr. Henry N. Wagner, Johns Hopkins University.

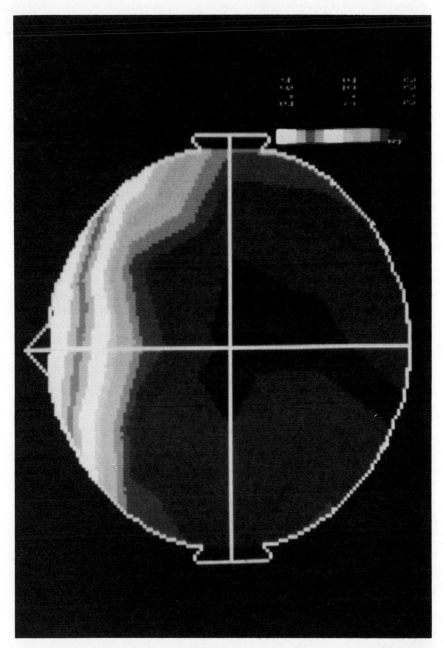

Figure 3. In this image, data from computed tomography (CT scan) and a computerized evoked potential mapping technique (brain electrical activity mapping) have been combined in a preliminary study of schizophrenia. This pilot data suggests that, in schizophrenia, definable gross anatomic pathology may be associated with regionally specific electrophysiological differences. Provided by Dr. John M. Morihisa, Georgetown University School of Medicine and the VA Medical Center, Washington, D.C.

stood. In addition, the very anatomy of the head conspires against the investigator of brain electrical activity. The skull varies in its thickness and has various holes inserted in it. In addition, the brain is folded into complex convolutions and lobes. Finally, despite ingenious research efforts (Elbert et al, 1985; Jervis et al, 1985), the sensitivity of computerized EEG and evoked potential mapping to movement artifacts, medication effects and the limited resolution provided by 20 to 28 data points represent a daunting set of hurdles. Fortunately, there is hope on the technological horizon in the form of an evolutionary advance in the mapping of brain electrical activity that characterize and localize the magnetic fields generated by neurons in order to provide measures of electrophysiologic function. This approach, magnetoencephalography (MEG) holds out the promise of three-dimensional measures of brain electrical activity and greater resolution with less of the distortion associated with detection from the cortical surface. However, at the present time these measurements must be made by Super Quantum Interference Devices (SQUID) that must be cooled to -260 degrees centigrade. In addition, special rooms must be constructed for SQUID studies in order to reduce the effect of other magnetic fields on recording.

Until such technologic advances are more fully realized, the use of computerized mapping of EEG and evoked potentials will remain an exciting and useful research tool. At the present time there are no clear indications in psychiatry for their application in clinical practice. Specifically, there is no evidence that clearly supports the use of computerized mapping approaches in preference to the standard EEG and evoked potential clinical laboratories presently in existence.

SINGLE PHOTON EMISSION COMPUTED TOMOGRAPHY (SPECT)

Single photon emission tomography is based upon the detection of gamma radiation from single photon emitting radionuclides such as I-123. In this technique an I-123 labeled radiopharmaceutical such as I-123-p-isopropyl-amphetamine (123-I-IMP) is administered to a subject. The gamma radiation emitted by this radiopharmaceutical can be measured by a variety of gamma detector systems using NAI(T1) scintillation crystals (Jaszczak and Coleman, 1985; Coleman et al, 1986). From this data a three-dimensional image of the distribution of the radiopharmaceutical can be obtained. In this manner a measure of brain blood flow can be obtained by using a radiopharmaceutical (for example, 123-I-IMP) whose distribution reflects cerebral blood flow (Kuhl et al, 1982). Rush and colleagues (in press) have reported a preliminary study using SPECT to study patients with affective disorders. In this report, patients with unipolar depression had decreased blood flow and patients with manic or mixed-phase bipolar illness had increased blood flows compared to controls.

Of greater potential utility is the possibility that SPECT will be able to provide quantitative measurements of the brain distribution of physiologically specific radiopharmaceuticals. For example, Holman and colleagues (1985) used an I-123 labeled radiopharmaceutical that bound to the muscarinic acetylcholine receptors in the brain to study a patient with Alzheimer's disease. This case study using 123-labeled 3-quinuclidinyl-4-iodobenzilate (123-I-QNB) reported a moderate impairment in muscarinic receptor binding function in this patient with Alzheimer's disease. This work demonstrates the use of "high-specific-activity radioisotope-labeled neurotransmitter antagonists" in SPECT research to assess receptor binding function in the living human.

While these new radiopharmaceutical applications hold great promise for the value of SPECT in psychiatric research, the clinical applications of this technique in psychiatry has yet to be determined.

MAGNETIC RESONANCE IMAGING (MRI)

As Dr. Andreasen described in Chapter 11 of this volume, magnetic resonance imaging is based upon the differential manner that certain elements can absorb and emit electromagnetic energy while subjected to a powerful magnetic field. This technique utilizes hydrogen nuclei to generate structural information, but it can also be used to investigate sodium, phosphorous, or carbon. In this manner, MRI techniques have the potential (James et al, 1982) to assess brain function as well as structure. For example, since the body stores energy as phosphate bonds, MRI has the potential to investigate the utilization of chemical energy in the living brain. This technique may present the greatest promise of all the functional approaches described here. However, significant technological and theoretical (Paans et al, 1985; Brownell et al, 1982) obstacles must be overcome before the functional potential of MRI can be available for clinical application. For example, the MRI technique is dependent upon the number of nuclei investigated for the quality of its measurement. Thus, hydrogen atoms, which are very numerous, are the easiest to use to create images. Phosphorous, which is less prevalent, requires the most powerful magnets, and such superconducting MRI systems require extremely low temperatures and highly sophisticated technical support. Even with these requirements, the resolution and technical quality of phosphorous imaging with MRI is not yet sufficiently developed for clinical application at this time.

REGIONAL CEREBRAL BLOOD FLOW (rCBF)

At present, regional cerebral blood flow (rCBF) can be measured by using inhaled radioactive xenon-133 gas (Obrist et al, 1967, 1971, 1975; Risberg et al, 1975) and measuring its clearance from the brain with an array of detectors. This data can then be used to construct two-dimensional maps of brain blood flow (Figure 4). Unlike positron emission tomography or SPECT, this particular technique has little ability to investigate subcortical structures. This technique is based upon a basic neuroscience principle which posits that regional cerebral blood flow is closely correlated to brain metabolism. Thus, by measuring regional differences in brain blood flow we can infer information concerning local differences in neuronal metabolism.

One of the first studies of cerebral blood flow in schizophrinia (Kety et al, 1948) used a nitrous oxide method and reported that whole brain blood flow was not significantly different between 22 schizophrenic subjects and normal controls. This finding has been replicated by Ingvar and Franzen (1974), Mubrin et al (1982), Gur and colleagues (1983), and Weinberger and colleagues (1986). Although two studies (Ariel, 1983 and Mathew, 1982) have reported significantly lower whole-brain blood flow in schizophrenia, both these studies failed to

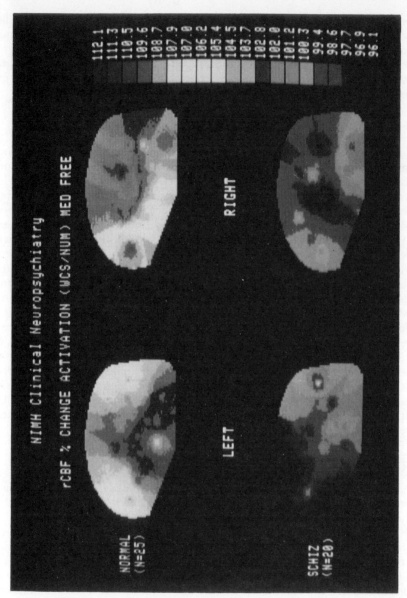

Figure 4. This picture depicts regional cerebral blood flow (rCBF) relationships in the left and right sides of the brain of patients with schizophrenia compared to normal controls. In this case, the values are based upon a ratio between a simple numbers task and the Wisconsin Card Sort, a cognitive activation task which places a demand upon a relatively specific part of the frontal lobes, the dorso-lateral prefrontal cortex. These pictures demonstrate the activation of this region in the normal controls when compared to activity during the number task. The schizophrenic patients fail to demonstrate this normal activation of this region during the task. These results provide evidence of dysfunction of the dorso-lateral prefrontal cortex in schizophrenia. Provided by Dr. Daniel R. Weinberger, NIMH.

correct for PCO_2, which can significantly influence measures of blood flow. In addition Gur (1984) has pointed out that some of the schizophrenic patients studied by Ariel had a history of some substance abuse.

The first regionally specific study of psychiatric patients by Ingvar and Franzen (1974a, 1974b) and Franzen and Ingvar (1975a, 1975b) used intra-arterial xenon injection and reported that medicated schizophrenic patients did not demonstrate the "hyperfrontal" pattern of blood flow seen in control subjects. Although a number of methodologic limitations have been pointed out (Berman et al, 1984) in this classical study, this work focused attention on the frontal lobes as a potential pathophysiologic site of dysfunction in schizophrenia.

This finding of "hypofrontality" in schizophrenia was not confirmed by Mathew (1982) or Gur and colleagues (1983). Using the xenon-133 inhalation technique, Gur and colleagues (1983, 1984) studied 15 medicated schizophrenic patients compared to 25 normal controls and a sample of 19 unmedicated schizophrenic patients compared 19 matched controls. In both studies all subjects were studied in three conditions, in random counterbalanced order: 1) resting state; 2) performing a verbal task; and 3) performing a spatial task. The results of the studies during cognitive activation revealed abnormalities in hemispheric changes during task performance. Specifically, the study provided evidence in support of a hypothetical overactivation of the left hemisphere in schizophrenia. In addition, significant effect of medication and gender were also demonstrated. This work extends Gur and colleagues' pioneering work on an organizing theory implicating left hemispheric dysfunction and left hemispheric overactivation in schizophrenia (Gur 1978). Gur (1984) has also studied 14 medicated patients with major depression compared to 25 controls and found that overall resting flows did not differ and no hemispheric or anteroposterior differences were found in this state. During cognitive activation differences were found between patients and controls and these abnormalities were different for male and female patients.

Most recently, Weinberger and colleagues (Weinberger et al, 1986; Berman et al, 1984), using the xenon-133 inhalation technique, have built upon these pioneering studies of regional brain blood flow in schizophrenia and focused upon a specific region of the frontal cortex (Figure 5). In this study, 25 drug-free chronic schizophrenic patients and 25 normal controls were studied under three conditions: 1) the resting alert state; 2) the cognitive activation state of the Wisconsin Card Sort test; and 3) the cognitive activation state of a number-matching test. The value of studying brain function during specific cognitive activation tests is emphasized by the fact that during the resting state, a subject's mental activities and any concomitant physiological reflection of this state are extremely variable. The value of the Wisconsin Card Sort is that it is felt to specifically examine the functional integrity of the dorsolateral prefrontal cortex (DLPFC) (Milner, 1963). The number-matching test was used to control for the effects of performing a cognitive activation test and experiencing an rCBF study. In the number match, no group specific regional differences were delineated. In the Wisconsin Card Sort, the patients demonstrated significantly decreased absolute and relative blood flow to the dorsolateral prefrontal cortex compared to controls (Figure 5). These results suggest a potential role for dysfunction in the dorsolateral prefrontal cortex in the pathophysiology of schizophrenia.

In a second study from this same laboratory (Berman et al, 1986), evidence is

PREFRONTAL CORTEX

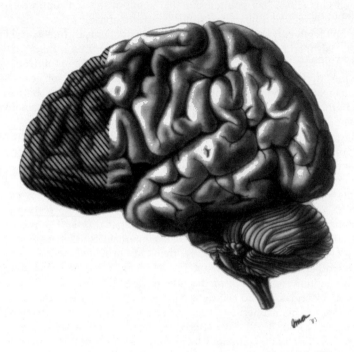

Figure 5. The prefrontal cortex, a region of the frontal lobes that recent brain imaging strategies have focused on in the study of schizophrenia. Provided by Dr. Daniel R. Weinberger, NIMH.

presented that argues against this finding being the result of medication state, attention, or effort. This study by Berman and colleagues suggests that dysfunction of the dorsolateral prefrontal cortex in schizophrenia is a "cognitively linked physiological deficit." Future studies may involve the use of single-photon-emission tomography (SPECT) or PET to provide three-dimensional information about brain activity (including subcortical structures) to complement the two-dimensional data from rCBF. Beyond the strength of addressing the contribution of medication effects and controlling for state factors such as attention, effort, and clinical status, this study also utilized an important basic strategy in functional brain imaging. These two studies (Weinberger et al, 1986; Berman et al, 1986), use to special advantage, several paradigms of cognitive activation, both to cognitively stress a specific functional brain region (Wisconsin Card Sort/ DLPFC) and to control for effort, attention, clinical state, and the effect of taking a cognitive test (number match, visual continuous performance task). Finally, these two studies provide the experimental basis for one of the most promising and exciting organizing theories of schizophrenia. Based upon neuroscience principles, this organizing theory suggests specific neurofunctional pathophysiology that may explain aspects of the clinical presentation of schizophrenia as well as the natural history of this devastating disorder.

ORGANIZING THEORIES AND THEIR USEFULNESS

The field of functional brain imaging is filled with a complex set of data that are often contradictory and sometimes all but impossible to even compare. In an attempt to provide a theoretical structure for our interpretation and assimilation of these complex data sets we have come to adopt a number of "organizing theories" of abnormal function in psychiatric research.

The dopamine theory of schizophrenia and theories of abnormal hemispheric lateralization or abnormalities of the left hemisphere (Nasrallah, 1986; Gur, 1978, 1984; Gur et al, 1983, 1984, in press; Flor-Henry et al, 1979; Guenther and Breitling, 1985; Guenther et al, 1986; Morstyn et al, 1983; Sheppard et al, 1983) and temporal lobe abnormalities (Andreasen, 1986; Flor-Henry 1969) were early "organizing theories."

One of the most interesting new "organizing theories" has been posited by Weinberger and his colleagues (Weinberger, 1986; Morihisa and Weinberger, 1986a) and involves a specific functional region of the frontal lobes, the dorsolateral prefrontal cortex. Its basis in functional brain imaging and its derivation from the neurosciences makes it of particular relevance to this discussion.

This theory begins with the observation that the clinical pathological presentation of patients with frontal lobe pathology (lack of initiative, poor insight, social withdrawal, flat affect, poor judgment) is quite reminiscent of a constellation of schizophrenic symptoms often termed negative symptoms or defect state. With the advent of our newly won capability to image brain function in the living human, an opportunity to investigate this apparent similarity of clinical presentation was obtained. Positron emission tomography studies have provided data consistent with frontal lobe pathology, and recently the work of Wolkin and colleagues (1985) has specifically demonstrated abnormalities of brain metabolism in the region of the frontal lobes. The sister structural imaging techniques of CT and MRI have also provided evidence for brain abnormalities in the frontal lobes of schizophrenic patients (Shelton and Weinberger, submitted for publication; Andreasen, 1986). Combining CT scans and computerized mapping of auditory and visual evoked potentials, Morihisa and McAnulty (1985) have reported abnormalities that also focus attention on the frontal lobes. Finally, the rCBF work of Weinberger and his colleagues (Berman et al, 1984; Weinberger et al, 1986; Berman et al, 1986) has refined our focus of suspicion to a specific region of the frontal lobes, the dorsolateral prefrontal cortex.

By demonstrating a physiological deficit in schizophrenia that does not appear to be explained by medication status, or state factors, Weinberger (in press) has provided a structural framework for organizing our thinking about the pathophysiology that might underlie schizophrenia. Drawing upon basic neuroscience findings concerning the neuroanatomic connections and functional interrelationships of the DLPFC as well as recently reported findings concerning the natural history of CNS dopamine systems, an "organizing theory of relevant anatomy and physiology" is developed implicating dorsolateral prefrontal cortex dysfunction in schizophrenia (Morihisa and Weinberger, 1986a; Weinberger, in press). First, the neuroscience studies of Fuster, Nauta, Goldman-Rakic, and others provide a richly fertile setting for such a theory. The prefrontal cortex is a highly evolved component of the neocortex and represents the largest functional subdivision of the cerebral cortex (Goldman-Rakic et al, 1983). Perhaps of greatest importance to this theory, the functional integrity of the prefrontal cortex is necessary for the organization and continuity of behavior required for achieving specific future goals (Goldman-Rakic et al, 1983), a fundamental element for adaptation to a changing world (Morihisa and Weinberger, 1986a). More specifically, the dorsolateral prefrontal cortex enjoys a diversity of connections with each type of association cortex (Nauta, 1971; Fuster, 1980) as well as behaviorally significant limbic, diencephalic, and mesencephalic nuclei that circumstantially implicate its importance to the regulation of behavior. Of special interest, the DLPFC is specifically linked to classically subcortical dopamine systems (Porrino and Goldman-Rakic, 1982). Moreover, animal studies with monkeys suggest that interruption of this structure causes the loss of the ability to perform tests (delayed-response) that assess the animal's ability to develop rules based upon the environment and then to change the rules to adapt to changing environmental conditions. If this basic and vital cognitive function were indeed crucially dependent upon this brain region, then the findings of abnormal DLPFC function associated with poor Wisconsin performance may be related to some of the clinical pathology seen in schizophrenia.

Pursuing this model, basic science studies also suggest that the dopamine input into the DLPFC may be the crucial element in this dysfunction (Brozoski et al, 1979; Goldman-Rakic et al, 1983). Furthermore, basic science studies suggest that prefrontal cortex glucose metabolism is enhanced following administration of dopamine agonists (McCulloch et al, 1982), which suggests that dopamine systems may augment DLPFC activity. If this were the case, a subtle lesion of dopamine innervation to the DLPFC could explain a number of the generally accepted but unexplained clinical phenomenology of schizophrenia. First, if there were an interruption of dopamine innervation to the DLPFC, this might explain the dysfunction of the frontal lobes that is reminiscent of a frontal lobe syndrome (negative symptoms). At the same time, loss of dopamine pathways in the prefrontal cortex could result in disinhibition of the subcortical dopamine system (Pycock et al, 1980), providing a tempting explanation for positive symptomatology. In addition, recent neuroscience findings suggest that there is an age-associated decrease in dopamine in the prefrontal cortex (McGeer and McGeer, 1981) which would enhance defect symptoms over time, and an age-related decrease of subcortical dopamine receptor activity (Wong et al, 1984; Bzowej and Seeman, 1985) that might ameliorate the disinhibitory effects of a prefrontal cortical lesion and thus lead to a decrease of positive symptoms. This could explain the clinically observed (Pfohl and Winokur, 1982) regression of positive symptoms over time and the predominance of negative symptoms with increasing age in schizophrenia.

Finally, several animal studies (Goldman and Alexander, 1977; Tucker and Kling, 1967; Goldman, 1971) suggest that the dysfunction associated with the DLPFC does not become functionally manifest until adulthood is attained and presumably certain brain systems become dedicated and committed. Thus, the usual appearance of schizophrenia in adolescence could also be partially explained by this theoretical model. The ability of this theory to organize our recent findings from in vivo brain imaging, its economic explanation of schizophrenic phenomena, and the fact that it is rooted in basic neuroscience findings provides a compelling lead to follow in our expanding investigations of the mind.

CONCLUSION: THE DANGERS AND SEDUCTIVE QUALITIES OF ORGANIZING THEORIES

There is a seductive attraction to organizing theories, in part engendered by the complexity and frustrating ambiguity of our brain imaging findings to date. The human mind desires order and meaning and, unfortunately, it may be too early to expect anything coherent to be permanently extractable from the present state of brain imaging research. We sometimes lose sight of the diversity of the forest because we focus upon what appears to be a meaning-laden tree of organizational theory. The immediate danger is to allow this theory too much control over our thinking, our interpretation of data, our development of research paradigms, and our decisions concerning future avenues of investigation to explore. Finally, there is a latent danger in any overenthusiastic embracing of specific unifying theories of psychiatric illness. This danger is the disappointment and anger we feel when the theories come up short or lead us down blind alleys or, perhaps most damning, merely go nowhere after promising so much. This is not an idle danger. Indeed, although the scientific advances have created a new substrate of technology, this is in many ways a repetition of the reaction to the failure of early psychiatry to define the underlying structural pathognomonic lesions of psychiatric illnesses that led to the rejection of biological causes and an embracing of environmental factors. Dr. Andreasen has alluded to this phenomenon as the "amnestic disorder" suffered by psychiatry and neurology during the middle of the 20th century, during which time the search for brain abnormalities in patients with mental illnesses was abandoned. Indeed, her words would seem to be already applicable to todays problems:

> . . . the notion of seeking for the causes of mental illness in brain structure seemed ludicrous and over-simplified. Evidence that had accumulated concerning neuropathological causes of schizophrenia and manic-depressive illness was conflicting rather than incisively convincing. (Chapter 11)

Although we now adopt a more reasonable, eclectic view of the causes of psychopathology, we are on the brink of a similar danger of overexpectation and overenthusiastic reductionism in our relationship with functional brain imaging. We must resist the temptation to demarcate apparent patterns of congruence to the exclusion of findings which do not fit our organizing theories. There is no question that organizing theories provide a useful and thought-provoking means of dealing with problematic oceans of conflicting information. Indeed, the organizing theory method of data interpretation may provide the most instructive manner of teaching the information of functional imaging available to us. However, we must also teach the ability to maintain an optimistic skepticism and an understanding, critical pessimism in our overall struggle with these massive and complex data sets. In the end we must take advantage of the very strengths that distinguish humans from other species, the ability to develop strategies and rules to obtain future goals that take into account past experiences but can modify these rules as changing conditions in the present mandate: Simply put, the ability to think and plan and rethink and then plan anew.

REFERENCES

Alexander GE, Goldman PS: Functional development of the dorsolateral prefrontal cortex: an analysis utilizing reversible cryogenic depression. Brain Res 143:233-249, 1978

Andreasen NC: Is schizophrenia a temporolimbic disease? in Can Schizophrenia be Localized in the Brain? Edited by Andreasen NC. Washington, DC, American Psychiatric Press, Inc., 1986

Andreasen NC (Ed): Brain Imaging for Psychiatrists. Washington, DC, American Psychiatric Press, Inc. (in press)

Andreasen NC, Nasralah HA, Dunn V, et al: Structural abnormalities in the frontal system in schizophrenia. Arch Gen Psychiatry 43:136-144, 1986

Ariel RN, Golden CJ, Berg PA, et al: Regional cerebral blood flow in schizophrenics. Arch Gen Psychiatry 40:258-263, 1983

Baron JC, Comar D, Zaritian E, et al: Dopaminergic receptor sites in human brain positron emission tomography. Neurology 35:16-24, 1985

Baxter CR, Phelps ME, Mazziotta JC, et al: Cerebral metabolic rates for glucose in mood disorders: studies with positron emission tomography and fluorodeoxyglucose F 18. Arch Gen Psychiatry 42:441-447, 1985

Berger H: Uber das elektrenkephalogramm des menschen, I. Arch Psychiatr Nervenkr 87:527-571, 1929

Berman KF, Weinberger DR, Morihisa JM, et al: Regional cerebral blood flow in psychiatry: application to clinical research, in Brain Imaging in Psychiatry. Edited by Morihisa JM. Washington, DC, American Psychiatric Press, Inc., 1984

Berman KF, Zec RF, Weinberger DR: Physiologic dysfunction of dorsolateral prefrontal cortex in schizophrenia, II: role of neuroleptic treatment, attention and mental effort. Arch Gen Psychiatry 43:126-135, 1986

Bickford RG, Brimm J, Berger L, et al: Application of compressed spectral array in clinical EEG, in Automation of Clinical Electroencephalography. Edited by Kellway P, Peterson J. New York, Raven Press, 1973

Brodie JD, Christman DR, Corona FJ, et al: Patterns of metabolic activity in the treatment of schizophrenia. Ann Neurol (suppl) 15:S166-S169, 1984

Brownell GL, Budinger TF, Lauterbur PC, et al: Positron tomography and nuclear magnetic resonance imaging. Science 215:619-626, 1982

Brozoski TJ, Brown RM, Rosvold HE, et al: Cognitive deficit caused by regional depletion of dopamine in prefrontal cortex of rhesus monkey. Science 205:929-932, 1979

Buchsbaum MS: Middle evoked potentials. Schiz Bull 3:93-104, 1977

Buchsbaum MS: Positron emission tomography (PET) in psychiatry, in Brain Imaging in Psychiatry. Edited by Morihisa JM. Washington, DC, American Psychiatric Press, Inc., 1984

Buchsbaum MS, Ingvar DH, Kessler R, et al: Cerebral glucography with positron tomography: use in normal subjects and in patients with schizophrenia. Arch Gen Psychiatry 39:251-259, 1982

Buchsbaum MS, DeLisi LE, Holcomb HH, et al: Anteroposterior gradients in cerebral glucose use in schizophrenia and affective disorders. Arch Gen Psychiatry 41:1159-1166, 1984

Buchsbaum MS, Awsare SV, Holcomb H, et al: Topographic differences between normals and schizophrenics: the N120 evoked potential component. Neuropsychobiology (in press)

Bzowej NH, Seeman P: Age and dopamine D2 receptors in human brain. Neuroscience Abstracts 11:889, 1985

Coleman RE, Blinder RA, Jaszczak RJ: Single photon emission computed tomography (SPECT), part II: clinical applications. Invest Radiol 21:1-11, 1986

Comar D, Zarifan E, Verhas M, et al: Brain distribution and kinetics of IIC-chloropromazine in schizophrenics. Psychiatry Res 1:23-29, 1979

Coppola R: Issues in topographic analysis of EEG activity, in Topographic Mapping of the Brain Electrical Activity. Edited by Duffy FH, Boston, Butterworths, 1986

Coppola R, Buchsbaum MS, Rigal F: Computer generation of surface distribution maps of measures of brain activity. Comput Biol Med 12:191-199, 1982

DeLisi LE, Buchsbaum MS, Holcomb HH, et al: Clinical correlates of decreased antero-posterior metabolic gradients in positron emission tomography (PET) of schizophrenic patients. Am J Psychiatry 142:78-81, 1985a

DeLisi LE, Holcomb HH, Cohen RM, et al: Positron emission tomography in schizophrenic patients with and without neuroleptic medication. J Cereb Blood Flow Metab 5:201-206, 1985b

Duffy FH: Topographic display of evoked potentials: clinical application of brain electrical activity mapping (BEAM). Ann NY Acad Sci 388:183-196, 1982

Duffy FH, Burchfield JL, Lombrosco CT: Brain electrical activity mapping (BEAM): a method for extending the clinical utility of EEG and evoked potential data. Ann Neurol 5:309-332, 1979

Elbert T, Lutzenberger W, Rockstroh B, et al: Removal of ocular artifacts from the EEG—biophysical approach to the EOG. Electroencephalogr Clin Neurophysiol 60:455-463, 1985

Estrin T, Uzgalis R: Computer display of spatio-temporal EEG patterns. IEEE Trans Biomed Eng 16:192-196, 1969

Farde L, Hall H, Ehrin E, et al: Quantitative analysis of D2 dopamine receptor binding in the living human brain by PET. Science 231:258-261, 1986

Farkas T, Wolf AP, Jaeger J, et al: Regional brain glucose metabolism in chronic schizophrenia. Arch Gen Psychiatry 41:293-300, 1984

Flor-Henry P: Psychosis and temporal lobe epilepsy: a controlled investigation. Epilepsia 10:363-395, 1969

Flor-Henry P, Koles ZJ, Howarth BG, et al: Neurophysiological studies of schizophrenia, mania and depression, in Hemispheric Asymmetries of Function in Psychopathology. Edited by Gruzelier JH, Flor-Henry P. New York. Elsevier, 1979

Franzen G, Ingvar DH: Abnormal distribution of cerebral activity in chronic schizophrenia. J Psychiatr Res 12:199-214, 1975a

Franzen G, Ingvar DH: Absence of activation in frontal structures during psychological testing of chronic schizophrenics. J Neurol Neurosurg Psychiatry 38:1027-1032, 1975b

Fuster J: The Prefrontal Cortex. New York, Raven Press, 1980

Garnett ES, Firnau G, Nahmias C: Dopamine visualized in the basal ganglia of living man. Nature 305:137-138, 1983

Goldman PS: Functional development of the prefrontal cortex in early life and the problem of neuronal plasticity. Exp Neurol 32:366-387, 1971

Goldman PS, Alexander GE: Maturation of prefrontal cortex in the monkey revealed by local reversible cryogenic depression. Nature 267:613-615, 1977

Goldman-Rakic PS, Isseroff A, Schwartz ML: The neurobiology of cognitive development, in Handbook of Child Psychology: Biology of Infancy Development. Edited by Mussen P. New York, Wiley, 1983

Gotman J, Gloor P, Ray WG: A quantitative comparison of traditional reading of the EEG and interpretation of computer extracted features in patients with supratentorial brain lesions. Electroencephalogr Clin Neurophysiol 38:623-639, 1975

Greenberg JH, Reivich M, Alavi A, et al: Metabolic mapping of functional activity in human subjects with the [18F] fluoro-deoxyglucose technique. Science 212:678-680, 1981

Guenther W, Breitling D: Predominant sensorimotor area left hemisphere dysfunction in schizophrenia measured by brain electrical activity mapping. Biol Psychiatry 20:515-532, 1985

Guenther W, Breitling D, Banquet JP, et al: EEG mapping of left hemisphere dysfunction during motor performance in schizophrenia. Biol Psychiatry 21:249-262, 1986

Gur RE: Left hemisphere dysfunction and left hemisphere overactivation in schizophrenia. J Abnorm Psychol 87:225-238, 1978

Gur RE: Regional cerebral blood flow in psychiatry: the resting and activated brains of schizophrenic patients, in brain imaging in psychiatry. Edited by Morihisa JM. Washington, DC, American Psychiatric Press, Inc., 1984

Gur RE, Skolnick BE, Gur RC: Brain function in psychiatric disorders, I: regional cerebral blood flow in medicated schizophrenia. Arch Gen Psychiatry 40:1250-1254, 1983

Gur RE, Skolnick BE, Gur RC, et al: Brain function in psychiatric disorders, II: regional cerebral blood flow in medicated unipolar depressives. Arch Gen Psychiatry 41:695-699, 1984

Gur RE, Gur RC, Skolnick BE, et al: Brain function in psychiatric disorders, III: regional cerebral blood flow in unmedicated schizophrenics. Arch Gen Psychiatry 42:329-334, 1985

Holman BL, Gibson RE, Hill TC, et al: Muscarinic acetylcholine receptors in Alzheimer's disease: in vivo imaging with iodine 123-labeled 3-quinuclidinyl-4-iodobenzilate and emission tomography. JAMA 254:3063-3066, 1985

Ingvar DH, Franzen G: Abnormalities of cerebral blood flow distribution in patients with chronic schizophrenia. Acta Psychiatr Scand 50:425-462 1974a

Ingvar DH, Franzen G: Distribution of cerebral activity in chronic schizophrenia. Lancet 2:1484-1486, 1974b

Itil TM, Saletu B, Davis S: EEG findings in chronic schizophrenics based on digital computer period analysis and analog power spectra. Biol Psychiatry 5:1-13, 1972

Jablonski T, Prohovnik I, Risberg J, et al: Fourier analysis of ^{133}Xe inhalation curves. Acta Neurol Scand 60 (Suppl 72): 216-217, 1979

James AE Jr, Price RR, Rollo FD, et al: Nuclear magnetic resonance imaging: a promising technique. JAMA 247:1331-1334, 1982

Jaszczak RJ, Coleman ER: Single photon emission computed tomography (SPECT), I: principles and instrumentation. Invest Radiol 20:897-910, 1985

Jernigan TL, Sargent T, Pfefferbaum A, et al: Fluorodeoxyglucose PET in schizophrenia. Psychiatry Res 16:317-329, 1985

Jervis BW, Nichols MJ, Allen EM, et al: The assessment of two methods for removing eye movement artifact from the EEG. Electroencephalogr Clin neurophysiol 61:444-452, 1985

Kety SS, Woodford RB, Harmel MH, et al: Cerebral blood flow and metabolism in schizophrenia. Am J Psychiatry 104:765-770, 1948

Kling AS, Metter EJ, Riegh WH, et al: Comparison of PET measurement of local brain glucose metabolism and CAT measurement of brain atrophy in chronic schizophrenia and depression. Am J Psychiatry 143:175-180, 1986

Kuhl DE, Barrio JR, Huang SC, et al: Quantifying local cerebral blood flow by N-Isopropyl-p (^{123}) iodoamphetamine (IMP) tomography. J Nucl Med 23:196-203, 1982

Lehman D: Multichannel topography of human alpha EEG fields. Electroencephalogr Clin Neurophysiol 31:439-499, 1971

Lemieux JF, Vera RS, Blume WT: Technique to display topographical evolution of EEG events. Electroencephalogr Clin Neurophysiol 58:565-568, 1984

Mathew RJ, Meyer JS, Francis DJ, et al: Cerebral blood flow in depression. Am J Psychiatry 137:1449-1450, 1980

Mathew RJ, Duncan GC, Weinman ML, et al: Regional Cerebral Blood Flow in Schizophrenia. Arch Gen Psychiatry 39:1121-1124, 1982

Mazziotta JC, Phelps ME, Carson RE, et al: Tomographic mapping of human cerebral metabolism: sensory deprivation. Ann Neurol 12:435-444, 1982

Mazziotta JC, Huang SC, Phelps ME, et al: A noninvasive positron computed tomography technique using oxygen-15-labeled water for the evaluation of neurobehavioral task batteries. J Cereb Blood Flow Metab 5:70-78, 1985

McCulloch J, Savaki HE, Sokoloff L: Distribution of effects of haloperidol on energy metabolism in the brain. Brain Res 243:81-90, 1982

McGeer PL: Brain imaging in Alzeheimer's disease. Br Med Bull 42:24-28, 1986

McGeer PL, McGeer EG: Neurotransmitters in the aging brain, in The Molecular Basis of Neuropathology. Edited by Darrison AM, Thompson RHS. London, Edward Arnold, 1981

McGeer PL, Kamo H, Harrop R, et al: Positron emission tomography in patients with clinically diagnosed Alzheimer's disease. Can Med Assoc J 134:597-607, 1986

Milner B: Effects of different brain lesions on card sorting. Arch neurology 9:100-110, 1963

Morihisa JM (Ed): Brain Imaging in Psychiatry. Washington, DC, American Psychiatric Press, Inc., 1984

Morihisa JM: Electrophysiological evidence implicating frontal lobe dysfunction in schizophrenia. Psychopharmacol Bull 22:885-889, 1986b

Morihisa JM: Computerized EEG and evoked potential mapping, in Brain Imaging for Psychiatrists. Edited by Andreasen N. Washington, DC, American Psychiatric Press, Inc. (in press)

Morihisa JM, McAnulty GB: Structure and function: brain electrical activity mapping and computer tomography in schizophrenia. Biol Psychiatry 20:3-19, 1985

Morihisa JM, Weinberger DR: Is schizophrenia a frontal lobe disease? an organizing theory of relevant anatomy and physiology, in Can Schizophrenia be Localized in the Brain? Edited by Andreasen N. Washington, DC, American Psychiatric Press, Inc., 1986a

Morihisa JM, Duffy FH, Wyatt RJ: Brain electrical activity mapping (BEAM) in schizophrenic patients. Arch Gen Psychiatry 40:719-728, 1983

Morstyn R, Duffy FH, McCarley RW: Altered P300 topography in schizophrenia. Arch Gen Psychiatry 40:729-734, 1983

Mubrin A, Knezvic S, Koretic D, et al: Regional cerebral flow patterns in schizophrenic patients. Regional Cerebral Blood Flow Bulletin 3:43-46, 1982

Nasrallah HA: Is schizophrenia a left hemisphere disease? in Can schizophrenia be Localized in the Brain? Edited by Andreasen NC. Washington, DC, American Psychiatric Press, Inc., 1986

Nauta WJH: The problem of the frontal lobe: a reinterpretation. J Psychiatr Res 8:167-187, 1971

Nilsson A, Risberg J, Johnson M, et al: Regional changes of cerebral blood flow during haloperidol therapy in patients with paranoid symptoms. Acta Neurol Scand 56 (Suppl 64):478-479, 1977

Obrist WD, Thompson HK, King HC, et al: Determination of regional cerebral flow by inhalation of ^{133}Xenon. Circulation Research, 20:124-135, 1967

Obrist, WD, Thompson HK, Wang HS, et al: A simplified procedure for determining fast compartment rCBF by ^{133}Xenon inhalation, in Brain and Blood Flow. Edited by Russell RWR. London, Pitman Publishing Co., 1971

Obrist WD, Thompson HK, Wang HS, et al: Regional cerebral blood flow estimated by ^{133}Xenon inhalation. Stroke 6:245-256, 1975

Paans AMJ, Vaalburg W, Woldring MG: A comparison of the sensitivity of PET and NMR for in vivo quantitative metabolic imaging. Eur J Nucl Med 11:73-75, 1985

Parfitt DN: The neurology of schizophrenia. Journal of Mental Sciences 102:671-718, 1956

Perlmutter JS, Larson KB, Raichle ME, et al: Strategies for in vivo measurement of receptor binding using positron emission tomography. J Cereb Blood Flow Metab 6:154-169, 1986

Persson A, Ehrin E, Eriksson L, et al: Imaging of [C]-Labelled RO 15-1788 binding to benzodiazepine receptors in the human brain by positron emission tomography. J Psychiatr Res 19:609-622, 1985

Petsche H: Topography of the EEG: survey and prospects. Clin Neurol Neurosurg 79:15-28, 1976

Pfohl B, Winokur G: The evolution of symptoms in institutionalized hebephrenic catatonic schizophrenics. Br J Psychiatry 141:567-572, 1982

Pfurtscheller G, Ladurner G, Maresch H, et al: Brain electrical activity mapping in normal and ischemic brain, in Brain Ischemia: Quantitative EEG and Imaging Techniques, Progress in Brain Research, Vol 62. Edited by Pfurtschellr G, Jonkman EJ, Lopes da Silva FH. New York, Elsevier Science Publishers, 1984

Phelps ME, Juhl DE, Mazziotta JC: Metabolic mapping of the brain's response to visual stimulation: studies in humans. Science 211:1145-1148, 1981a

Phelps ME, Mazziotta JC, Kuhl DE, et al: Tomographic mapping of human cerebral metabolism: visual stimulation and deprivation. Neurology 31:517-529, 1981b

Phelps ME, Mazziotta JC, Huang SC: Study of cerebral function with positron computed tomography. J Cereb Blood Flow Metab 2:113-162, 1982

Phelps ME, Mazziotta JC, Baxter L, et al: Positron emission tomography study of affective disorders: problems and strategies. Ann Neurol 15:s149-s156, 1984

Pockberger H, Rapplesberger P, Petsche H, et al: Computer-assisted EEG topography as a tool in the evaluation of actions of psychoactive drugs in patients. Neuropsychobiology 12:183-187, 1984

Porrino LJ, Goldman-Rakic PS: Brainstem innervation of prefrontal and anterior cingulate cortex in the rhesus monkey revealed by retrograde transport of HRP. J Comp Neurol 205:63-76, 1982

Pycock CJ, Kerwin RW, Carter CJ, et al: Effect of lesion of cortical dopamine terminals on subcortical dopamine in RATS. Nature 286:74-77, 1980

Remond A: Orientations et tendences des methodes topographiques dans l'etude de l'activité electrique du cerveau. Rev Neurol 93:399-410, 1955

Reivich M, Alavi A, Gur RC, et al: Determination of local cerebral glucose metabolism in humans: methodology and applications to the study of sensory and cognitive stimuli, in Brain Imaging and Brain Function. Edited by Sokoloff L. New York, Raven Press, 1985

Risberg J: Regional cerebral blood flow measurement by ^{133}Xe-inhalation: methodology and applications in neuropsychology and psychiatry. Brain Lang 9:9-34, 1980

Roth WT: Late event related potentials and psychopathology. Schizophr Bull 3:105-120, 1977

Rumsey JM, Duara R, Grady C, et al: Brain metabolism in autism. Arch Gen Psychiatry 42:448-455, 1985

Rush AJ, Schlesser MA, Stokey E, et al: Cerebral blood flow in depression and mania, in Brain Imaging in Psychiatry and Neurology: Positron Emission Tomography and Other Techniques. Edited by Buchsbaum MS, Usdin E, Bunney WE Jr, et al. Pacific Grove, CA, Boxwood Press (in press)

Shagass C: Early evoked potentials. Schizophr Bull 3:80-92, 1977

Shagass C, Roemer RA, Straumanis J, et al: Temporal variability of somatosensory, visual and auditory evoked potentials in schizophrenia. Arch Gen Psychiatry 36:1341-1351, 1979

Shagass C, Roemer R, Staumanis J, et al: Topography of sensory evoked potentials in depressive disorders. Biol Psychiatry 15:183-207, 1980

Sheppard G, Gruzelier J, Manchanda R, et al: O positron emission tomographic scanning in predominantly never-treated acute schizophrenic patients. Lancet 24-31, 1983

Smith RC, Calderan M, Ravichandran GK, et al: Nuclear magnetic resonance in schizophrenia: a preliminary study. Psychiatry Res 12:137-147, 1984

Sokoloff L: Relationships among local functional activity, energy metabolism and blood flow in the central nervous system. Fed Proc 40:2311-2316, 1981

Sokoloff L: The radioactive deoxyglucose method, in Advance in Neurochemistry 4. Edited by Agranoff BW, Aprison MH. New York, Plenum, 1982

Stump DA, Williams R: The noninvasive measurement of regional cerebral circulation. Brain Lang 9:35-46, 1980

Tucker TJ, Kling A: Differential effects of early and late lesions of frontal granular cortex in the monkey. Brain Res 5:377-389, 1967

Uytdenhoef P, Portelange P, Jacquy J, et al: Regional cerebral blood flow and lateralized hemispheric dysfunction in depression. Br J Psychiatry 143:128-132, 1983

Wagner HN, Burns HD, Dannals RF, et al: Imaging dopamine receptors in the human brain by positron tomography. Science 221:1264-1266, 1983

Walter WG, Shipton HW: A new toposcopic display system. Electroencephalogr Clin Neurophysiol 3:281-292, 1951

Weinberger DR: Implications of normal brain development for the pathogenesis of schizophrenia. Arch Gen Psychiatry (in press)

Weinberger DR, Berman KF, Zec RF: Physiological dysfunction of dorsolateral prefrontal cortex in schizophrenia, I: regional cerebral blood flow (rCBF) evidence. Arch Gen Psychiatry 43:114-124, 1986

White FJ, Wang RY: Comparison of the effects of chronic haloperidol treatment and A9 and A10 dopamine neurons in the rat. Life Sci 32:983-993, 1983

Whitehouse PJ: The concept of subcortical and cortical dementia: another look. Ann Neurol 19:1-6, 1986

Widen L, Blomgrist G, DePaulis T, et al: Studies of schizophrenia with positron CT. J Clin Neuropharmacol 7 (Suppl. 1):538-539, 1984

Wolkin A, Jaegar J, Brodie J, et al: Persistence of cerebral metabolic abnormalities in chronic schizophrenia as determined by positron emission tomography. Am J Psychiatry 142:564-571, 1985

Wong DF, Wagner HN Jr, Dannals RF, et al: Effects of age on dopamine and serotonin receptors measured by positron emission tomography in the living human brain. Science 226:1393-1396, 1984

Afterword to Section II

by John M. Morihisa, M.D., and Solomon H. Snyder, M.D.,
Section Editors

The same forces that spawned the neurosciences also gave birth to modern psychiatry, and they are now moving us closer to a synthesis of disciplines that seeks to understand the very nature of thought, action, and feelings. This convergence of multiple avenues of investigation represents a potential well-spring of knowledge about ourselves. Technological advances have brought us civilization but understanding of our own nature promises even more. Within this promise are many potential missteps and blind alleys. For example, in Chapter 12 we alluded to both the usefulness as well as the dangers inherent in our use of "organizing theories" in psychiatric research. In this dynamically evolving field we must adopt a complex stance that can assimilate both the enthusiasm for what we may achieve as well as the frustration and disappointment that we will surely suffer in this scientific odyssey.

Thus, we hope to promote a viewpoint in which the reader is sharply critical and skeptical of individual studies but optimistic and excited about the field in general. This is in no way a contradiction, and in fact will help guard against the temptation to too quickly endorse and embrace each finding as a basic principle of neuroscience, with the inevitable disappointment and anger when conflicting and confusing findings are reported and clinical applications are excruciatingly slow to develop.

This section has attempted to capture the excitement and wonder of some of the recent evolutionary advances in psychiatric research based on the neurosciences. At the same time, we have endeavored to highlight some of the difficulties, contradictions, seductive dangers, ambiguities, and limitations of this neuroscience-based psychiatric research, not as criticism of the field but as an indication of the youthful state of our tentative gropings along a new frontier of human knowledge. We will no doubt make mistakes and be led down promising paths that lead us full circle to our starting point. This must not deter us from the formidable task of developing new and clinically useful ways of measuring brain function to better understand the underlying pathophysiology of disorders of the mind.

Although the first flight of the Wright brothers was limited in scope and failed to resolve many of the most important issues of aerodynamics and none of the application issues of present day air travel, it still represented a promising and exciting beginning to a new world of opportunities to improve the human condition. In a similar manner we stand upon a new threshold of knowledge in the neurosciences and psychiatry that raises our hopes in our battle against mental illness, but which will require of us enormous determination, patience, wisdom, and luck to fulfill this promise.

III

Differential Therapeutics

Contents

Section III

Differential Therapeutics
Foreword

by John F. Clarkin, Ph.D., and Samuel W. Perry, M.D.,
Section Editors

The easiest way to practice psychiatry is to view all patients and problems as basically similar and to apply a standard therapy or standard mix of therapies in every treatment. Many practitioners continue to use such an approach. As this section attests, however, everything we have learned in recent decades indicates that this approach is misguided and no longer tenable—it deprives our patients of the most effective and specific treatment, and it wastes scarce resources.

FACTORS PROMPTING DIFFERENTIAL THERAPEUTICS IN PSYCHIATRY

Five factors have prompted an increasing recognition that the choice of therapy is best tailored to the specific needs of the individual patient:

Research in psychopharmacotherapy. Over the past 30 years countless studies have compared the relative and specific efficacies of various psychotropic medications for specific targeted symptoms and syndromes. By using carefully defined patient groups, well controlled designs with placebo controls, and systematic outcome criteria, these studies have provided a scientific model for differential therapeutics.

Reliable diagnostic system. Research in psychopharmacotherapy requires reliable diagnostic criteria. This requirement was one compelling force in the development of the *Diagnostic and Statistical Manual of Mental Disorders, Third Edition (DSM-III)* (American Psychiatric Association, 1980), which is specific in its criteria, reliable in its utilization, atheoretical in its conception, and relatively successful in separating different groups of patients not only in terms of their clinical syndromes (Axis I), but also in terms of their personality disorders (Axis II), medical problems (Axis III), prior functioning (Axis IV), and current stressors (Axis V). This reliable diagnostic system was catalyzed by the demands of prior research and, in turn, has facilitated current scientific investigation of both pharmacotherapy and psychotherapy.

Improvements in psychotherapy research design. Twenty years ago Kiesler (1966) noted that in most psychotherapy research, "patients" (who were not clearly specified) were assigned to "therapy" (also often taken as a uniform but unknown entity) and outcomes were judged by a global and nonspecific score. Because of these faulty methods, such studies yielded no scientifically valid data regarding which specific interventions produced which specific ends. As a result, the clinician was provided with little useful information to guide treatment planning. In recent years more sophisticated research designs have exploded this "uniformity myth." Psychotherapy research now involves careful selection of homogeneous subjects, manualization and monitoring of a specific therapeutic process, systematic descriptions of the therapists, and outcome measures that are standardized, targeted, and specific (Strupp and Bergin, 1969; Paul, 1967; and Bergin, 1971).

Specificity of psychiatric treatments. The advances in psychotherapy research have been complemented by the development of more specific psychiatric interventions. Whereas exploratory and supportive techniques previously encompassed the therapist's repertoire, the field has broadened remarkably with, for example, the introduction of specific behavioral, cognitive, and focal dynamic methods. There has also been a similar expansion of the possible settings, duration, and formats of treatment and the frequent use of medications and psychotherapy in combination. These developments have increased the options available to a specific patient, but have also placed a greater demand on the consultant to be informed about the growing number of therapeutic approaches.

Extramural pressure. Our "consumers" and third-party payers are understandably requesting, more and more often, that we provide the most effective and cost-efficient treatments and that we be able to explain (and at times justify) the decisions that we have made.

RESISTANCES TO DIFFERENTIAL THERAPEUTICS

The above factors prompting the development of differential therapeutics have been countered by a reluctance among mental health professionals to become more involved in the process of establishing the principles and empirical data upon which treatment decisions are made. These resistances stem from several sources:

Lack of supporting data. Although medication specificity has been fairly well established for a number of conditions, the specificity of psychotherapies has not yet been well documented. There are two possible reasons for this failure to find strong specific effects of different nonpharmacological treatments: the failure may reflect limitations in the specificity of available research; or the failure may reflect the relatively greater importance of shared or nonspecific factors in promoting change, such as the healing ritual, raised expectations, or the nature of the interpersonal relationship. To the degree that nonspecific factors are more important, differential treatment selection is less crucial.

Impracticality. Another source of the resistance is the experience that differential therapeutics in many settings may seem no more than an academic exercise. Those who administer an overworked and understaffed mental health clinic know that the facility can survive only if the hordes of new patients are assigned quickly enough to make room for the next wave of arrivals. While we appreciate the practical demands imposed by such settings, the selection of treatment should not be made expeditiously, unobtrusively, or as a matter of routine. When compromises are necessary, it should be recognized how and why they have been made.

Personal factors. Therapists are understandably unlikely to consider treatment modalities that they are not trained in or inclined to do. They have worked hard to become experts, but in most instances they are expert in only a few of the expanding variety of available treatment techniques. As a result, therapists tend to recommend preferentially those treatments they have to offer rather than to consider systematically each of the alternative possibilities.

Fears of premature standardization. A fourth resistance stems from the concern that any attempt to establish criteria for treatment selection is potentially dangerous. It is feared that guidelines for treatment selection are liable to encourage closure before available research data warrant anything approaching firm conclusions. Many practitioners worry that criteria will be carved in stone (on the basis of scanty evidence) and that clinical judgment will be overruled by bureaucratic procedure sanctified by pseudoscience: third-party payers will take advantage of any further treatment selection criteria in order to fund only the least expensive acceptable modality; and before long, clinical and intellectual issues will become primarily financial ones, and individual clinical creativity will be squelched.

FORGING AHEAD DESPITE LIMITATIONS

Although the above concerns must be recognized, there are at least three reasons for forging ahead into the difficult field of differential therapeutics:

Inevitable limitations of psychotherapy research. The complexities of psychotherapy outcome studies ensure that definitive findings will be extremely long in coming and will probably always be, to some extent, inconclusive. Research investigations generally measure the characteristics of whole populations and generate results that cannot be applied to any given individual without consideration of that patient's uniqueness. Furthermore, while the history of medicine reminds us that accepted clinical judgment is often very wide of the mark, an informed clinical decision is undoubtedly superior to blind chance as a guide to treatment. While we await more substantial data, decisions about treatment must be made—and, of course, are being made every day. Neither we nor our patients can wait indefinitely for results to accumulate before attempting to summarize the current state of differential therapeutics.

Inevitable fiscal constraints. It is naive to believe that the examination of differential therapeutics will have a detrimental effect on the support rendered by third-party payers and governmental funding agencies. The interest of outside agencies in regulating psychotherapy is already present and growing rapidly. There are clear signs both within and outside the psychiatric community that indicate differential therapeutics has received increasing attention during the past decade and simply cannot be avoided. The question is no longer *whether* to discuss and investigate treatment selection, but *how*.

Inevitable discourse. Although the material presented in this section will be new to many clinicians, in fact numerous authors have already attempted to systematize the indications, contraindications, and enabling factors for the various psychiatric treatments. Goldstein and Stein (1976) has articulated the indications of specific behavioral techniques for specific conditions. Beutler (1983) has written on the criteria for selecting specific treatments based on the patient's reactance, locus of control, and complexity of problem areas. Barlow (1985) has reviewed treatment planning for a number of prevalent adult disorders. And we (Frances et al, 1984; Perry et al, 1985) have reviewed the research and clinical wisdom in the area of differential therapeutics and, based on the available data, have formulated treatment planning along five axes: format, techniques, duration and frequency, medication, and setting. This section should therefore not be regarded as an *invention* of differential therapeutics, but rather as an *update* on the art and science of treatment selection.

GOALS AND ORGANIZATION OF THIS SECTION

The primary goal of this section is to provide a clear statement of what we know and what still remains to be investigated regarding treatment selection. In order to achieve this goal, this section will summarize the current research data and growing clinical acumen in a way that will be useful to all mental health professionals who are trying to integrate an overall approach to treatment planning. It will also point out the gaps in our knowledge to stimulate further discussion, refinement, and research.

The ideal way to organize a discussion on differential therapeutics would be around different psychiatric diagnoses; however, unlike many other fields of medicine, a specific diagnosis in psychiatry is rarely a clarion call to a specific treatment. Although the *DSM-III* has been helpful in providing a more reliable diagnostic system, numerous individuals can have the same multiaxial diagnosis, yet appropriately receive quite different treatments (Karasu, 1984; Perry et al, 1985). Furthermore, organizing this section around diagnoses could be misleading and suggest that guidelines for differential therapeutics are intended to be rigid and static, rather than, at this point in our knowledge, tentative and evolving.

We have therefore organized this section not around specific diagnoses, but around the five major decisions each clinician must make in formulating a treatment plan: setting (for example, inpatient, day hospital, outpatient); format (for example, family, group, individual); strategies and techniques (for example, exploratory, behavioral, cognitive); frequency and duration (for example, once a week sessions for 15 weeks); and medication (for example, anxiolytics, neuroleptics, antidepressants).

Howard Klar, M.D., reviews how the major *settings* relate to the goals of treatment.

Larry Beutler, Ph.D., surveys current data regarding treatment *strategies* as they apply to different diagnoses and to important variables of the patient.

Samuel Perry, M.D., discusses the "dosage" of therapy, that is, the *frequency and duration* of psychosocial interventions, including the thorny issue of when to prescribe no treatment for the patient.

Gretchen Haas, Ph.D., and John Clarkin, Ph.D., consider the choice of treatment *format*, recognizing both the independence and interdependence of this treatment variable with the strategies of treatment.

Carl Salzman, M.D., and Allen Green, M.D., summarize the current knowledge concerning the choice of a specific *psychotropic drug* for a specific problem in a specific patient.

And, finally, Allen Frances, M.D., Katherine Shear, M.D., and Mina Fyer,

M.D. raise the issues that arise in a *psychiatric clinic* and in a *training program* when one takes differential therapeutics seriously.

Although the choice of a specific treatment for an individual patient remains one of the most difficult tasks in clinical psychiatry, it is also one of the most challenging and interesting. We believe the following chapters reflect the excitement in this advancing field of differential therapeutics.

REFERENCES

American Psychiatric Association: Diagnostic and Statistical Manual of Mental Disorders, Third Edition, Washington, DC, American Psychiatric Association, 1980

Barlow DH (Ed): Clinical Handbook of Psychological Disorders. New York, Guilford Press, 1985

Bergin AE: The evaluation of therapeutic outcomes, in Handbook of Psychotherapy and Behavior Change: An Empirical Analysis. Edited by Garfied SL, Bergin AE. New York, Wiley, 1971

Beutler LE: Eclectic Psychotherapy: A Systemic Approach. New York, Pergamon Press, 1983

Frances A, Clarkin JF, Perry S: Differential Therapeutics in Psychiatry: The Art and Science of Treatment Selection. New York, Brunner/Mazel, 1984

Goldstein AP, Stein N: Prescriptive Psychotherapy. New York, Pergamon, 1976

Karasu T (Ed): American Psychiatric Association Commission on Psychiatric Therapies: The Psychiatric Therapies. Washington, DC, American Psychiatric Association, 1984

Kiesler DJ: Some myths of psychotherapy research and the search for a paradigm. Psychol Bull 65:110-136, 1966

Paul GL: Strategy of outcome research in psychotherapy. Journal of Consulting Psychology 31:109-118, 1967

Perry S, Frances A, Clarkin JF: A DSM-III Casebook of Differential Therapeutics: A Clinical Guide to Treatment Selection. New York, Brunner/Mazel, 1985

Strupp HH, Bergin AE: Some empirical and conceptual bases for coordinated research in psychotherapy: a critical review of issues, trends, and evidence. Int J Psychiatry 7:18-90, 1969

Chapter 13

The Setting for Psychiatric Treatment

by Howard Klar, M.D.

Where should psychiatric treatment take place? Often, this decision must be made under great pressure, quickly, and with limited clinical information. Paradoxically, the decision is frequently made by clinicians with limited experience and knowledge of the availability, virtues, and limitations of the available treatment options; that is, by psychiatric residents. Yet the answer to the question, "Where can this patient, with this particular syndrome, at this specific point in the course of an illness, with these predictors of response to a particular mode of treatment, be treated?", is the crystal upon which the lattice of future treatments and, possibly, clinical course and outcome will be built.

Failure to hospitalize patients who are potentially harmful to themselves and others can result in disastrous outcomes. Conversely, prematurely hospitalizing a patient because the dramatic presentation puts family and clinicians on edge can unduly stigmatize a patient—even in our relatively enlightened times—and distort a patient's future course of personal development and clinical care.

Treatment carries with it financial as well as human costs, which are frequently substantial. Psychiatric hospitalization in a major New York City hospital costs approximately $470.00 per day, exclusive of physicians' fees. Thus, a 30-day stay in an acute care inpatient setting costs someone (patient, insurance company, taxpayer, hospital) $15,000, not including the cost of lost wages to the patient and family, and disrupted family functioning. Strangely enough, owing to the nature of insurance reimbursement patterns, this expensive month in a hospital can be far less costly to the patient than a two-month stay in an intensive care partial hospital program that charges $125.00 per day. Such factors make the decision regarding treatment setting a complex one. It is not as simple as, "What is clinically indicated?"

Treatment settings are defined by their restrictiveness, structure, length of stay, goals (acute care, rehabilitation, maintenance), and cost (which, because of varying policies of third-party payers, may be difficult to assess). In selecting a treatment setting the clinician must try to match the clinical variables of the patient—age, diagnosis, severity and urgency of the problems, motivation, available resources, risks and benefits of utilizing a particular setting, and response to prior treatment—to the treatment setting that will most benefit that particular patient. The question that should guide this decision is, "What is the primary goal of treatment at this time?"

In order to try to provide some guidelines for these decisions—since the data are inadequate to provide more than some rules of thumb and best guesses—this chapter will describe three basic goals of treatment, for which there seem to be three well defined and established clinical settings. These settings are not necessarily available to all patients, at all times, in all places; however, it is my goal to describe the available options in a more or less ideal situation.

Acute care settings are for those patients who present as decompensating or disorganizing, whose symptoms pose a threat to life or property, who may require complex diagnostic tests or treatments. The goal of treatment is to protect the decompensating patient, rapidly diagnose the cause, and institute treatment to return the patient to his or her previous level of function. The settings that are best designed to accomplish this are intensive care inpatient psychiatric units, intensive care partial hospital programs (day hospitals), and outpatient crisis intervention, which also includes home care.

Rehabilitation programs are designed to elevate the patient's level of function beyond what it was when he or she presented for acute treatment, and most often to help the patient resume employment. The settings of rehabilitation programs include long-term inpatient reconstructive hospitals, long-term day hospitals or sheltered workshops, and outpatient psychotherapy.

Settings for maintenance therapy are designed to prevent acute exacerbations or debilitating deterioration in patients with chronic psychiatric illness. They are also designed to provide structure and humane living situations for patients who are so ill that they cannot function outside of an institutional setting. The settings for maintenance therapy include chronic care inpatient hospitals, chronic care day hospitals, and maintenance outpatient supportive therapy and pharmacotherapy.

These categories are designed to provide a broad outline of available choices. In clinical practice, the categories may not be so distinct, the fit between patient and setting not so tight, and some choices may not be available. Further, the goals of treatment change, sometimes by design, other times serendipitously. For example, a borderline patient who presents as acutely suicidal following the breakup of a romance may rapidly compensate in an acute care inpatient setting, and require rapid transition into a rehabilitative partial hospital. Indeed, one of the tasks of differential treatment planning is to be alert to the potential demands for changes in setting as the clinical situation changes.

Further, we need to avoid an unfortunate tendency toward rapidly prescribing specific settings for specific diagnoses, simply because it was the clinical tradition in which we were trained (Fink et al, 1979). While our knowledge of the efficacy of differential treatments is in its infancy, we do know that alternatives to the conventional wisdom of our training exist, have merit, and warrant consideration. Consequently, acute psychosis need not necessarily be treated on an inpatient basis, any more than chest pain necessarily warrants treatment in a coronary care unit. Rather, the clinician should have an open mind, be aware of and consider the alternatives, and discuss the possibilities with the patient and the patient's family, rather than respond reflexively. To some extent, the demands of caring for patients make us all creatures of habit—for the most part good ones—in treating our patients. In this chapter I will describe the various settings for each treatment goal in some detail, the relative indications for utilizing these settings, the variables to be weighed in making the choice, and the research data available to assist clinicians in making these choices. The goal is not to carve rules in stone, but to highlight options and to know when the utilization of one or another might maximize the outcome and quality of care.

ACUTE CARE SETTINGS

Intensive Care Inpatient Settings

Intensive care inpatient units have, with good reason, been the time-honored locus of care for acutely ill psychiatric patients. They are considered the safest and most obvious choice for treatment of severely ill patients. Critics, increasing in volume and number since the 1960s, have called the frequency with which this setting is chosen into question (Szasz, 1961). Of course, even the staunchest critic of acute inpatient care would acknowledge that certain conditions can best be managed in the highly structured, restrictive setting of an inpatient unit. Within this structure, the highly trained staff can most efficiently acquire diagnostic information, protect the patient from dangerous acting out (by restraint and seclusion if necessary), institute pharmacologic treatment (at times against the patient's will), and contemplate the next treatment step, secure in the knowledge that the patient is in treatment. Most often, these units are based on the medical model—the patient is "sick" and requires treatment. This can foster regressive behavior in patients (a major criticism by opponents of inpatient care) and disrupt social role functioning. This risk must be weighed against the benefit of providing the safest haven to a decompensating patient. Typically, patients stay on these units from 10-30 days before moving on to rehabilitative or maintenance programs.

Intensive Care Partial Hospital Programs

The community psychiatry movement of the 1960s rekindled interest in an already established but neglected treatment: partial hospitals. In the hopeful atmosphere of the 1960s, some predicted that partial hospitals in combination with medications were the harbingers of the demise of inpatient treatment (Mendel, 1968). This has not been the case (Klar et al, 1982). However, partial hospitals have dispelled the idea that "more is better"; that is, more structure, more time, and more restrictions; at least for some, "less is more and even better."

Although intensive partial hospital settings are like acute inpatient settings in the sense that they are highly structured, based on the medical model, and aimed at rapid diagnosis, and in the sense that they institute treatment to ameliorate symptoms, they are fundamentally different as well. The prevailing treatment attitude in these settings is far less accepting of the "sick-role," and encourages the patient's active participation in treatment. Since patients live at home, the acute partial hospital program is akin to a full-time job, and is consequently less disruptive to social and family roles and is less stigmatizing. Partial hospitalization is a less regressive treatment modality than inpatient care, asks more of the patient, and actively attempts to mobilize the patient's adaptive skills and support network in the treatment.

Most often these settings are within or closely affiliated with inpatient units. Ideally, patients can move easily between the two settings, with the partial hospital serving as an alternative for inpatient care, and the inpatient unit providing a safety net if the patient briefly deteriorates or if there are transient disruptions in the support network.

Under optimal conditions these units mirror inpatient units in their staffing patterns and allow relatively brief lengths of stay (a maximum of 60 days).

Outpatient Crisis Intervention

Crisis intervention is usually a brief, time-limited, intense treatment that requires frequent sessions, a well mobilized support network, a staff that is available and reachable (particularly if the crisis intervention team is not hospital based, where there is most often an emergency room), and a versatile, multidisciplinary staff.

A growing variation on the theme of crisis intervention is home care. Identified patients in crisis who have viable support networks are regularly visited by a team, often a physician and nurse clinician or social worker (sometimes all three), and treated at home. Such treatment places intense demands on the patient's family as well as on the visiting staff, but carries with it the benefit of being least disruptive to the patient, and is potentially far less traumatic to the patient's self-esteem. The team, the patients, and the families engaged in this treatment require ready access to the more restrictive settings should the situation deteriorate and demand emergency care. However, with compliant patients and solid support networks, home care is an important acute care consideration.

Clinical Considerations

Let us assume that the clinician has decided that a patient requires acute care. The patient has presented with an acute episode, is behaving in an uncharacteristically disturbed fashion which disrupts functioning or poses a serious threat to the patient's reputation or social network, is homicidal or suicidal, or requires supervised diagnostic tests or treatment (for example, electroconvulsive therapy). Let us also assume that the clinician has all three modalities of treatment available. How shall the choice of treatment setting be made?

A general rule of thumb is to opt for the least restrictive and regressive setting that will protect the patient and allow for the control of the patient's acute episode. Crisis intervention and home care ask the most of the acutely disturbed patient and family. Strong compliance, tolerance of symptoms, and motivation are required of all parties involved. A history or signs of rapid response to medication is also a strong prediction of good outcome in this treatment setting. Thus, a patient who is acutely disturbed with an obvious diagnosis, able to attend daily hospital treatment, living with a supportive and very involved social network, and highly compliant, is the best patient for crisis intervention or home care.

Intensive partial care settings are an underutilized, highly effective treatment for acutely ill patients. Many patients currently treated on inpatient units can be as effectively treated in partial hospitals (Klar et al, 1982). Acutely ill patients who pose no danger to themselves or others are capable of coming into and going out of the program, or who cooperate with family members willing to bring them, can and most often *should* be treated in intensive care partial hospitals. The most common obstacles to this choice are the clinician's reluctance to use outpatient treatment for a seriously ill patient (Washburn et al, 1976), inadequate third-party payment for partial hospital treatment which paradoxically makes more expensive inpatient care significantly less expensive for the patient than partial hospitalization (Fink, 1982) and lack of experience with this treatment setting on the part of referring clinicians (Fink et al, 1978). One can safely refer to partial hospitals a significant number of acutely ill, diagnostically complex patients who are now being referred for inpatient admissions. Indeed, in the absence of dangerous behavior, substance abuse, or serious medical problems, partial hospitalization would seem to represent the "best-fit" setting for the treatment of acutely ill patients who also have adequate social support systems.

The acute care inpatient unit represents the most restrictive, structured, and protective of treatment settings. It is a Janus-faced treatment, carrying lifesaving potential on the one hand, and possibly inducing severely regressive, stifling, maladaptive behavior patterns on the other. It carries enormous financial costs to society (someone, in fact, always pays), and can brand patients for life. Inpatient hospitalization should, therefore, be carefully weighed, and less potent treatments fully explored before admitting the patient.

The goal for the admission must be preeminent in the mind of the clinician. Acutely homicidal and suicidal patients, patients with deliria, or patients with dementia, who are acutely disturbed, obviously require immediate admission and care. Patients who are likely to destroy their reputations—for example, a manic physician with "the cure" for cancer who wishes to tell all his patients, or the mother with a severe postpartum depression that renders her unable to care for her infant—need rapid admission. For the most part, inpatient treatment should be the treatment of last resort for acute illness. While it may help us to sleep better in the short run, the long term impact on patients' self-esteem, finances, and attitude toward treatment can be harmful, particularly with first episode patients. Yet, when indicated, acute inpatient treatment, properly managed, is an extraordinarily potent and helpful treatment.

Research Data

Clinical judgment is the bedrock on which the determination to select the acute care setting rests. The research literature provides data supporting the use of outpatient treatment as the first time treatment for acute psychiatric illness. Interestingly, these studies, described below, imply that for some patients, outpatient care is *not* a viable alternative to inpatient treatment. However, even in cases where inpatient treatment is required, the use of acute care outpatient facilities to shorten the duration of inpatient care seems to be the better treatment.

Several studies have compared outcome results between patients randomly assigned to either acute day hospital treatment or inpatient care. The results of these studies can best be summed up by the statement of Herz and colleagues (1971): "On virtually every measure used to evaluate outcome, there was clear evidence of the superiority of day treatment" (p. 1379). These measures include symptom relief, level of social functioning, and even family burden. Furthermore, 18 months after treatment, the superior outcome of day treatment held up. Of course, not all patients presenting for acute care can be safely assigned to day treatment. Wilder and colleagues (1966) found, however, that in large municipal hospitals, serving a medically indigent population (patients least likely to have the stable social support required for day treatment), 66 percent could still be treated in day hospitals. Other studies report a range (22–59 percent) of patients who can safely be assigned to day treatment (Herz et al, 1971; Washburn 1976). In all of these studies the same point is made: Clinicians significantly underestimate the extent to which day treatment can be used as an alternative to inpatient care.

The reasons for this underutilization are many. They stem from deeply ingrained clinical reflexes regarding who we can treat with a given treatment (Hogarty, 1968); lack of experience with day treatment programs and their efficacy (Platt et al, 1980); greater direct cost to the patient from day treatment (Langsley et al, 1964); and a distressingly long time between the presentation of solid research findings and their integration into clinical practice (Luborsky, 1969).

The literature comparing crisis intervention and home care to acute inpatient treatment is less clear, but no less optimistic regarding the benefits of outpatient treatment. The confusion stems, in part, from multiple definitions of what is meant by "crisis intervention," unclear exclusion criteria for the different studies and, consequently, as in the case of partial hospitalization, nonspecific data regarding the number of patients who can be treated in an outpatient program. What unifies the studies, however, is the notion that a brief, highly focused, intensive outpatient treatment can, for a selected patient population, be enormously helpful to acutely disturbed patients and their families. Early studies by Langsley and associates (1968, 1969) demonstrate that in carefully selected patients deemed in need of hospitalization, family oriented crisis intervention could hasten the resumption of social and vocational functioning, and if hospitalization proved necessary, could curtail the length of stay.

Several studies advocate removing the patient from his or her usual living situation and commencing treatment in a "surrogate family" or "crisis home" (Mosher and Menn, 1978; Polak and Kirby, 1976). Such facilities are rather hard to find under usual circumstances, but when available, they do demonstrate that extremely ill patients can be effectively treated outside the hospital.

Home care provides an intriguing extension of the above, and a growing data base supports its utility as well. In an imaginative and innovative series of papers, Stein and Test (1980) reported the results of the program "Training in Community Living" (TCL). The study group, predominantly acutely ill schizophrenics, were randomly assigned to inpatient care or TCL. Training in Community Living entailed training in social skills, psychoeducation, medication at home or at work, and family treatment. The results, in keeping with all the data described, indicate clinical outcome benefits as well as enormous financial savings from TCL. However, these benefits were maintained only as long as the TCL team was available to the patient. Once the team was removed from the community, the outcome measures resembled those of patients treated on inpatient units. Fenton and Tessier (1979), in Canada, have demonstrated the benefits of home care in treating acutely ill schizophrenics. They underscore the need for a stable, cooperative family structure and the need for access to hospital treatment when indicated.

Despite all of the above, some patients will require acute hospitalization. What should the criteria be for using inpatient care? Some authors have described weighted scales in order to select patients for inpatient treatment. These scales have utilized symptoms, the nature of support systems, dangerousness, and prognosis as the major determinants of hospitalization (Warner, 1961; Warner et al, 1962; Skodal and Karasu, 1980). Others have described algorithms designed to help clinicians distinguish patients suitable for inpatient treatment from those suitable for outpatient care (Sherrill, 1971; Anderson and Kuehnle 1974), but to date these algorithms have not been quantitatively studied. Glick and associates (1984) have reviewed the literature on chronic psychiatric patients and recommended guidelines for hospitalizing these frequent consumers of inpatient treatment. They have emphasized the importance of having clearly defined goals for the hospitalization, and the importance of arranging rapid transition to outpatient treatment and inducing the patient into outpatient care while still hospitalized.

To summarize: Most studies emphasize the growing conviction that given appropriate social supports, a patient who, with the assistance of a network can manage life without alienating those who are most important to him or her, without damaging his or her reputation, and whose symptoms are not dangerous to self or others, can be managed outside the hospital. Furthermore, the number of these patients is far greater than we previously imagined. Researchers still need to refine these data, however; for example, to determine whether patients falling into certain diagnostic categories are more likely to benefit from inpatient treatment; and to identify the characteristics of social support systems that predict success of outpatient treatment, in order to enhance their influence.

Integrating these data into clinical practice will require the work of educators, who must disseminate this information; administrators, who will make hospital policy and conduct utilization review; third-party payers, whose reimbursement patterns will play a significant role in dictating the settings of mental health care in the future; and clinicians in the field, who will need the courage of the clinical researchers' convictions until time and experience make these convictions their own.

REHABILITATION SETTINGS

Most patients rapidly recover from acute episodes of psychiatric illness and require follow-up care. An even greater number of patients initially present with subacute disorders which, nevertheless, severely disrupt their vocational and social functioning. Much of the financial and social cost of psychiatric illness, particularly schizophrenia, derives from its indirect cost (lost wages, taxes, disruption of the family functioning), rather than the direct cost of caring for the patient (Gunderson and Mosher, 1975). Consequently, settings that help patients return to functioning at or above their prior level of functioning or settings that help patients adjust to the limitations that a psychiatric illness might impose ought to be a major area of clinical consideration.

The settings that most often concern themselves with long-term rehabilitative efforts have only recently become an object for clinical research and contemplation. This mirrors the tendency, now rippling through all of medicine, to place increasing emphasis on long-term care and management of chronic illness. In part, this is a direct extension of the effectiveness of the acute care interventions that psychiatry now has available; patients rarely have a rapid demise— the question now becomes, how can we use our resources to preclude a slow, steady decline?

Inpatient Rehabilitation

Undoubtedly the most controversial of all rehabilitation settings, reconstructive hospitals rest on the assumption that long-term involvement (usually six months or more) in a highly structured setting, with intensive psychological treatment, vocational rehabilitation, and gradual reintegration into the community will significantly alter the course of psychiatric illness. Clinicians who advocate the utilization of these facilities argue that for many patients, only a structured, closed setting can provide the safety necessary to help the patient grapple with the powerful emotions and deeply entrenched maladaptive patterns which are at the heart of his or her problem. Furthermore, these clinicians would argue that the enormous cost of hospitalizing patients for a year or more and the risk of prolonged regression is offset by the potential resumption of functioning in society. While most clinicians who have worked in these settings can point to great success stories, few can predict in advance which patients are likely to benefit from such expensive and potentially risky treatments. In the absence of data that facilitates the identification of these patients, and in the presence of data showing that many patients can benefit from less costly and regressive treatments, opponents argue that such settings are difficult to justify. In the current climate of "cost-benefit" preoccupation, advocates of such settings would do well to clarify and define those patients likely to benefit from them, and to demonstrate the benefits that accrue from this treatment.

Partial Hospital Rehabilitation Programs

The goal of partial hospital rehabilitation programs is to provide on an outpatient basis the structure necessary to help severely impaired but not acutely ill patients to endure the psychotherapeutic and vocational interventions necessary to help them get back on track. Programs are quite variable, but differ greatly from inpatient settings in their staffing patterns (with less emphasis on medical personnel and more on occupational, family, and rehabilitation therapy); time frames (most last four months to one year); and geography (most are outside the grounds of psychiatric hospitals). Clinicians in these programs emphasize interrupting the "sick-role" of the patient and treating the program as a job, albeit in a somewhat protected atmosphere. Traditional psychotherapeutic interventions (individual, group, and family) are largely viewed as adjuncts to the major task of helping the patient resume or begin his or her work life.

Outpatient Psychotherapy

Outpatient psychotherapy is the least well defined of the settings for rehabilitation. Duration varies from several weeks (for example, focal therapy, which helps a patient resume functioning after a sudden loss) to many years (as in psychoanalysis, which is designed to resolve subtle but disruptive patterns of behavior). In general, patients thought to require only outpatient psychotherapy are less impaired than those referred to either of the alternatives previously described. Chapter 16 will describe the format and goals of the various psychotherapies.

Clinical Considerations

All of the above programs share the goal of restoring or improving functioning, rather than simply resolving an acute problem. Thus, they presume that the patient brings a modicum of social and vocational skills to the treatment situation. These patient assets or enabling factors are the most significant variables in considering where the patient should receive rehabilitation (Frances et al, 1984).

Outpatient psychotherapy provides the least structure, most often little in the way of vocational rehabilitation or focused practice on social skills. It should be reserved for the patient who has many assets: for example, for patients who are compliant with medication, who regularly attend appointments, who have been able to maintain work and social relationships despite the psychological problems that bring them into treatment, and who can tolerate the emotional stress of treatment without destructive acting out. As psychopathology invades and disrupts broader areas of functioning, more highly structured and intensive settings become the best alternatives.

Partial hospital rehabilitation programs are best suited to the heterogeneous population of patients with severe vocational or social problems stemming from severe personality disorders or with the vestiges of acute episodes of Axis I disorders. A common clinical practice is to use partial hospitalization along with outpatient psychotherapy in order to maximize therapeutic gain. This combination of treatments is most often recommended for patients with severe personality disorders. The structure and low-symptom tolerance of the partial hospital setting provides both a buffer from, and organizing adjunct to, the emotional turmoil engendered by individual treatment, and precludes the regression that might develop as a result of long-term hospitalization (Hyland, 1979; Craaford, 1977).

Using hospitals for long-term inpatient rehabilitation creates a thicket of clinical, economic, and ethical dilemmas for both clinician and patient. Clinicians have serious reservations about inducing patients into the role of an "institutionalized" patient, making patients overreliant on hospitals, and inhibiting the development of adaptive skills by using inpatient rehabilitation treatment (Talbott and Glick, 1986). Still, most experienced clinicians feel that for some patients this costly, ambitious undertaking is rewarded by the enormous strides these patients make in this setting (Paul and Lentz, 1977). In the absence of clear-cut markers pointing to which patients are likely to benefit from this treatment, it should be reserved for those patients who have given evidence of previous levels of higher functioning, and have not improved in outpatient rehabilitation. There may also be a group of clinicians, very skilled in this area who, by dint of their experience, can identify patients who can thrive in this setting. One hopes that they will begin to clarify the criteria by which they arrive at these conclusions.

Research Data

Psychiatry has come a long way in its ability to quiet the acute symptoms of mental illness. The research already cited in this chapter attests to that. Do we now have data that suggest ways to use the settings just discussed to demonstrate an ability to do more than simply alleviate the worst symptoms? The answer is, unfortunately, not clear. There are may studies comparing the outcomes of long versus short hospitalizations; but these studies, for the most part, compared long-term stays in acute care settings to shorter stays with outpatient follow-up. There are no studies clearly comparing long-term inpatient rehabilitation settings to outpatient settings.

The many studies comparing long inpatient stays to briefer hospitalization follow-up suggest that briefer hospitalization is at least as effective in acute situations and may be superior over the long term. Herz and colleagues (1976) found that for inpatients living with their families, brief hospitalization with partial hospital follow-up is a superior treatment to lengthy inpatient care. Washburn and associates (1976) noted that although patients in rehabilitation programs may periodically require brief hospitalizations, partial hospital patients fare better on many measures of outcome (subjective distress, family burden, community functioning), and these differences hold up 18 months after the acute episode.

Several studies suggest that long-term hospitalization is beneficial for some patients. However, these hospitalizations were not specifically designed for social rehabilitation. As Swartzburg and Schwartz (1976) note, the most salient issue in evaluating therapeutic setting and length of stay is the tasks that were accomplished during the hospitalization. Thus, in reviewing the next cluster of studies, we should wonder what the goal of the inpatient treatment was, and whether the favorable outcome noted related to the accomplishment of this task. Mattes and associates (1977a, 1977b) reported that in a comparison of patients randomly assigned to shorter and longer hospitalizations, the long-term patients were found to have less pathology by their families three years after hospitalization. Burhan (1969) reported that patients hospitalized for a very brief stay (14.8 days) were four times more likely to be rehospitalized than were long stay patients (38 days). In these three studies, the benefits of the long-term treatments were isolated to those noted and did not include diagnosis as an outcome predictor.

Glick and colleagues (1976) conducted an extensive comparison of long-term and brief hospitalization. Their data suggest that a small population of high functioning schizophrenic patients seemed to fare better with long-term hospitalization. However, this population of patients were also most likely to begin and follow through on outpatient rehabilitation. Whether the superior outcome noted for these patients is attributable to the long-term hospitalization, to the effects of outpatient rehabilitation, or to patient variables remains an open question. This study by Glick and colleagues does, however, concur with other studies which emphasize that for most schizophrenic patients, brief hospitalization (less than 21 days), with aggressive follow-up care, appears to represent the most balanced, humane, and effective approach (Caton, 1982).

In a recently published series of papers, McGlashan (1984a, 1984b, 1986) has described the long-term outcomes of 446 patients in several different diagnostic categories who received long-term (an average 3 years 4 months) in-patient treatment, and were followed up approximately 15 years after discharge. Schizophrenic patients fared poorly. Roughly two-thirds were chronically ill or marginally functioning at follow-up; the remaining one-third did, however, achieve functional outcomes. Outcome for patients with affective disorder and borderline personality disorder was far better. The idiosyncracies of the Chestnut Lodge sample raises some question about the generalizability of these data; however, the highly functional outcomes of some of these patients suggest that long-term inpatient care does not necessarily induce regression and chronicity, and may indeed be the most effective treatment for certain subgroups of patients.

Two studies compare the effects of rehabilitation treatment and outpatient psychotherapy on a group of previously hospitalized patients. The authors randomly assigned discharged patients, with heterogeneous diagnoses, to either a rehabilitative partial hospital program or outpatient psychotherapy. In both studies, patients treated in the partial hospital had significantly better outcomes in terms of subjective distress, employment, and social functioning (Meltzoff and Blumenthal, 1966; Frances et al, 1979).

Research in the rehabilitation of psychiatric patients, at least in America, has lagged behind research efforts in unraveling the underlying causes and treatment of acute symptomatology. Morgan and Cheadle (1983) described an innovative rehabilitation program in England which rests on graded increments in social and vocational functioning. Patients gradually move from locked, tightly supervised wards to relatively unsupervised halfway houses. Throughout the lengthy treatment, the emphasis is on acquisition of skills, social role, and vocational functioning. Unfortunately, these authors did not provide the type of follow-up data to make their argument truly persuasive. However, a rehabilitative model akin to that advocated by Paul and Lentz (1977) would seem worthy of study, particulary if we hope to cut into the enormous human and financial cost generated by chronic psychiatric illness.

CHRONIC CARE

Some patients, despite our best efforts, never get well or even better. From the onset of their illness, they are plagued by symptoms, haunted and impaired by their lack of social and vocational skills, and taken advantage of in more ways than we can begin to enumerate. Some fortunate, chronically impaired patients have families, communities, or are part of organizations that can offer them asylum from their painful and tormented experience. Most are not so lucky; they don't respond to our most modern treatments, they thwart our therapeutic zeal, they live on our doorsteps and in train stations, and they consequently pose the greatest challenge to our compassion and wisdom, as well as to our care delivery system.

The growing impact of these patients on our resources, the dilemma they pose for society (not only psychiatry), the complex web of psychobiology and environmental interaction that underlie the illnesses that get patients into this awful predicament, are well reviewed elsewhere (Talbott, 1983), and beyond the scope of this discussion. Rather, I will review clinical settings which can provide treatment for these patients, realizing that this may beg the question of how to provide the social supports they require, since our treatments are currently ineffective.

Chronic Care Hospitals

The public and our profession sway back and forth in their attitudes toward chronic care hospitals. Once the "crown jewel" of moral treatment, these hospitals became repositories of neglect and abuse, and spurred the deinstitutionalization movement of late 1960s and early 1970s. As the difficulties and inadequacies associated with community care and deinstitutionalization became evident (Borus, 1981; Michels and Eth, 1986), the call for "reinstitutionalization" and refurbishing of these hospitals began and continues.

Obviously, some patients need chronic institutionalization. Their symptoms render them unable to survive independently in our society, or they pose too much of a danger to themselves or others to be allowed to live outside an institution. They require a lifetime of structured, supervised, and humane care. Currently chronic care hospitals are woefully understaffed and underfunded. Similarly, facilities other than inpatient hospitals—for example, "L-facilities" in California, designed to provide the functions of asylum, custody, and supervision—are inadequate for the numbers of patients who require such care (Talbott and Glick, 1986). The advent of community care and deterioration of the chronic care hospitals has not led to the widespread benefits to patients originally hoped for. The need for asylums is not obsolete; public planners and psychiatrists need to assess the need for such facilities and strenuously argue for their re-establishment and/or improvement.

Chronic Care Partial Hospitals

The majority of partial hospital patients are treated in chronic care programs. Shorter inpatient stays and deinstitutionalization have mandated the development of such programs to care for the burgeoning number of chronic patients in the community. Unlike other partial hospital programs, chronic care programs are modest in their goals, high in their tolerance of symptoms, and concrete and goal directed in their philosophies.

Staff to patient ratios are usually low, and staff make-up emphasizes rehabilitation and recreational therapy. Usually attendance requirements are flexible, and the staff tries to prevent these patients from "falling through the cracks" of the system. Length of stay is usually indefinite, and readmission following an acute episode is usually the rule.

Maintenance Outpatient Therapy

Many chronic patients are reluctant to be involved with defined programs of care. They are willing to attend monthly coffee groups, meet briefly with a therapist who monitors their clinical state, and can adjust and administer medications. Such patients often develop intense institutional transferences and are able to tolerate the inevitable comings and goings of therapists in clinic settings. Efforts to involve such patients in more intensive treatments—for example, chronic care or rehabilitative partial hospitals—are always worth a try, but often fall flat. Consequently, an ongoing relationship with a neutral, relatively pleasant, albeit superficially involved therapist allows for the patient to remain in touch and enhances medication compliance, without stressing the patient's interpersonal coping skills beyond their limits.

Clinical Considerations

Contemplating the care of severely and chronically disabled psychiatric patients is one of our most exasperating and painful therapeutic tasks. Often we wonder, "Is there anything at all out there for this patient?" Or, "Should we just give the revolving door another shove?" Certainly, the overriding concern in caring for these patients has to be to ensure their physical safety and humane care; and the safest and easiest way to do this is to admit the patient to a chronic care hospital. This decision, while theoretically the safest and likeliest to ensure the patient's well being, is, in practice, not so simple. Critics would argue that chronic care facilities are, first, not so safe or humane; and that shrinking budgets and inadequate staffing make these hospitals antithetical to the concept of asylum. Second, the argument goes, hospitalizing a patient for many months or years will only encourage deterioration and is a violation of civil rights (Szasz, 1968). It is, unfortunately, not easy to counter these arguments.

Chronic care partial hospitals are wonderful alternatives to chronic institutionalization, provided the patient has adequate shelter and support to provide protection while attending the program. Single room occupancy hotels or public shelters often fall short of these minimal standards. Thus, many patients are left to the unpredictable life of the streets, and all of the dangers and indignities that life there carries with it.

Outpatient maintenance psychotherapy is not a treatment for the most deteriorated and impaired patient. Rather, it is a treatment for the chronic patient who functions to some extent and is minimally compliant (that is, a patient who shows up once in a while and has adequate social supports, but is unable or unwilling to attend a more structured program).

The options are limited. Chronic patients pose an enormous challenge, and the review of the limited research in this area which follows implicitly argues for the need to expand our efforts to develop adequate facilities and techniques to treat these difficult patients.

Research Data

One of the great paradoxes of modern psychiatry is the relative lack of research, both theoretical and therapeutic, on chronic patients. Researchers have demonstrated the efficacy of drugs in quelling acute symptoms, and the advantages of acute care and rehabilitative partial hospitals in shortening or eliminating acute inpatient stays. But there are few well done studies defining the profiles of patients who require chronic hospitalization or the characteristics of chronic settings which can prevent deterioration. Such studies are difficult, time consuming, difficult to objectify and operationalize, and short of funds in a time of diminishing resources and wary funders.

Most studies concerned with the setting for chronic care have examined the relative cost differences between community and inpatient care for these patients. Murphy and Datel (1976) studied cost-effectiveness of treating mentally retarded patients in the community compared to treating them in institutions. Projected over a 10-year period, the community treated group was treated at a considerable savings. A study of 500 deinstitutionalized chronic schizophrenic patients (Cassell et al, 1972) demonstrated that a significant number of these patients, hospitalized for an average of 18 years, could work for reasonable periods of time, live independently, and be maintained at a savings of almost 25 percent of the cost of institutional care. Both of these studies, and others in a similar vein, suffer from significant methodologic difficulties, lack random assignment, lack control groups, and fail to adequately evaluate the quality of the patient's life in the community.

Weisbrod (1979) compared 130 chronic patients randomized into two treatment groups: In one, patients were hospitalized and assigned to community mental health care; and in the other, patients were assigned to an intensive community care program that aggressively tried to maintain patients in the community. In the four-year study period, costs for community care were somewhat higher, but were offset by the monies generated by the patients' employment and improved social role functioning. This study was conducted in a rural area with a relatively homogeneous patient population. It therefore may not be predictive of the needs and settings required for the care of most chronic patients in our country. Despite the methodologic problems with this and the other studies cited, the deinstitutionalization and cost-effectiveness bandwagon has rolled, and enormous numbers of patients requiring chronic care were discharged from institutions.

One extremely well done study suggests an approach for caring for these patients in a partial hospital setting. Linn and associates (1979) studied 10 Veterans Administration chronic-care partial hospital programs, identified the characteristics of centers likely to have good outcome results, and patients likely to benefit from treatment in these settings. Centers emphasizing occupational therapy and diminished stimulation, lower rates of patient turnover, and longer lengths of stay were associated with reduced symptoms, longer remissions, greater alterations in patient attitude, and generally operated at the lowest cost. Poor outcome was associated with more professional staff hours, more group therapy, and rapid patient turnover.

Studies conducted with predominantly schizophrenic patients, who undergo traditional psychodynamic outpatient maintenance therapy compared to drug therapy, underscore the relative inability of this approach to influence the course of the illness (May, 1968). While the humanity and caring implicit in this intensive approach has been one of the strongest arguments for its continuation, others have argued that the steady concern for the "whole patient" can be accomplished by carefully administered, well trained treatment teams (Carpenter and Heinrichs, 1982). Studies of maintenance family therapy, psychoeducation, and social skills learning have been far more optimistic in their findings regarding outpatient maintenance therapy.

Family treatment, particularly of chronic schizophrenic patients, has become an increasingly popular form of maintenance treatment. Data suggesting that high levels of criticism and overinvolvement (high expressed emotion) by relatives is harmful to schizophrenic patients (Vaughn and Leff, 1976; Brown et al, 1972) fostered several studies of the impact of altering these familial dynamics on the course of the illness. Leff (1982) reported that reduction of levels of expressed emotion in families was possible, and correlated with patient benefits.

Falloon and colleagues (1982) have reported that a prolonged family treatment emphasizing the acquisition of several skills could significantly reduce symptoms, relapse, and rehospitalization in a group of hospitalized schizophrenics. Other family approaches emphasizing psychoeducation have shown to be effective maintenance therapies for some chronic patients (Anderson et al, 1980; Heinrichs and Carpenter, 1983; Goldstein et al, 1978). These data argue strongly for considering outpatient family treatment as part of the maintenance psychotherapeutic program with chronic patients, particularly with schizophrenics.

Individual approaches to maintenance therapy that have proven effective also emphasize social learning. Hogarty and colleagues (1973) describe sociotherapy, a social learning, psychoeducative approach, which seems to enhance medication compliance and improve patients' living situations in the community.

Data from these studies suggest that for patients who can live outside an institution without posing an undue danger to themselves (perhaps fewer than we now imagine), maintenance therapy should emphasize social skills learning and psychoeducation. Such approaches, whether in partial hospitals, or family or individual meetings, seem most likely to enhance the patient's quality of life and improve the chances for living in the community.

CONCLUSION

It is hoped that this chapter has outlined the choices available to clinicians faced with determining an appropriate setting for psychiatric care. In some instances data argue for, and in other instances the lack of data argues against, making the same choices we've always made. Outpatient treatment may, in more cases than we imagined, be as effective as inpatient hospitalization for acute psychiatric illness. A patient's persistent inability to return to prior levels of function despite conventional outpatient psychotherapy may indicate a need for long-term rehabilitative hospitalization; however, a period of treatment in a rehabilitative partial hospital should be tried first. Finally, despite what many believe, the need for chronic psychiatric hospitals has not diminished. More patients than we can now adequately treat require humane custodial care and don't belong on the streets.

Beyond a new set of choices, there is another message nestled in this discussion. Psychiatrists and health policy makers need to become interested in levels of care for psychiatric patients. One treatment does not fit all, and a given patient may require several different settings in the course of an illness. Too often, public planning has been based on a current enthusiasm or despair for particular psychiatric treatments, without adequate attention being paid to the shifting nature of the illnesses we treat and the treatments they require. We can treat acute psychiatric illnesses very well, but the need for treatment doesn't end there. Psychiatry must turn its gaze and resources to developing the methods of treatment necessary to restore functioning, prevent relapse and deterioration, and to providing asylum when all else fails.

REFERENCES

Anderson CM, Hogarty GE, Reiss DJ: Family treatment of adult schizophrenic patients: a psycho-educational approach. Schizophr Bull 6:490-505, 1980

Anderson WH, Kuehnle JC: Strategies for the treatment of acute psychosis. JAMA 229:1884-1889, 1974

Brown GW, Birley JLT, Wing JK: Influence of family life on the course of schizophrenic disorders: a replication. Br J Psychiatry 121:241-258, 1972

Borus JF: Deinstitutionalization and the chronically mentally ill. N Engl J Med 305:339, 1981

Burhan AS: Short-term hospital treatment: a study. Hosp Community Psychiatry 20:369-370, 1969

Cassell WA, Smith CM, Grunberg F, et al: Comparing costs of hospital and community care. Hosp Community Psychiatry 23:197-200, 1972

Caton CLM: Effect of length of inpatient treatment for chronic schizophrenia. Am J Psychiatry 139:856-861, 1982

Craaford C: Day hospital treatment for borderline patients: the institution as transitional object, in Borderline Personality Disorders. Edited by Hartocollis P. New York, International Universities Press, 1977

Falloon IRH, Boyd JL, McGill CW, et al: Family management in the prevention of exacerbations of schizophrenia: a controlled study. N Engl J Med 306:1437-1440, 1982

Fenton F, Tessier L, Struening EA: A comparative trial of home and hospital care. Arch Gen Psychiatry 36:1073-1079, 1979

Fink EB: Encouraging third-party coverage of partial hospitals. Hosp Community Psychiatry 33:38-41, 1982

Fink EB, Longabaugh R, Stout R: The paradoxical underutilization of partial hospitalization. Am J Psychiatry 135: 713-716, 1978

Fink EB, Heckerman CL, McNeill D: An examination of clinician bias in patient referrals to partial hospital settings. Hosp Community Psychiatry 30:631-632, 1979

Frances A, Clarkin J, Weldon E: Focal therapy in the day hospital. Hosp Community Psychiatry 30:195-199, 1979

Frances A, Clarkin J, Perry S: Differential therapeutics, in Psychiatry: The Art and Science of Treatment Selection. New York, Brunner/Mazel, 1984

Glick ID, Hargreaves WA: Psychiatric Hospital Treatment for the 1980s: A Controlled Study of Short versus Long Hospitalization. Lexington, MA, D.C. Heath, 1979

Glick I, Klar H, Braff D: Guidelines for hospitalizing the chronic psychiatric patient. Hosp Community Psychiatry 35:934-936, 1984

Goldstein MJ, Rodnick EH, Evans JR, et al: Drug and family therapy in the aftercare treatment of acute schizophrenia. Arch Gen Psychiatry 35:1169-1177, 1978

Gunderson JG, Mosler LR: The Cost of Schizophrenia. Am J Psychiatry 132:901-906, 1975

Heinrichs DW, Carpenter WT: The psychotherapy of schizophrenia, in Psychiatry Update: The American Psychiatric Association Annual Review, Vol. 1. Washington, DC, American Psychiatric Press, 1982

Heinrichs DW, Carpenter WT: The coordination of family therapy with other treatment modalities for schizophrenia, in Family Therapy in Schizophrenia. Edited by McFarlane WR, Beels CC. New York, Guilford Press, 1983

Herz M, Endicott J, Spitzer R, et al: Day versus inpatient hospitalization: a controlled study. Am J Psychiatry 127:1371-1382, 1971

Herz M, Endicott J, Spitzer R: Brief versus standard hospitalization: the families. Am J Psychiatry 133:795-801, 1976

Hogarty G: Psychiatric day center: Baltimore City Health Department. Maryland State Medical Journal 17:84, 1968

Hogarty GE, Goldberg SC, and the Collaborative Study Group: Drug and sociotherapy in the aftercare of schizophrenic patients. Arch Gen Psychiatry 28:54-64, 1973

Hyland J: The day hospital treatment of the borderline patient, in Proceedings of the Annual Conference on Partial Hospitalization. Edited by Luber R, Maxey J, Lefkowitz P. Federation of Partial Hospitalization Study Groups, 1979

Klar H, Frances A, Clarkin JF: Selection criteria for hospitalization. Hosp Community Psychiatry 33:929-933, 1982

Langsley DG, Stephenson WF, MacDonald JM: Why not insure hospitalization? Mental Hospital 15:16-17, 1964

Langsley DG, Pittman FS, Machotka P, et al: Family crisis therapy: results and implications. Fam Proc 7:145-158, 1968

Langsley DG, Flomehaft K, Machotka P: Follow-up evaluation of family crisis therapy. Am J Orthopsychiatry 39:753-759, 1969

Leff J, Kuipers L, Berkowitz R, et al: A controlled trial of social intervention in the families of schizophrenic patients. Br J Psychiatry 141:121-134, 1982

Linn M, Caffey E, Klett J, et al: Day treatment and psychotropic drug aftercare of schizophrenic patients. Arch Gen Psychiatry 36:1055-1066, 1979

Luborsky L: Research cannot yet influence clinical practice. International Journal of Psychiatry 7:135-140, 1969

Mattes JA, Rosen B, Klein DF: Comparison of the clinical effectiveness of "short" vs. "long" stay in a psychiatric hospital, II: results of a three-year posthospital follow-up. J Nerv Ment Dis 165:387-394, 1977a

Mattes JA, Rosen B, Klein DF, et al: Comparison of the clinical effectiveness of "short" vs. "long" stay psychiatric hospitalization, III: further results of a three-year posthospital follow-up. J Nerv Ment Dis 165:395-402, 1977b

May PRA: Treatment of Schizophrenia: A Comparative Study of Five Treatment Methods. New York, Science House, 1968

McGlashan TH: The Chestnut Lodge follow-up study, I: follow-up methodology and study sample. Arch Gen Psychiatry 41:573-585, 1984a

McGlashan TH: The Chestnut Lodge follow-up study, II: long-term outcome of schizophrenia and the affective disorders. Arch Gen Psychiatry 41:586-601, 1984b

McGlashan TH: The Chestnut Lodge follow-up study, III: long-term outcome of borderline personalities. Arch Gen Psychiatry 43:20-30, 1986

Meltzoff J, Blumenthal RL: The Day Treatment Center: Principles, Application and Evaluation. Springfield, Illinois, Charles C. Thomas, 1966

Mendel WM: On the abolition of the psychiatric hospital, in Comprehensive Mental Health: The Challenge of Evaluation. Edited by Roberts LM. Madison, University of Wisconsin Press, 1968

Michels RM, Eth S: Ethical issues in psychiatry research on communities: a case study of the community mental health program, in Ethical Issues in Epidemiologic Research. Edited by Tancredi L. New Brunswick, Rutgers University Press, 1986

Morgan R, Cheadle J: Psychiatric Rehabilitation. 1983

Mosher LR, Menn AZ: Lowered barrier in the community: the soteria model, in Alternatives to Mental Health Treatment. Edited by Stein LI, Test MA. New York, Plenum, 1978

Murphy JG, Datel WE: A cost-benefit analysis of community versus institutional living. Hosp Community Psychiatry 27:165, 1976

Paul GL, Lentz RJ: Psychosocial Treatment of Chronic Mental Patients: Milieu versus Social Learning Programs. Cambridge, Harvard University Press, 1977

Platt S, Knights A, Hirsch S: Caution and conservatism in the use of a psychiatric day hospital: evidence from a research project that failed. Psychiatry Res 3:123-132, 1980

Polak PR, Kirby MW: A model to replace psychiatric hospital. J Nerv Ment Dis 162:13-22, 1976

Sherrill R: A hospitalization criteria checklist as an evaluation tool for an emergency service. Hosp Community Psychiatry 28:801-807, 1971

Skodol A, Karasu T: Toward hospitalization criteria for violent patients. Compr Psychiatry 21:162-165, 1980

Stein LI, Test MA: Alternative to mental hospital treatment, I: conceptual model, treatment program, and clinical evaluation. Arch Gen Psychiatry 37:392-397, 1980

Swartzburg M, Schwartz A: A five-year study of brief hospitalization. Am J Psychiatry 133:922-924, 1976

Szasz TS: The Myth of Mental Illness. New York, Harper and Row, 1961

Szasz TS: Law, Liberty and Psychiatry. New York, Collier Books, 1968

Talbott JA: The Chronic Mental Patient Five Years Later. Orlando, Florida, Grune & Stratton, 1983

Talbott JA, Glick ID: The inpatient care of the chronically mentally ill. Schizophr Bull 12:129-140, 1986

Vaughn CE, Leff JP: The influence of family and social factors on the course of psychiatric illness: a comparison of schizophrenic, neurotic and depressed patients. Br J Psychiatry 129:125-137, 1976

Warner SL: Criteria for involuntary hospitalization of psychiatric patients in a public hospital. Mental Hygiene 45:122-128, 1961

Warner SL, Fleming B, Bullock S: The Philadelphia program for home psychiatric evaluations, precare and involuntary hospitalization. Am J Public Health 52:29-38, 1962

Washburn S, Vannicelli M, Scheff BJ: Irrational determinants of the place of psychiatric treatment. Hosp Community Psychiatry 27:179-182, 1976

Weisbrod BA: Guide to benefit cost analysis, as seen through a controlled experiment in treating the mentally ill (discussion paper 559-79). Madison, WI, University of Wisconsin, Institute for Research on Poverty, 1979

Wilder J, Levin G, Zwerling I: A two-year follow-up evaluation of acute psychotic patients treated in a day hospital. Am J Psychiatry 122:1095-1101, 1966

Chapter 14

Differential Therapeutics and Treatment Format

by Gretchen L. Haas, Ph.D., and John F. Clarkin, Ph.D.

One of the primary considerations in differential treatment planning involves the selection of the treatment format, or mode of delivery (individual, group, or family/marital). The treatment format can be most simply understood as the interpersonal context (therapist/patient, dyadic/spousal, family, group) or paradigm within which the treatment is conducted. Each format is characterized by a rather specific set of treatment parameters—all determined largely by the number and identities of the participants and, most important, their relationship to the presenting problem and the identified patient (for example, parents, peers, spouse, or strangers).

Formats vary in terms of the specific roles and therapeutic contracts between therapist and patient. In an individual therapy, some form of contract, either explicit or implied, is drawn between therapist and patient alone—whereas in couples or family therapy, a conjoint contract is made contingent upon the involvement of multiple participants. In group, the contract is with multiple others—usually persons from outside of the patient's immediate social environment. Such basic structural differences in the therapist-patient relationship make for basic differences in the character and intensity of the transference (Mittleman, 1948; Slavson, 1964), the goals of treatment, and the nature of the working alliance between patient and therapist.

Treatment format is determined, in part, by the general perspective from which a presenting problem is initially defined. For example, the treatment of a patient with an eating disorder can vary significantly, depending upon whether it is viewed (etiology aside) as a current adaptation to a larger problem involving the family unit (suggesting a need for a family intervention) or as the patient's personal adaptation to the unique biological, social, and historical situation (in which case an individual or group treatment is more likely indicated). The goals of the treatment will vary accordingly.

Second, the conceptualization of the presenting problem and selection of a treatment format will determine the composition of the working unit; that is, who will be the active participants in the treatment. The therapeutic alliance between patient and therapist will differ markedly depending upon the structure and composition of the working unit—be it dyadic, triadic, or other.

Finally, although therapeutic strategies and techniques are influenced, in part, by the format of treatment, these can vary relatively independent of treatment format and in accordance with the particular theoretical model (for example, psychoanalytic, systems theory, behavioral, social learning) from which the therapist is working. Thus, within any therapeutic format, techniques vary, conforming with a particular theory of therapeutic intervention. As will be illustrated in this chapter, the consideration of each of these two dimensions can be of crucial importance in determining indications and contraindications for use of a particular therapy with a particular patient or disorder.

In this chapter we will address questions regarding the relative utility and specific merits of each major treatment format, with an eye to determining the most appropriate applications of each. We will review the empirical literature and clinical guidelines which currently inform the clinician's choice of treatment format. Finally, we will discuss recommendations for the selection of treatment format and questions for future research.

THE PARADIGM SHIFT—CHANGING FORMATS FOR CHANGING PERSPECTIVES: HISTORICAL CONSIDERATIONS

From a historical perspective, each of the major therapeutic formats (individual, group, and marital/family) reflects a paradigmatic shift in the conceptualization of psychiatric disorders and their associated treatments. From the perspective of social and technological evolution, each format offers a distinctive contribution to the development of a diversified therapeutic technology that can be adapted to the specific needs of a broad range of patients, presenting problems, and psychiatric disorders.

Individual Treatments

The individual therapy format has the longest tradition in 20th century psychiatry. Freud and Breuer's (1895) pioneering work in the psychoanalytic method was instrumental in establishing the individual format as the first generic mode of treatment. Freud's almost exclusive use of an individual format was consistent with his emphasis on an internal (intrapsychic) locus of conflict. For pragmatic reasons, too, he preferred to work with the patient alone, as evidenced in an experimental conjoint treatment of one patient with spouse. Upon premature termination of the couple's treatment, Freud remarked that he was "utterly at a loss" in the treatment of relationships; he noted that when the spouse's resistance was added to that of the patient, the process of therapy was obstructed and more likely to be prematurely broken off (Freud S, 1915).

Individual therapies continue to dominate the field of psychotherapy today. As we will discuss later in a review of the empirical literature on treatment formats, individual therapy remains the treatment of choice for several types of psychiatric disorders. In addition, certain personality disorders and specific types of adjustment disorder are found to prosper from an individual-based psychotherapeutic approach.

Family Treatments

It was not until the mental hygiene movement of the 1930s that interest in the family and group treatment formats first took hold (Broderick and Schrader, 1981). This occurred at a time when social service agencies in general, and child guidance clinics in particular, identified a broad-ranging need for more efficient and economical means of providing mental health services to the larger community. The exigencies of psychotherapy with children and adolescents forced practitioners to re-evaluate the individual treatment format. It was recognized that therapeutic success with children often necessitated some involvement of family members in the treatment, in order to ensure regularity of attendance as well as to promote maintenance of therapeutic outcomes. Initial interviews with parents and family members were instituted for purposes of gathering information about the family and establishing an alliance with the parents and/or other key members of the child's support system.

Nathan Ackerman, a child psychiatrist in the United States, was one of the first to work with the entire family in regular conjoint family therapy sessions. He began to define the family—in contrast to the child—as the appropriate unit for diagnosis and treatment. Concurrently, John Bowlby, working at the Tavistock Child Guidance Clinic in London, described the use of family interviews as an adjunct to individual therapy with children. He related the case of a male adolescent with whom he had come to an impasse in treatment. Frustrated with a lack of progress, it occurred to him to confront all of the presumed "actors" in the "drama"—that is, mother, father, and patient. Word spread of the apparent success of this interview technique. In 1951, John Bell, a professor of psychology at Clark University, heard an account of Bowlby's family interview and adopted the method as standard procedure in working with children and their parents (Broderick and Schrader, 1981).

A review of the early trends in the development of the family treatment format reveals that it served several adaptive functions within the social and historical context from which it evolved: 1) it was recognized to be an important adjunct to individual interventions with children and adolescents whose family environments contributed to their problems; 2) it helped to diminish family resistance to continuation of the child in treatment; and 3) it was particularly well suited to brief treatment of focal problems occurring in the context of the family or marital unit.

Historically, the use of a family format has derived in large part from etiological considerations and an emphasis on the contextual origins of the presenting problems; that is, how the family or marital dyad contributes to and maintains the disorder. More recently, family and marital treatments have been given broader application, with greater emphasis on their practical utility instead of a focus on the role of family/dyad in the etiology of the problem. Hence, we see family- and marital-based treatments for various medical (such as hypertension) and psychiatric disorders (such as agoraphobia, schizophrenia), wherein the spouse or family member is enlisted as adjunct therapist or to provide social support to the patient.

Group Treatments

The initial application of the group treatment format in the United States is attributed to Joseph Pratt (1907), a Boston internist who used a supportive/ didactic group intervention to treat patients with tuberculosis. Pratt met with patients in classes devoted to education in the treatment of the condition, and to mutual support via testimonial and weekly review of individual progress. Social facilitation factors appeared successful in reducing the depression and social isolation characteristic of the chronic illness. Pratt's group intervention resembles more contemporary group treatments which capitalize on the encouragement and support from involved others, and which utilize social forces to minimize neurotic secondary gains from illness (Lieberman, 1975). In more current parlance, Pratt used the supportive and educative functions of the group format to provide a form of psychoeducation in order to increase hope and effective coping with the illness. Lazell (1921) also used the group format to deliver a form of psychoeducation to patients with schizophrenia. Following the lead of Pratt, Lazell used a group psychoeducational approach to the treatment of institutionalized schizophrenic patients. He attributed the success of this work to the educative and socializing functions of the group didactic method.

Simultaneous with the child guidance movement was a growing emphasis on problem oriented approaches for remedial treatment of focal disorders (for example, "war neuroses" and psychosomatic illness). Such disorders suggested the need for specific treatments for focal disorders, with treatment provided in an economical fashion to multiple patients presenting with the same problem. Hence, the origin of homogeneous group treatments for such problems as alcoholism, "war neurosis," and antisocial behavior.

Second, the interpersonal and culturalist schools of psychoanalytic psychotherapy (represented by Harry Stack Sullivan and Karen Horney) emphasized the important influence of environmental variables in understanding the origins and functions of neurotic conditions. This changing view of the nature of psychiatric disorder, giving increasing recognition to interpersonal variables associated with the etiology and course of individual psychopathology, contributed to the exploration of interpersonally oriented treatments. Such treatments capitalized on the facilitative influence of a social group. There was also a growing recognition that strict reliance on the individual patient's perspective to the exclusion of the perspectives of important others (such as family and significant others) limited the pool of available information to guide diagnosis and treatment.

Moreover, the social psychology literature of the 1940s, represented by Kurt Lewin (1947) and Talcott Parsons (1937), and clinical observations of group dynamics specialists during the 1950s, suggested that substantial leverage could be gained by exposing the individual to the activity and verbal feedback of other persons, particularly persons outside of the patient's natural social sphere. Therapeutic intervention in a nonfamilial group format offered the advantages of such factors as identification with the group (Freud S, 1921; Yalom, 1975) (for example, serving an ego supportive function), circumvention of resistances which were seen to impede the establishment of a working alliance (as, for example, in the case of antisocial behavior), development of frustration tolerance and an awareness of the social consequences of impulsive and/or acting-out behavior (for example, in the treatment of parasuicidal patients and alcoholics), and social support functions provided by the other members of the group.

Hence, major concepts from the field of social psychology informed the application of group treatments, even those which were more clearly psychoanalytic in orientation. Such ideas can be traced in a review of the history of the group psychotherapy movement.

From a more traditional psychoanalytic framework, Burrow (1927), one of the leaders of the psychoanalytic movement in the United States, utilized the group format to circumvent patients' resistance and to promote frank confrontation of neurotic processes. Schilder (1936) emphasized the psychoanalytic technique of free association in a group format. He noted that the verbalizations of one member often stimulated the associations of another. Wender (1951) utilized the concept of transference and emphasized the role of the group in the re-enactment of family dynamics. With a similar emphasis on intrapsychic processes, the analyst Alexander Wolf (1950) incorporated a traditional psychoanalytic model in the group setting where identificatory and imitative functions were viewed as enhancing the analytic process and generalization of individual interpretation.

In contrast to this emphasis on the *intra*personal in applications of the group format, during the 1950s there developed a growing *inter*personal and functionalist orientation in the use of group treatments. Here the nature of the individual's in vivo interaction with others in the group was assumed to be an important experiential factor contributing to the psychotherapy process. Moreno (1957) saw the members of the group as therapeutic agents who participated in interactions that facilitated individual growth. From a more systems oriented perspective, Bion (1959) conceptualized individual behaviors as manifestations of group forces, and so emphasized interpretations to the group as a whole.

In summary, it appears that the historical impetus to the development of the group format was based, in part, on the functional advantages that it afforded: 1) an economical mode of delivering information; 2) an effective means of reducing or circumventing the resistances expressed in individual therapy; 3) adjunctive "ego" supports or ancillary therapists in the form of other patients; and 4) a setting in which interactional forces could be played out and examined.

REVIEW OF THE RESEARCH

Whereas evolutionary trends in the development of new technologies reflect the demands of the specific historical period and setting in which they arise, the value of any new development is ultimately assessed in terms of its utility and relative effectiveness—effectiveness as compared to the existing technologies.

Methodological Considerations

Empirical approaches to assessing the effectiveness of treatment formats clearly must take into account the therapeutic techniques, goals, and patient populations with which a particular format has been used. Studies which set out to assess the relative efficacy of treatment formats for a heterogeneous sample of patients, problems, and therapeutic strategies are methodologically flawed in that they offer limited power to detect significant effects.

Three different methods are currently used to combine information and arrive at generalizations from various psychotherapy outcome studies: the narrative review, the box score method, and meta-analysis. All three methods of data integration are helpful, and no one method is definitive. In assessing the differential effectiveness of treatment formats, narrative reviews (Parloff and Dies, 1977; Grunebaum, 1975), box score reviews (Luborsky et al, 1976; Gurman and Kniskern, 1978), and meta-analysis (Shapiro and Shapiro, 1982; Smith et al, 1980; Jacobson and Margolin, 1979; Wampler, 1982) all contribute to the overall picture.

Nonetheless, each treatment format has methodological shortcomings. The narrative review is open to considerable bias because it involves no systematic means of selecting and aggregating data. It is not surprising that, by using this method, two different reviewers of the same area can select an overlapping but somewhat different sample of research studies and, in so doing, arrive at different conclusions.

The "box score" method (Luborsky et al, 1976) was an attempt to quantify the process of research review and reduce the selection bias in narrative reviews. This approach is merited for its use of specific a priori criteria for inclusion of studies. For each category of treatment under study, a tally is made of the number of qualifying studies falling into each of three categories of outcome: positive correlation with outcome, negative correlation with outcome, or showing no significant relationship with outcome. One problem with this method is that no consideration is given to the number of subjects with which a specific outcome is found. A comparison is scored a tie when a nonsignificant trend prevails in favor of one treatment—a difference that might have been significant in a larger sample. For this reason, in the case wherein several small N studies show no significant treatment effect while a large N study shows a sizable treatment effect, the overriding conclusion, based on the outcome for the larger *number* of studies, is that the treatment shows no effect. Second, in most applications of the box score method, there is no effort to select studies on the basis of the quality of design. Thus, a well designed, large, and generalizable study is scored with equal weight to one that is poorly designed with a small N.

Many of the problems of the narrative and box score methods are mitigated using a method termed meta-analysis (Smith et al, 1980). One of the most desirable features of this approach is that it translates the quantitative findings from multiple studies into a common metric and thus permits integration of quantitative outcome data from several studies. Cases are described on each of several variables: type of experimental treatment, type of control treatment, age of subjects, length of treatment, and so on. The results of each study are described in terms of the experimental effect size statistic—an index of the magnitude of the treatment effect—computed as the difference between the average outcome scores for each of the two treatment groups, and adjusted using the standard deviation (a measure of variability of scores around the mean) for the control group. Using this standardization procedure, the raw data from different studies is combined to yield an overall quantitative measure of the relative efficacy of an experimental treatment in comparison with a standard or control treatment. Effect sizes can be calculated for different types of patients, therapists, study designs, treatment methods and formats, and so forth. Because the meta-analysis technique, unlike the box score method, retains the continuous quantitative characteristics of the outcome data, the two methods can yield different conclusions from the same group of studies (Wampler, 1982).

Nonetheless, one of the problems with meta-analytic comparison studies such as that of Smith and colleagues (1980) is that, when collapsing across multiple studies, the investigators can compromise statistical power by maximizing the heterogeneity of the treatments they are comparing. For example, studies included in these comparisons can vary substantially on such dimensions as the nature of the problem being treated, the outcome variables being measured, the nature of the therapeutic setting, and other descriptive characteristics of the treatment.

Given the heterogeneity of their sample, it is not surprising that Smith and colleagues' (1980) comparison of treatment formats (individual versus group versus family) using meta-analytic techniques failed to yield any significant differences across treatment formats, comparing as it did treatment studies which varied in terms of goals, techniques, and targeted problems. A more sophisticated approach to meta-analysis is illustrated by the work of Shapiro and Shapiro (1982), who controlled for major treatment variables such as therapeutic setting, therapist experience, and nature and severity of the disorder. These investigators found that treatment mode (individual, family, or group) *was* significantly related to the magnitude of treatment effects, with individual therapy appearing most effective, group therapy somewhat less effective, and family and couples therapy showing markedly smaller treatment effects.

Finally, in reviewing empirical studies of treatment formats, one should attend not only to the differential effects of treatment on the final goals or outcomes, but also to their effect on the mediating goals of treatment—those assumed to be predictive of long-term outcome and intrinsically related to the mechanism of change in that treatment. These goals would include such intervening variables as treatment drop-out and compliance rates, effects of treatment on various contextual (for example, interpersonal relationship, behavioral) variables. They also serve as intermediate or short-term outcome variables when assessing treatments assumed to show only long-term benefits or "sleeper effects."

DIRECT COMPARISON OF INDIVIDUAL TO OTHER FORMATS

The researcher who wants to compare directly the relative benefits of the three major treatment formats faces multiple problems, as illustrated in a recent study by Pilkonis and colleagues (1984). These investigators compared individual, group, and conjoint therapies administered to 64 outpatients over an average of 27 sessions. The patient sample was moderately homogeneous with respect to diagnosis and symptomatology. All patients were nonpsychotic outpatients with moderate degrees of symptomatology and impairment in functioning (mean Global Assessment Score of 57.5).

One of the major methodological flaws of this study was that patients were not randomly assigned to individual, marital, or group format, nor was assignment based on any assessment of the type of symptom or functional analysis of the presenting problem (for example, individual problem versus problem under control of marital interaction versus social relationship problem). Thus, for example, a patient with little or no marital conflict could have been assigned to marital treatment. Second, while therapists in the three formats reported some general commonality in treatment technique, the techniques or strategies ranged from psychoanalytic to "psychodynamic within systems context" to "eclectic-interactional-phenomenologic." Consequently, within the three formats of treatment, the techniques used were probably not uniform, thereby confounding any results attributable to format of treatment with variation due to treatment technique.

Significantly, an important attempt was made to measure the impact of treatment on the mediating goals specific to the three treatment formats. However, this effort to directly compare formats was compromised by the lack of equivalence of mediating goals and selected assessment instruments across the three treatment formats. For example, the Social Avoidance and Distress Scale and the Locus of Control of Interpersonal Relationships Scale were used to assess the unique impact of group therapy; the Family Concept Test was used to assess the special impact of conjoint therapy; and the Private Self-Consciousness Scale was selected to assess increase in self-awareness and self-exploration with individual therapy.

Given the above design problems, it is not surprising that outcomes were relatively similar across treatment formats. Differences in outcome were more clearly associated with therapist characteristics than with differences in format.

Nonetheless, as noted by the authors, the finding of differential treatment effects on various outcome domains was of some significance; for example, the advantage of individual therapy in heightening self-awareness in lower class patients, the advantage of group and conjoint therapy in lessening interpersonal problems with more chronically ill patients, and the benefits of conjoint therapy for older significant others. Another finding was the higher drop-out rate among individuals with more symptomatic and less supportive significant others. Such specific effects—and not global issues of general outcome—offer a more meaningful estimate of the effectiveness of treatment and are thus likely to be the focus of future controlled research.

MATCHING TREATMENT FORMAT TO DIAGNOSIS

One of the most frequently used means of selecting a treatment format begins with a consideration of the symptoms and/or diagnosis of the identified patient. We will review those diagnostic categories for which there is some empirical data available on the relative efficacy of contrasting formats of treatment.

Schizophrenia

Probably the most impressive series of treatment outcome studies in recent years have been those which compare family with individual or group formats for the treatment of schizophrenia. Accumulating evidence that the family environment plays an important role in the course of the illness (Brown et al, 1972; Vaughn and Leff, 1976) has given impetus to the development of family based treatments for schizophrenia. Controlled studies of family interventions demonstrate that they are effective in reducing family variables associated with exacerbation of symptoms and relapse (Falloon et al, 1982; Leff et al, 1982). Patients returning to live with families characterized by criticism of the patient, hostility, and overinvolvement (that is, high expressed emotion) (Vaughn and Leff, 1976) are more likely to relapse than are those returning to families that do not manifest these reactions to the patient.

Results of two recent controlled studies indicate that family intervention can be effective in reducing expressed emotion (EE) and subsequent rates of rehospitalization (Falloon et al, 1982; Leff et al, 1982). Leff and colleagues (Leff et al, 1982) randomly assigned schizophrenic patients with high EE relatives to an experimental family or control (routine outpatient) treatment. The experimental treatment package included an educational program for family members, a multifamily relatives' group with patients excluded, and family treatment with the patient. The aim in the multifamily group was for the families with the most effective coping strategies (presumably the low EE families) to teach or model these skills during interaction with the other families. In the family therapy (mean of 5.6 sessions), a range of strategies and techniques (dynamic interpretations, problem solving, structural approaches) was used with the aim of lowering EE. The experimental treatment was successful in reducing critical comments but not overinvolvement. Change in EE status was accompanied by a significant reduction in the relapse rate over a nine-month follow-up period.

In a study of lower class schizophrenic patients and families in the Los Angeles area, Falloon and colleagues (1982) compared individual treatment with behavioral family therapy for schizophrenics and their high EE relatives in a total of 40 sessions over a two-year period. Both the individual and family treatment groups received neuroleptic medication and rehabilitation counseling. The behavioral family therapy yielded significantly fewer exacerbations of symptoms, fewer episodes of depression, lower ratings of negative symptoms, and better role functioning. An important mediating outcome effect was that families involved in the family treatment showed fewer negative emotional responses, more effective coping behavior in handling life stresses, and less family burden than those for whom there was no family intervention.

Glick and colleagues (1985) found that the addition of family intervention during the inpatient phase of treatment for chronic schizophrenic patients resulted in more positive family attitudes toward the patient and the illness, and better long-term outcome for the patient.

A review of these three studies suggests that intervention with the family as well as the patient—of even limited duration—can be effective in reducing family environment stressors and the consequent likelihood of patient relapse. In this case, the family treatment format (that is, conjoint treatment of family and patient) may be more important than the specific techniques used (such as behavioral, dynamic, educational) in working with the schizophrenic patient.

Comparisons of groups with individual format for schizophrenia have yielded varied results showing a major juncture along the division between inpatient and outpatient treatments. As Keith and Matthews (1984) noted in their review of the literature on psychosocial treatments for schizophrenia, there is substantial evidence that the efficacy of interpersonal treatments such as group therapy is phase-specific. During the acute phase when positive symptoms are most severe and social functioning is most frankly disordered, a multiple stimulus intervention such as a group treatment can have a noxious influence on the patient.

In contrast, there is some evidence of specific benefits from group treatments during the nonacute phase of the illness. Although certain studies of group and individual formats in the aftercare treatment of schizophrenics yielded equivocal results (Levene et al, 1970; Herz et al, 1974), a second group of studies comparing individual with group therapy showed superior outcomes for patients treated in a group format (O'Brien et al, 1972; Donlon et al, 1973). O'Brien and colleagues (1972) showed that group therapy was more effective in terms of obtaining compliance with maintenance treatment, enhancing clinical outcome, and improving social effectiveness at the 24-month follow-up. Related findings from Malm (1982) suggest that communication oriented group intervention added to drug treatment and social skills training can be particularly effective in reducing negative symptoms—anhedonia, social withdrawal, and lethargy.

In summary, interpersonal treatments can be of particular value in the long-term treatment of schizophrenia. The use of family treatments in combination with standard drug treatments has demonstrated efficacy during both the inpatient and outpatient phase, although involvement of the patient may be limited during the phase of acute symptomatology. Group interventions seem to have less general application and appear to be most effective as an adjunct to drug treatments during the outpatient phase.

Affective Illness

An impressive literature has accumulated on the use of individual psychotherapy, often in combination with medication, for the treatment of depression. Review of the controlled studies of individual treatments for depression, including interpersonal therapy (Klerman et al, 1974; Weissman et al, 1979), cognitive therapy (Rush et al, 1977; Murphy et al, 1974; Shaw, 1977), and social skills training (Bellack et al, 1981), reveals the effectiveness of the individual format for this disorder.

Family and marital treatment formats have also gathered enthusiastic support in the treatment of affective disorders. Growing evidence that social factors can play a significant role in the etiology and course of affective disorders (as reviewed by Klerman et al, 1984) has contributed to the investigation of interpersonal (such as group, marital, and family) treatment formats for depression. Marital treatments tend to focus on marital adjustment problems which often precede, and may contribute to, the onset of depression (Jacobson and Margolin, 1979; Coyne, in press). In light of the strong theoretical arguments for marital and family treatments for depression, there have been few controlled studies that compare the marital/family format with alternate formats for the treatment of affective disorders. In a controlled comparison of marital versus individual treatments for married women with unipolar depression as defined in the *Diagnostic and Statistical Manual of Mental Disorders, Third Edition (DSM-III)* (American Psychiatric Association, 1980), superior outcome was found for patients who received a marital treatment (Beach and O'Leary, 1986). A controlled study of the comparative effects of marital therapy and antidepressant medication showed significant specific effects for both marital therapy and drug treatments (Friedman, 1975).

The rationale for group treatments for depression is based on evidence that social dysfunction often occurs during the acute phase of a depressive disorder, in association with marital stress or a lack of adequate social supports (Parker, 1978). These treatments capitalize on the apparent remedial influence of a close intimate relationship on depressive symptoms (see Haas et al, 1985).

There is some empirical support for the use of a group format in the treatment of depression (Steinmetz et al, 1983); however, in a controlled study comparing group and individual formats using a psychoeducational approach to treatment of depression (Brown and Lewinsohn, 1984), results suggest no differential benefit of one format over the other. Interestingly, it has been found that in a group treatment for Research Diagnostic Criteria (RDC) depressive disorders, individual patient outcomes are predicted, in part, by perceived family support (Steinmetz et al, 1983). What specific benefits accrue from a group treatment appear to be related to the social support provided by group members (Brown and Lewinsohn, 1984).

In summary, there is a growing interest in the use of family, marital, and group treatments to alter specific components of the interpersonal life of the depressive. To date, however, only a few studies attest to the relative efficacy of involving the marital partner or family in treatment (for example, Beach and O'Leary, 1986; Friedman, 1975; McLean et al, 1973; Glick et al, 1985).

The research on treatments for bipolar affective disorders is relatively sparse. The early clinical literature on family treatments urged an integrated presentation of psychoeducation and crisis management strategies (Fitzgerald, 1972; Greene et al, 1976). Subsequent controlled research has revealed evidence of specific benefits from including bipolar patients in a combination of couples group therapy and lithium treatment (Davenport et al, 1977). Other controlled studies of family treatments for bipolar patients suggest that individual (Cochran, 1984) and family (Glick et al, unpublished manuscript) interventions have particular value for enhancing compliance with long-term lithium treatment. Group therapies for bipolar patients have been, by-and-large, discouraged, based on clinical reports of the disruptive influence of the bipolar patient on the group process (Yalom, 1975). The benefits of homogeneous couples groups for treatment of the bipolar patient appear relatively more promising, possibly due to the mediating influence on marital stability (Davenport, 1977).

Agoraphobia

A recent review of the research on treatments for agoraphobia (Barlow and Waddell, 1985) indicates that 60 to 70 percent of those agoraphobics completing exposure-based treatment (regardless of format) will show significant clinical improvement that will be maintained for four years or more. However, the general efficacy of the treatment is reduced by such factors as drop-out, frequency of relapse, and failure to maintain treatment effects following the termination of treatment. Group and marital formats have been introduced by some investigators in an effort to alleviate these problems. Results for patients treated in a group format reveal that group cohesiveness was associated with a continuation of contact among group members following termination of the group and with post-termination improvement (Hand et al, 1974). Furthermore, there is evidence that agoraphobes treated as a group benefit from the social support elements of this format (for example, agoraphobes from the same neighborhood showed superior outcome to those from geographically distant locations (Sinnott et al, 1981). Presumably, those from the same area provided more social support.

Given that 75 percent of agoraphobics are women and many of them are married (Barlow and Waddell, 1985), it is not surprising that characteristics of the marital interaction may be associated with etiology, maintenance (Goldstein and Chambless, 1978), and response to treatment. For example, in a subgroup of cases, the agoraphobia appears to serve a function in the marriage. In such cases the spouse may show deterioration of functioning when the symptomatic spouse improves (Hafner, 1979). The correlation between symptomatology in the patient and functioning of the nonsymptomatic spouse raises the question of whether the symptoms of agoraphobia serve some function in these marriages (Cobb et al, 1984). Hafner (1979) documented observations of the spousal interaction of 36 married female agoraphobics treated by the author over a period of three years. In seven cases, husbands displayed abnormal jealousy which appeared to adversely influence the wives' response to treatment. In these cases, improvement in the wives' symptoms was associated with deterioration, sometimes quite dramatic, in their husbands.

The quality of the marital interaction may also influence the treatment outcome in terms of the extent to which the spouse typically provides support and encouragement. Agoraphobes with unsatisfactory marriages are less likely to improve following in vivo exposure treatment, and are also more likely to relapse during a six-month follow-up period than those with satisfactory marriages (Milton and

Hafner, 1979). Munby and Johnston (1980) followed up 66 agoraphobic patients five to nine years after completion of a behavioral treatment delivered in one of three independently assigned treatments: 18 patients were treated in an individual psychotherapy; 36 female agoraphobic patients were treated with various behavioral appraoches; and 12 married female agoraphobics were treated in a home-based program using treatment manuals with the husband as a co-therapist. There is some suggestion that the latter treatment was the most effective in that the patients seen in this group responded slightly better to treatment initially and had less recourse to other therapies during the follow-up period. The authors suggest that the apparent superiority of the couples treatment could be attributed to the strategy of teaching the patient and spouse to deal with the agoraphobic problem, resulting in less need for professional intervention.

A more direct and controlled comparison of treatment formats for agoraphobia showed some superiority of a marital over a group format. Barlow et al (1984) investigated the group treatment of agoraphobia. Married agoraphobic (*DSM-III* criteria) women were randomly assigned to either behavioral group treatment with their spouses participating in all sessions, or behavioral group treatment without spouses. Treatments in both conditions consisted of graduated exposure combined with instruction on panic management procedures and self-help statements. Those in the couples' condition were instructed to communicate during periods of anxiety and panic, and negotiated strategies for handling anxiety. Both intervention groups showed highly significant overall change on the symptoms. There was some evidence in favor of the couples' intervention, in that 9 of 11 patients who improved beyond a clinically relevant cut-off score had been given the couples treatment, while six of nine who showed less improvement were in the patient alone group.

Alcoholism

McCrady (1985) has summarized the clinical treatment decisions for choice of format, techniques, setting, and client-treatment matching for patients suffering from alcohol abuse and addiction. Prominent in these decisions are the nature of alcohol dependency, personal resources of the patient, social environment's support for alcohol, and psychological health. The reviewer notes that while few treatment approaches have stood out as definitively superior to others, those treatment packages that have shown the most success have actively involved the existing social network of the alcoholic, or helped the alcoholic construct a new social system that supports abstinence. For example, community reinforcement treatment (Hunt and Azrin, 1973), marital treatments (for example, Hedberg and Campbell, 1974; McCrady et al, 1979), and family treatments (Steinglass, 1976) have yielded better results than individually treated controls. Surveys (Leach and Norris, 1977) indicate that 70 percent of those involved in Alcoholics Anonymous (AA) for one year or more have sustained sobriety. The success of the AA self-help group has spawned multiple offspring, including the multiple family group approach of Al-Anon, and, more recently, the self-help group format for individuals with a familial history of alcoholism (Children of Alcoholics).

Sexual Dysfunction

A recent review of the evidence on the role of treatment format in the behavioral intervention with sexual dysfunctions (Lipman et al, 1985) indicated that group format, minimal therapist contact bibliotherapy, and standard couple format all have demonstrable effectiveness. Differences among the formats are subtle. However, the reviewers asserted that it is premature to conclude that all therapeutic formats are equally effective, and call for more rigorous comparative research in which homogeneous problem categories are used while holding the therapy content constant. They also point to the need for utilization of multidimensional outcome assessment.

Personality Disorders

There is a paucity of controlled research on indications and contraindications for the selection of a particular format in the treatment of personality disorders. The bulk of the clinical literature recommends individual treatments for personality disorders due to the notion that the chronic and ego-syntonic character of these disorders requires intensive interpretation of defenses and resistances. Certain of the disorders, however, have shown beneficial response to group interventions, particularly in the case of acute symptoms and/or impulsive and acting-out behaviors. Use of a group treatment with patients who are actively suicidal, self-injurious, or dangerous and/or noxious to other people takes advantage of the external limits, feedback, and social reinforcement value of the group. Linehan and colleagues (1983) have designed a group intervention component of a multiple treatment program for the parasuicidal patient. Herein, the group treatment capitalizes on training/application of social skills in the group context. Individual therapy is tapered off with the addition of group therapy, and there is an overt effort to promote generalization of interpersonal skills from the individual therapy to the group context. The explicit goal of achieving a successful transfer of alliance from the individual (patient/therapist) working relationship to a larger interpersonal context is viewed as an important mediating goal of treatment. The generalization of learned social skills to the individual's home and community is assumed to be more effective when treatment is delivered in a combination (two-phase) format including first, individual, and later, group treatment.

A more general review of the literature suggests that group treatments for antisocial personality disorders (Liebowitz, 1986) and some borderline conditions (Kernberg, 1983) may be indicated, particularly when used in combination with individual and/or milieu treatments.

Adjustment Disorders

Central to the understanding and treatment of developmental or life-stage related adjustment disorders is the role of psychosocial variables in the onset, adjustment, and recovery process. Life stage or situational problems related to events such as transition to adulthood, change in or retirement from a primary role, divorce, separation, or loss are usually psychosocial in nature and often call for a redefinition of roles and role relationships, a re-evaluation of perceptions of self in relation to others, and changes in the pattern of interpersonal interaction within the family, social group, or community at large. The assessment of such disorders necessarily calls for an evaluation of the temporal, situational, and social contextual variables that may be related to the presenting problems.

MATCHING TREATMENT FORMAT TO SITUATIONAL/LIFE-STAGE CONTEXT

Adaptation to a New Role Within the Family

Such life-stage and family related changes as marriage, child-rearing, divorce, and death usually have an impact on the entire family. Family systems theorists and strategic family therapists view the process of adaptation to a new role in the family as one which forces the redefinition of intrafamilial role relationships and interpersonal boundaries. At times of role transition and life-stage related change, a family (as a unit and including its individual members) is likely to experience greater stress and difficulty in coping with the problems of daily life (Haley, 1980). Patterns of communication and coping, which were quite adequate, may be at once dysfunctional, calling for radical interventions in an effort to resolve internal conflict and ameliorate stress.

Adjustment to New Living Situation

Exemplary of this type of problem are the difficulties experienced by some adolescents and young adults leaving the parental home for the first time. The stress of adjusting to a new environment and new role expectations (such as college, a new job, independent living) may provoke symptoms of depression, anxiety disorders, identity confusion, and more serious clinical disorders such as clinical depressions, psychotic disorders, substance abuse, or suicide. The educational, counseling, and guidance fields have been active in promoting the use of both individual and group interventions to deal with such problems. The less severe problems such as motivational and/or attitudinal problems, mild habit disorders, and social withdrawal are often treated successfully in a group format wherein the external social reinforcement provided by others (Levy, 1979), identification with a social group, and the social facilitation effects of conjoint behavior change appear to be particularly effective (Lieberman and Boreman, 1983). The more severe or chronic disorders include those which, although elicited by situational or life events, are, nevertheless, more seriously debilitating or of potential danger to the individual or others. Such disorders would most likely fall into the categories of *DSM-III* Axis I conditions, for which the principles discussed earlier would, of course, apply.

Divorce

Considerable attention has been given to the influence of divorce on both the marital partners and the children involved in the separation and restructuring of the family. Individual treatments are usually supportive and reality oriented, whereas family treatments tend to be used in dealing with the general impact on the parenting and companionship relations of family members (Block, 1983; Sager, et al, 1983). The clinical literature advocates group format for brief, focal treatments that are more psychoeducational in nature than directed to personality or behavioral change. There is some suggestion that the homogeneous group setting involving members of the same sex is most beneficial in treating divorcing couples (Block, 1983). In a random assignment, controlled comparison of group therapy with self-help treatments and a waiting list control condition, Johnson and Alevizos (1978) found that subjects receiving group therapy reported significantly better adjustments and satisfaction with treatment at the end of a brief (two-month) treatment for adjustment to marital separation.

Bereavement

Although little empirical data is available on specific treatments for bereaved adults (Lieberman et al, in press), the clinical literature reports a long history of individual treatments for individuals experiencing grief or melancholic reactions to the loss of a significant other. There is some evidence that mourning proper, referring to the natural process of grieving and adjustment to object loss (Freud S, 1957), can be effectively treated in a homogeneous group therapy where participants serve an important social support function. More serious depressive reactions to separation and loss necessitate more intensive treatments—usually medication in combination with an individual therapy or a brief, crisis oriented family treatment devoted to relief of the more acute symptomatology.

MATCHING TREATMENT FORMAT TO PRESENTING PROBLEMS

Several trends in contemporary psychiatry have led from a predominantly diagnosis-driven orientation in treatment planning to include a focus on presenting problems. Empirical support for a problem oriented approach comes from evidence that problems better predict long-term patient outcome than do diagnoses (Longabaugh et al, 1983). Second, the demonstrated efficacy of behavorial treatments for more focal disorders (for example, phobias, habit disorders, and so forth) has also contributed to more problem oriented treatment planning. Third, the growing popularity of homogeneous group treatments for a variety of relatively focal disorders, as adjunct treatment for medical disorders (such as hypertension and renal failure), as primary treatments for focal psychiatric disorders (such as alcoholism and substance abuse), and as the prominant format for self-help interventions (such as assertiveness training), has reinforced the trend toward problem oriented therapeutic interventions.

Child and Adolescent Behavioral Problems

As will be discussed later in this chapter, central to the treatment of any disorders of childhood or adolescence (whether focal or syndromal) is the reality that the child's developmental status necessitates a unique kind of dependency upon the family environment. The interaction of familial and social environmental variables with the biologically driven maturational processes makes consideration of the interpersonal context an essential prerequisite in the assessment of child and adolescent problems. Second, the relative vulnerability of the child to environmental forces and the possible influence of the family on the course of a childhood disorder (regardless of etiology) suggests the importance of including the family in treatment as well as assessment.

Perhaps most exemplary of the social and interpersonal nature of childhood problem behavior are aggressive behaviors which, by definition, imply some relationship to a social context (Ross, 1974). Thus, it is not surprising that some of the most sophisticated strategies for treatment of behavior disorders of childhood and adolescence focus directly upon social factors (Patterson and Brodsky,

1966; Thomas et al, 1968) and familial factors such as parental child rearing attitudes (Freud A, 1972) and practices (Patterson, 1982). Many of the more successful treatments deal *exclusively* with parental behaviors, based on the assumption that a mediating goal, namely change in dysfunctional patterns of parenting behavior, will ultimately result in modification of the child or adolescent's problem behavior. The efficacy of this approach is displayed in the examples from Patterson's (1982) and Patterson and Fleischman's (1979) work with the parents of acting-out children.

Such treatments also show evidence of important secondary benefits. Humphreys and colleagues (1978) studied the effects of parent behavior training on the behavior of siblings of noncompliant children. Eight cases of mothers and children, referred for treatment of noncompliant behavior, were followed in a home based behavioral treatment program that was designed to train the mother to be a more effective reinforcing agent with her children. Home observations indicated that without direct instructions from the therapists, mothers used the behavioral skills that they learned in the treatment not only with the problem child but also with the siblings. Sibling compliance to parental commands increased from pretreatment to posttreatment, as did the compliance of the problem child.

Other nontargeted beneficial effects of parent management training include reduction of maternal depression (Patterson and Flesichman, 1979) and increased maternal self-esteem (Eyberg and Robinson, 1982; Forehand et al, 1980; Patterson and Flesichman, 1979); and enhanced attitudes toward offspring (Forehand et al, 1980) have been shown to increase following behavioral intervention targeted at the behavioral problems of the adolescent. Mothers of deviant children have been shown to be less depressed following effective behavioral treatment and to begin to perceive their children as well adjusted.

Outstanding among the individual treatments for acting-out or aggressive behavior in children and adolescents are those which utilize a cognitive, problem-solving approach (Shure and Spivack, 1978; Spivack et al, 1976). The derivation of these treatments is based largely on a theoretical model which implicates cognitive processes, such as the child's reflective-impulsive cognitive style (Kagan, 1966) and ability to see the perspective of others (Feshbach, 1975) in the etiology of aggressive behavior. As Kazdin (1984) notes in his review of outcome studies of cognitive therapy with children, the majority of these studies have involved normal children who show a range of behavioral problems. Those which attempt to evaluate efficacy with clinical populations show equivocal results, revealing change in cognition but not in social behavior (Camp et al, 1977).

Direct empirical comparisons of the most prominent individual and family treatments for aggressive behavior in children have not been done. The most successful approaches call upon essentially different theoretical models of aggressive behavior (social learning/behavioral versus cognitive) and utilize intervention formats which derive most directly from these models. Thus, in the area of treatments for behavior disorders of children, comparisons of individual and family formats are complicated by the relative value of the individual versus family context for the specific model of therapeutic action and associated strategies of intervention.

Marital Conflict

Marital problems have in common with the problems of childhood and adolescence a focus on interpersonal variables, most obviously because of the intrinsic interpersonal nature of these problems, but also because of evidence that interpersonal variables may contribute to or maintain the dysfunctional interactions (Jacobson et al, 1984; Coyne et al, 1986). In a box score review of the research on treatments of marital problems, Gurman and Kniskern (1978) concluded that marital treatment is superior to individual treatment for problems of an interactional nature. However, it has been pointed out (Bennun, 1984) that this review collapsed studies in which one spouse had an individually diagnosed condition with those in which marital conflict alone was the issue.

Because the marital treatment format for marital problems has so much face validity, there is currently little controlled research which compares it with alternate formats, such as group and individual formats. Instead, there is some clinical literature on the situations in which one would use individual format for marital discord, including the not uncommon situation in which one partner wants treatment and the other does not (Bennun, 1984). There are also a number of studies of marital treatment, especially behavioral marital treatment (Jacobson et al, 1984), which document the effectiveness of marital therapy for marital conflict.

CURRENT GUIDELINES FOR TREATMENT FORMAT

Global comparisons of the three treatment formats are of limited value in that they show more commonalities than differences and fail to provide information regarding the relative utility of formats for specific disorders and/or problems. What is needed are more specific hypotheses as to which formats would be most beneficial in treating specific problems and disorders. Nonetheless, some leads do exist.

Disorders Involving the Social Sphere

For some disorders, the nature of the illness or problem may call for intervention involving significant others in the environment. Disorders such as these seem to fall into two general categories: a) those in which the illness is especially burdensome to the family or friends, and thus calls for supportive and educative efforts with those people on whom the illness has a negative impact; and b) those disorders that by their very nature are functionally related to the social context. For example, the deficit in schizophrenia may result in a need for low interpersonal stimulation, and family members vary in their sensitivity to this need. In contrast, those prone to depression may need unusual amounts of interpersonal support and encouragement. These may be illness conditions that call for treatment formats (family group, or family/marital), which have an impact on those important objects in the patient's environment.

The more the symptoms or behaviors are under the interactional or functional control of the interpersonal environment, the more likely effects will come from modifying that environment. Patterson's (1982) work with the interpersonal environment of the antisocial adolescent is most illustrative here.

When the difficulty is directly and solely interactional in nature and is causing distress in the family environment (for example, marital conflict with no diagnoses of Axis I conditions in either party), a marital or family treatment format involving the relevant parties certainly has face validity, and is probably at least as effective, if not more so, than other treatment formats (Gurman and Kniskern, 1978).

In contrast, in cases in which the etiology of the disorder is not viewed as social or environmental in nature and yet the disorder itself has a detrimental impact on the family or other social (for example, work) context, the use of a family or group treatment is indicated.

Third, in cases wherein neither etiology nor secondary effects of the disorder involve the family, consideration of the mechanisms of change or vicissitudes of the working alliance may suggest the need for a family or group intervention. For example, sexual dysfunctions may or may not involve the significant other (spouse) in contributing to the condition, but the spouse may be crucial in the practice of behaviors that lead to recovery (Masters and Johnson, 1979).

Social Systems Needed to Encourage Treatment

Given the multiple systems (biochemical, intrapersonal, marital, familial, social network, community, cultural) impinging upon the individual, treatment planning will be most efficacious when these multiple variables are taken into account in the selection of treatment format. What we know of the problem may be less important than knowing which troubled systems can most effectively and efficiently be treated and changed. Thus, there may be situations in which the nature of the condition does not call for change by significant others, but involvement of significant others in treatment will enhance the nature of the working alliance, circumvent the problems of an overly intense or negative transference to the therapist, and thereby reduce treatment drop-out and increase sustained patient work at the treatment itself. Agoraphobic disorders which are not intrinsically interpersonal in nature, referred to as "simple" (versus the "complex" type) (Hafner, 1986), are examples of this type.

In some cases of individual symptoms, the symptom may not be under the behavioral control of the environment, but the introduction of the significant other to the treatment may assist the patient in overcoming the problematic behaviors and in coping with the condition in the long run. The work in agoraphobia is most instructive here.

Certain mediating goals of treatment, such as medication compliance, compliance with psychosocial treatment, decrease in family burden concerning the illness of the individual, and so forth, may respond differentially to treatment formats. For example, treatment compliance, including medication compliance, can be adversely affected by the family environment (Pilkonis et al, 1984) and thus may necessitate family intervention (Glick et al, 1985; Haas et al, in press).

If the existing social system of the patient is insufficient and/or nonexistent, group treatment may provide a support system for the patient that encourages social relationships, sustains treatment involvement, and buffers the patient from future stressors.

Severity of Illness

The healthier and more independent the patient, the more likely the patient is to benefit from an individual-format therapy with mediating goals of changing that individual's cognition, emotional modulation and control, and behavior. Contrariwise, the more severe the symptoms and dysfunction of the patient, the more the patient is dependent upon a stable interpersonal network for support, guidance, structure, and direction. Therefore, the more severe the condition of the patient, the more likely some form of environmental intervention is needed in the treatment regimen. In addition, the more disturbed the family environment of the patient, the more likely family intervention will assist in the course of the ill family member. This is most evident in the current research in schizophrenia, and may be relevant to the very young and elderly.

Matching Treatment Format to the Phase of Treatment/Course of Illness

One of the most robust findings in the treatment of the major psychiatric disorders is that involvement of the family during the acute phase of illness may be instrumental in improving long-term course and outcome (Falloon et al, 1982; Leff et al, 1982; Glick et al, 1985). There is also a growing literature which suggests that psychotherapy (Keith and Matthews, 1982), group therapy (Shakir et al, 1979; Volkmar et al, 1980; Rosen, 1980; Cochran, 1984), and family therapies, in particular (Falloon et al, 1984), can be effective in enhancing patient compliance with the phase of continuation and maintenance medication treatments.

Partially based on the research that has been completed to date, McFarlane and Beels (1983) have organized a decision-tree model for integrating family and group formats when a family member has schizophrenia. Phase I involves an assessment of the family's ability to comply with treatment. It is suggested that noncompliant families be treated with strategic family therapy, while compliant families be sent to Phase II. In Phase II, the decision rests on number of previous episodes, with first episode families treated by a psychoeducational method (Goldstein et al, 1978) and the multiple episode families treated with the Connection and Survival Skills Workshop aspects of the Anderson approach (Anderson et al, 1980). Phase III is the follow-up phase, in which basic lessons of previous work are individualized and applied in a multiple family group format of either short-term or long-term duration. Phase IV involves strategic family therapy (Haley, 1980; Madanes, 1981) for families with younger, more responsive premorbid patients, when the family does not seem to have learned enough in the less directive multifamily groups. Phase V, systemic family therapy (Selvini-Palazzoli et al, 1978), is reserved for those families who fail in all other treatment formats. While this decision-tree model has no research to substantiate it, and includes some family treatments (such as strategic family therapy) that have no evidence of efficacy in clinical trials, the model is clinically helpful in attempting to integrate differential aims of treatment in sequence based on certain family characteristics.

Patient's Preference

There are numerous studies that yield little differential outcome due to format of treatment, at least where severity of illness is moderate or less. Thus, if one format of treatment is not working, the clinician should be flexible in considering another. If the patient has a strong preference for one format, that preference probably should be honored.

IMPLICATIONS FOR FUTURE RESEARCH

Controlled empirical investigations of the relative efficacy of individual, group, and family treatment formats are at present limited in number and scope of application. Those controlled comparisons that have been done focus on a few specific disorders; for example, affective disorders, schizophrenia, phobic disorders, and some behavior problems. Second, several of the studies which make direct comparisons across treatment formats lack the basic methodological and design features of controlled outcome research.

The remedy for this deficiency is not in systematic comparison of all formats for each and every disorder. Neither are global comparisons of the three treatment formats particularly helpful. Such comparison studies are relatively conservative tests of therapeutic efficacy, requiring powerful specific effects of substantial incremental value to outweigh the nonspecific effects common to the different treatments. It is not surprising that, to date, such studies more often reveal more commonality or equivalence of formats than differences.

What is needed are guidelines for the direction of further empirical investigation in this area. Research, as well as practice, stands to benefit from the principle of incremental gain, referring here to the differential value of pursuing a particular line of investigation. Differential therapeutics, with its revolutionary shift of focus—a deemphasis on etiology and a newly developing emphasis on the prognostic and functional characteristics of psychiatric disorders—represents a major paradigm shift in 20th century psychiatry. In parallel, research on therapeutic interventions should be guided by more specific hypotheses about the site of therapeutic action (for example, intrapsychic, behavioral, attitudinal, or cognitive) and the likely mechanism of change in the treatment of a particular disorder. (The complexities of this issue are illustrated by the competing theoretical models and therapeutic approaches to the treatment of aggressive behavior in children.)

In keeping with this paradigm shift, empirical investigations of treatment format should be guided by basic principles of psychopathology and change processes. Experimental psychopathology, which aims to identify the mediating processes and/or deficits associated with particular disorders, has particular potential for informing further work in this field. No less important is what can be learned from the clinical observations and theory of therapeutic action. Whether informed by empirical data, clinical observation, or a hypothetico-rational/deductive approach, attention to the hypothetical models of change and the prescribed mediating goals of treatment should guide us in the field of psychotherapy outcome research. Such an overarching principle need be applied in the design of controlled studies of particular formats for specific disorders. As the data suggest, some leads do exist. The call is now for a more systematic and rationally guided program of outcome research.

REFERENCES

Anderson CM, Hogarty G, Reiss DJ: Family treatment of adult schizophrenic patients. Schizophr Bull 6:490-505, 1980

Barlow DH, Waddell MT: Agoraphobia, in Clinical Handbook of Psychological Disorders. Edited by Barlow DH. New York, Guilford Press, 1985

Barlow DH, O'Brien GT, Last CG: Couples treatment of agoraphobia. Behav Ther 15:41-58, 1984

Beach SR, O'Leary KD: The treatment of depression occurring in the context of marital discord. Behav Ther 17:43-49, 1986

Bellack AS, Hersen M, Himmelhoch JM: Social skills training for depression: a treatment manual. J Supple Abstract Serv Catalog Selected Documents Psychol 10:92(MS 2156), 1980

Bennun I: Marital therapy with one spouse, in Marital Interaction: Analysis and Modification. Edited by Hahlweg K, Jacobson NS. New York, Guilford Press, 1984

Bion W: Experiences in Groups. London, Tavistock, 1959

Bloch DA: Family systems perspectives on the management of the individual patient, in Psychiatry Update: The American Psychiatric Association Annual Review, vol. 2. Edited by Grinspoon L. Washington, DC, American Psychiatric Press, Inc., 1983

Broderick C, Schrader S: The history of professional marriage and family therapy, in Handbook of Family Therapy. Edited by Gurman A, Kniskern D. New York, Brunner/Mazel, 1981

Brown GW, Birley JLT, Wing JK: Influence of family life on the course of schizophrenic disorder: a replication. Br J Psychiatry 121:241-258, 1972

Brown RA, Lewinsohn PM: A psychoeducational approach to the treatment of depression: comparison of group, individual and minimal contact procedures. J Consult Clin Psychol 52:774-783, 1984

Burrow T: The group method of analysis. Psychoanal Rev 14:268-280, 1927

Camp B, Blom G, Hebert F, et al: "Think aloud": a program for developing self-control in young aggressive boys. J Abnorm Child Psychol 5:157-169, 1977

Cobb JP, Mathews AM, Childs-Clarke A, et al: The spouse as co-therapist in the treatment of agoraphobia. Br J Psychiatry 144:282-287, 1984

Cochran SD: Preventing medical noncompliance in the outpatient treatment of bipolar affective disorders. J Consult Clin Psychol 52:873-878, 1984

Coyne JC: Strategic therapy with couples having a depressed spouse, in Family Intervention in Affective Illness. Edited by Clarkin JF, Haas GL, Glick ID. New York, Guilford Press (in press)

Coyne JC, Kahn J, Gotlib IH: Depression, in Family Interaction and Psychotherapy. Edited by Jacob T. New York, Plenum, 1986

Davenport YB, Evert MH, Adland ML, et al: Couples group therapy as an adjunct to lithium maintenance of the manic patient. Am J Orthopsychiatry 49:495-502, 1977

Donion PT, Rada RT, Knight SW: A therapeutic aftercare setting for "refractory" chronic schizophrenic patients. Am J Psychiatry 130:682-684, 1973

Eyberg SM, Robinson EA: Parent-child interaction training: Effects on family functioning. J Clin Child Psychol 11:130-137, 1982

Falloon IRH, Boyd JL, McGill CW, et al: Family management in the prevention of exacerbations of schizophrenia: a controlled study. N Engl J Med 306:1437-1440, 1982

Falloon IRH, Boyd JL, McGill CW: Family Care of Schizophrenia: A Problem-solving Approach to the Treatment of Mental Illness. New York, Guilford Press, 1984

Falloon IRH, Boyd JL, McGill CW, et al: Family management in the prevention of morbidity of schizophrenia: clinical outcome of a two-year longitudinal study. Arch Gen Psychiatry 42:887-896, 1985

Feshbach N: Empathy in children: some theoretical and empirical considerations. Counseling Psychologist 5:25-30, 1975

Fitzgerald R: Mania as a message: treatment with family therapy and lithium carbonate. American Journal of Psychotherapy 26:547-555, 1972

Forehand R, Wells KC, Griest DL: An examination of the social validity of a parent training program. Behav Ther 11:488-502, 1980

Freud A: The child as a person in his own right. Psychoanal Study Child 27:621-625, 1972

Freud S: General Introduction to Psychoanalysis. New York, Liveright, 1915

Freud S: Group Psychology and the Analysis of the Ego (1921), in Complete Psychological Works, Standard Edition, vol. 18. Translated and edited by Strachey J. London, Hogarth Press, 1959

Freud S: Mourning and melancholia (1917), in Complete Psychological Works, Standard Edition, vol. 14. Translated and edited by Strachey J. London, Hogarth Press, 1957

Freud S, Breuer J: Studies on hysteria (1895), in Complete Psychological Works, Standard Edition, vol. 2 Translated and Edited by Strachey J. London, Hogarth Press, 1955

Friedman AS: Interaction of drug therapy with marital therapy in depressive patients. Arch Gen Psychiatry 32:619-637, 1975

Glick ID, Clarkin JF, Spencer JH, et al: A controlled evaluation of inpatient family intervention. Arch Gen Psychiatry 42:882-886, 1985

Goldstein AJ, Chambless DL: A reanalysis of agoraphobia. Behav Ther 9:47-59, 1978

Goldstein MJ, Rodnick E, Evans JR, et al: Drug and family therapy in the aftercare treatment of acute schizophrenia. Arch Gen Psychiatry 35:1169-1177, 1978

Greene BL Lustig N, Lee RRL: Marital therapy when one spouse has a primary affective disorder. Am J Psychiatry 133:827-830, 1976

Grunebaum H: Soft-hearted review of hard-nosed research on groups. Int J Group Psychother 25:185-195, 1975

Gurman AS, Kniskern DP: Research on marital and family therapy: progress, perspective and prospect, in Handbook of Psychotherapy and Behavior Change, 2nd edition. Edited by Garfield S, Bergin A. New York, John Wiley, 1978

Haas GL, Clarkin JF, Glick ID: Marital and family treatment of depression, in Handbook of Depression: Treatment Assessment and Research. Edited by Beckham EE, Leber WR. Homewood, IL, Dorsey Press, 1985

Haas GL, Glick ID, Spencer JH, et al: The patient, the family and compliance with posthospital treatment for affective disorders. Psychopharmacol Bull (in press)

Hafner RJ: Agoraphobic women married to abnormally jealous men. Br J Med Psychol 52:99-104, 1979

Hafner RJ: Marriage and Mental Illness. New York, Guilford Press, 1986

Haley J: Leaving Home: The Therapy of Disturbed Young People. New York, McGraw-Hill, 1980

Hand I, Lamontagne Y, Marks IM: Group exposure (flooding) in vivo for agoraphobics. Br J Psychiatry 124:588, 1974

Hedberg AG, Campbell L: A comparison of four behavioral treatments of alcoholism. J Behav Ther Exp Psychiatry 5:251-256, 1974

Herz MI, Spitzer RL, Gibbon M, et al: Individual versus group aftercare treatment. Am J Psychiatry 131:808-812, 1974

Hogarty GE, Anderson CM, Reiss DJ et al: Family psychoeducation, social skills training, and maintenance chemotherapy in the aftercare treatment of schizophrenia. Arch Gen Psychiatry 43:633-642, 1986

Horowitz MJ, Marmar C, Weiss DS, et al: Brief psychotherapy of bereavement reactions: the relationship of process to outcome. Arch Gen Psychiatry 41:438-448, 1984

Humphreys L, Forehand R, McMahon R, et al: Parent behavioral training to modify child noncompliance: effects on untreated siblings. J Behav Ther Exp Psychiatry 9:235-238, 1978

Hunt GM, Azrin NH: A community-reinforcement approach to alcoholism. Behav Res Ther 11:91-104, 1973

Jacobson NS, Margolin G: Marital Therapy: Strategies Based on Social Learning and Behavior Exchange Principles. New York, Brunner/Mazel, 1979

Jacobson NS, Follette WC, Elwood RW: Outcome research on behavioral marital therapy: a methodological and conceptual reappraisal, in Marital Interaction. Edited by Hahlweg K, Jacobson NS. New York, Guilford Press, 1984

Johnson SM, Alevizos PM: Divorce Adjustment: Clinical and Survey Research (Preliminary Report). Eugene, University of Oregon, 1978

Kagan J: Reflection-impulsivity: the generality and dynamics of conceptual tempo. Journal of Educational Psychology 71:17-24, 1966

Kazdin AE: Treatment of conduct disorders, in Psychotherapy Research: Where Are We and Where Should We Go? Edited by Williams JBW, Spitzer RL. New York, Guilford Press, 1984

Keith SJ, Matthews SM: Group family and milieu therapies and psychosocial rehabilitation in the treatment of the schizophrenic disorders, in Psychiatry Update: The American Psychiatric Association Annual Review, vol. 1. Edited by Grinspoon L. Washington, DC, American Psychiatric Press, Inc., 1982

Keith SJ, Matthews SM: Schizophrenia: a review of psychosocial treatment strategies, in Psychotherapy Research: Where Are We and Where Should We Go? Edited by Williams BW, Spitzer RL. New York, Guilford Press, 1984

Kernberg O: Psychoanalytic studies of group processes: theory and applications, in Psychiatry Update: The American Psychiatric Association Annual Review, vol. 2. Edited by Grinspoon L. Washington DC, American Psychiatric Press, Inc., 1983

Klerman GL, Dimascio A, Weissman M: Treatment of depression by drugs and psychotherapy. Am J Psychiatry 131:186-191, 1974

Klerman GL, Weissman MM, Rounsaville BJ, et al: Interpersonal Psychotherapy of Depression. New York, Basic Books, 1984

Lazell E: The group treatment of dementia praecox. Psychoanal Rev 8:168-179, 1921

Leach B, Norris JL: Factors in the development of Alcoholics Anonymous (A.A.), in The Biology of Alcoholism, vol. 5. Edited by Kissin B, Begleiter H. New York, Plenum, 1977

Leff J, Kuipers L, Berkowitz R, et al: A controlled trial of social intervention in the families of schizophrenic patients. Br J Psychiatry 141:121-134, 1982

Levene HL, Patterson V, Murphey BG, et al: The aftercare of schizophrenics: an evaluation of group and individual approaches. Psychiatr Q 44:296-304, 1970

Levy LH: Processes and activities in groups, in Self-Help Groups for Coping with Crises: Origins, Members, Processes and Impact. Edited by Lieberman MA, Borman L. San Francisco, Jossey-Bass, 1979

Lewin K: Frontiers in group dynamics. Human Relations 1:5, 1947

Liebowitz MR, Stone MH, Turkat ID: Treatment of personality disorders, in Psychiatry Update: The American Psychiatric Association Annual Review, vol. 5. Edited by Frances AJ, Hales RE. Washington, DC, American Psychiatric Press, Inc., 1986

Lieberman MA: Group methods, in Helping People Change. Edited by Kanfer FH, Goldstein AP. New York, Pergamon Press, 1975

Lieberman MA, Videka-Sherman L: The impact of self-help groups on the mental health of widows and widowers. J Orthopsychiatry (in press)

Lieberman MA, Borman L: Self-Help Groups for Coping with Crises: Origins, Members, Processes, and Impact. San Francisco, Jossey-Bass, 1979

Lipman E, Fichten C, Brender W: The role of therapeutic format in the treatment of sexual dysfunction: a review. Clin Psychol Rev 5:103-117, 1985

Longabaugh R, Fowler R, Stout R, et al: Validation of a problem-focused nomenclature. Arch Gen Psychiatry 40:453-461, 1983

Luborsky L, Singer B, Luborsky L: Comparative sutdies of psychotherapy. Arch Gen Psychiatry 132:995-1008, 1976

Madanes C: Strategic family therapy. San Francisco, Jossey-Bass, 1981

Malm U: The influence of group therapy on schizophrenia. Acta Psychiatr Scand (Suppl) 297:2-65, 1982

Masters WH, Johnson VE: Human Sexual Inadequacy. Boston, Little, Brown, 1979

McCrady BS: Alcoholism, in Clinical Handbook of Psychological Disorders. Edited by Barlow DH. New York, Guilford Press, 1985

McCrady BS, Paolino TJ, Longabaugh RL, et al: Effects on treatment outcome of joint admission and spouse involvement in treatment of hospitalized alcoholics. Addict Behav 4:155-165, 1979

McFarlane WR, Beels C: Family research in schizophrenia: a review and integration for clinicians, in Family Therapy in Schizophrenia. Edited by McFarlane W. New York, Guilford Press, 1983

McLean PD, Ogston K, Grauer L: A behavioral approach to the treatment of depression. J Behav Ther Exp Psychiatry 4:323-330, 1973

Milton F, Hafner J: The outcome of behavior therapy for agoraphobia in relation to marital adjustment. Arch Gen Psychiatry 36:807-811, 1979

Mittleman B: The concurrent analysis of married couples. Psychoanal Q 17:182-197, 1948

Moreno J: The First Book on Group Psychotherapy. New York, Beacon House, 1957

Munby M, Johnston DW: Agoraphobia: the long-term follow-up of behavioral treatment. Br J Psychiatry 137:418-427, 1980

Murphy GE, Woodruff RA, Herjanic K, et al: Variability of the clinical course of primary affective disorder. Arch Gen Psychiatry 30:757-761, 1974

O'Brien CP, Hamm KB, Ray BA, et al: Group vs. individual psychotherapy with schizophrenics: a controlled outcome study. Arch Gen Psychiatry 27:474-478, 1972

Parker G: The Bonds of Depression. Sydney, Australia, Angus & Robertson, 1978

Parloff M, Dies R: Group psychotherapy outcome research 1966-1975. Int J Group Psychother 27:281-319, 1977

Parsons T: The Structure of Social Action. New York, Free Press, 1937

Patterson GR: The aggressive child: victim and architect of a coercive system, in Behavior Modification and Families. Edited by Mash EJ, Hamerlynck LC. New York, Brunner/Mazel, 1976

Patterson GR: Coercive Family Process. Eugene, Oregon, Castalia Publishing Co, 1982

Patterson GR, Brodsky G: A behavior modification programme for a child with multiple problem behaviors. J Child Psychol Psychiatry, 7:277-295, 1966

Patterson GR, Fleischman MJ: Maintenance of treatment effects: some considerations concerning family systems and follow-up data. Behav Ther 10:168-185, 1979

Pilkonis P, Imber S, Lewis P, et al: A comparative outcome study of individual, group, and conjoint psychotherapy. Arch Gen Psychiatry 41:431-437, 1984

Pratt JH: The class method of treating consumption in the homes of the poor. JAMA 49:755-759, 1907

Rosen AM: Group management of lithium prophylaxis. Paper presented at the 133rd Annual Meeting of the American Psychiatric Association, San Francisco, 1980

Ross AO: Psychological Disorders of Children: A Behavioral Approach to Theory, Research and Therapy. New York, McGraw-Hill, 1974

Rush AJ, Beck AT, Kovacs M, et al: Comparative efficacy of cognitive therapy and pharmacotherapy in the treatment of depressed outpatients. Cognitive Therapy Research 1:17-37, 1977

Sager CJ, Brown HS, Crohn H, et al: Treating the Remarried Family. New York, Brunner/Mazel, 1983

Schilder P: The analysis of ideologies as a psychotherapeutic method, especially in group treatment. Am J Psychiatry 93:601-617, 1936

Selvini-Palazzoli M, Boscolo L, Cecchin G, et al: Paradox and Counterparadox: A New Model of the Therapy of the Family in Schizophrenic Transaction. New York, Jason Aronson, 1978

Shakir SA, Volkmar FR, Bacon S, et al: Group psychotherapy as an adjunct to lithium maintenance. Am J Psychiatry 136:455-456, 1979

Shapiro D: Recent applications of meta-analysis in clinical research. Clinical Psychology Review 5:13-34, 1985

Shapiro D, Shapiro D: Meta-analysis of comparative therapy outcome studies: a replication and refinement. Psychol Bull 92:581-604, 1982

Shaw BF: Comparison of cognitive therapy and behavior therapy in the treatment of depression. J Consult Clin Psychol 45:543-551, 1977

Shure MB, Spivack G: Problem-solving techniques in child-rearing. San Francisco, Jossey-Bass, 1978

Sinnott A, Jones RB, Scott-Fordham A, et al: Augmentation of in vivo exposure treatment for agoraphobia by the formation of neighborhood self-help groups. Behav Res Ther 19:339-347, 1981

Slavson SR: A Textbook in Analytic Group Psychotherapy. New York, International Universities Press, 1964

Smith ML, Glass GV, Miller TI: The Benefits of Psychotherapy. Baltimore, Johns Hopkins University Press, 1980

Spivack G, Platt JJ, Shure MB: The Problem-Solving Approach to Adjustment. San Francisco, Jossey-Bass, 1976

Steinglass P: Experimenting with family treatment approaches to alcoholism 1950-1975: a review. Fam Process 15:97-123, 1976

Steinmetz JL, Lewinsohn PM, Antonuccio DO: Prediction of individual outcome in a group intervention for depression. J Consult Clin Psychol 51:331-337, 1983

Thomas DR, Becker WC, Armstrong M: Production and elimination of disruptive classroom behavior by systematically varying teacher's behavior. J Appl Behav Anal 1:35-45, 1968

Vaughn CE, Leff JP: The influence of family and social factors on the course of psychiatric illness: A comparison of schizophrenic and depressed neurotic patients. Br J Psychiatry 129:125-137, 1976

Volkmar FR, Shakir SA, Bacon S, et al: Group therapy as an adjunct to lithium maintenance. Paper presented at the 133rd Annual Meeting of the American Psychiatric Association, San Francisco, 1980

Wampler K: Bringing the review of literature into the age of quantification: meta-analysis as a strategy for integrating research findings in family studies. Journal of Marriage and the Family Nov: 1009-1023, 1982

Weissman MM, Prusoff BA, DiMascio A, et al: Research directions on comparisons of drugs and psychotherapy in depression. Psychopharmacol Bull 15:19-21, 1979

Wender L: Current trends in group psychotherapy. Am J Psychother 3:381-401, 1951

Wolf A: The psychoanalysis of groups. Am J Psychother 4:16-50, 1950

Yalom ID: The Theory and Practice of Group Psychotherapy, 2nd edition. New York, Basic Books, 1975

Chapter 15

Strategies and Techniques of Prescriptive Psychotherapeutic Intervention

by Larry E. Beutler, Ph.D., and Marjorie Crago, Ph.D.

New ideas and theories arising directly from empirical, scientific inquiry have always been fewer, less startling, and sometimes contradictory when compared to those arising from clinical observation. As a result, the allegiance between psychotherapy and empirical science has been a shaky one and most therapeutic approaches have relied little upon scientific confirmation (Barlow, 1981). Empirical investigators base their distrust of clinical developments on the observation that clinical theories proliferate at a rate which threatens the credibility of the psychotherapy enterprise, and certainly at a faster rate than controlled research can provide confirmation. Well over 200 psychotherapy theories and philosophies are present in the armamentarium of the mental health professions (Corsini, 1981) and, with few exceptions, these treatments exist without a single, empirical investigation to verify them (Smith et al, 1980; Beutler, 1979).

On the other hand, clinicians are also skeptical of scientific developments in psychotherapy, and not always without reason. For example, when Eysenck (1952) proposed that psychotherapy research had failed to demonstrate observable effects beyond those which could be anticipated from spontaneous recovery, the subsequent skepticism on the part of most clinicians finally proved to be warranted some 30 years later (Smith et al, 1980). Such examples leave the clinician in the very difficult position of distrusting controlled, scientific findings. This distrust is likely to reach critical levels if the current trend of public and political pressures continue to insist that scientific methods should be the basis for verifying psychotherapy's worth. The public's response to the rising costs of health services emphasizes the failure of the psychotherapy community to establish public credibility, and sharpens the differences that exist between conclusions based upon clinical and empirical knowledge. One of the clearest differences in clinical and empirical wisdom exists in regard to the belief in the prescriptive specificity of psychotherapy.

Most clinicians argue in favor of maintaining theoretical and/or technical diversity in the application of psychotherapy, and emphasize that psychotherapy's effects must be understood as a complex interplay among particular procedures, philosophies, and therapists, on one hand, and particular conditions and patients, on the other. This belief in the specificity of psychotherapeutic effects often finds itself at variance with those who are knowledgeable in research literature and who suggest that all psychotherapies produce approximately equal effects (Smith et al, 1980; Luborsky et al, 1975). Is this discrepancy another instance of research lagging behind clinical intuition, or is it an example of clinicians placing faith in the unproven or unprovable? In this chapter we will explore current literature on this topic in order to clarify some of the issues and, where applicable, to provide some answers to the question of how well psychotherapy serves as a specific treatment for specific problems or patients.

A SEARCH FOR RESOLUTIONS

The discrepancy between the nonspecificity of findings suggested by most research and the prevalent belief in the specific effects of particular psychotherapy interventions may be a function of three major problems inherent in current psychotherapy research methods.

The Masking Influence of Patient and Therapist Variables

In research paradigms which utilize large samples of heterogeneous patient groups, the influence of therapist and patient variables may be so great that they mask the relative effects of specific interventions. Certainly, there is evidence to indicate that patient and therapist variables are very strong precipitators of therapeutic change, independent of the type of intervention provided (Garfield, 1980). Some would argue that there is little variance of outcome remaining once the variance attributable to patient and therapist factors is taken into consideration (Lambert and DeJulio, 1978). This position would logically support the contention that therapeutic outcome may be enhanced if the *right* therapist variables are matched with the *right* patient variables. This reasoning underlies one of the directions in which the search for specificity has been focused.

Inadequacies of Measurement

Those who are committed to the importance of tailoring specific approaches to specific individuals draw attention to the difficulty of assessing the complexities of psychotherapy induced changes with unidimensional, self-report measures (Waskow and Parloff, 1975). Group based measures, they argue, are insensitive to the fine nuances and needs of each individual patient. In response to this concern, numerous methods have been developed to target changes which are relevant to the rationales of different psychotherapies (Malan, 1976). Authors who are committed to the search for specificity maintain that while treatments may have no particular advantage over one another when evaluated by means of global and very general measures of change (Beutler and Hamblin, 1986; Mintz and Kiesler, 1982), these differences may be revealed when the specific outcomes of particular treatments are known.

Lack of Treatment Reliability

Finally, those who argue for the importance of treatment specificity observe that there is more variation among clinicians of the same therapeutic school but of dissimilar levels of experience than there is among therapists of different therapeutic schools and comparable levels of experience (Fiedler, 1950). If therapists of a given orientation do not resemble one another in practice, how can research hope to determine whether one intervention is different or better than another? Indeed, Strupp (1981) has observed that even highly experienced therapists are surprisingly inflexible in modifying their interventions from patient to patient.

He suggests that therapists must be trained very specifically in order to learn to adjust their procedures to fit the needs of specific patients.

Researchers have responded to this criticism by emphasizing the importance of developing reliable interventions, based upon therapy manuals. Numerous manuals have evolved by which therapeutic approaches and philosophies can be implemented with a relatively high degree of reliability. Cognitive therapy (Beck et al, 1979), interpersonal therapy (Klerman et al, 1984), psychodynamic therapy (Strupp and Binder, 1984), as well as many other approaches have been condensed into treatment manuals. These various theoretical approaches have also been extended to a variety of modalities including group and family treatments (Freeman, 1983). The reliability of manualized therapies has been established, and external judges are able to discriminate among various approaches when observing therapists who follow these manuals (Luborsky et al, 1982).

While clinicians may be somewhat loathe to apply cookbook therapies, there is evidence to suggest that the more faithfully one complies with the treatment structure suggested by these manuals, the more effective the treatment, regardless of the theoretical basis which underlies it (Beutler et al, 1986). Moreover, the development of treatment manuals has forced clinicians to specify more clearly than ever before the activities which constitute and distinguish the application of their philosophies. This type of specificity has paved the way for a clear test of the specific effects of therapeutic procedures, and of the ways in which these therapeutic procedures interact with patient characteristics (Elkin et al, 1985).

From the foregoing perspectives, one can conclude that: 1) a valid prescriptive protocol for the implementation of psychological treatment has not yet been devised; and 2) in order to establish psychotherapy as a prescriptive treatment, there is a need to understand the interrelationships among specific patient, treatment, therapist, and outcome variables. In response to these conclusions, research has pursued three promising approaches for making psychotherapy more specific to patient needs.

PRESCRIPTIVE PSYCHOTHERAPY METHODS

The most *acceptable* methods for developing prescriptive approaches to psychotherapy may not be the most efficacious ones. Since personal characteristics of the patient and therapist seem to be more potent contributors to treatment outcome than are either treatment techniques or patient diagnoses (Lambert and DeJulio, 1978), it would seem that the most efficacious, prescriptive approach to psychotherapy would be to match particular patient qualities with certain identifiable qualities of therapists. However, external pressures have been exerted to encourage the development of prescriptive interventions based upon patient diagnosis and therapist orientation, even though neither of these variables has shown great promise for predicting outcome when considered alone. Matches based upon treatment "brand" and patient diagnosis are more easily accepted by clinicians and more easily comprehended by the public than are those based upon personally focused variables such as belief, personality, and value similarities. A compromise position has been to utilize prescriptive formulations based upon specific and isolated therapy technologies, on the one hand, and personal, nondiagnostic patient characteristics, on the other. In the following pages we will explore some of the evidence for each of these three methods of assigning prescriptive psychological interventions.

Matching Patient and Therapist Personal Characteristics

The idea that one may be able efficaciously to match specific patients with specific therapists has been particularly intriguing to psychotherapy researchers over the past three decades. A variety of potential matching variables have been explored in this process, ranging from demographic characteristics to attitudes and values. One of the early efforts to define compatible matching dimensions evolved from the work of Whitehorn and Betz (1960), who observed that therapists whose interests were verbal and philosophically oriented (A-types) produced larger gains among schizophrenic patients than did therapists whose interests were more task oriented and practical (B-types). For 20 years, matching therapist A-B type with patient diagnosis has been explored as a potentially effective method of assigning psychotherapy. The results have been inconsistent, however, and the most reliable current conclusions suggest that matching on such broad variables as therapist interest patterns and patient diagnosis provides relatively little of value in predicting the outcome of specific therapy relationships (Beutler et al, 1986).

While relatively extensive efforts to evaluate demographic characteristics as suitable matching variables (Luborsky et al, 1980) have also largely failed to find long-term outcome benefits, similarity of ethnic background, age, and sex may have some important implications for maintaining a patient in treatment (Beutler et al, 1986). Certain personality and attitudinal matches have shown more promise for enhancing long-term benefit than have demographic matches (Beutler et al, 1986). For example, in a well controlled series of studies of therapist and patient personality matches, Berzins (1977) demonstrated that patients who were relatively dependent and needy of external support and structure responded best to therapists who were autonomy oriented and quite independent. The reverse also proved to be true, and an a priori application of an empirically defined algorithm to an independent sample of clinical clients resulted in patient-therapist matches which substantially improved the effectiveness of psychotherapy compared to alternatively matched subsamples.

From a review of personality and attitude matching studies, Beutler (1981) concluded that: 1) similarity in certain attitudes and belief systems is a relatively strong predictor of the changes in belief systems and values which occur during psychotherapy; and 2) the degree to which the patient acquires the therapist's belief system is predictive of the amount of improvement realized in the treatment process. Compared to the estimated 10 percent of total outcome variance which is attributable to therapist technique and philosophy (Lambert et al, 1978), matching studies suggest that as much as 30 percent of the outcome variance can be attributed to a facilitative match of compatible belief systems and personality patterns (Beutler, 1983; Berzins, 1977).

While more precise specification of matching patterns is still needed, matching patient and therapist belief and personality variables is a clearly promising direction for more research on therapy efficacy. Unfortunately, it is unlikely that clinicians will readily accept these procedures if they require that one's personal beliefs about sex, discipline, aggression, and dependency be revealed. These variables do not fit well within the established theoretical structures of practicing clinicians.

Matching Diagnoses to Global Orientations

By far the most favored approach to prescriptive treatment research is matching global psychotherapy orientations (for example, psychodynamic, cognitive, behavioral, and so on) to patients with clearly defined and diagnosed syndromes. In spite of its apparent simplicity, research in this area has been plagued by the lack of reliability both in applying various treatment interventions and in defining the patient populations to which these interventions are to be applied. While many clinicians differentiate among psychotherapies only in terms of intensity (for example, supportive versus long-term) or modality (group versus individual), the varieties of specific approaches number over 200 (Corsini, 1981). An analysis of the procedures employed by therapists who represent these schools suggests that most can be adquately represented by five approaches which are distinguishable in application: *behavioral, experiential, cognitive modification, interpersonal,* and *psychodynamic* (Beutler, 1983). While the clinical efficacy of these five categories of psychological intervention has been demonstrated, their relative utility for specific diagnostic subgroups is hard to demonstrate from available research. This point is exemplified by reviewing the status of knowledge regarding those disorders for which the clinical efficacy of specific treatments has been explored.

PHOBIC DISORDERS. Phobias represent the diagnositc entity for which there is the most consistent evidence that a specific intervention (that is, exposure treatment) has a specific relationship to outcome. While there is variation in the effectiveness of behavioral exposure treatments, depending on a variety of extra-diagnostic variables, few patient or therapist variables have emerged as more powerful determiners of improvement than the procedure of repeated exposure to the feared object itself. However, research in this area has increasingly focused on developing ways in which simple exposure may be effectively enhanced. From these efforts, it seems that the addition of paradoxical injunctions (Michelson and Mavissakalian, 1985), anxiety management strategies (Butler et al, 1984; Emmelkamp et al, 1985), and modeling procedures (Ladouceur, 1983) all increase the effectiveness of basic exposure methods (Williams et al, 1984).

While exposure therapies have consistently been found to be effective (and cost effective) interventions for monosymptomatic phobias (Emmelkamp et al, 1985; Butler et al, 1984; Minor and Leone, 1984), results with more complex disorders such as agoraphobia have been less consistently positive. Anxiolytics and antidepressants have produced remarkable effects in some patient groups and are considered by some to be "treatments of choice" among individuals with these complex phobias (Liebowitz and Klein, 1982). However, recent literature suggests that there may be distinguishing features among some patients with complex phobias which may make them better candidates for particular psychological interventions than for chemical ones (Goldstein, 1982). With this point in mind, Michelson and Mavissakalian (1985) found that a highly structured exposure treatment is as effective as a tricyclic antidepressant regimen among agoraphobics, and Mavissakalian (1984) persuasively argues that in vivo exposure treatments continue to be the simplest and most cost effective interventions for these patients.

ANXIETY DISORDERS.   A wide variety of psychological interventions also are effective in ameliorating other forms of anxiety (Haynes-Clement and Avery, 1984; Hekmat et al, 1984; Ricketts and Galloway, 1984). While studies usually have failed to find differences among treatment types, recent data have suggested that relaxation training may be particularly beneficial in reducing mild situational anxiety when compared to cognitively or psychoeducationally oriented treatments (Ricketts and Galloway, 1984). Differential treatment effects appear to depend on the type of anxiety experienced; for example, task or performance anxiety as opposed to social anxiety (Stravynski et al, 1982; Haynes-Clement and Avery, 1984), and the use of simultaneous, multiple interventions seems to increase the effectiveness of any individual treatment (Cappe and Alden, in press). Clearly, characteristics other than the symptomatic manifestation of anxiety itself appear to be relevant to the treatment process and, to the degree that different treatments produce different outcomes, a refinement of these distinguishing variables is still to be accomplished.

DEPRESSION.   By far the most prescriptive, clinical trials research in recent years has been directed at the treatment of nonpsychotic depressive disorders. Interpersonal therapies (Klerman et al, 1984), cognitive modification therapies (Beck et al, 1979), and behavior therapies (Lewinsohn et al, 1978) have all been demonstrated to have clinical efficacy for depressive disorders. Researchers investigating the cognitive therapies have been particularly active (Rush, 1984), and sound, methodologically oriented research has demonstrated the relative value of these approaches when contrasted both with conventional antidepressant regimens (Simons et al, 1984; Beck et al, 1979) and other psychotherapies (Teasdale et al, 1984). This finding has been sufficiently consistent to conclude that, at least among individuals who have exogenous and reactive depressions, cognitive modification therapies are effective and may be especially useful if patients are unable to tolerate the negative side effects of tricyclic or other antidepressants.

In spite of its effectiveness, the mechanism of action of cognitive therapy does not appear to be in the amount of actual cognitive change induced by the treatment (Simons et al, 1984), and this fact has led to the speculation that any psychotherapy which is structured, specifically trained, and closely monitored may do well among depressed patients. Steinbrueck and colleagues (1983) argue convincingly that the relative effectiveness of traditional psychotherapies has been underestimated as applied to depression. Indeed, meta-analysis of the results obtained by various forms of psychotherapy fail to reveal significant differences in treatment outcomes among depressed populations, although cognitive and behavioral therapies consistently produce remarkably strong effects (Smith et al, 1980). Structured psychoeducational approaches (Brown and Lewinsohn, 1984) and social skills training (Thase et al, 1984) have all made positive showings as interventions for depressive conditions. Behavioral methods which are designed to enhance clients' social skills are especially helpful and produce results that are equivalent to cognitive change therapies among depressed individuals (McKnight et al, 1984). Indeed, the clear superiority of cognitive change therapies over relationship oriented psychotherapies when therapists have received equal amounts of training and supervised practice also is yet to be demonstrated (Kornblith et al, 1983).

Recent evidence suggests that the effect of various psychotherapies depends much more upon how consistently one follows the prescribed treatment protocol than upon the specific interventions themselves (Beutler et al, 1986). Moreover, after reviewing the literature in some depth, Steinmetz and colleagues (1983) emphasize the importance of nondiagnostic patient factors in determining the relative value of various treatment interventions. Likewise, Williams (1984) concludes that, although cognitive therapy is at least as effective as antidepressant medications for the treatment of nonpsychotic depression, the relative efficacies of even closely related treatments may be a function of nondiagnostic patient characteristics, such as stylistic patterns of functioning and coping (McKnight et al, 1984).

EATING DISORDERS. Cognitive, hypnotic, behavioral, psychodynamic, interpersonal, and family interventions have all been advocated and have garnered empirical support for their clinical efficacy in the treatment of eating disorders. As in most other symptom based syndromes, however, little can be said beyond the observation that most treatments seem to work. Most studies which have compared traditional therapies with psychoeducational (Connors et al, 1984), behavioral (Straw and Terre, 1983), and bibliotherapy (Abramson, 1985) treatments fail to show differential rates of effectiveness in the treatment of various eating disorders.

Clinical researchers seem to be increasingly drawn toward the study of cognitive and behavioral interventions, which frequently involve family oriented contacts and multiple modalities of treatment. Ordman and Kirschenbaum (1985) have demonstrated the value of such a multimodal approach among a group of bulimic patients when compared with a briefer and unimodal intervention. While some evidence also supports the relative, positive effects of cognitive and behaviorally oriented treatments when compared to psychodynamic and nondirective interventions (Kirkley et al, 1985), this effect may be an artifactual reflection of differing amounts of expertise among the practitioners of these procedures.

Upon reviewing this literature, one is persuaded to conclude that most interventions are modestly effective and the more interventions one receives, the greater the likelihood of improvement. Since all treatments seem to work with some clients and at the same time to be equally ineffective with others, one is again required to explore the probable importance of patient and therapist dimensions that are not captured within "brand name" therapies or syndrome labels.

SLEEP DISORDERS. Sleep disorders represent a broad set of behavioral patterns, frequently complicated by the presence of medical conditions such as seizures, narcolepsy, or respiratory impairment (Williams and Karacan, 1978). The psychological treatment of many of these disorders has been widely touted and researched. However, difficulties continue to exist in defining the various disorders for the purposes of research, and systematic comparisons among various treatments with respect to specific disorders is still lacking.

Among sleep disorders, behaviorally and cognitively oriented treatments are generally considered to be the treatments of choice. Most research has compared one type of behavioral or cognitive treatment with another of the same variety, however (Miller and Dipilato, 1983; Woolfolk and McNulty, 1983). While such comparisons suggest that both behavioral and cognitive change treatments are effective in ameliorating functional sleep disturbances, they do not yield clear evidence that more traditional psychotherapeutic interventions would not be equally effective.

In reviewing the foregoing dilemma, Hauri and Sateia (1984) conclude that behavioral and cognitive therapies are effective, but that greater specificity of both the nature of the patient population and the nature of the treatment is required in order to develop true indicators and contraindicators for specific interventions. This point can be extended to relationship oriented treatments, and serves again to remind the reader that the dimensions on which symptomatic diagnoses are based are frequently not the dimensions which are most relevant in predicting the probable effectiveness of different psychological interventions.

SEXUAL DISTURBANCES.   Many writers tacitly assume that behavioral treatments are the interventions of choice for most sexual dysfunctions (Zilbergeld and Kilmann, 1984). This conclusion emanates largely from the seminal work of Masters and Johnson (1970) in which these treatments were initially described and related to specific patient disorders. However, a careful review of the research on which such conclusions are based reveals that the evidence for the relative value of these treatments is not as persuasive as one might hope. Research has largely failed to systematically and methodologically compare behavioral and nonbehavioral treatment outcomes (Reynolds, 1977). For example, research on the relative value of treatments for psychogenic female sexual dysfunctions consists largely of case analyses (Sotile and Kilmann, 1977). In the absence of sound, comparative research, the relative advantage of behavioral treatments can only be justified with respect to certain kinds of sexual conditions (LoPiccolo and Stock, 1986). Behavior therapy achieves its most consistent and clearest results in cases of premature ejaculation and primary orgasmic dysfunction in women (Zilbergeld and Kilmann, 1984). The advantage of sex therapy over alternative psychological interventions for the treatment of erectile problems and situational orgasmic complaints is less well established (Zilbergeld and Kilmann, 1984; Barlow, 1986; LoPiccolo and Stock, 1986). In addition to behavior therapy, there is, in the literature, some support for the effectiveness of psychoanalytically oriented interventions, brief sexual counseling, and couples therapy for these latter conditions (Reynolds, 1977).

Variations among the outcome rates of various therapies appear to be, at least in part, a function of the severity of the patient's disturbance, how compliant patients are with the prescribed regimen, how many additional areas of functioning are affected or contribute to the sexual dysfunction, the stability of corollary marital or sexual relationships, and a host of other nondiagnostic variables (Sotile and Kilmann, 1977; Barlow, 1986). While behavioral interventions appear to be at least as good as alternative therapies in treating sexual dysfunctions, it may be a mistake to consider any particular treatment as the treatment of choice until further evaluation and comparative assessment can be undertaken.

CHRONIC MEDICAL COMPLAINTS.   The application of psychological interventions to medical problems and to chronic pain suggests that tension headaches tend to respond relatively well to such behavioral interventions as biofeedback and relaxation training when compared with control (Hart, 1984) or relationship oriented (Bell et al, 1983) treatments. However, this research also suggests that biofeedback procedures exert their effects because they induce positive expectancies and facilitate patient confidence as much as because of the technical aspects of the feedback itself (Holroyd et al, 1984). Similar findings with regard to the use of behavioral interventions for coronary-prone individuals (Levenkron et al, 1983) raise the possibility that the effectiveness of these interventions reflect the fact that they can easily be presented in a way that is consistent with the patient's view of his or her condition, thus meeting preexisting expectations. The observation that the effects of various behavioral interventions depends, in part, on the patient's personality style, expectancies, severity of disturbance, and characteristic defenses (Beutler, 1983) again underlines the importance of attending to these characteristics and variables as much as to symptomatic presentations in developing prescriptive interventions.

Matching Nondiagnostic Patient Characteristics to Psychotherapy Interventions

Since the symptomatic dimensions on which diagnoses are based may not be the most relevant ones for designing psychotherapy programs, other paradigms for developing individualized treatments are increasingly being advocated (Brooker et al, 1984; Glass, 1984). Even within such a specific treatment paradigm as cognitive therapy, emphasis is being placed upon defining a framework for selecting among specific procedures. These proposals emphasize the function of patient and problem characteristics that are largely independent of the specific symptoms presented (Murphy, 1985; Rush, 1984).

One of the major problems facing the investigator who attempts to determine the way in which nondiagnostic variables contribute to the effects of specific interventions is the sheer number of such variables from which one must select. Without any clear theoretical structure by which to determine or to preassign the significance of various nondiagnostic patient variables, the task of finding the most relevant variables to match with specific therapeutic approaches becomes unwieldy.

The effort to match patient variables to various therapeutic procedures has been described as "technical eclecticism" (Norcross, 1986). Norcross and Prochaska (1982) have suggested that this approach characterizes approximately 30 percent of those who practice psychotherapy. Yet, there is no unifying theory and no agreed upon set of dimensions either to characterize relevant patient variables or therapeutic interventions. In response, some authors have developed a theoretical structure within which to consider the relevance of psychotherapeutic interventions (Prochaska, 1984; Lazarus, 1980). Others have attempted to take an empirical approach in selecting the most relevant patient dimensions and matching these to specific therapies (Beutler, 1983).

Norcross (1986) observes that those who advocate integrating psychotherapeutic theories to nondiagnositc aspects of patient problems do so in very diverse ways. A few examples of the most promising of these eclectic approaches bear special consideration.

MULTIMODAL PSYCHOTHERAPY. Lazarus (1980) has approached the task of matching therapeutic technique to patient variables by advocating a host of interventions within a general cognitive-behavioral theory. His approach has been to focus on patterns among various realms of patient functioning. These functional areas are identified by the acronym, BASIC ID. This acronym represents Behavior, Affect, Sensory, Imagery, Cognitive, Interpersonal, and Biological (identified in the acronym as *D*, for drugs) experiences. The therapist's task is to identify the areas of concern, prioritize their importance to the patient's functioning, and to direct a focused intervention at each of the relevant areas in order to achieve maximal change. While the interventions emphasize behavioral procedures, they are not restricted to these treatments. Lazarus advocates a variety of experiential, analytical, and interpersonal procedures in order to facilitate resolution of the conflict identified within each functional area.

Multimodal therapy has become the most visible of the technical eclectic interventions, and perhaps one of the most promising. A number of studies have suggested that clearly focused interventions based upon these principles increase treatment effectiveness and facilitate improvement, especially in classroom settings (Smith and Southern, 1980; Gerler, 1981). The relative effects of this intervention in traditional, adult psychotherapy relationships has been less clearly demonstrated. It is apparent, nonetheless, that interventions which address themselves to a variety of behaviors facilitate treatment gain over unimodal interventions for such things as social phobias (Butler et al, 1984), eating disorders (Ordman and Kirschenbaum, 1985), alcoholism (Oei and Jackson, 1984), and anxiety disorders (Hoshmand et al, 1985).

TRANSTHEORETICAL PSYCHOTHERAPY.   Prochaska (1984) has approached the problem of defining relevant patient characteristics through a series of rather intensive investigations of problem-solving skills. Through these studies, Prochaska and his colleagues have identified four stages which characterize the process of change across populations and problems. These stages include, in sequence: 1) precontemplation or preparation, 2) contemplation and active assessment, 3) action on the problem, and 4) maintenance/reinforcement of change.

Concomitantly, Prochaska has identified 10 change processes which function at five different levels. The levels of change include: 1) symptom or situational, 2) cognitive, 3) intrapersonal, 4) among or within systems, and 5) within interpersonal relationships. The processes of change are thought to distinguish among various therapeutic approaches, and range from consciousness raising, self-inspection, evaluation, counterconditioning, contingency management, to reliance upon helping relationships. Through naturalistic studies of the problem-solving process, Prochaska proposes that certain kinds of processes are suited to each stage and level of change. By matching the stages and level of change to the most relevant processes, it is anticipated that therapeutic effectiveness will be enhanced.

Unfortunately, this particular approach to prescriptive psychotherapy has not been systematically evaluated within the psychotherapeutic relationship itself. While the stages of change are well defined, both within normative populations and populations of pathologically distressed individuals, the processes of change are relatively broad and may not be specific enough to form a basis for the prescription of the specific procedures which characterize psychotherapy relationships. However, given the success that Prochaska and his colleagues (namely, Norcross, 1986) have had in identifying the dimensions of change within various populations, one must consider the approach to be a promising one which deserves further exploration.

SYSTEMATIC ECLECTIC PSYCHOTHERAPY.   In contrast to the rational and theoretical approaches to defining patient variables advocated by Lazarus (1980) and Prochaska (1984), Beutler (1983) has attempted to define relevant patient variables on an empirical basis. By assessing the body of literature in which one type of psychotherapy has been compared to another, and by systematically exploring the types of patient populations on which the comparisons were made, Beutler proposes that three major dimensions can be used to predetermine the probable response of patients to different therapy procedures. The first of these dimensions is that of symptom complexity, a dimension which is thought to differentiate the effectiveness of symptom- and conflict-focused interventions. The second dimension is the patient's level of interpersonal reactance against external control, a dimension which is thought to predict the degree to which interpretive and directive therapeutic procedures will be fruitful. The third dimension emphasizes the role of patient defensive style and sets the relevant focus of treatment on behavioral, cognitive, or affective realms of experiences. Using a task analysis procedure, Beutler (1983) has catalogued a large number of specific procedures from various therapies in terms of these dimensions, and has formulated hypotheses about the potential impact of these procedures on patients representing various combinations of the dimensions. Beutler has proposed that increased efficacy of intervention can be achieved by matching patients both to relevant beliefs held by a specific therapist about issues which characterize patient conflict, and to the technical interventions themselves.

Given the complexity of this proposal, it is likely that the verification process will take place in small steps and over a long period of time. To this point, however, there is a body of evidence to support the importance of matching therapist directiveness to patient interpersonal reactance (Beutler et al, 1986). Indeed, matching directiveness of therapy and patient reactance to external control may be a sufficiently potent variable to be predictive both of positive change and of deterioration effects (Forsyth and Forsyth, 1982).

Beutler and colleagues (Beutler and Mitchell, 1981; Calvert et al, in press) have also found that patient defensive style differentiates both between the value of specific interventions, and global, theoretical applications. When compatible matches of patient and therapist are defined prior to treatment, treatment outcome is significantly enhanced in those relationships where the patient utilizes internalizing defensive styles and the therapy is insight-focused. Less precise outcome predictions have been obtained for matches in which patients who utilize externalized defenses are treated with behavioral procedures (Beutler et al, 1986). While the model proposed by Beutler appears to be promising, there is considerable need for greater definition of the predictive variables and more research into the mode and process of their effect.

DIFFERENTIAL THERAPEUTICS. Frances and colleagues (1984) have approached differential treatment assignment from a clinical perspective. This approach is quite different from those considered in the foregoing paragraphs, primarily because of the inclusion of nonpsychotherapeutic interventions under the prescriptive umbrella. This model effectively addresses the differential application of diverse therapeutic procedures to the patient, based upon such variables as setting, anticipated duration, and format of treatment. The approach defines a decision tree by which to determine the restrictiveness and nature of the medical treatment to be applied, even before psychotherapy may be offered. Decisional criteria for assessing the suitability of the patient for psychotherapy are applied in the same way as decisions about hospitalization, the use of psychoactive medications, and the assignment of other primary or adjunctive treatments. Indeed, nonpsychotherapy interventions are assigned with greater specificity than is psychotherapy. In the latter arena, the authors differentiate among three general classes of therapy and provide limited information to support their differential assignment.

Relatively modest research efforts have been applied to this broad ranging prescriptive model. Like systematic eclectic psychotherapy, the model itself is relatively complex and difficult to research within a single program. In order to verify its accuracy, a long-term, complex, and sequential research effort will be required. Nonetheless, this approach has a significant advantage over other eclectic models in its breadth of application and its reliance upon clinical wisdom. By combining it with theoretical systems which are more specific in dictating particular psychological interventions, a very detailed treatment program could be defined which might have application far beyond psychotherapy.

SUMMARY AND CONCLUSIONS

While most clinicians adopt an "eclectic" philosophy in their desire to apply specific procedures to specific patients, the meaning of this term is unclear. To many, "eclecticism" reflects only a reliance upon the common, nontechnical ingredients of psychotherapy and a belief in the substantial equivalence of all forms of psychological intervention (Garfield, 1980). To others, a belief in prescriptive or eclectic psychotherapies assumes the specificity of certain technical procedures for facilitating certain outcomes and processes.

In the midst of the concern for specificity in defining patient, therapy, therapist, and outcome variables, certain political realities and social expectations have both facilitated and inhibited the search for prescriptive interventions. Research suggests that effective patient and therapist matching is perhaps the most promising of the efforts to make treatment more controllable, specific, and efficacious. Unfortunately, therapists are resistant to considering the role of their own cognitive, value, and belief systems as this approach requires. Also, the task of cataloging each therapist's beliefs and matching these to those of each prospective patient is sufficiently onerous as to make the approach less compelling than one based on global patient and treatment variables. Nevertheless, therapists are well advised to capitalize on the client benefits deriving from similarity of world views and expectations, and dissimilarities on views of interpersonal needs (for example, dependency patterns).

Matching therapeutic procedures to patients representing various diagnostic entities has received the greatest amount of attention but is probably the least likely to provide effective prescriptive formulations. The dimensions on which primary (Axis I) diagnoses are based do not appear to be the dimensions which determine efficacy of specific types of psychotherapy. There are a few exceptions to this rule, however, with phobic disorders clearly being responsive to exposure treatments, and symptom oriented disorders (such as sexual dysfunction) being quite responsive to behaviorally oriented therapies. The more multisymptomatic the condition, the less diagnostic labels seem to differentiate among efficacy rates of various psychological interventions, and the safer one is in relying upon familiar and preferred procedures.

An emerging effort to derive prescriptive interventions is based upon the identification of a compatible match between specific interventions and nondiagnostic patient variables. Characteristics related to personality, coping style, and social and cognitive functioning seem to hold promise for determining, predicting, and controlling the value of relatively specific psychotherapy interventions. This line of investigation is very new, however. While many of the approaches appear sound and the research seems to be promising, much yet needs to be done to clarify the nature of the patient population, the relevant patient dimensions, the psychotherapeutic interventions of choice, and the outcomes which are associated with each of the prescriptive formulations.

A number of very promising approaches are emerging for prescribing the application of psychotherapies, and it is probably unwise to conclude that all therapies are equally effective with all conditions under all circumstances. New methods of assessing therapies, determining outcomes, analyzing data, and applying therapeutic procedures themselves are increasingly suggesting that: 1) the benefits of psychotherapy are much greater than previously thought (Steinbrueck et al, 1983; Smith et al, 1980); 2) some technical interventions are better than others; and 3) the efficacy of these interventions may be enhanced by attending to compatible patient variables, such as severity of disruption and resistence to external control (Beutler et al, 1986).

One can distill from the foregoing pages that there are certain problems that continue to plague the effort to define prescriptive psychotherapeutic interventions. Among these are the tendency for theorists to adhere to myths of therapy and patient and therapist uniformity. Equally unfortunate is a contrasting tendency to develop an ever-increasing proliferation of theoretical formulations, which claim to be accompanied by uniquely different and new interventions. These new theories are propounded, practiced, and advocated without external support or verification.

Collectively, the problem facing the field, both clinically and empirically, is to make practitioners as well as scientists aware that efforts to develop indicators and contraindicators for various treatments are only as good as the assumptions that: 1) different thoretical philosophies are accompanied by different therapy procedures, and 2) the interventions advocated produce some unique influence on the nature of therapeutic change. While current literature can only tentatively accept the validity of the foregoing assumptions, it is possible to establish some general recommendations for the implementation of prescriptive psychotherapeutic interventions, based upon current understandings of research findings. These recommendations apply to the following areas:

1. the assessment of indicators and contraindicators for psychotherapy
2. the evaluation of nondiagnostic and therapy relevant patient characteristics
3. the development of a psychotherapy plan
4. the preparation of patients for assuming psychotherapeutic roles
5. the planned implementation of maximally successful psychotherapy procedures

1. Indicators for Psychotherapy. Both research and clinical impression suggests that there are a variety of patient characteristics which either assume the status of prerequisites or serve as positive indicators for successful psychotherapy. Frances and colleagues (1984) have described many of these indicators succinctly, and the interested reader is referred to this source for greater explication of their significance. The indicators include, in order of importance:

a. ability to function in the absence of externally imposed, protective controls or environmental structure (such as hospitalization, constraint, and so on)
b. sufficient discomfort to motivate attendance and participation in the therapeutic process
c. a history of at least some good interpersonal relationships and accompanying social skills
d. willingness to evaluate personal behavior and to perceive this behavior as self-driven or modifiable (for example, psychological mindedness)

2. *Nondiagnostic Patient Characteristics.* While it is conventional and appropriate to establish a formal *DSM-III* diagnosis, at least Axis I diagnoses seem to be more relevant for the application of medical interventions than psychological ones. A diagnosis of active psychosis, for example, may indicate the need for confinement and the applications of phenothiazines, while a diagnosis of bipolar affective disorder may indicate the requirement for lithium therapy. Beyond these requirements of diagnosis, however, current literature suggests that there are a variety of nondiagnostic indicators which are more relevant than diagnostic ones to the development of a specific psychotherapy plan. While these are represented in different ways, the interested reader is referred to the writings of Lazarus (1980) and Beutler (1983) for further details on the development of such a plan. Among the considerations of greatest relevance are the following:

a. a determination of how seriously disturbed and broad ranging the patient's symptoms are in producing a disruption of life activities (for example, school, family, work)
b. a determination of how the patient is likely to respond to external controls and directives (for example, how defensive and resistant to authority the patient may be)
c. an assessment of the patient's expectations regarding the roles of patient and therapist, the length of the treatment, and the mode of psychotherapy to be applied (such as group, individual, family, marital)
d. a determination of the patient's treatment objectives for symptomatic relief, personality change, or interpersonal conflict resolution

3. *Develop a Treatment Plan.* From the foregoing information, the therapist should work to prioritize treatment objectives, develop a working formulation that includes the dynamic themes or interpersonal patterns that have theoretical meaning for the therapist, and define markers by which effective change can be indicated (Malan, 1976; Strupp and Binder, 1984). Research is beginning to emphasize that treatment outcomes, in part, reflect how consistently therapists develop a treatment plan and how closely this plan is followed (Beutler et al, 1986). Relevant treatment plans should include the following considerations:

a. the selection of an appropriate format or mode (individual, family, group therapy, and so forth) *b.* a delineation of how the initial therapeutic procedures can be made to be compatible with patient expectations for treatment duration and format

c. a predetermined method for establishing a collaborative relationship by emphasizing relative value and belief compatibilities and by empathizing with patient dilemmas and conflicts

d. a plan by which the therapeutic focus (interpersonal conflict, dynamic theme, or symptomatic complaint) can be maintained, and change can be evaluated, anticipating the probable pitfalls and conflicts

e. a determination as to whether cotherapeutic or adjunctive therapeutic procedures also will be required, based upon the therapeutic procedures required and those within the therapist's own armamentarium (for example, the implementation of exposure therapy for phobic disorders, the use of sexual or marital therapy for sexual dysfunctions, the implementation of cognitive change procedures for major anxiety and depressive disorders)

In delineating the therapeutic plan, the therapist is advised to keep in mind 1) the power of the collaborative and empathic relationship; 2) the power of specific therapeutic procedures for well defined and circumscribed symptoms (such as phobic disorders, sexual dysfunction, and so forth); 3) the value of being consistent with one's own preferences; 4) the presence of specific indicators for the use of directive and nondirective procedures (for example, patients whose history suggests resistance to external authority do poorly with directive procedures); and 5) the relative advantages of a symptom-focused or conflict-focused orientation, depending upon the degree of disruption in patient life functions and activities created by the problem (Beutler, 1983).

4. Preparing the Patient for Treatment. Considerable research has suggested that advanced preparation (that is, role induction) of the patient enhances both treatment duration and treatment effectiveness (Beutler et al, 1986). Role induction has been implemented in a variety of ways, including the use of video tapes to illustrate therapy roles, written instruction about the therapeutic process and procedures, and direct instruction by the therapist. In preparing the patient for treatment, the following points should be addressed:

a. a definition of the treatment objectives, based upon the treatment plan and the pretherapy assessment of the nature of the patient's symptoms, the conflictual or interpersonal theme, the nature of the patient's environment and support system, and so forth

b. a definition of the markers by which the patient can assess the changes experienced in the course of treatment (for example, changes in feelings, changes in environments, changes in symptoms, changes in the nature of the patient-therapist relationship)

c. a definition of the probable length and mode of treatment (in long-term treatments it is advisable to present a time marker at the end of which to reassess the usefulness of treatment)

d. presentation of the therapist's philosophy of change and of the philosophy which will guide the therapeutic process

e. a definition of the roles expected of both therapist and patient (for example, the requirement for patients to engage in homework assignments, the nature of free association, the anticipation of role playing exercises, and so on)

Within the context of defining each of the foregoing parameters, assessment of the patient's acceptance of the treatment rationale is relevant in order to ensure that the patient's expectancies are consistent with those of the therapist.

5. *Implementation of the Treatment Plan.* Consistency in the implementation of the treatment plan is increasingly observed to be a prerequisite for effective psychotherapy. This entails the maintenance of a strict focus upon the predetermined conflict, symptom, or interpersonal pattern. While this focus, as well as the treatment plan itself, can and should be re-evaluated constantly and periodically throughout the course of treatment, these changes should be presented to the patient in order to ensure continuing collaboration, patient involvement, and consistency of treatment. The specifics of implementing the treatment plan should probably include the following considerations:

a. persistent attention to maintaining both the treatment alliance and the patient's sense of collaborative involvement in treatment decisions
b. retention of the treatment focus, as befits the therapist's preferred orientation and the patient's needs
c. thoughtful and consistent adoption either of an actively directive or relatively nondirective stance, based upon the patient's historical relationship with authorities (that is, patients with strong resistance to external authorities tend to respond poorly to authoritative therapists, while those with strong dependency needs and a history of reliance upon external authorities respond quite well to directive and active interventions)
d. continuing process diagnosis to assess change in the patient's patterns and to alter the treatment format, objectives, or methods is required (for example, making specific decisions about changing the use of active directive interventions, the change of focus from conflict to symptom or vice versa, and the role of adjunctive or specific technical procedures)
e. ongoing and consistent feedback to and from patients regarding changes indexing improvement or deterioration.

While the foregoing recommendations provide reasonable guidelines for the practice of prescriptive psychotherapies, there is much research yet to do in making interventions more specific than they currently are, and in defining ways in which the treatment relationship can be enhanced and facilitated among those individuals who are not usually considered to be the most ideal or appropriate candidates for psychotherapy. As this research expands and becomes refined, the practitioner can anticipate a broadening of the powers of psychotherapy and increasing opportunities to expand the range of human functioning.

REFERENCES

Abramson EE: Dismantling the behavioral treatment of obesity. International Journal of Eating Disorders 4:107-111, 1985

Barlow DH: On the relation of clinical research to clinical practice: current issues, new directions. J Consult Clin Psychol 49:147-155, 1981

Barlow DH: Causes of sexual dysfunction: The role of anxiety and cognitive interference. J Consult Clin Psychol 54:140-148, 1986

Beck AT, Rush AJ, Shaw BF, et al: Cognitive Therapy of Depression. New York, Guilford, 1979

Bell NW, Abramowitz SI, Folkins CH, et al: Biofeedback, brief psychotherapy and tension headache. Headache 23:162-173, 1983

Berzins JI: Therapist-patient matching, in Effective Psychotherapy: A Handbook of Research. Edited by Gurman AS, Razin AM. New York, Pergamon Press, 1977

Beutler LE: Toward specific psychological therapies for specific conditions. J Consult Clin Psychol 47:882-897, 1979

Beutler LE: Convergence in counseling and psychotherapy: a current look. Clinical Psychology Review 1:79-101, 1981

Beutler LE: Eclectic Psychotherapy: A Systematic Approach. New York, Pergamon Press, 1983

Beutler LE, Hamblin DL: Individualized outcome measures of internal change: methodological considerations. J Consult Clin Psychol, special edition 54:48-53, 1986

Beutler LE, Mitchell R: Differential psychotherapy outcome among depressed and impulsive patients as a function of analytic and experiential treatment procedures. Psychiatry 44:297-306, 1981

Beutler LE, Crago M, Arizmendi TG: Therapist variables in psychotherapy process and outcome, in Handbook of Psychotherapy and Behavior Change, 3rd Edition. Edited by Garfield SL, Bergin AE. New York, Wiley, 1986

Brooker AE, Becnel HP Jr., Mareth TR: Psychotherapy: developing a treatment paradigm. Psychol Rep 54:251-261, 1984

Brown RA, Lewinsohn PM: A psychoeducational approach to the treatment of depression: comparison of group, individual, and minimal contact procedures. J Consult Clin Psychol 52:774-783, 1984

Butler G, Cullington A, Munby M, et al: Exposure and anxiety management in the treatment of social phobia. J Consult Clin Psychol 52:642-650, 1984

Calvert SJ, Beutler LE, Crago M: Psychotherapy outcome as a function of therapist-patient matching on selected variables. Journal of Social and Clinical Psychology (in press)

Cappe RF, Alden LE: A comparison of treatment strategies for clients functionally impaired by extreme shyness and social avoidance. J Consult Clin Psychol (in press)

Connors ME, Johnson CL, Stuckey MK: Treatment of bulimia with brief psychoeducational group therapy. Am J Psychiatry 141:1512-1516, 1984

Corsini RJ: Handbook of Innovative Psychotherapies. New York, Wiley, 1981

Elkin I, Parloff MB, Hadley SW, et al: NIMH treatment of depression collaborative research program. Arch Gen Psychiatry 42:305-316, 1985

Emmelkamp PMG, Mersch PP, Vissia E, et al: Social phobia: a comparative evaluation of cognitive and behavioral interventions. Behav Res Ther 23:365-369, 1985

Eysenck HJ: The effects of psychotherapy: an evaluation. Journal of Consulting Psychology 16:319-324, 1952

Fiedler FE: The concept of an ideal therapeutic relationship. Journal of Consulting Psychology 14:239-245, 1950

Forsyth NL, Forsyth DR: Internality, controllability, and the effectiveness of attributional interpretations in counseling. Journal of Counseling Psychology 29:140-150, 1982

Frances A, Clarkin J, Perry S (Eds): Differential Therapeutics in Psychiatry. New York, Brunner/Mazel, 1984

Freeman A (Ed): Cognitive Therapy with Couples and Groups. New York, Plenum, 1983

Garfield SL: Psychotherapy: An Eclectic Approach. New York, Wiley, 1980

Gerler ER: The multimodal counseling model: 1973 to the present. Elementary School Guidance and Counseling 15:285-294, 1981

Glass RM: Psychotherapy: scientific art or artistic science? Arch Gen Psychiatry 41:525-526, 1984

Goldstein AJ: Agoraphobia: treatment successes, treatment failures, and theoretical implications, in Agoraphobia. Edited by Chambless DL, Goldstein AJ. New York, Wiley, 1982

Hart JD: Predicting differential response to EMG biofeedback and relaxation training: the role of cognitive structure. J Clin Psychol 40:453-457, 1984

Hauri PJ, Sateia MJ: Nonpharmacological treatment of sleep disorders, in Psychiatry Update: The American Psychiatric Press Annual Review, vol. 3. Edited by Grinspoon L. Washington, DC, American Psychiatric Press, Inc., 1984

Haynes-Clement LA, Avery AW: A cognitive-behavioral approach to social skills training with shy persons. J Clin Psychol 40:710-713, 1984

Hekmat H, Lubitz R, Deal R: Semantic desensitization: a paradigmatic intervention approach to anxiety disorders. J Clin Psychol 40:463-466, 1984

Holroyd KA, Penzien DB, Hursey KG, et al: Change mechanisms in EMG biofeedback training: cognitive changes underlying improvement in tension headache. J Consult Clin Psychol 52:1039-1053, 1984

Hoshmand LT, Helmes E, Kazarian S, et al: Evaluation of two relaxation training programs under medication and no-medication conditions. J Clin Psychol 41:22-29, 1985

Kirkley BG, Schneider JA, Agras WS, et al: Comparison of two group treatments for bulimia. J Consult Clin Psychol 53:43-48, 1985

Klerman G, Weissman M, Rounsaville BJ, et al: Interpersonal Psychotherapy of Depression. New York, Basic Books, 1984

Kornblith SJ, Rehm LP, O'Hara MW, et al: The contribution of self-reinforcement training and behavioral assignments to the efficacy of self-control therapy for depression. Cog Ther Res 7:499-528, 1983

Ladouceur R: Participant modeling with or without cognitive treatment for phobias. J Consult Clin Psychol 51:942-944, 1983

Lambert MJ, DeJulio SS: The relative importance of client, therapist, and technique variables as predictors of psychotherapy outcome: the place of therapist "nonspecific" factors. Presented at the meeting of the American Psychological Association, Scottsdale, AZ, March, 1978

Lazarus AA: The Practice of Multimodal Therapy. New York, McGraw-Hill, 1980

Levenkron JC, Cohen JD, Mueller HS, et al: Modifying the Type A coronary-prone behavior pattern. J Consult Clin Psychol 51:192-204, 1983

Lewinsohn PM, Munoz R, Youngren M, et al: Control Your Depression. Englewood Cliffs, NJ, Prentice-Hall, 1978

Liebowitz MR, Klein DF: Agoraphobia: Clinical features, pathophysiology, and treatment, in Agoraphobia. Edited by Chambless DL, Goldstein AJ. New York, Wiley, 1982

LoPiccolo J, Stock WE: Treatment of sexual dysfunction. J Consult Clin Psychol 54:158-167, 1986

Luborsky L, Singer B, Luborsky L: Comparative studies of psychotherapies: is it true that "everyone has won and all must have prizes?" Arch Gen Psychiatry 32:995-1008, 1975

Luborsky L, Mintz J, Auerbach A, et al: Predicting the outcome of psychotherapy: findings of the Penn Psychotherapy Project. Arch Gen Psychiatry 37:471-481, 1980

Luborsky L, Woody GE, McLellan AT, et al: Can independent judges recognize different psychotherapies? an experience with manual-guided therapies. J Consult Clin Psychol 50:49-62, 1982

Malan DH: Toward the Validation of Dynamic Psychotherapy. New York, Plenum Press, 1976

Masters WH, Johnson VE: Human Sexual Inadequacy. Boston, Little, Brown, 1970

Mavissakalian M: Exposure treatment of agoraphobia, in Psychiatry Update: The American Psychiatric Association Annual Review, vol. 3. Edited by Grinspoon L. Washington, DC, American Psychiatric Press, Inc., 1984

McKnight DL, Nelson RO, Hayes SC, et al: Importance of treating individually assessed response classes in the amelioration of depression. Behav Ther 15:315-335, 1984

Michelson L, Mavissakalian M: Psychophysiological outcome of behavioral and pharmacological treatments of agoraphobia. J Consult Clin Psychol 53:229-236, 1985

Miller WR, DiPilato M: Treatment of nightmares via relaxation and desensitization: a controlled evaluation. J Consult Clin Psychol 51:870-877, 1983

Minor SW, Leone C: A comparison of in-vivo and imaginal participant modeling. J Clin Psychol 40:717-720, 1984

Mintz J, Kiesler DJ: Individualized measures of psychotherapy outcome, in Handbook of Research Methods in Clinical Psychology. Edited by Kendall PC, Butcher JN. New York, Wiley, 1982

Murphy GE: A conceptual framework for the choice of interventions in cognitive therapy. Cognitive Therapy and Research 9:127-134, 1985

Norcross JC: Eclectic psychotherapy: An introduction and overview, in Handbook of Eclectic Psychotherapy. Edited by Norcross JC. New York, Brunner/Mazel, 1986

Norcross JC, Prochaska JO: A national survey of clinical psychologists: characteristics and activities. The Clinical Psychologist 35:1-8, 1982

Oei TPS, Jackson PR: Some effective therapeutic factors in group cognitive-behavioral therapy with problem drinkers. J Stud Alcohol 45:119-123, 1984

Ordman AM, Kirschenbaum DS: Cognitive-behavioral therapy for bulimia: an initial outcome study. J Consult Clin Psychol 53:305-313, 1985

Prochaska JO: Systems of Psychotherapy: A Transtheoretical Analysis, second edition. Homewood, IL, Dorsey Press, 1984

Reynolds BS: Psychological treatment models and outcome results for erectile dysfunction: a critical review. Psychol Bull 84:1218-1238, 1977

Ricketts MS, Galloway RE: Effects of three different one-hour single-session treatments for test anxiety. Psychol Rep 54:115-120, 1984

Rush AJ: Cognitive therapy, in Psychiatry Update: The American Psychiatric Association Annual Review, Vol. 3. Edited by Grinspoon L. Washington, DC, American Psychiatric Press, Inc., 1984

Simons AD, Garfield SL, Murphy GE: The process of change in cognitive therapy and pharmacotherapy for depression. Arch Gen Psychiatry 41:45-51, 1984

Smith ML, Glass GV, Miller TI: The Benefits of Psychotherapy. Baltimore, MD, Johns Hopkins University Press, 1980

Smith RL, Southern S: Multimodal career counseling: an application of the "BASIC ID." Vocational Guidance Quarterly 29:56-64, 1980

Sotile WM, Kilmann PR: Treatments of psychogenic female sexual dysfunctions. Psychol Bull 84:619-633, 1977

Steinbrueck SM, Maxwell SE, Howard GS: A meta-analysis of psychotherapy and drug therapy in the treatment of unipolar depression with adults. J Consult Clin Psychol 51:856-863, 1983

Steinmetz JL, Lewinsohn PM, Antonuccio DO: Prediction of individual outcome in a group intervention for depression. J Consult Clin Psychol 51:331-337, 1983

Stravynski A, Marks I, Yule W: Social skills problems in neurotic outpatients. Arch Gen Psychiatry 39:1378-1385, 1982

Straw MK, Terre L: An evaluation of individualized behavioral obesity treatment and maintenance strategies. Behavior Therapy 74:255-266, 1983

Strupp HH: Toward the refinement of time-limited dynamic psychotherapy, in Forms of Brief Therapy. Edited by Budman SH. New York, Guilford Press, 1981

Strupp HH, Binder JL: Psychotherapy in a New Key: A Guide to Time-Limited Dynamic Psychotherapy. New York, Basic Books, 1984

Teasdale JD, Fennell MJV, Hibbert GA, et al: Cognitive therapy for major depressive disorder in primary care. Br J Psychiatry 144:400-406, 1984

Thase ME, Hersen M, Bellack AS, et al: Social skills training and endogenous depression. J Behav Ther Exp Psychiatry 5:101-108, 1984

Waskow IE, Parloff MB (Eds): Psychotherapy Change Measures (publication no. 74–120). Rockville, MD, National Institute of Mental Health, 1975

Whitehorn JC, Betz BJ: Further studies of the doctor as a crucial variable in the outcome of treatment with schizophrenic patients. Am J Psychiatry 117:215-223, 1960

Williams JMG: Cognitive-behavior therapy for depression: problems and perspectives. Br J Psychiatry 145:254-262, 1984

Williams RL, Karacan I: Sleep Disorders: Diagnosis and Treatment. New York, Wiley, 1978

Williams SL, Dooseman G, Kleifield E: Comparative effectiveness of guided mastery and exposure treatments for intractable phobias. J Consult Clin Psychol 52:505-518, 1984

Woolfolk RL, McNulty TF: Relaxation treatment for insomnia: a component analysis. J Consult Clin Psychol 51:495-503, 1983

Zilbergeld B, Kilmann PR: The scope and effectiveness of sex therapy. Psychotherapy 21:319-326, 1984

Chapter 16

The Choice of Duration and Frequency for Outpatient Psychotherapy

by Samuel W. Perry, M.D.

By dividing this section on differential therapeutics into separate chapters representing the components of psychotherapy (setting, format, technique, time, and psychotropic medication), the editors have structurally indicated that each of these components has a potential therapeutic valence of its own and that no single component sufficiently describes a psychiatric treatment. Terms such as "psychiatric hospitalization" or "group therapy" or "behavioral modification" or "maintenance neuroleptics," while suggestive, are not adequate descriptions of what the therapeutic process involves. For the clinician confronted with the challenge of selecting the best treatment for a particular patient and for the investigator interested in studying the efficacy of a particular form of psychotherapy, a multiaxial categorization is necessary.

This perspective is especially applicable to the component discussed in this chapter: time. A growing and exciting literature indicates that how long a treatment lasts may powerfully affect the therapeutic process; however, in reviewing this literature, we must be cognizant that duration itself does not sufficiently describe a given treatment. When we read about the impressive results, for example, of the new brief therapies, of marathon sessions, of abbreviated hospitalization, or of single interviews, we should always ask what were the other features of the treatment (What format? What technique? What setting? What medication?) that influenced the outcome besides the prescribed time.

Traditionally, time has not been viewed as a separate component of psychotherapy with its own therapeutic impact. Instead, the duration of treatment has generally been considered as being dependent upon countless other co-variables (see Table 1). In short, psychotherapy of whatever persuasion simply continued until it was over—with expected negotiations and renegotiations along the way regarding whether termination was in sight. However, during the past decade the issue of time in psychotherapy has been challenged by forces from both within and outside the mental health professions. The extramural impetus has been the increasing concern of third-party payers about the cost-effectiveness of psychotherapy, and the wishes of our consumers who, while not necessarily seeking a magical "quick cure," are understandably eager for a treatment that can get the job done sooner.

But the challenge from within the profession is in many ways more interesting, for here the impetus for change stems not from imposed demands but from accumulating data and from innovative approaches that have encouraged us to re-examine our traditional handling of time. This chapter will first present a brief review of that data; that is, the available research regarding the relationship

Table 1. Relationship of Co-variables to Duration of Psychiatric Treatment*

Co-variable	Factors Increasing Duration	Factors Decreasing Duration
Diagnosis	Chronic (e.g., schizophrenia; bipolar affective; Axis II)	Acute (e.g., adjustment disorder; brief reactive psychosis)
Precipitating stress	Less likely	More likely
Treatment goals	Ambitious (e.g., character reconstruction)	Limited (e.g., relief of focused conflict or acute symptoms)
Premorbid functioning	Poor	Good
Patient's desire	Enduring relationship	Brief contact
Patient's expectations	Change takes a long time	Change should occur quickly
Patient's time/money	Extensive	Limited
Therapist's stance	Reflective, neutral	Active, authoritative
Therapist's training/orientation	Psychodynamic	Biomedical
Therapist's availability	Open	Limited
Geographical accessibility	Easy	Difficult
Life cycle	25–50 years old	Child, adolescent, elderly
Technique	Exploratory	Behavioral/directive
Setting	Maintenance (e.g., chronic state hospital)	Reparative (e.g., crisis intervention program)
Format	Heterogeneous group	Family/marital therapy

*Modified from Frances A, Clarkin J, Perry S: Differential Therapeutics in Psychiatry: The Art and Science of Treatment Selection. New York, Brunner/Mazel, 1984 of time to outcome in outpatient psychotherapy; it will then discuss the rationale for treatments of various intensities and lengths. (The relationship of time to inpatient care is discussed in Chapter 13.)

RESEARCH ON DURATION AND FREQUENCY

Most comparative studies have failed to demonstrate a significant advantage of longer treatment. Three large and respected reviews (Butcher and Koss, 1978; Luborsky et al, 1975; Smith et al, 1980), despite using very different methods, have independently arrived at this conclusion. However, by looking more closely at the individual outcome studies used in these reviews (Frances et al, 1984), one sees how the design of the compiled studies tends to favor the initial impact of brief treatment: first, the severity of impairment is often uncontrolled; second, brief treatments are favored by regression to the mean (patients are seen at their worst and bound to improve); third, the studies measure symptom relief rather than character change; and fourth, some studies use instruments that measure changes that are statistically significant but not clinically meaningful.

Furthermore, as stated at the beginning of this chapter, duration cannot easily be separated from other variables. Brief therapies, whatever their orientation, tend to be more active, directive, and focused; therefore, the comparison of brief and longer treatments may be more a comparison of different techniques than of different time schedules. This fact may explain the findings of Smith and colleagues (1980); because their meta-analysis consisted predominantly of behavioral studies, it is not surprising they found that the peak therapeutic effect occurred somewhere between the first and seventh sessions and that there was no simple relationship between the duration and effect of therapy. In contrast, Orlinsky and Howard (1978) reviewed studies of treatments that, overall, were more varied in techniques; these investigators concluded that the total number of sessions is generally correlated with more positive results and, to a somewhat lesser extent, the total duration of treatment also significantly correlates with greater therapeutic benefits. More recently, Howard and his colleagues (1986) did a meta-analysis of 15 diverse sets of data from studies involving over 2,400 patients covering a period of over 30 years of research. Their analysis indicated that 15 percent of patients improve before attending the first session; by 8 sessions of psychodynamic or interpersonal therapies approximately 50 percent of patients are measurably improved; and approximately 75 percent are improved by 26 sessions. One implication of this study is that if patients have not improved by the 26th session (for example, once weekly for six months), a clinical review may be indicated. Another implication is that 26 weeks might be used as a rational time limit for time-limited psychotherapy.

Orlinsky and Howard (1978) reviewed 16 studies that measured how treatment outcome was affected by frequency of sessions; they concluded that, in general, no harm came from more intensive therapies and that some studies showed advantages if the patients were seen more than once a week. This conclusion is consistent with earlier studies that showed that neurotic patients did significantly better if seen twice a week as opposed to once a week (Graham, 1958) and that weekly individual or group therapy was superior to seeing patients for half an hour once every two weeks (Imber et al, 1957). However, here again, this positive relationship between frequency and outcome is not generalizable to all treatments for all patients; for example, Graham (1958) documented that adult psychotic outpatients did less well if seen twice rather than once a week, supporting the clinical impression that severely disturbed patients may have difficulty with a therapeutic relationship that is too intense. Though not showing this negative effect, a study of VA clinic patients by Lorr and colleagues (1962) did find that improvement was not related to frequency of sessions, a conclusion that has been reached by at least six other studies performed with diverse patients in very different settings (Heilbrunn, 1966; Heinicke, 1969; Kaufman et al., 1962; Rosenbaum et al., 1956; Van Slambrouck, 1973; Zirkle, 1961). The noteworthy study at Menninger Clinic comparing psychoanalytically oriented psychotherapy with psychoanalysis also found no relationship between outcome and frequency of sessions (Kernberg et al, 1972).

Newman and Howard (1986), having struggled for years over the relationship between time and therapeutic outcome, recently proposed that rather than examining the effectiveness of different frequencies or durations, we should measure "therapeutic effort," one component being "dosage" (that is, the amount of treatment administered in a clinical episode). They point out that despite the recent acclaim for time-limited psychotherapy (usually 15 to 20 sessions), the more traditional time-*un*limited therapy usually requires a lower "dosage." For example, Taube and colleagues (1984) found that the median dosage of outpatient psychotherapy is approximately five or six sessions.

Given the confusing and at times contradictory results of the many studies that have compared outcome with duration and frequency, the clinician is tempted to dismiss this research and, confronted with the individual patient, intuitively struggle with the confounding variables as best one can while waiting for more definitive studies that will clearly indicate who shall be given what treatment and for how long. The danger of ignoring this area of research (aside from the fact that third-party payers are heavily invested in the results) is that the clinician will become so focused on other features of the patient and the treatment— diagnosis, symptoms, resistance, goals, dose and type of medication, whatever—that the duration and frequency will not be given necessary attention. The therapy then simply proceeds at its own familiar pace "until it is over"; the opportunity is lost to potentiate the therapeutic process by re-examining and possibly changing the treatment's intensity or expected length.

In this spirit of re-examining our traditional use of time, we will briefly look at the chosen length and frequency of sessions, then discuss in more detail the rationale behind four common treatment durations: 1) "continuous or intermittent psychotherapy," in which treatment is always available to the patient and a definite termination is neither explicitly nor implicitly prescribed; 2) "long-term psychotherapy," which may last for years but from which an eventual termination is expected; 3) "brief therapy," which may last for weeks or perhaps months and in which the goals are more focused and limited; and 4) "consultation" of one or two sessions without further treatment. The intention in suggesting the rationale for each of these four overlapping durations is not to be dogmatic but, on the contrary, to stimulate further discussion and research so that dogmatism will not reign.

LENGTH OF SESSIONS

The reasoning behind the conventional "hour" is not very convincing. For logistical and personal reasons, Freud saw his patients on the hour with very little time in between patients for a breather and notetaking (Jones, 1953). Even therapists using nonanalytic techniques have been influenced by this precedent as well as by a wealth of accumulated clinical experience that has indicated it usually takes somewhere around an hour "to get the job done" and that patients benefit from having a designated time period to structure their involvement and regression—though some therapists, both for convenience and financial reasons, have shortened Freud's "hour" to 50 or even 45 minutes. When the therapist is not getting paid directly for the service, such as in clinical or general hospital settings, the length of sessions tends to be more flexible. Castelnuovo-Tedesco (1965) has suggested the value of the "20-minute hour" in conducting supportive psychotherapy, a time consistent with what patients expect for follow-up visits from nonpsychiatric physicians; and Zirkle (1961) has even advocated "five-minute psychotherapy." Patients requiring maintenance on lithium, neuroleptics, or methadone are frequently allotted very brief sessions; although such scheduling may appear cost-effective, the risk is that a therapeutic relationship will not be formed, psychosocial issues will not be sufficiently addressed, and noncompliance with medication will eventually lead to more extensive (and expensive) treatment.

At the other end of the spectrum are those situations which often require more than the conventional "hour." Marital, family, and group formats, particularly in the early phases of treatment, often take more time to allow all participants to express their views and interact. Initial consultations also frequently require more time to engage the patient, gather data, and begin to form a therapeutic alliance. This is especially true for consultations in the general hospital where additional time is necessary to discuss the patient with the staff and to write an informed note. For these reasons, an initial consultation is best scheduled at the end of the day or when a "free" hour follows the session and can be used if necessary. Proponents of crisis intervention (Bellak and Small, 1978; Caplan, 1964; Ewing, 1978) have stressed the need to tailor the length of sessions to fit the individual's requirements; and some authors have suggested "marathon" sessions to wear down defenses and defensiveness on the unproven assumption that months or even years of treatment can be compressed into a relatively short period. The most provocative suggestion has been that patients in an exploratory psychotherapy be "dismissed" after a few minutes if the therapist feels additional time on that day will not be productive (Lacan, 1978). While few would go to that extreme, the point is well taken that the therapist should not adhere too rigidly to the conventional "hour" and should adjust fees according to the time–effort and not simply to the number of sessions.

FREQUENCY OF SESSIONS

As with length of sessions, the choice of session frequency is based more on tradition, logistics, and accumulated clinical experience than on systematic research. However, most therapists—whatever their theoretical and technical persuasion—would agree on four general principles: First, sessions that are scheduled at regular intervals provide an organizing structure in the patient's life and treatment. Second, the actual structure provided by regular scheduling is greatly enhanced by the transferential meaning a patient gives to having "his time" predictably assigned. Third, a certain intensity is necessary to facilitate change ("If you bake a cake at 200 degrees, you don't end up with a cake"). And fourth, sessions that are scheduled too frequently at some point become no longer cost-effective and may even iatrogenically induce a harmful regression and dependency.

Beginning therapists, understandably eager to have rules to deal with the ambiguities of psychotherapy, tend to be more rigid in determining the frequency of sessions: maintenance psychopharmacotherapy once per month, supportive psychotherapy once per week, behavioral modification or exploratory psychotherapy twice per week, psychoanalysis four or five times per week, and so on. Experienced psychotherapists tend to be more flexible; they have learned that the choice of frequency depends more on the patient than on the type of treatment. For example, some patients are capable of doing intensive psychoanalytic work with sessions scheduled less than four times per week; and some patients remain unmotivated to change or experience no sense of balance in their lives with sessions scheduled only once a week. In the absence of scientific data to alter these clinical impressions, one is left with only the modest suggestions that the frequency of sessions be based on an independent determination of the patient's assets and needs, and that a given frequency not be routinely prescribed because it "goes with" a particular kind of duration, format, technique, or diagnosis.

CONTINUOUS OR INTERMITTENT PSYCHOTHERAPY

The rationale for continuous or intermittent psychotherapy has been underemphasized in training and in the psychiatric literature, leading to a confusion about its indications and goals. Few would argue that patients with a chronic and severe "neurochemical" illness, such as schizophrenia or bipolar affective disorder, often require continuous treatment. The understanding is that the frequency of sessions will depend on illness severity, on capacity for self-monitoring of symptoms and medication, and on available support from family and other resources. More intensive therapy is prescribed during crises and exacerbations of the underlying disease. Furthermore, the assumption is that such disorders are treatable but not curable, and for this reason, therapy will continue indefinitely.

More controversial is the choice of continuous psychotherapy for patients with disorders that appear more functional in origin and are not so severe, yet by all indications are chronic. This group is comprised most prominently by certain patients with Axis II personality disorders, but also with Axis I diagnoses— such as the milder but persistent affective disorders, refractory anxiety disorders, somatoform disorders, psychosexual paraphilias, substance abuse, and intermittent explosive disorders.

It is obvious that many patients with these disorders do not require continuous psychotherapy, but it is also obvious from clinical experience that some of these patients do in fact benefit from a treatment that is more or less always available. There is an understandable reluctance among such patients to acknowledge that their treatment will never be completely terminated. This reluctance may be shared by the therapist, perhaps out of a concern that such an acknowledgement will diminish the patient's hope. However, without such an acknowledgement, the risk is that the "endless" psychotherapy will not be viewed as a consequence of the underlying disorder and the limitations of available treatment, but rather as a failure of the patient or therapist.

This defeatist view of continuous psychotherapy can be side-stepped if one applied the model of standard medical practice. There, an open-ended "life-long" continuous or intermittent time arrangement is commonly prescribed not just for more serious chronic illnesses (like diabetes or essential hypertension), but also for chronic illnesses that are milder and not life-threatening. Like psoriasis, arthritis, and headaches, many functional disorders may be relatively mild, recurrent, or chronic, and benefit from intermittent or sustained symptomatic and supportive care. However, because of the nature of psychotherapy and psychiatric symptoms, this medical model cannot always be easily applied. Before concluding that a continuous or intermittent treatment is indicated, the therapist must address several difficult questions: Is the therapy fostering an unnecessary regression and dependency that makes an absolute termination appear less feasible than it is? Is the patient simply avoiding the inevitable anxiety, sadness, anger, and disappointment that commonly accompany a lasting termination? Is the therapist postponing a definite termination for countertransferential reasons? And has there been a failure to distinguish treatment goals from those life goals that are outside the purview of psychotherapy (Ticho, 1972)? In ambiguous situations, a consultation may be helpful to determine whether intermittent or sustained support is indicated, or whether this "crutch" is iatrogenically causing a potentially healthy function to become weak or even wasted.

LONG-TERM PSYCHOTHERAPY

Long-term psychotherapy is a label often used synonymously with exploratory techniques, such as psychoanalytically oriented psychotherapy; but actually supportive and directive therapies are frequently "long-term" as well (Perry et al, 1985). Regardless of technique, the rationale for this duration is that some psychiatric disorders are so engrained, complex, and diffuse that an extended period of time is necessary for both the dissection and resolution of the problems, and for the patient to assimilate and apply the new solutions into his or her daily life. Empirically, this time period has been found to require at least several months, but more often years. However, long-term psychotherapy is not really "open-ended" if both patient and therapist expect that at some point a termination date will be set, that a distinct ending to treatment will then occur, and that this process is a mutually desired goal.

The distinction between continuous and long-term psychotherapy is subtle, but important. Although an established termination does not mean that the patient may thereafter never return, the process and expectations of treatment are different if an eventual ending is anticipated. As opposed to continuous psychotherapy, a statement is being made that the therapist-patient relationship will be different from the traditional relationship offered by physicians, priests, and advisors who are available indefinitely to lend an ear and give advice as the situation requires. The implication is that at some point the patient will be capable of separating and dealing with future problems alone.

When the long-term therapy proceeds more or less successfully and an eventual termination appears likely, the distinction between continuous and long-term therapy becomes clear. But there are occasions when this distinction becomes blurred: Month after month, and year after year, at regularly scheduled appointments, the patient and therapist struggle with the underlying disorder without openly accepting that a definitive and sustained termination is unlikely. These stalemated situations pose at least four potential dangers. First, the patient's failure to resolve the chronic problems and to terminate treatment may erroneously be attributed to resistance, to an unconscious wish to defeat the therapist, to a "negative therapeutic reaction" (Freud, 1923), or, more sweepingly, to a lack of motivation or will. Second, the inherent limitations of psychotherapy will remain unacknowledged and therefore will not be examined and worked through. Third, the therapist may become more frustrated and the patient more hopeless because the anticipated termination has not been achieved. And fourth, the stalemated therapeutic situation may ferment frustration and bitterness in both parties to the point that treatment ends by default on a dyspeptic note.

In addition to changes in technique, format, setting, or medication to avoid these dangers, a change in the time structure of treatment can also be helpful. One option is for the therapist to explicitly change the duration from long-term to continuous, explaining that the patient's chronic disorder will require a treatment that continues indefinitely, but that the intensity of that treatment can be adjusted according to current need. This explanation may not only instill more hope and reassurance, but may actually be more cost-effective: confident that treatment will not end, the patient may tolerate sessions that are scheduled far less frequently (Bennett and Bennett, 1984). An alternative approach is for the therapist to prescribe "treatment holidays" of several weeks or months so that the benefits of previous treatment can be consolidated, the patient can acquire more autonomy and confidence, and a clearer determination can be made between what treatment is or is not currently accomplishing. After this assessment, an eventual termination may be feasible; or if not, the therapist and patient may agree upon a series of brief treatments (that is, intermittent psychotherapy) for those times when conflicts are most pressing and accessible for change.

These suggestions for a stalemated long-term psychotherapy are made primarily to remind us that the component of time can have a therapeutic impact of its own and is not simply dependent on the patient's pathology or on other treatment variables. This point is especially germane to long-term psychotherapies that are routinely, perhaps even automatically, prescribed for "support" or "character change." Some patients may experience more "support" when the therapist indicates continuous availability rather than implying, however subtly, that one day treatment will end. Conversely, character change may not require the traditionally prescribed extensive treatment; such change may not only be possible but facilitated by a briefer therapy (as discussed below). The closing point to be made here is that because regularly scheduled long-term psychotherapy is expensive, is discrepant with traditional medical practice, and is weakly supported by available research, the prescription of this duration requires the most thoughtful assessment of indications, contraindications, and enabling factors (Perry et al, 1983).

BRIEF PSYCHOTHERAPY

The rationale and indications for briefer treatments have been modified by the "brief dynamic therapies," a label that generally refers to studies of Malan (1976) at the Tavistock Clinic in London, to the work of Davanloo (1978) in Canada, and to the reports of Sifneos (1972) and Mann (1973) in the United States. Although these brief dynamic therapies are often referred to collectively, there are some differences. Sifneos restricts "focal therapy" to somewhat healthier patients with oedipal problems and tends to use more directive and cognitive techniques. Mann emphasizes that separation-individuation problems are present in all patients and that "time-limited" treatment is therefore an especially apt paradigm to explore such problems. Davanloo and Malan are far more flexible in their selection criteria and techniques. Despite these differences, these brief dynamic treatments share many common features: The therapist and patient engage quickly, focus attention more or less on one event or symptom or conflict, agree that interpretations and decisions will be made with incomplete data, and that the goals of treatment will be limited; then by using both a psychodynamic understanding and frequent confrontations, the therapist actively helps the patient resolve the underlying conflict within a period of time that either implicitly or explicitly will be brief, usually somewhere between 20 and 40 sessions.

Certain misconceptions have already developed about the origins and intent of brief dynamic therapy (Perry and Michels, 1986). One pervasive misconception is that these treatments are innovative because they are brief. Actually, most psychotherapies have always been brief in private practice as well as in psychiatric clinics (Butcher and Koss, 1978; Koss, 1979). Frances and colleagues (1984) reviewed over 100 articles regarding treatment duration and concluded that most psychotherapies fit quite naturally into a short period of time. These authors found that proponents of crisis intervention, problem solving, behavioral therapy, marital therapy, sexual therapy, family therapy, and cognitive therapy all described treatments that on the average required less than 15 sessions, and that this recommended brief duration was used in actual practice.

A second misconception is that the brief dynamic therapies were conceived as a response to pressure from consumers and third-party payers. This is not the case. While not impervious to current fiscal needs, those who developed these treatments have not been primarily concerned with cost-effectiveness. Their search has been to find a more effective treatment, not simply a shorter one.

A third misconception is that the brief treatments were conceived as yet another attempt to find a way of using psychodynamic concepts for those patients who do not have the necessary attributes for more ambitious exploratory treatments. On the contrary, the major advocates of these new treatments, however else they may differ, prescribe methods that have stringent enabling factors (Perry et al, 1983).

The fourth misconception is in some ways just the opposite of the third; namely, that the brief dynamic therapies attempt (but fail) to be a compressed form of long-term exploratory treatments. The contention is that the limited duration of treatment leaves large and perhaps malignant areas of the patient's character unexplored and also precludes the arduous but necessary working through, the "assimilation" that only time can provide (Bibring, 1954). Proponents of this view further argue that "premature" interpretations can lead to a "wild analysis" (Shafer, 1985) and that by controlling the therapeutic process, the therapist controls the patient as well; the therapist thereby departs from the psychoanalytic tradition and deprives the patient of the confidence and autonomy that can only come from finding one's own way through the maze of conflicts as they are revealed in the transference (Shafer, 1983). Thinly disguised in these arguments is the suggestion that brief therapists for countertransferential reasons may have little tolerance for ambiguity and uncertainty, and therefore have an unconscious need to impose their wills on others (Perry and Michels, 1986).

These contentions, though persuasive, reflect a slight misunderstanding about the origins, techniques, and intent of these new, briefer treatments. From a historical perspective, brief dynamic therapy is not the recently conceived child of psychoanalysis. Most of the early psychoanalytic cases were relatively brief, and the psychoanalytic movement was quite mature before "classical" psychoanalysis (Valenstein, 1979) took its place beside treatments of shorter duration. In terms of technique, brief dynamic therapy adheres tightly to many fundamental tenets of psychoanalysis. Interpretations are based on fantasies, dreams, associative trends, symptom formation, transference material, and other manifestations of unconscious conflict; they are not unreasonable or unsubstantiated (that is, "wild"). Brief therapists point out that passivity must not be confused with neutrality (Perry and Viederman, 1981) and that interpretations are most mutative when the therapeutic atmosphere is intense, as many highly regarded analysts have maintained (Freud, 1914; Starchey, 1934; Gill, 1979). Brief dynamic therapists further point out that although their methods are often associated with analysts in the past who were interested in shortening treatment, they do not advocate the nonabstinent "active" therapy of Ferenczi and Rank (1925), nor the transferential manipulation and "corrective emotional experience" of Alexander and French (1946). In terms of intent, brief dynamic therapists make explicit that, like the duration of treatment, the goals of treatment are limited; that is, to resolve specific difficulties and not to achieve the more global ambitions of psychoanalysis.

Having addressed these common misconceptions, we can now better appreciate how brief dynamic therapy has altered our traditional view of time in psychotherapy. Four ways will be mentioned. First, these treatments have demonstrated that the use of exploratory techniques does not automatically mean that therapy will be prolonged. In the past, it was commonly felt that unlike cognitive or behavioral approaches, psychodynamic methods required extended periods of time. This view derived in part from an evolving psychoanalytic belief in the overdetermination of symptoms and in the need for regression and "timelessness" to work through a transference neurosis. Brief dynamic therapy has challenged these assumptions.

Second, and closely related to this first point, these innovative briefer treatments have presented convincing evidence that the resolution of intrapsychic conflict can occur far more rapidly than formerly believed. Moreover, on follow-up many years later, these circumscribed character changes are sustained (Malan, 1976). Following Lindemann's (1944) pioneer work on crisis intervention, Caplan (1964) and Ewing (1978) noted that coping with an overwhelming stress could foster maturation and even lead to a higher level of functioning. But brief dynamic therapists go one step further; they indicate that even in the absence of a profound crisis, an intense confrontational therapy can catalyze a lasting improvement of ingrained character problems, at least within a focused area of unconscious conflict.

Third, brief dynamic therapy has established that the prescription of a more or less defined period of time can in itself be a powerful therapeutic intervention. Although Freud himself used this approach in his treatment of the Wolf Man (1918), and Rank elaborated this idea by rather artificially imposing his theory of birth anxiety (Ferenczi and Rank, 1925), the advocates of brief dynamic therapy have examined this technique more systematically. Mann (1973), for instance, describes the way in which setting the specific date of termination at the start of treatment highlights issues of separation-individuation as they relate to the patient's chief complaint and individual character structure. Although other brief therapists do not advocate demarcating a time frame so explicitly, they share a view that by implicitly conveying that treatment will be brief, they force (and enable) the patient to achieve the defined task more quickly. Infantilization and unnecessary dependency are thereby discouraged.

Fourth, and most important, these briefer dynamic therapies have stimulated others to investigate more systematically the process and outcome of dynamic treatments, especially concerning their time-effectiveness. Malan (1976), for example, found that patients with high motivation and low focality of conflict did well in therapy but often required longer treatment than those with high motivation and a circumscribed problem. Those with low motivation did poorly regardless of how focused their presenting problems were or how long the treatment lasted. The point here is not that these findings challenge existing clinical impressions, but rather that an effort is being made by psychodynamic therapists to document these impressions in a scientific manner.

CONSULTATION WITHOUT FURTHER TREATMENT

Having begun with a discussion of psychotherapies that may last a lifetime, we have now reached the other extreme: the prescription of only one or two sessions. Clinicians have appreciated the sustained therapeutic impact of a consultation, and the efficacy of these very brief treatments has been described (Bloom, 1981; Malan et al, 1975). Moreover, a very abbreviated treatment does not preclude the use of psychodynamic techniques. Viederman and Perry (1980), for example, have recommended that a "psychodynamic life narrative" be presented to a patient after only one or two sessions as a way of increasing self-esteem, communicating an empathic understanding, and providing an organizing structure to help master the distress associated with physical illness or other crises.

If a brief consultation appears sufficient, few would argue for recommending further treatment at that time—but what about the recommendation of no further treatment for those patients who have *not* sufficiently improved after one or two sessions? This decision, the recommendation of no treatment as the prescription of choice, may be the most difficult for any consultant to make. The guidelines for this recommendation have only recently been described (Frances and Clarkin, 1981; Frances et al, 1984; Perry et al, 1985); and little systematic data are available to guide the decision. Furthermore, this recommendation must often be given to patients who desperately want relief from their suffering and who may well continue to do poorly if left to their own devices.

Given the difficulty in recommending no further treatment, the consultant is often inclined to defer this decision and give treatment a try under the erroneous decision that "it may not help, but it can't hurt." However, psychotherapy is analogous to any potent medicine: On the average it is more effective than no treatment (Smith et al, 1980; Luborsky et al, 1975; Andrews and Harvey, 1981), but it does have its own particular brand of side-effects, dependency and over-dosage, and, for some, it either does not work or is not necessary.

Once a treatment begins—even on a trial basis—it gathers momentum. As expectations become mobilized and time and money are invested, both therapist and patient often find it easier to continue their involvement with one another than to cut their losses, limit their goals, and acknowledge that no treatment might have been and might still be a preferred choice. In addition, no matter what kind of treatment is performed, strong transference feelings develop which then make the recommendation of no treatment much more difficult to accept in a realistic way. This situation is even more unsettling when the patient has actually gotten worse during the course of treatment. Feeling at least partly responsible for this deterioration, the therapist may attempt to assuage his or her guilt by increasing therapeutic zeal. At that point, the recommendation of no treatment is even harder to consider.

In appreciation of this difficulty, I will now describe four relative indications for the recommendation of no further treatment beyond one or two sessions. Though somewhat schematic, this discussion may at least remind the consultant of this option and may stimulate further research in this area.

Patients at risk for negative response. Little information is available on the specific patient attributes that predict a negative response. Uncontrolled studies suggest that severely disturbed patients may deteriorate in some exploratory individual and group therapies (Aronson and Weintraub, 1968; Fairweather et al, 1960; Kernberg et al, 1972; Weber et al, 1965); however, because these same patients might conceivably have benefited from another form of treatment, they do not necessarily constitute a group for whom no treatment would have been pref-erable. In a survey of experienced therapists (Strupp et al, 1969; Strupp et al, 1977), negative responses were related to borderline and masochistic features as well as to the patient's low ego strengths and motivation, and to the thera-pist's relative lack of skill. The most extensive review of negative responses summarized data from 40 reports (Bergin and Lambert, 1978); but as Frances and colleagues have described (1984), some of the best studies in this review failed to distinguish a negative response from a nonresponse, or assumed a negative response only on the basis of differential variance and outcome, or did not distinguish whether the negative response was due to psychotherapy or was due to other interventions. The humble conclusion based on available data is that researchers must make greater efforts to measure negative results and the factors that predict them.

Patients at risk for no response. The rate of various positive responses to psycho-therapy and psychotropic medications tends to cluster at roughly 60–70 percent (Smith et al, 1980). The 30–40 percent who did not show positive results fall into three hypothetical categories: 1) patients who would have gotten worse except for the beneficial effects of treatment, and who are able to maintain the status quo only because of treatment (these are really veiled positive responders); 2) patients who are untouched by treatment and who continue to follow the natural course of their disorder (these are the true nonresponders); and 3) patients who would have gotten better except for the noxious effects of treatment and are held in stalemate because of it (these are veiled negative responders). Whereas treatment would be recommended and continued for apparent "nonresponders" in the first category, the recommendation of no treatment should be strongly considered for those patients in the second and third.

Patients likely to have spontaneous improvement. Once a patient is in treatment, spontaneous improvement is impossible to measure; studies therefore have used groups receiving no treatment as controls and have found that spontaneous improvement depends upon the diagnosis: only nine percent of borderline and schizophrenic patients appear to improve spontaneously, whereas up to 54 percent of patients with other diagnoses improve (Endicott and Endicott, 1963). A summary of 17 well controlled studies (Bergin and Lambert, 1978) found a median rate of 43 percent for spontaneous remissions; however, some of these patients may not have been improving "spontaneously," but rather responding to waiting lists, initial evaluations, or other research procedures (Malan et al, 1975). Furthermore, the treated group of patients may have improved in ways that the intake-outcome measures did not assess.

Recommendations of no treatment as a therapeutic intervention. Since I began this chapter by discussing how the prescription of time can in itself be a therapeutic intervention, it is important not to end by discussing how the prescription of "no time" can also have a therapeutic impact. Included in this category would be the oppositional patient who needs treatment but, because of false pride or a need to defy, is likely to refuse it. When this patient is told that treatment is likely to be useless or too expensive or too difficult or not necessary, he or she may respond by angrily trying to convince the consultant that treatment must be provided. With this maneuver, admittedly manipulative, an oppositional patient who might otherwise take pride in fighting for a way out of treatment may now take pride in fighting for a way into it.

The recommendation of no treatment as a specific therapeutic intervention is also indicated for those patients who can function on an adequate level, but who want treatment to justify regression or an escape from the responsibilities in the real world. Refusing to provide treatment supports the healthier aspects of their functioning and improves their sense of mastery and competence. Closely related to this group are those patients who are in a never-ending chain of therapies and never allowed fully to experience any of the separations or to integrate the impact of any one treatment before beginning another. The recommendation of no treatment—or at least an extended delay before beginning the next treatment—can help these patients consolidate their gains and increase their confidence.

SUMMARY

I end this chapter in a tone less cautious than when I began. In the past, the frequency and duration of treatment was largely determined by other co-variables in the patient, the therapist, or the type of psychotherapy (see Table 1). However, because of forces from both within and outside our profession, this traditional view is being challenged and increasingly time is being appreciated as a more independent component of psychotherapy.

In the spirit of this re-examination and on the basis of existing studies, some tentative conclusions and recommendations can be made:

1. Despite their reputation, most outpatient psychotherapies are relatively brief (less than 15 sessions) both in their theoretical description and in their actual practice; these include crisis intervention, problem solving, behavioral therapy, marital therapy, sexual therapy, family therapy, and cognitive therapy.

2. Most comparative studies as well as large reviews of these studies have failed to demonstrate the value of longer treatments. Although this general conclusion is contaminated by methodological problems both in the studies themselves and in their cumulative reviews, nevertheless the onus is now on the therapist who recommends a longer psychotherapy as an initial approach for any "neurotic" patient.

3. The traditional "hour" session (45–50 minutes) is based on convention, logistics, finances, and clinical experience and not on any controlled studies. Although patients and therapists both benefit from having a pre-arranged time period for a given session, more flexibility is necessary in establishing what that time period should be for consultations and for all types of continuing psychotherapies.

4. The frequency of sessions should be determined more by the needs and capacities of a given patient and less by the type of psychotherapy being prescribed. For example, some patients in "supportive psychotherapy" experience no benefit if seen only once per week, whereas other patients in "psychoanalytically oriented psychotherapy" can do intense exploratory work when seen at weekly intervals.

5. The value of continuous or intermittent "life-long" psychotherapy for non-psychotic disorders has been underemphasized in training and in the psychiatric literature, but is consistent with the medical model for treating chronic or recurrent illnesses that are not life threatening but benefit from sustained or intermittent symptomatic care. This duration may be considered for certain patients with Axis II personality disorders, milder but persistent affective disorders, refractory anxiety disorders, somatoform disorders, psychosexual paraphilias, substance abuse, and intermittent explosive disorders.

6. In contrast to point number 5 above, long-term psychotherapy (in which a final and absolute termination is expected) is discrepant with traditional medical practice, is weakly supported by available research, is expenseive, and can iatrogenically induce stalemates, frustration, and hopelessness. For these reasons, this duration is rarely recommended as an initial approach.

7. Brief dynamic psychotherapies have indicated that implicit or explicit prescription of a limited time period can catalyze rather than impede the patient's involvement.

8. These new brief therapies have also demonstrated that in certain patients (with rather demanding enabling factors) exploratory techniques can be used within a limited time frame and produce lasting character change, at least within a focal area of conflict; however, the favorable results of these treat-

ments may stem more from the prescribed techniques than from the relatively short duration.

9. Consultation consisting of only one or two sessions can produce a sustained therapeutic impact. Furthermore, these very brief "treatments" do not preclude the use of psychodynamic techniques, including clarification and interpretation.

10. The prescription of no treatment, though one of the most difficult recommendations, is indicated for patients at risk for a negative response (for example, certain borderline personalities), at risk for no response (for example, antisocial personalities), likely to have spontaneous improvement (for example, normal bereavement), or likely to experience the recommendation of no treatment as therapeutic (for example, a college freshman reassured that he can handle his situational anxiety without therapy).

In the absence of more systematic studies, these 10 conclusions cannot be taken as dogma but rather as a reminder that when confronted with the task of selecting a particular treatment for a particular patient, the consultant cannot simply let other variables determine the therapy's duration and frequency. The prescription of time in itself can have a powerful therapeutic impact.

REFERENCES

Alexander F, French T: Psychoanalytic Therapy. New York, Ronald Press, 1946

Andrews G, Harvey R: Does psychotherapy benefit neurotic patients? Arch Gen Psychiatry 38:1203-1208, 1981

Aronson H, Weintraub W: Patient changes during clinical psychoanalysis as a function of initial status and duration of treatment. Psychiatry 31:369-379, 1968

Bellack L, Small L: Emergency Psychotherapy and Brief Psychotherapy, second edition. New York, Grune & Stratton, 1978

Bennett MI, Bennett MB: Uses of hopelessness. Am J Psychiatry 141:559-562, 1984

Bergin AE, Lambert MV: The evaluation of psychotherapeutic outcomes, in Handbook of Psychotherapy and Behavior Change: An Empirical Analysis. Edited by Garfield SL, Bergin AE. New York, John Wiley, 1978

Bibring, E: Psychoanalysis and the dynamic psychotherapies. J Am Psychoanal Assoc 12:745-770, 1954

Bloom BL: Focused single-session therapy: initial development and evaluation, in Forms of Brief Therapy. Edited by Budman SH. New York, Guilford Press, 1981

Butcher JN, Koss MP: Research on brief and crisis-oriented psychotherapies, in Handbook of Psychotherapy and Behavior Change, second edition. Edited by Garfield SL, Bergin AE. New York, John Wiley, 1978

Caplan G: Principles of Preventive Psychiatry. New York, Basic Books, 1964

Castelnuovo-Tedesco P: The Twenty Minute Hour. Boston, Little, Brown, 1965

Davanloo H: Basic Principles and Techniques in Short-Term Dynamic Psychotherapy. New York, Spectrum, 1978

Endicott NA, Endicott J: "Improvement" in untreated psychiatric patients. Arch Gen Psychiatry 9:575-585, 1963

Ewing CP: Crisis Intervention as Psychotherapy. New York, Oxford University Press, 1978

Fairweather G, Simon R, Gebhard ME, et al: Relative effectiveness of psychotherapeutic programs: a multicriteria comparison of four programs for three different treatment groups. Psychological Monographs: General and Applied 74 (5, whole no. 492), 1960

Ferenczi S, Rank O: The Development of Psychoanalysis. New York, Nervous & Mental Disease Publication Company, 1925

Frances A, Clarkin J: No treatment as prescription of choice. Arch Gen Psychiatry 38:542-545, 1981

Frances A, Clarkin J, Perry S: Differential Therapeutics in Psychiatry: The Art and Science of Treatment Selection. New York, Brunner/Mazel, 1984

Freud S: Remembering, repeating and working through (1914), in Complete Psychological Works, Standard Edition, vol. 12. Translated and edited by Strachey J. London, Hogarth Press, 1958

Freud S: From the history of an infantile neurosis (1918), in Complete Psychological Works, Standard Edition, vol. 17. Translated and edited by Strachey J. London, Hogarth Press, 1958

Freud S: The ego and the id (1923) in Complete Psychological Works, Standard Edition, vol. 19. Translated and edited by Strachey J. London, Hogarth Press, 1958

Gill MM: The analysis of the transference. J Am Psychoanal Assoc 27:263-288, 1979

Graham SR: Patient evaluation of the effectiveness of limited psychoanalytically-oriented psychotherapy. Psychol Rep 4:231-234, 1958

Heilbrunn G: Results with psychoanalytic therapy and professional commitment. Am J Psychother 20:89-99, 1966

Heinicke CM: Frequency of psychotherapeutic sessions as a factor affecting outcome: analysis of clinical ratings and test results. J Abnorm Psychol 74:553-560, 1969

Howard KI, Kopta SM; Krause MS, et al: The dose-effect relationship in psychotherapy. Am Psychol 41:159-164, 1986

Imber SD, Frank JD, Nash EH, et al: Improvement and amount of therapeutic contact: an alternative to the use of no-treatment controls in psychotherapy. Journal of Consulting Psychology 21:309-315, 1957

Jones E: The Life and Work of Sigmund Freud. New York, Basic Books, 1953

Kaufman I, Frank T, Freind J, et al: Success and failure in the treatment of childhood schizophrenia. Am J Psychiatry 118:909-913, 1962

Kernberg OF, Bernstein CS, Coyne R, et al: Psychotherapy and psychoanalysis: final report of the Menninger Foundation's psychotherapy research project. Bull Menninger Clin 36:1-276, 1972

Koss, MP: Length of psychotherapy for clients seen in private practice. J Consult Clin Psychol 47:210-212, 1979

Lacan J: The Four Fundamental Concepts of Psychoanalysis. New York, W.W. Norton, 1978

Lindemann E: Symptomatology and management of acute grief. Am J Psychiatry 101:141-148, 1944

Lorr M, McNair D, Michaux W, et al: Frequency of treatment and change in psychotherapy. Journal of Abnormal and Social Psychology 64:281-292, 1962

Luborsky L, Singer B, Luborsky L: Comparative studies of psychotherapy: is it true that "everyone has won and all must have prizes"? Arch Gen Psychiatry 132:995-1008, 1975

Malan DH, Heath ES, Bascal HA, et al: Psychodynamic changes in untreated neurotic patients, II: apparently genuine improvements. Arch Gen Psychiatry 32:110-126, 1975

Malan DH: The Frontier of Brief Psychotherapy. New York, Plenum, 1976

Mann J: Time Limited Psychotherapy. Cambridge, Harvard University Press, 1973

Newman FL, Howard KI: Therapeutic effort, treatment outcome, and national health policy. Am Psychol 2:181-187, 1986

Orlinsky DE, Howard KI: The relation of process to outcome in psychotherapy, in Handbook of Psychotherapy and Behavior Change: An Empirical Analysis, second edition. Edited by Garfield SL, Bergin AE. New York, John Wiley, 1978

Perry S, Michels R: Countertransference in the selection of brief therapy, in Countertransference and Transference. Edited by H Myers. Hillsdale, NJ, Analytic Press, 1986

Perry S, Viederman M: Adaptation of residents to consultation-liaison psychiatry. Gen Hosp Psychiatry 3:141-147, 1981

Perry S, Frances A, Klar H, et al: Selection criteria for individual dynamic psychotherapies. Psychiatr Q 55:3-16, 1983

Perry S, Frances A, Clarkin J: A DSM-III Casebook of Differential Therapeutics: A Clinical Guide to Treatment Selection. New York, Brunner/Mazel, 1985

Rosenbaum M, Friedlander J, Kaplan S: Evaluation of results of psychotherapy. Psychosom Med 18:113-132, 1956

Shafer R: The termination of brief psychoanalytic psychotherapy. Int J Psychoanal Psychother 2:135-148, 1983

Shafer R: Wild Analysis. J Am Psychoanal Assoc 33:275-300, 1985

Sifneos PE: Short-Term Psychotherapy and Emotional Crisis. Cambridge, Harvard University Press, 1972

Smith ML, Glass GV, Miller TI: The Benefit of Psychotherapy. Baltimore, Johns Hopkins University Press, 1980

Strachey J: The nature of the therapeutic action of psychoanalysis. Int J Psychoanal 15:127-159, 1934

Strupp HH, Fox RE, Lessler K: Patients View Their Psychotherapy. Baltimore, Johns Hopkins University Press, 1969

Strupp HH, Hadley SW, Gomes-Schwartz R: Psychotherapy for Better or Worse: An Analysis of the Problem of Negative Effects. New York, Jason Aronson, 1977

Taube CA, Burns BJ, Kessler L: Patients of psychiatrists and psychologists in office-based practice: 1980. Am Psychol 39:1435-1447, 1984

Ticho EA: Termination of psychoanalysis: treatment goals, life goals. Psychoanal Q 41:315-333, 1972

Valenstein AF: The concept of "classical" psychoanalysis. J Am Psychoanal Assoc 27:113-136, 1979

Van Slambrouck S: Relation of structural parameters to treatment outcome. Dissertation Abstracts International 33:5528, 1973

Viederman M, Perry S: Use of a psychodynamic life narrative in the treatment of depression in the physically ill. Gen Hosp Psychiatry 3:177-185, 1980

Weber JJ, Elinson J, Moss LM: The application of ego strength scales to psychoanalytic clinic records, in Developments in Psychoanalysis at Columbia University: Proceedings of the 20th Anniversary Conference. Edited by Goldman GS, Shapiro D. New York, Columbia Psychoanalytic Clinic for Training and Research, 1965

Zirkle GA: Five-minute psychotherapy. Am J Psychiatry 118:544-546, 1961

Chapter 17

Differential Therapeutics: Psychopharmacology

by Carl Salzman, M.D., and Alan I. Green, M.D.

Psychopharmacology is a continuously evolving discipline. The practicing clinician faces an ever-increasing task just to keep abreast of the new agents available, new uses for old agents, and side effects of them all. The further problem of how to handle the patient who does not respond to a standard, accepted treatment becomes yet another hurdle that may require consultation with an expert psychopharmacologist. This chapter attempts to simplify the general psychiatrist's burden by reviewing the practical clinical aspects of some of the new strategies in psychopharmacology.

Until recently, two of the cardinal rules of psychopharmacology were: 1) use a drug only for the specific purpose for which it was intended (for example, use an anticonvulsant only for a seizure disorder); and 2) avoid concurrent medications for the same disorder (polypharmacy). Recent research and clinical experience, as outlined in this chapter, however, now suggest a broader range of therapeutic activity for some psychotropic drugs such as antidepressants and anticonvulsants. In addition, judicious use of concurrent medications now seems warranted for the treatment of resistant depression and for the management of schizophrenia with behavioral disruption.

The following chapter reviews some of the new indications and dosages for standard psychotropic drugs as well as appropriate use of polypharmacy. Organized according to clinical syndrome, the treatment approaches include: 1) affective disorders: delusional depression, lithium resistant affective disorder, and treatment resistant depression; 2) anxiety disorders: general anxiety disorder and panic anxiety; and 3) schizophrenia.

AFFECTIVE DISORDERS

Delusional Depression

For more than a decade, it has been recognized that depressed patients with delusions of somatic dysfunction, delusions of hopelessness and untreatability (nihilism), or delusions of persecution (paranoia) are less responsive than nondelusional patients to treatment with cyclic antidepressants (Glassman et al, 1975). Recent research studies have demonstrated an improved therapeutic efficacy of amitriptyline when combined with perphenazine in patients who have delusional depressions (Spiker et al, 1985). Clinical experience has confirmed this research observation and suggests that many different combinations of neuroleptic and cyclic antidepressants will provide therapeutic results superior to that of the antidepressant alone. On the basis of both the research and clinical observations, the addition of a neuroleptic to cyclic antidepressant treatment should now be considered a standard therapeutic approach for patients with delusional depression. Lithium has been reported to further potentiate the neuroleptic-cyclic antidepressant combination (Price et al, 1983), especially in patients with bipolar disorder (Nelson and Mazure, 1986), although these observations await further confirmation.

Traditionally, delusionally depressed patients have been treated with ECT and many clinicians are still convinced that ECT is superior to all other treatments including the neuroleptic–antidepressant combination (NIMH, 1986). An early study demonstrated a nearly 96 percent response rate of "psychotic depression to ECT" (Greenblatt et al, 1962). More recently, Nelson and Mazure (1986) found ECT especially helpful for psychotically depressed unipolar patients who were resistant to an antidepressant–neuroleptic combination. However, a rigorously designed study, employing contemporary diagnostic and outcome criteria comparing ECT to the neuroleptic–antidepressant combination in delusionally depressed patients, has never been performed. Therefore, clinical lore, rather than research evidence, is often cited by advocates of one or the other approach. Proponents of ECT for delusional depression point to a more rapid response, with fewer immediate side effects. Although relapse may occur following ECT, maintenance treatment with cyclic antidepressants or with lithium often prevents a return of symptoms. Proponents of the drug combination, however, note the greater patient (and doctor) acceptance of drugs versus ECT, the lower likelihood of long-term toxic consequences, and the more ready transition to maintenance drug treatment.

Other factors that have not yet been studied in research programs may help the clinician decide between these two treatment approaches. These factors include the severity of the depressive symptoms, especially the delusions, and the age of the patient. Young patients, and those whose depressive symptoms are not life threatening, probably should be treated with a cyclic antidepressant–neuroleptic combination. In these patients, speed of response is not critical, drug side effects are usually well tolerated, and treatment acceptability is often a factor. However, in older patients, or in those whose depression is severe, ECT may be the preferred approach. This is especially true when vegetative symptoms threaten to compromise physiological function or, when, as a result of the delusions, the depressed patient refuses all sustenance, treatment, and assistance. In very elderly patients (who often have the most severe depressions and delusions), drug treatment may be considerably slower and more toxic than ECT. For these severely ill elderly patients, ECT may still remain the antidepressant treatment of choice.

Lithium Resistant Affective Disorder

Since the initial reports of Takazaki and Hanacka (1971) and Ballenger and Post (1978), carbamazepine has been reported to be effective for the treatment of lithium resistant mania, for manic patients who have incompletely responded to lithium, or for those who are prone to lithium toxicity. Carbamazepine has proved helpful for the rapid cycling bipolar patient (with more than three affective episodes in a 12-month period) and for patients with severe manic episodes (Post, 1986). Carbamazepine also has antidepressant activity although this effect is considerably less reliable and predictable than its anti-manic properties (Post, 1986).

For most patients, carbamazepine is a safe, nontoxic drug. Although 25 percent of recipients experience some form of side effects, these are predominantly mild and subside after one week (Okuma, 1984). Neurologic side effects are the most common and include dizziness, drowsiness, incoordination, and ataxia. Gastrointestinal disturbances are also common and include nausea, vomiting, abdominal pain, diarrhea, and constipation. Pruritic skin rash has been reported in eight percent of patients (Ballenger and Post, 1978), but more severe dermatologic conditions, including the potentially fatal Stevens-Johnson syndrome (Patterson, 1985), occur considerably less frequently. Many patients who take carbamazepine may develop a drop in their blood count. This does not usually indicate serious bone marrow supression; it usually returns to normal when the drug is withdrawn. However, potentially fatal hematologic reactions including aplastic anemia (Kwentus et al, 1985), thrombocytopenic purpura, and agranulocytosis (Piscotta, 1975) have been described. Therefore, if the white blood count drops below 3,000–4,000, or if the drop is accompanied by decreases in other blood cell indices (red count, platelets), carbamazepine should be discontinued.

Although the clinical efficacy of carbamazepine seems to have been convincingly demonstrated among bipolar patients as a group, some clinicians are still doubtful about the therapeutic reliability of carbamazepine's effects for individual patients. Lithium, therefore, remains the treatment of choice for both acute mania and for the prevention of recurrent manic episodes. Carbamazepine is considered a second-line drug. When used, it is prescribed in 200 mg dosage increments, starting with 200 mg once a day and increasing by 200 mg every third day according to the individual patient's needs. Many patients will respond at doses of 200 to 600 mg/day; others may require 1,000 mg/day. An occasional patient who has had a partial response to 1,000 mg/day may require higher doses for complete response. Although the therapeutic plasma level for carbamazepine's anticonvulsive effect is between 8–12 ng/ml, no therapeutic range has been established for its antimanic effect.

Carbamazepine induces the hepatic microsomal enzyme system lowering plasma concentrations of many other drugs (Jann et al, 1985). It has been reported to cause a delirium when combined with neuroleptics (Yerevanian and Hodgeman, 1985). The combination of carbamazepine with lithium may be more therapeutic than either drug alone in some lithium resistant bipolar patients (Lipinski and Pope, 1982). However, neurotoxicity in patients taking lithium and carbamazepine has been reported (Shukla et al, 1984). Carbamazepine has been safely prescribed in conjunction with monoamine oxidase inhibitors but must not be combined with isoniazid (Ayd, 1986). Erythromycin increases carbamazepine levels (Yong et al, 1983).

Treatment Resistant Depression

Over the years, numerous studies of cyclic antidepressants have reported an overall response rate in depression of approximately 70 percent. In an effort to improve the therapeutic efficacy of these drugs, research has been directed toward the remaining 30 percent who either do not respond to antidepressant treatment or respond incompletely. As a result, a stepwise plan to guide the clinician in the therapeutic approach to this group of treatment resistant patients has been developed. The steps include: 1) review the diagnosis for accuracy;

2) question treatment compliance, dosage adequacy, and duration of treatment at therapeutic doses; 3) switch to another antidepressant; 4) use adjunctive therapy.

In some cases, the reason for treatment failure with the cyclic antidepressants may be erroneous diagnosis. Not all sadness, grief, or dysphoria is true depression, and not all patients who use the word "depression" to describe their mood are suffering from a major depressive disorder. The distinction between true major depression and other forms of unhappiness is of critical importance in patients who are elderly or suffer from physical illness, since only minimal therapeutic response to cyclic antidepressants is likely in patients without a major depressive disorder, whereas the likelihood of toxicity is quite high. (Salzman and van der Kolk, 1984). In addition, as noted above, patients with delusional depressions require the use of both an antidepressant and a neuroleptic, or ECT.

Assuming that the patient has a major depressive disorder without delusions, the next step is to determine if the medication has been taken as prescribed. Estimates of cyclic antidepressant noncompliance run as high as 30 percent (especially in older patients), probably as a result of side effects (Salzman, 1984b). Even if the cyclic antidepressant is taken in adequate dosages, there is a wide range of therapeutic blood and tissue levels due to differences among individuals in absorption, protein binding, and clearance. Measuring the cyclic antidepressant blood level may serve as an approximate guide to the therapeutic range, but reliable correlation between blood level and therapeutic response has only been demonstrated for imipramine, nortriptyline, and, in some laboratories, desipramine. Widening of the QRS complex on the EKG serves as a sensitive monitor for antidepressant cardiotoxicity (Salzman, 1985).

In most cases, a four-week course of at least 300 mg of imipramine (or equivalent cyclic antidepressant) constitutes a therapeutic trial; recent data suggest that a therapeutic failure cannot be assumed unless six weeks have passed (Quitkin et al, 1984).

Assuming the depressed patient has had an adequate trial of a cyclic antidepressant, the next therapeutic step is to consider the use of a second cyclic antidepressant. Here, clinical experience diverges. Some clinicians have observed that a failure to respond to adequate treatment with one cyclic antidepressant is evidence that the patient is a cyclic antidepressant nonresponder; they will, therefore, either switch to a monoamine oxidase (MAO) inhibitor or use adjunctive therapy (see below). Others elect to try a "second generation" antidepressant such as amoxapine, maprotiline, or trazodone. There are few data to support the switch from a so-called norepinephrine re-uptake blocking antidepressant to a serotonin re-uptake blocking antidepressant.

Another therapeutic approach to treatment resistant depressions is the use of adjunctive medication. There is a growing body of research data, as well as clinical experience, to suggest that when lithium is added to a cyclic antidepressant regimen, a nonresponsive patient may improve dramatically. It has been suggested that the improvement may be due to a lithium-induced release of presynaptic serotonin, although the exact mechanism of therapeutic augmentation is unknown (DeMontigny et al, 1983; Heninger et al, 1983). Doses of lithium sufficient to produce a blood level of approximately 0.8 Meq/1 (doses of

900–1200 mgs per day) are usually sufficient to augment the cyclic antidepressant response. Approximately 50 percent of treatment resistant patients with true nondelusional major depressive disorder may have a therapeutic response to the drug combination (Charney, personal communication, 1986).

Depressed patients who are resistant to cyclic antidepressants and who have either not responded to lithium augmentation or are unable to tolerate the side effects of lithium may be candidates for thyroid supplementation. Research evidence has suggested that l–triiodothyronine (T3) when added to imipramine, augments therapeutic response (Rabkin et al, 1983; Prange et al, 1984; Goodwin et al, 1982; Schwartz et al, 1984). Daily doses of 25–50 mcgs of T3 have been used. Unfortunately, in contrast to the research data, clinical experience suggests that, at present, the antidepressant augmentation by T3 is neither as effective nor as predictable as the response produced by the addition of lithium.

Early reports documented the potential usefulness of combining cyclic antidepressants with monoamine oxidase inhibitors. Clinical experience as well as recent evidence, however, suggests that this combination may not enhance efficacy in a cyclic antidepressant nonresponder. Although not as toxic as once believed, the combination is not recommended for general clinical use. The use of MAO inhibitors alone, however, in the treatment of cyclic resistant patients is sometimes surprisingly successful. Although MAO inhibitors traditionally have been reserved for use with patients having a so-called "atypical depression" [a depression that is characterized by a considerable degree of anxiety, and which does not meet the *Diagnostic and Statistical Manual of Mental Disorder, Third Edition (DSM-III)* criteria for Major Depressive Disorder], clinicians have observed that when platelet monoamine oxidase levels have been inhibited by at least 80 percent, patients with major depressive disorder sometimes also show a therapeutic response. For patients who can tolerate the side effects of monoamine oxidase inhibitors, the switch to this class of antidepressants constitutes another step in the therapeutic approach to the cyclic antidepressant resistant depressed patient.

Most clinicians who have been unsuccessful in treating a patient with a major depressive disorder with cyclic antidepressants, second generation antidepressants, monoamine oxidase inhibitors, or adjunctive therapy turn to ECT. As already noted, ECT is one of the treatments of choice for delusional depression. It is also a treatment of choice for patients with severe major depressive disorder who have not responded to any pharmacotherapy. Although some controversy still surrounds the use of ECT, its therapeutic effectiveness in major depressive disorder is well known. Many clinicians, in fact, would recommend ECT as the *first* treatment in severe, life-threatening depressions, and as the second-line treatment for antidepressant resistant patients (that is, given instead of exposing the patient to further drug toxicity with drug combinations).

ANXIETY DISORDERS

Generalized Anxiety Disorder

Most clinicians, sharing a concern about benzodiazepine tolerance and dependence, usually attempt to prescribe these drugs only for brief periods. This is typically accomplished during times of acute stress or crisis. Unfortunately, since anxiety tends to recur, many patients, especially those with chronic physical illness (Mellinger et al, 1984), cannot be managed with short-term benzodiazepine use and take the drugs on a regular basis for long periods.

In most patients, tolerance to the antianxiety effect of benzodiazepines does not seem to develop with chronic use (Rickels et al, 1983), although tolerance to the sedative effect does occur. The development of abstinence symptoms upon abrupt cessation of benzodiazepine suggests physiological dependence. In general, these withdrawal symptoms are more severe when the benzodiazepines have been taken in high doses, or for a long period of time, or both. In one study, withdrawal reactions occurred in 43 percent of patients treated for 8 months, but in only 5 percent of patients treated for less than 8 months (Rickels et al, 1983). Withdrawal symptoms include sleep disturbance, irritability, tension, anxiety, panic, hand tremor, profuse sweating, decreased concentration, dry retching, nausea, weight loss, palpitations, muscular pains, stiffness, seizures, psychosis, dry mouth, choking feelings, "legs like jelly," decreased appetite, occasional morning vomiting, and mild depression (Lader and Petersson, 1983; Lader, 1983; Salzman, 1984a). The short acting benzodiazepines (oxazepam, Serax; lorazepam, Ativan; alprazolam, Xanax) are more likely to produce severe withdrawal symptoms upon abrupt cessation.

Although many patients are prescribed benzodiazepines for relief of both physical and emotional symptoms, not all of these patients actually need ongoing antianxiety treatment. In one study, at least one-third of patients had their medication discontinued without clinical worsening (Rickels et al, 1983). Considering the likelihood of drug dependence, it may be useful for clinicians to attempt a trial of gradual benzodiazepine withdrawal in all chronically medicated patients in order to identify the substantial proportion who may not require continuous chronic drug therapy (Rickels et al, 1984). Successful intermittent benzodiazepine treatment may prevent the development of drug dependence.

Panic Disorder

Panic disorder is a common crippling illness (Marks and Lader, 1973). In milder forms, it inhibits freedom of movement and quality of life of the sufferer. In its more extreme forms, the sufferer may be phobic and able to function only in severely proscribed circumstances. Because the panic attack is an overwhelming and usually terrifying experience, sufferers also constantly expect, and attempt to guard against, future attacks. This leads to a severe secondary anticipatory anxiety. In addition, a variety of coping strategies arise that include regression, interpersonal manipulation, magical thinking, and rationalization. Psychotherapy is of limited usefulness and traditional antianxiety medication offers no substantial relief. Behavioral treatment is often only partially effective in reducing the symptoms.

There have been many theories about the development of panic disorder, including those based on psychodynamic or behavioral principles. Recent evidence has suggested that patients with panic disorders have a dysregulation of the norepinephrine neurotransmission system and that the psychological and behavioral components of the syndrome may be secondary to this or other biological dysfunctions (Charney et al, 1984; Nesse et al, 1984).

One of the more extraordinary developments in modern psychopharmacology has been the successful treatment of panic disorder using "antidepressant" drugs. These drugs have been so successful that many clinicians now consider them to be the first choice treatment for this disorder. There are three classes of drugs utilized: tricyclic antidepressants, especially imipramine; MAO inhibitors, especially phenelzine; and alprazolam, a new benzodiazepine (suggested to have antidepressant properties). Each drug has clear advantages and drawbacks.

Imipramine was the first drug to be used successfully for the treatment of panic anxiety. Approximately 80–85 percent of patients with panic anxiety have been estimated to show significant therapeutic response to imipramine. No cyclic antidepressant has been shown to be more efficacious than imipramine, and some authors consider it as the drug of first choice (Klein, 1985). Doses of imipramine to treat panic are comparable to those used for depression, 150–300 mg/day (Liebowitz, 1985). Lower starting doses, however, are generally recommended, averaging 25–50 mgs at bedtime with gradual dosage increments of 25–50 mgs until panic is alleviated. If the patient has not completely responded, imipramine blood levels should be checked and the dosage should be increased until a blood level of at least 200 ngs/ml is achieved. The side effects of imipramine treatment of panic disorder includes the familiar triad of tachycardia, orthostatic hypotension, and anticholinergic symptoms. Some panic disorder patients experience over-stimulation, even at low doses; for some, weight gain is a potential unwanted side effect.

Like imipramine, the MAO inhibitors are very effective in suppressing panic attacks. Clinical experience has suggested that phenelzine may actually be slightly superior to imipramine (Sheehan et al, 1980). The side effects of phenelzine are well known: potential hypertensive crisis, orthostatic hypotension, weight gain, and anorgasmia. The weight gain may be substantial in some cases. Although several drugs, including cyproheptadine (Sovner, 1984) and bethanocol have been suggested for the treatment of anorgasmia, there is no consistently successful treatment for this side effect other than dose reduction or drug discontinuance. Less frequent side effects include edema and myoclonic jerks. The edema sometimes partially responds to diuretics; there may be a partial response of the myoclonic jerks to vitamin B_6 or to low doses of clonazepam.

For some patients, the side effects of phenelzine outweigh the therapeutic effect and limit the usefulness of this drug. For others, however, the side effects actually occur less frequently and are less severe than with imipramine. Furthermore, most patients who respond to the panic blocking effect of phenelzine do not find the dietary restrictions onerous or the side effects overwhelming.

Alprazolam has demonstrated antipanic effects in doses of 3–10 mg/day (Sheehan et al, 1984), although maximum daily doses of 4–6 mg are more usual. Patients are usually started on 0.25–0.5 mgs three times daily with meals, and dosage increments of 0.25–0.5 mg every one to two days are usually well tolerated. There may be dosage plateaus during the initial weeks of treatment until a stable antipanic dose is reached (Sheehan, 1985). The antipanic effect of alprazolam may be most noticeable in patients whose panic is mild to moderate in severity. In patients with very severe panic disorder, alprazolam may reduce or attenuate the panic episodes, but may not eliminate them entirely. Alprazolam may also be very effective as an adjunctive agent for use in patients treated with imipramine or phenelzine, should there be only a partial therapeutic response. The typical side effects of alprazolam include sedation, unsteadiness, and slurring of speech. Occasional forgetfulness, irritability, and an impairment of motivation has also been noticed (Sheehan, 1985). Dependence on this drug is common; clinical experience suggests that withdrawal symptoms upon abrupt cessation are particularly severe.

Whichever drug is chosen, patients should be treated for at least six symptom-free months before a dose tapering or drug discontinuation is considered. During this six-month period, many clinicians encourage their patients to place themselves in settings which had previously been associated with a panic attack. If the patient has remained symptom-free for six months during which time re-exposure to panic stimuli has occurred, then dosage tapering may begin. Relapse figures are variable and are, at best, estimates. Typically, however, many patients show a return of panic episodes even after continuous drug treatment for two or more years. Drug withdrawal from alprazolam is often more difficult than from tricyclics or monoamine oxidase inhibitors. As with other benzodiazepines, withdrawal from alprazolam produces heightened anxiety and insomnia. Relapse rates may be as high as 80 percent during alprazolam withdrawal (Klein, 1985).

Given the efficacy of all three drugs in patients with panic disorder, the clinician must select among them on the basis of a number of factors. Severity of panic symptoms; the patient's cardiovascular status; the patient's potential sensitivity to anticholinergic, orthostatic hypotensive, and cardiac side effects; the use of concomitant medication; and the ability to follow an MAO inhibitor diet must all be considered.

For many patients, imipramine is probably the best first choice antipanic drug. Most patients will respond and if doses are kept within a modest range, side effects should be mild. Imipramine should not be prescribed to patients who are likely to be sensitive to anticholinergic side effects, who have cardiac conduction disorders, or who are taking medication known to interact with imipramine. Blood levels of imipramine may be monitored to guide the dosage, and, as noted, widening of the QRS on the EKG is a signal of impending cardiac toxicity (Salzman, 1985).

Alprazolam is suggested for patients with mild to moderate panic, but should be prescribed with caution to patients who are taking other benzodiazepines, other central nervous system (CNS) sedatives, or who cannot voluntarily restrict their alcohol intake. Patients who take alprazolam should be told of the high likelihood of developing physiological dependence, and should be instructed not to abruptly discontinue the drug. If no therapeutic response occurs at doses between 4–6 mg/day, or if sedation or other side effects compromise daily functioning, then the patient should be switched to imipramine or phenelzine.

For patients with severe, crippling panic disorder, or for those patients who have not responded to other antipanic medication, or who cannot tolerate imipramine or alprazolam side effects, phenelzine should be prescribed. A pretreatment platelet monoamine oxidase level is necessary. Most patients will respond at doses between 45–75 mg/day. In nonresponding patients, the dose should be increased until platelet monoamine oxidase levels have been suppressed to at least 80 percent of the pretreatment level, unless side effects become too intense. Patients should be told about the diet and warned about the weight gain, dizziness, anorgasmia, edema, and myoclonic jerks. In responsive patients who develop intolerable side effects, a switch from phenelzine to tranylcypromine may be helpful (Klein, 1985).

Whichever drug is used, patients should be maintained on their therapeutic regimen for 6–12 symptom-free months, with panic-stimulus challenges. At the end of this period, very slow tapering should be initiated. A return of clinically significant panic suggests the need for ongoing treatment.

SCHIZOPHRENIA

Although no new drugs have become available for the treatment of schizophrenia, several new strategies for the use of neuroleptics have recently been developed. The stimulus for these strategies has been twofold. First, there has been a growing realization among clinicians that high dose neuroleptic treatment has only limited usefulness in schizophrenia (Donlon et al, 1980) and actually may be potentially very dangerous (Salzman and Hoffman, 1982). Second, it has become clear that various neuroleptic side effects, including tardive dyskinesia and akathisia, may both compromise the therapeutic effect of the drugs themselves (van Putten, 1974; Ratey and Salzman, 1984) and interfere with a patient's participation in other therapeutic programs (Rifkin and Kane, 1984). Thus, the new strategies are all designed to provide for optimal control of psychosis and disruptive behavior while using the lowest possible dosages. The strategies are reviewed below: One is particularly useful in the treatment of acutely ill schizophrenic patients; the other two have been designed for use in patients with chronic schizophrenia.

Strategy for the Low Dose Management of Acute Behavioral Disruption in Schizophrenia

Agitation, restlessness, assaultiveness, and rage can be seen in either an acute schizophrenic process or in an exacerbation of a more chronic illness. In the past, such symptoms have often been treated by giving sedating "low-potency" neuroleptics (such as chlorpromazine or thioridazine) until the patient is calmed, sedated, or even asleep. An alternative approach has employed very high doses of nonsedating high-potency neuroleptics generally given parenterally until behavior control is achieved. Both of these traditional treatment approaches are associated with the development of common neuroleptic side effects such as orthostatic hypotension and acute extrapyramidal reactions.

A new strategy for the control of behavioral disruption accompanying the schizophrenic process involves the use of intramuscular benzodiazepines, given together with low doses of high potency intramuscular neuroleptics (Koster van Groos, 1973); Modell et al, 1985; Salzman et al, 1986). The combination of 5 mgs of intramuscular haloperidol (or another parenterally administered nonsedating neuroleptic) in combination with 1 or 2 mg of intramuscular lorazepam has been especially successful in producing immediate control of disruptive behaviors in patients. Early data suggests that most patients require only one or two such double injections; oral neuroleptic treatment without benzodiazepines may then be instituted or continued (Salzman et al, 1986). Although further research is being conducted, this combined approach holds promise as an effective but relatively nontoxic method of managing acute behavioral problems associated with schizophrenia.

Strategy for the Maintenance Treatment of Chronic Schizophrenia

As stated above, lower dose neuroleptic treatment of chronic schizophrenic patients is being attempted in certain groups of patients. There have been several strategies employed. The first involves simply a reduction of the neuroleptic dose. While it is generally agreed that significant neuroleptic dose reduction may result in increased rates of relapse in chronic schizophrenic patients (Davis, 1975; Herz and Melville, 1980; Kane, 1984), not all patients relapse. Recently, a carefully controlled dose reduction study, while confirming the data about increased likelihood of relapse, also noted that the chronic schizophrenic patients whose neuroleptic doses had been reduced had better social adjustment in the community (Rifkin and Kane, 1984). This study suggested, therefore, that although risk of relapse might be increased, neuroleptic dosage reduction brought about enough gains in other aspects of the quality of the schizophrenic patient's life to justify careful use of this strategy.

Other studies have suggested that imminent relapse following dose reduction can be predicted by an increase in thought disturbance, paranoia, tension, and anxiety (Herz et al, 1982; Marder et al, 1984). These data, in light of the observation that chronic schizophrenic patients may function better on lower doses, have stimulated the development of an alternative dose reduction strategy. Called intermittent or targeted treatment, it involves using medication only when psychotic or prodromal symptoms appear and withdrawing or reducing doses when no psychosis is present. Careful observation of the patients for signs of prodromal symptoms enables drugs to be rapidly reinstituted, if necessary (Herz et al, 1982; Carpenter et al, 1984).

Most clinicians would probably agree that the use of the lowest possible dose of neuroleptic to maintain a reasonable level of functioning in patients with chronic schizophrenia is a worthwhile goal. Finding this optimal low dose, whether on a continuous dose or intermittent treatment basis, however, requires frequent contact with the patient and complete cooperation between patient, family, and treating physician. A stable treatment environment without rotation of prescribing psychiatrists is also necessary. Unfortunately, many patients with chronic schizophrenia, as well as their families, cannot meet these criteria; many outpatient mental health clinics, community mental health centers, and medication clinics are not sufficiently staffed to provide the close medication supervision and personal continuity that may be necessary for these approaches to be successful. This raises questions about the practical application of these dosage reduction strategies in nonresearch settings. Nevertheless, the clinical lesson to be learned from these dose reduction studies is clear and deserves wide broadcast: Some patients with schizophrenia, when treated with reduced doses of neuroleptics, or intermittently with neuroleptics, may actually have their quality of life improved even though their risk of relapse is increased.

CONCLUSION

The practicing psychiatrist may, at times, feel overwhelmed by the plethora of recently published information regarding new psychotropic drugs or drug prescribing techniques. Nevertheless, basic issues of diagnostic assessment and differential toxicity continue to be the most significant determinants of psycho-pharmacological treatment for two reasons. First, an accurate diagnosis is essential for effective treatment and is often the best predictor of treatment response. In all cases of treatment failure (so-called treatment resistance) the diagnosis should be questioned and re-evaluated. Second, since different therapeutic indications have generally not been established for drugs within the same class (for example, neuroleptics, cyclic antidepressants, benzodiazepines), the selection of a particular drug is usually based on side effect profiles. If one drug in the class, when prescribed, causes unacceptable side effects, another should be tried.

When a psychotropic drug has been ineffective and the diagnosis is thought to be correct, two other prescribing principles should be remembered. First, an adequate dosage and treatment period must be utilized. Frequently, subtherapeutic dosages and/or inadequate length of treatment are misread as treatment resistance. Second, even though one drug at adequate dosage and length of treatment does not work, another drug of the same class often may work and should be tried.

In addition to applying these basic pharmacotherapeutic principles, the practicing clinician must attempt to learn about new combinations of drugs or new strategies of drug treatment, some of which are reviewed in this chapter, that offer an expanded selection of treatments for the difficult patient. However, when reading the psychopharmacology literature, the practicing clinician must remember that single case reports or nonblind comparisons may often be misleading; new techniques must be evaluated in a patient sample large enough to justify conclusions regarding therapeutic efficacy and toxicity. Only after a cautious evaluation (which may take years) should new treatment techniques be accepted into general clinical practice.

REFERENCES

Ayd FJ Jr: Carbamazepine therapy for manic depresive illness: an update. International Drug Therapy Newsletter 21:9-12, 1986

Ballenger SC, Post RM: Therapeutic effects of carbamazepine in affective illness: a preliminary report. Psychopharmacology 2:159-175, 1978

Carpenter WT Jr; Heinrichs DW: Intermittent pharmacotherapy of schizophrenia, in Drug Maintenance Strategies in Schizophrenia. Edited by Kane JM. Washington, DC, American Psychiatric Press Inc., 1984

Charney DS, Heninger GR, Brier A: Noradrenergic factors in panic anxiety. Arch Gen Psychiatry 41:751-763, 1984

Davis JM: Overview—maintenance therapy in psychiatry, I: schizophrenia. Am J Psychiatry 132:1237-1245, 1975

de Montigny C, Cournoyer R, Morisette R, et al: Lithium carbonate addition in tricyclic antidepressant-resistant unipolar depression. Arch Gen Psychiatry 40:1327-1334, 1983

Donlon PT, Hopkin JT, Tupin JP, et al: Haloperidol for acute schizophrenic patients: an evaluation of three oral regimens. Arch Gen Psychiatry 37:691-695, 1980

Glassman AH, Kantor SJ, Shostak M: Depression, delusions, and drug response. Am J Psychiatry 132:716-719, 1975

Goodwin FK, Prange AJ, Post RM, et al:Potentiation of antidepressant effects by L–triiodothyronine in tricyclic non-responders. Am J Psychiatry 139:34-38, 1982

Greenblatt M, Grosser GH, Wechsler HA: A comparative study of selected antidepressants medication and ECT. Am J Psychiatry 119:144-153, 1962

Heninger GR, Charney DS, Sternberg DE: Lithium carbonate augmentation of antidepressant treatment. Arch Gen Psychiatry 40:1335-1342, 1983

Herz MI, Melville C: Relapse in schizophrenia. Am J Psychiatry 137:801-805, 1980

Herz MI, Szymanski HV, Simon JC: Intermittent medication for stable schizophrenic outpatients: an alternative to maintenance medication. Am J Psychiatry 139:918-922, 1982

Jann MW, Ereshefsky L, Sakland SR, et al: Effects of carbamazepine on plasma haloperidol levels. J Clin Psychopharmacol 5:106-109, 1985

Kane JM: Dosage reduction strategies in the long term treatment of schizophrenia, in Drug Maintenance Strategies in Schizophrenia. Edited by Kane JM. Washington, DC, American Psychiatric Press Inc., 1984

Klein DF: An update on panic disorders. Currents 4:5-10, 1985

Koster van Groos GA: Treatment of neurotic and psychotic anxiety with lorazepam. Curr Med Res Opin 1:288-290, 1973

Kwentus JA, Qureshi GD, Lingon N, et al: Aplastic anemia: a complication of carbamazepine in a psychotic patient. J Clin Psychopharmacol 5:183, 1985

Lader M: Dependence on benzodiazepines. J Clin Psychiatry 44:121-127, 1983

Lader M, Petersson H: Abuse liability of anxiolytics, in Anxiolytics: Neurochemical, Behavioral and Clinical Perspectives. Edited by Malick ES, Yamayura HJ. New York, Raven Press, 1983

Liebowitz MR: Imipramine in the treatment of panic disorder and its complications. Psychiatr Clin North Am 8:37-48, 1985

Lipinski JF, Pope HG Jr: Possible synergistic action between carbamazepine and lithium carbonate in the treatment of three acutely manic patients. Am J Psychiatry 139:948-949, 1982

Marder SR, van Putten T, Mintz J, et al: Maintenance therapy in schizophrenia: new findings, in Drug Maintenance Strategies in Schizophrenia. Edited by Kane JM. Washington, DC, American Psychiatric Press Inc., 1984

Marks I, Lader M: Anxiety states (anxiety neurosis): a review. J Nerv Ment Dis 150:3-18, 1973

Mellinger GD, Balter MB, Uhlenhuth EH: Prevalence and correlates of the long-term regular use of anxiolytics. JAMA 251:375-379, 1984

Modell JG, Lenox RH, Weiner S: Inpatient clinical trial of lorazepam for the management of manic agitation. J Clin Psychopharmacol 5:109-113, 1985

National Institute of Mental Health: Consensus Development Conference Statements VOC, 1986

Nelson JC, Mazure CM: Lithium augmentation in psychotic depression refractory to combined drug treatment. Am J Psychiatry 143:363-366, 1986

Nesse RM, Cameron OG, Curtis GC, et al: Adrenergic function in patients with panic anxiety. Arch Gen Psychiatry 41:771-776, 1984

Okuma T: Therapeutic and prophylactic effects of carbamazepine in bipolar disorders. Psychiatr Clin North Am 41:771-776, 1984

Patterson JF: Stevens-Johnson syndrome associated with carbamazepine therapy. J Clin Psychopharmacol 5:185, 1985

Piscotta AV: Hematologic toxicity of carbamazepine. Adv Neurol 11:423-439, 1975

Post RM: Carbamazepine (Tegretol) and affective disorders. Currents 5:5-10, 1986

Post RM, Ballenger JC, Uhde TW, et al: Efficacy of carbamazepine in manic-depressive illness: implication for underlying mechanism, in Neurobiology of the Mood Disorders. Edited by Post RM, Ballenger JC. Baltimore, Williams and Wilkins, 1984

Prange AJ, Loosen PT, Wilson K, et al: The therapeutic use of hormones of the thyroid axis in depression, Neurobiology of Mood Disorders. Edited by Post RM, Ballenger JC. Baltimore, Williams and Wilkins, 1984

Price LH, Conwell Y, Nelson JC: Lithium augmentation of combined neuroleptic-tricyclic treatment in delusional depression. Am J Psychiatry 140:318-322, 1983

Quitkin FM, Rabkin JG, Ross D, et al: Duration of antidepressant drug treatment. Arch Gen Psychiatry 41:238-245, 1984

Rabkin JG, Klein DF, Quitkin F: Somatic treatment of acute depression, in Schizophrenia and Affective Disorders. Edited by Rifkin A. Bristol, England, John Wright & Sons Ltd., 1983

Ratey JJ, Salzman C: Recognizing and managing akathesia. Hosp Community Psychiatry 35:975-977, 1984

Rickels K, Case GW, Downing RW, et al: Long-term diazepam therapy and clinical outcome. JAMA 250:767-771, 1983

Rickels K, Case GW, Winnoker A, et al: Long-term benzodiazepine therapy: benefits and risks. Psychopharmacol Bull 20:608-615, 1984

Rifkin A, Kane JM: Low dose neuroleptic maintenance treatment of schizophrenia, in Drug Maintenance Strategies in Schizophrenia. Edited by Kane JM. Washington, DC, American Psychiatric Press Inc., 1984

Salzman C: Benzodiazepine habituation and withdrawal. Family Pract 6:39-47, 1984a

Salzman C: Overview, in Clinical Geriatric Psychopharmacology. Edited by Salzman C. New York, McGraw-Hill, 1984b

Salzman C: Clinical use of antidepressant blood levels and the electrocardiogram. New Engl J Med 313:512-513, 1985

Salzman C, Hoffman SA: Rapid tranquilization. Hosp Community Psychiatry 33:346, 1982

Salzman C, van der Kölk BA: Treatment of depression, in Clinical Geriatric Psychopharmacology. Edited by Salzman C. New York, McGraw-Hill, 1984

Salzman C, Green AI, Rodriguez-Villa F, et al: Benzodiazepines combined with neuroleptics for acute and severe disruptive behavior. Psychosomatics 27 (suppl):17-21, 1986

Schwartz G, Halanis A, Baxter L, et al: Normal thyroid function in desipramine nonresponders converted to responders by the addition of L–triiodothyronine. Am J Psychiatry 141:1614-1616, 1984

Sheehan DV: Monoamine oxidase inhibitors and alprazolam in the treatment of panic disorder and agoraphobia. Psychiatr Clin North Am 8:49-62, 1985

Sheehan DV, Ballenger J, Jacobsen G: Treatment of endogenous anxiety with phobic hysterical and hypochondriacal symptoms. Arch Gen Psychiatry 37:51-59, 1980

Sheehan DV, Coleman JH, Greenblatt DJ, et al: Some biochemical correlates of panic attacks with agoraphobia and their response to a new treatment. J Clin Psychopharmacol 4:66-75, 1984

Shukla S, Godwin CD, Long LEB, et al: Lithium carbamazepine neurotoxicity and risk factors. Am J Psychiatry 141:1604-1606, 1984

Sovner R: Treatment of tricyclic antidepressant-induced orgasmic inhibition with cyproheptadine (letter). J Clin Psychopharmacol 4:169, 1984

Spiker DG, Weiss JC, Dealy RS, et al: The pharmacological treatment of delusional depression. Am J Psychiatry 142:430-436, 1985

Takazaki H, Hanacka M: The use of carbamazepine (tegretol) in the control of manic-depressive states. Seishu-Igaku 13:1310-1318, 1971

van Putten T: Why do schizophrenic patients refuse to take their drugs? Arch Gen Psychiatry 31:67-72, 1974

Yerevanian BI, Hodgman CH: A haloperidol-carbamazepine interaction in a patient with rapid-cycling bipolar disorder. Am J Psychiatry 142:785-786, 1985

Young YY, Ludden TM, Bell RD: Effect of erythromycin on carbamazepine kinetics. Clin Pharmacol Ther 33:460-464, 1983

Chapter 18

Differential Therapeutics: Clinical, Teaching, Research, and Administrative Issues

by Allen J. Frances, M.D., M. Katherine Shear, M.D., and Minna Fyer, M.D.

A systematic attention to differential therapeutics of the sort suggested in previous chapters of this section will necessarily impact on every aspect of psychiatric clinical, educational, research, and administrative practice. Surprisingly little has been written about these implications of differential therapeutics and, in many settings, relatively little thought is given either to the process of treatment selection or to its consequences. The purpose of this chapter is to highlight the various factors that lead to optimal patient/treatment matchups. Although, for clarity of presentation, we will present separate sections for the clinical, educational, research, and administrative issues that are involved, in actual practice these are inextricably intertwined and are best considered together and in an integrated fashion. We hope that this chapter will help psychiatrists and other mental health professionals, whether they be clinicians, educators, researchers, or administrators (or all of these), and whether they are in private, hospital, or agency practice, to think through the many practical issues that render differential therapeutics a difficult, but also fascinating, endeavor.

CLINICAL ISSUES

Careful attention to differential therapeutics results in a fairly dramatic change in the methods used in evaluating patients for treatment. It is often desirable to clarify for the potential patient, during the very first phone contact, that the initial visits will be used to provide a psychiatric consultation and are not necessarily the beginning of the psychiatric treatment. The psychiatric consultation will consist of data gathering, discussions about diagnosis, and joint negotiations to determine whether, what kind, and with whom treatment is indicated. Unless this is made explicit before the data gathering actually begins, most patients will naturally assume that the person doing the consultation will also provide the treatment, and most consultants will slip easily into their favorite forms of treatment without a careful consideration of the choices involved in treatment selection. We believe that this is an error which reduces the attention to differential treatment selection as perhaps the most important function of the evaluation. The key to good treatment selection is a good consultation.

The best descriptions of the consumer oriented approach to psychiatric evaluation have been provided by Lazare and Eisenthal (1979). These authors have demonstrated the great value of engaging the patient in an active collaboration and negotiation throughout the consultation period. This results in improved data gathering and decision making (in many instances the patient does know best). Moreover, an informed consumer is much more likely subsequently to follow through upon whatever plans are made and to participate more intelligently and enthusiastically in the treatment endeavor.

There has also been a recent upsurge of interest in the development of psychoeducational programs for affective (Beck et al, 1981), anxiety (Mathews et al, 1981), schizophrenic (Anderson et al, 1986), and other disorders. This is in recognition of the fact that patients usually begin the psychiatric consultation quite ignorant about the nature, course, prognosis, and treatment of their condition and are likely to feel confused, demoralized, and isolated by their symptoms. It is enormously reassuring to discover that one is not alone—that the symptoms are common enough to be well understood and that effective treatments are available. For many patients it is also a pleasant surprise to have a doctor explain what is happening in a detailed and straightforward fashion. The most frequent complaints voiced by patients about the treatment they receive from doctors (of all specialties) is that they don't discuss in enough detail the diagnosis, cause, and treatment of the presenting symptoms and don't leave sufficient time for answering the many questions that arise. In many instances, it is wise to include the family in at least some of the discussions.

After educating the patient about the condition, the next step in the consultation is to lay out the treatment options. These should cover whichever aspects of the treatment decision tree are most pertinent in the given clinical situation (that is, setting, format, orientation, duration and frequency, use of medication, the possibility of no treatments, and so on). This should be done with sufficient detail, clarity, and simplicity so that the patient (and perhaps family) can become informed consumers choosing among the alternative treatments that might be offered. There are, of course, a small minority of patients who are too anxious, disorganized, or dependent to participate meaningfully in such an educational and decision making process, and who will therefore be offered less education and less responsibility for the choices made. This is a matter to be determined by the clinical judgment of the consultant. We would caution, however, that our experience suggests that consultants consistently underestimate their patients' interest in and capacity for learning about their conditions and helping to make treatment decisions.

The next step in the consultation consists of a negotiation between consultant and patient (and sometimes also family members) concerning what steps will be taken next. The nature of the negotiation, and the relative contribution made by patient and consultant, will vary depending on the urgency of the situation, the capacity of the patient, and the seeming clarity of the best next step. At the extreme of minimal negotiation is an involuntary commitment to the hospital for a dangerous manic patient who has an urgent condition, little capacity, and a clearcut optimal treatment. At the extreme of maximal patient choice is the frequent situation in outpatient practice in which there is little urgency, the patient is fully competent, and a number of different treatments are close possible contenders. In this latter situation, the consultant should carefully explain the nature, goals, setting, demands, and techniques of each intervention (perhaps providing some educational comment about the specific advantages and disadvantages of each for the particular patient) and then let the patient make the final decision.

In many instances, the consultant may not feel expert enough to describe one (or more) of the possible treatment choices in a way that would do it justice. This is an indication for the patient to have additional consultations with therapists who can provide data on these other possible treatment options. This allows the patient to determine how professionals with different experience and training each formulate the problem, and to learn firsthand the ways in which the treatment might be conducted within the other models.

Another advantage of multiple consultations before deciding with whom to begin treatment is that it provides the patient with a wider selection of therapist personalities as well as of alternative methods. There is good evidence that the therapeutic alliance measured early in treatment is the best predictor of treatment outcome (Hartley, 1985). It therefore makes great sense to increase the odds of a good therapist/patient personality match by allowing the patient to interact with several different therapists before choosing the one preferred for the treatment. All of us generally like to exercise this kind of freedom of choice before selecting a car mechanic, an accountant, or a mentor. The chemistry of the interpersonal matching is probably even more crucial for psychiatric patients and their therapists. Patients usually welcome this suggestion, although they do not always act on it. The fact that the consultant is flexible enough to encourage them to meet with other therapists often has the paradoxical result of increasing the patient's desire to be treated by the consultant. Private practitioners who understandably are interested in increasing the rate at which patients in consultation become treatment patients may thus paradoxically achieve this by providing the opportunity for such patients to see other potential therapists before deciding with whom they want to work. We have also organized our hospital outpatient clinic to allow for such choice of therapist for those patients who want or need it (Andrews et al, in press).

A question that consistently arises in negotiating and choosing a treatment is the degree to which patients should have modest or ambitious goals for the treatment. More ambitious goals usually require more commitment, time, and money. In most instances, it is the consultant's job to lay out the possible benefits and demands of the different treatment options and the patient's job to decide amongst them. The choice of the sex of the therapist is often related to the ambitiousness of the treatment. Most patients have an obvious preference regarding whether the therapist should be male or female. If the treatment is meant to be supportive and quickly to ameliorate symptoms, it is usually best for the patient to have a therapist of the sex that comes most naturally, since this will reduce the risk of dropout and make for an easier and faster working relationship. If the treatment goals include character change, it generally makes more sense for the patient to select the therapist whose sex will more thoroughly smoke out transference problems, even if this makes the initial work together more difficult.

Even beyond the initial consultation period, a concern for differential therapeutics will often continue to inform important treatment decisions. If a treatment becomes stalemated, it may be wise to have a consultation and to consider adding or subtracting other treatment possibilities. All too often patient and therapist wait patiently and endlessly for a light at the end of the tunnel in a treatment that just isn't likely ever to work.

A lack of response is the best indication for trying a different approach. A patient who has previously received a long duration of unsuccessful individual treatment should probably try a group or family treatment, and vice versa. Many of our treatment decisions in psychiatry (perhaps most) are no more than best guesses and need not be adhered to forever if there are no signs of progress. Almost always there are effective alternatives, and flexibility is the better part of valor in recommending them. The best predictor that something will not work in the future is its failure to have worked in the past (Frances H, et al, 1984a). The same may be said for problems in the interpersonal chemistry of the patient/therapist match. In some instances, such difficulties are no more than the result of the expected transference evolution and require interpretation and working through. Often, however, patients and therapists are so encumbered by an interpersonal mismatch that they cannot form an effective therapeutic alliance to resolve whatever (perhaps mutual transference difficulties) accounts for their friction. Our experience in such situations suggests strongly that a no-fault switch of therapists is often desirable and results in much better "second marriages" of patients and therapists (Andrews et al, in press).

A concern about the knowledge of differential therapeutics is likely to decrease clinical dogmatism and increase therapist and patient resourcefulness in finding a treatment approach that will work. There is usually an effective treatment available if both parties look hard enough for it.

EDUCATIONAL ISSUES

There is no single or best method of teaching differential therapeutics. An integrated program combining didactic and clinical approaches is more effective than the sum of the individual parts. We will discuss the following educational components, as they might interact in a psychiatric residency program: the curriculum, the clinical experience, the treatment planning conference, and the supervisors.

The Curriculum

The didactic curriculum should include a course that focuses specifically on differential therapeutics and also require that instructors teaching courses on the various psychiatric treatments emphasize the issue of criteria for patient selection. The course on differential therapeutics at the Payne Whitney Clinic consists of five sessions given during the summer of the third year of the psychiatric residency. The first session is an overview of psychotherapy outcome research and its relationship to differential therapeutics. The most pertinent findings from the literature are summarized, emphasizing those reviews that aggregate results across studies. The methodological limitations of the available research are identified, especially those that may explain why findings do not yet demonstrate specific outcome differences for different treatments. There is a discussion outlining the designs for the ideal research studies for answering questions about differential therapeutics, and an exploration of the ways in which the findings generated by such studies might be used to guide clinical practice.

The next three meetings are devoted to a study of the clinical and research literature concerning each of the steps that comprise the decision tree discussed in previous chapters of this section: 1) the setting of treatment (for example, inpatient, partial hospital, or outpatient); 2) the format (individual, group, or family); 3) the orientation (psychodynamic, learning, systems, or biological) 4) the frequency and duration; and 5) the match of therapist to patient and so on.

For each of the choices on each step of the algorithm, the pertinent systematic research (if there is any), the variety of clinical opinions reported in the literature, and our own clinical experience are combined to arrive at a set of indications, contraindications, and enabling factors. There is then a discussion of how recommendations are made from among the competing alternatives and the ways in which different approaches may best be combined. The last meeting of the course is used for a detailed discussion of illustrative cases (Perry et al, 1985). The class is encouraged to share opinions, and often differences, on how to apply the data presented in the previous sessions to the complexity of the clinical situation. It is this part of the course that is in many ways the most interesting.

The Clinical Experience

Because we believe that the evaluation of a new patient is the most crucial of all psychiatric skills, we provide a number of different clinical experiences throughout the training program to ensure that all graduates are widely experienced and thoroughly supervised in this activity. Virtually all mental health professionals, however else they spend their time, are engaged throughout their careers in doing consultations. Training in consultations and differential therapeutics should occur in every year of the training program at progressively increasing levels of sophistication.

Experiences in evaluation alone are not sufficient for differential therapeutics to come fully alive. Trainees should also have supervised clinical experiences delivering a number of the different treatments they are recommending for their patients. We believe that trainees should have a varied mix of somatic, psychodynamic, behavioral, cognitive, and system treatments, provided individually and in group and family contexts, and in varied contexts and settings, and they should become familiar with both brief and long-term work. Furthermore, the discussion of differential treatment choices between supervisor and trainee will have maximum impact to the extent that it leads to a real decision. This implies that the clinic be prepared to expand its treatments to provide previously lacking services when a need for them has been identified (an issue addressed again below, under the heading "Administration").

The Conference

A weekly Treatment Planning Conference provides an opportunity to review and advise on all dispositions made on patients evaluated during that week. The conference serves various purposes. In some instances, the evaluating trainee, the patient, and the supervisor have already made what seems to them to be the obvious decision, and the trainee comes to the conference hoping to receive fairly quick confirmation. We usually, but not always, find ourselves in agreement, and in cases of disagreement we must decide whether it is worth reopening the issue with the patient. In many instances, however, the evaluating clinician, the patient, and supervisor are unsure of what to choose, and the conference offers a fascinating opportunity to ponder the uncertainties occasioned by tough treatment decisions. The conference also serves as a clinical clearinghouse matching patient need with agency resources. It provides an in vivo opportunity to teach residents and staff the principles of differential therapeutics and their practical application within the art of the possible. The discussion of treatment decisions provides an excellent opportunity to evaluate trainee and staff performance and clinical judgment, and to focus on areas for additional training.

The Teachers

If a clinic is to provide the wide range of services that enlivens differential therapeutics, it needs practitioners to deliver these services; and, more importantly, it needs teachers to instruct these practitioners and the new trainees. How to get these teachers? One major avenue is the careful and energetic recruitment of full time, part time, and voluntary faculty. It is highly desirable that departments of psychiatry be pluralistic and versatile in their faculties (and not do what comes more naturally in recruiting). If recruitment of individuals skilled in a particular modality is not possible for reasons of finances or availability, it is often helpful to call in an expert consultant on a time limited basis to train the cadre of local teachers who can then maintain and expand the program by teaching others.

Another important issue that arises in regard to the teachers has to do with supervisor–trainee assignments. Some supervisors are excellent teachers, but only within the narrow compass of one therapy, done one particular way, with one group of very highly selected patients. Trainees must also be exposed to supervisors who serve as role models for flexibility and the integration of a variety of models. We also encourage trainees to seek multiple opinions rather than assume that any of their supervisors has any special monopoly on the truth. Moreover, we convey to trainees that they (in conjunction with their service director) are ultimately responsible for whatever decisions are made and cannot beg off by saying "My supervisor told me to do this." Differences of opinion between supervisor and trainee should be aired and settled in coordination with the service director. This is often an interesting learning experience for all involved.

The Results

What are the possible gains and risks of a training program that pays considerable attention to differential therapeutics? Perhaps we should face the risks first. Might we not train a cohort of broadly based and flexible know-nothings who possess a confused hodgepodge of half fact, and such great openess to new developments in the field, that they are prey to every new fad? Is this result any better than the risk in the other direction of producing narrow adherents to a rigid, dogmatic orthodoxy? Obviously either extreme is undesirable and different programs are more likely to succumb to one or the other risk. We believe that the ideal of every training program should be that its graduates are widely knowledgeable, broad as well as deep in their interests, and sufficiently curious to keep learning and growing professionally. Our sense is that a careful attention to differential therapeutics furthers this goal and makes good programs better.

RESEARCH ISSUES

Much of the available treatment outcome literature (especially for the psychotherapies) is relatively uninformative in guiding differential therapeutic decisions because of the failure of studies to demonstrate optimal treatment–patients matchups (Smith et al, 1980). This has been interpreted by some commentators to mean that the various treatments, however different they may appear on the surface, are in fact effective by virtue of shared active ingredients; that is, the so-called nonspecific effects of treatment (Frank, 1978). An alternative interpretation is that most studies have lacked sufficient specificity and refinement to demonstrate the optimal patient/therapy/therapist matchups that do exist. In general, outcome studies have included relatively undefined patient samples; treated them with relatively undefined and possibly overlapping interventions; which are delivered by inexperienced and unsupervised therapists; outcome is assessed with global and relatively nonspecific measures; and, finally, the design aims primarily to find out which treatment is the overall winner rather than asking the more interesting question of which treatment is specifically better in which situation (Frances, et al, 1984b).

Fortunately, a number of recent refinements in the methods of outcome research promise to enhance its relevance to the question of differential treatment selection. This increased specificity of outcome research may increase its resolution sufficiently so as to detect the different specific effects of the alternative treatments. Patient selection, guided by *DSM-III* and other available assessment instruments, is now reliable and clearly specified. Treatments are explicitly targeted for specific patient problems, standardized in operational manuals, distinguished from one another, and carefully supervised and monitored to minimize overlap. A large number of reliable, valid, and specific instruments to access outcome have been developed, allowing the investigator to assess the specific kind of change aimed for by the different treatments delivered in the populations selected. Finally, and in some ways most importantly, research attention has advanced beyond the two primary questions—Does this treatment work? Is it better, in some global way, than the alternatives? Studies are now often designed to determine the more important clinical questions—What are the mechanisms and the active ingredients of the various treatments, and in which particular patients and situations are they least or most effective (Waskow, 1984)?

Another encouraging emerging trend in the outcome research literature is the awareness that for many conditions (particularly affective and anxiety disorders) there are effective medication treatments, but also effective psychotherapies. In these instances, studies are necessary to compare the outcome, side effects, and compliance of drugs versus psychotherapy, to determine the patient characteristics that predict best response to one or another approach, and to determine the nature of the interaction when both types of treatment are used together (so far, results suggest that combined treatment produces additive results). It is important not to regard drugs and psychotherapy as competitors in some sort of horse race. Rather, the comparative studies are meant to define the specific indications for each, as well as for combinations of both.

Despite the reasonable optimism just expressed that outcome research will become increasingly specific and incisive in its approach and will increasingly inform differential treatment selection in psychiatry, certain caveats are definitely in order. The biggest problem is the sheer magnitude of the task. The previous chapters in this section have discussed treatment selection decisions concerning setting, format, orientation, duration and frequency, and the use of medications. Within each of these steps of a treatment selection decision tree there are many alternative possibilities from which to choose (in fact, for orientations perhaps more than 250 types of psychotherapy have been identified) and there are almost endless possible interactions, combinations, and permutations linking the choices made on each of the steps with one another. It would take almost an eternity and an unrealistic disposition of scarce resources to test the differential effectiveness of more than a small fraction even of those choices that seem clinically reasonable. We must recognize that outcome research in psychiatry can target only the most obvious and important differential therapeutic questions. Moreover, each patient represents a complex interaction of hundreds of possibly pertinent predictor variables which would have to be understood in interaction with hundreds of possibly pertinent therapist and therapy variables. Treatment selection, for the foreseeable future, will continue to rely heavily on clinical experiences, patient preference, and common sense. Clinical intuition and clinical judgment can be informed, but not replaced, by our advancing treatment outcome research effort.

ADMINISTRATIVE ISSUES

The explosion of new and specific psychiatric treatments has created a serious administrative dilemma that must be faced in both clinic and private practice settings. Many clinics and private practitioners are expert at delivering just one or a few treatments. Patients who are evaluated under such circumstances are likely to receive whatever treatment is more or less routinely offered to everyone, even if this does not represent what the literature suggests might be the specific optimal choice. All sorts of examples come to mind in this regard. Many patients who would benefit most from a day hospital must be admitted to inpatient services because no day hospital is available. Delusionally depressed patients who are often responsive only to electroconvulsive treatment (ECT) may not receive ECT because many (especially public) hospitals do not provide it. Agoraphobic patients who would benefit from a behavior therapy regimen often cannot find a program or practitioner expert in delivering this form of treatment, and some states have only a handful of psychoanalytically trained therapists.

Granted that not every form of psychiatric treatment can be conveniently located for ready access everywhere, and that not every clinic or practitioner can be expert in everything; but the crucial administrative question regarding differential therapeutics remains—How can we ensure that the treatment delivery system in psychiatry is designed to meet the wide variety of specific patient needs, rather than that patients routinely receive the treatment that is the one preferred by the treatment delivery system?

The previous sections of this chapter, on the clinical, educational, and research aspects of differential therapeutics, all contribute to an answer to this administrative question. Insofar as a clinician or practitioner carefully distinguishes the process of consultation from the beginning of treatment, it becomes less likely that all patients will receive more or less uniform treatments. This is reinforced further to the degree that evaluating clinicians are taught about the availability of different psychiatric treatments, their differential indications, and the research suggesting specific patient/therapy matches.

Our own emerging interest in the topic of differential therapeutics over the last decade has had an obvious impact on our administrative practices in both our clinic and private practice settings. It became clear that our outpatient department would have to expand and increase the variety of its services if it were to meet the wide-ranging needs of its constituents. This led to the recruitment of specialists in treatments previously underrepresented in our clinic faculty (for example, behavioral, cognitive, family, and group psychotherapies) and the development of a number of specialty clinics especially designed to meet targeted patient problems (affective, anxiety, schizophrenic, substance abuse, psychophysiologic geriatric, and sexual disorders). In our private practices, such concerns led us to increase our training, experience, and expertise with treatments previously not part of our repertoires, and also to develop referral networks with other private practitioners who had those skills we decided that we couldn't or wouldn't acquire. We recognize that such a course may not be within the resources of all clinics and practitioners and that there are clear financial implications consequent to the decisions to expand the variety of one's services or refer out patients whose needs cannot be met within those that exist. Differential therapeutics is the art of the possible. However such questions are ultimately decided, and often compromises are inevitable, they must be asked. It is perfectly reasonable for a clinic or practitioner to choose to offer only a limited array of treatments, but it is unreasonable to do this out of ignorance that other choices exist and unfair not to let patients know about the other possible approaches.

A further administrative implication is also clear. Insofar as it is possible, it makes great sense to separate the evaluation and treatment services. A centralized evaluation system helps to ensure that recommendations about treatments are not unduly influenced by the expertise, needs, biases, and countertransferences of the treators. An evaluation service is likely to develop special expertise in differential therapeutics and to be more catholic and impartial in its recommendations. In our clinic, we have also been impressed with the value of the Treatment Planning Conference which regularly and systematically reviews and endorses all treatment assignments made by the evaluation service. This conference ensures quality control and helps in recruitment of patients for specialty programs.

CONCLUSIONS

Treatment selection in psychiatry relies upon a subtle combination of clinical art and clinical science. This is an area that has received far too little clinical, educational, research, and administrative attention. A number of suggestions emerge from our review of these issues. The careful consideration of differential therapeutic possibilities requires that a central emphasis be placed on the psychiatric consultation. The consultative process should be separated clearly from the onset of treatment and should be charged with the responsibility not only for making a psychiatric diagnosis, but also with providing psychoeducation about diagnosis and treatment, and negotiating a treatment plan with the patient as informed consumer. In order to ensure that this consultation process is done well, it is necessary to provide training in differential treatment selection, to systematically keep abreast of research in this area, and to provide an administrative structure that allows for the variety of appropriate treatment choices. These are certainly not easy tasks, but they are necessary if we are to provide our patients with the specific treatment most tailored to their needs.

Differential therapeutics is a relatively new consideration in psychiatry and clearly we have a long way to go before it can be performed with a satisfying specificity. In the meantime, it is best to be flexible and humble in our recommendations, respectful of our patient's wishes and opinions, and to know the research literature, but also to trust in clinical intuition and judgment.

REFERENCES

Anderson C, Reiss D, Hogarty G: Schizophrenia in the Family: A Practitioner's Guide to Psychoeducation and Management. New York, Guilford, 1986

Andrews S, Leavy A, de Chilo N, et al: Patient therapist mismatch: we would rather switch than fight. Hospital Community Psychiatry (in press)

Beck AT, Rush AJ, Shaw BF, et al: Cognitive Thearpy for Depression. New York, Guilford, 1981

Frances A, Clarkin J, Perry S: Differential Therapeutics in Psychiatry: The Art and Science of Treatment Selection. Brunner/Mazel, 1984a

Frances A, Sweeney J, Clarkin J: Does psychotherapy have specific effects? Am J Psychother 39:159-174, 1984b

Frank J: Persuasion and Healing. Johns Hopkins University Press, 1973

Hartley DE: Research on the therapeutic alliance in psychotherapy, in Psychiatry Update: The American Psychiatric Association Annual Review, Vol. 4. Edited by Hales R, Frances A. Washington, DC, American Psychiatric Press, Inc., 1985

Lazare A, Einsenthal S: Negotiated approach to the clinical encounter, in Outpatient Psychiatry: Diagnosis and Treatment. Edited by Lazare A. Baltimore, Williams and Wilkins, 1979

Mathews AM, Gelder MG, Johnson DW: Agoraphobia: Nature and Treatment. New York, Guilford Press, 1981

Perry S, Frances A, Clarkin J: The DSM-III Guide to Differential Therapeutics. New York, Brunner/Mazel, 1985

Smith M, Glass G, Miller T: The Benefits of Psychotherapy. Baltimore, Johns Hopkins University Press, 1980

Waskow IE: Specification of the technique variable in the NIMH treatment of repression collaborative research program, in Psychotherapy Research: Where Are We and Where Should We Go? Edited by Williams J, Spitzer R. New York, Guilford Press, 1984

Afterword

by John F. Clarkin, Ph.D., and Samuel W. Perry, M.D.

We concluded the foreword of this section by stating that the selection of a specific treatment for a specific patient was one of the most interesting yet one of the most difficult tasks confronting the clinical psychiatrist. All these chapters have supported this statement. In both tone and content, they have conveyed the stimulating growth in the rich field of differential therapeutics, but also the enormous problems facing both the researcher and the clinician.

In recent decades we have benefited from the naming of hundreds of psychiatric diagnoses and the proliferation of hundreds of promising treatments, but with these benefits has come a burden. The permutations of possible diagnostic-treatment interactions could keep researchers busy for eternity. Conclusive studies documenting treatment selection criteria for even the most common diagnoses would take years to accomplish.

This situation has been appreciated by the chapters' authors, all of whom have indicated that the clinician—confronted with the complexities and uniqueness of a particular patient and asked to recommend the best treatment—must continue to rely upon an informed consumption of the relevant scientific literature and on clinical judgement (Perry et al, 1985).

Four other common themes are either explicitly or implicitly shared by all the authors. First, they all recognize that the clinician must remain flexible in approach, educating the patient about a range of therapeutic possibilities, then negotiating for an acceptable and accepted treatment. Second, all authors appreciate the bias in any clinician's treatment selection, biases that arise from one's training, temperament, sex, style, locale, and all the other systematic and unsystematic experiences that influence the clinician. Third, all authors indicate a reluctance to rely too heavily on diagnosis alone when selecting the best treatment. Beutler, for example, in choosing a particular therapeutic technique, considers several nondiagnostic issues, such as symptom complexity and defensive style. Perry, in discussing treatment duration and frequency, describes the poor correlation between the seriousness and severity of an illness and the length and intensity of treatment; for example, a major depressive episode (Axis I) even when severe (Axis V) may require a treatment that is relatively brief; whereas a patient with a personality disorder (Axis II) though mild (Axis V) may require intermittent interventions throughout his or her life. Haas and Clarkin emphasize that the format of treatment will be influenced by the patient's interpersonal situation, an axis not included in the *DSM-III* (Frances et al, 1984a).

A fourth theme shared by all authors is a willingness, despite ambiguity and uncertainty, to make specific recommendations to guide treatment selection. Based on our reading of the chapters in this sections as well as on our review of the literature (Frances et al, 1984b) and our own clinical experience (Perry et al, 1985), we believe some recommendations are worth highlighting:

Regarding treatment setting: (1) Inpatient psychiatric hospitalization is used too often and too soon; more patients should be treated in day hospitals, halfway houses, and crisis intervention settings. (2) Deinstitutionalization has its limits;

inpatient settings, for both acute and custodial care, will always be necessary for some patients. (3) Because many crucial decisions must be made in the emergency room, more systematic studies are needed to investigate this setting. (4) As the general hospital has become increasingly important for psychiatric care, the range of effective interventions for both patients and staff in this setting has been expanded.

Format: (1) Psychiatric problems that traditionally were assigned to an individual treatment can effectively be treated with marital, family, or group formats. (2) Different formats can be used for a single case, either concurrently or sequentially (for example, individual and family; marital then group). (3) A particular technique or a particular setting does not automatically determine the format (for example, a family treatment for a psychiatric inpatient, a group format using psychoanalytic techniques). (4) Spouses and families have a lot to tell us, often things that the individual patients cannot or will not reveal; the benefit of marital or family formats at times may stem from this additional information as well as the interpersonal process. (5) Marital or family therapy is the treatment of choice when the presenting complaint is a marital or family problem. (6) The homogeneous group is often the treatment of choice for specific target problems (for example, substance abuse, bulimia, hypochondriasis, agoraphobia). (7) "Self-help" groups (for example, Alcoholics Anonymous, Gamblers Anonymous, Weight Watchers) treat more emotional problems than the entire psychiatric profession, yet this format is probably an underutilized source of referral and is certainly a format that has not been sufficiently studied. (8) The heterogeneous group is particularly useful for treating interpersonal problems and for establishing social skills and networks, but careful role induction is often necessary to reduce dropouts; otherwise patients feel they are placed in the paradoxical and untenable position of having to overcome interpersonal problems and inhibitions in order to get treatment for these very problems. (9) Individual treatment is the best format for intrapsychic problems of longstanding duration. (10) For the patient in crisis, a combination of individual and family treatment is usually best.

Duration and Frequency: (1) Briefer therapies increasingly have become the treatment of choice for even longstanding problems; they can also serve as a trial at treatment to guide longer term recommendations. (2) Treatment does not need to be continuous; consistent with the medical model, patients can enter an active treatment phase and leave to return months or sometimes years later for another active treatment as stresses and conditions change. (3) The recommendation of no treatment always warrants consideration; put simply, like other medical treatments, psychotherapy can make some patients worse, or does not help, or is not necessary. (4) Long-term intensive psychotherapy with the expectation of an absolute termination is expensive and the least consistent with the medical model; it should most often be reserved for character change or for supportive treatments with chronic conditions.

Technique: (1) Psychoeducation is useful across all conditions and at times may be the treatment of choice; (2) Supportive techniques are the most common and most versatile in reversing demoralization, buttressing defenses, and teaching coping skills. (3) Although scientific studies have not yet documented that specific emotional problems require specific therapeutic approaches, the state of the art suggests that certain marriages work particularly well: psychodynamic techniques for character change, behavioral techniques for targeted symptoms (for example, phobias, eating disorders), strategic techniques for oppositional behaviors, and cognitive techniques for anxiety disorders and mild-to-moderate depressions.

Somatic Treatments: (1) To increase compliance and to enhance the placebo effect, somatic treatments should always be provided within the context of a therapeutic relationship. (2) Within a given family of psychotropic medication, the particular choice of drug is usually based on the different profile of side effects rather than on the differential effectiveness. (3) For patients with serious psychiatric disorders that have not previously responded to medication, it is important to ensure that their medications' trials were adequate in both dosage and duration; if so, a different family of psychotropic drugs can be prescribed for the disorder sequentially until an effective one is found. To reduce demoralization, the patient should be an informed participant in this thorough and serial trial.

Additional Suggestions: (1) Although some schools of therapy (for example, psychoanalytic, behavioral) have at times emphasized a rigid adherence to one approach, many patients require a treatment that interweaves strategies and techniques from different theoretical orientations. (2) The suggestion that combinations are useful is not an endorsement for "shotgun" prescriptions; combined treatments require a rationale. (3) The sex of the therapist, although insufficiently studied, is very likely to influence transference manifestations and treatment outcome. Therapies aimed at character change should probably be conducted by a therapist whose sex presents the most difficulties for the patient, whereas therapies designed to alleviate symptoms should most often be conducted by a therapist whose sex poses the least problems for the patient. (4) Consultation during a psychiatric treatment is generally used too little or too late. If a treatment seems stalemated, consultation should be arranged. Even if the stalemate is secondary to a particular transference paradigm that is amenable to working through with the present therapist, a consultation more often catalyzes rather than disrupts this process. In other kinds of stalemates, transfer to another therapist is indicated if the consultant cannot provide specific and mutually acceptable advice that will improve the therapeutic situation.

A Final Word: Given the inherent clinical and research difficulties in the area of differential therapeutics, it is fitting that we conclude with one more humbling recommendation. No psychiatrist can expect to be competent in all the effective treatments currently available. Therapists must know not only what they do well but also what they don't, and be willing and able to refer patients to another therapist either from the start, concurrently during the treatment, or in sequence after one part of the treatment has been completed. To convey this possibility to the patient, psychiatrists can indicate that the initial clinical encounter will be designed in part to determine if treatment is necessary and if so, what kind of treatment and by whom.

REFERENCES

Frances A, Clarkin JF, Perry S: DSM-III and family therapy. Am J Psychiatry 141:406-409, 1984a

Frances A, Clarkin JF, Perry S: Differential Therapeutics: A Guide to the Art and Science of Treatment Planning in Psychiatry. New York, Brunner/Mazel, 1984b

Perry S, Frances A, Clarkin JF: A DSM-III Casebook of Differential Therapeutics: A Clinical Guide to Treatment Selection. New York, Brunner/Mazel, 1985

IV

Violence and the Violent Patient

IV

Violence and the Violent Patient

Section IV

Violence and the Violent Patient
Foreword

by Kenneth Tardiff, M.D., M.P.H., Section Editor

Psychiatrists must be prepared to evaluate and treat violent patients, but also are expected to serve as informed commentators regarding violence in society. A number of studies emphasize that violence among psychiatric patients is frequent enough to merit concern, and the ability to manage these patients is necessary. For example, approximately 10 percent of the patients admitted to private as well as public hospitals manifested violent behavior toward others prior to admission to these hospitals (Tardiff and Sweillam, 1980; Craig, 1982; Tardiff, 1984), and seven percent of patients residing in state hospitals for long periods of time were assaultive (Tardiff and Sweillam, 1982). Of patients presenting for evaluation in two private hospital outpatient clinics, three percent had manifested recent assaultive behavior toward others (Tardiff and Koenigsberg, 1985).

The evaluation and treatment of the violent patient presents a special set of concerns. First there is concern for one's own safety, which may be justified in light of reports that 40 percent of psychiatrists have reported being assaulted at least once during their careers (Madden et al, 1976; Tardiff and Maurice, 1977), and that 48 percent of psychiatric residents in a training program were assaulted at least once during residency (Ruben et al, 1980). A second concern is the legal liability of the professional in terms of *Tarasoff*-like decisions, which require the professional to protect potential victims from their violent patients (Beck 1985). The issue of one's safety and the safety of others, added to one's past experiences with violence, generate feelings and reactions within the therapist which must be recognized and taken into consideration in the care of the violent patient.

This section focuses on the evaluation and treatment of the violent patient, although this clinical information is preceded by two chapters which provide a broad view of the determinants and patterns of violence in society, and is followed by a chapter describing the legal framework in which the clinician works. Given constraints of space, there are notable areas of violence not covered in this section. For example, we have not covered the evaluation and treatment of victims of violence. As is reported in Chapter 20, the National Crime Survey found that the rate of assault was 24.1 per 1,000 persons over 12 years of age in 1983. The frequency of physical or sexual violence aimed at psychiatric patients appears to be much higher—for example, 22 percent of outpatients (Herman, 1986) and 48 percent of inpatients (Carmen et al, 1984)—in two studies. Neither have we covered the dynamics or treatment in specific types of violence such as child abuse, rape, arson, terrorism, spouse abuse, and other domestic violence. All of these subjects merit consideration in subsequent editions of the *Annual Review*.

In Chapter 19 I begin by sketching the landscape of violence in terms of the interaction of factors within the individual and the environment in the causation of violence. This chapter illustrates the complex, multifactorial nature of violent behavior, and should serve as a framework for both evaluation and treatment of the violent patient. Biological factors seem to be nonspecific in the way they affect violence. Rather than a specific mechanism, they tip the balance toward violence by impairing a person's ability to achieve goals through nonviolent means or by increasing impulsivity, irrationality, irritability, or disorganization of behavior. The individual is affected by physical factors in the environment such as heat, noise, and overcrowding; by psychological factors such as conflict with others and the effects of television violence and other mass media violence; and by social factors such as culture and poverty.

In Chapter 20 Park Dietz presents quantitative information from the annual *Uniform Crime Reports* of the F.B.I. and the periodic *National Crime Survey Report* conducted by the Bureau of the Census. He has selected three types of violent crimes—nonlethal attacks, homicides, and robberies—to illustrate the differing characteristics of offenders and victims, as well as to give us an appreciation of their frequencies.

These crimes range from the instrumental or economically motivated violent crime, to the violent crime expressive of some underlying psychopathology. In addition, Dietz presents his observations and analyses of a number of special or notorious offenses such as assassination, mass murder, serial murder, bombing, and skyjacking. Although the clinician will be called upon to see only a small portion of the persons perpetrating these violent crimes, he or she should be familiar with statistics on criminal violence as an informed member of society.

Chapter 21, by William Reid and George Balis, addresses the evelution of the violent patient. It considers the physical setting, particularly in terms of the safety of the clinician. In addition to the usual elements of the history and physical and mental status examinations, it presents areas that deserve special attention; for example, awareness of substance induced violence and the need for routine urine and blood screens for alcohol and drugs, as well as the need for an exhaustive neuropsychological and medical evaluation of the patient. It presents guidelines for using a decision tree approach to arrive at the differential diagnosis of the violent individual. Finally, there are guidelines for the short-term prediction of violent behavior.

In Chapter 22 Paul Soloff describes the emergency management of the violent patient. This involves the rapid assessment and swift intervention against target symptoms of violent behavior so as to insure the safety of the patient and others. Although a more definitive diagnosis will result from extensive evaluation of the patient, a rapid differential diagnosis must be made for purposes of management in the emergency situation. One must rule out an organic brain disorder, since management involves treatment of the underlying etiology and the patient is rarely amenable to verbal intervention. Likewise the functional psychoses must be ruled out, since the patient is rarely amenable to verbal intervention. Having done so, often the remaining diagnostic groups—that is, the nonpsychotic, nonorganic types—may be approached in terms of verbal intervention. The decision as to whether verbal intervention, medication, seclusion, or restraint is used in the emergency management is based on clinical considerations; that is, on the specific patient and circumstances rather than on any legal concept of degree of restrictiveness. This chapter provides specific practical guidelines for the use of all of these techniques of managing the violent patient in the emergency situation.

In Chapter 23 John Lion and I discuss the long-term treatment of the violent patient, about which little has been written. Long-term treatment covers aftercare of the seriously disabled violent patient, as well as the long-term psychotherapy of the more intact violent patient and his or her family. There is discussion of problems with aftercare of the violent patient. We state the goals of psychotherapy, which include development of self-control, increase of verbal ability and affective awareness, appreciation of the consequences of violent behavior, and insight regarding the dynamics of violence. We emphasize the importance of dealing with transference and countertransference issues. In addition to psychotherapeutic techniques, there is brief mention of the need for social intervention, as well as a longer discussion of the medications that have been tried in the long-term treatment of violent patients. Special concerns are the safety of the therapist, and what the therapist should keep in mind in fulfilling a duty to protect potential victims from patients in outpatient treatment.

In Chapter 24 Paul Appelbaum presents the legal implications of violence occurring in inpatient and outpatient treatment settings. He discusses the need to balance the patient's right to be free from assault with the right to be free of unnecessary restraint within psychiatric facilities. He stresses that decisions in limiting freedom should be based on generally prevailing standards of clinical care. He discusses the complex legal environment concerning the use of involuntary medication and the somewhat more straightforward parameters for the use of seclusion and restraint. The legal liability of patients and staff on inpatient units is reviewed and considered to be minimal. This is in contrast to the liability of professionals for violence committed by patients following release from hospitals or while patients are in ongoing outpatient treatment. Of greatest concern is the question of how and when the professional should warn potential victims when an assessment of violence potential reveals a significant danger. Yet other means of protecting a potential victim—that is, commitment of the patient—is not without problems. Finally, there are limitations on ways of insuring compliance among violent patients once they are discharged into the community.

Given the societal expectation that psychiatrists manage violent patients and protect society while respecting the rights of violent patients, the guidelines presented in this section should be given serious attention.

REFERENCES

Beck JC (Ed): The Potentially Violent Patient and the *Tarasoff* Decision in Psychiatric Practice. Washington, DC, American Psychiatric Press Inc., 1985

Carmen E, Rieker P, Mills T: Victims of violence and psychiatric illness. Am J Psychiatry 141:378-383, 1984

Craig TJ: An epidemiological study of patterns associated with violence among psychiatric inpatients. Am J Psychiatry 139:1262-1266, 1982

Herman JL: Histories of violence in an outpatient population: an exploratory study. Am J Orthopsychiatry 56:137-141, 1986

Madden DJ, Lion JR, Penna MW: Assault on psychiatrists by patients. Am J Psychiatry 133:422-425, 1976

Ruben I, Wolkon G, Yamamoto J: Physical attacks on residents by psychiatric patients. Diseases of the Nervous System 38:13-16, 1980

Tardiff K: Characteristics of assaultive patients in private psychiatric hospitals. Am J Psychiatry 141:1232-1239, 1984

Tardiff K, Koenigsberg H: A study of assaultive behavior among psychiatric outpatients. Am J Psychiatry 142:960-963, 1985

Tardiff K, Maurice W: The care of violent patients by psychiatrists: a tale of two cities. Canadian Psychiatric Association Journal 22:83-86, 1977

Tardiff K, Sweillam A: Assault, suicide and mental illness. Arch Gen Psychiatry 37:164-169, 1980

Tardiff K, Sweillam A: The occurrence of assaultive behavior among chronic psychiatric inpatients. Am J Psychiatry 139:212-215, 1982

Chapter 19

Determinants of Human Violence

by Kenneth Tardiff, M.D., M.P.H.

In this chapter I will review a broad spectrum of studies aimed at determining why some people manifest violent behavior toward others. My goal is to present possible etiological factors which, of course, would be related to the evaluation, treatment, and, it is hoped, to the prevention of human violence. Because of space constraints, this review will not include studies on nonhuman violence. Animal studies have demonstrated the complexity of aggression as a behavior. It appears to have a genetic-biologic substrate, but is also greatly influenced by the physical environment and interaction with other animals. A variety of neurotransmitters appear to be related to aggressive behavior in animals. As Singhal and Telner (1983) have pointed out, it is difficult to integrate animal studies because of the different models of aggression used in the laboratory. The reader is referred to a number of other sources for reviews of animal studies (Brain and Benton, 1981; Valzelli, 1981; Hamburg and Trudeau, 1981; Simmel et al, 1983). The applicability of animal models to the complex phenomena of human behavior, particularly if one is addressing clinical issues, should be approached with caution, since often animal aggression is expressed in a noninjurious form as ritualized behavior, as opposed to the human form of aggression that often leads to injury and, at times, death (Coe and Levine, 1983).

In considering the causes of human violence, as any other aspect of human behavior, one must use a multifactorial model. Although somewhat artificial, one may conceptualize a group of internal or innate factors within the individual as increasing or decreasing that individual's predisposition to violence. These factors may be present at the time of birth—for example, genetic factors, hormones, neurotransmitters—or factors acquired during childhood development. These internal factors interact with external factors, which may tip the balance toward violent behavior—for example, socioeconomic factors, the mass media, provocation, and the availability of weapons.

NEUROPHYSIOLOGICAL FACTORS

In the search for a biological basis for violent behavior researchers have explored the limbic system of the brain. Building on a number of their own previous studies and studies done by others, Mark and Ervin (1970) and Monroe (1970) called attention to the role of neurophysiological dysfunction of the brain; the former investigator in terms of temporal lobe epilepsy (now called partial complex seizures), and the latter investigator in a more subtle sense, that of limbic ictus and episodic dyscontrol. Mark and Ervin's advocacy of neurosurgical procedures to manage violence in some temporal epileptic patients has provoked a strong reaction by some members of the profession and the public, who fear that the role of abnormal physiology of the brain would be exaggerated and that other factors, such as socioeconomic ones and others discussed later in this chapter would not be addressed.

A decade later, in 1980, a large international collaborative study confirmed that significant violence defined as "directed exertion of extreme and aggressive physical force which, if unrestrained, would result in injury, destruction or abuse." For this study significant violence was rare among epileptic patients during seizures. Furthermore, aggressive behavior during seizures was usually stereotyped, unsustained, and not purposeful in nature (Delgado-Escueta et al, 1981, p. 715). Leicester (1982) looked at 500 cases referred to a neurologist and found that of the 17 patients referred for temper tantrums, none had organic factors (that is, epilepsy or episodic dyscontrol syndrome). Rather, the violent episodes were the results of psychological factors. Finally, Hermann and Whitman (1984) reviewed 64 studies conducted since 1962 that assessed the relation among temporal lobe epilepsy, aggression, and other forms of psychopathology. They focused on studies of the interictal period in terms of irritable, aggressive, or hostile behavior using neurosurgical and nonneurosurgical patients, as well as surveys of prison populations. They concluded that controlled investigations showed no overall differences in the levels of violence between persons with and without epilepsy. Among individuals with epilepsy, other factors were found to be associated with violence per se, such as low socioeconomic status, sex, age, and problems with the earlier development of the individual.

Lewis (1982) found that of 97 delinquent, adolescent boys in correctional schools, 18 had psychomotor epilepsy, and that the more violent boys were those with this disorder. Five boys committed violent acts during seizures, but violence was interictal as well. The violent boys with temporal lobe epilepsy were more likely to report impaired or distorted memory and to have low IQs, a frequent history of head trauma, and paranoid ideation and/or hallucinations, all of which were associated with poor impulse control and were not directly related to seizures. Thus, the individual may manifest violence secondary to seizure activity on one occasion, and as a result of other factors associated with poor impulse control on other occasions.

Devinsky and Baer (1984) have continued to emphasize the importance of temporal lobe epilepsy in violence, and have illustrated various forms of violence that one may encounter through the use of case histories. They did not address the prevalence of violent behavior among temporal lobe epileptic patients compared to the general epileptic population or to the general nonepileptic population. They did criticize studies that used patients with generalized seizures in control groups, since a primary limbic focus may be obscured by general seizure activity, or a secondary limbic focus of the seizure activity may result from the generalized seizure activity. Likewise, Monroe (1985) has continued to maintain that episodic dyscontrol is often associated with limbic ictus but is not detected because the surface electroencephalogram (EEG) is an insensitive procedure for measuring subcortical activity. He points out that support for his theory of limbic ictal phenomena rests with the response of individuals with dyscontrol syndrome to anticonvulsant regimes.

In conclusion, it would appear that the story of epilepsy and the more subtle aberrations of neurophysiological activity in violence is not complete. There are probably some persons with temporal lobe epilepsy who manifest hostility and violence in the interictal period as well as nonpurposeful violence during their seizures. However, their number is probably not great among other persons with epilepsy and infinitesimal in relation to violence in general. Violent persons with epilepsy have other conditions that are associated with poor impulse control independent of seizure activity; thus, careful attention must be paid to the selection of subjects as well as controls in future studies which, it is hoped, will use more sensitive procedures for recording subcortical neurophysiological activity. In terms of evaluation of patients, the EEG and other measures of neurophysiological dysfunction are standard, and consideration must be given to anticonvulsants in the treatment of violent patients.

HORMONAL FACTORS

Violence may be associated with endocrine diseases such as Cushing's syndrome or hyperthyroidism, but this review will explore the more subtle possible contributions of hormones in violence, namely, recent studies of androgens, hypoglycemia, and the premenstrual syndrome.

Androgens

Olweus et al (1980) in Sweden looked at 58 normal adolescent boys 16 years of age, using a battery of inventories and scales. There were significant associations between plasma testosterone levels and self-reports of physical and verbal aggression, which mainly reflected responsiveness to provocation and threat. However, these findings should be viewed with caution, in light of the small number of significant correlations and the large number of variables analyzed in relation to testosterone levels. Rada et al (1976) measured plasma testosterone levels in 52 rapists and 12 child molesters. The rapists were classified according to the degree of violence during the commission of rape. The plasma testosterone levels were related to the degree of violence manifested by the rapist, as well as to self-reports on the Buss-Durkee Hostility Inventory (BDHI).

However, a number of studies have not found a relation between androgens and violence. Matthews (1979) found no differences in mean testosterone levels between prisoners with a history of violent crime and prisoners at the same institution incarcerated for nonviolent crime. Mattsson et al (1980) compared 40 male delinquent recidivists with a group of normal adolescents of the same age and pubertal stage. The delinquent recidivists had slightly higher, although not statistically significant, mean levels of plasma testosterone. Neither staff ratings nor psychiatric ratings of aggression were correlated with plasma testosterone levels. In a second study by Rada and his colleagues (1983) of 18 rapists, 26 child molesters, and 11 controls from the treatment staff of a state hospital, there were no significant differences among these groups in terms of plasma testosterone levels, and no hormonal differences among the offenders in relation to the degree of violence involved in their offenses or to ratings of violence using the BDHI. There have been few studies in which the level of androgen has been controlled. Money and Dalery (1977) found that the administration of synthetic progesterones or estrogens for sex offenders, in essence a hormonal castration, had no effect on aggressive behavior. Davidson and colleagues (1979) found that androgen treatment of hypogonadal men had no effect on aggressive behaviors.

In summary, the evidence supporting a causative link between androgens and violence is not convincing. This author believes the increased rates of violence by men in society is accounted for by other factors such as socioeconomic ones. In my study of thousands of patients residing in state hospitals for long periods of time, there was no difference between men and women in terms of rates of violent behavior toward other persons (Tardiff and Sweillam, 1982).

Hypoglycemia

Hypoglycemia has been studied as a cause of aggressive and violent behavior. By arbitrary definition, hypoglycemia in adults has been equated with values of blood sugar below 40 mg per 100 ml. Although a detailed discussion of the medical aspects of hypoglycemia is not warranted, a brief differentiation of hypoglycemia disorders that occur in the fed state, as opposed to the fasting state, is in order. In the fed state, hypoglycemia is the result of temporary excessive release of insulin following eating, and lasts for a limited period of time. In over two-thirds of the cases, hypoglycemics in the fed state are "functional"; that is, without demonstrable etiology. The diagnosis is made by a five-hour glucose tolerance test. Distinct from hypoglycemia in the fed state, fasting hypoglycemia is a more prolonged condition and is caused by insulin excess, most commonly by islet cell tumors, although the administration of excess insulin and hypoglycemia secondary to a chronic alcoholic ingestion must be considered.

A number of studies have shown an association between pathological aggression and hypoglycemia. Frederichs and Goodman (1969) examined 600 hypoglycemia patients and found that 89 percent were highly irritable, and 45 percent demonstrated overt antisocial behaviors. Virkkunen (1982) studied hypoglycemia among habitually violent offenders and found that habitually violent offenders had hypoglycemia to a greater degree than the control population, which consisted of psychiatric personnel. The reactive hypoglycemic phase lasted longer among violent offenders with antisocial personality as opposed to those with intermittent explosive disorders.

In conclusion, although hypoglycemia may be implicated in extreme cases of violence, its role in the common, often mild disorder of "functional" hypoglycemia, is unclear. Perhaps in some individuals with certain personality and environmental precipitants, the hypoglycemic state may tip the balance toward aggressive behavior. Nevertheless, the clinician who suspects hypoglycemia as a factor in violence should consider a glucose tolerance test with measurement of plasma epinephrine and norepinephrine.

Premenstrual Syndrome

Although for centuries there has been recognition of physical and psychological changes in the premenstrual period, recently the premenstrual syndrome has become the focus of attention because it may form the basis of a temporary insanity plea in relation to criminal responsibility. Already, in France and England, severe premenstrual syndrome has been accepted as a contributing factor in crimes of manslaughter, arson, and assault (Dalton, 1980). The premenstrual syndrome includes a variety of symptoms and a range of severity from mild to incapacitating, depending on the individual involved. Some of these symptoms include feelings of irritability, tension, fatigue, or depression. A study by d'Orban and Dalton (1980) has shown that of 50 women charged with crimes of violence, 44 percent committed their offense during the premenstrual period, and there was significant lack of offenses during the ovulatory and post-ovulatory phases of the menstrual cycle. Yet one must be cautious in extrapolating these findings to "normal" individuals. Progesterone has been recommended as a treatment for the premenstrual syndrome including any associated criminal activity (Dalton, 1980, 1984).

Critics of this approach argue that studies have not utilized placebos and controls, and that other aspects of intervention such as recommendations to avoid alcohol and to maintain a stable diet, as well as the interpersonal attention given the patient, account for any apparent emotional or behavioral change. Reid and Yen (1981) have done an extensive review of the literature with 305 citations in regard to the etiology of premenstrual syndrome. They have concluded that there is a lack of evidence to support theories of etiology or treatment in the areas of estrogen excess, progesterone deficiency, vitamin deficiencies, hypoglycemia, endogenous hormone allergy, fluid retention, or primary psychosomatic causes.

In conclusion, the concept of premenstrual syndrome as a psychiatric disorder is controversial (premenstrual dysphoric disorder in *DSM-III-R*). The implication for women is a two-edged sword to be approached with caution; that is, if it is used to excuse a few for acts of violence, this may raise unsubstantiated concerns about the abilities of women in positions of power and responsibility.

Overall, there are many problems with studies of the role of hormones in human aggression. There are differing definitions and levels of aggression, ranging from self-reports of aggressive traits and feelings, to extreme criminal violence. Even in extreme cases, the evidence that androgens, hypoglycemia, or premenstrual syndrome are factors in violence is inconclusive.

GENETIC DETERMINANTS

In terms of specific genetic defects, there has been a flurry of interest and research over the past two decades in sex chromosome abnormalities. Obviously, a link with specific genetic abnormalities and homicide and other acts of violence would be important in terms of criminal responsibility. There have been a number of surveys of men in prisons and other correctional institutions showing that XYY men are disproportionately represented. More recent studies have attempted to eliminate the sampling bias inherent in obtaining subjects from the institutionalized population. Schiavi and his colleagues (1984) have reviewed that literature and conducted a double blind, controlled study in Copenhagen. They found no association between the XYY or XXY chromosomal abnormalities and violence. It appears that the specific role of these sex chromosome abnormalities is doubtful, and that any association with arrests for crimes is probably linked to other factors, such as the low intelligence of these men. The role of XXX karyotype in a homicidal woman has been reported, but again other factors such as low IQ and early development seemed to be major determinants (Kazamatsuri et al, 1985).

There is some evidence that genetic inheritance is related to criminal acts. Mednick and Volavka (1980) have pointed out that earlier twin studies showing increased criminal behavior in monozygotic twins as compared to dizygotic twins were subject to a number of sampling problems; however, more recent studies using better methodology also have found increased criminal behavior in monozygotic as compared to dizygotic twins. Given that twins share the same environmental as well as genetic backgrounds, further investigation has turned to adoption studies. In two such studies in Scandinavia, there was no support for a genetic basis of homicide, and some support for an association in crimes involving property (Hutchings and Mednick, 1977; Bohman, 1978). A later paper by Bohman (1982) reported that a study of adopted men in Sweden committing violent crimes showed that their crimes were related to their own alcohol abuse, but not to violence in their biological or adoptive parents, although nonviolent petty property crimes did seem to have a genetic predisposition.

In summary, there appears to be no specific chromosomal abnormality that accounts for violent behavior, and studies of inheritance support only a genetic relationship for economic, property crimes, not for violence.

NEUROTRANSMITTERS

Earlier studies of neurotransmitters have implicated increased levels of norepinephrine and dopamine in aggressive behavior (Eichelman et al, 1981); however, the most promising work has involved the serotonergic system. Brown and colleagues (1979, 1982) conducted two studies of men with a history of aggressive behavior, excluding those with a history of primary affective disorders, schizophrenia, or severe brain syndromes, as well as those ingesting drugs or alcohol 10 days preceding the study. They found that a history of aggressive behavior and a history of suicidal behavior were both related to decreased cerebrospinal fluid (CSF) 5–HIAA levels. They believe that altered serotonin metabolism may be a highly significant contributing factor to these behaviors in whatever diagnostic group they occur. Lidberg and colleagues (1985) studied the CSF–5–HIAA levels in a group of men convicted of criminal homicide and a group of men who attempted suicide, and found that these groups had lower levels of 5–HIAA in spinal fluid than did male controls. They did not, as Brown did, exclude alcoholics or patients with schizophrenia or affective illness. Linnolia et al (1983) studied violent offenders, excluding schizophrenics or those with major affective disorders, but not alcoholics. All of the subjects had killed or attempted to kill with unusual cruelty. They found that impulsive offenders had significantly lower CSF–5–HIAA concentrations than nonimpulsive offenders, the latter group defined as those who had premeditated their crimes. Furthermore, those offenders with a history of suicide attempts had lower CSF–5–HIAA levels than those without a history of suicide. This is in agreement with other studies of suicide and serotonin metabolism (Linkowski, 1985). Thus, low CSF–5–HIAA concentration may be a marker of impulsivity rather than of a specific type of violence; that is, suicide or externally directed aggression.

PSYCHIATRIC DISORDERS

Although many acts of violence, particularly related to economic motives, are not committed by psychiatric patients, the role of psychiatric disorders in violent behavior has been a subject of study for decades. Rabkin (1979) has extensively reviewed a number of studies and concluded that arrest and conviction rates for violent crimes among psychiatric patients exceed those for the general population, and that there has been a pronounced, relative, as well as absolute, increase in these rates over time. This recent increase in rates may be related to policies which have increasingly discharged patients into the community. Rabkin noted that psychiatric patients come disproportionately from the poor, uneducated populations, and questioned whether this as well as psychiatric illness may be responsible for violent criminal acts.

Yet, psychiatric patients should not be regarded as a homogeneous group. Tardiff has found that violent patients admitted to and residing in both public and private hospitals are more likely to have diagnoses of schizophrenia, mania, mental retardation, and organic mental disorders than nonviolent patients (Tardiff and Sweillam, 1980, 1982; Tardiff, 1984). Taylor examined 203 male prisoners and found that 46 percent were directly driven to commit violent offenses by their psychotic symptoms and, if indirect consequences of the psychosis were taken into account, 82 percent of their offenses were probably attributable to their illness. Within the psychotic group, those driven to offend by their delusions were more likely to have been seriously violent (Taylor, 1985). A recent review of the literature including these and other studies of violence among psychiatric inpatients confirms that diagnosis and course of the illness are important factors in predicting the incidence of violence in hospitals (Krakowski et al, 1986).

However, if one looks at a different treatment setting—that is, the outpatient clinic rather than the inpatient psychiatry unit or prison—psychiatric patients with increased rates of assault are not in the psychotic diagnoses, but rather have diagnoses of childhood, adolescent, and personality disorders (Tardiff and Koenigsberg, 1985).

Menuck (1983) has reviewed the literature on some of these personality disorders, including the borderline as well as the over-controlled types of personality disorders. In addition, he has reviewed studies relating violence to alcohol, with its concurrent releasing of inhibitions against antisocial and violent behavior, and decreasing perceptual and cognitive alertness with resulting impairment of judgment. There are a number of epidemiological studies that have found a strong link between alcohol use and certain types of homicide involving disputes (Goodman et al, 1986; Tardiff et al, 1986). A number of street drugs of abuse are found to be associated with violent behavior, including amphetamines, cocaine, hallucinogens, and minor tranquilizers-sedatives (Menuck, 1983; Nurno et al, 1985). In our study of homicides in Manhattan, we found that opiate drug abuse was related to violence indirectly and not in terms of a primary psychopharmacologic effect. Narcotics play a key role because of the activities aimed at obtaining these drugs. One-third of male homicide victims died in drug-related homicides (Tardiff et al, 1986).

DEVELOPMENTAL FACTORS

Some factors impact on the development of the individual and shift the balance of one's character toward violence as an adult. Kempe and Helfer (1980) have reported that being abused as a child is related to becoming a physically abusive adult; that is, a child abuser or otherwise violent adult. Furthermore, child abuse is not infrequent and there are reports that one percent of children are physically abused each year (Heins, 1984). This rate reflects actual reports of child abuse and since only serious physical abuse is reported, the real incidence of child abuse is probably higher than this. There is evidence that not only being abused as a child is related to adult violence, but that witnessing intrafamily violence—for example, spouse abuse—is related to increased problems with violence among children, especially boys, such as being hyperactive, cruel, bullying, and having temper tantrums (Jaffe et al, 1986). There are indications that domestic violence directed toward spouses is a common problem in the United States; for example, of 492 male and female patients interviewed in a general hospital emergency room, 22 percent reported being pushed around, hit, or hurt by their spouses or by boyfriends or girlfriends (Goldberg and Tomlanorich, 1984).

Thus we see that child and spouse abuse are significant problems in the United States, and that being abused as a child or being in a family where a spouse is abused both tip the balance toward being violent as an adult. Of course, child and domestic violence is not a primary cause of adult violence, but is in a chain of causation. Other factors affect whether there is violence in a family, many of which have been covered in this chapter; for example, the presence of psychiatric disorders, alcohol and drug abuse, or other pathology in the perpetrator, or socioeconomic factors such as poverty, unemployment, education, or culture. Other characteristics of the child are also important in child abuse such as being premature, being a sick child, or demonstrating behavior or physical appearance which generates a violent reaction by the parent because of the parent's own psychopathology (Kempe and Helfer, 1980; Spinetta, 1978).

TELEVISION AND MASS MEDIA

Yet, violence need not actually take place in the home to influence the development of the child and adolescent. Television viewing and other mass media have been suspected as factors in violence. A recent report by the National Institute of Mental Health focused on entertainment programming and reviewed approximately 2,500 studies conducted since 1970. It concluded that most of these studies demonstrated a relation between televised violence and later aggressive behavior (NIMH, 1982). Freedman (1984) criticized this report, pointing out that few of the studies reviewed have been concerned with the relatively long-term effects of television, or that they have not involved natural settings. In his review of field experiments and correlational studies, he concluded that there is a consistent, small correlation between television violence and aggressiveness, but that there is little convincing evidence in natural settings that viewing television violence causes people to be more aggressive.

Thus, future research should be done in naturalistic settings and the long-term effect of television news reports depicting violence, as well as motion pictures and television music videos, should be studied.

SOCIOECONOMIC DETERMINANTS

Focusing not on the individual, early studies have pointed to an association between violence and major social factors. The high rates of homicide and other types of violence in the South have led some to believe that violence is part of the southern culture and tradition. An alternative explanation has suggested that poor economic conditions in the southern states accounted for their higher rates of violence, while others have explained that there are greater numbers of blacks in the south, who have higher crime rates than whites. Criminal violence in black ghettos has been explained in terms of the necessity to fight rather than to be able to achieve through verbal or legitimate means. Added to this is the break-up of families, alienation, discrimination, and frustration. Thus, some have hypothesized that blacks live in a violent subculture (Silberman, 1980; Wolfgang and Ferracuti, 1967; Wolfgang, 1981), while others have found that for domestic violence, there is no difference between blacks and whites if socio-economic status is controlled in the analysis (Centerwall, 1984).

In a study of large Standard Metropolitan Statistical Areas (SMSAs) that compared rates of violent crime, including homicide as reported by the F.B.I., Blau and Blau (1982) found that racial inequality and stress were associated with rates of homicides. However, they found that the increased rates of violent crime for blacks and for southern regions of the country were both based on economic inequality. Economic inequality was not merely poverty, but rather relative income differences among individuals. Thus, the theory says that violence occurs because of hostility in one person who perceives that he or she is disadvantaged relative to other persons (Vold, 1979). Some studies have found that economic inequality is not related to violence, but that absolute poverty is related to violence and other criminal behavior; for example, the percentage of persons below the poverty line of the United States Social Security Administration (DeFronzo, 1983; Williams, 1984).

The contradictory results are probably due to the use of large metropolitan areas as units of analysis. These areas are often heterogeneous; for example, one SMSA contains suburban Long Island and central Manhattan. A recent study by Messner and Tardiff used neighborhoods as smaller units of analysis, which were more naturalistic, to test the hypothesis that economic inequality is related to homicide. We found that economic inequality and race were not related to homicide, but rather that the prime determinants were absolute poverty and marital disruption. (Messner and Tardiff, in press.) Obviously, in this formula is the effect of massive unemployment, which has been found to have a causal relationship with crime (Thornberry and Christenson, 1984).

Thus, the social determinants of violence are linked in a cycle in terms of poverty and the inability to have basic necessities of life, disruption of marriages, production of single parent families, unemployment, and further difficulty in maintaining interpersonal ties, family structures, and social control.

OTHER ENVIRONMENTAL FACTORS

Bystanders

There is evidence that social control of crime by members of society other than law enforcement officials may deter violence and other crimes. Shotland and Goodstein (1984) have found that the number of bystanders available for surveillance and intervention may prevent the commission of crime and, in a cyclical way, fear of crime may reduce the number of bystanders available for surveillance. This suggests that under certain circumstances crime causes crime, and implies that an important factor in the social control of crime is the relative balance between offenders' fear of surveillance and the bystanders' fear of crime.

The relative strength of each of these forces determines whether a neighborhood will be either a safe or a hostile and dangerous setting in terms of violence. This is consistent with findings in studies by Messner and Tardiff (1985) which analyzed homicide patterns in New York City in relation to a routine activities approach to explain direct contact predatory violations that have three components: an offender motivated to commit the violation, a suitable target to be victimized by the offender, and the absence of guardians capable of preventing the violation. In our study, we found that the probability of "capable guardians" being present was related to the decreased incidence of homicide.

Thus, the effect of bystanders or capable guardians on the level of violence in a community has implications in terms of programs such as "crime watch" and other efforts at community organization.

Physical Environment

Physical crowding may be related to homicide and violent crime; yet, there are conflicting studies as to whether density defined by the number of buildings in a geographic area or the number of inhabitants in a building is related to violent crime. Some contend that there is increased contact, decreased defensible space, and increase of violence in high density areas, while others argue that increased density is related to increased social control and decrease of violent crime (Anderson, 1982; Sampson, 1983).

Metropolitan areas with central cities have had the highest rates of homicide, followed by nonmetropolitan counties, and last by metropolitan areas without central cities. It appears that there is less difference between urban and rural areas in primary homicides as opposed to secondary homicides; that is, secondary to crime, which are increased in urban areas (Jason et al, 1983). A major deficit of environmental density studies is that they do not take economic factors mentioned above into consideration. Bell and Baron (1981) have reviewed a number of ecological and ethnological studies as well as laboratory studies which correlated the ambient temperature of the environment with violent crime and riots. They concluded that there is a relation between heat and aggression that is curvilinear; that is, moderately uncomfortable ambient temperatures produce an increase of aggression, while extremely hot temperatures decrease aggression and lead to flight rather than fight.

In conclusion, the clinician should appreciate the social and economic setting in which the violent patient lives for purposes of evaluation and treatment. Furthermore, the environmental determinants of violence in society—for example, overcrowding, heat, and the role of others around the potentially violent individual—have direct relevance to violence by patients in an inpatient hospital setting. A number of studies have noted that inpatient violence is related to the number of patients in relation to the number of staff, as well as to the education, experience, and attitudes of the staff on the unit. Patients must have the opportunity to participate in their environment and to interact with staff members and other patients if isolation, anger, and violence are to be avoided (Depp, 1983; Gutheil, 1984; Tardiff, 1983).

Firearms

Firearms are important since they probably turn what would have been an assault into homicide. Nationally, Jason and colleagues (1983) found that more than two-thirds of homicides in the period from 1976 to 1979 involved firearms; and there is evidence that there has been a significant increase in the number of homicides associated with firearms in this century, particularly since 1960. Determining whether this increase is due to increased availability of firearms is complex and not easily achieved. Some measures of availability have included information about the manufacture, import, and sales of guns, but imports are not measured accurately and there is little available data on exports and the rate at which all guns are removed from circulation. In addition to difficulty in quantifying availability of guns, the overall availability of guns may not reveal much about the relation of firearms to violence (Kleck, 1979; Cook, 1982).

With this confusion about the definition of availability and the difficulty of linking availability of guns to homicide rates, some researchers have turned to evaluation of the impact of gun control legislation. Findings concerning state gun control legislation are not consistent. The Gun Control Act of 1968 was found to have no effect on homicide in New York and Boston (Zimring, 1975), but both the Bartley-Fox Amendment in Massachusetts and the District of Columbia's Firearms Control Act of 1975 have been shown to be related to a decrease of homicides involving firearms (Deutsch, 1980; Jones, 1981).

The availability of a gun in the home is of obvious importance, as we will see in the evaluation of violence potential in our patients. What we do not know is the availability of guns by criminals in the illegitimate market, and whether their use in homicide-related crimes would be decreased by gun control legislation.

CONCLUSION

Human violence is the result of a complex interaction of the characteristics of the individual with influences in the environment. To date, biological or innate predisposing factors such as neurophysiological dysfunction, some hormones, inheritance, neurotransmitter abnormalities, or certain psychiatric disorders are nonspecific in the way they cause violence. Rather than a specific mechanism, they tip the balance by impairing the individual's ability to achieve goals by more appropriate nonviolent means or by increasing impulsivity, irritability, irrationality, or disorganization of behavior.

The influence of the environment and persons around the individual exert their effects during development of the individual, and more immediately preceding the violent episode. Influences during development include having been subjected to physical abuse as a child, witnessing violence either in a real sense within one's family or subculture, or through television and other mass media. Environmental factors that precede the violent episode include the setting of poverty and other adverse social conditions, which have a damaging effect on the family and social network, as well as on the individual and the more immediate influence of alcohol and drug abuse and availability of weapons.

For the individual patient, some biological and environmental factors may be more important than others, but it is the responsibility of the clinician to weigh all of these in the evaluation of the individual, in the determination of the danger he or she poses to others, and, of course, in the planning and implementation of treatment.

REFERENCES

Anderson AC: Environmental factors and aggressive behavior. J Clin Psychiatry 43:280-283, 1982

Bell PA, Baron RA: Ambient temperature and human violence, in Multidisciplinary Approaches to Aggression Research. Edited by Brain PF, Benton D. Amsterdam, Elsevier/North Holland Biomedical Press, 1981

Blau JR, Blau PM: The cost of inequality: metropolitan structure and violent crime. American Sociological Review 47:114-129, 1982

Bohman M: Some genetic aspects of alcoholism and criminality. Arch Gen Psychiatry 35:269-276, 1978

Bohman M, Cloninger R, Sigvardsson S, et al: Predisposition to petty criminality in Swedish adoptees. Arch Gen Psychiatry 39:1233-1241, 1982

Brain PF, Benton D (Eds): Multidisciplinary Approaches to Aggression Research. Amsterdam, Elsevier/North Holland Biomedical Press, 1981

Brown, GL, Goodwin FK, Ballenger JC, et al: Aggression in humans correlates with cerebrospinal fluid amine metabolites. Psychiatry Res 1:131-139, 1979

Brown, GL, Ebert MH, Goyer PF, et al: Aggression, suicide and serotonin: relationship to CSF amine metabolites. Am J Psychiatry 136:741-746, 1982

Centerwall BS: Race, socioeconomic status and domestic homicide: Atlanta, 1971-72. Am J Public Health 74:813-815, 1984

Coe CC, Levine S: Biology of aggression. Bull Am Acad Psychiatry Law 11:131-148, 1983

Cook PJ: The role of firearms in violent crime: an interpretive review of the literature, in Criminal Violence. Edited by Wolfgang ME, Weiner NA. Beverly Hills, Sage, 1982

Dalton K: Cyclical criminal acts in premenstrual syndrome. Lancet 2:1070-1071, 1980

Dalton K: The Premenstrual Syndrome and Progesterone Therapy. Chicago, Yearbook Medical Publishers, 1984

Davidson JM, Smith ER, Levine S, et al: Treatment of hypogonadal men with androgens. Clinics in Endocrinology and Metabolism 48.955-958, 1979

DeFronzo J: Economic assistance to impoverished Americans: relationship to incidence of crime. Criminology 21:119-136, 1983

Delgado-Escueta AV, Mattson RH, King L, et al: The nature of aggression during epileptic seizures. N Engl J Med 305:711-716, 1981

Depp FC: Assaults in a public mental hospital, in Assaults Within Psychiatric Facilities. Edited by Lion JR, and Reid WH. New York, Grune & Stratton, 1983

Deutsch SJ: Intervention modeling: analysis of changes in crime rates, in Frontiers in Quantitative Criminology. New York, Academic Press, 1980

Devinsky O, Baer D: Varieties of aggressive behavior in temporal lobe epilepsy. Am J Psychiatry 141:651-656, 1984

d'Orban PT, Dalton J: Violent crime and the menstrual cycle. Psychol Med 10:353-359, 1980

Eichelman B, Elliott GR, Barchas J: Biomedical, pharmacological and genetic aspects of aggression, in Biobehavioral Aspects of Aggression. Edited by Hamburg DA, Trudeau MB. New York, Alan Liss, 1981

Frederichs C, Goodman H: Low Blood Sugar and You. New York, Constellation International, 1969

Freedman JL: Effect of television violence on aggressiveness. Psychol Bull 96:227-246, 1984

Goldberg WG, Tomlanovich MC: Domestic violence victims in the emergency room: new findings. JAMA 251:3259-3268, 1984

Goodman RA, Mercy JA, Loya F, et al: Alcohol use and interpersonal violence: alcohol detected in homicide victims. Am J Public Health 76:144-149, 1986

Gutheil TG: A review of quantitative studies, in The Psychiatric Uses of Seclusion and Restraint. Edited by Tardiff K. Washington, DC, American Psychiatric Press, Inc., 1984

Hamburg DA, Trudeau MD: Biomedical Aspects of Aggression. New York, Alan R. Liss, 1981

Heins M: The 'battered child' revisited. JAMA 251:3295-3300, 1984

Hermann BP, Whitman S: Behavioral and personality correlates of epilepsy: a review, methodological critique and conceptual model. Psychol Bull 95:451-497, 1984

Hutchings B, Mednick SA: Criminality in adoptees and their biological parents: a pilot study, in Biosocial Bases of Criminal Behavior. Edited by Mednick SA, Christiansen KO. New York, Gardner Press, 1977

Jaffe P, Wolfe D, Wilson SK, et al: Family violence and child adjustment: a comparative analysis of girls' and boys' behavioral symptoms. Am J Psychiatry 143:74-77, 1986

Jason J, Strauss LT, Tyler CW: A comparison of primary and secondary homicides in the United States. Am J Epidemiology 117:309-319, 1983

Jones ED: The District of Columbia's Firearms Control Regulations Act of 1975: the toughest handgun control law in the United States—or is it? Annals of the American Academy of Political and Social Sciences 5:135-139, 1981

Kazamatsuri H, Nanko S, Mako Y: Homicidality in a woman with 47, xxx karyotype. J Clin Psychiatry 46:346-347, 1985

Kempe CH, Helfer R (Eds): The Battered Child Syndrome, third edition. Chicago, University of Chicago Press, 1980

Kleck G: Capital punishment, gun ownership and homicide. American Journal of Sociology 84:882-910, 1979

Krakowski M, Volavka J, Brizer D: Psychopathology and violence: a review of the literature. Compr Psychiatry 27:131-148, 1986

Leicester J: Temper tantrums, epilepsy and episodic dyscontrol. Br J Psychiatry 141:262-266, 1982

Lewis DO, Pincus JH, Shanok SS, et al: Psychomotor epilepsy and violence in a group of incarcerated adolescent boys. Am J Psychiatry 139:882-887, 1982

Lidberg L, Tuck JR, Asberg M, et al: Homicide, suicide and CSF 5–HIAA. Acta Psychiatr Scand 71:230-236, 1985

Linkowski P: Editorial: Suicide and biochemistry. Biol Psychiatry 20:123-124, 1985

Linnolia M, Virkkunen M, Scheinin M, et al: Low cerebrospinal fluid 5–hydroxyindoleacetic acid concentration differentiates impulsive from nonimpulsive violent behavior. Life Sci 33:2609-2614, 1983

Mark VH, Ervin FR: Violence and the Brain. New York, Harper & Row, 1970

Matthews R: Testosterone levels in aggressive offenders, in Psychopharmacology of Aggression. Edited by Sandler M. New York, Raven Press, 1979

Mattsson A, Schalling D, Olwens D, et al: Plasma testosterone, aggressive behavior and personality dimensions in young male delinquents. J Am Acad Child Psychiatry 19:476-490, 1980

Mednick SA, Volavka J: Biology and crime, in Crime and Justice: An Annual Review of Research, vol II. Edited by Morris N, Touny M. Chicago, University of Chicago Press, 1980

Menuck M: Clinical aspects of dangerous behavior. Journal of Psychiatry and Law 11:277-304, 1983

Messner S, Tardiff K: The social ecology of urban homicide: an application of the 'routine activities' approach. Criminology 23:241-267, 1985

Messner S, Tardiff K: Economic inequality and levels of homicide: an analysis of urban neighborhoods. Criminology (in press)

Money J, Dalery J: Sexual disorders: hormonal and drug therapy, in Handbook of Sexology. Edited by Money J, Musaph H. Amsterdam, Elsevier/North Holland Biomedical Press, 1977

Monroe RR: Episodic Behavioral Disorders. Cambridge, Harvard University Press, 1970

Monroe RR: Episodic behavioral disorders and limbic ictus. Compr Psychiatry 26:466-479, 1985

NIMH: Television and Behavior: 10 Years of Scientific Progress and Implications for the Eighties. Washington, DC, U.S. Government Printing Office, 1982

Nurco DN, Ball JC, Shaffer JW, et al: The criminality of narcotic addicts. J Nerv Ment Dis 173:94-102, 1985

Olwens D, Mattsson A, Schalling D, et al: Testosterone, aggression, physical and personality dimensions in normal adolescent males. Psychosom Med 42:253-269, 1980

Rabkin JG: Criminal behavior of discharged mental patients: a critical review of the research. Psychol Bull 86:1-27, 1979

Rada RT, Laws DR, Kellner R, et al: Plasma testosterone levels in the rapist. Psychosom Med 38:257-268, 1976

Rada RT, Kellner R, Stivastava C, et al: Plasma androgens in violent and nonviolent sex offenders. Journal of the American Academy of Psychiatry and Law 11:149-158, 1983

Reid RL, Yen SSC: Premenstrual syndrome. Am J Obstet Gynecol 139:85-104, 1981

Sampson RJ: Structural density and criminal victimization. Criminology 21:276-293, 1983

Schiavi RC, Theilgaard A, Owen DR, et al: Sex chromosome abnormalities, hormones and aggressivity. Arch Gen Psychiatry 41:93-99, 1984

Shotland RL, Goodstein LI: The role of bystanders in crime control. Journal of Social Issues 40:9-26, 1984

Silberman CE: Criminal Violence, Criminal Justice. New York, Vintage, 1980

Simmel EC, Hahn ME, Wathers JK: Aggressive Behavior: Genetic and Neural Approaches. Hillsdale, N.J., Lawrence Erlbaum Associates, 1983

Singhal RL, Telner JI: A perspective: psychopharmacological aspects of aggression in animals and man. Psychiatr J Univ Ottawa 8:145-153, 1983

Spinetta JJ: Parental personality factors in child abuse. J Consult Clin Psychol 46:1409-1414, 1978

Tardiff K: A survey of assault by chronic patients, in Assaults Within Psychiatric Facilities. Edited by Lion JR, Reid WH. New York, Grune & Stratton, 1983.

Tardiff K: Characteristics of assaultive patients in private psychiatric hospitals. Am J Psychiatry 141:1232-1235, 1984

Tardiff K, Koenigsberg HW: Assaultive behavior among psychiatric outpatients. Am J Psychiatry 142:960-963, 1985

Tardiff K, Sweillam A: Assault, suicide and mental illness. Arch Gen Psychiatry 37:164-169, 1980

Tardiff K. Sweillam A: The occurrence of assaultive behavior among chronic psychiatric inpatients. Am J Psychiatry 139:212-215, 1982

Tardiff K, Gross E, Messner S: A study of homicide in Manhattan, 1981. Am J Public Health 76:139-143, 1986

Taylor PJ: Motives for offending among violent and psychotic men. Br J Psychiatry 147:491-498, 1985

Thornberry TP, Christenson RC: Unemployment and criminal involvement: an investigation of reciprocal causal structures. American Sociological Review 49:398-411, 1984

Valzelli L: Psychobiology of Aggression and Violence. New York, Raven Press, 1981

Virkkunen M: Reactive hypoglycemia tendency among habitually violent offenders: a further study by means of the glucose tolerance test. Neuropsychobiology 8:35-40, 1982

Vold GV: Theoretical Criminology. New York, Oxford Univ Press, 1979

Williams K: Economic sources of homicide: reestimating the effects of poverty and inequality. American Sociological Review 49:283-289, 1984

Wolfgang ME: Sociocultural overview of criminal violence, in Violence and the Violent Individual. Edited by Hays JR, Roberts TK, Solway KS. New York, S.P. Medical and Scientific Publications, 1981

Wolfgang ME, Ferracuti F: The Subculture of Violence: Toward an Integrated Theory in Criminology. New York, Methuen, 1967

Zimring F: Firearms and federal law: the Gun Control Act of 1968. Journal of Legal Studies 4:133-198, 1975

Chapter 20

Patterns in Human Violence

by Park Elliott Dietz, M.D., M.P.H., Ph.D.

Psychiatrists are routinely called upon to treat violent patients and those who have been victims of violence and to assess dangerousness to others. This work and the more specialized tasks of forensic and correctional psychiatrists can be enhanced by a knowledge of criminology, a field that few psychiatrists have the time or inclination to master. This chapter draws on criminological information, including national crime statistics and large-scale victim surveys, to review current information about specific violent crimes.

The crime-specific approach taken here has both advantages and disadvantages. The principal advantages stem from the fact that there is considerable specificity to certain aspects of violent behavior, such as the role of weapons in converting assaultive incidents and robberies into homicides, or the role of sexual sadism in the behavior of lust murderers and serial killers. The principal disadvantage of a crime-specific approach is the risk of losing sight of the commonalities among offenses. The review of determinants of violent behavior in Chapter 19 counters this disadvantage by showing that the social and biological determinants of violent behavior (and many psychological determinants as well) are by and large not associated with particular criminal acts, but rather are correlated with antisocial behavior or criminality in general. Contrary to popular belief, specialization in particular crimes is the exception and not the rule among violent offenders.

The violent patients most often encountered in psychiatric practice are those whose violence is expressive of transient states of intoxication or emotional arousal, and is reflective of maladaptive relationships with family members or of psychopathology. The most common offenses in this population are threats and nonfatal attacks, which often represent expressive violence. These behaviors are therefore considered first. At the other end of the expressive–instrumental continuum are those who commit robbery, which is always at least partially financially motivated. To highlight those contrasts to be found between those who threaten and attack without financial motive and those whose violence is partially financially motivated, and because of its high incidence, robbery is also reviewed, despite the fact that robbers are more likely to be career criminals who eschew psychiatric treatment and that robbers are less often referred for psychiatric evaluation (probably because their motives usually seem obvious). Homicide is intermediate between these two extremes on the expressive–instrumental continuum and is treated in detail, despite its much lower incidence, because of the high proportion of murderers who are referred for psychiatric examination after the offense. Finally, a few special offenses that are too often presumed to reflect mental illness—assassination, mass murder, serial murder, bombing, and skyjacking—are treated in summary fashion. This chapter does not deal with the subjects of rape and other sexual assaults, arson, or kidnapping, even though they constitute criminal violence, or with lawful violence such as judicial executions, self-defense, martial arts, or contact sports. Terrorism is considered only in the sections on bombing and skyjacking because of the relatively small number of terrorist incidents in the United States to date.

THREATS

Despite their potential for provoking or foreshadowing violent harm to others, threats are not ordinarily regarded as violent behavior. Verbal behavior may express an intent to harm with great clarity. Yet even where the intent is conveyed and the threat is capable of execution, we hesitate to call the behavior violent. It is as if we accept the childhood adage, "Sticks and stones can break my bones, but words can never hurt me." Whether violent or not, patients' threats command attention from psychiatrists because we know that threats reflect thoughts, desires, and emotions and that they are sometimes carried out, and because some jurisdictions have imposed a legal duty on therapists to take action which might avert the threatened harm.

In some jurisdictions, threats are charged as simple assault (which under common law was an attempt or offer to commit a battery), while in others they are charged as terroristic threats, harassment, or under such general provisions as disorderly conduct statutes. Threats are an element of other crimes, such as rape, robbery, and kidnapping, but are rarely charged when these more serious charges can be brought. Conditional threats in which the threatener specifies the means by which the offered harm may be avoided can, in some instances, be prosecuted as extortion or coercion.

The few existing studies of threats by mental patients have produced a few findings that can help guide clinical decision-making but which do not, taken as a whole, provide clear guidance about the management of threatening patients. When compared with attacks, threats are more likely to be directed toward authority figures, while attacks are more likely to be directed toward peers (Dietz, 1981). Of 100 patients committed to a mental hospital because of homicidal threats (81 verbal and 19 by actions), four subsequently committed suicide, two killed someone whom they had threatened, and one killed someone other than the threatened person within the follow-up period of more than five years (Macdonald, 1968). Twenty percent of 43 schizophrenic murderers in South Korea who were referred by the courts for psychiatric evaluation had made homicidal threats to their families and neighbors prior to the murder (Yoon et al, 1973). Thirty-two percent of 25 murderers referred by the courts for psychiatric evaluation had made one or more homicidal threats prior to the murder, and 28 percent had done so within three months of the murder; of these latter seven men, only two killed the person whom they had threatened, and the other five killed someone else (Dietz, 1985). Thus, the probability of a homicidal threat by a mentally disordered person being carried out is much lower than the probability of a mentally disordered murderer having made a homicidal threat. Moreover, the person against whom a threat is directed is not necessarily the person at greatest risk of being victimized.

One special problem that arises from time to time in clinical practice is the discovery that a patient has threatened a public figure. The temptation in such instances is to assume that the patient has no access to the public figure and that the threat is symbolic or expressive of some more diffuse grievance. In research in progress at the University of Virginia, we have found that at least 10 percent of the persons writing threatening letters to nongovernmental public figures physically approach the person whom they have threatened by attending a public appearance or by traveling to their homes, offices, agencies, studios, or other haunts. While the clinician may be aware that threats to the president or to presidential candidates should be reported to the Secret Service, few know where to report other public figure threats. Threats to U.S. senators, members of congress, and officials of federal agencies are dealt with by the F.B.I.; threats to federal judges, prosecutors, or witnesses, by the U.S. Marshals Service; threats to state officials, by the state police or its equivalent; and threats to local officials are dealt with by the local law enforcement agency. No centralized agency handles threats to entertainment or sports figures, but studios and television networks will sometimes provide a mailing address or forward urgent communications.

ATTACKS

The most prevalent forms of violence with which psychiatrists must deal are attacks that are neither sexually nor financially motivated and that do not result in death. Ironically, they are the least studied of the prevalent violent crimes. Referred to colloquially as "assaults," these attacks fall within a variety of social science and legal definitions for which there has been minimal standardization. Assault, which under common law was an attempt or offer to commit a battery, is often confounded with battery, the unlawful use of force on another person, especially in the psychiatric literature. Attacks include all manner of unlawful touching, from throwing water to barroom brawls to surgery without consent to nonfatal grenade launchings and a variety of potentially injurious behaviors such as attempting to punch, kick, stab, shoot, or burn someone.

The definitional problems arise partly from a lack of standardization among jurisdictions in the names given to particular types of offensive behavior. For example, identical behaviors could be charged as assault and battery, simple assault, and aggravated assault in three different jurisdictions. Within a given jurisdiction, the legal definitions of these offenses are designed to provide a gradation of seriousness that simultaneously takes account of intent and harm. For example, attempts to harm someone with a lethal weapon that result in no injury are typically graded identically to beatings resulting in serious injury. This is illustrated in the definition of aggravated assault in the Model Penal Code (Section 210.1), which forms the basis of many state statutes: "A person is guilty of aggravated assault if he: a) attempts to cause serious bodily injury to another, or causes such injury purposely, knowingly or recklessly under circumstances manifesting extreme indifference to the value of human life; or b) attempts to cause or purposely or knowingly causes bodily injury toward another with a deadly weapon" (American Law Institute, 1980, p. 174).

For methodological and logistical reasons, researchers have generally focused either on attacks within a single type of institution (most notably the family, hospitals, prisons, or schools) or attacks reported to the police (which include some of the more serious attacks occurring within institutions). Studies of violence within psychiatric facilities are of particular interest to psychiatrists and have recently been reviewed and compiled in a single volume (Lion and Reid, 1983).

The family violence literature (for example, Gelles, 1974; Pagelow, 1981; Straus et al, 1980) and the now overwhelmingly large body of literature on child abuse (see, for example, Wells, 1980) also contain a wealth of information on intrafamilial attacks, most of which are never reported to the police, and which should be of particular interest to psychiatrists. A review of studies of violence within the family or within other institutions is beyond the scope of this chapter.

National data on attacks are available from only two sources. The first and most longstanding is the annual *Uniform Crime Reports* of the Federal Bureau of Investigation, which deal only with aggravated assault incidents reported to the police and which are published under the title *Crime in the United States*. Data from this source are meant to be a complete enumeration of all of the offenses reported to the police in jurisdictions submitting their data, which in 1984 encompassed 94 percent of the population (Federal Bureau of Investigation, 1985). The second is the periodic *National Crime Survey Report*, based on victimization surveys conducted for the Bureau of Justice Statistics by the Bureau of the Census, which deal with several categories of attacks reported to census takers conducting household interviews and which are published under the title *Criminal Victimization in the United States*. In 1983, the most recent year for which data have been published, a representative sample of some 127,000 persons living in about 60,000 households was included in the survey (Bureau of Justice Statistics, 1985). Both sources include data on aggravated assaults, defined roughly in accordance with the Model Penal Code language quoted above. Only the *National Crime Survey Reports* include data on simple assault, which is defined for this purpose as "[a]ttack without a weapon resulting either in minor injury (e.g., bruises, black eyes, cuts, scratches, swelling) or in undetermined injury requiring less than two days of hospitalization [or] attempted assault without a weapon" (Bureau of Justice Statistics, 1985).

Types of Offenses and Offenders

The typologies of offenses and offenders that have been proposed to date are based either on apparent motivation or on psychological characteristics of the offender. None of these has been adopted for widespread use. A classification of offenses analogous to that proposed below for homicides would have the virtues of mutual exclusivity, comprehensiveness, and comparability to homicide:

1. *Primary assaults* arising between persons who, prior to the offense, had established a relationship, however brief, without criminal purposes. Assaults within the family and most assaults occurring within other institutions or in the context of arguments are included here.
2. *Secondary assaults* arising in the course of criminal transactions between persons without a preexisting, noncriminal relationship. In urban areas today, drug transactions and robberies are the most common situations in which secondary assaults occur.
3. *Tertiary assaults* in which no interaction between victim and offender precedes the attack, as occurs in attacks on strangers in public places, many arsons, bombings, and sniper incidents, and most failed assassination attempts.
4. *Mixed assaults* involving elements of more than one of the above types, as in robbery-assaults within families, bombings in which the offender had a rela-

tionship with one of multiple victims, or attacks by arson on criminal associates and innocent victims who happen to be present.

Assaultive behavior is so nearly universal that any effort to classify offenders must either ignore those persons whose assaultive acts ceased in adolescence or become a typology of mankind. For psychiatrists, the classificatory task will most often amount to an effort to determine the degree to which a particular assault was reflective of organic pathology, intoxication, irritability, thought disorder, emotional state, character pathology, and purposive efforts to achieve identifiable goals. The results of such inquiries most often do not permit classification of the patient so much as classification of one instance of the patient's behavior, because a single individual will often commit multiple assaults as a result of differing combinations of factors.

Epidemiology of Offenses

Tables 1 and 2 give the most recent data available on the incidence of various types of assaults. As with most other crimes, underrecognition of the offense by victims and underreporting to the police lead to many offenses not being investigated. Thus, the true incidence of the behavior is better estimated from victimization survey data than from police report data. It is likely that many offenses, particularly those within families and other institutions, are neither reported to the police nor revealed in victimization surveys. In general, the larger the city, the higher the rates of aggravated assault.

In the United States, aggravated assault rates are lowest in the winter and highest in the summer (Federal Bureau of Investigation, 1985). Aggravated assaults occur at higher rates on Fridays, Saturdays, and Sundays than on other days (Pittman and Handy, 1964). In 1983, approximately one-half of all assaults occurred between 6:00 P.M. and 6:00 A.M., and the more serious assaults tended to occur at night somewhat more often than the less serious assaults (Bureau of Justice Statistics, 1985). Victimization survey data show that approximately one-half of

Table 1. Frequencies and Rates per 1,000 Population of Violent Crimes Reported to the Police in the United States in 1984

Offense	Frequency	Rate
Aggravated assault	685,349	2.90
Robbery	485,008	2.05
Murder and nonnegligent homicide	18,692	0.08
Forcible rape[1]	84,233	0.36
Arson[1]	101,836[2]	0.53

[1]These data are provided for comparative purposes only, as rape and arson are not reviewed in this chapter.
[2]This figure is based on reports from fewer police departments than the other frequencies tabulated here.
Source: Federal Bureau of Investigation, 1985

Table 2. Frequencies and Rates of Victimization per 1,000 Persons Age 12 and Over by Violent Crime in the United States in 1983[1]

Offense	Frequency	Rate	Percent Reported to the Police
Assault	4,600,090	24.1	45.8
Aggravated assault	1,517,310	8.0	56.5
Completed with injury	537,120	2.8	62.8
Attempted with weapon	980,190	5.1	53.0
Simple assault	3,082,770	16.2	40.6
Completed with injury	824,070	4.3	49.4
Attempted without weapon	2,258,710	11.9	37.4
Robbery	1,149,170	6.0	52.6
Completed robbery	709,550	3.7	63.6
With injury	252,450	1.3	73.7
Without injury	457,090	2.4	58.1
Attempted robbery	439,630	2.3	34.7
With injury	124,940	0.7	51.3
Without injury	314,690	1.7	28.1

[1]These data are estimates derived from a survey of some 60,000 representative households and are the most recent data available. Note that more than one victimization may occur in a single incident of violent crime. Thus, the number of offenses may be lower than the number of victimizations.

Source: Bureau of Justice Statistics, 1985

all assaults by strangers occur in the street and other public places, and that the most common site of assaults by nonstrangers is in or near the victim's home (Bureau of Justice Statistics, 1985).

Characteristics of Offenses

In 1983, weapons were used in 32 percent of all assaults and 95 percent of the aggravated assaults by strangers, and in 26 percent of all assaults and 90 percent of the aggravated assaults by nonstrangers. A firearm was used in 24 percent and a knife in 29 percent of all aggravated assaults by armed offenders. In 1983, 67 percent of aggravated assaults were committed by a single offender, 14 percent by pairs of offenders, four percent by three offenders, and eight percent by four or more offenders. Simple assaults involved a single offender somewhat more often (77 percent). Members of assaulting groups were all white in 64 percent and all black in 23 percent (Bureau of Justice Statistics, 1985).

In their study of 241 aggravated assaults in St. Louis, Pittman and Handy (1964) reported that approximately one-fourth of the offenders and approximately one-fourth of the victims had been drinking alcohol at the time of the offense. No data are available on the specific role, if any, of other drugs in the commission of assaults because violent offenses are aggregated in all of the major studies of drug use. Pittman and Handy (1964) found that verbal arguments preceded 75 percent of the assaults.

In 1983, 53 percent of all assaults reported to surveyers were known not to have been reported to the police (Bureau of Justice Statistics, 1985). As shown in Table 2, reporting was more likely for the more serious assaults, but even for aggravated assaults more than two-fifths go unreported. Of those assaults reported, some are regarded as unfounded by the police on the basis of preliminary investigation. Approximately 60 percent of aggravated assaults considered by the police to be founded result in an arrest (Federal Bureau of Investigation, 1985). Thus, approximately one-third of the most serious assaults acknowledged in surveys result in an arrest.

Offender Characteristics

As with other violent crimes, males predominate among offenders. In 1983, 89 percent of the single-offender aggravated assault victimizations were committed by males, 11 percent by females; for simple assaults the respective proportions were 86 percent male and 14 percent female (Bureau of Justice Statistics, 1985). Except for victims under 20, two-thirds of whose offenders are estimated to be younger than 21, more than 80 percent of all single-offender-assault offenders are estimated by the victims to be 21 or older (Bureau of Justice Statistics, 1985). In 1984, 61 percent of aggravated assault arrestees were white, and 38 percent were black (Federal Bureau of Investigation, 1985). National data on social status, education, or employment among offenders are unavailable.

Although there have been many studies of violent offenders referred for psychiatric evaluation, most do not disaggregate data by type of offense. The only data available on the prevalence of mental disorder among assaultists who committed their offenses in the community derive from a single study of 56 men charged with nonsexual batteries of various kinds who were committed to a maximum security institution for psychiatric evaluation. In this highly selected population, approximately one-half of the men received diagnoses of alcoholism and approximately one-half received diagnoses of schizophrenia according to the criteria of Feighner and colleagues (1972); 20 percent received diagnoses of affective disorders; and the next most common diagnoses, each of which was made in nine percent of the men, were antisocial personality disorder and other personality disorders (Dietz, 1985). No diagnostic data are available for a representative group of offenders.

Victim Characteristics

Population groups vary substantially in their rates of assault victimization. Rates vary by age, with age-specific victimization rates highest for those aged 16–19 and lowest for those aged 65 or older. Rates are higher for males than for females and higher for the unemployed than for the employed. Although the overall assault rate is similar among blacks and whites, the rate of aggravated-assault victimization is higher among blacks and the rate of simple assault higher among whites (Bureau of Justice Statistics, 1985).

In 1983, 54 percent of assault victims were attacked by strangers. Victims offered some resistance to offenders in 81 percent of assaults, including evasion, using physical force, threatening or reasoning with the offender, trying to get help or frighten the offender, or using or brandishing a weapon. Approximately 80 percent of all age, sex, and racial groups of victims offered resistance, except for decreasing proportions above the age of 50 (Bureau of Justice Statistics, 1985).

In 30 percent of all assaults the victim receives some injury. Physical injury occurs more often among black victims than white victims, more often in the younger age groups, more often among the lowest income victims, and more often in nonstranger assaults (Bureau of Justice Statistics, 1985). Assault victims sometimes suffer posttraumatic stress disorder or other psychological sequelae, but the frequency of such responses is unknown.

ROBBERY

Robbery is the stock and trade of the violent career criminal and one source of cash for drug addicts, delinquents, and other opportunists. While other violent crimes rarely yield immediate financial gain, robbery is the prototype of violent crime for profit. Robbery is often confounded with burglary (the entering of a dwelling place during the night with intent to commit a felony) and theft (the taking of the property of another), from which it differs in the requirement that robbery involves force or threat of force. Definitions of robbery vary somewhat among the states, but many statutes are based on the Model Penal Code (Section 222.1) definition: "A person is guilty of robbery if, in the course of committing a theft, he: a) inflicts serious bodily injury upon another; or b) threatens another with or purposely puts him in fear of immediate serious bodily injury; or c) commits or threatens immediately to commit any felony of the first or second degree" (American Law Institute, 1980, p. 96).

Types of Offenses and Offenders

No adequate typology of robbery offenses has gained acceptance. Most of those proposed are flawed by the use of categories that are not mutually exclusive. Nearly all robberies fall into one and only one of the following five categories:

1. *Commercial robberies* in which the victims are at work or are patrons of the commercial concern in which the robbery occurs
2. *Street robberies of strangers* in which the victims are not at work and the robbery occurs in a public place
3. *Home robberies of strangers* in which the robbery occurs in the dwelling of one or more of the victims or their host
4. *Confidence robberies* in which the robber or an accomplice has lured the victim into a vulnerable position after a brief acquaintance (for example, robberies of clients by prostitutes or drug dealers and the converse)
5. *Nonstranger robberies* in which the victim and offender have a preexisting relationship

The best-known typology of robbers was developed by Conklin (1972) on the basis of his interviews with 67 imprisoned robbers in Massachusetts, all of whom were adult males and three-fifths of whom were black:

1. *The professional robber* is committed to crime as a career, tends to specialize in robbery, plans the crimes, and seeks money to support a hedonistic lifestyle. This robber usually carries a weapon and targets commercial establishments. Although gaining $500 or more per robbery, this robber spends the money quickly. Accomplices assigned to particular functions may be used for particular robberies, but do not comprise a stable gang. Professional robbers are usually from middle class origins, white, and in their mid-20s. Most drink, but few use drugs.
2. *The opportunist robber* selects vulnerable and accessible victims (such as elderly women, taxi drivers, and drunks), carries no weapon, and gains small amounts of cash for extra spending money. This robber generally operates with a group, but the members do not have specialized functions. Opportunist robbers are usually from lower-class origins, black, and in their teens or early 20s. This is the most prevalent type of robber found among prisoners.
3. *The addict robber* is committed to theft because of the lower risk of violence and apprehension but resorts to robbery, usually unarmed, as a last resort to support his drug habit.
4. *The alcoholic robber* commits seemingly random and unplanned robberies, often as an afterthought to assault and battery.

Based on interviews with 33 female robbers imprisoned in Florida, Fortune and colleagues (1980) differentiated two patterns: *career robbers*, who have long criminal records and actively participated in robberies, and *situational robbers* without extensive criminal records, who robbed in response to severe economic need or peer pressure or while intoxicated.

Epidemiology of Offenses

Frequencies and rates of robbery according to police reports and a victimization survey are shown in Tables 1 and 2. As with most other crimes, underrecognition of the offense by victims and underreporting to the police lead to many offenses not being investigated. Both sources of data show increasing rates of robbery from the mid-1970s until 1981, and decreasing rates since then. Population-based rates are highest in the northeastern states and lowest in the southern states. In general, the larger the city, the higher the rates of robbery.

In the United States, robbery rates are lowest in the spring and highest in the winter, usually peaking in December (Federal Bureau of Investigation, 1985). Macdonald (1975) has suggested that the winter increase reflects the longer hours of darkness, greater financial need during the holidays, and the ability of robbers in some climates to wear ski masks without arousing suspicion. Robberies occur up to twice as often on Fridays and Saturdays as on other days of the week (Normandeau, 1968; Macdonald, 1975). Local variations depend on paydays and the day of arrival of Social Security and other government benefit checks. In 1983, 55 percent of all robberies and 61 percent of armed robberies occurred between 6:00 P.M. and 6:00 A.M. (Bureau of Justice Statistics, 1985).

Victimization survey data that do not specifically address commercial robberies show that approximately 70 percent of robberies by strangers occur in the street or other public areas, and that the most common site of robberies by nonstrangers is in or near the victim's home (41 percent) (Bureau of Justice Statistics, 1985). Police-report data show that 20 percent of all robberies occur in commercial establishments, gas stations, and convenience stores (Federal Bureau of Investigation, 1985). This figure overestimates the proportion of commercial robberies because they are more likely to be reported. Offenses within institutions such as hospitals, prisons, and schools are particularly likely to go unreported. For example, only one-sixth of the robberies and attacks in schools known to principals were reported to the police (National Institute of Education, 1981).

Characteristics of Offenses

Weapons were used in 50 percent of the stranger robberies and 36 percent of the nonstranger robberies surveyed in 1983. A firearm was used in 32 percent and a knife in 38 percent of all armed robberies (Bureau of Justice Statistics, 1985). The less vulnerable the victim, the more likely is the robber to wield a firearm (Cook, 1982). In 1983, 49 percent of robberies were committed by a single offender, 25 percent by pairs of offenders, 13 percent by three offenders, and 10 percent by four or more offenders. Members of robbing groups were all black in 57 percent and all white in 26 percent (Bureau of Justice Statistics, 1985).

As suggested earlier, 47 percent of the incidents recognized by the victims as robberies are not reported to the police. Of those reported, some are regarded as unfounded by the police on the basis of preliminary investigation (Block and Block, 1980). Of those not considered unfounded, only 26 percent result in an arrest (Federal Bureau of Investigation, 1985). Thus, approximately 14 percent of robberies in the nation result in an arrest. The attrition of cases in the criminal justice system has been better studied for robbery than for other offenses and illustrates the low certainty of punishment for violent offenders.

In a study of robberies in Washington, D.C., Williams and Lucianovic (1979) determined that four percent of all robberies and 34 percent of robberies in which there was an arrest resulted in at least one conviction of an adult. Nearly one-half of the cases in which there was an arrest but no conviction were screened out by a prosecutor or dismissed by a judge who decided that the charge could not be proved. Over 90 percent of the indicted defendants entered a guilty plea to some offense (not always robbery), and 75 percent of the small fraction going to trial were convicted. Of those robbers convicted, 62 percent were sentenced to some period of incarceration. Thus, only about 2.5 percent of robberies resulted in a sentence of incarceration.

Greenwood (1982) also found high rates of attrition among 650 robbery cases processed through the criminal justice system in four counties in southern California in 1973. Police did not seek a complaint against 23 percent of the people arrested for robbery, presumably because of victim unwillingness to testify or lack of evidence. Of the cases brought to the prosecutor, 18 percent were rejected, 67 percent were filed as felonies, and 15 percent were filed as misdemeanors. Of those filed as felonies, 34 percent were dismissed and one percent reduced to misdemeanors by the judge; 65 percent were held to answer. Of the latter, 12 percent were dismissed or acquitted, and 88 percent were convicted of some charge. Of those convicted, 37 percent were sentenced to incarceration in prison, 55 percent were sentenced to jail terms or committed to the California Youth Authority, and eight percent were given noncustodial sentences. Overall, 11 percent of arrested robbers received a prison sentence and 15 percent received some other custodial sentence. If the proportion of offenses resulting in arrest was comparable to that for the nation, Greenwood's data would suggest that approximately three percent of robberies result in a prison sentence, and another four percent result in some other custodial sentence.

Given that robbery is more likely to have a rational economic motive than other violent crimes, the fact that fewer than 10 percent of robberies lead to imprisonment (2.5 percent in one study and approximately seven percent in the other) gives offenders ample opportunity to learn from criminal associates and from their own experience that the supposed sanctions against robbery are not likely to be imposed. The attrition studies also underscore the likelihood that the highly selected subgroup of offenders who find their way to prison are unrepresentative of those offenders at large who have managed to avoid detection, arrest, prosecution, or conviction. The fact that most offenses do not result in an arrest highlights the fact that criminal records represent only a minimum estimate of an individual's criminal behavior.

Offender Characteristics

As with other violent crimes, males predominate among offenders. In 1983, 94 percent of the single-offender robbery victimizations were committed by males, six percent by females (Bureau of Justice Statistics, 1985). In 1984, 67 percent of robbery arrestees were younger than 25 (Federal Bureau of Investigation, 1985). Official police statistics are fairly accurate in representing the age distribution of robbers, because the lower likelihood of young offenders coming to the attention of the police is counterbalanced by the greater likelihood of arrest of those who do (Green, 1985). Victims of single-offender robberies in 1983 reported that 54 percent of their offenders were black and 41 percent were white (Bureau of Justice Statistics, 1985). The number of blacks committing robberies is inflated by the fact that young blacks so often rob in gangs. Blacks are disproportionately likely to be arrested. In 1984, 37 percent of robbery arrestees were white and 61 percent were black (Federal Bureau of Investigation, 1985). Like other violent offenders, robbers, on the average, have completed approximately 10 years of school and have high rates of unemployment. Williams and Lucianovic (1979) found that a higher proportion of robbers (62 percent) than of other adult defendants (50 percent) were unemployed.

Compared to other defendants, those charged with robbery were more likely to have a history of prior arrests, prosecutions, and convictions, more likely to have been on conditional release for another offense at the time of their robbery arrest, and more likely to be rearrested within the next four years, usually for crimes other than robbery (Williams and Lucianovic, 1979). Peterson and Braiker (1980) found that 60 percent of incarcerated armed robbers had also committed assaults, 52 percent had committed burglary, and 37 percent had sold drugs. The average rate of armed robbery among these men was 4.6 per year, with a median of 1.5 per year. Ten percent of the men averaged over 30 crimes annually.

Robbery has attracted little attention among psychiatrists, in part because the motive in robbery is usually so obvious that only a small proportion of robbers is referred for pretrial psychiatric evaluation. Fortune and colleagues (1980) found high frequencies of troubled family backgrounds, alcohol abuse, and drug abuse among female robbers, as is characteristic of most offender groups. Robbers referred for psychiatric examination had the same distribution of *DSM-III* diagnoses as other offenders referred to the same court clinic (Bluestone and Mallela,

1979). Harry (1985) studied a small group of male robbers (most of whom suffered psychotic disorders) referred for psychiatric examination to a maximum-security hospital and found two patterns for these men: 1) substance abusers in their 20s who used weapons to commit noncommercial robberies as an afterthought to other offenses; and 2) men in their 30s without substance abuse who most often attempted to rob commercial establishments without a weapon.

Victim Characteristics

Population groups vary substantially in their rates of robbery victimization. Rates vary by age, with age-specific victimization rates highest for those aged 16–24 and lowest for those aged 65 or older. Rates are higher for males than for females, higher for blacks than for whites, and higher for the unemployed than for the employed. Moreover, the risk of victimization varies inversely with income (Bureau of Justice Statistics, 1985). Cohen and colleagues (1981) showed that various combinations of these sociodemographic characteristics are associated with extreme variations in the risk of robbery. For example, among unemployed, low income blacks aged 16–29 who live alone, the relative risk is 9.85 times greater than average; among home-centered, high income whites aged 50 and over who do not live alone, the relative risk is 0.13 times the average. Teenagers are at greatest risk of robbery during school, where one percent of secondary school students are robbed each month, as are one-half as many of their teachers (National Institute of Education, 1981).

In 1983, 78 percent of robbery victims were robbed by strangers. Victims offered some resistance to offenders in 63 percent of robberies, including using physical force, trying to get help or frighten the robber, evasion, threatening or reasoning with the robber, or using or brandishing a weapon. Resistance was somewhat more common among women than men, among whites than blacks, and among younger than older victims (Bureau of Justice Statistics, 1985.)

According to the best estimates available, approximately one percent of gun robberies leads to a victim death (Cook, 1980; Zimring, 1977) as compared with a fatality ratio about one-fifth as high for nongun armed robberies (Cook, 1980). Gun robberies are less likely than other robberies to result in nonfatal injury to victims, but more likely to result in the victim's death (Block, 1981; Conklin, 1972; Cook, 1980; Zimring, 1977), presumably because the victims are less likely to resist a robber with a gun than those armed with other weapons but more likely to suffer fatal injuries from the use of a gun than from other weapons. In 31 percent of all robberies the victim receives some injury. Physical injury occurs more often among female victims than male victims, more often among white victims than black victims, more often in nonstranger robberies, and somewhat more often among the higher income victims (Bureau of Justice Statistics, 1985). Victim resistance is associated with victim injury, but no data are available that would tend to show which of these is causal to the other. Conklin (1972) found that victims were more likely to require hospitalization if their offenders were young, black, multiple, or a combination of these, which may reflect the greater vulnerability of their victims, their less frequent brandishment of weapons to intimidate victims, or efforts to impress peers. Robbery victims sometimes suffer posttraumatic stress disorder or other psychological sequelae, but the frequency of such responses is unknown.

HOMICIDE

The tendency of researchers to treat homicide as if it were a distinct pattern of behavior has been the source of considerable misunderstanding. It is as if we had an enormous body of research on sudden death due to myocardial infarction which made only passing reference to the fact that cardiovascular disease often precedes such deaths, and that sudden death is only one of the many possible outcomes of cardiovascular disease. Homicide is but one outcome of a variety of interpersonal processes, not all of which are criminal, violent, aggressive, or intended to cause death. Common law definitions of homicide are highly complex and vary somewhat among the states, but many state statutes are based on the Model Penal Code (Section 210.1) definition: "A person is guilty of criminal homicide if he purposely, knowingly, recklessly, or negligently causes the death of another human being" (American Law Institute, 1980, p. 4). Thus, murder, manslaughter, and negligent homicide are all types of criminal homicide.

Types of Offenses and Offenders

Many authors have proposed typologies of homicide that are based on legal elements, on the circumstances surrounding the offense, on the victim–offender relationship, or on offenders' apparent motives. Most of those proposed are flawed by the use of categories that are not mutually exclusive. A typology based on the work of Smith and Parker (1980), Jason et al (1983), and Tardiff et al (1986) that would encompass all homicides in a reasonable number of categories is:

1. *Primary homicides* arising from assaultive acts between persons who, prior to the offense, had established a relationship, however brief, without criminal purposes. Most homicides arising from arguments, brawls, and intrafamilial violence are included here.
2. *Secondary homicides* arising in the course of criminal transactions between persons without a preexisting, noncriminal relationship. In urban areas today, drug transactions and robberies are the most common situations in which secondary homicides occur.
3. *Tertiary homicides* in which no interaction between victim and offender precedes the killing, as in most assassinations, mass murders of strangers, contract killings, and sniper incidents, and many murders by arson or bombing. Though commanding the greatest public attention, this group results in the fewest deaths.
4. *Mixed homicides* involving elements of more than one of the above types, as in robbery-murders within families, bombings in which the offender had a relationship with one of multiple victims, or murders by arson of criminal associates and innocent victims who happen to be present.

Morrison (1973) has proposed a four-group typology of homicide offenders that reflects much of the current understanding of offenders and is an advance over many of the less carefully constructed typologies, but which is flawed by the fact that multiple categories may apply to a single offender:

1. *Mentally ill homicide offenders*, including "psychotic homicide offenders," "psychopathic assaultists," and "violent sex offenders"

2. *Deliberate antisocial lifestyle homicide offenders*, including "felony homicide offenders," "professional hired assassins," and "political assassins"
3. *"Square John" homicide offenders*, including "personal offender one-time losers" and "accidental homicide offenders"
4. *Subcultural assaulter homicide offenders*, including "victim-precipitated homicide offenders," "violent subculture homicide offenders," and "mob riot homicide offenders"

Although there is considerable diversity among the subset of homicide offenders who are referred for pretrial forensic psychiatric examination, the most common patterns observed are:

1. *Rebellious homicide offenders* who commit primary, secondary, or mixed homicides, and who evidence antisocial personality disorder, alcoholism, substance abuse disorders, or a combination of these
2. *Inadequate homicide offenders* who commit primary homicides in a context of unmet dependency needs, often accompanied by anxiety, depression, and alcohol abuse, and often associated with claimed amnesia for the killing which is variously interpreted as the product of repression, dissociation, or malingering
3. *Psychotic homicide offenders* who commit primary homicides (and occasionally other kinds) while psychotic because of a lack of treatment or a failure to take prescribed medication

Epidemiology of Offenses

The frequency and rate of murder and nonnegligent homicide shown in Table 1 underestimate the incidence of homicide because 1) these data exclude negligent and justifiable homicides; 2) some homicides are mistaken for natural deaths, accidents, and suicides; 3) the manner of death remains undetermined for a proportion of violent deaths; and 4) the concealed bodies of some homicide victims are never discovered. Klebba (1975) found that total homicide rates per 100,000 population (including criminal and noncriminal homicides) increased from 1.2 in 1900 to 9.7 in 1933, fell to 5.0 during World War II, rose to 6.5 immediately after the war, declined gradually to 4.7 in 1960, and rose to 9.8 in 1973. Annual *Uniform Crime Reports* data from 1970 to 1984 on murder and nonnegligent homicide show an increase from a rate per 100,000 population of 7.8 in 1970 to 9.8 in 1974, a decline to 8.8 in 1976 and 1977, an increase to 10.2 in 1980, and a decline to 7.9 in 1984. Population-based rates are highest in the southern states and lowest in the northeastern and midwestern states. In general, large metropolitan areas have the highest homicide rates, rural areas a lower rate, and small cities the lowest rates.

Although a number of studies of single cities and the national data in many years show somewhat higher homicide rates in the summer and in December, the pattern by month for the nation as a whole shows less seasonal variation than observed for aggravated assault or robbery. This probably reflects the fact that the somewhat opposite trends observed for these two offenses tend to cancel each other out when homicides stemming from both of these types of offense are aggregated with other homicides. Older single-area studies found higher rates of homicide on weekend days than on other days of the week (Constantino et al, 1977; Munford et al, 1976; Wolfgang, 1958), but the most recent New York study (in which there were many drug-related homicides) showed little variation by day of the week (Tardiff et al, 1986). Lester (1979), studying mortality data for 1973, found a significant increase in homicides on major national holidays (New Year's Day, Memorial Day, Thanksgiving, and Christmas), when the average daily homicide frequency was 64, as compared to other days of the year, when the average was 47 homicides. Approximately one-half of all homicides occur between 8:00 P.M. and 2:00 A.M. (Tardiff et al, 1986; Wolfgang, 1958).

Within cities, homicide rates vary by neighborhood and census tract (Wolfgang, 1958), with the highest rates of homicides within the home tending to occur in poor areas and the highest rates of homicides in public tending to occur in downtown business areas (Munford et al, 1976). Approximately 40 to 50 percent of all homicides occur in the victim's home, and 20 to 30 percent in the street (Constantino et al, 1977; Wolfgang, 1958). One-third of male victims are killed on the street, and approximately one-third of male offenders kill on the street; one-third of female victims are killed in the bedroom, and approximately one-third of female offenders kill in the kitchen (Wolfgang, 1958).

Characteristics of Offenses

Although the proportion of homicides involving firearms, particularly hand-guns, increased dramatically in the 1960s and 1970s, the proportions of homicides committed with various weapons have been stable within a few percentage points in recent years. In 1984, 59 percent were committed with firearms; 21 percent with cutting or stabbing instruments; six percent with hands, feet, and other bodily weapons; six percent with blunt objects; two percent by strangulation; one percent by fire; fewer than one percent each by other forms of asphyxiation, drowning, narcotics, explosives, and poison; and three percent by other or unspecified weapons. Of the firearms used in these homicides, 74 percent were handguns, 12 percent shotguns, eight percent rifles, and six percent unspecified (Federal Bureau of Investigation, 1985). The weapons used in homicide vary according to urbanization. In remote rural areas, the rate of homicides by beating is approximately twice that in cities, but the rates of homicide by firearms, by cutting or stabbing, and by strangulation are lower (Baker et al, 1984).

The frequency and quantity of alcohol and other drug ingestion among offenders and victims at the time of the homicide are difficult to ascertain because of delays in arrest, infrequency of offender screening, exaggeration of intoxication claims to reduce culpability, survival of victims prior to death, selective screening of victims, and postmortem production of alcohol by fermentation. Alcohol has been detected in one-third to three-quarters of homicide victims (Budd, 1982; Constantino et al, 1977; Hollis, 1974; Loya et al, 1986; Tardiff et al, 1986; Wolfgang, 1958). Loya and colleagues (1986) reported the presence of alcohol in 46 percent of Los Angeles homicide victims from 1970 to 1979; alcohol was detected in 34 percent of white non-Hispanics, in 48 percent of blacks, and in 57 percent of Hispanic victims. Tardiff and colleagues (1986) reported that 30 percent of male victims and 20 percent of female victims of homicide in Manhattan in 1981 had one or more drugs other than alcohol in their bodies at the time of death.

Opiates were found in 11 percent, sedatives and minor tranquilizers in four percent, cocaine in three percent, and other drugs in three percent. Approximately seven percent of the victims had taken more than one drug. No reliable and generalizable data are available on the proportion of homicide offenders using alcohol or other drugs at the time of the offense.

Wolfgang (1958) found that the police-recorded motive was a trivial altercation in 35 percent of homicides. These killings stemmed from such events as "a jostle, a slightly derogatory remark, or the appearance of a weapon in the hands of an adversary" (p. 188). Although some such events seem trivial to middle and upper class observers, they represent challenges to which lower class men are expected to respond with "physical combat as a measure of daring, courage, or defense of status" (Wolfgang, 1958, p. 188). In 1984, 45 percent of homicides stemmed from arguments, 24 percent from established or suspected felonies (of which robbery was the most common), and 16 percent from other circumstances; in 15 percent the circumstances were unknown (Federal Bureau of Investigation, 1985).

A higher proportion of homicides than of any other violent crime is cleared by arrest. In 1984, 74 percent of homicides resulted in an arrest. Unsolved homicides in which no arrest occurs are more likely than solved homicides to involve a victim aged 65 or older, a motive of robbery, and death by beating, and are more likely to occur on weekends and in the street (Wolfgang, 1958). Greenwood (1982) found that of 1,813 homicide arrests in California in 1979, a conviction was eventually secured in 61 percent, and 58 percent of the arrestees eventually received a custodial sentence.

Offender Characteristics

As with other violent crimes, males predominate among homicide offenders. In 1984, 84 percent of the single-offender, single-victim homicides were committed by males, and 15 percent by females (Federal Bureau of Investigation, 1985). In 1984, seven percent of murder arrestees were aged 17 or younger, and 34 percent were aged 18 to 24 (Federal Bureau of Investigation, 1985). The median age of offenders is 25 for those killing strangers, 29 for those killing acquaintances, and 32 for those killing family members (Reidel et al, 1985). In 1984, 54 percent of homicide arrestees were white and 45 percent were black; 16 percent of the total number of arrestees were Hispanic (Federal Bureau of Investigation, 1985). Offense rates were consistently higher among blacks than among whites from 1968 to 1978 for the nation as a whole and in eight cities studied (Reidel et al, 1985). Like other violent offenders, homicide offenders on the average have completed about 10 years of school (Deiker, 1974) and have high rates of unemployment.

No adequate diagnostic studies of a representative group of homicide offenders are available. Many studies have been published of offenders referred for psychiatric evaluation, but most do not use standardized diagnostic criteria. In one study applying the criteria of Feighner and colleagues (1972) to 25 psychiatrically referred murderers, the most prevalent diagnostic findings were: alcoholism (14); antisocial personality disorder (11); no diagnosis (4); affective disorders (3); and other personality disorder (2) (Dietz, 1985). The victims of mentally disordered murderers are less likely to be strangers than are the victims of murderers in general (Dietz, 1985; Mowat, 1966).

Victim Characteristics

Homicide victimization rates vary dramatically by age, race, and sex. Age-specific rates decrease from the first year of life (infanticides) to a prepubescent trough, increase sharply to a peak at ages 20–29, decrease linearly to age 85, and increase slightly thereafter (Baker et al, 1984). Rates are significantly higher among blacks compared to whites and among men compared to women. The highest victimization rates are found among young black males (Loya, 1986; Munford, 1976; Pokorny, 1965; Voss and Hepburn, 1968; Wolfgang, 1958). Homicide is the leading cause of death among blacks aged 20–34 (Baker et al, 1984). Among both blacks and whites, the homicide rate is higher among persons with low income (Constantino et al, 1977). Child victims, who are most often killed by family members, are particularly likely to have been illegitimate and to have teenage mothers, even when compared to children in other public welfare families (Kaplun and Reich, 1976). Homicide victimization rates vary by marital status, with the highest rates observed among divorced persons and the lowest rates among young widows (Humphrey et al, 1981–1982).

In 1984, 18 percent of homicide victims were relatives of the offender; nine percent were friends and neighbors; 30 percent were acquaintances; 18 percent were strangers; and in 26 percent the relationship was not known (Federal Bureau of Investigation, 1985). Men are most likely to be killed by friends or acquaintances, women by their husbands (Loya et al, 1986). A large majority of homicides occurs between members of the same racial or ethnic group. In 1984, 91 percent of U.S. homicides involving blacks or whites were intraracial. In Houston, 81 to 91 percent of Hispanic victims in various years studied were killed by other Hispanics (Pokorny, 1965). In one study, homicide victims were more likely than the general population to have received institutional psychiatric care for alcoholism, sociopathy, and drug addiction (Herjanic and Meyer, 1976).

SPECIAL OFFENSES

Assassination

The term "assassin" derives from the Arabic word for an Islamic mystical sect that terrorized its enemies by sudden attacks committed under the influence of hashish (Lewis, 1968). No offense of assassination is defined by law, but one federal statute suggests the range of victims whose murder might be regarded by Congress as assassination. This statute (18 U.S.C. 1751, 351) provides for federal prosecution of one who kidnaps, assaults, or "assassinates" a president, a cabinet official, a member of congress, or a justice of the Supreme Court. Social scientists have defined assassination more broadly, in some instances including nonfatal attacks and a much larger group of officeholders. Kirkham and colleagues (1969), for example, define assassination as a deadly attack upon a public officeholder or one actively aspiring to public office.

Crotty (1971) identified five types of assassinations, some of which have not occurred in the United States:

1. *Anomic assassinations*, committed by irrational individuals for personal reasons
2. *Elite substitutions*, in which a member of the ruling elite is replaced without changing the structure or prevailing ideology of the society

3. *Tyrannicide,* in which a despot is murdered
4. *Terroristic assassinations,* reflecting the systematic use of mass terror by an organized group or government
5. *Propaganda by deed,* in which the assassination is designed to raise public consciousness about a particular political issue

On the basis of his careful study of assassins in the United States, Clarke (1982) suggested that the offenders represent the following types, which he recognized were not mutually exclusive:

1. *Type I offenders* view the assassination as a sacrifice on behalf of political ideals. Their extremism is "rational, selfless, principled and without perversity," as in the cases of Czolgosz, Booth, Collazo, and Torresola.
2. *Type II offenders* exhibit extreme needs for "acceptance, recognition and status," but rationalize their acts as serving a larger public purpose and political ideal, as in the cases of Oswald, Byck, Moore, and Fromme.
3. *Type III offenders* are antisocial individuals without political motives for whom the destruction of others is an end in itself, as in the case of Zangara.
4. *Type IV offenders* suffer from severe emotional and cognitive disabilities which render them incapable of grasping the ramifications of their actions (and are presumably psychotic), as in the cases of Lawrence, Schrank, and Guiteau.

Persons holding the office of president of the United States are at higher risk of death by homicide than any other occupational group. Ten percent of presidents have been assassinated. Of 40 presidents, 10 (25 percent) have been attacked at least once. Simon (1969) calculated the odds of an officeholder in the United States from 1790 to 1968 experiencing an attack as 1:6 for presidents, 1:143 for senators, 1:167 for governors, and 1:1000 for congressmen. The risks have risen subsequently. Of 12 attacks on presidents, six have occurred in the fall (September through November), three in the winter, two in the spring, and one in the summer.

All assassination attempts have taken place in an exposed and open setting, usually a public appearance, in a major urban area. All but two of the presidential assassination attempts have involved handguns. The two exceptions are Oswald's use of a rifle and Byck's attempt to skyjack a plane with which to crash into the White House. Among presidential assailants, only Booth is known to have consumed alcohol immediately prior to the attack, although Sirhan did so as well. Of the 13 presidential assailants, at least nine traveled extensively before the attack and at least five recorded their plans in diaries.

Six of the 13 presidential assailants were in their 20s, five in their 30s, and two in their 40s, with an age range of 24–45. Two of the 13 have been women. Two were Hispanics and 11 Caucasian. Four were unemployed, six blue-collar workers, and three white-collar workers. None of the presidential assailants had a prior history of known criminal violence, but James Earl Ray had been convicted of armed robbery. Felthous (1985) reported that all six assassins who killed another person during the attack were themselves killed or executed. None of the unsuccessful assassination attempts has resulted in imposition of the death penalty, and three have resulted in findings of not guilty by reason of insanity (Lawrence, Schrank, and Hinckley).

Mass Murder

Although the term "mass murder" has been applied to events as dissimilar as the Whitman Texas Tower shootings, the series of lust murders attributed to Jack the Ripper, the mass poisonings in Jonestown, current abortion policy in the United States, the Holocaust, and the Bhopal industrial disaster, it is preferable for behavioral science purposes to restrict the term to incidents in which a single offender willfully injures five or more persons, of whom three or more are killed (Dietz, in press).

Mass murders occur with a frequency that is too low to permit the ordinary research habits of psychiatrists or criminologists to elucidate their characteristics. These murders generate an extreme degree of publicity that leads to unusual media influences (both beneficial and detrimental) on criminal investigation, on the processing of cases through the criminal justice system, and on the behavior of offenders, would-be offenders, and others. In the face of this publicity, mass murders typically evoke a premature and sometimes erroneous conclusion that the offender must have been psychotic. These features also characterize the serial murders taken up below.

Mass murders in the United States with the largest numbers of victims (10 or more) have all been committed by men with paranoid symptoms of some kind. James Huberty and his wife, who routinely abused one another, treated their home as an armed fortress. Mrs. Huberty once threatened neighbors with a gun, and James Huberty, an admirer of Hitler, blamed President Carter for the economic conditions that caused his unemployment. Depressive symptoms predominate among those who kill at least three, but fewer than 10, victims in a single incident. The most common of these cases are those in which depressed men, sometimes drinking excessively, kill their families and sometimes themselves. If these cases make the national news, it is a brief appearance. Even when the man does not kill himself, thereby allowing his story to become public at the trial, these cases do not capture the national imagination. They seem to be regarded as family business and are perhaps too close for comfort.

I have stated elsewhere (Dietz, in press) that mass murderers fit unambiguously into one of the following three categories:

1. *Family annihilators,* usually the senior man of the house, who is depressed, paranoid, intoxicated, or a combination of these. He kills each member of the family who is present, sometimes including pets. He may commit suicide after killing the others, or may force the police to kill him.
2. *Pseudocommandos,* who are preoccupied by firearms and commit their raids after long deliberation. James Huberty carried a rifle, a shotgun, and a pistol, and hundreds of rounds of ammunition (Levin and Fox, 1985). Charles Whitman hauled to the top of the tower a footlocker containing a rifle, a shotgun, two pistols, a revolver, 700 rounds of ammunition, food, water, a radio, and toiletries (Sifakis, 1982). The murderer may force the police to kill him.
3. *Set-and-run killers,* who employ techniques allowing themselves the possibility of escape before the deaths occur. Examples include those who bomb buildings or vehicles on which they are not traveling, who set fires, or who tamper with food or products, as in the Tylenol poisonings. While the offender may have one or more particular victims in mind, he considers the indiscriminate

killings of bystanders an unimportant cost in relation to the enhanced probability of escape provided by these methods. As with bombings generally (Federal Bureau of Investigation, 1983), the most common motives are anger or revenge toward persons or institutions, but extortion, insurance fraud, and ideological motives are also observed.

Serial Murder

Serial killers are defined by the FBI Academy Behavioral Science Unit as those who kill others in three or more separate incidents. Without exception, these offenders kill more strangers than family members. This fact is almost tautological, however, since it is unlikely that one could kill three family members, one at a time, without someone noticing a pattern. Serial killers are sometimes able to kill dozens of victims before being caught, which generally requires either careful execution and an acceptable public persona (as in the John Wayne Gacy case), or high mobility (as in the case of Lucas and Toole), or both (as in the case of Ted Bundy). While every serial killer is mentally disordered, nearly all are psychopathic sexual sadists, and few, if any, are psychotic. Psychotic offenders rarely have the wherewithal to repeatedly escape apprehension.

In contrast to murder generally, the victims of serial killers are most often strangled, beaten, or knifed, rather than shot. I attribute this fact to the greater intimacy of contact weapons over projectile weapons, reflecting the sexual component of the killers' motivation. Like other sexual sadists, they often pursue occupations and hobbies that bring them in contact with injured and suffering persons, or persons over whom they have control. Ambulance services, hospitals, mortuaries, correctional facilities, police agencies, and specialized military combat units prove attractive to them but sometimes have standards that they cannot meet. The single most prevalent job is probably that of a security guard. Their interest in police-related activities and their inability to become legitimate police officers (due to a criminal record, lack of discipline, or other factors) reveals itself in such behaviors as collecting police paraphernalia, using police badges or equipment to gain access to victims, monitoring police radio frequencies, and, most strikingly, inserting themselves into the investigation of their own crimes.

Highly inflated estimates of the number of serial killers and their victims have appeared in the press. The number of identifiable serial killers at large or in custody in 1985 was approximately 35. Claims to the contrary notwithstanding, there is no empirical evidence that the frequency of serial killers is increasing or is higher in the United States than in other countries. Improved communications among police agencies, new recognition of the phenomenon, and centralized reporting to the F.B.I. Academy Behavioral Science Unit in recent years all increase the probability of a series of murders being attributed to a single offender, leading to increased detection. The true rate of occurrence is not known for any country at any time, so it is not yet possible to study temporal trends or to make international comparisons.

Offenders who have killed five or more victims in five or more killing incidents fall within the following categories (Dietz, in press):

1. *Psychopathic sexual sadists*, for whom the killing is a source of sexual excitement. Among those who kill a series of 10 or more victims in 10 or more

separate killing incidents, this is the most common and possibly the only type. Although these men have oddities of fantasy and worldview that lead some psychiatrists to label them "borderlines," this most often reflects the psychiatrists' unwillingness or inability to face the fact that these men enjoy killing people, as in the older tendency to label men like Albert Fish "ambulatory" or "latent" schizophrenics. Examples include Ted Bundy, Edmund Kemper, Dean Corll, John Wayne Gacy, Wayne Williams, and Henry Lee Lucas.

2. *Crime spree killers*, who kill repeatedly during a series of crimes motivated by the search for excitement, money, and valuables. The most famous cases in this category are those of Bonnie Parker and Clyde Barrow and of Charles Starkweather. Less familiar examples occur among men who kill repeatedly during robberies less sensational than those of Bonnie and Clyde.

3. *Functionaries of organized criminal operations*, including traditional organized crime (La Cosa Nostra), ethnic gangs, prison gangs, and street gangs. Contract killers, illegal mercenaries, and terrorists are subsumed by this category.

4. *Custodial poisoners and asphyxiators*, most of whom are caretakers of the debilitated, of children, or of both. On ample evidence, physicians and nurses have been suspected of serial killings of patients in hospitals in New Jersey, Michigan, Texas, and Ontario. The recent cases in which cause of death has been established have involved the administration of curare-like agents, digitalis compounds, and insulin, but analogous cases which would pose greater postmortem detection problems may involve administration of potassium or other electrolytes, or various forms of mechanical asphyxiation. Similar cases have occurred in the homes of babysitters, foster parents, and, of course, the baby farms of 19th-century England.

5. *Supposed psychotics*, who claim to be acting at the direction of command hallucinations or under the influence of compelling delusions. In some of the best known cases, examining psychiatrists have disagreed as to whether the offender was psychotic. For example, David Berkowitz (known as Son of Sam or the .44 Caliber Killer) was said by some commentators to have maintained that he killed his six murder victims at the direction of a dog and in keeping with the interpreted content of delusions of reference, but by others to have been malingering mental illness. Angelo Buono (the Hillside Strangler), John Linley Frazier, and Herbert Mullin are additional examples.

Bombing

Bombings are incidents in which an explosive device is unlawfully detonated or an incendiary device is unlawfully ignited, including those in which detonation or ignition occurs prematurely as a device is prepared, transported, or placed. Explosive devices are constructed with explosive materials, such as dynamite; incendiary devices, such as Molotov cocktails, are constructed with flammable materials designed to have a burning effect (also known as "firebombs"). Other bomb-related crimes include the unlawful possession of explosive or incendiary devices, offenses involving hoax devices, and bomb threats.

The Federal Bureau of Investigation (1983, 1984), which has collected nationwide data on bombings since 1972, is the source of the data reported here. During the years for which data are available (1972–1984), bombings reached a nationwide peak in 1975 (2,074), declined in each year except 1980 to a low of

687 bombings in 1983, and increased to 803 in 1984. In 1984, four-fifths of the devices were explosive and one-fifth incendiary. Bombings show no stable pattern from year to year in the month or day of occurrence. Most bombings occur at night, with the highest number between midnight and dawn. The leading targets of bombings in 1983 were residences (226), commercial operations (136), vehicles (129), individuals (62), and schools (49), with smaller numbers of bombings directed toward postal facilities and equipment, government property, public safety agencies, churches, and other targets. Three bombings in 1983 and 15 in 1984 were directed at medical facilities, an increase reflecting organized bombings of abortion clinics. Large cities and western states experience the highest numbers of bombings, but population-based rates have not been calculated.

Although there was a time when bombings were principally the work of extremist groups, in the United States today bombings are most often used by vengeful individuals as retaliative instruments. One-half to three-fifths of the bombings for which a motive can be established involve mischief, animosity, or revenge, and few involve monetary gain or intimidation. The Federal Bureau of Investigation's Terrorist Research and Analytical Center recorded 22 terrorist bombings in 1983 and 13 in 1984, and these resulted in no casualties.

Although there is no reason to believe that they account for more than a small fraction of bombers, two classes of repetitive bombers are of particular psychiatric interest. The first consists of those whose motives are based in delusions which, if true, would be grounds for animosity, a desire for revenge, or other motives found among nonpsychotic bombers. The second consists of those who are obsessed with explosive devices, go to great lengths to secure materials and technical information, demonstrate inordinate fascination with explosives, and occasionally report sexual or other emotional arousal or gratification associated with explosions. Macdonald (1977) uses the term "compulsive bomber" to refer to individuals with these characteristics who engage in repetitive bombings. This term tends to foreclose inquiry into why some individuals obsessed with explosives actually construct and detonate them, while others do not. In my view, the underlying obsessive-compulsive psychopathology, which is common to all those obsessed with explosives, cannot be used to explain why only some such persons actually construct and detonate bombs. Like those obsessed with firearms, fire, violence, or particular sexual acts, some factor other than the obsession must operate to convert intense interest to unlawful action, and this additional factor is most often sociopathy, intoxication, life stress, or intense emotional states.

In 1984, six persons were killed and 112 others injured in bombings. Of those killed, three were the offenders, two the intended victims, and one a bystander. The other casualties were incurred by 52 bystanders, 35 intended victims, 24 offenders, and one law enforcement officer. The estimated value of property damaged in these incidents was $5.6 million, of which one-half occurred in commercial operations and medical facilities.

Skyjacking

Skyjacking is the seizure of control of an aircraft by the threat or use of force or violence while the aircraft is in flight or in the preflight stages. It is proscribed by the federal air piracy statute (46 U.S.C. Section 1472, 1982). From 1961 through 1984 there were 282 attempted or completed skyjackings in the United States.

The largest number of offenses was initiated in New York, the second largest in Miami. Of 151 successful offenses, 79 percent terminated in Cuba. Attempts peaked at 40 (33 of which succeeded) in 1969 and abruptly declined as of 1973 after the introduction of blanket screening and the signing of the U.S.–Cuba extradition treaty. In the last decade there have been annual averages of 12 attempts and five successes. Firearms are the most commonly used weapons (47 percent of incidents), followed by real or alleged bombs and explosives (28 percent), and knives (13 percent).

For lack of an empirically derived classification of skyjackers, they are usually classified according to their principal motives. Personal-ideological skyjackers act individually to express political or other ideological views. Fugitive skyjackers act to flee prosecution, but often claim political motives. Terrorist skyjackers conduct their offenses as members of organized groups with a predetermined objective. Only one terrorist skyjacking occurred in the United States from 1971 through 1979. Extortion-skyjackers, who demand money, demanded and used parachutes to escape until several models of commercial aircraft were modified to preclude opening the rear doors in flight (Landes, 1978). Mentally ill skyjackers harbor deluded, suicidal, or other idiosyncratic motives.

Of 382 offenders, 94 percent have been male. For 344 skyjackers whose ethnicity is known, 46 percent were white, 33 percent Latin, 18 percent black, two percent Arab, and one percent other. The high number of Latin offenders derives from efforts of U.S. skyjackers to reach Cuba, particularly during the 1968–1972 peak. Skyjackers have ranged in age from 14–73; 37 percent are younger than age 25, 37 percent aged 25–34, and 26 percent aged 35 and over (Federal Aviation Administration, 1985).

No adequate diagnostic studies of skyjackers are available, but estimates of the proportion who are mentally ill range from 16 percent (the proportion of prosecuted U.S. skyjackers committed to mental hospitals) to 36 percent (the proportion of international skyjackers believed to be "mentally disturbed" according to an INTERPOL study (Eustace, 1976). Of 49 offenders studied by the Department of Justice, 14 (29 percent) had previous criminal histories; the remaining 35 included six persons "discontented" with their lives in the United States, four fugitives, three military deserters, and two persons with domestic problems (Evans, 1969). In U.S. skyjackings, 12 offenders have been killed and three have committed suicide during the offense, and the number of passengers and crew members killed is probably on the same order of magnitude.

The Federal Aviation Administration began developing a skyjacker "profile" in the late 1960s, before magnetometer screening was routine. The profile consists of a dozen characteristics, most of which are kept secret, that can aid in selecting passengers for more intensive searches. Among the characteristics that have been included in the profile at some stage of its use are particular age ranges, male sex, paying for tickets in cash, and purchasing a one-way ticket (Landes, 1978). Excluding passengers apprehended at the gate with weapons, 67 percent of those actually attempting or completing skyjackings were said to definitely fit the profile, 13 percent were said to probably fit, and 20 percent did not fit (Federal Aviation Administration, 1985).

ACKNOWLEDGEMENTS

Source materials for portions of this chapter were obtained in part through literature reviews written for the author's seminar on Crimes of Violence at the University of Virginia School of Law by the following students: Anne E. Cowley (robbery); Susan Hankin Denise and Jeff Guyton (homicide); David Liss (assassination); and Cyril V. Smith (skyjacking).

REFERENCES

American Law Institute: Model Penal Code. Philadelphia, American Law Institute, 1980

Baker SP, O'Neill B, Karpf RS: The Injury Fact Book. Lexington, MA, Lexington Books, 1984

Block R: Victim–offender dynamics in violent crime. Journal of Criminal Law and Criminology 72:743-761, 1981

Block R, Block CR: Decisions and data: the transformation of robbery incidents into official robbery statistics. Journal of Criminal Law and Criminology 71:622-636, 1980

Bluestone H, Mallela J: A study of criminal defendants referred for competency to stand trial in New York City. Bull Am Acad Psychiatry Law 7:166-178, 1979

Budd RD: The incidence of alcohol use in Los Angeles County homicide victims. Am J Drug Alcohol Abuse 9:105-111, 1982

Bureau of Justice Statistics: Criminal Victimization in the United States, 1983. Washington, DC, U.S. Department of Justice, 1985

Clarke J: American Assassins. Princeton, Princeton University Press, 1982

Cohen LE, Cantor D, Kluegel JR: Robbery victimization in the U.S.: an analysis of a nonrandom event. Social Science Quarterly 62:644-657, 1981

Conklin JE: Robbery and the Criminal Justice System. Philadelphia, JB Lippincott, 1972

Constantino JP, Kuller LH, Perper JA, et al: An epidemiologic study of homicides in Allegheny County, Pennsylvania. Am J Epidemiology 106:314-324, 1977

Cook PJ: Reducing injury and death rates in robbery. Policy Analysis 6:21-45, 1980

Cook PJ: The role of firearms in violent crime: an interpretive review of the literature, in Criminal Violence. Edited by Wolfgang ME, Weiner NA. Beverly Hills, CA, Sage, 1982

Crotty WJ: Assassinations and their interpretation within the American context, in Assassinations and the Political Order. Edited by Crotty WJ. New York, Harper and Row, 1971

Deiker TE: Characteristics of males indicted and convicted of homicide. J Soc Psychol 93:151-152, 1974

Dietz PE: Threats or blows? observations on the distinction between assault and battery. Int J Law Psychiatry 4:401-416, 1981

Dietz PE: Mentally Disordered Offenders (report to the Center for the Interdisciplinary Study of Criminal Violence). Philadelphia, University of Pennsylvania, 1985

Dietz PE: Mass, serial, and sensational homicides. Bull NY Acad Med (in press)

Eustace MD: Aerial Hijacking: Stimulus to International Collaboration (National Security Series No. 6). Kingston, Ontario, Queen's University Centre for International Relations, 1976

Evans AE: Aircraft hijacking: its cause and cure. American Journal of International Law 63:695-710, 1969

Evans AE: Aircraft hijacking: what is being done? American Journal of International Law 67:641-671, 1973

Federal Aviation Administration: Aircraft Hijackings and Other Criminal Acts Against Civil Aviation: Statistical and Narrative Reports. Washington, DC, U.S. Government Printing Office, 1985

Federal Bureau of Investigation: Bomb Summary. Washington, DC, U.S. Department of Justice, 1983

Federal Bureau of Investigation: Bomb Summary. Washington DC, U.S. Department of Justice, 1984

Federal Bureau of Investigation: Crime in the United States: 1984. Washington, DC, U.S. Department of Justice, 1985

Feighner JP, Robins E, Guze SB, et al: Diagnostic criteria for use in psychiatric research. Arch Gen Psychiatry 26:57-63, 1972

Felthous A: Fates of assailants of U.S. presidents. J Forensic Sci 30:31-36, 1985

Fortune EP, Vega M, Silverman I: A study of female robbers in a southern correctional institution. Journal of Criminal Justice 8:317-325, 1980

Gelles RJ: The Violent Home: A Study of Physical Aggression Between Husbands and Wives. Beverly Hills, CA, Sage, 1974

Green GS: The representativeness of the Uniform Crime Reports: ages of persons arrested. Journal of Police Science and Administration 13:40-52, 1985

Greenwood PW: The violent offender in the criminal justice system, in Criminal Violence. Edited by Wolfgang ME, Weiner NA. Beverly Hills, CA, Sage, 1982

Harry B: A diagnostic study of robbers. J Forensic Sci 30:50-58, 1985

Hollis WS: On the etiology of criminal homicide—the alcohol factor. Journal of Police Science and Administration 2:50-53, 1974

Herjanic M, Meyer DA: Psychiatric illness in homicide victims. Am J Psychiatry 133:691-693, 1976

Humphrey J, Hudson RP, Cosgrove S: Women who are murdered: an analysis of 912 consecutive victims. Omega: Journal of Death and Dying 12:281-287, 1981–1982

Jason J, Strauss LT, Tyler CW: A comparison of primary and secondary homicides in the United States. Am J Epidemiology 117:309-319, 1983

Kaplun D, Reich R: The murdered child and his killers. Am J Psychiatry 133:809-813, 1976

Kirkham J, Levy S, Crotty W: Assassination and Political Violence: A Report to the National Commission on the Causes and Prevention of Violence. Washington, DC, U.S. Government Printing Office, 1969

Klebba AJ: Homicide trends in the United States, 1900–74. Public Health Rep 90:195-204, 1975

Landes WH: An economic study of U.S. aircraft hijacking, 1961–1976. Journal of Law and Economics 21:1-31, 1978

Lester D: Temporal variation in suicide and homicide. Am J Epidemiology 109:517-520, 1979

Levin J, Fox JA: Mass Murder: America's Growing Menace. New York, Plenum Press, 1985

Lewis B: The Assassins: A Radical Sect in Islam. New York, Basic Books, 1968

Lion JR, Reid WH (Eds): Assaults within Psychiatric Facilities. New York, Grune & Stratton, 1983

Loya F, Allen NH, Vargas LA: Homicide—Los Angeles, 1970–1979. Morbidity and Mortality Weekly Report 35:61-62, 1986

Macdonald JM: Homicidal Threats. Springfield, IL, Charles C Thomas, 1968

Macdonald JM: Armed Robbery: Offenders and Their Victims. Springfield, IL, Charles C Thomas, 1975

Macdonald JM: Bombers and Firesetters. Springfield, IL, Charles C Thomas, 1977

Morrison WA: Criminal homicide and the death penalty in Canada: time for re-assessment and new directions: toward a typology of homicide. Canadian Journal of Criminology and Corrections 15:367-396, 1973

Mowat RR: Morbid Jealousy and Murder. London, Tavistock, 1966

Munford RS, Kazer RS, Feldman RA, et al: Homicide trends in Atlanta. Criminology 14:213-231, 1976

National Institute of Education: Violent schools—safe schools, in Perspectives on Crime Victims. Edited by Galaway B, Hudson J. St. Louis, CV Mosby, 1981

Normandeau A: Trends and Patterns in Crimes of Robbery (with Special Reference to Philadelphia, Pennsylvania, 1960 to 1966). Ph.D. dissertation, Philadelphia, University of Pennsylvania, 1968

Pagelow MD: Woman-Battering: Victims and Their Experiences. Beverly Hills, CA, Sage, 1981

Peterson MA, Braiker HB: Doing Crime: A Survey of California Prison Inmates. Santa Monica, CA, Rand Corp, 1980

Pittman DJ, Handy W: Patterns in criminal aggravated assault. Journal of Criminal Law, Criminology and Police Science 55:462-470, 1964

Pokorny A: A comparison of homicides in two cities. Journal of Criminal Law, Criminology and Police Science 56:479-487, 1965

Reidel M, Zahn MA, Mock LF: The Nature and Patterns of American Homicide. Washington, DC, US Department of Justice, 1985

Sifakis C: The Encyclopedia of American Crime. New York, Facts on File, 1982

Simon R: Deadly attacks upon public officeholders in the United States, in Assassination and Political Violence: A Report to the National Commission on the Causes and Prevention of Violence. Edited by Kirkham J, Levy S, Crotty W. Washington, DC, US Government Printing Office, 1969

Smith MD, Parker RN: Types of homicide and variation in regional rates. Social Forces 59:136-147, 1980

Straus M, Gelles R, Steinmetz S: Behind Closed Doors: Violence in the American Family. New York, Doubleday, 1980

Tardiff K, Gross EM, Messner SF: A study of homicide in Manhattan, 1981. Am J Public Health 76:139-143, 1986

Voss HS, Hepburn JR: Patterns in criminal homicide in Chicago. Journal of Criminal Law, Criminology and Police Science 59:499-508, 1968

Wells DP: Child Abuse: An Annotated Bibliography. Metuchen, NJ, Scarecrow Press, 1980

Williams KM, Lucianovic J: Robbery and Burglary (Publication No. 6, PROMIS Research Project). Washington, DC, Institute for Law and Social Research, 1979

Wolfgang ME: Patterns in Criminal Homicide. Philadelphia, University of Pennsylvania, 1958

Yoon SH, Kan GSH, Lee JN: Homicide in schizophrenics. Neuropsychiatry (Seoul, Korea) 12:189-201, 1973

Zimring FE: Determinants of the death rate from robbery: a Detroit time study. Journal of Legal Studies 6:317-332, 1977

Chapter 21

Evaluation of the Violent Patient

by William H. Reid, M.D., M.P.H., and George U. Balis, M.D.

The psychiatrist or other clinician who takes responsibility for evaluation of the violent individual, particularly one who sees patients in an emergency setting, must possess not only skill in psychiatric assessment, but competence—even expertise—in crisis management, social assessment, and general medicine. Staff who deal with the patient before and during the evaluation should have formal training in many of the clinical issues that are likely to arise, as well as in prevention and management of violence (Jacobs, 1983; Lehmann et al, 1983).

This chapter will discuss some of the clinical and training needs for adequate evaluation, including the things necessary for staff and patient safety, arriving at case formulation and diagnosis, and beginning treatment. Specific issues of control of violence and treatment of the patient are addressed in Chapter 22.

Violence is not a symptom of any single disorder. In fact, violence of some kind may accompany dozens of named and unnamed psychiatric, general medical, and social conditions (Jacobs, 1983). It may be related to chronic lack of impulse control, or to apparent emotional overcontrol (from which violent episodes may explode only very occasionally and without warning) (Tupin, 1983). Our purpose is to help the clinician narrow the almost overwhelming number of etiologic and treatment choices.

AVAILABILITY AND USE OF RESOURCES

Evaluation of the violent patient varies with, and is related to, the facilities and resources available. Similarly, available facilities and resources dictate to some extent the kinds of patients who will come, or be brought, for evaluation.

In a city with many facilities, each facility (such as a public hospital emergency room, an acute-care psychiatric hospital, a substance abuse detoxification center, and a private general hospital) may specialize in treating specific types of violent patients. For example, police will take belligerent alcoholics to the detoxification center, while aggressive schizophrenics will be brought to the psychiatric hospital, and so on. Some facilities, however, must be prepared for a variety of potentially violent referrals; in smaller communities, the general hospital serves this multifunction role.

THE EVALUATION SETTING

No matter what the source of referral, or of potential violence, the interview setting contributes to one's ability to perform a good evaluation. Fortunately, the setting requirements are neither complex nor expensive. Think about privacy without isolation, security without constriction, comfort without fragility, and respect without vulnerability.

Privacy Without Isolation

The interview–evaluation process should take place in relative privacy. The patient and family must be able to talk freely with the clinician. The setting should not be so isolated, however, that either therapist or patient feels in danger should the interview get out of control. The presence of security personnel either in the room or visible nearby is not a detriment to the evaluation; indeed, their presence often calms and reassures the patient.

Security Without Constriction

In some settings, and with many patients, the possibility of assault or injury dictates physical measures of security: one or more attendants in or near the room; physical separation of examiner and patient, as by bars; or physical restraint of the patient. To the extent consistent with safety for all concerned, one should make the setting—and patient—free of constrictions during the evaluation process. Bear in mind that violence, such as assault by the patient, is most often sudden and rarely predictable.

Most authors agree that some control of the patient must be accomplished before the evaluation can proceed (Tupin, 1983). Sometimes the two, evaluation and control, begin simultaneously; sometimes control is the beginning of treatment. All forms of restraint, including chemical, may significantly diminish the accuracy of the examination. Evaluations of sedated patients are rarely reliable. Conclusions reached on the basis of acute evaluation should be rechecked later, when more nearly complete data are available.

A few authors suggest that calls for security be coded (for example, "Dr. Armstrong to the Emergency Room"), and imply that the primary reason for this is to avoid upsetting the patient (Dubin, 1981). Others, such as Lion, see less need for caution (or even secrecy) about the issue of the patient's need for control. We agree. There is usually no real danger of upsetting or frightening the patient. Indeed, communicating that the patient's behavior is not acceptable, and that the patient will not be allowed to hurt himself or others, is often an important part of reassurance and management (Lion et al, 1968).

Comfort Without Fragility

Whenever feasible, the patient—who is likely to be confused, frightened, anxious, humiliated, and/or in physical pain—should be made comfortable. One may provide amenities such as a soft chair or something to eat, and express concern for the patient's comfort. This can be done in even the most spartan setting to some extent. It need not mean using fragile furniture or easily damaged equipment.

Respect Without Vulnerability

The offering of food or comfort implies respect for the patient, who may be in a situation of great embarrassment and disdain by others. One can best evaluate, and eventually treat, such individuals by beginning with the respect due patients, and not by treating them as criminals, incompetents, or objects of disgust.

PERSONNEL

The personnel who participate in the evaluation should have some training and interest in working with violent patients, and should have some understanding of the dangers and rewards involved. One should try to eliminate clinicians and support people who are either overly optimistic or overly pessimistic, particularly those with omnipotent thoughts such as "I can handle any violent patient," or "I can sense danger." Of course, the sadistic person, who may use the patient's violence as an excuse to harm him, should be eliminated as well.

Clinicians who evaluate such patients must be competent in both the psychological and the medical aspects of emergency and acute-care psychiatry. They should be comfortable with their own conflicts regarding violence, assailants, and victims. Wishes to punish, fears of retaliation, and identification with the assailant or victim are routine among evaluators, but should not be acted upon.

Social awareness and an understanding of the contributions of setting and culture to violence are crucial, since most violence is at least as intimately bound up in the relationship between assailant and victim(s)—triggering stimuli within the environment, and cultural norms and expectations—as it is in the patient's individual pathology.

MEDICAL AND OTHER BACKUP

The range of medical backup and collateral resources that might be recommended is as broad as the ranges of patients, types of violence, and kinds of institutions in which the evaluation may take place. At minimum, for emergency workup, one requires the clinical and technical means to spot acute danger to self or others, related acute physical illness, and rapidly progressing medical conditions which may be misperceived as "psychological."

If one sees patients in a large urban emergency room, the personnel and equipment needed for extensive examination, rapid laboratory tests, specialty consultations, radiography, rapid treatment, and restraint should be available. Even in a facility in which only a narrow group of patients is seen, laboratory, x-ray, and physical examination facilities must be nearby.

THE EVALUATION

History

As mentioned above, the history is a primary part of the evaluation. "History" implies not only psychiatric history—present illness, medical background, family, and social information—but also a careful exploration of obvious, and sometimes very subtle, hints to mental, physical, and social *precipitants*, *settings* of violence, and *gratifications* or "relief" associated with violence. Each of these provides one or more facets of multideterminism and multiple consequences for the assailant.

Crain (1979) suggests that the clinician develop a sort of "dramatic script" of violent incidents in the patient's history, which will lead to a complete formulation for a given patient. Time and place, surroundings, preceding events, warnings or provocations, thoughts and feelings of the assailant, careful description of the incident, injuries or damage which result, and subsequent feelings of the patient often come together to quickly clarify the violent situation and the patient characteristics that are involved with it.

Whether the violence is "instrumental" or "expressive" is important to one's interpretation. That is, did the violence accomplish something, or was it apparently an end in itself? Other topics highlighted by Crain are level of impulsivity, extent of disruption of "homeostasis" before the incident, presence of dysphoria, "cognitive pathology" (organic or functional), personality style, psychodynamics, and the interpersonal and sociocultural environment.

Lion's work of over a decade ago is consistent with more modern lists of important symptoms and signs in the history (Lion, 1972; Lion et al, 1968). He suggests attending to neurologic "clues" such as headache, altered states of consciousness, recent personality or sexuality changes, infections, traumata, and repetitive behaviors (both classic seizures and repeated rages). Among psychosocial factors that must be considered are the usual psychiatric items, with particular attention to ways the patient's difficulty may be escalated. For example, does the patient have a job that places others in danger? Does the patient own weapons? Has the patient been involved in other kinds of impulsive, destructive activity (such as automobile recklessness or suicide attempts)?

Some patients seem to provide volumes of excellent data in a clear way that appears sincere. Others seem incoherent, with communication that the evaluator finds unintelligible. In both cases, a caveat is required. The apparently sincere, helpful patient may well be omitting crucial information, consciously or not. Doctors are accustomed to honest patients, who provide helpful information and work with the clinician; the violent patient, or one who has recently been violent, may not do any of these. On the other hand, the speech of even an incomprehensible patient may contain important hints for evaluation or treatment.

Corroborating and Supporting Information

Since the patient is often in a crisis or acute situation in which protective and/ or therapeutic action is mandatory, one must seek a complete history in every way possible. Collateral interviews are very important, and usually easy to obtain, provided the evaluator insists that they are necessary. Some patients should not be accepted for examination (in part because beginning the examination often incurs legal responsibility for management) unless witnesses and other sources of information are available for interview as well. For example, police, who may have observed a violent person very soon after the incident, must not be allowed merely to drop that person at the door of the emergency room. Similarly, family members, previous counselors, teachers, co-workers, and victims often provide important data that is either inaccessible to or hidden by the patient. Even the "good historian," upon whom clinicians might rely in some medical settings, must not be taken at face value (although his or her comments should be respected).

Information gathered in the heat of crisis, in which everyone involved may be anxious and upset, is often insufficient foundation for long-term planning. Whoever eventually manages the patient must see that reevaluation, with new interviews of the patient and others involved, takes place when things have stabilized.

Interview

In the interview itself, the clinician uses the skills that are appropriate in most other acute evaluation settings: observation, doctor–patient relationship, thoughtful and organized interrogation, eliciting of all possible biopsychosocial information, drawing on past experience, and synthesis of available data into a coherent, useful formulation. He or she must do this in an atmosphere of 1) potential danger to others; 2) potential legal issues (criminal or civil); 3) countertransference issues surrounding violence; and 4) crisis, with the expectation that the situation must be managed quickly.

The evaluator's feelings about the patient and the patient's violent behavior—some of which is countertransference and some not—figure prominently in the accuracy and completeness of the evaluation, and eventually in the career of the clinician. The literature is filled with advice about the dangers of certain patients, and proscriptions against turning one's back on them, trusting them, frightening them, upsetting them, or even negotiating with them. There is room, however, for some normalization of our relationships with the violent patient. It should be possible, without being foolhardy, to talk *with* the patient, without conveying the expectation that the patient will attack or the impression that the patient is a terrifying or shameful person. While we advocate safety above all else during the evaluation, the fact remains that most potentially violent patients will not harm anyone within the near future, and that the resources of the institution and its personnel can prevent serious injury should the patient lose control. The patient deserves our reassurance and an explanation for our actions whenever possible. Like our other patients, the violent patient deserves to have the clinician stand beside him, literally and figuratively, against the common problem of violent behavior.

Physical Examination

In an emergency room setting, the physical examination of a currently violent patient begins with a quick global assessment of the patient's physical condition. One should focus on information that can be readily obtained by direct observation (such as body posture, gait, speech, respiration, pupil size, skin condition, odors) or by simple clinical procedures (such as pulse rate, blood pressure, temperature).

Special attention should be given to signs that suggest substance induced organic brain syndromes (OBSs) (intoxication, withdrawal, delirium, hallucinosis, and delusional affective disorders). Obvious physiologic signs of intoxication include: *dysarthria* (seen with alcohol, barbiturates, and phencyclidine [PCP], for example); *incoordination and unsteady gait* (seen with alcohol, barbiturates, and hallucinogens); *nystagmus* (seen with alcohol, barbiturates, and PCP); *dilated pupils* (seen with amphetamine, cocaine, hallucinogens, and anticholinergics); *flushing* (seen with alcohol); *perspiring* (seen with amphetamine, cocaine, and hallucinogens); *dry skin and mucus membranes* (seen with anticholinergics and antihistamines); *tachycardia* (seen with amphetamine, cocaine, hallucinogens, and anticholinergics); and *elevated blood pressure* (seen with amphetamine, cocaine, and PCP).

Lacrimation, rhinorrhea, dilated pupils, piloerection, sweating, tachycardia, and fever are typical of opioid withdrawal. Coarse tremor of the hands, irritability, sweating, tachycardia, elevated blood pressure, nausea, and vomiting are common in withdrawal from alcohol, barbiturates, or similarly acting sedative-hypnotics. Needle marks, tracks of thrombotic veins, and scars from old infections on the arms suggest intravenous drug abuse.

Other easily observable signs that suggest an organic etiology include characteristic odors, incontinence, poor hygiene, exophthalmos, uneven pupil size, facial assymmetries, cushingoid facies, purple striae of the skin, congenital stigmata, ocular palsy, lymphadenopathy, skin lesions, tremor, twitching, and abnormal movements, posture, or gait.

After the violent behavior is brought under control, a systematic physical and neurological examination is performed. Special care may be needed to avoid provoking further violence and to maximize the patient's cooperation. A professional, reassuring attitude should help allay fears associated with reality distortion. Some distancing by the clinician, perhaps deferring optional procedures that might be seen as assaultive (for example, rectal exam), is often necessary. Paranoid or delirious patients, especially, may be confused and frightened, and may misinterpret medical intervention.

Consultation, Laboratory and Other Backup

Many of the items below are carried out after the initial evaluation, when acute control has been established and history and physical examination have narrowed diagnostic probabilities.

CONSULTATION. If organic factors are suggested, consultation is advisable when evaluating the violent patient, especially when homicidal or serious assaultive behavior is involved. Consultations—in neurology, internal medicine, endocrinology, epileptology, and additional fields—may be sought, depending on historical, physical and laboratory findings.

LABORATORY TESTS. In addition to routine complete blood count (CBC), blood chemistry, and urinalysis, a diagnostic battery for violent patients must include screens of serum and urine for drugs and alcohol, electroencephalogram (EEG), brain computerized tomographic (CT) scan or magnetic resonance imaging (MRI) if available, serum B_{12} and folate, thyroid function tests, and serologic tests for syphilis.

A toxic screen should be done for all assaultive patients. Blood and urine samples must be taken as soon as possible. It is very important to document the time since ingestion of possible intoxicating or addictive substances. For certain intoxicants, such as PCP, which rapidly become bound to tissues and disappear from the bloodstream, a negative report is not sufficient. The toxic screen should include alcohol, barbiturates, and other sedative-hypnotics, amphetamines, cocaine, tetrahydrocannabinol (THC), hallucinogens, PCP, and their metabolites. One may also wish to search for other drugs, either over-the-counter or prescribed (such as anticholinergics, antihistamines, or diet pills).

An EEG with a sleep record is an important part of the complete evaluation, especially if there are symptoms of an episodic dyscontrol syndrome. Nasopharyngeal and sphenoidal electrode placements may increase positive findings. The major limitations of the EEG are high rates of both false negative and false positive findings, and low specificity of patterns obtained. Thus, while the EEG can be normal in a significant number of patients with obvious cerebral dysfunction (for example, 30 percent of epileptics), it is abnormal in 10–15 percent of the general population (Kuger, 1964). These limitations are even more pronounced in psychiatric populations (Ellingson, 1954; Tucker et al, 1965; Balis, 1985; Woods and Short, 1985).

The brain CT scan is used to rule out structural brain lesions such as atrophy, hydrocephalos, and tumors. Magnetic resonance imaging (MRI) has significant advantages over CT. A number of experimental imaging methods may prove useful in the diagnosis of the violent patient. These include positron emission tomography (PET), single-photon emission computerized tomography (SPECT), regional cerebral blood flow (rCBF), and brain electrical activity mapping (BEAM).

Routine endocrine, metabolic, and serologic screens should include serum B_{12} and folate for pernicious anemia, thyroid function tests, and serologic tests for syphilis. Patients at high risk for Acquired Immune Deficiency Syndrome (AIDS) should be screened for HTLV-III antibodies as part of a dementia workup. Additional tests that may be required include glucose tolerance with concomitant measurement of plasma epinephrine and norepinephrine (for hypoglycemia attacks), lumbar puncture, serum ceruloplasmin (for Wilson's disease), urine porphobilinogen (PBG), and chromosomal studies.

PSYCHOLOGICAL TESTS. Some psychological tests are useful in the evaluation of the violent patient. Intelligence tests are required for patients suspected of subnormal intellectual functioning, and may help assess organic brain syndrome. Routine structural (for example, Minnesota Multiphasic Personality Inventory [MMPI]), and simple neuropsychological measures (Bender Gestalt and Wechsler Memory Scales) are useful aids in experienced hands. The Halsted-Reitan and Luria-Nebraska batteries provide highly specific information about neurologic deficits and localization of the disease process (Filskov and Boll, 1981; Lezak, 1985).

Although a number of structural and projective tests have been developed or modified to predict violence or dangerousness, none has proved satisfactory in individual cases, especially when used alone. The Overcontrolled Hostility scale of the MMPI may prove useful in the chronically overcontrolled person who may commit an isolated violent act (Megargee, 1970).

DIFFERENTIAL DIAGNOSIS AND THE DECISION TREE APPROACH

One should note that it is not our purpose to imply that most of the disorders below always, or even usually, give rise to violence. Rather, we assume the clinician is faced with a violent patient and must search for the cause of his or her symptoms.

Neither *The Diagnostic and Statistical Manual of Mental Disorders, Third Edition (DSM-III)* (American Psychiatric Association, 1980) nor the draft of its revision, *DSM-III-R* (American Psychiatric Association, 1985) is sufficient for evaluating violent behavior in terms of diagnostic labels. The psychiatrist is the expert professional who can best determine whether or not violent behavior is a symptom of a mental disorder and make clinical judgments regarding management, treatment, and prognosis. In this chapter, terminology from *DSM-III* is used; this will be carried into its revision, *DSM-III-R*, with one important exception. Intermittent explosive disorders and isolated explosive disorders will be subsumed under "Organic personality syndrome (explosive type)," since the *DSM-III* requirement that "there be no signs of aggressiveness between episodes is rarely met and signs of central nervous system (CNS) damage are common" (American Psychiatric Association, 1985).

Table 1 lists the *DSM-III* diagnoses according to the frequency with which violence is a symptom in the disorders. Disorders with violent behavior as a

Table 1. *DSM-III* Diagnoses Associated with Violent Behavior

A. Violent Behavior as an Essential Feature
   Intermittent explosive disorder
   Isolated explosive disorder
   Undersocialized conduct disorder, aggressive
   Socialized conduct disorder, aggressive
   Antisocial personality disorder, aggressive
   Borderline personality disorder
   Sexual sadism
B. Violent Behavior as an Associated Feature
   Substance use disorders
   Organic mental disorders
   Mental retardation
   Attention deficit disorder
   Brief reactive psychosis
   Schizophrenic disorder
   Schizoaffective disorder
   Paranoid disorder
   Bipolar disorder
   Posttraumatic stress disorder
C. Violent Behavior as an Infrequent Feature
   Atypical psychosis
   Major depression
   Dysthymic disorder
   Cyclothymic disorder
   Atypical depression
   Paranoid personality disorder
   Histrionic personality disorder
   Schizoid personality disorder
   Schizotypal personality disorder
   Psychogenic fugue
   Adjustment disorder with Disturbance of Conduct

required feature include intermittent explosive disorder; isolated explosive disorder; conduct disorder, undersocialized, aggressive; and conduct disorder, socialized, aggressive. Diagnoses listing violent behavior among choices of essential symptoms are antisocial personality, borderline personality, and sexual sadism. Disorders in which violent behavior is an associated feature, but not invariably present, include certain organic mental disorders (especially substance induced organic brain syndrome; Table 2), mental retardation, attention deficit disorder with hyperactivity, various psychotic disorders, bipolar disorder (manic), and posttraumatic stress disorder. Violence may occur as an infrequent symptom in other affective disorders; paranoid, borderline, schizoid, schizotypal, and histrionic personality disorders; psychogenic fugue, and adjustment disorder with disturbance of conduct.

Table 2. Organic Mental Disorders Associated with Violent Behavior

Etiologic Factor	Organic Brain Syndromes
1. *Substance Induced*	
Alcohol	Intoxication, idiosyncratic intoxication, withdrawal delirium, hallucinosis, dementia
Barbiturates, other Hypnotic–sedatives	Intoxication, withdrawal delirium
Amphetamines, other	Intoxication, delirium, delusional disorder
Cocaine	Intoxication, delusional disorder
Phencyclidine (PCP)	Intoxication, delirium, mixed mental disorder
Hallucinogens	Hallucinosis, delusional disorder
Anticholinergics	Intoxication, delirium
Hydrocarbons (e.g., glue)	Intoxication, delirium
Other drugs (e.g., steroids)	Intoxication, delirium, delusional disorder, personality disorder, affective disorder
2. *Central Nervous System Disorders*	
Traumatic brain injuries	
Intercranial infections (e.g., encephalitis)	
Space-occupying lesion (e.g., tumors)	
Cerebrovascular disorders (e.g., strokes)	
Degenerative disorders (e.g., Alzheimer's)	Delirium
Wilson's disease	Dementia
Multiple sclerosis	Organic personality syndrome
Normal pressure hydrocephalus, etc.	Organic delusional syndrome
3. *Systemic Disorders Affecting Central Nervous System*	Organic affective syndrome
	Hallucinosis
	Mixed or other organic brain syndrome
Metabolic disorders (e.g., hypoglycemia)	Hallucinosis
Endcocrinopathies (e.g. Cushing's)	Mixed or other organic brain syndrome
Vitamin deficiencies (e.g., B_{12}, folate)	
Systemic infections	
Systemic lupus erythematosus	
Porphyria	
Industrial poisons (e.g., lead)	
4. *Seizure Disorders*	
Ictal episodes	Partial complex seizures
Postictal episodes	Postseizure encephalopathy, delirium
Interictal episodes	Temporal lobe epilepsy, personality disorder
"Limbic syndrome"	"Episodic dyscontrol," Intermittent explosive disorder

In the emergency room, most patients with violent behavior carry diagnoses of schizophrenia and other psychoses, substance induced organic brain syndrome, and to a lesser extent mania, borderline personality, seizure disorder, mental retardation, and antisocial personality (Skodol, 1978; Rada, 1981; Suh and Carlson, 1979; Jacobs, 1983; Lion et al, 1969). Violence on psychiatric wards is unusual; schizophrenic and manic patients constitute the majority of those displaying assaultive behavior (although not proportionately more when compared to patients with other diagnoses) (Reid et al, 1985). On general medical/surgical wards, violence is rare. When it appears, the patient usually has an acute organic brain syndrome (metabolic or drug induced delirium) or dementia (Reid et al*). In children and adolescents, disorders commonly associated with violence include conduct disorders, substance use disorders and related organic brain syndrome, attention deficit disorder, mental retardation, and epilepsy (Lewis and Bella, 1976; Lewis et al, 1979; Stewart et al, 1980; Pfeffer et al, 1983).

Table 3 summarizes the differential diagnosis on the basis of a "decision tree" approach. The first step in this process is to differentiate organic mental disorders from functional ones.

Organic Mental Disorders

This category is chosen when organic etiology is known or inferred from history, clinical examination, and/or testing. Substance related disorders are the most common and may present with any type of organic brain syndrome: intoxication, delirium, dementia, withdrawal, hallucinosis, delusional disorder, affective disorder, personality disorder, and mixed or other organic brain syndrome.

Delirium and dementia can be diagnosed on the basis of the clinical picture (for example, cognitive deficit), while the remaining organic brain syndromes should be chosen only if other evidence is present. Delirium is characterized by impaired levels of awareness with disturbances of attention, orientation, and memory, which develop quickly and fluctuate over time. Attempts to restrain the delirious patient may precipitate further assaultiveness, but may be necessary if the etiology of the violence is unknown. Ordinary intoxication must be differentiated from idiosyncratic intoxication (for example, with alcohol in certain individuals); both are often associated with aggressiveness. A toxic screen is required.

The next step is to consider organic mental disorders with other causes. Many present with delirium, dementia, delusional or affective disorder, explosive personality, hallucinosis, and mixed or other organic brain syndrome. Possible central nervous system (CNS) pathology includes trauma, infection, space-occupying lesion, cerebrovascular disorders (stroke, multi-infarct dementia), degenerative disorders (Alzheimer's dementia), Wilson's disease, multiple sclerosis, and normal pressure hydrocephalos. Many systemic problems affect the CNS, including metabolic disorders (hypoglycemia, acidosis, hypoxemia, uremia), endocrinopathies (hypo- or hyperthyroidism, Cushing's syndrome, hyperinsulinism), vitamin deficiencies (pellagra, pernicious anemia, Korsakoff's syndrome), infections and toxins, systemic lupus erythematosis, porphyria, Sydenham's chorea, and environmental and induced poisons (Balis, 1983).

Epilepsy deserves special mention. Violent behavior in an epileptic may be

---

*Manuscript available from Dr. Reid

Table 3. Differential Diagnosis of Violent Behavior

		Violent, Aggressive Behavior Predominant Clinical Feature
		↓
Organic Mental Disorders		
Substance intoxication,	yes	Organic etiology, known or from
organic personality disorder, etc.	←	history or clinical picture
		↓ no
Psychotic Disorders		
Schizophrenic disorder,	yes	Psychotic features (delusions, halluci-
schizoaffective disorder, etc.	←	nations), bizarre behavior
		↓ no
Affective Disorders		
Bipolar disorder,	yes	Depressed, irritable or expansive mood
cyclothymic disorder, etc.	←	predominant clinical feature
		↓ no
Personality Disorders		
Antisocial, borderline,	yes	Inflexible and maladaptive personality
paranoid, schizotypal	←	trait features
		↓ no
Conduct Disorder		
Undersocialized, aggressive social-	yes	Habitual delinquency with antisocial or
ized, aggressive	←	dyssocial features
		↓ no
Attention Deficit Disorder		
With hyperactivity,	yes	Developmentally inappropriate inat-
without hyperactivity	←	tention and impulsivity
		↓ no
Disorders of Impulse Control		
Intermittent explosive disorder,	yes	Ego-dystonic assaultive or destructive
isolated explosive disorder	←	episodes on little or no provocation
		↓ no
Dissociative Disorder		
Psychogenic fugue, multiple person-	yes	Sudden, transient alteration in
ality	←	consciousness and identity
		↓ no
Posttraumatic Stress Disorder		
Acute, chronic or delayed	yes	Traumatic event followed by symp-
	←	toms of reexperiencing the trauma
		↓ no
Adjustment Disorder		
With disturbance of conduct, with	yes	Maladaptive reaction to a psychosocial
mixed emotional features	←	stressor
		↓ no
Antisocial Behavior		
(V code)	yes	No evidence of psychopathology
	←	

ictal, postictal, or interictal (between seizures). Ictal violence (for example, part of an automatism of a partial complex seizure) occurs but is rare (Mark and Ervin, 1970; Gunn and Fenton, 1971; Ashford et al, 1980). Violence in the ictal state with other epilepsies is rare; for example, only five patients out of 5,400 cases reviewed by Delgado-Excueta and his colleagues. In the postictal state, especially after status epilepticus, violence may be part of a prolonged confusional state (Somerville and Bruni, 1983).

The concept of an interictal "epileptic personality, explosive type" remains controversial (Balis, 1978). A number of investigators have challenged the notion of a specific epileptic personality in noninstitutionalized patients, and/or have maintained that epileptics do not differ significantly from other patients with chronic disease in incidence or severity of psychopathology. Several studies suggest that temporal psychomotor epileptics are more likely to be emotionally disturbed than patients with centrencephalic (idiopathic) seizures. Patients with complex partial seizures and a focus of abnormality in the temporal lobe (spikes, focal slow waves) appear to be at some risk for impulse dyscontrol associated with irritability, aggressiveness, explosiveness, and rage reactions (Mignone et al, 1970; Bear, 1977). This is particularly linked to dominant hemisphere involvement.

Although ictal or subictal mechanisms have been postulated to account for the explosive violence of some temporal lobe epileptics, it is likely that the epilepsy, violence, and personality changes may be epiphenomena of limbic pathology, with the resulting deep brain dysfunction causing the manifest symptoms (Balis, 1978; Stevens and Herman, 1981). The nosological concept of episodic dyscontrol, as defined by Mark and Ervin (1970), describes seizure-like outbursts of explosive anger in patients who have no history of epilepsy. The attacks are minimally provoked or unprovoked, are often preceded by an aura, are often associated with amnesia for the episode, and are followed by symptoms which suggest postictal depression. Patients feel remorseful after the attack. Many have histories of childhood hyperactivity, idiosyncratic intoxication, many traffic tickets and accidents, and (occasionally violent) sexual impulsiveness (Maletsky, 1973).

Functional Mental Disorders

Following the decision tree approach (Table 3), one must first rule out psychotic disorders, based upon absence of delusions, hallucinations, and bizarre behavior. In the presence of such features, proceed with the differential diagnosis of schizophrenic, schizophreniform, schizoaffective, and paranoid disorders; brief reactive psychosis, and atypical psychosis.

Next, consider the affective disorders on the basis of criterion symptoms related to depression, irritability, or expansive mood. Psychotic affective disorders usually produce a mood-congruent psychosis. Patients with bipolar disorder (manic) may show hyperirritability that can escalate into assaultive behavior. The association between depression of any type and violent behavior is often underestimated (Rada, 1981). Irritability and excessive anger can be prominent features of both major depression and dysthymic disorder, and may occasionally progress to outbursts, especially in psychotic depressions. Murder of loved ones, often presenting as murder-suicide, is a well known but fortunately rare event. Some assaultiveness in children has been described as a "depressive equivalent" masking covert depression (Glaser, 1967).

Differential diagnosis of personality disorders is largely based upon evidence of inflexible, maladaptive characteristics of adults. Conduct disorders in children and adolescents are associated with habitual delinquency with antisocial (undersocialized) or dyssocial (socialized) features. Antisocial personality disorder presents a high risk for serious assaultive behavior in some settings, although rarely in hospitals. Patients with unstable borderline personality disorder are sometimes violent and very occasionally homicidal, in addition to being often self-mutilating and self-destructive (as can be seen by their polydrug abuse and suicide attempts). Patients with paranoid personality may become violent during brief psychotic decompensation.

In children and adolescents, conduct disorders, specific developmental disorders, and mental retardation are the most common diagnoses associated with violence (Pfeffer et al, 1983). Many assaultive delinquents have histories of violent behavior from early childhood (Lewis and Bella, 1976). Past inappropriate aggressive behavior, absence of anxiety or depression, and parental assaultiveness are the best predictors of adolescent violence (Pfeffer et al, 1983). Juvenile delinquents have a disproportionate incidence of neurological abnormalities (Lewis et al, 1979).

Assaultive adults often have childhood histories of temper tantrums, fighting, disobedience, hyperactivity, inattention, learning difficulties, anhedonia, and insensitivity to pain and punishment (Balis, 1986). Attention deficit disorder (ADD) with hyperactivity is developmentally linked to undersocialized conduct disorder in adolescence, antisocial and borderline personality in adulthood, mental retardation, intermittent explosive disorder, and residual ADD in adults. Aggressiveness, low frustration tolerance, and temper outbursts all may escalate into violence.

Evidence for disorders of impulse control (intermittent explosive disorder, isolated explosive disorder) is based on ego-dystonic assaultive or destructive episodes of little or no provocation, in the absence of interepisodic signs of generalized impulsivity or aggressiveness. The ICD–9 has retained "explosive personality"; DSM-III has not, apparently preferring to refer to such violent episodes as "state" rather than "trait" features.

The dissociative disorders are characterized by sudden alteration in consciousness or identity. In psychogenic fugue, the patient may have occasional outbursts against persons or property. In multiple personality disorder, the personality which is dominant at a particular time may be assaultive.

In posttraumatic stress disorder, the diagnostic evidence is based on a history of significant physical or emotional trauma followed by symptoms related to reexperiencing it. Increased irritability may be associated with sporadic and unpredictable explosions with little or no provocation. Violence in patients with adjustment disorder with disturbance of conduct, a diagnosis related to maladaptive reaction to psychosocial stressors, is rarely directed at other people. Mental retardation, subnormal intellectual and adaptive functioning with onset before the age of 18, is diagnosed whether or not there is a coexisting mental disorder. Its placement in the hierarchy described here cannot be clearly delineated. Explosive behavior with assaultive or destructive episodes is an occasional feature.

Failure to diagnose any of the above disorders should lead one to conclude that clinical pathology is unlikely. The patient's aggression should then be considered a probable reflection of simple antisocial behavior or situational violence.

EVALUATION OF RISK AND PREDICTION OF DANGEROUSNESS

A complete discussion of risk evaluation and prediction of dangerousness is not possible in this chapter. We can, however, briefly address a number of important principles that are consistent with clinical experience and recent research in the field. Table 4 lists risk factors in propensity for violence, as reported in the literature.

Current Risk of Violence

The most important concept to be learned about the risk of violence in the acute phase of evaluation or treatment is that accurate prediction is difficult and often goes against commonly accepted clinical axioms. The authors particularly caution against interviewers or other staff assuming they can tell when they are in danger. This often leads to a false sense of control of the situation, and vulnerability to surprise assault or other incident. In fact, most violence in hospitals is not well predicted and takes place without warning (Reid et al, 1985).

Although one may not be able to estimate accurately the possibility of further violence by the patient, certain conditions make preventive measures important. These are usually well understood by experienced emergency personnel, but may be overlooked by the clinician who rarely deals with violent patients. They include acute psychosis, confusion or agitation; paranoia with need to protect oneself against imagined attack; intoxication of any kind; explosive or episodic violence in the history; clouded consciousness or other conditions that impair the patient's ability to perceive accurately the environment; psychopathy and/or criminal allegations in which escape may be important to the patient; acute mania or hypomania, and any situation in which there is little information available about the patient.

One often thinks of violent patients as being forced to come for evaluation; however, many potentially violent individuals come to clinics and physicians of their own accord. When a patient presents with fears of hurting someone, or perhaps with only a vague feeling that "something's going to happen and I need to come into the hospital," the clinician must take these comments seriously. Such patients usually know far more about their needs than the evaluator, even if the details are not immediately obvious. In spite of emphasis on cost control, need for carefully documented admission symptoms, and encouragement of outpatient care, one should be very cautious when denying admission to such a patient.

The use of seclusion, restraint, sedative medications, or additional personnel during the evaluation must be carefully considered. If medication is administered, it should be in line with accepted guidelines (Tardiff, 1984). Safety for all concerned must be the primary consideration; in fact, the evaluation should not proceed until this is assured. Then, issues such as the patient's rights and medical needs can be appropriately weighed. The choice of a method of physical control, if used, should take into account the patient's medical and emotional status, the patient's anxiety and fears, probable diagnosis, and the likelihood that the control measure (for example, medication) will interfere with important evaluation or treatment later. Sedative neuroleptics, for example, are quite calmative, but their effects last for hours or days, their side effects may mask

Table 4. Risk Factors in Propensity for Violence

A. Aggressive, Violent Behavior
  1. Current hyperirritability, hostility, short fuse
  2. Recent history of assaultive behavior
  3. Past history of recurrent violent, assaultive behavior
  4. Childhood history of persistently aggressive, destructive behavior
  5. History of repeated traffic violations (reckless driving, etc.)
B. Developmental Antecedents
  6. Violence (brutality) in early home environment
  7. Severe psychopathology in the parents (alcoholism, sociopathy)
  8. History of child abuse and child neglect
  9. Perinatal and early childhood brain insult
  10. History of brain injury (head trauma, encephalitis, etc.)
  11. Childhood history of serious inattention and learning problems
  12. Severe and persistent nonsubmissiveness to authority of early onset
  13. Childhood history of severe hyperactivity, restlessness
  14. Juvenile delinquency with undersocialized features
C. Psychopathology
  15. Habitual alcohol abuse and dependence
  16. Polydrug abuse–dependence (barbiturates, opioids, cannabis, hallucinogens)
  17. Pathologic alcohol intoxication
  18. Partial complex seizures
  19. Recurrent fugues and other amnestic episodes not related to drug use
  20. Repeated suicidal attempts and gestures
  21. Intense paroxysmal affects and sudden mood swings
  22. Severe or pervasive psychopathology, with prominent persecutory delusions
  23. Hypersexuality
D. Personality Traits
  24. Impulsivity (absence of reflective delay)
  25. Emotional lability, excitability, intense interpersonal emotions
  26. Low frustration tolerance, inability to delay gratification
  27. Cathectic lability (labile object relationships, nonsustained pursuits)
  28. Egocentricity (self-centeredness, social unconcern, entitlement)
  29. Propensity for acting out dysphoric feelings
  30. Low self-esteem and failure to achieve
  31. Inability to tolerate criticism
  32. Inability to examine one's own behavior

(or mimic) symptoms, and although specific for psychotic episodes, they are not indicated for all types of confusion or agitation. Similarly, prolonged restraint or seclusion of patients without adequate monitoring may lead to worsening of serious organic illness, self-injury, or suicide.

Assault on staff during evaluation has not been well studied, although there are now good data on the incidence and severity of assaults on treatment units (Tardiff and Sweillam, 1982; Reid et al, 1985). In spite of occasional media reports of serious assaults in evaluation settings such as emergency rooms and outpatient clinics, there is little evidence that the actual rate of significant assault is particularly alarming. Training and common sense appear to offer good protection against injury to staff and other patients.

Prediction of Dangerousness

In some cases, the evaluator is asked to predict the future behavior of a violent patient. Is it safe to send the patient home? Does the patient meet criteria for commitment? Can the patient be housed in a jail cell with other prisoners?

No matter what one's philosophical position with respect to the currently controversial issue of prediction of dangerousness, the fact remains that the psychiatrist must often make decisions that involve potential danger to the patient, danger to others, and liability for the clinician and the institution. In an emergency room, faced with real people—patient, family, potential victims— one cannot skirt issues; decisions must be made based upon the best available information and the competence of the evaluator. Fortunately, we have tools and knowledge that allow adequate short-term prediction in many cases, although a number of caveats apply. Dubin (1981) discusses evaluating and predicting dangerousness, naming several of the same predictors as Lion and Crain, already mentioned. He implicates drug or alcohol intoxication, drug or alcohol withdrawal, acute organic brain syndromes (delirium), acute psychosis, paranoid character, borderline personality, and antisocial personality. This list does not discriminate with respect to likelihood or type of violence, however. The person with antisocial personality, for example, is unlikely to be acutely out of control during evaluation or treatment. For assessment in a crisis setting, Hackett (1977) has suggested observing the patient's posture, speech, and motor activity for tension, stridor, and agitation, respectively.

Dubin and others occasionally suggest that the interviewer rely upon whether or not he or she "thinks the patient poses an extremely high potential for violence" (Dubin, 1981, p. 482). We suggest a more conservative approach, in which the penalty for being wrong about dangerousness is merely embarrassment, and not injury. Unobtrusive back-up personnel or humane restraint, provided in a reassuring and protecting manner, will not interfere with the evaluation.

Psychiatric predisposition is an important determinant. If, for example, violence is related to paranoid psychosis, continuing psychosis should give rise to caution. If use of a particular drug or alcohol is associated with losing control, use great caution if it is available to the patient.

The introduction of a setting in which violence has previously occurred markedly increases the likelihood that the violence will recur (for example, domestic quarrels in which the spouse humiliates the patient). One can see that the patient's behavior in a hospital or interview room may offer little of use for predicting violence outside the clinical setting.

In spite of evidence for statistical accuracy in clinical prediction of dangerousness, the real-life usefulness of such efforts is limited. Violent episodes are almost always rare events in the patient's overall existence; that is, most very dangerous people are not violent for more than a few minutes a day. Paranoid patients are usually paranoid a great deal of the time, but assaultive only rarely. Patients with potentially homicidal emotional conflicts involving family members are very hard to separate from many more patients with obvious similar, but not lethal, conflicts. A violent episode, such as a matricide, may be the first clear indication that covert fantasy has become overt action.

It goes without saying that one of the most important things the clinician can do is to document his or her reasons for taking clinical actions and the factors that went into making the decisions. The medical record is a vital communication to other clinical personnel, as well as a legal document. Opinions, findings, and even uncertainties are important to the continuing care of the patient. Judgments made in good faith, after reasonable consideration of available facts and alternatives, are very unlikely to return to haunt the doctor, in court or elsewhere. Undocumented actions, on the other hand, may lead to an embarrassing need to explain months later some decision that was eminently logical at the time.

AGENCY: WHOM DOES THE DOCTOR REPRESENT; TO WHOM IS THE DOCTOR RESPONSIBLE?

The question of agency—that is, the legitimate allegiances and responsibilities attached to the evaluator—is sometimes an obvious one, and sometime quite subtle. The psychiatrist who is working for a police department, a security agency, or one of the Armed Services must be concerned with agency every day. In the case of a military evaluator, for example, he or she has duties to the patient, to potential victims, to the patient's military unit, to the clinician's commanding officer, and to the Service itself, some of which are codified in regulations or guidelines. Confidentiality is quickly, and legitimately, compromised by notification of the patient's unit commander, and sometimes by reporting procedures that will eventually cause the patient to lose his or her job, regardless of the clinical outcome of the case.

In the civilian sector, one usually does not notify an employer as a matter of course. Although there is a vaguely worded "duty to warn" potential victims, the clinician may think that his or her primary agency is to the patient, with some unclear responsibility to the hospital or society. He or she may resist disclosure of information in the name of the patient's privilege.

In fact, however, agency enters almost every evaluation of a violent patient to some extent. The prisoner and prison psychiatrist may both understand that confidentiality in the institution is a relative matter. The forensic or police psychiatrist must be very cautious and understand, and communicate to the patient, the extent of his or her responsibility to the courts or law enforcement officials. The medical director, administrator, or even the board members of a hospital are usually entitled to information about patients whose behavior may affect the institution (for example, through damage, lawsuit, or unusual drain on resources). In addition, these bodies of which the evaluator is an agent—the prison warden, chief of police, or hospital board—may legitimately influence the outcome of one's evaluation. It is thus important to be aware of the factors that influence the clinician's activities, and to explain them to the patient whenever necessary for his or her complete understanding of the situation.

REFERENCES

American Psychiatric Association: Diagnostic and Statistical Manual of Psychiatric Disorders, Third Edition. Washington, DC, American Psychiatric Association, 1980

American Psychiatric Association: DSM-III-R in Development. Washington, DC, American Psychiatric Association, 1985

Ashford JW, Schultz SC, Walsh FO: Violent automatism in a partial complex seizure. Arch Neurol 39:120-122, 1980

Balis GU: Behavior disorders associated with epilepsy, in The Psychiatric Foundations of Medicine, vol. 4. Edited by Balis GU, McDaniel E, Wurmser L, et al. London, Butterworth, 1978

Balis GU: Organic Mental Disorders, in Treatment of the DSM-III Psychiatric Disorders. Edited by Reid WH. New York, Brunner/Mazel, 1983

Balis GU: Electroencephalographic correlates of psychopathology (abstract). Proceedings of the Fourth World Congress of Biological Psychiatry, Philadelphia, 1985

Balis GU, Monopolis S: Developmental behavioral antecedents of violence, in Proceedings of the APA Annual Meeting. Washington, DC, American Psychiatric Association, 1986

Bear DM, Fedio P: Quantitative analysis of interictal behavior in temporal lobe epilepsy. Arch Neurol 34:454, 1977

Crain PM: Clinical approaches to assaultive behavior, 1: evaluation. Psychiatr J Univ Ottawa 4:224-228, 1979

Delgado-Excueta AV, Mattson RH, King L, et al: The nature of aggression during epileptic seizures. N Engl J Med 305:711, 1981

Dubin WR: Evaluating and managing the violent patient. Ann Emerg Med 10:481-484, 1981

Ellingson RJ: The incidence of EEG abnormality among patients with mental disorders of apparently nonorganic origin: a critical review. Am J Psychiatry 111:263-275, 1954

Filskov SB, Boll TJ (Eds): Handbook of Clinical Neuropsychology. New York, John Wiley & Sons, 1981

Glaser K: Masked depression in children and adolescents. Am J Psychiatry 21:567-574, 1967

Gunn J, Fenton G: Epilepsy, automatism and crime. Lancet 1:1173-1176, 1971

Hackett T: Management of the violent patient, in Syllabus, Massachusetts General Hospital CME course in emergency psychiatry and crisis intervention. Boston, Massachusetts General Hospital, 1977

Jacobs D: Evaluation and management of the violent patient in emergency settings. Psychiatr Clin North Am 6:259-269, 1983

Kuger J: Electroencephalography in Hospital and General Consulting Practice. Amsterdam, Elsevier, 1964

Lehmann LS, Padilla M, Clark S, et al: Training personnel in the prevention and management of violent behavior. Hosp Community Psychiatry 34:40, 1983

Lewis DO, Bella DA: Delinquency and Psychopathology. New York, Grune & Stratton, 1976

Lewis DO, Shanok SS, Pincus JH, et al: Violent juvenile delinquents. J Am Acad Child Psychiatry 18:307-319, 1979

Lezak M: Neuropsychological Assessment. New York, Oxford University Press, 1985

Lion JR: Evaluation and Management of the Violent Patient. Springfield, IL, Charles C Thomas, 1972

Lion JR, Bach-y-Rita G, Ervin FR: The self-referred violent patient. JAMA 205:91-93, 1968

Lion JR, Bach-y-Rita G, Ervin FR: Violent patients in the emergency room. Am J Psychiatry 125:1706-1711, 1969

Maletsky BM: The episodic discontrol syndrome. Diseases of the Nervous System 34:178, 1973

Mark VH, Ervin FR: Violence and the Brain. New York, Harper & Row, 1970

Megargee EI: The prediction of violence with psychological tests, in Current Topics in Clinical and Community Psychology, vol. 2. Edited by Spielberger CD. New York, Academic Press, 1970

Mignone RJ, Donnelly EF, Sadowsky D: Psychological and neurological comparisons of psychomotor and nonpsychomotor epileptic patients. Epilepsia 11:345-359, 1970

Pfeffer CR, Plutchik R, Mizruchi MS: Predictors of assaultiveness in latency age children. Am J Psychiatry 140:31-35, 1983

Rada RT: The violent patient: rapid assessment and management. Psychosomatics 22:101-109, 1981

Reid WH, Bollinger M, Edwards G: Assaults in hospitals. Bull Am Acad Psychiatry Law 13:1-4, 1985

Shwed H: Teaching emergency room psychiatry. Hosp Community Psychiatry 31:558-562, 1980

Skodol AE: Emergency psychiatry and the assaultive patient. Am J Psychiatry 135:202-204, 1978

Somerville ER, Bruni J: Tonic status epilepticus presenting as confusional state. Ann Neurol 13:549, 1983

Stevens JR, Herman BP: Temporal lobe epilepsy, psychopathology and violence: the state of the evidence. Neurology 31:1127, 1981

Stewart MA, DeBlois S, Meardon J, et al: Aggressive conduct disorder in children. J Nerv Ment Dis 168:604-610, 1980

Suh M, Carlson RA: A socio-psychiatric profile of emergency service patients. Can J Psychiatry 24:219-223, 1979

Tardiff K, Sweillam A: The occurrence of assaultive behavior among chronic psychiatric inpatients. Am J Psychiatry 139:212-215, 1982

Tardiff K (Ed): The Psychiatric Uses of Seclusion and Restraint. Washington, DC, American Psychiatric Press, 1984

Tucker GJ, Detre T, Harrow M, et al: Behavior and symptoms of psychiatric patients and the electroencephalogram. Arch Gen Psychiatry 12:278, 1965

Tupin JP: The violent patient: a strategy for management and diagnosis. Hosp Community Psychiatry 34:37-40, 1983

Woods BT, Short MP: Neurological dimensions in psychiatry. Biol Psychiatry 20:192-198, 1985

Chapter 22

Emergency Management of Violent Patients

by Paul H. Soloff, M.D.

Violence is endemic in the mental health treatment setting and constitutes a real if unacknowledged occupational hazard. Physical assaults upon psychiatrists, psychotherapists, and mental health professionals have been reported from all clinical settings, including inpatient wards, outpatient clinics, public, and private facilities (Lion, 1983). Ironically, the most extreme examples, in which patients murder their psychiatrists, are often reported from the least suspect settings, the private offices of community psychiatrists (Danto, 1982–1983). Estimates of the incidence of assault on mental health personnel are drawn from retrospective questionnaires or reviews of incident reports. These studies describe the career experience of clinicians, violent episodes recorded within a given time frame, or percentage of overall assaults directed at staff within an institution. The reported incidence of assaults varies with the profession sampled, the setting, and the survey methods.

Using a survey questionnaire, Madden (1976) found that 42 percent of psychiatrists had been assaulted at some point in their careers, generally in their younger years when working with more impaired patients. One-half of psychiatric residents in one program experienced an assault during their years of training (Ruben, 1980). Hatti and colleagues (1982) compared the lifetime experience of psychiatrists in Philadelphia to a group in London. Among the respondents, 20 percent of psychiatrists in Philadelphia and 24 percent of those in London had been assaulted at least once during their careers. Bernstein (1981) surveyed psychiatrists, psychologists, clinical social workers, and marriage counselors in inpatient and outpatient settings. Of the responding clinicians, 14.2 percent reported actual assaults on at least one occasion. Thirty-three percent of incidents occurred in an inpatient setting, 26 percent in an outpatient setting, and 21 percent in a private practice situation. Over a one-year time period, 24 percent of therapists surveyed by Whitman and colleagues (1976) reported actual physical assault. Forty-three percent were personally threatened during the study year.

Within institutional settings, Depp (1976) found that 12 percent of 379 documented assaults by patients at St. Elizabeths Hospital over an eight-month period were directed at staff. Lion reported 203 incidents of assault against staff in a one-year period in a Maryland state hospital, with as many as five times that number of assaults unreported to administration (Lion et al, 1981). On a still larger institutional scale, there are more than 12,000 violent incidents reported each year in the 28 psychiatric facilities in New York State (Edwards and Reid, 1983).

Assault is an occupational hazard in all mental health settings. It is important for each facility to examine its own experience and define policies and procedures appropriate to meet the presenting problems of its own patient population. Policy should be reviewed, approved, and supported at the highest level of clinical administration, and procedures rehearsed by staff on a regular basis to facilitate the safe care of the violent patient. It is necessary for all mental health professionals to learn and practice the steps needed for emergency management of the violent patient. This review will focus on the emergency management of the violent patient using verbal, chemical, and physical control techniques.

CHOICE OF INTERVENTION

Emergency management of the violent patient clearly differs from the customary process of clinical diagnosis and treatment. Emergency care implies rapid assessment and swift symptomatic relief through immediate intervention. Treatment is directed against the target symptoms of agitated and violent behavior regardless of cause, often with little time for diagnostic sophistication. The primary goal of emergency management is to ensure "the safety of the patient, yourself, and others" (Hanke, 1984). Until the threat of violence or actual physical assault is "contained, controlled, and concluded," neither patient nor staff can work on causes (Soreff, 1984). The immediacy of the situation requires a rapid assessment of potential danger through the use of behavioral, diagnostic, and historical cues, leading to a clinical decision among three levels of intervention: verbal, chemical, or physical controls. Each of these interventions will be discussed separately, although in practice, each may be used to facilitate the other. The choice of intervention will depend upon many factors, including the setting, degree of violent threat, and underlying cause.

The nature of the setting, its staff, and security resources largely determine the kind of patient and presentation that can be safely managed, and the level of immediate response. Practice will obviously differ among emergency departments, outpatient clinics, general hospital wards, inpatient psychiatric units, and locked forensic facilities. The sophistication and experience of staff and the philosophy of care will often determine the choice of verbal, chemical, or physical controls for the patient, given identical violent threat. Experience suggests that the more secure the setting and experienced the staff, the less aggressive and restrictive the preferred intervention will be.

The choice of intervention will vary with the nature and gravity of the violent threat; for example, the waving cane of an elderly patient prompts a different response than the fist of an angry young man. At the extreme, a threat with deadly force will require expert police intervention *before* the patient's problem can be considered by the mental health team. Systematically assessing the degree of risk in every threatening situation is a basic clinical skill of emergency care and is critical to choosing an appropriate response to the violent patient. A commonsense concern for safety should prevail.

It is assumed throughout this chapter that violence is but a presenting complaint of a clinical problem which will receive closer attention under calmer conditions. The violent patient may be psychotic or nonpsychotic, have a functional or organic disorder, or be suicidal or homicidal as part of an affective, schizophrenic, paranoid, or drug related disorder. The patient may be intoxicated or withdrawing from drugs. Not all violent persons are mentally ill, nor is all violence in mental patients a product of their illness (Rada, 1981). The differential diagnosis of the violent patient (examined in Chapter 21) will lead eventually to treatments specific to each disorder; however, in the interim, interventions for acute violence must be rapid and directed toward immediate behavioral control. Within the limitations of emergency management, certain well defined techniques for the assessment of the violent patient are common to all settings and assist the choice of intervention among verbal, chemical, and physical controls. These principles involve the use of behavioral, diagnostic, and historical cues to judge the need for external control of behavior.

ASSESSMENT

Whenever possible, *prevention* of a violent episode is the first consideration of an emergency intervention. The preventive management of the violent patient depends upon the successful prediction of imminent danger, a prediction based upon clear and unequivocal behavioral cues found in speech, affect, posture, and motor activity (Dubin, 1981; Hanke, 1984). The escalating, agitated patient is tense in posture, paces the floor, and is unable to sit. This patient speaks in a loud, strident, threatening manner. The affect is extreme, marked by lability, with predominantly anxious or angry expression. There is poor modulation of affect or movement, suggesting little control over impulse. Violent episodes are generally not sudden or unprovoked, but develop around a focal point, a target provided by interaction with staff or others. The degree of impulse control demonstrated by the patient is a critical factor in the clinician's decision concerning the need for external controls (Hanke, 1984). Clear behavioral standards are used for this assessment. Is the patient directable—verbally responsive? Will the patient comply with requests; will the patient sit down; can the patient "talk about it" instead of "acting it out?"

The degree of impulse control in an emergency room setting can often be measured through the patients' behavior around the simple administrative routines of registration, giving financial information, and waiting for the doctor. On the inpatient service, the patient's ability to listen and respond to fellow patients or staff gives some assurance of impulse control. A commonsense approach is often safest. If the staff feels uncomfortable and threatened, they are most likely feeling the brunt of behavioral cues signaling imminent loss of control and danger. Immediate attention is indicated to abort a violent episode. The escalating patient cannot wait long for relief.

In addition to behavioral cues, diagnostic impressions may be readily apparent and assist decision making. Is the patient grossly intoxicated, delirious, pressured, or loose? Although angry, is the patient rational or seriously deluded? Available history is quickly integrated into this data base. Any previous history of violence? Of admissions to mental hospital? To jail? Is the patient "well known to the system" or a diagnostic unknown? Utilizing behavioral, diagnostic, and historical cues, the clinician decides 1) whether external controls are needed to assure safety for further assessment; and 2) whether this intervention will be at the level of verbal, chemical, or physical controls, or a combination of all three.

Verbal Interventions

Talk is the time-honored tool of the mental health professional. A generation has been raised with the psychodynamic perspective that even the "barricaded battler" can be "rendered quickly cooperative by someone who is trained and who knows what he is doing" (Barton, 1966). The violent patient is often presented sympathetically as an individual frightened of his or her own impulses and seeking help to prevent loss of control (Lion, 1972). The success or failure of talk as an interpersonal restraint to violence depends on both patient and therapist variables. The experience and skill of the interviewer is clearly important in defusing violent threat with *directable* and *responsive* patients. For such patients, struggling with conflicts over power, dependency, or self-esteem, the psychodynamic verbal tradition—in the form of crisis intervention—remains the treatment of choice. The skillful clinician may calm the agitated paranoid, borderline, or mildly psychotic patient by supportively clarifying their grievances and encouraging the patient to "talk it out" while emphasizing behavioral controls. In such cases, a violent outcome may be due, in part, to unskilled management on the part of the clinician.

Knowledge about the clinician's contribution to assault is derived primarily from inpatient or outpatient settings in which the patient is well known. Violence erupting in the course of psychotherapy is often attributed to errors in technique, transference, or countertransference factors. Hatti and colleagues (1982) reported that 24 percent of episodes of assaults in psychiatrists were precipitated by conflicts in psychotherapy, and 10 percent by transference problems. Madden and colleagues (1976) noted that 53 percent of psychiatrists who were assaulted felt they had contributed to the assault by acting in a provocative manner, by making comments or interpretations that were not well received. In the study by Ruben et al (1980), 11 of 15 resident psychiatrists who were assaulted during their training felt they had contributed to the attack. Residents who were attacked were more willing to show feelings, either verbally or physically, when angry and had higher scores on the irritability scale of a psychiatric evaluation (PSE).

Staff contribution to violent episodes on inpatient services has been discussed at length in the literature and includes factors such as denial or countertransference feelings toward violent patients (Lion and Pasternak, 1973); racial tensions (Kalogerakis, 1971); or treatment structures characterized by authoritarianism, underinvolvement by medical staff, and a lack of program clarity (Moos, 1974). In institutional settings, patients may be encouraged to act out overtly the covert conflicts of the staff. Thus, epidemics of fire-setting or riots have occurred when staff was struggling to deal with their feelings over the loss of a clinical director (Boling and Brotman, 1975; Erickson and Realmuto, 1983).

A study of the contribution of victims of assault is always a useful exercise in that it offers hope of lessening future provocations through better preparation. Nonetheless, the utility of psychodynamic interaction with many violent patients is severely limited by the underlying disease process. Many violent patients are beyond the reach of verbal intervention by virtue of intoxication, delirium, or psychosis. Where the basic cognitive preconditions to understanding are impaired, efforts at "talking down" the violent patient are doomed to failure and may lead to escalation despite the best efforts of a skillful staff. A more balanced behavioral and cultural perspective of the violent patient recognizes the fact that, for all too many patients, violence is a customary response to frustration, an adaptive and even expected response in some social settings. Contrary to our psychodynamic theories, many patients are neither frightened by their angry impulses or particularly interested in seeking help for control. It is a basic tenet of this discussion that violent behavior is a symptom motivated by many causes, that safe management must rely more upon observed behavior and measured response than upon preconceived psychodynamic formulations concerning violence. Thus, any discussion of verbal technique must begin with the understanding that the clinician will continually assess and assure himself or herself of the safety of the setting through monitoring the behavioral state of the patient throughout the verbal encounter.

TECHNIQUE

The many texts defining emergency interventions advocate similar behavioral and verbal styles for approaching potential aggressors. Indeed, the *form* of the verbal exchange with an agitated, aggressive patient may be as important as the content. Not surprisingly, these guidelines resemble an ethologist's formula for inhibiting "intraspecific aggression in man." Although primarily developed in the emergency room, the principles are generally applicable in other settings:

1. To avoid provoking aggression, the clinician *speaks softly, moves slowly*, and *sits down*. Personal space ("body-buffer zone") is respected. A passive, nonthreatening posture and manner avoid intimidation. The patient should not be interrupted or abruptly left alone. The clinician should not hide his or her hands or turn his or her back on an agitated patient. Formal introductions, use of titles, and full explanations maintain respectful psychological distance and preserve the patient's self-esteem.
2. Display of the clinician's physical size and psychological (administrative) power should be minimized. Concretely, the clinician should behave deferentially and think "small." The patient's power to make choices should be respected whenever possible. (Feelings of powerlessness and helplessness provoke violent defense.)
3. The clinician *listens uncritically, shows empathy*, and *avoids any entanglement* in delusional projections (Soreff, 1981; Jacobs, 1983). The interview should be *unhurried* so long as it is calming.
4. *Food and drink* may be offered, a cultural symbol of help, assurance, and nurturance.
5. A woman may be present to assure the patient of a male therapist's nonaggressive intent or further inhibit his aggression, especially where homosexual concerns are suspected. Often the smallest woman ("underwhelming force") is the best deterrent against the violent impulse of an angry male (Romoff, 1985). Other potentially inhibiting forces may include family or friends.
6. The setting for the talk should be somewhat private and quiet but structurally open to allow rapid and separate exit by *either* party. In this regard, concern for safety dictates that there be no closed doors or objects which could be used as weapons.
7. Dynamic exploration is often provocative and should be limited initially to obtaining history, principally the patient's own account of the grievance. The therapist's replies are limited to clarification and reassurance that help is at hand. It is often necessary to remind the angry patient that the doctor is not the legitimate object of the patient's anger (Soreff, 1981). Lion (1972) notes the importance of helping the patient identify the "correct" targets of the

anger rather than allowing the anger to remain global and unfocused or directed at the clinician. A specific focus allows exploration of issues and some defusing of affect. Verbalizing affect with behavioral controls is a therapeutic experience that relieves the need for physical action. The clinician must communicate "positive expectations" about the patient's ability to exercise self-control over violent impulses (Guirguis, 1978), and "expect the best but be prepared for the worst" (Resnik and Ruben, 1975). In cases in which the clinician is frightened, this is the *first* topic to resolve before further evaluation.

8. Medication may be offered to assist the patient to maintain control. Security officers may be asked to "sit in" on the session. The need for medication or security personnel arises when talk is no longer sufficient to defuse anger. Each setting must have its own well rehearsed protocol for changing the level of intervention, which may include display of force, medication, and seclusion or restraint.

MEDICATION INTERVENTION

When talk alone is insufficient to calm an agitated and escalating patient, consideration must be given to the use of psychotropic medication. The specific aims of this intervention vary with the clinical problem, but always involve the related functions of treatment and restraint. Treatment is directed at those acute affective or cognitive symptoms suggesting imminent loss of behavioral controls. These include agitation, hostility, belligerence, and suspiciousness regardless of the underlying process. The goal is to provide sufficient symptom relief that the patient can utilize his or her own internal controls and continue the interpersonal process toward a resolution of the crisis. This is most effective in dealing with the transient stress-related reactions of primitive character types (such as borderline, schizotypal, and paranoid). In other cases, where symptoms reflect acute exacerbation of psychotic pathology, as in schizophrenia, manic-depression, or paranoid delusional disorders, medication offers some emotional distance from hallucinations and delusions, and some relief of symptom severity. In the extreme, the use of medication may be as a final "chemical restraint" for violence-in-progress. It is at times reassuring to remember that even the most violent episode can be concluded by intravenous anesthesia! A role may be defined for antianxiety agents, neuroleptics, and sedative-hypnotic drugs, depending on the degree and cause of the violent behavior. For general discussion, it is assumed that antianxiety medications of the benzodiazepine class are generally offered electively and taken orally by agitated nonpsychotic patients, that neuroleptic agents are more properly reserved for psychotic patients and may be used, electively or coercively, orally or parenterally, and that intravenous sedative-hypnotics (such as sodium amytal) are reserved for extreme violence-in-progress, when other medications are less effective.

Medication Strategies

ANTI-ANXIETY AGENTS. Most authors agree that the decision to use medication in emergency situations is based on clear and present evidence of escalation toward violent loss of control. In the case of the cooperative but agitated outpatient, especially the nonpsychotic individual in crisis, antianxiety agents are often recommended for acute management. The clinical assumption is that the patient will be better able to control his or her own behavior once anxiety and its accompanying disruption of thought and judgment are under control (Lion, 1979).

The benzodiazepines have clear utility and efficacy in the treatment of acute anxiety disorders; however, their efficacy in the acute management of the anxious violent patient is somewhat controversial. Differences among drugs and patient populations produce apparently contradictory findings. For example, chlordiazepoxide is widely used as an effective antianxiety agent; however, in an experimental setting in which college students try to solve difficult problems following ingestion of the drug, chlordiazepoxide is associated with an *increase* in group hostility in response to experimentally planned provocation (Salzman et al, 1974). Oxazepam reduces hostility to provocation in the same experimental setting. "Librium rage" has been described in several case reports as a drug related disinhibition of hostility and aggression; yet, given to patients attending a violence clinic, with histories of temper outbursts, belligerence, assaultive and impulsive behavior, Librium (chlordiazepoxide) is not associated with aggravation of hostility despite daily doses of up to 200 mg (Lion, 1979). An analogous situation has been described for alprazolam. This medication is widely used for relief of anxiety, yet in patients with borderline personality disorder, it has been associated with marked disinhibition of self- and other-directed violence, including suicide attempts and mutilation (Gardner and Cowdry, 1985). Nonetheless, the general efficacy of antianxiety agents, their rapid absorption from oral administration and widespread acceptance and familiarity to the public, all contribute to their usefulness in the emergency outpatient department. A pill "to take the edge off" may well prevent escalation of the anxious patient to violent action and facilitate further interpersonal work.

NEUROLEPTIC MEDICATION. Although there may be circumstances in which neuroleptic medication is offered electively in the spirit of facilitating evaluation, the more typical indication—progressive agitation—requires prompt intervention and is not an elective procedure. At this point, the patient's treatment is no longer entirely voluntary. Once the decision to medicate is made, the patient is calmly but firmly told that his or her behavior is slipping out of control, that medication is needed now to prevent further loss of control so that the evaluation can continue. While the "offer" cannot be refused, the patient may be given a choice of oral (elixir) or parenteral medication to preserve self-esteem. The clear assumption is that therapeutic work will continue after administration of medication; however, further escalation will remove all possibility of useful verbal interaction and raise the need for a show of force, physical restraint, and/or seclusion. Faced with hostility, agitation, and the threat of imminent violence, the method of rapid tranquilization with parenteral neuroleptics may be considered.

Rapid neuroleptization. Rapid neuroleptization is defined as the "careful titrated administration of parenteral high potency antipsychotic drugs" (Anderson and Kuehnle, 1980). Twenty years of experience with this technique in acutely psychotic patients has demonstrated both general safety and efficacy as an emergency treatment. An extensive literature covering a multiplicity of open and double blind clinical trials demonstrates efficacy in agitated psychotic patients for drugs as diverse as chlorpromazine, mesoridazine, perphenazine, chlorprothixene, haloperidol, thiothixene, trifluoperazine, and fluphenazine (enanthate, decanoate, and HCL) (Mason and Granacher, 1980). For haloperidol alone, Donlon and colleagues (1979) reviewed a literature involving approximately 650 patients receiving parenteral rapid tranquilization. Although developed primarily with schizophrenic or manic patients in acute psychotic states, rapid tranquilization is effective for the relief of affective or behavioral dyscontrol manifested by excitement, agitation, hostility, belligerence, assaultive, or destructive behavior. Systematic study demonstrates some improvement in core symptoms of mania and schizophrenia, including flight of ideas, delusions, hallucinations, and disorganized thought. Medication protocols for rapid neuroleptization vary widely in unit dose, frequency of administration, and maximum daily dose limits, agreeing only on the superiority of the parenteral route over the oral because of speed of absorption and increased bioavailability (for example, the intramuscular route for haloperidol produces a tenfold greater plasma level for a single acute dose over the oral route in the first half-hour, a twofold advantage remaining as long as 24 hours later) (Donlon, 1979).

Clinical response with this method is rapid. Improvement in hostility and belligerence has been noted within 20 minutes of an initial injection of haloperidol 10 mg (Firling, 1978), with marked improvement—including core symptoms of thought disorder, delusions, and hallucinations—within six hours (Donlon et al, 1980) and symptom remission for many acutely psychotic patients within 24–72 hours (Danik, 1963; Oldham and Bott, 1971). Empirical studies demonstrate efficacy in a large proportion of acutely psychotic patients using rapid tranquilization techniques. Response rates from 50 to 95 percent have been reported in acutely psychotic patients within 48 hours of treatment using modest medication doses (Slotnick, 1971; Fitzgerald, 1969). Studies using the Brief Psychiatric Rating Scale (BPRS) or other research assessment measures have reported 40–50 percent in BPRS scores within two to three hours with repeated parenteral administration of high and low potency neuroleptics (Man and Chen, 1973; Reschke, 1974; Anderson and Kuehnu, 1974).

The important variables in this technique involve the choice between high and low potency neuroleptics, loading dose, frequency of injection, and time frame for titration. The decision concerning high versus low potency neuroleptics addresses the clinician's intent in rapid tranquilization. Early investigators, utilizing combinations of oral and intramuscular chlorpromazine (a low potency neuroleptic), achieved doses as high as 1500–3500 mg daily within 48 hours for rapid control of psychotic behavior (Mountain, 1963; Klein and Davis, 1969), making use of the sedative properties of the drug. Nilson (1969) advocated the adjunctive use of sodium amytal (125–250 mg IM) with chlorprothixene (25–75 mg IM QID) to produce sleep for three to six days as initial treatment. In cases where the clinician's intent is "chemical restraint," excessive sedation and parkinsonian slowing, generally undesirable in routine treatment, are regarded as useful elements of physical control by these authors (Fann, 1972; Nilson, 1969). When the goal is continuation of assessment or psychological intervention, preference must be given to high potency, nonsedating neuroleptics.

The "loading dose" in rapid tranquilization varies widely from study to study. Haloperidol, for example, has been given in single doses from 2.5 mg to 30 mg IM, with a frequency from every 20 minutes to once daily, and in total daily maximum doses of up to 100 mg (Sangiovanni et al, 1973; Oldham, 1971; Carter, 1977; Donlon et al, 1980). Studies of low versus high dose medication protocols (for example, haloperidol 15 mg versus 60 mg daily) indicate optimal efficacy in a middle range (15–45 mg daily) for most patients, demonstrating a need for flexibility in titration against clinical symptoms (Anderson et al, 1976). While there may be some slight advantage against acute symptoms with higher doses in the first 24–48 hours (such as sedation), the overall efficacy for high dose strategies is not significantly superior to lower dose strategies. Ericksen and colleagues (1978) compared a high dose regimen of haloperidol (60 mg IM for five days followed by oral taper to 15 mg daily over the next week) to a standard dose (15 mg orally) in 42 acutely decompensated schizophrenic patients. There was no significant difference between groups on BPRS scores of improvement despite great differences in plasma levels of haloperidol. Using oral haloperidol, Donlon and associates (1980) compared a high dose strategy (20 mg increments from day 1 to a maximum of 100 mg daily by day 5) to a moderate dose strategy (10 mg increments each day from day 1 to a maximum of 100 mg daily by day 10) to a fixed 10 mg oral dose for 10 days in 63 acutely schizophrenic patients. There was no significant difference in outcome among groups using the BPRS. Similar proportions of each group showed side effects, though drowziness was more prominent in the high dose strategy. In these studies, marked and parallel improvement in both high and low dose challenges the strategy of high dose "loading" with neuroleptics. Baldessarini and colleagues (1984) have recently described a disturbing trend toward chronic massive dosing with high potency neuroleptics—far in excess of equivalent therapeutic doses with low potency agents. The popularity of rapid neuroleptization would appear to be one cause of this trend. Following rapid neuroleptization, oral doses given as maintenance may remain far in excess of actual clinical need. Addressing the problem of excessive dosing, Salzman and colleagues (1986) recommend the simultaneous use of parenteral haloperidol and parenteral lorazepam to reduce the total neuroleptic dosage used for emergency management. A ratio of 5 mg of haloperidol to 1 or 2 mg of lorazepam was found effective for acute control of disruptive and violent patients, and "spared" the use of higher doses of neuroleptic medication.

Risks. The risks of rapid neuroleptization relate to the usual spectrum of side effects for each class of drug and to the potential for adverse interactions with underlying disorders responsible for the behavioral dyscontrol. Recall that the technique is often used in acute emergencies to treat violent behavior irrespective of cause. Thus, the sedative or anticholinergic effects of neuroleptics may mask or aggravate certain delirious or toxic metabolic confusional states. For this reason, intoxication with alcohol or sedative-hypnotic drugs is a relative contraindication to rapid tranquilization until it is clear that the patient's level of consciousness is not progressively worsening (as might be true with rising blood alcohol levels). Similarly, overdose with strongly anticholinergic drugs can produce a delirium which would be aggravated by some neuroleptics. In such circumstances, physical controls alone are preferred while medical investigation proceeds. Ironically, the rapid relief of symptoms with neuroleptics may deprive the clinician of an opportunity to establish an accurate diagnosis. One must weigh the long-term prognostic value of an accurate diagnosis against the short-term advantage of rapid behavioral control. In new or unusual presentations, physical control alone may be preferred to allow medication-free study of the patient. The rapid relief of agitation and hostility may lull the staff into a false and premature sense of security. Anderson and Kuehnle (1980) remind us that depressed patients remain at high risk for suicide despite rapid resolution of psychotic content. Staff may lessen their surveillance with the passing of acute agitation, not recognizing the severity of the underlying affective disorder.

The side effects of rapid neuroleptization include the sedation, orthostatic hypotention, and anticholinergic effects common to the lower potency neuroleptic agents and the extrapyramidal symptoms of the high potency drugs. Life threatening hypotensive crises have been reported by Man (1973) in two patients receiving parenteral chlorpromazine (50 mg IM) in the course of rapid tranquilization. One patient in the same study developed status epilepticus (Man, 1973). A test dose of 10–25 mg chlorpromazine IM has been used to test sensitivity to severe orthostasis prior to embarking on an aggressive medication protocol. Using low potency drugs such as chlorpromazine requires large volumes of medication to be injected (for example, 25 mg/cc), resulting in local tissue irritation. Good nursing technique proscribes individual volumes larger than 3cc per site, limiting the amount of medication for each injection. A high concentration, high potency neuroleptic may be preferred for this practical reason alone.

A paradoxical effect of rapid tranquilization may be an increase in agitation as the patient first experiences extrapyramidal symptoms (EPS) or sedation. More subtle manifestations of akathesia have been associated with exacerbations of psychosis in patients receiving fluphenazine enanthate or trifluoperazine (Van Putten et al, 1974). Paranoid patients, in particular, may fear loss of control and loss of ability to defend themselves, resulting in greater initial agitation. Appleton (1965) and Lion (1983) caution against excessive sedation, euphemistically termed "snowing" the patient, as this practice may provoke increased defensive combativeness in the drugged, confused, and disoriented patient.

The potential also exists for other rare but serious disorders attributable to high potency neuroleptics (not necessarily limited to rapid tranquilization). Gelenberg (1977) has described cases of neuroleptic induced catatonia together with Parkinson's syndrome in eight patients treated with fluphenazine or haloperidol. The neuroleptic malignant syndrome, a potentially lethal syndrome of neuromuscular rigidity and high fever, is associated with high potency neuroleptics, as is the rare laryngeal dystonic reaction, with potential for serious airway obstruction (Kaskey and Nasr, 1979; Salzman and Hoffman, 1982). The use of prophylactic anticholinergic drugs is advocated by many authors to minimize the potential for severe EPS and behavioral toxicity attributable to these side effects.

In light of the empirical data challenging the need for high doses of potent neuroleptics, and the evidence that such high doses are often needlessly prescribed beyond acute management (for example, Baldessarini et al, 1984), Tupin (1985a) has suggested redefining the rapid tranquilization process as "focal neuroleptization," emphasizing its use as "a short-term therapy aimed at controlling specific symptoms," using *small* repeated doses of high potency neuroleptics to initiate treatment or to achieve control of emergent symptoms.

Technique.   Rapid neuroleptization is an intensive care procedure to be conducted only with adequate staff and monitoring of vital signs and behavior. Choice of drug and technique may vary with the setting, the urgency of the clinical presentation, and the experience of the staff. Ideally, the patient's medical and psychiatric history should be reviewed, including previous response to medication. A brief physical examination should be performed as an initial test dose of medication given, with proper monitoring for special sensitivity to sedation, EPS, or orthostatic hypotension. While these steps are feasible for violence erupting in the course of an inpatient hospitalization, they are difficult if not impossible to follow under the most acute conditions in the emergency room setting. At the very least, a diagnosis of delirium or toxic metabolic origin for violence should be ruled out and a measure of vital signs (including level of awareness) obtained prior to the first injection. In the most extreme cases, where violence is either imminent or in progress, physical restraint must precede medication and provide a safe "holding action" for emergency medical evaluation. With the patient in restraints, a brief exam can be performed and blood drawn for needed toxic or metabolic screens. *Indeed, at the clinician's discretion, the risks of rapid tranquilization may be avoided entirely through the appropriate use of physical controls (restraint or seclusion).*

There are many medication protocols for rapid neuroleptization (see Table 1). For the high potency neuroleptics, a useful low dose strategy may prescribe haloperidol 5 mg (1 cc) IM every four to eight hours, for a daily maximum of 15–30 mg (Feldman, 1969; Fitzgerald, 1969). A typical high dose strategy utilizing haloperidol prescribes 10 mg IM every 30 minutes with a 24 hour maximum of 45–100 mg (Carter, 1977). Mason and Granacher (1976) suggest that most patients treated for acute psychosis with parenteral haloperidol will require 20–60 mg over a two- to six-hour period.

While the more sedating, low potency neuroleptics are less often used, the clinician may still prefer the sedation available with drugs such as chlorpromazine. For chlorpromazine, a test dose of 10–25 mg IM is generally recommended, looking for excessive sensitivity to orthostatic hypotension. If orthostasis is not a problem after one hour, chlorpromazine may be given as 25 mg IM (1cc) every four hours (low dose strategy), or up to 75 mg IM (3cc) every four hours (high dose strategy) for daily maximum ranges up to 400 mg IM in 24 hours (Hamid and Wertz, 1973; Brauzer, 1970). Because of the low concentration–high volume injections required, oral doses should be offered as soon as is clinically feasible. Severe orthostatic hypotension is a relative contraindication to continuing rapid tranquilization with chlorpromazine. In the extreme case, a hypotensive crisis (for example, systolic BP ≤ 80 mm/Hg on rising) may require urgent treatment with I.V. support and the use of vasopressors such as metaraminol bitartrate (Aramine injection) or levarterenol bitartrate (Levophed). Recall that epinephrine (Adrenalin) is contraindicated, as it may paradoxically lower blood pressure further in neuroleptic induced orthostatic hypotension (Mason and Granacher, 1976).

The total daily dose of parenteral medication required to effect control over disruptive symptoms provides the basis for calculating conversion to oral doses in the ensuing days. Some authors recommend a mg-for-mg translation, using the 24-hour maximum as their guide and allowing further parenteral "PRN" doses in case of relapse. Others suggest oral doses equivalent from ⅔ to 1½ times the parenteral dose administered in the first 24 hours (Polak and Laycob, 1971; Mason and Granancher, 1980). This oral dose should be given as elixir

Table 1. Medication Interventions for Emergency Management

	Parenteral (IM) Unit Dose[†]	Usual Daily Range	Side Effects and Complications
I. Neuroleptic			
A. High Potency (Conc.)			EPS: dystonia, akathesia, parkinsonian symptoms Sedation, anticholinergic symptoms, orthostatic hypotension, painful injection site
Haloperidol (5 mg/ml)	2.5–10 mg IM	15–60 mg	
Thiothixene (2 mg/ml)	4–8 mg IM	16–60 mg	
Fluphenazine HCL (2.5 mg/ml)	5 mg IM	20–60 mg	
			Rare complications: laryngeal dystonia, neuroleptic malignant syndrome, drug induced catatonia, behavioral toxicity
B. Low Potency			
Chlorpromazine (25 mg/ml)	25–75 mg IM	100–400 mg	
Mesoridazine (25 mg/ml)	25 mg IM	25–200 mg	
II. Anti-anxiety			Sedation, potentiates CNS depressants, respiratory depression, paradoxical increase in hostility ("librium rage")
Diazepam (10 mg/2 ml)	5–10 mg P.O./IM*/IV**	5–40 mg	
Chlordiazepoxide (100 mg/2 ml)	50 mg P.O./IM	200–500 mg	
III. Sedative-Hypnotic			Potentiates CNS depressants, respiratory depression, paradoxical excitement, bronchospasm, laryngo-spasm
Sodium Amytal	2.5 or 5% Solution IV**—1 cc/min.	150–300 mg	

[†]Generally given IM q 30–60 min.
*IM absorption may be slow and incomplete
**Generally reserved for violence in progress

and may be divided into two or more doses depending upon clinical need (for example, the use of sedation). Titration downward should be the rule as soon as the patient's clinical condition is stable.

SEDATIVE-HYPNOTIC AGENTS. At the extreme end of the behavioral spectrum is the situation of violence-in-progress. Confrontation and physical control obviously precede consideration of medication. With the acutely violent patient under temporary physical control or in restraints, the clinician may choose to use sedative-hypnotics over neuroleptics if the goal is immediate sedation. In some settings, where leather restraints or seclusion techniques are not available or allowed, intravenous amytal may be administered while the patient is physically restrained by staff. Sodium amytal in doses of 200–500 mg may be given by slow intravenous push (as a 2.5 or 5 percent solution) at the rate of 1cc per minute until sleep is induced. The advantage is rapid and total control of behavior through sedation. Complications include potentiation of excitement if insufficient doses are given, laryngeal spasm, or respiratory depression. Barbiturates will also potentiate the effects of other central nervous system (CNS) depressants present, including alcohol or other sedative-hypnotics (that is, taken in overdose). Where leather restraints are applied, or a seclusion area is available to "buy time," the intramuscular route may be utilized. As a creative alternative to barbiturate narcosis in a situation requiring rapid sedation, Tupin (1975) suggests intravenous diazepam (5–10 mg).

PHYSICAL INTERVENTION: SECLUSION AND RESTRAINT

When verbal intervention and voluntary medication are refused or fail to calm the progressively escalating, aggressive patient, seclusion and restraint remain the final measures available to assure safety and treatment. These traditional methods of physical control must be viewed as intensive care treatments for the acutely violent patient. As defined by the American Psychiatric Association Task Force on Seclusion and Restraint, this treatment is indicated: 1) to prevent imminent harm to the patient or other persons when other means of control are not effective or appropriate; 2) to prevent serious disruption of the treatment program or significant damage to the physical environment; 3) for treatment as part of an ongoing plan of behavior therapy; 4) to decrease the stimulation a patient receives; 5) at the request of a patient (American Psychiatric Association Task Force Report No. 22).

The therapeutic principles that underlie the use of physical controls include: 1) containment of the violent impulse; 2) isolation from frightening or confusing external stimuli; and 3) definition of disrupted ego boundaries (Gutheil, 1978; Rosen, 1978). Seclusion and restraint have been advocated in all disorders presenting acute violence, including schizophrenia, mania, organic brain syndromes, acute intoxication, personality disorders, and episodic dyscontrol syndromes. They are occasionally requested by patients fearful of their own destructive urges (Lion, 1972; Bursten, 1976). Aside from the obvious safety considerations, the use of physical controls "buys time" for staff to conduct diagnostic maneuvers or to begin parenteral medication under controlled conditions.

In an emergency room setting, where patients may be brought in by police in handcuffs, restraint may provide a temporary measure of security and control while assessment and treatment begin. Telintelo and colleagues (1983) reported that 60 percent of restrained patients seen in a university hospital emergency department arrived in restraints, but that 42 percent of those restrained were able to be released following treatment and were referred to outpatient care. On the inpatient service, restraint may be required for medical treatment of an uncooperative, psychotic patient, or for treatment of acute violent exacerbations of the psychiatric illness.

Physical controls are utilized when the patients' behavior exceeds the tolerance of the setting, a tolerance which is defined by staff patterns, experience, patient population, and philosophy of care. Thus, the "threshold" for using physical controls may vary from the emergency room to the inpatient divisions of the same hospital. With rare exception, mechanical restraint or seclusion is an involuntary treatment, requiring the use of force and suspension of the patient's right to refuse. In some states, legislation or judicial rulings may define the allowable indications for physical restraint, yet all agree on its legitimate use as an acute emergency management technique for violence. A review of the empirical literature on seclusion and restraint offers a valuable perspective on actual practice in diverse settings, defining precipitating factors, diagnostic considerations, duration, risks, and benefits of these procedures.

Review of Empirical Literature

Empirical studies of seclusion and restraint followed the first serious judicial reviews of the practice and provided concrete clinical evidence on the incidence of seclusion and restraint in diverse settings, the diagnostic and demographic characteristics of secluded patients, the precipitating behaviors, duration, and effectiveness of seclusion as an emergency treatment. Sixteen empirical studies have been reported on the use of seclusion or restraint in adult inpatient settings (Table 2). Comparison among studies is made difficult by the diversity of treatment settings, patient populations, and even definitions of seclusion or restraint. Methodologic differences among studies include retrospective versus prospective designs, correction of data for "days at risk," the use of concomitant medications to shorten the duration of seclusion, and institutional policies that regulate implementation and duration of seclusion procedures. A summary of findings from such diverse studies can yield only an approximation of current definable practice. Nonetheless, a review of the patterns of use for physical controls reveals that the most important variables governing the incidence of seclusion and restraint are the nature of the patient population (acute versus chronic), the hospital setting (public versus private), the patient's legal status (voluntary versus involuntary), and the treatment philosophy of the unit (Soloff et al, 1985). These factors are amply documented in a summary of descriptive research in Table 2.

Less apparent but equally relevant are systems issues involving staff morale, public and administrative support, adequacy of training, and security of the setting (Gutheil, 1984). The incidence of seclusion and restraint in adult inpatient settings ranges from a low of 1.9 percent in the chronic state hospital population studied by Tardiff (1981) to a high of 66 percent on an NIMH research unit where schizophrenic patients were treated without medication (Wadeson and Carpenter, 1976). In general, public facilities accepting acute admissions of both voluntary and involuntary patients tend to have the highest seclusion rates (Table 2). Any prescreening selection of patient admissions for financial, diag-

Table 2. Incidence of Seclusion/Restraint in Adult Inpatient Settings

Senior Author	Inpatient Setting	Population Served	Incidence of Seclusion/Restraint (% patients)
Tardiff (1981)	State hospital	Chronic, public, voluntary/involuntary	1.9
Soloff (1978)[+]	Military hospital	Acute, active duty, voluntary/involuntary	3.6
Wells (1972)	Psychiatric unit	Acute, private/public, unknown (locked unit)	4.0
Ramchandani (1981)	Psychiatric unit, general hospital	Acute, unknown, voluntary/involuntary	4.7
Bornstein (1985)[+*]	Psychiatric unit, general hospital	Acute, private/public, voluntary/involuntary	5.3
Mattson (1978)	Psychiatric unit, general hospital	Acute, private, voluntary only	7.2
Gerlock (1983)	University psychiatric hospital	Acute, public, voluntary/involuntary	10.0
Soloff (1981)*	University psychiatric hospital	Acute, public, voluntary/involuntary	10.5
Oldham (1983)	University psychiatric hospital	Acute, private, voluntary/involuntary	18.0
Convertino (1980)	CMHC	Acute, public, voluntary/involuntary	21.0
Telintelo (1983)[+]	Emergency room	Acute, public, voluntary/involuntary	24.0
Plutchik (1978)	Municipal psychiatric hospital	Acute, public, voluntary/involuntary	26.0
Schwab (1979)*	Psychiatric unit, university general hospital	Acute, public/private, unknown (locked unit)	36.6
Binder (1979)	Crisis intervention unit	Acute, public, voluntary/involuntary	44.0
Phillips (1983)	State hospital (research institute)	Acute, public, voluntary/involuntary	51.0
Wadeson (1976)	NIMH research unit	Acute, public, unknown	66.0

*Prospective study
[+]Restraint study

nostic, or legal criteria is reflected in a reduced incidence of seclusion and restraint. Research philosophies requiring long periods of medication-free observation also result in higher than usual seclusion rates (Schwab and Laymeyer, 1979). Similarly, philosophies of care regarding thresholds of tolerance for violence relate directly to the rate of seclusion (Okin, 1985).

Most studies agree on the type of patient likely to require seclusion or restraint. In acute adult treatment units, the young, schizophrenic, or manic patient is primarily responsible for the majority of seclusion events. Such patients are generally psychotic at the time of seclusion and are secluded early in their hospital stay, presumably before the maximal effects of medication and milieu have been achieved. Nonpsychotic patients who require restraint demonstrate a high proportion of acting out impulsive borderline disorders (Soloff, 1978). In the chronic state hospital population, the greatest proportion of seclusion events is attributable to patients with mental retardation and nonpsychotic disorders, though the largest absolute number of patients secluded are schizophrenic (Tardiff, 1981). In most studies, race and sex are not directly related to the incidence of physical controls, though the question of systematic bias in treatment has occasionally been raised (Kuhlman, et al, 1982; Flaherty and Meagher, 1980). In contrast, chronicity of illness and legal status on admission are both correlated with increased incidence of seclusion. Committed patients are secluded for similar behaviors as are their voluntarily admitted peers, though the incidence of seclusion for committed patients is significantly higher, suggesting that committed patients may be secluded as much for their status and attribution of dangerousness as for their actual behavior. The greatest use of seclusion and restraint is for a behavior pattern defined as "escalating agitation," "agitated uncontrolled behavior," or "behavior disruptive to the therapeutic milieu." As noted in Table 3, actual physical violence generally ranks second to the preventive use of seclusion as a precipitating event in most empirical studies. Exceptions to this rule include two prospective studies involving direct contact with the staff responsible for each seclusion-restraint event (Soloff and Turner, 1981; Bornstein, 1985). In these two prospective studies, actual physical violence toward staff was the predominant cause of seclusion or restraint, leading one to speculate as to whether the prospective research design inhibits staff in their preventive use of physical controls. The method of chart review, utilized in the majority of studies, has been faulted by Lion and colleagues (1981), who demonstrated a fivefold underreporting of actual violence in hospital records. Dietz and Rada (1983) add that "underdetection" by staff may also constitute a source of underestimating the incidence of assault in hospital incident reports.

The duration of locked seclusion varies widely within and between studies, from a brief time-out of 10 minutes, to a protracted period of 120 hours within the same setting (Soloff and Turner, 1981). Mean durations range from 4.1 hours in a municipal hospital psychiatric unit (Plutchik et al, 1978) to 15.7 hours in a crisis intervention unit (Binder, 1979). Duration of seclusion and restraint is partly determined by staff and milieu factors not directly related to the individual patient's clinical progress. Soloff and Turner (1981) found the duration of seclusion to be statistically independent of diagnosis, mental status (psychotic versus nonpsychotic), legal status, and precipitating behavior. It is the independence of cause and duration in the application of physical controls which most disturbs

Table 3. Precipitants to Seclusion/Restraint in Rank Order

Soloff (1978)[+]	#1	Violation of community or administrative limits	35.1%
	#2	Patient escalating, unable to control behavior	16.2%
	#3	Physical attack or threat on staff—physical contact	14.4%
			of episodes
Ramchandani (1981)	#1	Agitated, loud, and shouting	54.3%
	#2	Combined violent threat/attack	41.3%
			of patients secluded
Mattson (1978)	#1	Behavior disruptive to threapeutic environment (nonviolent)	34.4%
	#2	Assaultive to others	25.1%
			of episodes
Soloff (1981)*	#1	Physical attack on staff with physical contact	34.6%
	#2	Patient escalating, unable to control behavior	24.3%
			of episodes
Oldham (1983)	#1	Escalating/agitation	38.0%
	#2	Threats to others	25.0%
	#3	Assaultiveness	21.0%
			of episodes
Convertino (1980)	#1	Disruptive or agitated behavior	38.0%
	#2	Violent behavior	31.0%
			of episodes
Plutchik (1978)	#1	Agitated, uncontrolled behavior	21.0%
	#2	Physical aggression toward other patients	15.3%
			of episodes

Table 3. Precipitants to Seclusion/Restraint in Rank Order (Continued)

Schwab (1979)*			
	#1	Destimulation	28.0%
	#2	Agitation	17.0%
	#3	Poor impulse control	15.0%
			of all reasons cited
Binder (1979)			
	#1	Agitation	16
	#2	Uncooperativeness	14
	#3	Violent behaviors	14 times
			cited in seclusion record
	#1	"Other" (violence toward self, public nudity, screaming, medical procedures, etc.).	39.0%
Phillips (1983)			
	#2	Agitation, overstimulation, poor impulse control	31.0%
	#3	Actions or threats of violence toward others	30.0%
			of episodes
Bornstein (1985)†*			
	#1	Physical activity against staff or physician	39.5%
	#2	Unknown	22.0%
	#3	Verbal threat to staff or physician	18.4%
			of episodes

†Restraint study
*Prospective study

legal scholars, raising issues of seclusion as a punitive or administrative sanction analogous to solitary confinement in penal institutions.

With the application of physical controls, *restraint is treatment*. The potential for abuse of this treatment is widely discussed in sensationalized accounts in the media and in scholarly reviews by the judiciary. The relation between ideal treatment for the individual—both medically and legally—and the preservation and safety of a therapeutic milieu are, at times, in apparent conflict. The hospital has a duty to provide a therapeutic setting and protection for the safety of all its patients, and must balance this duty against the needs of an individual patient who is violent and disruptive by virtue of illness. Each setting defines its own limits to disruptive behavior and acts in defense of the social milieu when limits are exceeded. Psychotic behavior may prompt seclusion, while willful and malicious behavior requires administrative discharge. When the use of seclusion serves *only* the purpose of social control and not the needs of the individual patient, the legitimacy of this treatment may be challenged. Seclusion and restraint are never condoned for punishment, for the convenience or comfort of staff, or for social control alone.

Technique

The physical techniques for controlling agitated psychiatric patients require training and regular review in a manner analogous to the efforts given to cardiopulmonary resuscitation (CPR). In this modern era of pharmacologic sophistication, psychiatric residents are rarely trained or prepared to physically handle violent or disruptive patients. Nurses, attendants, and security staff do not fare much better. To meet this need, experienced persons have developed workshops to teach physical methods of nonaggressive confrontation and noninjurious control. Lion and his colleagues have developed a model program for the State of Maryland to teach physical techniques to mental health personnel, who are then tested and certified for competence in the application of these techniques (Lion and Soloff, 1984). While physical technique may vary from program to program, several important general principles apply to all clinical settings and warrant specific review.

The decision to use seclusion and restraint is typically made by nursing staff observing behavior that exceeds accepted limits for that particular unit. Once the clinical decision has been made to proceed with seclusion, a seclusion "leader" is chosen among available clinical staff. The leader designates the roles to be played by the remaining participants and directs all steps in the seclusion and restraint process. All communication between staff and patient is initiated by the seclusion leader. This individual need not be the most senior member of the staff present, but may be chosen for familiarity with the patient, physical characteristics such as sex, size, or general bearing. (Often the least intimidating member of a nursing staff may win the cooperation of an agitated and violent patient sooner than the largest or toughest authoritarian on the staff.) A show of force *must* be available from the beginning of any confrontation with the agitated and potentially violent patient. Even if force is not ultimately employed, it is important for patients to perceive clearly that there is sufficient force to control their behavior. Sufficient personnel must be present to overwhelm the patient safely with minimum risk to all. Ideally, there should be one staff member present for each limb and one to monitor the head, neck, and airway. Whenever possible, a staff member is designated as the seclusion "monitor" to clear the area of other patients and physical obstructions to the seclusion room. The monitor stands clear of physical action, obtains medication when needed, and notes any and all injuries or difficulties with physical technique, allowing for an accurate critique of the seclusion process after the event.

The confrontation begins with deployment of the "show of force" around the patient in such a manner as to allow rapid access to the patient's extremities. The patient should be given few and clear behavioral options without undue verbal threat or provocation. Since control of behavior is the predetermined goal of the confrontation, psychodynamic negotiation is superfluous and defeats the purpose of setting limits. The patient should be told clearly and directly the purpose of the seclusion and given the behavioral option to walk quietly to the seclusion room accompanied by staff. ("Your behavior is out of control. You must take a time-out in seclusion to regain control over your behavior.") The patient's behavioral options are spelled out clearly, with every effort made to allow a safe and orderly retreat to the seclusion room, avoiding humiliation or threat to the patient's self-esteem.

The attitude of staff at this point is critical. Rather than appear "combat ready," staff should convey an air of confidence and calm, a measured control that indicates both the ability to control the patient if necessary and, conversely, a professional approach to a routine and familiar procedure. The time allotted for the patient's decision is brief, seconds rather than minutes. If the patient agrees to walk to seclusion, staff members on either side firmly but supportively hold his or her arms to minimize risk should the patient lose control en route. If the patient fails to indicate compliance quickly, physical force must commence at a signal given by the seclusion leader. One method of "take down" requires each staff member to seize and control the movement of one extremity and, using backward movement, bring the patient to the ground. The patient's head must be supported and controlled by a fifth staff member (positioned behind the patient) to prevent striking the ground during the "take down" procedure. This staff member then controls the head to prevent biting. (Where fewer staff are available, a single individual may control the patient's head by crossing the patient's arms over the head, creating a vise.)

The use of noninjurious technique is critical from both a practical and clinical perspective. The use of force to contain violent behavior early in a hospital course must not be so traumatic that it precludes a therapeutic alliance with the patient once the issue of violence is resolved. With the patient completely restrained on the ground, additional staff may be called to secure the limbs and prepare to move the patient to the seclusion room or apply mechanical restraints. In the most violent cases, staff may choose to inject medication at this time. The agitated, uncooperative patient may require to be physically carried in the recumbent position with arms pinned to sides, legs held tightly at knees, head controlled, with lift applied uniformly to the back, hips, and legs. More compliant patients may be walked to seclusion with adequate control over both arms. Once in seclusion, the patient is changed into a hospital gown and all potentially destructive objects such as rings, belts, shoes, and so forth, are removed. The staff exit from seclusion requires coordination as well. The patient is positioned on his or her back with the head toward the seclusion door and feet pointing in the opposite direction. Staff exit in coordinated fashion, one at a time, releasing legs first and arms last, with the final staff member moving backward out of the seclusion door, which is quickly secured. A face-down position is not recommended because of the possibility of compromising respiration, especially in an extremely obese individual. It is useful for staff to review each seclusion or restraint maneuver after the fact. The seclusion monitor critiques the event, allowing an emotional release of tension from the staff.

Each facility should develop and rehearse a specific set of physical techniques to be used for seclusion and restraint and provide regular in-service training for staff. The methods to be used should be approved at the highest level of hospital administration and specified in the hospital policy manual. Documentation of required in-service training and faithful implementation of prescribed procedures is critical from a medico-legal perspective should a serious, untoward event occur in the course of restraining a patient.

Basic principles for monitoring the patient in seclusion or restraint have been recommended by the American Psychiatric Association Task Force and apply to all settings:

1. Although seclusion and restraint are generally initiated by "on line" nursing staff, a physician's review and order for continuation should be obtained as soon as possible. The APA Task Force recommends that a physician should see the patient *within three hours and preferably within one hour* following the first episode of seclusion of a given patient. The physician's order for continuation must be documented as well as the result of his or her personal examination, giving the reasons for continuation of physical controls. (Termination of the episode must also be by physician order.)
2. A minimum of two visits a day by the responsible physician is recommended, ideally 12 hours apart. Depending upon the patient's clinical condition, it is understood that monitoring may be much more intensive; for example, if the patient is receiving rapid neuroleptization, medical treatment, or observation for withdrawal of drugs.
3. The order for seclusion is generally valid for 12 hours with adequate documentation of an examination and justification for continuation required. If the patient is continuously secluded/restrained for 72 hours or longer, the hospital director or designee defined in hospital policy must review and approve the continuation of seclusion.
4. Nursing observation should be made at least every 15 minutes to document the patient's clinical condition. An effort to engage the patient verbally should be made at least every two hours, and toiletting accomplished at least every four hours. Requests for fluids, food, or other measures of bodily comfort should be promptly met with documentation of intake. As each entry into seclusion may require a display or even use of force, mealtimes, medication, and change of bedpan (or change of room when needed) must be coordinated.
5. The patient will have to be debriefed concerning the experience. It is important that a clear explanation be given as to why the procedure was utilized. All too often patients are left with a distorted picture of their experience, colored by psychotic percepts and misunderstandings (Binder and McCoy, 1983; Wadeson and Carpenter, 1976).

Seclusion versus Restraint: Risks and Benefits

A choice between seclusion or restraint as a means of physical control is all too often made on the basis of legislated prejudice rather than clinical need. Both have advantages and disadvantages. The clinician should be familiar with both, and, where permitted by law, choose according to immediate need. Total physical restraint, accomplished by means of four-point leather cufflets or cold wet pack, requires skilled and constant nursing care for fluids, feeding, and toiletting in bed. For the patient in four-point leather restraints, circulation must be checked at least every 15 minutes. The circulation of the extremities may be easily compromised, or abrasions may occur as a result of struggling against the cuffs. The more restrictive cold wet pack causes the patient to shiver and generate heat. Struggling causes the patient to become fatigued in a warm, cocoon-like wrapper. In the presence of phenothiazine medication and dysregulation of temperature, the insulation of the wet sheets can cause alarming elevation of body temperature and a potentially dangerous hyperthermia (Greenland and Southwick, 1978). For this reason, cold wet packs must be opened approximately every two hours or converted to four-point restraints for some period prior to reapplication. Struggling against physical restraints has been associated with rhabdomyolysis in a patient with phencyclidine intoxication (Lahmeyer, 1983).

The psychological impact on staff and patient of total physical restraint is responsible for much resistance against the method. The cultural and psychological indignity of being "tied down" and "defenseless" must be weighed against the benefit of free and safe access to the patient for medication, assessment, and reassurance. Physical restraint allows direct continuous contact between patient and staff, an important advantage lost in the use of the seclusion room. It may also prove valuable for medical treatments requiring close monitoring in agitated patients. Lion and Soloff (1984) describe the use of partial or ambulatory restraint devices, which allow the patient to mix safely with the patient population and minimize the isolation of seclusion.

The chief advantage of the locked seclusion room—physical autonomy for the patient—creates its chief liability, the possibility of self-directed violence or attack on staff upon entry. The patient has the freedom and dignity of self-toiletting and self-feeding—and the freedom to engage in fecal soiling, smearing, and throwing of food or other objects (such as mattress and bed pan). Feeding and medicating the secluded patient provides an opportunity for the patient to display self-control, or, alternatively, provides an occasion for renewed attack on staff. Some psychotic patients feel safe behind the locked door, while others pound the wall for hours, inflicting injury on themselves. In the extreme case, patients must be removed from seclusion for head pounding or self-mutilation—and placed in total body restraint.

Neglect is the principle "evil" of seclusion. Once "locked away," the patient may be viewed as a management problem rather than a person with profound psychological needs. The stigma of the seclusion experience follows the patient's reintegration into the milieu and may prejudice further psychodynamic work. Routinization of use of physical controls inevitably leads to abuse (Greenblatt et al, 1955; Guirguis, 1978).

Rarely, severe and untoward events occur in the seclusion process. Staff injury occurs more frequently during the seclusion process than from any other cause

(Lion, 1983). Patient death has occurred following struggles in the seclusion process and in the course of prolonged periods of seclusion. Nelson and colleagues (1983) has recently described a 20-year-old man with paranoid schizophrenia who tore open the vinyl cover of his mattress, "crawled head first to below his shoulders inside the mattress," and died of asphyxiation. The isolation of the patient from staff or patient observation may contribute to such tragic outcomes. The inability of staff to respond quickly to a patient in seclusion who is banging the head, gouging the eyes, or biting himself or herself adds to the potential liability of the method. The construction and thermal regulation of the room must be carefully designed for patient safety.

Recognizing that seclusion and restraint are intensive care treatments reinforces the need for rapid intervention with medication (where indicated), careful nursing surveillance, and release from restriction as soon as behavior is under control.

CONCLUSION

A review of verbal, chemical, and physical techniques in the acute management of the violent patient demonstrates a substantial body of knowledge concerning the safe and effective treatment of these difficult patients. Lessons derived from experience in emergency rooms and inpatient units can be generalized and adapted to specific treatment settings. *What is needed most in any approach to the violent patient is preparation for the inevitable;* that is, a defined policy and program of training and rehearsal specific to each setting on the use of verbal, chemical, and physical controls in the emergency management of the violent patient.

REFERENCES

American Psychiatric Association: Report of the Task Force on Psychiatric Uses of Seclusion and Restraint of the Council on Governmental Policy and the Law of the American Psychiatric Association (Task Force Report No. 22). Washington DC, American Psychiatric Association, 1985

Anderson WH, Kuehnu JC: Strategies for the treatment of acute psychosis. JAMA 229:1884-1889, 1974

Anderson WH, Kuehnle JC, Catanzano DM: Rapid treatment of acute psychosis. Am J Psychiatry 133:1076-1078, 1976

Anderson WH, Kuehnle JC: Treatment of psychosis by rapid neuroleptization: update 1980, in Haloperidol Update 1958-1980. Edited by Ayd FJ. Baltimore, Ayd Medical Co., 1980

Appleton WS: The snow phenomenon: tranquilizing the assaultive. Psychiatry 28:88-93, 1965

Baldessarini RJ, Katz B, Cotton P: Dissimilar dosing with high-potency and low-potency neuroleptics. Am J Psychiatry 141:748-752, 1984

Barton W: A study of patterns of service, in The Psychiatric Emergency. Edited by Glasscote R. Washington, DC, American Psychiatric Association, 1966

Bernstein HA: Survey of threats and assaults directed toward psychotherapists. Am J Psychother 35:542-549, 1981

Binder RL: The use of seclusion on an inpatient crisis intervention unit. Hosp Community Psychiatry 30:266-269, 1979

Binder RL, McCoy SM: A study of patients' attitudes toward placement in seclusion. Hosp Community Psychiatry 34:1052-1054, 1983

Boling L, Brotman C: A fire-setting epidemic in a state mental health center. Am J Psychiatry 139:946-950, 1975

Bornstein PE: The use of restraints on a general psychiatric unit. J Clin Psychiatry 46:175-178, 1985

Brauzer B, Goldstein BJ: The differential response to parenteral chlorpromazine and mesoridazine in psychotic patients. J Clin Psychopharmacol 10:126-131, 1970

Bursten B: Using mechanical restraints on acutely disturbed psychotic patients. Hosp Community Psychiatry 26:757-758, 1976

Carter RG: Psychotolysis with haloperidol: rapid control of the acutely disturbed psychotic patient. Diseases of the Nervous System 38:237-239, 1977

Convertino K, Pinto RP, Fiester AR: Use of inpatient seclusion at a community mental health center. Hosp Community Psychiatry 31:848-850, 1980

Danik JJ, Goverdam M: Haloperidol in the treatment of 120 psychotic patients. Am J Psychiatry 120:389-391, 1963

Danto BL: Patients who murder their psychiatrists. Am J Forensic Psychiatry 3:120-134, 1982–1983

Depp FC: Violent behavior patterns on psychiatric wards. Aggressive Behavior 2:295-306, 1976

Dietz PE, Rada RT: Seclusion rates and patient census in a maximum security hospital. Behavioral Sciences and the Law 1:89-93, 1983

Donlon PT, Meadow A, Tupin JP, et al: High vs. standard dosage fluphenazine HCL in acute schizophrenia. J Clin Psychiatry 39:800-804, 1978

Donlon PT, Hopkin J, Tupin JP: Overview: efficacy and safety of the rapid neuroleptization method with injectable haloperidol. Am J Psychiatry 136:273-278, 1979

Donlon PT, Hopkin JT, Tupin JP, et al: Haloperidol for acute schizophrenic patients: an evaluation of three oral regimens. Arch Gen Psychiatry 37:691-695, 1980

Dubin WR: Evaluating and managing the violent patient. Ann Emerg Med 10:481-484, 1981

Edwards JG, Reid WH: Violence in psychiatric facilities in Europe and the United States, in Assaults Within Psychiatric Facilities. Edited by Lion JR, Reid WH. New York, Grune & Stratton, 1983

Ericksen SE, Hurt SW, Chang S, et al: Haloperidol dose, plasma levels and clinical response: a double blind study. Psychopharmacol Bull 14:1 5-16, 1978

Erickson WD, Realmuto G: Frequency of seclusion in an adolescent psychiatric unit. J Clin Psychiatry 44:238-241, 1983

Fann WE, Linton PH: Use of perphenazine in psychiatric emergencies: the concept of chemical restraint. Current Therapeutic Research 14:478-482, 1972

Feldman P, Bay AP, Baser AW, et al: Parenteral haloperidol in controlling patient behavior during acute psychotic episodes. Current Therapeutic Research 11:362-366, 1969

Firling RJ: Acutely disturbed psychotic patients treated with parenteral haloperidol. IMJ 153:117, 1978

Fitzgerald CH: A double-blind comparison of haloperidol with perphenazine in acute psychiatric episodes. Current Therapeutic Research 11:515-519, 1969

Flaherty JA, Meagher R: Measuring racial bias in inpatient treatment. Am J Psychiatry 137:679-682, 1980

Gardner DL, Cowdry RW: Alprozalam-induced dyscontrol in borderline personality disorder. Am J Psychiatry 142:98-100, 1985

Gelenberg AJ, Mandel MR: Catatonic reactions to high-potency neuroleptic drugs. Arch Gen Psychiatry 34:947-950, 1977

Gerlock A, Solomons HC: Factors associated with the seclusion of psychiatric patients. Perspect Psychiatr Care 22:47-53, 1983

Greenblatt M, York R, Brown E: From Custodial to Therapeutic Patient Care in Mental Hospitals. New York, Russell Sage Foundation, 1955

Greenland P, Southwick WH: Hyperthermia associated with chlorpromazine and full-sheet restraint. Am J Psychiatry 135:1234-1235, 1978

Guirguis EF: Management of disturbed patients: an alternative to the use of mechanical restraints. J Clin Psychiatry 39:295-303, 1978

Guirguis EF, Durost HB: The role of mechanical restraints in the management of disturbed behaviour. Canadian Psychiatric Association Journal 23:209-218, 1978

Gutheil TG: Restraint vs. treatment: seclusion as discussed in the Boston State Hospital case. Am J Psychiatry 137:718-719, 1980

Gutheil TG: Observations on the theoretical basis for seclusion of the psychiatric inpatient. Am J Psychiatry 135:325-328, 1978

Gutheil TG: Review of individual quantitative studies, in The Psychiatric Uses of Seclusion and Restraint. Washington, DC, American Psychiatric Press, Inc., 1984

Hamid TA, Wertz WJ: Mesoridazine vs. chlorpromazine in acute schizophrenics: a double blind investigation. Am J Psychiatry 130:689-692, 1973

Hatti S, Dubin WR, Weiss KJ: A study of circumstances surrounding patient assaults on psychiatrists. Hosp Community Psychiatry 33:660-661, 1982

Hanke N: Handbook of Emergency Psychiatry. Lexington, MA, DC Heath, 1984

Jacobs D: Evaluation and management of the violent patient in emergency settings. Psychiatr Clin North Am 6:259-269, 1983

Kalogerakis MG: The assaultive psychiatric patient. Psychiatr Q 45:372-381, 1971

Kaskey GB, Nasr S: A side effect of rapid neuroleptization (letter). Am J Psychiatry 136:1232, 1979

Klein DF, Davis JM: Diagnosis and Drug Treatment of Psychiatric Disorders. Baltimore, Williams & Wilkins, 1969

Kuhlman T, Telintelo S, Winget C: Restraint use with emergency psychiatric patients: a new perspective on racial bias. Psychol Rep 51:343-347, 1982

Lahmeyer HH: PCP, physical restraints, and rhabdomyolysis. J Clin Psychiatry 44:239, 1983

Lion JR: Evaluation and Management of the Violent Patient. Springfield, IL, Charles C Thomas, 1972

Lion JR: Benzodiazepines in the treatment of aggressive patients. J Clin Psychiatry 40:70-71, 1979

Lion JR, Snyder W, Merrill GL: Underreporting of assaults on staff in state hospitals. Hosp Community Psychiatry 32:497-498, 1981

Lion JR: Special aspects of psychopharmacology, in Assaults Within Psychiatric Facilities. Edited by Lion JR, Reid WC. New York, Grune & Stratton, 1983

Lion JR, Pasternak SA: Countertransference reactions to violent patients. Am J Psychiatry 130:207-210, 1973

Lion JR, Reid WC, (Eds): Assaults Within Psychiatric Faculties. New York, Grune and Stratton, 1983

Lion JR, Soloff PH: Implementation of Seclusion and Restraint, in The Psychiatric Uses of Seclusion and Restraint. Edited by Tardiff K. Washington, DC, American Psychiatric Press, Inc, 1984

Lion JR, Snyder W, Merrill GL: Underreporting of assaults on staff in a state hospital. Hosp Community Psychiatry 32:497-498, 1981

Madden DJ, Lion JR, Penna MW: Assaults on psychiatrists by patients. Am J Psychiatry 133:422-425, 1976

Man PL, Chen CH: Rapid tranquilization of acutely psychotic patients with intramuscular haloperidol and chlorpromazine. Psychosomatics 14:59-64, 1973

Mason AS, Granacher RP: Basic principals of rapid neuroleptization. Diseases of the Nervous System 37:547-551, 1976

Mason AS, Granacher RP: Rapid tranquilization methods, in Clinical Handbook of Antipsychotic Drug Therapy. New York, Brunner/Mazel, 1980

Mattson MR, Sacks MH: Seclusion: uses and complications. Am J Psychiatry 135:1210-1213, 1978

Moos RH: Evaluating Treatment Environments: A Social Etiological Approach. New York, John Wiley & Sons, 1974

Mountain HE: Crash tranquilization in a milieu therapy setting. Journal of the Fort Logan Mental Health Center 1:43-44, 1963

Nelson SH, McKinney A, Ludwig K, et al: An unusual death of a patient in seclusion. Hosp Community Psychiatry 34:259-260, 1983

Nilson JA: Immediate treatment expedites hospital release. Hosp Community Psychiatry 20:36-38, 1969

Okin RL: Variation among state hospitals in use of seclusion and restraint. Hosp Community Psychiatry 36:648-652, 1985

Oldham AJ, Bott M: The management of excitement in a general hospital psychiatric ward by high dosage haloperidol. Acta Psychiatr Scand 47:369-376, 1971

Oldham JM, Russakoff LM, Prusnofsky L: Seclusion: patterns and milieu. J Nerv Ment Dis 171:645-650, 1983

Phillips P, Nasr SJ: Seclusion and restraint and prediction of violence. Am J Psychiatry 140:229-232, 1983

Plutchik R, Karasu TB, Conte HR, et al: Toward a rationale for the seclusion process. J Nerv Ment Dis 166:571-579, 1978

Polak P, Laycob L: Rapid tranquilization. Am J Psychiatry 118:300-307, 1971

Rada RT: The violent patient: rapid assessment and management. Psychosomatics 22:101-109, 1981

Ramchandani D, Akhtar S, Helfrich J: Seclusion of psychiatric inpatients: a general hospital perspective. Int J Soc Psychiatry 27:225-231, 1981

Reschke RW: Parenteral haloperidol for rapid control of severe, disruptive symptoms of acute schizophrenia. Diseases of the Nervous System 35:112-115, 1974

Resnik HLP, Ruben HL: Emergency Psychiatric Care: The Management of Mental Health Crises. Maryland, Charles Press, 1975

Romoff V: Management and control of violent patients at the Western Psychiatric Institute and Clinic, in: Clinical Treatment of the Violent Person. Edited by Roth L. DHHS Publ. (ADM) 85–1425. Washington, DC, U.S. Government Printing Office, 1985

Rosen M, DiGiacomo JN: The role of physical restraint in the treatment of psychiatric illness. J Clin Psychiatry 39:228-232, 1978

Ruben I, Wolkon G, Yamamoto J: Physical attacks on psychiatric residents by patients. J Nerv Ment Dis 168:243-245, 1980

Salzman C, Hoffman SA: Rapid tranquilization (letter). Hosp Community Psychiatry 33:346, 1982

Salzman C, Kochansky GE, Shader RI: Chlordiazepoxide induced hostility in a small group setting. Arch Gen Psychiatry 31:401, 1974

Salzman C, Green AI, Rodriguez-Villa F, et al: Benzodiazepines combined with neuroleptics for management of severe disruptive behavior. Psychosomatics 27(Suppl):17-26, . 1986

Sangiovanni F, Taylor MA, Abrams R: Rapid control of psychotic excitement states with intramuscular haloperidol. Am J Psychiatry 130:1155-1156, 1973

Schwab PJ, Laymeyer CB: The uses of seclusion on a general hospital psychiatric unit. J Clin Psychiatry 40:228-231, 1979

Slotnick VB: Management of the acutely agitated psychotic patient with parenteral neuroleptics: a comparative symptom effectiveness profile of haloperidol and chlorpromazine. Paper presented at the Fifth World Congress of Psychiatry, Mexico City, Nov. 1971

Soloff PH: Behavioral precipitants of restraint in the modern milieu. Compr Psychiatry 19:179-184, 1978

Soloff PH: Physical restraint and the non-psychotic patient: clinical and legal perspectives. J Clin Psychiatry 40:302-305, 1979

Soloff PH: Seclusion and restraint, in Assaults Within Psychiatric Facilities. Edited by Lion JR, Reid WH. Orlando, Florida, Grune & Stratton, 1983

Soloff PH, Turner SM: Patterns of seclusion: a prospective study. J Nerv Ment Dis 169:37-44, 1981

Soloff PH, Gutheil TG, Wexler DB: Seclusion and restraint in 1985: a review and update. Hosp Community Psychiatry 36:652-657, 1985

Soreff SM: Management of the Psychiatric Emergency. New York, John Wiley and Sons, 1981

Soreff SM: Violence in the emergency room, in: Phenomenology and Treatment of Psychiatric Emergencies. Edited by Comstock BS, Fann WE, Pokorny AD, et al. New York, Spectrum Publications, 1984

Star B: Patient violence/therapist safety. Social Work 29:225-230, 1984

Tardiff K: Emergency control measures for psychiatric inpatients. J Nerv Ment Dis 169:614-618, 1981

Telintelo S, Kuhlman TL, Winget C: A study of the use of restraint in a psychiatric emergency room. Hosp Community Psychiatry 34:164-165, 1983

Tupin JP: Management of violent patients, in Manual of Psychiatric Therapeutics. Edited by Shader RI. Boston, Little, Brown, 1975

Tupin JP: The violent patient: a strategy for management and diagnosis. Hosp Community Psychiatry 34:37-40, 1983

Tupin JP: Focal neuroleptization: an approach to optimal dosing for initial and continuing therapy. J Clin Psychopharmacol 5(Suppl):15S-21S, 1985a

Tupin JP: Psychopharmacology and aggression, in Clinical Treatment of the Violent Person. Edited by Roth LH. DHHS Publ No. (ADM) 85-145. Washington, DC, U.S. Government Printing Office, 1985b

Van Putten T, Mutalipassi LR, Malkin MD: Phenothiazine-induced decompensation. Arch Gen Psychiatry 30:102-105, 1974

Wadeson H, Carpenter WT: Impact of the seclusion room experience. J Nerv Ment Dis 163:318-328, 1976

Wells DA: The use of seclusion on a university hospital psychiatric floor. Arch Gen Psychiatry 26:410-413, 1972

Whitman RM, Armao BB, Dent OB: Assault on the therapist. Am J Psychiatry 133:426-431, 1976

Wing JK, Cooper JE, Sartorius N: The measurement and classification of psychiatric symptoms. Cambridge, England, Cambridge University Press, 1974

Chapter 23

The Long-Term Treatment of the Violent Patient

by John R. Lion, M.D., and Kenneth Tardiff, M.D., M.P.H.

CHARACTERISTICS OF VIOLENT OUTPATIENTS

The principles of long-term treatment of the violent patient addressed in this chapter pertain primarily to the outpatient setting, although some may have relevance for the long-term treatment of the institutionalized violent patient; for example, mentally retarded or psychotic inpatients. Assaultive behavior is less frequently seen as a problem for patients presenting for outpatient treatment than for inpatient treatment. A recent study by Tardiff and Koenigsberg found that three percent of patients presenting to the clinics at two private psychiatric hospitals in New York had manifested recent violence toward other persons (Tardiff and Koenigsberg, 1985). This is less than 10 percent of patients with a history of recent violence presenting to private and public hospitals for admission (Tardiff and Sweillam, 1980; Tardiff, 1984; Lion and Reid, 1983).

Although, as with the admission studies, males are more likely than females and younger patients are more likely than older patients to manifest violent behavior, diagnostic characteristics of violent outpatients differed from those of violent inpatients. Violent patients presenting to outpatient clinics were more likely to be in the nonpsychotic diagnostic categories—for example, personality, child, or adolescence disorders—rather than psychotic disorders. Among violent psychiatric outpatients, the spouse, mate, or other family members were targets of violence in approximately 60 percent of the cases.

TYPES OF LONG-TERM OUTPATIENT TREATMENT

There are two basic forms of long-term treatment of violent outpatients: aftercare, with a heavy reliance on medication and social intervention; and psychotherapy, predominantly with patients with personality disorders, perhaps with some medication and social intervention. The first will be dispensed with and most of this chapter will be concerned with the second. Aftercare may involve treatment of manic-depressive patients with a history of violence who are stabilized on lithium carbonate. Compliance with medication may be a problem. Psychotherapy may be indicated in terms of couples therapy to address other dynamic issues in the marriage and the effect of the manic depressive illness on the marriage.

Another type of aftercare patient is the schizophrenic with a history of violence. A prime concern with this type patient is a continuation of neuroleptic medication. Depot fluphenazine may be used for problem patients in terms of compliance, for example paranoid schizophrenics. It is not unusual to see the violent paranoid schizophrenic patient stabilize with medication in the hospital and be deemed appropriate for discharge. In the community, compliance is a problem, and subsequent deterioration results in violence and readmission. To address the problem of noncompliance with medication among formerly violent patients, legislation for mandatory aftercare programs has been passed in some states, for example in North Carolina and Hawaii. In the practical sense, mandatory aftercare is problematic to implement since most health professionals are reluctant to see themselves in a police role, and have legitimate fears about approaching a patient whom they suspect has not been taking medication and who, for example, may be paranoid and armed.

Most outpatient treatment will involve psychotherapy with patients with a variety of personality disorders. Personality disorders such as the borderline type often display self-mutilation and temper outbursts, while antisocial personalities are usually violent toward others, not themselves. The passive-aggressive personality may display anger and rage, while the weakening of control in the compulsive personality may manifest itself in a violent outburst. Paranoid and narcissistic personalities may show outbursts of aggression when challenged, and histrionic personalities as well may react to stress with dramatic shows of violence. Violence, then, may be a prominent part of character pathology and form the basis for therapy; however, the best candidate for outpatient treatment is the patient with episodic violence who manifests remorse and guilt following these violent episodes.

Group and family therapies are the usual modes of outpatient psychotherapy for the violent patient for several reasons. First, most violence goes on within families, and thus to treat the patient in isolation is ineffective, particularly if the victim and patient are engaged in a provocative interaction. This is also the case with violent adolescents who operate within a family unit. Second, group process often allows violent patients to discuss issues that they are too frightened to bring up in a one-to-one setting. When structured to treat the impulse character disorder, group therapy allows participants to see other patients troubled by recurring temper outbursts and low self-esteem. As these types of patients often have an impoverished ability to view their own pathology, confrontation by other members of the group becomes more effective and less threatening than if done by the therapist.

GOALS OF PSYCHOTHERAPY

There are five major goals in the psychotherapy of the violent patient.

Motivation of the Patient

First the therapist must evaluate the motivation of the patient and the reasons for a request for psychotherapy and treatment. A reason such as wanting to impress the court in an impending trial for a violent offense is not as promising a reason as remorse by the patient or pressure from a spouse in terms of divorce.

Achieving Self-Control

The second goal is the development of self-control. Often this is not difficult in the beginning phases of therapy. In the treatment of aggressive patients, there is often an initial "honeymoon" phase wherein aggression appears to cease.

The therapist is endowed with powerful attributes which represent the opposite of the patient's inner state. Accordingly, strength is gleaned by contact with the therapist and the patient finds, transiently, the ability to function without becoming aggressive. Sooner or later, however, this relationship becomes tested and the patient encounters some conflict outside of the treatment setting to which he or she responds with violence. Both the patient and the family are sharply disappointed, and this is when the real work of psychotherapy begins.

Dealing with Transference and Countertransference

Change in the nature of the transference is the most critical and potentially dangerous aspect of work with aggressive patients. The therapist must continually monitor this set of feelings, for it can change as a function of the patient's primitiveness. Paranoid and borderline patients, or those with a history of psychotic illness, are prone to handle the burgeoning intimacy of therapy with threats of violence or actual violent or destructive acts. Playful gestures within the therapy hour that suggest such rages should spark discussion, as should letters or notes, or messages on answering machines that can be interpreted as threatening or indicative of aggressive thoughts on the part of the patient. "Can this patient hurt me?" should be a dominant question in the clinician's mind. The purchase of weapons at home should be naturally monitored; in the context of the transference, it should give the therapist pause for thought.

The countertransference, likewise, requires evaluation (Lion and Pasternak, 1973). It is the most important indicator of the relationship between patient and therapist, though one easily subject to distortion in the case of violence. Aggression usually mobilizes fear in the clinician, who can respond by projecting anxieties onto the patient and seeing the latter as more violent and threatening than the patient really is. Conversely, denial of fear can lead to the false perception of the patient as "interesting" instead of a potential danger to society. One way of guarding against such errors is to have the patient seen in consultation. Forensic institutions operate on the principle of shared responsibility, whereby several clinicians make judgments about the patient's violent propensities. In clinical practice, the therapist should likewise think about having the violent patient seen from another viewpoint. This is particularly important when the clinician is excessively worried or ruminative about the risks the patient poses to society, and when the clinician becomes frightened for his or own safety. Consultation also has legal implications for the more formal assessment of risk, as will be described later.

Development of Affective Awareness and Insight

There should be development of affective awareness. It is critical for a violent patient to be cognizant of when he or she is becoming angry so that the patient is neither flooded with affect, or so little aware of it that he or she cannot respond appropriately to events. The patient must come to realize when he or she is getting angry and must identify the physiological state of anger. If the patient is aware of the anger, the patient can at least try and talk about it.

There should be the development of insight regarding the dynamics of violence for the individual patient and spouse, other family members, and friends. This involves creating some awareness within the patient by sensitization to the precipitating insults. Such a tactic involves repetitive attempts on the clinician's part to draw the patient's attention to issues of self-esteem and their challenge. The patient must develop insight into vulnerabilities, whether they be size, sexuality, abandonment, or other recurring themes. The clinician's role is always to inquire why the patient became aggressive, since violence is not a random event but occurs in response to a perceived insult. A wife's provocative comment, a statement of ridicule by a fellow worker, or a sick child's relentless crying may variably evoke rage by kindling inner sensitivities that bespeak fragility and weakness defended against by violence. Weakness is a key dynamic in the violent patient, and long-term therapy must constantly focus on the violent patient as helpless and brittle. As the patient comes to grips with these inner frailities and accepts them, he or she will develop a greater tolerance and elasticity with regard to human relationships and self. Such growth takes time and thus makes therapy long term. Violence is a most difficult behavior to treat, for it so often reflects grave internal misperceptions of the self.

Appreciation of the Consequences of Violence

Another goal of psychotherapy involves the elucidation of fantasy with the intent of increasing the patient's ability to predict and appreciate emotionally the sequellae of his or her acts. The patient should come to realize that if he hits his wife, he may end up in jail. To this end, he must fantasize what it is like to end up in jail with its steel doors and concrete floors. "What would happen if . . ." is the method used to get patients to think about the outcome of their behaviors. This tactic is mundane, but crucial to a successful therapy. An anticipation of consequences is a powerful cognitive way to stop one's self from being violent.

SOCIAL INTERVENTIONS

The role of social intervention is obvious in terms of aftercare; for example, assisting with the patient's basic needs such as housing, food, and transportation. In addition, aspects of a patient's life outside the office setting must be considered so as to understand the dynamics of violence and/or to intervene as an advocate for the patient. These aspects may involve education in terms of understanding that a patient with poor education lacks legitimate nonviolent means of achievement, and helping the patient improve educationally (for example, through vocational schooling). It may be necessary to intervene in terms of the patient's employment if a job is threatened. Consideration should be given to housing in terms of crowding and stress, the patient's subculture, peers, and neighborhood along the lines indicated in Chapter 19 on determinants of violence. If intervention is not warranted, at least therapy should be done keeping in mind what patients are subjected to in the environment once they leave a session in one's office.

MEDICATIONS

There is no one drug for the treatment of aggression just as there is no one etiology for violent behavior (Lion, 1975). A variety of drugs have been touted as useful for violent patients but each one is specific to an underlying etiology.

Neuroleptics

Neuroleptics are obviously used for schizophrenia and mania and in some organic disorders, where the etiology is known, for delusional thinking or control of violence. Haloperidol is particularly popular because of its ability to be administered rapidly in high doses on inpatient units, and its safety in use with epileptic patients (Donlon et al, 1979). Oral fluphenazine should be considered for inpatient treatment, which could be followed by depot fluphenazine during aftercare for problems with compliance, as in paranoid schizophrenic patients. Daily neuroleptic medication for violent mentally retarded patients as long-term treatment is not advised unless there is concurrent psychosis. Studies have found that many more mentally retarded patients are on neuroleptics than are indicated. This is a problem not only in terms of side effects such as tardive dyskinesia, but because neuroleptics decrease learning in a group of patients in whom learning is a major problem (Kuehnel and Slama, 1984).

Lithium

Lithium is of prime effectiveness when used for aggression and hypersexuality of mania and for prophylaxis of manic-depressive disorders. Sheard (1985) has reviewed earlier studies on lithium and the treatment of aggression in patients other than those with manic-depressive disorders. There appeared to be some effectiveness in nonblind trials in decreasing aggression in severely mentally retarded patients (Dostal and Zvolsky, 1970). Prison studies using placebos with single blind designs (Martoramo, 1972; Tupin et al, 1973) and double blind designs (Sheard, 1975, 1976) demonstrated a decrease of assaultive and other violent behaviors among prisoners treated with lithium. The prisoners did not have psychotic or bipolar illnesses or brain damage. The response in terms of decreased assaultive behavior was seen in a variety of personality disorders except for schizoid personality disorder. The effectiveness of lithium in chronic psychotic patients in terms of decreasing aggression is not convincing, and there is suspicion that some of the patients who responded in these studies had atypical bipolar illness (Martoramo, 1972; Van Putten and Sanders, 1975). There is little or no evidence that lithium is effective in the treatment of aggression associated with epilepsy (Jus et al, 1973).

Campbell and colleagues (1984) have reviewed the use of lithium in children and adolescents. One study of particular interest was a double blind study of 61 children of normal intelligence who manifested chronic aggressive behavior with conduct disorders of the undersocialized aggressive type (Campbell et al, 1982). Dosages of lithium ranged from 500 to 2,000 mgs a day and the mean serum level of lithium was 1.0 mEq/L. Lithium did decrease aggressive behavior. There was no difference between lithium and haloperidol in decreasing aggressive behavior; however, lithium did have fewer side effects than haloperidol. Although there was no history of affective illness, it was observed that the best results were obtained if there was a strong affective component to the aggression.

There have been no long-term studies of lithium and the treatment of aggressiveness in children and adults, or of lithium in the outpatient setting for long-term treatment of the violent individual. It should be noted that lithium is not currently approved for use in other than manic depressive illness, and it is not recommended for children under 12 years of age. Lithium is contraindicated in individuals with history or evidence of renal, hepatic, cardiac, or thyroid disease and should be administered with caution to patients at risk of pregnancy. Lithium administration requires very careful clinical and laboratory monitoring.

Carbamazepine

Carbamazepine has been reviewed recently by Evans and Gualtieri (1985). It is approved as an anticonvulsant for complex partial seizures as well as generalized clonic-tonic seizures and other types of partial seizures. Even though it is not recommended as the anticonvulsant of first choice, it is becoming increasingly used due to fewer side effects, such as sedation, compared to phenytoin and barbiturates. Earlier fears concerning thrombocytopenia, agranulocytosis, and aplastic anemia have been discovered to be unfounded and rare. Nevertheless, some researchers have continued to advise weekly blood counts, especially in the first three months of treatment (Schmidt, 1982).

Schmidt reports that approximately one-third of all patients treated with carbamazepine report side effects such as nausea, drowsiness, vertigo, ataxia, blurred vision, and diplopia, which are usually mild and decrease when the dosages decrease. There are other less frequent toxic consequences of treatment such as jaundice, renal effects, nystagmus, skin reactions, and thyroid effects. In approximately five percent of patients, carbamazepine is discontinued due to toxic reactions. Dyskinetic movements such as dystonia, dyskinesias, and other extrapyramidal reactions are rare and self-limited if the medication is withdrawn or the dosage is decreased.

For an anticonvulsant response in the therapeutic range, the serum levels are from 4–12 ng/ml. The usual method for treatment of seizures is to prescribe 100 to 200 mg twice a day for one week, and then to increase the dose by 100 to 200 mg increments and to measure serum levels when daily doses of 400 to 600 mg are achieved. It is not uncommon for patients with seizure disorders to take up to 1,200 mg a day. The onset of therapeutic effects is within the first days or weeks after treatment is initiated (Evans and Gualtieri, 1985).

In terms of treating aggression in psychiatric patients without epilepsy, there have been some uncontrolled studies showing that psychotic patients, predominantly schizophrenics with aggression, benefited from carbamazepine at doses of approximately 600 mg a day (Hakola and Laulumsa, 1982; Luchins, 1983). A controlled study by Neppe (1981) of chronic psychiatric inpatients, predominantly schizophrenics, showed that they did improve in terms of aggressive behavior. Although they did not have epileptic disorders, many did have temporal lobe abnormalities on the electroencephalogram (EEG). Luchins (1984) studied a group of schizophrenics without EEG abnormalities and found that carbamazepine was effective in decreasing aggression. Although concurrent neuroleptics were used, he found that the effect was not related to the dose of the neuroleptics. Caution should extent to its use in patients with gross brain damage and/or mental retardation. There have been reports of paradoxical worsening of aggression in this group of patients (Dalby, 1975).

Although phenytoin has been recommended for a long time in the treatment of episodic dyscontrol syndrome (Monroe, 1970, 1985) recent studies show that carbamazepine may be effective for this disorder in terms of decreasing aggressiveness and emotional liability (Girgis and Kiloh, 1980; Mattes et al, 1984; Stone et al, 1986). Further research is needed on the effectiveness of carbamazepine in episodic dyscontrol syndrome, since studies to date are not controlled and there is ambiguity in terms of diagnostic criteria for episodic dyscontrol syndrome. As was pointed out in Chapter 19, there are problems in terms of current degree of sophistication in EEG methodology in measuring epileptic activity in deep limbic areas of the brain. Nevertheless, for a patient with episodic violent behavior, given caution in terms of the side effects of carbamazepine, a clinical trial of this medication would be in order even if the EEG reveals no abnormalities.

Propranolol

Silver and Yudofsky (1985) reviewed 10 case studies of the successful use of propranolol for aggression in patients with head trauma, seizures, Wilson's disease, mental retardation, minimal brain dysfunction, Korsakoff's psychosis, and other organic mental disorders. Effective dosages were generally lower than 640 mgs a day and the response time varied from less than two days to more than six weeks. Side effects included lower blood pressure, decreased pulse rate and, rarely, respiratory difficulty such as wheezing or bronchospasms, nightmares, ataxia, and lethargy. Most of these patients were on concurrent neuroleptic medications, although a number were not taking these medications at the time of the propranolol treatment. There have been some reports of adverse central nervous system (CNS) and cardiovascular reactions when propranolol is used with neuroleptics (Miller and Rampling, 1982; Alexander et al, 1984).

Silver and Yudofsky recommend that a careful medical examination be done so as to exclude patients with bronchial asthma, chronic obstructive pulmonary disease, insulin dependent diabetes, cardiac disease, significant peripheral vascular disease, severe renal disease, and hyperthyroidism. Hypertensive patients should be given propranolol with caution, since sudden discontinuation of propranolol may result in rebound hypertension. They recommend that propranolol be given initially 20 mg three times a day and be increased by 60 mg every three to four days, usually to no more than 640 mg per day. Severe dizziness, wheezing, or ataxia are indications for decreasing the dose. The patient should be maintained on the highest dose of propranolol necessary for at least one month before concluding there is no response. It is advisable to monitor plasma blood levels of neuroleptics and anticonvulsants, particularly thioridazine, because plasma levels may increase three to four times when propranolol is added, thus increasing the risk of pigmentary retinopathy. The authors understand that prospective controlled studies on the effects of propranolol on the treatment of aggressive disorders currently are being carried out by Silver and Yudofsky as well as other researchers.

SPECIAL CONCERNS

There are special concerns about the treatment of violent patients, particularly in an outpatient setting. There are countertransference and inappropriate reactions by the therapist, legitimate concerns about one's safety, and the responsibility under *Tarasoff*-like rulings to protect potential victims from violence by one's patients.

Countertransference and Inappropriate Reactions

As Lion and Pasternak (1973) have pointed out, it is natural to have anxiety regarding violent patients—for example, the "Texas Tower Fantasy"—or excessive concern about ourselves as victims. Thus, it is important that the therapist analyze his or her reactions, particularly negative ones, to violent patients. As in other areas of psychiatry it is not necessarily wrong to have negative or inappropriate reactions to patients, but it is wrong not to have insight about these and to inappropriately act upon them. Therapists have experienced a wide variety of defense mechanisms in terms of violent patients; for example, projection in terms of anger at a patient for lack of progress and exaggeration of the patient's violence potential. There may be defense mechanisms of displacement from one violent patient to another who may not pose a danger, as well as reaction formation or identification with the aggressor in terms of treating attractive patients who are viewed as not as dangerous when in fact they are.

Coupled with the need for alertness on the part of the therapist is the need to avoid denial, the most prominent reaction to violence in a practice situation. Questions need to be asked about the ownership of weapons, about the existence of a victim, about previous violence toward the victim, about the patient's attitude toward his or her children, pets, spouse, and level of destructiveness within the household. When a patient indicates that he lost his temper, he should be queried in depth, lest both he and the therapist dismiss the event in mutual denial. This type of endeavor in the context of therapy may appear unsavory, but it is critical to the successful outcome of treatment. Knowledge of violence is too easily suppressed in the service of liking and identifying with a patient or avoiding confrontation with the patient or the patient's anger.

Safety of the Therapist

Irrespective of the type of patient seen, the clinician in an outpatient setting should establish the firmest contract regarding the patient's behavior. Most therapists practice in relative isolation, away from security personnel and other institutional safeguards, and thus must carefully screen their patients' ability to be manageable. Patients who have shown a capacity to be violent should be assessed for their capacity to tolerate verbal exploration in an office setting without agitation. The strictest limits should be set on the use of disinhibiting agents such as alcohol prior to an office visit. If a crisis occurs, the therapist might wish to consider seeing the patient in the emergency room, or in a setting where help can be monitored. Here, appropriate intervention can be made in the matter of hospitalization, and an assessment can be made regarding the role of the victim.

The safety of the office in the outpatient setting merits consideration. There should be a means of communicating both ways in case of trouble: that is, for the receptionist to inform the therapist and the therapist to inform the outside staff of problems with violent patients. If the receptionist senses that the patient poses a threat—for example, appears agitated, angry, or has been drinking—this should be communicated to the therapist before the therapist and patient enter the office and close the door. This may be done by code words or some other prearranged signal. Likewise, if the therapist is in danger inside the office—for example, from a patient who is becoming threatening, or one who perhaps produces a weapon—then the therapist should be able, through a code word by telephone or even a buzzer system, to alert the staff outside the office of the situation. The safety of the therapist is a prime consideration, since even feeling unsafe will impair evaluation and treatment.

A more subtle aspect of insuring the safety of the therapist is the response to a threat made by a patient. There is no such thing as a harmless threat; and clinicians threatened by former patients or those in active therapy must respond, lest the patient feel ignored and impotent, dynamics already operative in those who threaten. Threats will not go away. A therapist must demand to meet with the threatening patient in a safe place, with colleagues or security personnel available and alerted. The therapist can state that the threats are frightening, but that the therapist wishes to resolve what is going on between himself or herself and the patient. It is permissible—indeed, therapeutic—for a clinician to admit fear to a patient, for the latter is utilizing the very threat to create an aura of strength and power. At the same time, however, the appropriate comment about the threat involves some acknowledgment about its illegality and the response the therapist will take. "Your threats frighten me and I don't like being frightened. I want to straighten this out between us but I want you to know that I won't allow these threats to continue . . ." Violent patients who make verbal threats wish for intervention, and controls furnish this intervention.

Duty to Protect Potential Victims

Since the *Tarasoff* ruling in California in 1976, wherein a burden was placed on the therapist to protect any victim of the intended and imminent danger a patient posed, most clinicians have been sensitized to the matter of a patient's risk in society. The legal parameters of this and subsequent *Tarasoff*-like decisions are covered in Chapter 24. There will be some discussion of clinical parameters from the perspective of the therapist in that chapter. Additional discussion of legal and clinical issues can be found in a recent monograph by Beck and his colleagues (1985). Colliding conflicts here revolve around the violation of confidentiality versus the need to truly inform a victim of a real risk. Generally speaking, the therapist who decides that a patient is genuinely dangerous to a specific person is under some legal pressure to intervene, though such intervention can include, say, a period of hospitalization. To adopt a rigid position of informing all victims is to render a disservice to both the patient and victim; one tries, in all instances, to work the problem through in some therapeutic manner. Thus, the therapist can tell the patient that he or she is concerned about the latter's propensity for harm, and asks permission to bring in a potential victim for intervention. Patients usually welcome such efforts on some level, for they, too wish resolution to the unpleasant and highly charged affair. In some cases, a period of hospitalization allows patient–victim therapy to proceed or medication to reduce the intensity of the patient's rage. If done sensibly, rarely does the attempt to contact victims lead to a break of confidentiality.

Long-term therapy allows for the formation of transference, and in the case of violent patients, can lead to the development of violent ideation directed at the therapist, or at other figures on the outside of therapy. The clinician must be attuned to such occurrences, particularly in the case of patients with more primitive character disorders, who may translate feelings for or against the therapist into "acting out" behaviors at home or in the workplace. Warning victims may be less important than working with the patient to develop an understanding of whom he is really angry at. Or, to put the matter another way, the notification of victims takes place only when insight and introspection fail and the situation cannot be controlled any other way. Collegial consultation may be useful in assessing when the patient is truly dangerous, and when the therapist may be overreacting.

As Appelbaum (1985) emphasizes, a basic requirement in *Tarasoff*-like situations is that there be an assessment of violence potential which involves the gathering of data relevant to making a decision about a patient's danger to others. We believe this can be done by an experienced psychiatrist with reasonable accuracy for the near future—that is, within a week or so—the same as is done in terms of suicide potential. In fact, the evaluation of violence potential parallels the evaluation of suicide potential in a number of ways. In determining a patient's violence or homicide potential, it is important to determine how well planned the threat is; for example, a vague threat to "kill someone" is not as serious as a threat to "kill my boss because of (a particular reason)." Available means should be evaluated; for example, the possession of or a recent purchase of a gun. Past history of violence should enter the equation of violence potential and one should consider the degree of past violence; for example, broken bones or lacerations, as well as evaluation of past victims and circumstances leading to violence. A history of other impulsive behavior such as reckless driving, suicide, destruction of property, and sexual acting out increases the risk of violence. As was pointed out in Chapter 21 on evaluation, alcohol or drug abuse increases the risk of violent behavior. Last, psychosis, especially involving paranoid delusional thinking or command hallucinations, tips the balance toward increased risk of violence.

LONG-TERM ISSUES

Few therapists can carry many violent patients in extended therapy without discomfort, for the anxieties attendant to the care of these patients is significant. As patients slowly give up becoming violent, a risk of despondency ensues, similar to the phenomenology of the postpsychotic depressive state seen in the long-term therapy of schizophrenic patients. Aggressive patients value being aggressive and to relinquish such behaviors is to be confronted with passivity and dependency, as well as with the helplessness inherent in being weak. This therapeutic task is large, and violent patients, irrespective of etiology, tax the best clinician's capacity for patience and optimism. Such patients also can evoke within the therapist conflicts about the latter's own aggressions and inhibitions. Forensic psychiatrists are often more comfortable with the handling of dangerous patients and criminals than the clinicians in a more traditional psychiatric practice. An ability on the part of the therapist to discuss his caseload with colleagues and subject decisions and problems to peer scrutiny is crucial.

REFERENCES

Alexander HE, McCarty K, Giffen MD: Hypotension and cardiopulmonary arrest associated with concurrent haloperidol and propranolol therapy. JAMA 252:87-88, 1984

Appelbaum PS: *Tarasoff* and the clinician: problems in fulfilling the duty to protect. Am J Psychiatry 142:425-429, 1985

Beck JC (ed): The Potentially Violent Patient and the *Tarasoff* Decision in Psychiatric Practice. Washington, DC, American Psychiatric Press Inc., 1985

Campbell M, Small AM, Green WH, et al: Lithium and haloperidol in hospitalized aggressive children. Psychopharmacol Bull 18:126-130, 1982

Campbell M, Perry R, Green WH: Use of lithium in children and adolescents. Psychosomatics 25:95-106, 1984

Dalby MA: Behavioral effects of carbamazepine, in Advances in Neurology, vol. 11. Edited by Perry JK, Doly DD. New York, Raven Press, 1975

Donlon PT, Hopkin J, Tupin JP: Overview: efficacy and safety of the rapid neuroleptization method with injectable haloperidol. Am J Psychiatry 136:273-278, 1979

Dostal T, Zvolsky P: Antiaggressive effects of lithium salts in severely mentally retarded adolescents. International Journal of Pharmacopsychiatry 5:203-207, 1970

Evans RW, Gualtieri CT: Carbamazepine: a neuropsychological and psychiatric profile. Clin Neuropharmacol 8:221-241, 1985

Girgis M, Kiloh LG: Limbic Epilepsy and the Dyscontrol Syndrome. Amsterdam, Elsevier, 1980

Hakola HPA, Laulumsa VA: Carbamazepine in treatment of violent schizophrenics. Lancet 8285:1358, 1982

Jus A, Villeneuve A, Gautier J, et al: Some remarks on the influence of lithium carbonate on patients with temporal lobe epilepsy. Int J Clin Pharmacol Ther Toxicol 7:67-74, 1973

Kuehnel TG, Slama KM: Guidelines for the developmentally disabled, in The Psychiatric Uses of Seclusion and Restraint. Edited by Tardiff K. Washington, DC, American Psychiatric Press, Inc., 1984

Lion JR: Conceptual issues in the use of drugs for the treatment of aggression in man. J Nerv Ment Dis 160:72-82, 1975

Lion JR, Pasternak SA: Countertransference reactions to violent patients. Am J Psychiatry 130:207-210, 1973

Lion JR, Reid WH (Eds): Assaults Within Psychiatric Facilities. New York, Grune & Stratton, 1983

Luchins DJ: Carbamazepine for the violent psychiatric patient. Lancet 1:766, 1983

Luchins DJ: Carbamazepine in psychiatric syndromes: clinical and neuropharmacological properties. Psychopharmacol Bull 20:569-571, 1984

Martoramo JT: Target symptoms in lithium carbonate therapy. Compr Psychiatry 13:533-537, 1972

Mattes JA, Rosenberg J, Mays D: Carbamazepine versus propranolol in patients with uncontrolled rage outbursts: a random assignment study. Psychopharmacol Bull 20:98-100, 1984

Miller FA, Rampling D: Adverse effects of combined propranolol and chlorpromazine therapy. Am J Psychiatry 139:1198-1199, 1982

Monroe RR: Episodic Behavioral Disorders. Cambridge, MA, Harvard University Press, 1970

Monroe RR: Episodic behavioral disorders and limbic ictus. Compr Psychiatry 26:466-479, 1985

Neppe VM: Carbamazepine as adjunctive treatment in nonepileptic chronic inpatients with EEG temporal lobe abnormalities. J Clin Psychiatry 44:326-331, 1981

Schmidt D: Adverse effects of antiepileptic drugs. New York, Raven Press, 1982

Sheard MH: Lithium in the treatment of aggression. J Nerv Ment Dis 160:108-118, 1975

Sheard MH: Review: clinical pharmacology of aggressive behavior. Clin Neuropharmacol 7:173-183, 1985

Sheard MH, Marini JL, Bridges CI, et al: The effect of lithium in impulsive aggressive behavior in man. Am J Psychiatry 133:1409-1413, 1976

Silver JM, Yudofsky S: Propranolol for aggression: literature review and clinical guidelines. International Drug Therapy Newsletter 20:9-12, 1985

Stone JL, McDaniel KD, Hughes JR, et al: Episodic dyscontrol disorder and paroxysmal EEG abnormalities: successful treatment with carbamazepine. Biol Psychiatry 21:208-212, 1986

Tardiff K: Characteristics of assaultive patients in private hospitals. Am J Psychiatry 141:1232-1239, 1984

Tardiff K, Koenigsberg H: A study of assaultive behavior among psychiatric outpatients. Am J Psychiatry 142:960-963, 1985

Tardiff K, Sweillam A: Assault, suicide and mental illness. Arch Gen Psychiatry 37:164-169, 1980

Tupin JP, Smith DB, Clanon TL, et al: The long-term use of lithium in aggressive prisoners. Compr Psychiatry 14:311-317, 1973

Van Putten T, Sanders DG: Lithium in treatment failures. J Nerv Ment Dis 161:255-264, 1975

Chapter 24

Legal Aspects of Violence by Psychiatric Patients

by Paul S. Appelbaum, M.D.

Psychiatrists become involved with violence and its legal consequences in a variety of ways. In the criminal justice system, psychiatrists are often called upon to assess violent persons with regard to their state of mind at the time of a violent act, their potential for future violent behavior, and their capacities to participate in the adjudication and punishment process. In the civil justice system, similar questions arise as courts attempt to assess whether the harm caused by an act of violence should result in the assignment of liability and assessment of damages. Finally, psychiatrists routinely interact with violent persons in the mental health system, as they provide evaluation and treatment services.

The enormous scope of the interaction between the legal and mental health systems with regard to violent behavior places consideration of this topic as a whole well beyond the scope of this chapter. Thus, the chapter will focus on those legal aspects of violence that are likely to be of greatest concern to the majority of psychiatric clinicians: legal implications of violence occurring in the treatment setting. Specifically, consideration will be given to clinicians' potential for liability as a result of patient violence and the efforts of the state to regulate clinicians' responses to violence and its threat. Since the analysis of each of these issues differs for violence committed by inpatients and outpatients, the issues will be examined separately for those groups.

LEGAL ASPECTS OF VIOLENCE IN PSYCHIATRIC FACILITIES

Clinicians' Potential Liability

Although violence on inpatient psychiatric units is not a rare phenomenon (Lion and Reid, 1983), lawsuits derived from such episodes are less common than one might think. In part, this reflects the fact that most violence produces little or no injury (see, for example, Shader et al, 1977), and in part that psychiatric patients are not likely to have access to legal mechanisms that might allow them to pursue such cases. Nontheless, lawsuits do arise as a result of these episodes.

In general, these suits are based on clinicians' obligations to respect two sets of patients' rights, each with common law and constitutional dimensions, which at times may be in conflict with each other: the right to be free of violent assault and the right to be free of unnecessary restraint. The potential for liability arises when psychiatrists fail to balance these rights appropriately. In addition, members of the facility staff may also have a more limited right not to be subjected to violent assault, which may also give rise to litigation.

THE RIGHT TO BE FREE FROM VIOLENT ASSAULT. Patients' right to be free from violent assault when caused by negligence of the treating staff has long been recognized as a matter of common law (Annotation [a]). Clinicians who assume the duty to care for patients are considered to accept the responsibility of doing so in a nonnegligent manner. Since negligence is determined by comparing the behavior in question to the "standard of care" in the profession as a whole—that is, how other reasonable clinicians, similarly situated, would have responded in those circumstances—the profession itself is responsible for the creation of standards in this area. If deviation from those standards results in injury to a patient as a result of another patient's assault, liability may ensue.

An example of the application of these principles was seen in a case in which an adolescent girl, diagnosed as suffering from paranoid schizophrenia, was twice raped while she was an inpatient in a state hospital, because of inadequate supervision by hospital personnel (*Alphonso v. Charity Hospital of New Orleans*, 1982). Following discharge, the patient received a letter from her assailant, threatening to attack her again. In an attempt at self-protection, she slashed most of her body with a razor, hoping this would make her sexually unattractive. A court, in imposing liability, concluded that the failure to provide adequate supervision had constituted negligence, and that the negligence was causally linked to the harm the patient later inflicted on herself.

The question in cases such as this (alleging negligence in failing to prevent assaults on patients) is usually not merely whether some measures were not taken that might have been useful in preventing violent assault, but whether those measures would have been taken by other reasonable clinicians. Of course, individual clinicians may sometimes be helpless to provide protection when facility staffing patterns or physical designs render patients vulnerable. In such cases, the facility itself may be held liable for failing to meet the standard of care of similar facilities; in states that permit suits to be filed for negligent actions of the state government, the state may become the defendant when its practices result in injuries at state hospitals (Annotation [a]). Failure to abide by existing hospital policies for the protection of patients, whether because of clinical or administrative negligence, may constitute powerful evidence that the standard of care was not observed (*Cucalon v. State*, 1980).

Staff members, not only patients, may have a common law right to be protected from the effects of negligence with regard to violent assaults. Direct care personnel, who are frequently the target of patients' assaults (Lion et al, 1981), may initiate suit if injury occurs. Such suits have been infrequent in the past, and their resolution has generally turned on the question of whether the facility should have known the patient was dangerous and therefore should have warned the staff member or taken other appropriate actions (Annotation [a]). Suits alleging improper or inadequate staff training for dealing with violent patients as a cause of injury can be envisioned, although the author is unaware of any actions of this type to date. Staff injuries may often be covered by workmen's compensation statutes, which in providing monetary compensation will usually preclude further litigation by the injured worker.

Patients' rights to be free from assault may also have a constitutional basis. The leading decision on this subject is the U.S. Supreme Court's opinion in *Youngberg v. Romeo* (1982). The patient in the case, Nicholas Romeo, was a 33-year-old retarded man with an I.Q. of less than 10. In the 2½ years following his commitment to a Pennsylvania state facility for the retarded, he suffered injuries on 63 occasions, as a result both of self-abuse and of attacks by other residents, who often were responding to his provocative acts. The assaults resulted in fractures of an arm and a finger, human bites, injuries to his sexual organs, and numerous lesser injuries. Looking to the patient's "substantive liberty interests under the Fourteenth Amendment," which "are not extinguished by lawful confinement, even for penal purposes," the Court unanimously affirmed the unconstitutionality of the state's confining patients in unsafe conditions. Although the case dealt explicitly with the mentally retarded, the principles should apply equally to the mentally ill. It is of note, however, that the constitutional rationale rests on the obligations the state assumes when it deprives a citizen of liberty; voluntary patients, who are free to leave if conditions are poor, and patients in private facilities may not have similar constitutional rights. Members of the staff also lack constitutional protection for their right to be free from assault; they, too, are presumed to be able to leave if they find conditions too threatening.

THE RIGHT TO BE FREE OF UNNECESSARY RESTRAINT. The rights of staff and patients to be free of assault are tempered by the right of patients to be free of unnecessary restraint. Just as clinicians and facilities may be subject to suit for negligently allowing patients to be harmed, so may they be liable for overreacting to the threat of harm by imposing uncalled-for limitations on the freedom of movement of either potential victims or potential perpetrators. On a common-law basis, such actions as oversedating troublesome patients or excessively restricting their ability to move around may violate the standard of care and thus open clinicians to charges of negligence.

The constitutional dimensions of this issue were again defined by the decision in *Youngberg v. Romeo* (1982). Following the initiation of a suit on his behalf by his mother, Romeo was allegedly restrained for prolonged periods on a routine basis to prevent him from provoking other patients to assault him. The Court found that his interest in liberty from bodily restraint, which it described as "the core of the liberty protected by the Due Process Clause from arbitrary governmental action," survived his involuntary commitment. Not only could the state not restrain Romeo unnecessarily, but the Court found that he had a right to sufficient treatment (or "habilitation") to help him progress to the point where his own behavior no longer endangered his safety or the safety of others. Before the Supreme Court acted, a number of lower federal courts had found that patients' constitutional right to treatment (a right never embraced by the Supreme Court until *Romeo*, and then only in the limited way described above) entitled them to be free of unnecessary limitations on their freedom of movement (*Davis v. Hubbard*, 1980; *Wyatt v. Stickney*, 1972).

BALANCING PATIENTS' RIGHTS. It is clear from this description of patients' rights to be protected from assault and to be free of unnecessary restraint that these rights will often be in conflict. Since each set of rights carries the potential for clinician liability if violated, clinicians and facilities walk something of a tightrope here. Nonetheless, the courts have not been unreasonable in their suggestions as to how these conflicting rights might both be accommodated.

The constitutional dimensions of these rights are most easily balanced. In *Romeo* itself, the U.S. Supreme Court recognized the conflict and provided guidance. "An institution cannot protect its residents from all danger of violence if it is to permit them to have any freedom of movement," noted the Court. The

Court resolved this dilemma for constitutional purposes by holding that patients' Fourteenth Amendment rights entitle them only to a decision on balancing these rights by a professional "competent . . . to make the particular decision at issue." Thus, "liability may be imposed only when the decision by the professional is such a substantial departure from accepted professional judgment, practices or standards as to demonstrate that the person responsible actually did not base the decision on such a judgment." This is a standard that gives maximal deference to the opinions of treatment staff as to what degree of restrictions are necessary to protect the patient and others from the danger of assault.

The balance is more difficult to achieve when the common-law negligence standard is at issue. Since here the clinician and facility are under the obligation to live up to the generally prevailing standard of care, a more careful inquiry may be necessary. Evidence of the standard of care can be sought via consultation with experts from other facilities, reviews of the published literature on the prevention of violence, and inspection of applicable state regulations. Indeed, deviation from the latter may create a *de facto* presumption that the standard of care was violated.

Some general principles regarding standards in this area can be considered. Clinicians' responses to the threat of violence or its occurrence should always be nonpunitive. Any actions taken in a therapeutic setting should be designed to protect the patient or others; punishment is for the courts. Although this caveat is simple to state, normal human emotions often lead to a desire for retaliatory behavior, which staff members must firmly resist. In addition, written protocols should be developed for responding to violence or its threat. Staff members need to be educated about the protocols, taking into account the rapid turnover that often occurs among line staff in psychiatric facilities, and must be provided with whatever additional training is necessary to implement them. There are now a number of private organizations that will assist psychiatric facilities in the development of protocols and training programs for dealing with violent patients.

Unfortunately, although it is not difficult to resolve on paper the conflict between patients' rights to protection and freedom of movement, psychiatrists and other staff members may feel paralyzed in practice. There is a tendency in such circumstances to feel that whatever approach one takes opens the door to liability. Remembering that suits alleging infringement of either set of rights are rare may help in this regard. In addition, a useful rule of thumb can be stated: When in doubt as to whether a particular course of action that appears to be useful in preventing violence may actually be unnecessarily restrictive, it is better on several counts to err on the side of preventing violence. On ethical and clinical grounds, the harm of restricting freedom of movement, assuming it is a relatively short-term measure, will almost always be less than the harm that results from permitting an assault to occur. And from the point of view of preventing liability, a suit for violation of the right to freedom from restraints, even if successful, is likely to warrant much lower damages than a successful suit alleging severe injury or death as a result of clinicians' negligence in failing to impose restrictions.

Regulation of Clinicians' Responses to Patient Violence

The balancing process described above, in which freedom from assault and freedom of movement are weighed against each other, is not the only calculation in which clinicians must engage. Even when these rights have been set off against each other and a determination has been made that action to prevent violence is called for, there may be a variety of limitations placed by the state on the options that psychiatrists can select in responding to the threat or occurrence of violence by inpatients.

REGULATION OF INVOLUNTARY ADMINISTRATION OF MEDICATION. Until the mid-1970s, it was taken as a matter of course that medication, including neuroleptics, could be administered to committed patients, even over their objections. In fact, many clinicians routinely treated voluntary patients as well without their consent. This is no longer the case. A series of lawsuits, followed by statutory and regulatory initiatives, have defined a "right to refuse treatment" that restricts clinicians' discretion in this area.

All courts that have considered the issue have agreed at a minimum that voluntary patients have a clear right to refuse any treatment offered, although they may then be asked to leave the facility (see, for example, *Rogers v. Commissioner*, 1983). Similarly, there has been near unanimity that involuntary patients have a right to refuse treatment with neuroleptic medications, based on their right to privacy, which is not abrogated by commitment (Winick, 1986; for exceptions, see *R.A.J. v. Miller*, 1984; *Stensvad v. Reivitz*, 1985). The U.S. Supreme Court came to this conclusion in *Mills v. Rogers* (1982), but left definition of the parameters of the right to the lower federal and state courts. The result has been a diverse set of mechanisms constructed to protect, and in appropriate cases to override, the right to refuse treatment.

Approaches fall into two basic categories, which can be classified by their degree of conformance to the principles of informed consent. Some states, whether judicially, administratively, or legislatively, have recognized that the rights of committed patients to consent to or refuse medication, based on their right to privacy, are no different than those of any other medical or psychiatric patient. In those states, patients' refusal of medication can be overridden only when patients have been found to be incompetent to make their own treatment decisions (*A.E. and R.R. v. Mitchell*, 1980; Callahan and Longmire, 1983; *Davis v. Hubbard*, 1980; *Gundy v. Pauley*, 1981; *In re K.K.B.* 1980, *Jamison v. Farabee*, 1983; *Opinion of the Justices*, 1983; *People v. Medina*, 1985; *Rogers v. Commissioner*, 1983). The mechanisms by which competency and such additional criteria as the appropriateness of treatment are determined range from formal judicial hearings (for example, *Rogers v. Commissioner*, 1983) to administrative inquiries (for example, Zito et al, 1984) to reviews by administrators or consulting psychiatrists (for example, *Jamison v. Farabee*, 1983).

Alternatively, some states implicitly recognize that civil commitment alters the ground rules for informed consent. Patients' right to privacy is interpreted in these jurisdictions as conferring a right to object to treatment on the grounds of inappropriateness, but not a true right to refuse (*Anderson v. Arizona*, 1982; Callahan and Longmire, 1983; *Project Release v. Prevost*, 1983; *Rennie v. Klein*, 1985). Patients' refusal of treatment can be overridden by administrative mechanisms for reviewing the appropriateness of treatment, without regard to patients' competency.

Regardless of the interpretation of patients' right to refuse medication—and a number of jurisdictions still lack any definitive guidance on this question—there is complete agreement that medication can always be administered in emergencies, even without patient consent. The definitions of emergency differ widely, ranging from narrow requirements for a likelihood of immediate and serious physical harm, to less stringent notions focusing on the likelihood of patient deterioration and distress (compare *Rogers v. Commissioner*, 1983, with Pennsylvania Mental Health Bulletin, 1985). Yet all would concur that when violence appears imminent and medication might prevent its occurrence, at least short-term use of neuroleptics and other medications is permitted.

Thus, the impact of the spreading right to refuse treatment is seen less in emergency situations than in nonurgent cases, in which patients, even those with a history of provoking or committing violent acts, might have to go untreated for some time, thereby increasing the risk of violence. Solid empirical data on how often violent acts occur in such situations is lacking, although existing data suggest that long-term refusal is relatively infrequent and violence an even rarer outcome (Appelbaum and Hoge, 1986). Nonetheless, regulation of the previously unfettered administration of neuroleptic medications represents one of the most significant limitations on clinicians' repertoire of responses to violence.

REGULATION OF THE USE OF SECLUSION AND RESTRAINT. All states have enacted some regulations on the employment of seclusion and restraint for psychiatric inpatients. Usually the motivations behind these rules reflect both the belief expressed by the U.S. Supreme Court in *Romeo* that patients' freedom of movement must be protected even within the hospital, and a concern that restraints may be employed punitively or as a substitute for adequate treatment. Statutes and regulations typically limit the indications for seclusion and restraint (often requiring an imminent threat of violence); specify the amount of time over which these modalities can be employed; restrict their use with particular classes of patients (for example, the mentally retarded or children); mandate certain conditions that must accompany seclusion or restraint (for example, regular periods of relief, opportunities to use toilet facilities, and continuous staff observation); require physician involvement in decisionmaking about initiating restraints; and establish documentation and reporting requirements that facilities must fulfill (Tardiff and Mattson, 1984). After review of state regulations and deliberating for three years, a Task Force of the American Psychiatric Association recommended reasonable national guidelines which were approved by that organization for the safe and appropriate use of seclusion and restraint in relation to other means of managing violent behavior (APA, 1985).

Some of the earlier right to treatment cases in the 1970s found that the use of seclusion and restraint implicated patients' constitutional rights, foreshadowing the analysis in *Romeo*. These lower courts, however, went well beyond the U.S. Supreme Court in holding that seclusion and restraint cannot be used in nonemergencies solely for the purpose of behavior control (*Romeo v. Youngberg*, 1980), and that even in emergencies, they must constitute the least restrictive means available for protecting the patient and others (*Davis v. Hubbard*, 1980; *Wyatt v. Stickney*, 1972). Some courts established guidelines for the use of seclusion and restraint similar to those now found widely in state statutes and regulations (*Davis v. Hubbard*, 1980; *Eckerhart v. Hensley*, 1979; *Negron v. Preiser*, 1974; *Wyatt v. Stickney*, 1972). In fact, although the decision in *Romeo* casts doubt on the continued viability of the broad interpretation of patients' rights on which these decisions rest, their major impact may have been in stimulating states to establish their own standards for the use of these modalities.

As with the right to refuse treatment, it is difficult to identify with any degree of precision the outcomes of regulation of seclusion and restraint on the effectiveness of clinicians' responses to violence. Since, again, use in true emergencies is usually not restricted, the effect of these regulations must be seen, if at all, in the limitations they place on clinicians' discretion as to how situations of imminent danger might be prevented in the first place. Seclusion of patients as a therapeutic measure, designed to limit sensory stimulation and thus prevent escalation and potential violence, has been particularly hard hit by current regulations, which generally consider seclusion and restraint simply as means of controlling behavior, without any therapeutic benefits. Here, too, data on the effects of these regulations are lacking.

LIMITATIONS ON RECOURSE TO CRIMINAL SANCTIONS. The usual response to violence in our society involves arrest and prosecution. Indeed, some psychiatrists argue that violent episodes in psychiatric facilities should not be exempt from these sanctions, whatever other measures are also taken to protect patients and staff and to treat assaultive patients (Phelan et al, 1985; Schwarz and Greenfield, 1978).

Reasons for favoring arrest and prosecution include their presumed therapeutic benefits and efficacy in deterring future violent acts, and a more abstract belief that society ought to be aware of violent acts wherever they occur. Those who oppose widespread use of this option express concern about its effect on the psychiatrist–patient relationship, its actual efficacy in preventing the recurrence of violence, and the possibility that clinicians' motivations in suggesting arrest and prosecution may stem more from punitive impulses than from any of the other justifications offered (Appelbaum, 1983; Gutheil, 1985).

For those clinicians who want to prosecute patients for violence, however, there are substantial legal obstacles. Many of the key decisionmakers in the criminal justice system see mental health facilities and the treatment they offer as legitimate alternatives to criminal prosecution for mentally disordered persons. Psychiatrists who reject this "mad-bad" dichotomy may be looked on as punitive in their attitudes toward the mentally ill, and as unwilling to assume their responsibilities with regard to caring for these patients. Thus, psychiatrists who have been involved in attempts to prosecute violent patients report that police and court personnel are often reluctant to accept reports of violent incidents involving inpatients or to initiate the formal process of filing charges. Prosecutors, whose dockets are already clogged with cases they consider more important, may be similarly reticent about pursuing the charges. At every stage of the process, up to and including the trial stage, clinicians may be the objects of sarcasm, scorn, or anger for using the criminal justice process in a manner that many other of the participants consider to be inappropriate.

When, despite these pressures, cases proceed to trial, violent patients may escape punishment by means of a defense based on their lack of criminal responsibility for their actions as a result of their mental state, or because of judicial beliefs about the inappropriateness of prosecution. One New Jersey court responded to a case of this sort by noting that "to convict the involuntarily committee of a quasi-criminal offense for displaying the symptoms of his illness while in a place intended to treat that illness and upon the complaint of one whose duty it is to have the care and custody of such patient imposes punishment where none can either constitutionally or morally be justified" (*New Jersey v. Cummins*, 1979).

On the other hand, these widely held beliefs about the inappropriateness of criminal sanctions stemming from behavior within psychiatric facilities also apply to the behavior of staff members. Physical contact with patients that might constitute assault and battery in the outside world is often considered privileged because it is an essential part of psychiatric care. Thus, a Michigan court dismissed a patient's suit alleging that he had been assaulted by an attendant on the basis that the scuffle was precipitated by the patient's "repeated violations of the hospital rules against smoking, his refusal to leave his room with other patients for breakfast, and his physical aggression towards the attendant when the latter ordered the plaintiff to leave his room" (*Jacobs v. State*, 1979). For better or worse, except in egregious cases of injury or death, psychiatric facilities are often considered "asylums" that reside outside of the usual legal constraints on assaultive behavior.

LEGAL ASPECTS OF VIOLENCE BY PSYCHIATRIC PATIENTS IN THE COMMUNITY

Clinician's Potential Liability

In contrast to the uncommon prospect of liability for the acts of patients within psychiatric facilities, the potential for suits arising from assaults by patients in the community has grown considerably in recent years, and gives strong indications of continuing to do so. Much of the reason for this growth stems from a major alteration of traditional legal approaches to the question of psychiatrists' and other clinicians' liability in these cases.

RELEASE AND ESCAPE CASES. For at least several generations now, psychiatrists have faced the possibility of liability for violent and destructive acts committed by patients who were negligently released or permitted to escape from psychiatric facilities. The premise for liability in these cases rests on the tort law maxim that those who assume responsibility for controlling potentially dangerous persons can be held liable if they exercise their control negligently, so that harm occurs (*Restatement (Second) of Torts*). Until recently, however, a number of factors have combined to restrict the level of concern that such cases evoke among psychiatrists.

First, psychiatrists were clearly on notice as to the scope of their obligations. Only the actions of patients who had been hospitalized could invoke liability. In addition, the actions that psychiatrists were expected to take were both readily apparent and well within the compass of their usual interventions. If patients might present danger to persons outside the institution, psychiatrists were expected to take the necessary steps to keep them confined. This was an obligation with which psychiatrists had grown comfortable over the years.

Second, imposition of liability was generally a rare event. Courts that reviewed these cases tended to inquire faithfully about the standard of care of the profession, and to impose liability only when significant deviations had occurred. Psychiatrists' decisions that were seen in retrospect to have been erroneous, but which did not represent lapses from the standard of care, were dismissed as mere errors in judgment that did not warrant a finding of negligence (for example, *St. George v. State*, 1954). The opinions recognized that chances must often be taken with potentially violent patients for the sake of ultimate rehabilitation, and they generally encouraged such behavior (for example, *Eanes v. U.S.*, 1968). Furthermore, a finding of negligence usually required that the patient's behavior have been "foreseeable," which the courts interpreted narrowly as requiring evidence of past violence (Annotation [b]). Some states, in addition, afforded governmental immunity to release decisions made by psychiatrists at state facilities; a handful of states still do (*Cairl v. State*, 1982; *Sherrill v. Wilson*, 1983). These factors combined to limit rulings that psychiatrists had been negligent to situations in which truly egregious conduct had occurred.

Thus, the traditional release-and-escape cases, although a long-standing source of potential liability, were generally not of great consequence to most psychiatrists.

LIABILITY FOR THE ACTS OF OUTPATIENTS. This equilibrium was disrupted in 1974 with the initial decision of the California Supreme Court in *Tarasoff v. the Regents of the University of California* (see, generally, Beck, 1985). In this case, a court ruled for the first time that psychotherapists could be held liable for violence perpetrated by patients who had never been hospitalized. The rationale for the extension of liability to the actions of outpatients was that psychotherapists had a "special relationship" with their patients sufficient to impose on them the obligation to protect potential victims. The nature of this special relationship was never clearly defined, but seemed to derive from both the potential to exercise control over the patient in applying the civil commitment laws, and the presumed superior knowledge of the psychotherapist in detecting impending danger.

The effect of *Tarasoff* and the cases that have adopted it as precedent is to make the imposition of liability on clinicians much more likely. The large number of psychiatric outpatients increases the pool from which violent acts leading to liability might be drawn. Furthermore, when confronted with patients whom they think might be dangerous, psychotherapists (now no longer just psychiatrists) have only ambiguous guidance as to the measures they should take. The *Tarasoff* court, for example, held that "whatever steps are reasonably necessary under the circumstances" to prevent the violence from occurring must be taken. This might include such measures outside the usual scope of psychiatric practice as warning potential victims, involving family members in efforts to control the patient's behavior, or involving the police. Since in retrospect it will often appear that some measure that was not taken would in fact have prevented the violent act, juries now have much wider leeway for finding that the clinician's duty has not been met, than in the older cases in which the sole duty was to maintain custody.

Courts' latitude in applying the duty first enunciated in *Tarasoff* has also contributed to the perceived burden of the doctrine for clinicians. Although the courts still nominally require only that psychotherapists conform to the standards of their professions in evaluating patients, predicting dangerousness, and selecting treatment methods, the lack of standards for dealing with dangerous patients—particularly regarding prediction—have permitted idiosyncratic definitions of standards of care to be offered by plaintiffs' experts and accepted by juries sympathetic to the victims. In some cases, prevailing standards are simply ignored, such as those that encourage the use of less restrictive alternatives for patients who might pose some minimal risk of violence. When it comes to predicting dangerousness, the determination that a patient's violence was foreseeable is no longer predicated on the presence of previous violence, but can be established on seemingly the most tenuous of evidence (Appelbaum, 1984b).

The requirements drawn from the *Tarasoff* opinion, known generally as the "duty to protect," have been adopted as law by judicial decision in almost all of the jurisdictions in which cases have arisen, although the exact form has differed. Some courts have framed narrow definitions of the duty, requiring psychotherapists to protect only identifiable victims of their patients (for example, *Furr v. Spring Grove State Hospital*, 1983; *Leedy v. Hartnett*, 1981), while other courts have imposed broader obligations, which include protecting anyone who is likely to be harmed (*Lipari v. Sears, Roebuck and Co.*, 1980; *Petersen v. Washington*, 1983). In some cases, evidence of threats of violence or commitability was deemed necessary to invoke the duty (*Brady v. Hopper*, 1983; *Hasenei v. U.S.*, 1982), but most courts have rejected this limitation. One court found no obligation to protect victims who already knew of the patient's threats toward them (*Heltsley v. Votteler*, 1982), but another court disagreed (*Jablonski v. U.S.*, 1983). Although only a minority of states have yet had appellate court decisions recognizing the duty to protect, most commentators agree that clinicians are best advised to assume that, given the opportunity, their state's courts would adopt some version of the *Tarasoff* obligation, and to act accordingly.

California, where *Tarasoff* originated, has also been the first state to move legislatively to limit the duty to protect. California psychiatrists were successful in having a statute passed that clearly defines the situations in which psychotherapists are obligated to protect potential victims when an overt threat of violence has been made—and the duty they then have—to make reasonable efforts to warn the potential victim and the police (A.B. 1133, 1985). Similar action in other states may occur in response to the high level of clinicians' concern about their potential liability.

ACCOMMODATING THE LEGAL REQUIREMENTS. Evidence suggests that even before the imposition of the legal duty to protect, psychiatrists and other clinicians felt an ethical obligation to protect potential victims of their patients. Nonetheless, the cases that have turned this ethical obligation into a legal one have formalized and structured clinicians' roles. Viewed in its most reasonable interpretation, the duty to protect requires clinicians to undertake four tasks (Appelbaum, 1985a). Failure at any of these levels may result in the imposition of liability. First, the clinician is obligated to gather sufficient information to assess patients' dangerousness. For most patients, for whom the risk of violence is slight, the routine questioning usually performed in the initial evaluation concerning past acts of violence and present violent impulses will be sufficient. When clinicians' suspicion is triggered by these data or other evidence suggesting that patients may in fact represent a future danger, a more thorough evaluation is indicated. The factors to be sought in this evaluation include demographic and other patient characteristics that are known to be associated with a higher risk of violence (Monahan, 1981), and clinical factors that, although as yet unvalidated, are believed to be associated with violent acts (Gutheil and Appelbaum, 1982; see also Chapters 21 and 23 in this volume).

Once the information is gathered, clinicians must use the data to make a determination as to whether patients are sufficiently likely to commit future violent acts that some intervention to protect potential victims is warranted. This is the most difficult of the obligations imposed by the duty to protect. Available evidence has yet to demonstrate that psychiatrists have any meaningful ability to predict future violence, although predictions of violence in the immediate future may be more accurate than predictions over longer periods of time (Monahan, 1984). The best advice one can give at this time is for clinicians to follow a procedure for predicting dangerousness that relies on some consistent theoretical basis, even if an unvalidated one, and that has support in the professional literature. Such a procedure maximizes the chance of being able to demonstrate in court that the unfortunately nebulous standard of care relating to prediction was not violated.

With a prediction in hand, clinicians must select an appropriate course of action. Many practitioners are unaware that the duty imposed on them can be fulfilled in a variety of ways (Givelber et al, 1984). Although attorneys who defend malpractice cases favor warning potential victims as the most easily defended action, clinicians are often uncomfortable breaching the confidentiality of the therapeutic relationship as a first step. An approach that is more protective of the interest in continuing with treatment views such a rupture of confidentiality as a last resort. Means that are less intrusive on the therapeutic relationship should be tried first. In roughly ascending order of intrusiveness, psychiatrists can consider altering the focus of therapy, adding medication or raising the dosage, bringing the potential victim (if an intimate) into the therapy, hospitalizing the patient, asking family members or friends to watch over the patient to prevent access to weapons or contact with likely victims, notifying police, and notifying potential victims. Any of these choices may be appropriate in a particular situation, assuming it is likely to be effective in reducing the risk to potential victims.

The final stage of the duty to protect requires that the action chosen be implemented appropriately. This means, for example, that effective means must be selected of notifying authorities or potential victims. Follow-up should assure that referrals were in fact made, medications taken, and appointments kept. This is the easiest component of the duty to protect, requiring only the ordinary level of diligence that clinicians usually exercise.

It cannot be denied that the duty to protect is a burdensome one. The willingness of the courts to apply the duty broadly and to stretch the facts of particular cases, in accord with their desire to award compensation to sympathetic victims, increases the likelihood that liability will be imposed on clinicians whenever their patients commit violent acts. Nonetheless, even in an environment of uncertainty, one can only respond as best as is possible under the circumstances and leave the rest to fate. There is no need for psychotherapists to feel paralyzed by the risk of liability; reasonable guidelines for handling these cases, as described above, can reduce anxiety in that regard.

Regulation of Clinicians' Responses to Violence in the Community

Just as the law regulates and thereby limits the options available to psychiatrists for responding to violence by inpatients, so too do similar limitations apply to actions outside of psychiatric facilities.

LIMITATIONS ON INVOLUNTARY HOSPITALIZATION. Historically, standards according to which mentally ill persons could be hospitalized against their will were broad—the modal criterion being whether the patient was mentally ill and in need of treatment. The procedures employed alternated between analogues of the criminal justice model (for example, utilizing formal hearings and judicial decisionmakers) and more relaxed rules with relatively informal review of medical decisions (Appelbaum, 1985a). Since the early 1970s, however, most states have adopted both criminalized procedures and narrow criteria, the latter focusing on the patient's presumed dangerousness to self or others.

The most frequent critique of the current commitment system is that by focusing exclusively on dangerousness and demanding rigorous adherence to procedural norms, many severely ill people who would benefit from care, but cannot be persuaded to accept it voluntarily, are excluded from treatment (Appelbaum, 1985a). It might be thought, however, that the system is less problematic in dealing with potentially violent people, who presumably represent its target population. Unfortunately, this turns out not to be the case.

Although standards differ widely from jurisdiction to jurisdiction (reviewed in Beis, 1983), there are substantial barriers in most state statutes to the commitment even of patients whom the clinician believes may represent a danger to others. These barriers are both substantive and procedural, and have generally been erected in the name of insuring the accuracy of the commitment process. Looking at substantive criteria, for example, many states require that patients commit an "overt act" of violence before commitment may occur. Some add the requirement that the act have occurred within a particular period of time, such as the last 30 days. Similarly, the predicted act of violence must, in some jurisdictions, meet certain requirements of imminence. All of these requirements are designed, given the acknowledged difficulty psychiatrists have in predicting future violence, to limit predictions to a population with a relatively high probability of continued violent behavior.

On the procedural side of the ledger (reviewed in Van Duizend et al, 1984), many states have adopted formal rules of evidence, which require the exclusion of hearsay testimony from commitment hearings, even if that testimony might strongly suggest the patient's dangerousness. Some states require that evaluating psychiatrists warn patients that anything they say might be used to effect their commitment, and exclude from introduction into evidence all data gathered in the absence of such warnings. Patients may be granted a similar right in some jurisdictions to remain silent at the commitment hearing itself, thereby depriving the judge of any opportunity to see the patient exhibit the symptoms of mental illness under discussion. These rules, and many analogous ones, have been imported from the criminal system for the avowed purposes of insuring reliability of evidence and maintaining the fairness of the proceedings.

Endless arguments are possible as to whether the substantive and procedural limitations in fact increase or decrease the accuracy of commitment determinations. What is clear is that they represent substantial limitations on clinicians' discretion to respond to perceived threats of violence. This is ironic in that one of the major justifications for the duty to protect stems from the purported ability of psychiatrists to take action to detain potentially violent patients, thus giving them, in the law's eyes, the obligation to do so. The duty to protect cases make clear, however, that the impossibility of having a patient committed does not relieve the clinician of the obligation of taking further steps to protect the potential victim, such as issuing warnings.

Recent proposals to relax commitment criteria and, to a lesser extent, procedures, may offer some relief here. A number of states, for example, have made it easier to commit patients who are not dangerous, but are otherwise likely to deteriorate or undergo suffering (Alaska Statutes, Sec. 47.30.725; North Carolina General Statutes, Sec. 122–58, 1981; Texas Mental Health Code, Sec. 5547–50, 1984; Washington Revised Code, Sec. 71.05, 1982). Although not aimed at the potentially violent patient, these provisions may allow such persons to be committed more easily, since many of them would meet broader, treatment oriented criteria.

LIMITATIONS ON INVOLUNTARY OUTPATIENT TREATMENT. The majority of states make some mention in their commitment laws of the possibility of commitment to outpatient care (Keilitz and Hall, 1985). This approach would seem to be suited ideally to patients who present little risk of violence as long as they continue taking medications, but who may become dangerous if they stop their medications and decompensate. Unfortunately, outpatient commitment provisions in most states are structured so awkwardly that they are infrequently used, even for this group. The two major problems most statutes face concern the criteria for outpatient commitment and the mechanisms for enforcement of the commitment order.

In most states with outpatient commitment provisions in their statutes, the criteria for involuntary outpatient treatment are identical to those for inpatient commitment. Since, as noted, the latter require dangerousness to self or others of some substantial degree and imminence, it is unlikely that many patients who meet these criteria will be appropriate for outpatient care. Yet, it is precisely those patients who are not currently dangerous, but may become so if left untreated, for whom outpatient commitment may be most useful. This problem has been recognized recently in Hawaii and North Carolina, each of which has distinguished its outpatient and inpatient commitment criteria, allowing the former to be implemented for patients who have deteriorated in the past without treatment and are likely to do so again (Hawaii Revised Statutes, Sec. 334–12, 1984; North Carolina General Statutes, Sec. 122–58.4, 1983).

Even if the problem with the criteria is solved, however, enforcement remains a major issue. Unless the mental health system is given some leverage over committed outpatients to ensure that appointments are kept and medications taken, resistant patients will continue to frustrate efforts to provide care. Most current statutes are entirely silent on this issue, or provide that a hearing can be held and the patients hospitalized if they meet the usual, inpatient commitment criteria. Neither option insures treatment of patients who refuse care. On the other hand, our society shies away from the idea of creating "mental health police," who would track down delinquent patients and forcibly inject them with medications. A reasonable compromise might be to allow short-term—

perhaps three- to five-day—hospitalization for patients who fail to abide by outpatient commitment orders, during which time medication could be administered. That might provide both an incentive for patients to comply with treatment orders, and a means of evaluating their condition and instituting at least short-term treatment. Civil libertarians may offer constitutional objections to such a plan, but if the criteria for outpatient commitment are properly constructed, emphasizing the likelihood of deterioration without treatment, they should not be insuperable (Appelbaum, 1984a).

CONCLUSION

The demands placed on psychiatrists and other clinicians today with regard to the control of violence by patients do not make their lot an enviable one. Society now expects clinicians effectively to control their patients' violent proclivities and threatens liability if clinicians' efforts are unsuccessful. Yet, the tools available for this purpose are themselves limited by regulations that seek to promote other ends that society deems important.

The situation is difficult, but it is not hopeless. Appropriate legal reforms—limiting liability, as exemplified by California's recent modifications of the duty to protect and related proposals (Appelbaum, 1985b), and expanding clinicians' options, as broader commitment criteria might—would help ease things somewhat and should certainly be sought. In the meantime, psychiatrists need to give careful attention to their obligations and to the best available means for fulfilling them.

REFERENCES

A.E. and R.R. v. Mitchell, No. C78–466 (D. Utah, June 16, 1980)

Alphonso v. Charity Hospital of New Orleans, 413 So.2d 982 (La. Ct. App. 1982)

American Psychiatric Association: *Seclusion and Restraint: The Psychiatric Uses*, Task Force Report No. 22, Washington, DC, American Psychiatric Association, 1985

Anderson v. State of Arizona, 663 P.2d 570 (Ariz. Ct. App. 1982)

Annotation [a]: Liability of hospital for injury caused through assault by a patient. 48 ALR3d 1288

Annotation [b]: Liability of one releasing institutionalized mental patient for harm he causes. 38 ALR 3d 699

Appelbaum PS: Legal considerations in the prevention and treatment of assault, in Assaults Within Psychiatric Facilities. Edited by Lion JR, Reid WH. New York, Grune & Stratton, 1983

Appelbaum PS: Is the need for treatment constitutionally acceptable as a basis for civil commitment? Law, Medicine and Health Care 12:144-149, 1984a

Appelbaum PS: The expansion of liability for patients' violent acts. Hosp Community Psychiatry 35:13-14, 1984b

Appelbaum PS: Civil commitment, in Psychiatry. Edited by Michels R, Cavenar J, Brodie HKH, et al. Philadelphia, J.B. Lippincott, 1985a

Appelbaum PS: Rethinking the duty to protect, in The Potentially Violent Patient and the Tarasoff Decision in Psychiatric Practice. Edited by Beck J. Washington, DC, American Psychiatric Press, Inc., 1985b

Appelbaum PS: Tarasoff and the clinician: problems in fulfilling the duty to protect. Am J Psychiatry 142:425-429, 1985c

Appelbaum PS, Hoge SK: Empirical research on the effects of legal policy on the right to refuse treatment, in The Right to Refuse Antipsychotic Medication. Edited by Parry J. Washington, DC, American Bar Association, 1986

Beck J (Ed.): The Potentially Violent Patient and the Tarasoff Decision in Psychiatric Practice. Washington, DC, American Psychiatric Press, Inc., 1985

Beis E: State involuntary commitment statutes. Mental Disability Law Reporter 7:358-369, 1983

Brady v. Hopper, 570 F. Supp. 1313 (D. Colo. 1983)

Cairl v. State, 323 N.W.2d 20 (Minn. 1982)

Callahan LA, Longmire DR: Psychiatric patients' right to refuse psychotropic medication: a national survey. Mental Disability Law Reporter 7:494-499, 502, 1983

Cucalon v. State, New York Law Journal, April 14, 1980, p. 7, col. 4 (N.Y. Ct. Cl., Apr., 1980)

Davis v. Hubbard, 506 F. Supp. 915 (W.D.Ohio, 1980)

Furr v. Spring Grove State Hospital, 454 A.2d 414 (Md. Ct. Spec. App. 1983)

Eanes v. U.S., 280 F. Supp. 151 (E.D.Va. 1968)

Eckerhart v. Hensley, 475 F. Supp. 908 (W.D.Mo. 1979)

Giverber D, Bowers W, Blitch C: *Tarasoff*, myth and reality: an empirical study of private law in action. Wisconsin Law Review 1984:443-497

Gundy v. Pauley, 619 S.W.2d 730 (Ky.App. 1981)

Gutheil TG, Appelbaum PS: *Clinical Handbook of Psychiatry and the Law*. New York, McGraw-Hill, 1982

Gutheil TG: Prosecuting patients (letter). Hosp Community Psychiatry 36:1320–1321, 1985

Hasenei v. U.S., 541 F.Supp. 999 (1982)

Heltsley v. Votteler, 327 N.W.2d 759 (Iowa 1982)

In re the Mental Health of K.K.B., 609 P.2d 747 (Okla. 1980)

Jablonski v. U.S., 712 F.2d 391 (9th Cir. 1983)

Jacobs v. State of Michigan, Department of Mental Health, 276 N.W.2d 627 (Mich. App. 1979)

Jamison v. Farabee, No. C–78–0445–WHO (N.D. Cal. Apr. 26, 1983)

Keilitz I, Hall T: State statutes governing involuntary outpatient civil commitment. Mental and Physical Disability Law Reporter 9:378-397, 1985

Lion JR, Snyder W, Merrill G: Under-reporting of assaults on staff in a hospital. Hosp Community Psychiatry 32:497-498, 1981

Lion WR, Reid WH (Eds): Assaults Within Psychiatric Facilities. New York, Grune & Stratton, 1983

Leedy v. Hartnett, 510 F. Supp. 1125 (M.D. Pa. 1981)

Lipari v. Sears, Roebuck and Co. 497 F. Supp. 185 (D. Neb. 1980)

Mills v. Rogers, 457 U.S. 291 (1982)

Monahan J: The Clinical Prediction of Violent Behavior. Rockville, MD, NIMH, 1981

Monahan J: The prediction of violent behavior: toward a second generation of theory and policy. Am J Psychiatry 141:10-15, 1984

Negron v. Preiser, 382 F. Supp. 535 (S.D.N.Y.1974)

New Jersey v. Cummins, 403 A.2d 67 (N.J. Super. Ct. 1979)

Opinion of the Justices, 465 A.2d 484 (N.H. 1983)

Pennsylvania Mental Health Bulletin, 99–85–10, March 11, 1985

People v. Medina, 705 P.2d 961 (Col. 1985)

Petersen v. Washington, 671 P.2d 230 (Wash. 1983)

Phelan LA, Mills MJ, Ryan JA: Prosecuting psychiatric patients for assault. Hosp Community Psychiatry 36:581-582, 1985

Project Release v. Prevost, 551 F. Supp. 1298 (E.D.N.Y. 1982); 722 F.2d 960 (2nd Cir. 1983)

R.A.J. v. Miller, 590 F. Supp. 131a (N.D. Tex. 1984)

Rennie v. Klein, 462 F. Supp. 1131 (D.N.J. 1978), 476 F. Supp. 1294 (D.N.J. 1979), *aff'd in* part, 653 F.2d 836 (3rd Cir. 1981), *vacated and remanded*, 102 S. Ct. 3506 (1982), 700 F.2d 266 (3rd Cir. 1985)

Restatement (Second) of Torts, Section 319

Rogers v. Commissioner of the Department of Mental Health, 458 N.E.2d 308 (Mass. 1983)

Romeo v. Youngberg, 644 F.2d 147 (3d Cir. 1980)

St. George v. State, 127 N.Y.S.2d 147 (N.Y. App. Div. 1954)

Schwarz CJ, Greenfield GP: Charging a patient with assault of a nurse on a psychiatric unit. Can Psychiatr Assoc J 23:197-200, 1978

Shader RI, Jackson AH, Harmatz JS, et al: Patterns of violent behavior among schizophrenic inpatients. Dis Nerv Syst 38:13-16, 1977

Sherrill v. Wilson, 653 S.W.2d 661 (Mo. 1983)

Stensvad v. Reivitz, 601 F. Supp. 128 (W.D. Wis 1985)

Tarasoff v. Regents of the University of Califorina, 131 Cal. Rptr. 14, 551 P.2d 334 (1976)

Tardiff K, Mattson MR: A survey of state mental health directors concerning guidelines for seclusion and restraint, in The Psychiatric Uses of Seclusion and Restraint. Edited by Tardiff K. Washington, DC, American Psychiatric Press, 1984

Van Duizend R, McGraw BD, Keilitz I: An overview of state involuntary civil commitment statutes. Mental and Physical Disability Law Reporter 8:328-335, 1984

Winick B: The law of the right to refuse treatment, in The Right to Refuse Antipsychotic Medication. Edited by Parry J. Washington, DC, American Bar Association, 1986

Wyatt v. Stickney, 325 F. Supp. 781 (M.D.Ala. 1971), 344 F. Supp. 373 (M.D.Ala. 1972)

Youngberg v. Romeo, 102 S. Ct. 2452 (1982)

Zito JM, Lentz SL, Routt WW, et al: The treatment review panel: a solution to treatment refusal? Bull Am Acad Psychiatry Law 12:349-358, 1984

Afterword

by Kenneth Tardiff, M.D., M.P.H.

This section has, it is hoped, fulfilled its mission of: 1) giving psychiatrists an overview of violence in society; 2) providing detailed clinical guidelines for the evaluation and the emergency and long-term treatment of violent patients; and 3) reviewing the current legal environment concerning the treatment of violent patients. Yet, more remains to be done in the areas of research, development of programs of intervention, and further written clinical guidelines concerning the management of violence.

Future research should use clear phenomenological definitions of violence; that is, specific behaviors rather than subjective definitions of violence—for example, verbal aggression. Research on the biology of violence should involve more sensitive measures of neurophysiological and biochemical dysfunction of the brain, particularly subcortical activity. New technology should be used with nuclear magnetic resonance (NMR), positron emission tomography (PET), single-photon emission computerized tomography (SPECT), regional cerebral blood-flow (rCBF), and brain electrical activity mapping (BEAM). Studies of neuro-transmitters should go beyond use of cerebrospinal fluid to the use of autopsy material from violent individuals, and new localization techniques such as digital subtraction autoradiography for brain dopamine and serotonin receptor sites (Altar et al, 1985).

Epidemiological studies should use more sophisticated techniques and data systems concerning crime and violence, especially in terms of the underreported domestic violence and child abuse. Linkage of data systems may detect patterns of homicides in terms of serial murderers. There should be naturalistic, long-term studies of the impact of television and other mass media in terms of the production of violence (Freedman, 1984). There should be prospective studies of the ability to predict violence in the near and distant future, using factors described in the previous chapters dealing with evaluation of the violent individual as well as long-term treatment.

Intervention programs should be developed based on existing knowledge of violence in terms of its determinants and treatment. Programs of intervention for child abuse and spouse abuse are essential for early intervention as well as for prevention of future violence (Kempe and Helfer, 1980; Sherman and Berk, 1984; Felthous, 1983). Social programs should aim not only at relieving poverty and unemployment but look to community organization. Projects such as those of the Eisenhower Foundation have sought to rehabilitate neighborhoods in the inner city by developing positive family and neighborhood structures and attitudes, as well as jobs supported by the local business community (Curtis, 1985). Such projects should be evaluated. Any legislation that decreases drug and alcohol use will decrease the incidence of violence; for example, legislation aimed at drug enforcement or raising the drinking age must be given attention. Efforts to control guns or even to eliminate handguns, which serve no legitimate purpose in society, should be strengthened.

Attention should be given to the treatment facilities to insure they are safe for violent patients, as in seclusion rooms, and safe for therapists and their patients, whether it is the inpatient unit or office setting. There should be security procedures in terms of weapon searches and hostage-taking procedures. Staff should be trained in terms of verbal intervention and the prevention of violence, as well as the practice of seclusion and restraint for violent patients. Mandatory aftercare programs for violent patients should be studied. Further written guidelines should be developed for the use of involuntary medication and the control of violent behavior along the lines of the American Psychiatric Association Task Force on the Use of Seclusion and Restraint (American Psychiatric Association, 1985). There should be guidelines as to what is reasonable in terms of protecting an intended victim of violence.

Last there should be future coverage in *Annual Reviews* of important areas not covered in this section. This includes rape, child, and spouse abuse, with special emphasis on the evaluation and treatment of the victims of these and other violent acts.

REFERENCES

Altar CA, O'Neil SO, Walter RJ, et al: Brain dopamine and serotonin receptor sites revealed by digital subtraction autoradiography. Science 228:597-600, 1985

American Psychiatric Association: Seclusion and Restraint: The Psychiatric Uses. Task Force Report No. 22. Washington, DC, American Psychiatric Press, 1985

Curtis L: American Violence and Public Policy. New Haven, Yale University Press, 1985

Felthous AR: Crisis intervention in interpartner abuse. Bull Am Acad Psychiatry Law 11:249-260, 1983

Freedman JL: Effect of television violence on aggressiveness. Psychol Bull 96:227-246, 1984

Kempe CH, Helfer R (Eds): The Battered Child Syndrome, third edition. Chicago, University of Chicago Press, 1980

Sherman CW, Berk RA: The specific deterrent effects of arrest for domestic assaults. American Sociological Review 49:261-272, 1984

V

Psychiatric Epidemiology

Section V

Psychiatric Epidemiology
Foreword

by Myrna M. Weissman, Ph.D., Section Editor

The appearance of this section on psychiatric epidemiology in *The American Psychiatric Association Annual Review* is timely, and represents the increased relevance of the epidemiologic approach to psychiatric disorders for clinical psychiatry. Psychiatric epidemiology in the United States is undergoing a major shift from study of the prevalence of general psychiatric impairment to study of the prevalence and incidence of specific psychiatric disorders and a range of risk factors associated with their onset. In this focus, psychiatric epidemiology shares many of the same methods and promises of epidemiologic studies of the major chronic diseases such as coronary artery disease, hypertension, or lung cancer.

The improvements in diagnostic definition and reliability of psychiatric disorders have accelerated the developments in psychiatric epidemiology. In 1980, the National Institute of Mental Health Epidemiologic Catchment Area Program (ECA), the first large-scale, multi-site epidemiologic study of adult psychiatric disorders in the United States to incorporate these new diagnostic approaches, was initiated. There are many examples of the increasing dialogue between psychiatric epidemiology and clinical psychiatry.

This section is meant to acquaint the psychiatric clinician with the variety of epidemiologic approaches currently yielding data of relevance. The emphasis is generally on substantive findings from a range of epidemiologic approaches, rather than on general principles and methods in epidemiology. There have been many excellent texts on epidemiologic design and statistical methods for chronic diseases. These methods for chronic diseases, in general, are applicable to the study of psychiatric disorders.

Chapter 25 presents the definitions and conceptual framework of epidemiology and an overview of the historical developments in psychiatry as they have had an impact on current epidemiologic psychiatry. Chapter 26 describes the epidemiologic perspective on psychiatric diagnosis and the relevance of the new diagnostic tools to clinical practice. Chapter 27 reviews the first results of the magnitude and risks of psychiatric disorders using survey methods from the Epidemiologic Catchment Area Study. Chapter 28 describes the merging of two disciplines, genetics and epidemiology, which share common methods and interest in causes of familial resemblance of disorders and together broaden the notion of inheritance. Chapter 29 examines the continuities between adult and child psychiatric disorders using the high-risk paradigm with consideration of the range of possible reasons for the association. Chapter 30 moves the discussion of risk factors for psychiatric disorders to a consideration of their implications for preventive interventions, and also asks what disorders may be prevented or modified by the reduction or modification of known risk factors. Chapter 31 describes how devastating accidents of nature (for example, floods, fires, nuclear accidents) can provide clinically useful information on the effect of stress in the development of psychiatric disorders in adults and children.

While these chapters are diverse both in approach (community surveys, family–genetic and high risk studies, preventive trials, and natural experiments) and in the populations studied, they have several common themes:

1. They are clearly rooted in clinical psychiatry. The diagnostic approaches and the implications of findings are of relevance to practice.
2. They are clearly rooted in clinical medicine. The epidemiologic approaches used in the study of psychiatric disorders are identical to those used in the study of any chronic disease.
3. They are not ideologically wedded to any one narrow view of etiology. A range of potential risk factors are acknowledged, although no one study can justifiably include all.

Chapter 25

Epidemiology Overview

by Myrna M. Weissman, Ph.D.

Epidemiologic topics have always been popular in the lay press. Statements about an increase in suicide, cocaine use, or AIDS are made as social commentary on what goes on in our society. Epidemiology as a scientific method, however, has usually been associated with epidemics of infectious diseases and, more recently, with prevalent chronic illnesses such as heart disease or hypertension. Epidemiology has rarely been associated with psychiatric disorders. When discussed in psychiatry it has been almost exclusively within the context of surveys of communities. The purpose of this chapter is to describe basic concepts and methods in epidemiology and its history in psychiatry, and to illustrate the broad scope of epidemiology and its utility for understanding psychiatric disorders.

At best, a brief chapter can only give the flavor of a discipline. Persons whose interests are whetted should examine the several excellent textbooks available on epidemiology (Feinstein, 1985; Kleinbaum et al, 1982; Mausner and Bahn, 1974; MacMahon and Pugh, 1970; Lilienfeld, 1976; Lowe and Kostrzewski, 1973). While these texts are about general epidemiology with no specific focus on psychiatry, the conceptual and analytic approaches used in studying the epidemiology of any chronic disease are directly applicable to the study of psychiatric disorders.

METHOD AND SCOPE

Definition

Epidemiology traditionally has been defined as the study of the distribution of diseases or disorders in populations and the factors which influence that distribution (Gruenberg and Turns, 1975; MacMahon and Pugh, 1970). The underlying assumption is that disorders are not randomly distributed among populations, and that by identifying the variations and then isolating the characteristics of the population which may be related to the variations (the risks), a mode of intervention to reduce the risk and break the causal link producing the disorder will be suggested, and an understanding of etiology may be forthcoming.

Thus, the purpose of epidemiology is threefold: 1) to describe the occurrence of disorders; 2) to determine the factors which are associated with the onset of

This research was supported, in part, by grant MH 30929, the Yale Mental Health Clinical Research Center, National Institute of Mental Health; by the John D. and Catherine T. MacArthur Foundation Mental Health Research Network on Risk and Protective Factors in the Major Mental Disorders; and by the Epidemiologic Catchment Area Program, MH 34224, from the National Institute of Mental Health, Rockville, MD.

the disorder; and 3) to control the distribution of disorders in populations by intervening in the risks which produce the disorder (Kleinbaum et al, 1982).

Epidemiology has been called the basic science of preventive medicine. Although the understanding of the mechanism and etiology of disorders is a major goal, the strategy is to obtain practical control over highly prevalent disorders until there is elucidation of basic etiology. Moreover, the demonstration of associations between disorder and risk may suggest fruitful areas for pursuing etiologic research.

The recent interest in epidemiology is due, in part, to its success, not in psychiatry, but in the identification of risk factors for cardiovascular disease (for example, smoking, high cholesterol, and lack of exercise), which have been amenable to change or intervention. The adaptation of life style to modify these risk factors in large segments of the population has led to a remarkable reduction of mortality from cardiovascular disease, even without a comparable accelerated understanding of etiology.

Basic Concepts

Case, population at risk, and risk-factor are base epidemiologic concepts (Schwab and Schwab, 1978). *Case* can denote a disease, disorder, abnormal laboratory finding, or a symptom referable to persons from a defined population. The *population at risk* indicates the reference group from which case has been derived and is the number of persons in the reference group who could possibly be affected by the specific phenomena under study. The population at risk can be a community (see Chapter 27); family (see Chapters 28 and 29); survivors of a disaster (see Chapter 31); or any systematically defined group, including groups of patients. Although the epidemiologist often studies patients, the focus is not, as in clinical practice, on the individual case but on aggregates of cases in the population at risk. The epidemiologist may begin with a study of a population at risk and identify cases, or may begin with cases and refer back to a population. Whatever the starting point, the epidemiologist ends up with some estimate of cases per population or some assessment of the distribution of the factor(s) of interest in a population. These factors are called risks.

The *risk-factor* (exposure or hazard) concept is central to epidemiologic thinking. A risk factor is a specific characteristic or condition whose presence is associated with an increased likelihood that a specific disorder is present, or will develop at a later time. The risk-factor concept is based on the finding of a statistically significant association between a disorder and a factor (for example, lung cancer and smoking; cardiovascular disease and high cholesterol level; hypertension and race; major depression and recent life events; bipolar disorder and family history; schizophrenia and eye tracking).

The risk can be as variable as a particular time (for example, month, year, generation), place (such as urban, rural, developing countries), or person. Personal characteristics can be demographic, such as age, sex, social class, ethnicity, or marital status; biological, such as physiological functioning of an organ or biochemical levels; or social, such as personal living habits, diet, or exercise (Lilienfield, 1976).

The strategy for investigating the association may begin either with the risk factor or with the disorder. In the first instance, a representative sample of a population with the factor of interest is compared to a comparable population without the factor, and the rate of occurrence of disorder in each group is calculated. A statistically significant difference in outcome (that is, differential rate of occurrence of disorder in each group) would suggest an association.

In the second instance, a representative sample of persons with the disorder of interest (the cases) and a comparable sample of persons without the disorder (noncases or controls) are selected. The two groups are then compared on the rate of occurrence of the factor of interest. A statistically significant difference in the outcome (that is, differential rate of occurrence of the risk factor in each group) would suggest an association. The factor under study may not necessarily be causative. It may increase risk via correlation with other risk factors or may be found to be the consequence of the disorder.

Inferring that a given factor is a risk involves many uncertainties. The association is strengthened by evidence for a temporal association of the factor and the onset of the disorder, as well as the consistency, specificity, strength and coherence, or biological plausibility of the association (Lilienfeld, 1976).

Measures

Measures of disease frequency and of association are fundamental to epidemiology. A basic quantitative unit in epidemiology is a rate, which is the number of cases (the numerator), the number in the population from which the cases derive (the reference population or denominator), and the time in which the cases are observed. The numerator and denominator must be similarly restricted; that is, if the numerator is confined to a certain age, then the denominator should be similarly confined. For example, a typical rate may be expressed as: 5/100 females during a one-year period experience a major depression.

The most common measures include, but are not limited to:

1. *Incidence*, the rate of the new cases of a disorder in the population at risk during a defined period of time (typically one year) divided by the population at risk. Sometimes the term incidence is used to include new onsets of previously remitted cases; that is, recurrent, as well as new cases.
2. *Prevalence*, the rate of both new and old (existing) cases in a population for a defined period of time; for example, six-month prevalence.
3. *Morbid risk, disease expectancy*, and *lifetime prevalence* have been used to define the lifetime risk of acquiring a disorder. However, these terms are defined imprecisely in the literature. Lifetime risk for a particular disorder would develop if all individuals lived to some specified age. As a way of estimating the lifetime risk of disorders, some studies calculate the proportion of subjects in the general population who ever had the disorder; that is, *lifetime prevalence*. Other studies age-correct the denominator of this proportion by weighting each unaffected person by the proportion of the age of risk through which he or she has passed at the time that the person ceased to be observed; that is, *morbid risk or disease expectancy*. Morbid risk and disease expectancy measures are problematic in psychiatry because of the ambiguity about the length of the risk period.

Efforts to understand the cause of a disorder focus on incidence rates, since causal factors should operate before the onset of the disorder. However, with any chronic disease, especially where there are numerous causes and a prodromal phase, it is difficult to define the precise onset; for example, should the onset of schizophrenia be dated as the first hallucination, or the first signs of social withdrawal?

The two most commonly used measures of the degree of association between the putative risk factor under study and the disorder are relative risk and attributable risk. *Relative risk* is the ratio of the rate of disorder among the exposed and nonexposed persons. *Attributable risk* is the rate of the disease in exposed individuals that can be attributed to the exposure. This measure is derived by subtracting the rate of the disorder among the nonexposed persons from the corresponding rate among exposed individuals. A brief overview cannot begin to do justice to the range of sophisticated quantitative approaches that are widely used in epidemiologic research (Fleiss, 1973).

Designs

The method of investigation in epidemiology includes techniques to identify the characteristics of populations, to appropriately classify and divide them into groups, to compare the results obtained in the defined groups, and to analyze the importance of any observed differences (Feinstein, 1985).

Close attention is paid to the representativeness of the cases selected from the reference population (sampling frame), the strategies of the observations and comparisons (the design), the accuracy of classification (the case definition or diagnosis) (see Chapter 26), and the significance of the observed association groups (the quantitative measures).

Sampling, study design, and classification are central components of epidemiologic strategies. No amount of statistical manipulation will salvage a study at the end which has had problems in these aspects at the beginning.

Epidemiologic studies generally fall into three broad strategies (Mausner and Bahn, 1974):

1. *Descriptive*: study of the amount and distribution of a disorder within a population; who is affected, and where and when cases occur
2. *Analytic*: study of the determinants of disease or the reasons for relatively high or low associations
3. *Experimental*: manipulation of the study factor to determine effect on the disease or its components

Descriptive data provide the first step in elucidating the causes of a disorder by identifying groups with high or low rates of a specific disease. Once such identification has been made, the next step is to question why the rates are high or low in a particular group, place, or time. These observations lead to hypotheses which can then be tested through more focused analytic or experimental studies. The analytic or etiologic studies are conducted when enough is known about a disorder to test specific hypotheses.

In the experimental approach, the study factor is manipulated by experiments of nature or of events; for example, floods, fires, hurricanes, closing of a factory, or nuclear accidents (see Chapter 31; Hearst et al, 1986); or by the investigator, as in clinical trials or laboratory experiments, and the like.

While there are numerous variations, the basic study design under these three approaches can be broadly classified as cross-sectional, cohort, case control (see

Table 1). (See Kleinbaum and colleagues (1982) for a detailed discussion of design.)

Cross-sectional studies, also called survey and prevalence studies, employ a naturalistic sampling frame that selects samples from a larger population and then determines the frequency of the disorder and the variation in distribution by person, time, place, and so forth. The measurement of the disorder and its variation are done at the same time. While basic descriptive associations can be made, it is not possible to determine the temporal sequence between the factor and the disorder or, more important, whether the factor(s) associated with the disorder was present before the onset and thus related etiologically to the disorder. The cross-sectional design can answer questions about the frequency of the disorder, the ages, groups, and segments of a community affected; the proportion of known cases under medical care; the range of the clinical phenomena; and the similarity between cases seen in treatment and those who never seek care. The Epidemiologic Catchment Area study, which estimated rates of psychiatric disorders in adults selected by probability sampling from five urban communities, is an example of a cross-sectonal study (see Chapter 27). The major obstacle to such large-scale descriptive studies in psychiatry has been the unreliability of psychiatric diagnosis. The ability to carry out the ECA is directly related to improvements in diagnostic reliability.

Cohort studies (also called follow-up, incidence, or prospective studies) follow a population at risk of developing the disease for a given period of time during which new cases are identified. A cohort can also be defined as a group of patients, and information on the clinical course and natural history of the disease can be obtained. A cohort study is expensive and inefficient for rare diseases. The follow-up can be either prospective or retrospective. In a prospective study, the investigator follows a healthy cohort over a period of time (for example, Vaillant's 1983 study of a Harvard University class to determine their health and social functioning over a 40-year period).

In a retrospective cohort study, the investigator selects a study group and then goes back in time and traces the factor of interest in these groups over time. Robins' (1966) follow-up of more than 500 persons 30 years after they were first identified as attending a child guidance clinic is an example of a cohort study in retrospect. In the Vaillant study, the investigators followed the cohort over the 40-year study period. The Robins study identified the cohort after 30 years had elapsed, and then traced back (in retrospect) their history since the event of interest (referral to a child guidance clinic).

Case-control studies (also known as retrospective studies) follow a paradigm that proceeds from effect to cause (Schlesselman, 1982). This strategy involves the study of a predetermined number of individuals with the disorder of interest (the cases), who are compared to individuals who are similar to the cases in as many ways as possible, but for whom the disorder of interest is absent (the controls). Cases and controls are compared with respect to attributes considered relevant to the disorder under study. The controls provide an estimate of the frequency of exposure expected in persons free of disease (see Schlesselman, 1982, for a detailed discussion of case-control studies). The ratio of the rates in exposed persons and unexposed persons is the relative risk or odds ratio. The Weissman et al (1984) study, which examined differential risk of psychiatric

Table 1. Epidemiologic Designs

Type and Purpose of Study	Design
Descriptive Estimate frequency of a disorder and generate hypothesis	Cross-sectional (surveys–prevalence studies): estimate disease frequency and variations by person, place, time in a sample from a reference population at one point in time (See Chapter 27) Cohort (follow-up, incidence or prospective studies): follow a sample over time and observe development of new disorders or recurrence of new episodes (See Chapter 27)
Analytic Identify risk factors and estimate their effect; test hypothesis	Case control (retrospective): compare a sample with a particular disorder (case), to a sample who are similar to the cases with respect to the factor of interest but without the disorder (controls) (See Chapters 28 and 29)
Experimental Manipulate a factor, by experiments of nature or by the investigators, and observe the effect	Natural experiments: study outcome of experiments of nature (floods, nuclear accidents, fires, etc.) to determine their effect (See Chapter 31) Laboratory experiments: estimate acute responses and their effect on components of the disorder (See Chapter 28) Clinical trial: test the efficacy of treatment in the prevention of the disorder (prophylactic) or in the reduction of the disorder (therapeutic) Community interventions: test the efficacy of an intervention at the community level to modify a risk factor (See Chapter 30)

illness in families of psychiatrically ill patients as compared to families of non-psychiatrically ill normal controls, is an example of a case-control study.

There is some controversy over the range of experimental studies to be included under the rubric of epidemiology. Kleinbaum and colleagues (1982), in their outstanding textbook of epidemiology, include: laboratory experiments that estimate the effect of some biological or behavioral response believed to be a risk factor for disease; clinical trials that include random assignment of an intervention or treatment for a disorder; for example, Prien et al (1984) studies of maintenance pharmacologic treatment for prevention of relapse of a recurrent depression. The purpose is to test the efficacy of an intervention either as therapy or as prophylaxis. The treatment can be at the individual or at the community level (see Chapter 30).

HISTORY

General Epidemiology

While there has not been a definitive review of the history of epidemiology, the literature is replete with excellent reviews of selected aspects or areas relevant to psychiatric epidemiology to which the reader can be referred (Schwab and Schwab, 1978; Grob, 1985; Rosen, 1958; Millbank Memorial Fund, 1950, 1961; Shepherd, 1978, 1985; Shepherd and Cooper, 1964; Winslow et al, 1952; Susser, 1985; Dohrenwend et al, 1980; Cooper and Morgan, 1973; Robins, 1978; Regier and Burke, 1985; Gruenberg, 1973; Group for the Advancement of Psychiatry, 1961; Hare and Wing, 1970; Goldberg and Huxley, 1980; Jablensky, in press; Leighton, 1979).

John Graunt's *Bills of Mortality*, published in 1662, is usually credited with establishing the field of epidemiology (Rothman, 1981), since his systematic approach identified facts about disease that previously had not been appreciated. While collecting information on causes of death, Graunt was the first to notice that males had higher rates of both births and deaths, and that there was a high mortality among children. For example, more than one-third of the population died by the age of five. "Teeth" was recorded as a leading cause of death. Rickets had increased to epidemic and fatal proportions.

Modern epidemiology originated in England, where record keeping provided the means for monitoring deaths (Lilienfeld, 1980; Rothman, 1981). However, the field did not develop in England until William Farr's appointment in 1838 as Compiler of Abstracts to the General Registry Office. Farr systematized the collection of mortality data, outlined certain occupational risks, developed mathematical models for complex epidemiologic phenomena such as epidemic curves, and demonstrated an association between altitude and mortality from cholera. This, Rothman (1981) noted, set the stage for John Snow's investigation in 1854 of the role of the water supply in the transmission of cholera. Realizing that cholera was being spread by water from a particular pump, Snow dismantled the pump and retarded the epidemic. This was the first published demonstration of preventive intervention into a risk factor. (See Lilienfeld, 1980, for an interesting description of the French, English, and American schools of epidemiology and their development.)

The early successes in the field of epidemiology were in infectious disease, where the specific etiologic agent was not known. For example, Jenner's discovery, around 1800, that cowpox infection protected against smallpox, led to the eradication of smallpox once mass vaccination became feasible. The discovery of the importance of bacteria in disease by Pasteur in the mid-19th century led to the development of infectious disease epidemiology. For a number of years concern was almost exclusively on microbiological etiology and the control of etiologic agents through immunization. The most dramatic was the control of poliomyelitis in 1955, and the most recent, the procedures against measles. However, it was obvious that there were many diseases for which the model of infection did not fit the case. Moreover, it was recognized that even in infectious diseases, not all exposed individuals developed the disease, and the course of a disease was variable among individuals. Tuberculosis was the disease which precipitated the interest in the host factors or multifactorial etiology in vulnerability. For tuberculosis, exposure to the mycrobacterium constituted only a portion of the total etiology. However, this model was applicable to a variety of noninfectious disorders of a chronic nature (such as cardiovascular disease, arteriosclerosis, arthritis, and schizophrenia) where no single cause is evident, multiple causes are undoubtedly involved, and the disorders are likely to be etiologically heterogeneous.

Furthermore, in studying chronic disorders with multiple etiologies, the classic measures of infectious disease epidemiology (the length of time between exposure and onset of disease and the study of the shape of epidemic curves) were no longer useful (Cassel, 1964). In chronic diseases, the onset is slow and causative factors may act over a long period of time; rates may change slowly over time. It is often difficult to determine the precise onset. The study of populations and the variation of risk within populations for chronic disease has proven powerful. Findings on the association of cigarette smoking with lung cancer, the exposure to carcinogens in certain occupations, the health effect of low-level radiation, and so forth, have had implications for improving the health of large numbers of persons.

Following World War II, several large-scale studies of chronic disease were initiated in the United States. Most notable among them was the Framingham study, a longitudinal study of a healthy population to determine risk factors for cardiovascular disease (Snowden et al, 1982). This study identified diet and cholesterol and, more recently, estradiol as risks. Psychiatric disorders were, with few exceptions, excluded from these studies.

Psychiatric Epidemiology

According to Grob (1985), the history of psychiatric epidemiology had a different tradition. Although 19th-century psychiatrists (most of whom were employed as superintendents in institutions) kept statistics of demographic and geographic characteristics of their inpatients, this information was used for the purpose of policy advocacy and not for research. The status of psychiatric nosology also hindered inquiry. While direct etiologic classifications were not far advanced for other areas of medicine, the behavioral symptoms used to describe psychiatric disorders were even more vague and unreliable.

The first partially completed attempt to investigate the true prevalence of mental disorders, including both treated and untreated cases in a community study in the United States, was conducted in Massachusetts in 1855. Jarvis surveyed community leaders, as well as hospital and other official records, to determine the frequency of "insanity" and "idiocy," the major nosological distinction at that time. The U.S. census of 1880 also incorporated this distinction and provided the first national estimates of mental disorder (Weissman and Klerman, 1978, 1985).

Indirect procedures of ascertaining information from medical records and key informants characterized subsequent pre-World War II studies conducted in the United States, such as those reported by Lemkau (1958) in the Eastern Health District of Baltimore in 1933 and 1936, and by Roth and Luton (1943) in Williamson County, Tennessee, in 1935. Lemkau et al (1942) supplemented these procedures with data obtained from direct interviews determining the frequency of "nervousness" that had been conducted coincidentally by the National Health Survey in the same district.

Although not a community survey, Faris and Dunham (1967) examined the ecological distribution of first admissions to mental hospitals in Chicago in the 1930s. Diagnoses from hospital records were related to the area of residence of the patients. The highest rates of hospitalization for mental illness occurred in residents from areas with the highest social disorganization. This careful study demonstrated the importance of social variables in mental illness.

These studies, although advanced for their time, had two major limitations: Case ascertainment was incomplete, and clinical diagnoses were taken at face value with little attention to their reliability or validity. There were, however, examples of the contributions of epidemiologic approaches to understanding the etiology of psychiatric illness. For example, pellagra, at the turn of the century, accounted for 10 percent of admissions to mental hospitals in the South. The work of Goldberger in 1914, using a case-control method and careful observation in mental hospitals, demonstrated that pellagra psychosis was due to nutritional deficiency. The identification of the risk factor—a deficient diet—led to the intervention of change in diet, and to the elimination of the disease. This occurred even though the chemical structure of nicotinic acid was not characterized until 1939.

The period after World War II in the United States was also one of high activity in community surveys of mental impairment and health. The classic epidemiologic studies of this period included the work of Hollingshead and Redlich (1958) showing the relationship between social class and mental illness. The studies of Leighton et al (1963) in Nova Scotia, Srole et al (1962) in Manhattan, and Myers and Bean (1968) in New Haven demonstrated the importance of poverty, urban anomie, social stress, and rapid social change in the development of impairment. These studies introduced rigor to community surveys by giving attention to sampling, use of standardized questionnaires to systematize the collection of data, and sophisticated statistical techniques. They did not generate rates of psychiatric disorders and, therefore, did not have a major impact on clinical psychiatry. The studies of that period, because of diagnostic unrealiability, used measures of overall mental impairment that were independent of diagnosis and could not be translated into equivalent clinical diagnostic categories. These studies also showed high rates of impairment. From the point of view of policy, if so many persons were affected, the possibility of interventions seemed unlikely. As a result, no rates of treated and untreated specific psychiatric disorders were available in the United States in the 1970s. Large-scale studies of families were lacking. There was a separation between psychiatric epidemiology and clinical psychiatry.

In the 1960s, psychiatric research was flourishing. Psychopharmacology research used double blind, placebo-controlled clinical trials to test the efficacy of the new psychopharmacologic agents. Family–genetic studies of schizophrenia used cross-rearing adoptive techniques (Heston, 1966; Mednick et al, 1974; Kety et al, 1968) to examine the rate and diagnosis in children of biological parents with schizophrenia, adopted away from birth, and living with adoptive parents without schizophrenia. Psychopathologic studies, using uniform and comparable methods, examined whether reported differences between patients admitted to mental hospitals in the United States and the United Kingdom were mainly a function of different diagnostic nomenclature. While these studies were widely recognized in clinical psychiatry and used epidemiologic methods, they were not usually identified with epidemiology as a method. The major community studies in psychiatry that were identified as epidemiologic studies, with rare exception, did not generate rates of specific psychiatric diagnosis similar to those used in clinical psychiatry, and were not widely appreciated in clinical psychiatry.

Psychiatric epidemiology, clinical psychiatry, and research did not begin to converge until the mid-1970s, with the introduction into psychiatry of specified diagnostic criteria, improved diagnostic reliability, and standardized methods of assessing signs and symptoms of psychiatric disorders by direct interview or by family history. These new diagnostic techniques were needed for case identification in epidemiologic studies. Their availability served to bridge the gap between epidemiology and clinical psychiatry. They were first applied in 1975 to community samples in a small study of 500 subjects living in New Haven, Connecticut, and were shown to be feasible and reliable (Weissman and Myers, 1978).

Psychiatric epidemiology was also accelerated by social and political developments. In 1977, President Carter established the first President's Commission on Mental Health. Among its many endeavors, leading mental health researchers documented the lack of data on the magnitude and risk of psychiatric illness in the community based on clinical psychiatric diagnoses. Although the 1975 New Haven community study of 500 subjects had demonstrated the reliability of a structured diagnostic interview—the Schedule for Affective Disorders and Schizophrenia–Lifetime (SADS–L)—to assess psychiatric illness in the community, the administration of the SADS required clinically trained persons, which would not be feasible if large-scale community epidemiologic studies were to be undertaken. While there were several excellent structured diagnostic interviews available (Wing et al, 1974; Endicott and Spitzer, 1978; Helzer et al, 1981), none was completely suitable for use in epidemiologic studies (Dohrenwend et al, 1978; Regier and Burke, 1985).

In the late 1970s, the National Institute of Mental Health (NIMH) sponsored the development of a diagnostic instrument, the Diagnostic Interview Schedule (DIS), suitable for use in large-scale epidemiologic studies of psychiatric disorders (Robins et al, 1981). Soon after, in 1980, the Epidemiologic Catchment Area Study was initiated.

When the first ECA results were published in the October, 1984 issue of *Archives of General Psychiatry*, they were introduced by Chief Editor Daniel X.

Freedman in an editorial punningly entitled "Psychiatric Epidemiology Counts." This editorial and the papers it introduced put psychiatric epidemiology, at least temporarily, in the limelight. While the limelight is useful for attracting students and funding, it also represents an opportunity to extend the concept of epidemiology beyond descriptive studies of the community in an effort to demonstrate the variety of strategies possible and their utility in clinical psychiatric research.

Over the next few years, questions such as: "Why does it count? Is it accurately counting? Does it count for the clinician?" will be legitimately raised by the scientific and clinical community. Many of these questions will best be answered by the alternate epidemiologic design described.

EPIDEMIOLOGY, CLINICAL RESEARCH, AND PSYCHIATRY

The current limitations of epidemiology in psychiatric research are limitations inherent in our understanding of psychiatric disorders and not in the method (Editorial, 1983). As is well known, diagnostic classifications are based on manifest criteria rather than etiology, and the validity for most diagnoses has not been established. No biological risk factors have been unequivocally demonstrated for any of the disorders. The pathophysiology has not yet been demonstrated for any of the symptoms of the major mental disorders (Jablensky, 1984). Psychiatric disorders, like many chronic diseases, undoubtedly are due to more than one cause. Even in one of the most serious mental disorders, schizophrenia, where genetic heritability is supported by twin and adoption studies, a large part of the variance is unaccounted for.

These limitations, however, are not the end but a challenge to the development of epidemiologic designs which can yield testable hypotheses. As discussed by Jablensky (1984), many research designs in biologic psychiatry have low statistical power, ill-conceived controls, and samples of convenience. The result is a host of unreplicated studies. Alternately, epidemiologic studies have not proceeded beyond demonstrating a range of demographic (sex, age, social class) variables associated with major mental illness, which do not elucidate the mechanism by which the factors operate. Clearly, there is a need to integrate the search for biological markers and risk factors (see Chapter 28).

This outline of epidemiologic research strategies, which has included laboratory experiments and clinical trials as well as the designs traditionally associated with epidemiology, may raise questions about the boundaries between epidemiologic and clinical research. This overlap between epidemiologic and clinical research has been recently emphasized by Feinstein (1985), who describes epidemiology as the architecture of clinical research and defines a new collaboration, termed clinical epidemiology. Editorial debates about the linking of these domains, unfortunately, have also occurred. As the designs and strategies of epidemiologic research are defined in clinical disciplines, it is quite clear that boundaries are artifactual. Epidemiologic and clinical research has much to be gained by a marriage (Sackett, 1969; Orchard, 1980; Editorial, 1980). A host of unreplicated biological studies could be avoided by careful attention to sampling, diagnostic assessment, and use of appropriate comparison groups. These concerns are the basis of epidemiologic methods. Alternatively, the integration of epidemiology with clinical practice may reduce the number of well-designed epidemiologic studies with findings of little utility to the health of sick people.

In terms of clinical practice, epidemiologic studies thus far have yielded information of direct clinical utility which can be used by the clinician for more accurate diagnosis, earlier intervention, and to clarify prognosis. For example, one recent contribution to clinical psychiatry has been an awareness that information about disorders deriving solely from patients referred to clinical practice may not represent the full spectrum of the disorder and its prognosis. As shown by Cohen and Cohen (1984), the clinician's sample is biased toward cases of longer duration, of high co-morbidity, and of poor prognosis. Epidemiologic studies have shown that episodes of panic symptoms of short duration are common (Von Korff et al, 1985); that schizophrenia is not universally a chronic, unremitting disease; that heroin abuse is not incurable (Cohen and Cohen, 1984); and that agoraphobia can occur without panic attack (Weissman et al, in press, a). This epidemiologic information should sharpen clinical diagnosis and case finding, and help to provide more accurate information to patients and their families. While our ability to identify a population, person, and situation of risk for many psychiatric disorders and to provide treatment has outstripped our understanding of etiology, this is no less true in other areas of medicine. Epidemiologic surveys have shown the majority of persons with a psychiatric disorder do not seek treatment from a psychiatrist or any mental health professional (Shapiro et al, 1984). Many ill persons come to health care facilities, where their psychiatric symptoms are unrecognized and/or untreated. Epidemiologic studies have demonstrated the value of structured diagnostic interviews as screening techniques for case finding (Dohrenwend et al, 1980) and have pointed to places where persons who might benefit from treatment can be found.

In summary, the epidemiologic data have contributed to specifying the full range of psychiatric disorders, their high co-morbidity, and variable prognosis, including information on persons who recover from disorders and don't come for treatment. The data have also contributed to identifying persons at high risk for becoming ill, as well as the situations or times associated with the increased risk of illness. Recent studies have introduced diagnostic and other screening methodology which has wide utility for improving diagnostic precision and early case finding in clinical practice (Weissman et al, in press, b).

REFERENCES

Cassel J: Social science theory as a source of hypotheses in epidemiological research. Am J Public Health 54:1482-1488, 1964

Cohen P, Cohen J: The clinician's illusion. Arch Gen Psychiatry 41:1178-1182, 1984

Cooper B, Morgan HG: Epidemiological Psychiatry. Springfield, Illinois, Charles C Thomas, 1973

Dohrenwend BS, Krasnoff L, Askenasy AR, et al: Exemplification of a method for scaling life events: the PERI life events scale. J Health Soc Behav 19:205-229, 1978

Dohrenwend BP, Dohrenwend BS, Gould MS, et al: Mental Illness in the United States: Epidemiological Estimates. New York, Praeger Scientific, 1980

Editorial: A plea for clinical epidemiology. Br Med J 281:1163, 1980

Editorial: Diagnosis and classification of mental disorders, alcohol and drug related problems: a research agenda for the 1980s. Psychol Med 13:907-921, 1983

Endicott J, Spitzer RL: A diagnostic interview: the schedule for affective disorders and schizophrenia. Arch Gen Psychiatry 35:837-844, 1978

Faris REL, Dunham HW: Mental Disorders in Urban Areas: An Ecological Study of Schizophrenia and Other Psychoses. Chicago, The University of Chicago, 1967

Feinstein AR: Clinical Epidemiology: The Architecture of Clinical Research. Philadelphia, WB Saunders, 1985

Fleiss JL: Statistical Methods for Rates and Proportions. New York, John Wiley & Sons, 1973

Freedman DX: Psychiatric epidemiology counts. Arch Gen Psychiatry 41:931-933, 1984

Goldberg D, Huxley P: Mental Illness in the Community: The Pathway to Psychiatric Care. London, Tavistock Publications, 1980

Grob GN: The origins of American psychiatric epidemiology. Am J Public Health 75:229-236, 1985

Group for the Advancement of Psychiatry: Problems of Estimating Change in Frequency of Mental Disorders; Report No. 50. New York, Group for the Advancement of Psychiatry, 1961

Gruenberg EM: Progress in psychiatric epidemiology. Psychiatr Q 47:1-11, 1973

Gruenberg EM, Turns DM: Epidemiology, in Comprehensive Textbook of Psychiatry, vol. 1, second edition. Edited by Freedman AM, Kaplan HI, Sadock BJ. Baltimore, Williams & Wilkins, 1975

Hare EH, Wing JK (Eds): Psychiatric Epidemiology. London, Oxford University Press, 1970

Hearst N, Newman TB, Hulley SB: Delayed effects of the military draft on mortality: a randomized natural experiment. N Engl J Med 314:620-624, 1986

Helzer JE, Robins LN, Croughan JL, et al: Renard diagnostic interview: its reliability and procedural validity with physicians and lay interviewers. Arch Gen Psychiatry 38:393-398, 1981

Heston LL: Psychiatric disorders in foster home reared children of schizophrenic mothers. Br J Psychiatry 112:819 825, 1966

Hollingshead AB, Redlich FD: Social Class and Mental Illness. New York, John Wiley & Sons, 1958

Jablensky A: Epidemiological and clinical research as a guide in the search for risk factors and biological markers. J Psychiatr Res 18:541-554, 1984

Jablensky A: Epidemiological surveys of mental health of geogrphically-defined populations in Europe, in Community Surveys. Edited by Weissman MM, Myers JK, Ross C. New Brunswick, New Jersey, Rutgers University Press (in press)

Kety SS, Rosenthal D, Wender PH, et al: The type and prevalence of mental illness in the biological and adoptive families of adopted schizophrenia, in Transmission of Schizophrenia. Edited by Rosenthal D, Kety SS. London, Pergamon Press, 1968

Kleinbaum DG, Kupper LL, Morgenstern H: Epidemiologic Research: Principles and Quantitative Methods. Belmont, California, Wadsworth, Inc, 1982

Kurtzke JF: Neuroepidemiology. Ann Neurol 16:265-277, 1984

Leighton AH: Research directions in psychiatric epidemiology. Psychol Med 9:235-247, 1979

Leighton DC, Harding JS, Macklin DB, et al: The Character of Danger: Stirling County Study No. 3. New York, Basic Books, 1963

Lemkau PV: The epidemiological study of mental illnesses and mental health. Am J Psychiatry 111:801-809, 1958

Lemkau PV, Tietze C, Cooper H: Complaint of nervousness and the psychoneuroses. Am J Orthopsychiatry 12:214-223, 1942

Lilienfeld AM: Foundations of Epidemiology. New York, Oxford University Press, 1976

Lilienfeld AM (Ed): Times, Places, Persons: Aspects of the History of Epidemiology. Baltimore, John Hopkins University Press, 1980

Lowe CR, Kostrzewski J: Epidemiology: A Guide to Teaching Methods. London, Churchill Livingstone, 1973

MacMahon B, Pugh T: Epidemiology: Principles and Methods. Boston, Little, Brown, 1970

Mausner J, Bahn A: Epidemiology: An Introductory Text. Philadelphia, WB Saunders, 1974

Mednick SA, Schulsinger F, Higgins J, et al (Eds): Genetics, Environment, and Psychopathology. New York, North Holland Publishing Co, 1974

Millbank Memorial Fund: Epidemiology of Mental Disorder. New York, Millbank Memorial Fund, 1950

Millbank Memorial Fund: Cases of Mental Disorders: A Review of Epidemiologic Knowledge. New York, Millbank Memorial Fund, 1961

Myers JK, Bean LL: A Decade Later: A Follow-Up of Social Class and Mental Illness. New York, John Wiley & Sons, 1968

Orchard TJ: Epidemiology in the 1980s: need for a change. Lancet 2:845, 1980

Prien RF, Kupfer DJ, Mansky PA, et al: Drug therapy in the prevention of recurrences in unipolar and bipolar affective disorders. Arch Gen Psychiatry 41:1096-1104, 1984

Regier DA, Burke JD: Epidemiology, in Comprehensive Textbook of Psychiatry, vol. 1. Edited by Kaplan HJ, Sadock BJ. Baltimore, Williams & Wilkins, 1985

Regier DA, Myers JK, Kramer M, et al: The NIMH epidemiological catchment area program: historical context, major objectives, and study population characteristics. Arch Gen Psychiatry 41:934-941, 1984

Robins LN: Deviant Children Grown Up: A Sociological and Psychiatric Study of Sociopathic Personality. Baltimore, Williams & Wilkins, 1966

Robins LN: Psychiatric epidemiology. Arch Gen Psychiatry 35:697-702, 1978

Robins LN, Helzer JE, Croughan J, et al: National Institute of Mental Health diagnostic interview schedule: its history, characteristics, and validity. Arch Gen Psychiatry 38:381-389, 1981

Rosen G: A History of Public Health. New York, MD Publications, Inc, 1958

Roth WF Jr, Luton FH: The mental health program in Tennessee. Am J Psychiatry 99:662-675, 1943

Rothman KJ: Sounding boards: the rise and fall of epidemiology, 1959–2000 A.D. N Engl J Med 2:600-602, 1981

Sackett DL: Commentary: clinical epidemiology. Am J Epidemiol 89:125-128, 1969

Schlesselman JJ: Case-Control Studies: Design, Conduct, Analysis. New York, Oxford University Press, 1982

Schwab JJ, Schwab ME: Social Roots of Mental Illness: An Epidemiologic Survey. New York, Plenum, 1978

Shapiro S, Skinner EA, Kessler LG, et al: Utilization of health and mental health services: three epidemiologic catchment area sites. Arch Gen Psychiatry 41:971-978, 1984

Shepherd M: Epidemiology and clinical psychiatry. Br J Psychiatry 133:289-298, 1978

Shepherd M: Psychiatric epidemiology and epidemiological psychiatry. Am J Public Health 75:275-276, 1985

Shepherd M, Cooper B: Epidemiology and mental disorder: a review. J Neurol Neurosurg Psychiatry 27:277, 1964

Snowden CB, McNamara PM, Garrison RJ, et al: Predicting coronary heart disease in siblings: a multivariate assessment—the Framingham heart study. Am J Epidemiology 115:217-222, 1982

Srole L, Langer TS, Michael ST, et al: Mental Helath in the Metropolis: The Midtown Manhattan Study, vol. 1. New York, McGraw-Hill, 1962

Susser M: Epidemiology in the United States after World War II: the evolution of technique. Epidemiol Rev 7:147-177, 1985

Vaillant GE: The Natural History of Alcoholism. Cambridge, Massachusetts, Harvard University Press, 1983

Von Korff M, Eaton W, Reyl P: The epidemiology of panic attacks and disorder: results from three community surveys. Am J Epidemiol 122:970-981, 1985

Weissman MM, Klerman GL: The epidemiology of mental disorders: emerging trends. Arch Gen Psychiatry 35:705-712, 1978

Weissman MM, Klerman GL: Epidemiology: purpose and historical overview, in Psychiatry, vol. 3. Edited by Michels R, Cavenar JO Jr. Philadelphia, JB Lippincott, 1985

Weissman MM, Myers JK: Affective disorders in an urban community: the use of research diagnostic criteria in an epidemiological survey. Arch Gen Psychiatry 35:1304-1311, 1978

Weissman MM, Myers JK, Harding PS: Psychiatric disorders in a U.S. urban community. Am J Psychiatry 135:459-462, 1978

Weissman MM, Gershon ES, Kidd KK, et al: Psychiatric disorders in the relatives of probands with affective disorders: The Yale–NIMH collaborative family study. Arch Gen Psychiatry 41:13-21, 1984

Weissman MM, Leaf PJ, Blazer DG, et al: The relationship between panic disorder and agoraphobia: an epidemiologic perspective. Psychopharmacol Bull (in press, a)

Weissman MM, Merikangas KR, John K, et al: Family–genetic studies of psychiatric disorders: developing technologies. Arch Gen Psychiatry (in press, b)

Wing JK, Cooper JE, Sartorius N: The Measurement and Classification of Psychiatric Symptoms. London, Cambridge University Press, 1974

Winslow CEA, Smillie WG, Doull JA, et al: The History of American Epidemiology. Edited by Top FH. St. Louis, CV Mosby, 1952

Chapter 26

The Assessment of Psychiatric Diagnosis in Epidemiological Studies

by Lee N. Robins, Ph.D.

In the last 20 years, American psychiatry has shown a remarkable resurgence of interest in diagnosis, at least in part as a result of the development of a number of effective treatments that are diagnosis-specific. Along with this resurgence has come increased concern that there may be large numbers of cases in the population who would benefit from these treatments, but are not currently known to any treatment facility. There is also a recognition that further success in identifying causes and describing the course of specific disorders may depend on studies that utilize representative samples of all those who develop the disorder of interest, not only those who happen to come for treatment. Both treatment and research goals, therefore, have given new impetus to attempts to accurately assign diagnoses to members of the general population, whether treated or untreated.

In this chapter I review the traditions in American and European psychiatric epidemiology that have led to attempts to marry opinion survey and clinical assessment strategies to make possible accurate identification of cases of specific disorders in large general population surveys. In this chapter, I contrast the data generated by this marriage with results available with prior methods—surveys that made global assessments of mental health without specific diagnoses, and assessments of population prevalences of specific diagnoses through record linkages.

These advances have not been made without being challenged as to whether such an endeavor is truly feasible. It is difficult to prove that these new techniques actually do—or do not—produce reasonably accurate estimates of the prevalence of specific diagnoses. This chapter explains why these decisions are so difficult to make.

Finally, I summarize what useful information standardized diagnostic interviews can produce in addition to the diagnoses themselves, and how these

This research was supported by the Epidemiological Catchment Area Program (ECA). The ECA is a series of five epidemiologic research studies performed by independent research teams in collaboration with staff of the Division of Biometry and Epidemiology (DBE) of the National Institute of Mental Health (NIMH). The NIMH Principal Collaborators are Darrel A. Regier, Ben Z. Locke, and Jack D. Burke, Jr.; the NIMH Project Officer is Carl A. Taube. The Principal Investigators and Co-Investigators from the five sites are: Yale University, U01 MH 34224—Jerome K. Myers, Myrna M. Weissman, and Gary L. Tischler; The Johns Hopkins University, U01 MH 33870—Morton Kramer and Sam Shapiro; Washington University, St. Louis, U01 MH 33883—Lee N. Robins and John E. Helzer; Duke University U01 MH 35386—Dan Blazer and Linda George; University of California, Los Angeles, U01 MH 35865—Marvin Karno, Richard L. Hough, Javier I. Escobar, and M. Audrey Burnam. This work was also supported by Research Scientist Award MH 00334, USPHS Grants MH 17104 and MH 31302, and the MacArthur Foundation Risk Factor Network.

interview protocols, designed for use in epidemiological surveys, might be useful in clinical practice.

EPIDEMIOLOGIC SURVEYS WITHOUT DIAGNOSES

Surveys of mental disorder in the general population that estimate rates of specific diagnoses are newcomers to the scene of American psychiatric epidemiology. Among the famous studies that have done without diagnosis are Gurin and colleagues' *Americans View Their Mental Health* (1960), which asked about "nervous breakdowns" and 19 other symptoms suggesting depression or anxiety; studies using the Cornell Medical Index (Brodman et al, 1954), which gave numerical mental health scores; the Midtown Manhattan study (Srole et al, 1962), the Stirling County study, which assessed "caseness" (Leighton et al, 1963); studies using the Langner 22-item scale derived from the Midtown Manhattan study (Dohrenwend and Dohrenwend, 1969); counts of children's symptoms by Lapouse and Monk (1959); Langner et al's factor scores for children (1969); syndrome scores in studies using the PERI (Dohrenwend and Dohrenwend, 1982); and the Hopkins Symptom Checklist (Uhlenhuth et al, 1974).

High Prevalence Estimates

While the newer studies without diagnoses have compromised by scoring syndromes, the older studies usually attempted only to count the number of mentally ill persons in the population, and sought correlates of "caseness." They found very few persons in excellent mental health, and large numbers currently impaired. Such high rates of impairment have been looked upon with skepticism. The scoring methods may explain why they occur. These studies used one of two ways of deciding whether a respondent was a case: either a summary of interview responses was given to a psychiatrist, who was asked how surprised he or she would have been to see such a respondent in a clinical setting; or, a fixed number of positive answers was identified by a statistical method, such as discriminant analysis, as best distinguishing patients from community residents. From then on, people above that threshold were called cases and people below it were called well.

The first method asked the psychiatrist to make a decision based on information that he or she was almost certain to consider inadequate, and which the psychiatrist had no opportunity to amplify or elaborate. A list of yes–no answers to an incomplete set of symptom questions, with no follow-up for yes answers, was not the kind of evidence used in daily clinical practice. The psychiatrist had no choice but to assume that the limited information received would have stood up to cross-examination, and so an excess of positive cases was likely.

The second method, which assigns respondents to "case" status on the basis of the total number of positive responses, equates having a sprinkling of symptoms across many diagnostic categories with having all the symptoms of a single disorder, and treats severe and mild symptoms alike. Patients often have almost all the symptoms of a single disorder in a severe form, but no more symptoms of other disorders than do members of the general population. Since the interview asked about only a small sample of the symptoms of any patient's presenting disorder, patients' number of positive answers could be modest. Consequently, the cutting point that identified most patients as positive would also encompass members of the general population with a scattering of positive responses to symptoms of a variety of disorders, none representing severe symptoms. As a result, many persons in the general population who had a reasonably high level of personal distress but no psychiatric disorder would be counted as cases.

Demographic Correlates

In addition to producing high rates of mentally disordered persons in the community, these studies also agreed on what the demographic correlates of mental disorder were. The groups with the highest rates were found to be the elderly, women, the poor, the urban, and the divorced or separated.

While common findings obtained by studies using different interviews can be a powerful argument for the validity of findings, the conclusions with respect to the elderly and women of these early nondiagnostic studies have recently been challenged by results of studies that are diagnosis-specific (Robins et al, 1984). The agreement among these studies apparently stems from the core of common symptoms selected.

The common pattern of symptoms stemmed in part from the fact that many of these interviews are lineal descendants of the Army Neuropsychiatric Screening Adjunct (Star, 1950), a self-administered brief collection of questions adapted from the Minnesota Multiphasic Personality Inventory (MMPI) toward the end of World War II to predict which men eligible to serve would not make satisfactory soldiers. In each interview, anxiety and depressive disorders are the disorders best represented. Symptoms of substance abuse and personality disorders, disorders of impulse control, organic syndromes, and other disorders requiring psychotic symptoms are either omitted or represented by only one or two questions. It is this emphasis on anxiety and depression (disorders particularly common in women) at the expense of substance abuse and antisocial personality (disorders more common in men) that probably accounts for the consistent findings of the early studies that women are at especially high risk for psychiatric disorder.

These interviews also made no attempt to rule out physical explanations for these symptoms. The confounding of psychological symptoms with the physical symptoms that increase with age appears to explain why the elderly were found to have high rates.

The one finding from the early studies that has survived the introduction of diagnostic interviews into epidemiology is the finding that the divorced and separated have more mental disorders than other groups, but whether this is the cause of mental disorder or its consequence remains uncertain.

Demographic correlates are useful for suggesting etiological hypotheses. When disorders have different demographic correlates, as depression and alcohol abuse do, it is unlikely to be useful to talk about the etiology of mental disorder as a whole, because their distinct demographics suggest that they have different etiologies.

Use in Planning and Therapy

For many years, epidemiologic studies that measured "caseness" but not specific disorders were the best available basis for estimating the size of unmet treatment needs in the community. Because they identified a very large proportion of the general population as mentally ill, there appeared to be an almost unlimited demand for psychiatric services. Even if the total number of untreated mentally ill were correct, it would not be possible to calculate manpower requirements accurately from such studies, because not all disorders benefit equally from treatment and because the intensity of treatment required varies according to disorder. Contact with a psychiatrist is indicated for treatable disorders likely to be misdiagnosed if not referred, and for disorders that are easy to recognize but for which only a psychiatrist is likely to provide proper treatment. It is not clear that psychiatrists are needed to carry out routine treatment of disorders that can be easily recognized and successfully treated by nonspecialists, or of disorders for which no successful therapies are currently available. Studies that do not estimate the number of untreated persons with specific diagnoses in the population do not tell us what proportion of the population would benefit from specialist care.

Despite their disadvantages, surveys that lacked diagnoses have made a valuable contribution in sensitizing primary care physicians to the high rate of depression in their patients, and have provided interviews that can screen for these symptoms so that treatment for depression is provided as needed (Eastwood, 1975). Unfortunately, because of their limited coverage of symptoms of other disorders, they have not done the same for substance abusers. Yet the new diagnostic epidemiologic surveys have shown alcohol and drug abuse to be as common as affective and anxiety disorders combined (Robins et al, 1984), and much less likely than depression to present for treatment.

Thus, diagnostic surveys have much to offer in providing guides to the breadth of services needed, and to diagnostic areas where priorities for research in treatment and prevention should be increasing.

Why Diagnoses Were Omitted

PHILOSOPHICAL OBJECTIONS. Given the usefulness of diagnostic information for the general population in planning services and setting research agenda, one may wonder why it was so long in appearing on the American epidemiological scene. Part of the reason was probably a matter of philosophy. The "golden age" of the first large-scale American studies was from the end of World War II through the 1960s, a period during which diagnosis was not popular with many psychiatrists and most social scientists in the United States. During this heyday of psychodynamics, many influential psychiatrists felt no need for diagnosis because it would add nothing to their decision about what therapy to offer. Psychotherapy was always the preferred treatment, with full-scale psychoanalysis for the chosen few. Indeed, many psychiatrists disapproved of diagnosis, seeing it as derogatory in much the same way that giving an ethnic label is; as nihilistic, because they thought that associating psychiatric problems with disease suggested that the patient might be incurable; and as dehumanizing, because diagnosis would lead to treating the patient as an example of a disease rather than attending to the patient's uniqueness as a human being.

PRACTICAL OBJECTIONS. But the opposition was not only philosophical. Many clinicians doubted that diagnosis could be achieved in community samples on the scale needed for epidemiological studies. Some believed that accurate diagnoses required multiple contacts during which rapport could be built and defenses overcome. Some believed that direct questioning about symptoms would not work because people were suggestible, and would report symptoms they did not have if asked; or worse, might develop symptoms because they were asked about them. On the other hand, some believed that community samples would be so eager to impress the interviewer as competent, virtuous, and psychologically healthy that they would deny symptoms directly asked about, particularly symptoms such as drinking, fighting, and promiscuity that clearly could not be attributed to physical illness. And finally, there was the problem of recall. Psychiatric diagnosis requires providing a history of symptoms. Many thought that recall beyond very brief periods is so faulty that the oral history collected by interview, unsupported by medical records contemporaneous with the symptoms, would be so error-ridden as to be useless.

THE HISTORY OF CATEGORICAL DIAGNOSIS IN EPIDEMIOLOGY

Beginnings Abroad

Outside of the United States, diagnostic epidemiological studies conducted by personal interview were flourishing while they were being avoided in the United States (for example, Essen-Moller, 1956; Helgason, 1964; Lin, 1953). These studies overcame some of the objections outlined above by concentrating on geographically circumscribed areas such as islands or rural communities, in which populations were stable and their psychiatric problems were well known to neighbors and local authorities. Interviews were conducted by psychiatrists, who may also have had the responsibility for the care of a large proportion of the patients in the area. Key informants, such as the local doctor, were often interviewed, as well as or instead of the affected person, thereby providing the access to medical records and intimate knowledge of the respondent missing in the one-chance personal interview. Diagnostic assessment was a global evaluation of the data gathered, and was made by the psychiatrist who had conducted the interview.

Developments from Clinical Interviews in the United States

In the United States during this period, the problems of large scale diagnostic research in the community were being approached indirectly. The standardized interviews that would later be used for diagnostic epidemiological studies were being designed, but they were being written to carry out clinical research, not epidemiologic studies.

In the 1940s and 1950s at Harvard and Washington University, systematic diagnostic interviews were developed to be used in a series of descriptive follow-up studies of patients, aimed at clarifying psychiatric nosology. Originally, each study covered only a single diagnostic category, such as anxiety neurosis (Wheeler et al, 1950) or hysteria (Cohen et al, 1953). The applicability of these interviews to members of the general population, and therefore to epidemiologic studies, was discovered when they worked well with control subjects selected to compare with the clinical cases from factory employee rosters, school records, voter registration lists, and from the patients' relatives and acquaintances. Even their effectiveness with clinical cases was reassuring because assessing these clinical cases was remarkably like assessing a general population sample. The patients were followed up so long after their contact with psychiatric services (up to 30 years) that many had forgotten their earlier treatment and no longer thought of themselves as patients.

Washington University researchers' experience with these nonpatients and expatients refuted many of the arguments that had been offered for omitting diagnoses in epidemiologic studies. The symptom questions necessary for diagnosis were generally answered correctly by these nonpatients and relatives of patients, even when symptoms had not been experienced for years, as verified by the original treatment records that formed the basis for patient selection and by the records gathered at follow-up from hospitals, police, and social agencies for both patients and nonpatients (Robins, 1966, 1974). Supposedly "discreditable" information appeared to be freely given. Refusal to answer questions was rare, even when the topic was as intimate as promiscuity and homosexual experiences. The consistent rank order of symptoms of a disorder across study populations, and across changes in wording and order of questions, suggested that answers were not unduly influenced by the interview climate, and therefore probably not the product of suggestion or embarrassment. Indeed, there were hints that the information obtained during a single follow-up contact by an interviewer previously unknown to the respondent might not be inferior to what could have been obtained by a doctor with a long-standing clinical relationship to the respondent. Refusal rates were lowest when interviews were conducted out of town, where the respondent realized that chances of ever having to confront the interviewer again were very small (Robins, 1963). Patients still in treatment sometimes asked whether their answers would be shared with their doctors, and agreed to reply only when assured that they would not be.

With the encouraging discovery that diagnostic material was accessible and reasonably valid in single interviews conducted by persons with no clinical relationship to the respondent, and as questions were improved or added with each successive study to broaden the range of diagnoses covered, researchers at Washington University moved into studies that lacked even a tenuous connection to clinical samples, although those surveyed were not random samples of the population. They included bereaved persons identified through burial permit reports in the newspapers and neighborhood controls for them (Clayton et al, 1968); relatives of suicides identified through coroners' records (Robins E et al, 1959); young black men identified in elementary school records (Robins et al, 1971); Vietnam soldiers identified from Department of Defense active duty rosters, and civilian controls identified from Selective Service records (Robins, 1974); and members of the Teamsters' union (Robins et al, 1977).

As the sample sizes grew, and as collecting follow-up interviews required travel to distant cities, use of lay interviewers was initiated. Their use meant that questions had to be entirely specified, so that lack of clinical training did not prevent their acquiring the necessary information. At first, diagnoses were made by consensus between two psychiatrists reviewing the interview protocol, but in time the psychiatrists helped to design computer programs that followed the decision rules they had themselves been using.

Eventually the diagnostic criteria shared by these studies were written down and a comprehensive diagnostic interview written to implement them. The criteria became the Feighner Criteria (Feighner et al, 1972) and the fully specified set of questions was the Renard Diagnostic Interview (RDI) (Helzer et al, 1981). The RDI provided a set of questions to ascertain each criterion item and a computer program to produce diagnoses. The Feighner Criteria were the basis from which the Research Diagnostic Criteria (RDC) were developed (Spitzer et al, 1978), which in turn served as a major source for the *Diagnostic and Statistical Manual of Mental Disorders (Third Edition) (DSM-III)*, published by the American Psychiatric Association in 1980.

At Columbia University, Robert Spitzer and Jean Endicott also drafted an interview, the Psychiatric Status Schedule (PSS), which had an associated diagnostic computer program, DIAGNO, for use in clinical studies, including the United States–United Kingdom study seeking to explain why rates of schizophrenia in hospitals on the two sides of the Atlantic differed so greatly (Spitzer and Endicott, 1968). This was followed by their coauthorship of the Schedule for Affective Disorders and Schizophrenia (SADS) (1977) for the NIMH Collaborative Study of Depression. The SADS provided the information necessary to make diagnoses according to the Research Diagnostic Criteria. In the course of that study, the SADS was used not only with patients, but also with their (nonpatient) relatives and their control subjects. For nonpatients, a special form of the interview was developed—SADS–L (L = lifetime)—because they often had no current episode to evaluate. Weissman and Myers (1978) then adapted the SADS–L interview for use in an epidemiologic study of the general population in New Haven, using well trained clinicians as interviewers. That study appears to have been the first American study to attempt diagnosis in a random sample of the general population.

While full-scale diagnostic interviews were rarely used in epidemiologic studies in the United States during the 1970s, like clinical psychiatry years earlier, interviews written to detect single diagnoses were being used. Particularly popular was the CES–D (Radloff, 1977) to detect depression (Husaini et al, 1979).

The Diagnostic Interview Schedule

The first broad spectrum diagnostic interview written specifically for use in large epidemiologic studies was the NIMH Diagnostic Interview Schedule (DIS) (Robins et al, 1979), designed for the Epidemiologic Catchment Area study, described in Chapter 27 of this volume. It covered criteria not only of the Feighner and RDC systems (as had its predecessors, the RDI and the SADS), but it added coverage of a considerable part of *DSM-III*. The coverage of *DSM-III* was broadened in successive editions to cover 43 diagnoses. The DIS could be given by lay interviewers and scored by computer. It provided standard sets of probes to be used when a symptom was found to have occurred. These allowed the lay interviewer to imitate, in part, a physician's usual pursuit of positive responses to determine their clinical significance and the circumstances in which they occurred.

The DIS provided a richer variety of data than had previous interviews, a richness that has increased in successive versions of the interview. Its most recent version (Robins and Helzer, 1986), with its accompanying computer programs, produces explanation for *why* each negative symptom was *not* positive (not present, not clinically significant, always physically explained), and dates the first and most recent occurrence of each positive symptom, and the first and most recent episode for episodic disorders. Diagnoses are reported both for the lifetime of the respondent and currently, with "current" defined for four different time periods: the last two weeks, the last month, the last six months, and the last year. Diagnoses are reported both with and without a variety of exclusion criteria, such as the presence of preempting diagnoses; for schizophrenia, the absence of current impairment; and for depression, the requirement that all episodes are not attributable to "uncomplicated" bereavement.

The Composite International Diagnostic Interview

The many researchers who have used the DIS in English or translated into their native languages have suggested the addition or modification of some symptom questions to fit local requirements. Some of their modifications have been incorporated into a new diagnostic interview for epidemiology that merges the DIS with the PSE to form the Composite International Diagnostic Interview, or CIDI (Robins et al, 1985). This interview was constructed at the request of the ADAMHA/WHO Task Force on Nosology for use in cross-national studies to determine empirically whether American and European diagnostic systems select the same or different cases for the same diagnoses. After the addition of necessary questions, it will also be used to show how the so-called culture-specific disorders are handled by the major national and international systems; that is, the diagnostic categories to which they are assigned and the frequency with which they fall through each system's diagnostic net.

Modifications of Clinical Interviews for Epidemiologic Use

While no other comprehensive diagnostic interview has been written for use in the general population, in Europe, the PSE (originally written for the two World Health Organization (WHO) initiated studies described above) has been adapted for use in the general population (Brown et al, 1977). While the PSE's chief author, John Wing, keeps reminding its users that it is not truly a general diagnostic interview because it is restricted to syndromes present in the last four weeks and covers fully only a limited number of diagnostic syndromes, Brown's adaptation has expanded the interval covered to the last year, while restricting its coverage essentially to depression and anxiety for use in the general population.

Currently, two new interviews are under construction for use in clinical populations. John Wing is writing the SCAN to cover *DSM-III* diagnoses as well as the diagnoses covered in PSE, and Robert Spitzer and Janet Williams are writing the Structured Clinical Interview for DSM-III-R (SCID) (which is similar to the SADS but will make diagnoses according to the revision of *DSM-III*, *DSM-III-R*, to be published in 1987). If history repeats itself, these two interviews will eventually be modified for use in the general population, perhaps along with another comprehensive interview written only for clinical use, the Psychiatric Diagnostic Interview (PDI) (Othmer et al, 1981).

DIAGNOSTIC EPIDEMIOLOGY WITHOUT SURVEYS

We have recounted the history of diagnostic epidemiologic interviews as though population surveys were our sole source of diagnostic information. While the ascertainment of diagnoses by personal interview in general populations in the United States has had a relatively short history and a remarkable recent flourishing, diagnostically informed epidemiology based on treatment records has a long and distinguished history in the United States and elsewhere. Epidemiologic results are achieved by linking comprehensive sets of clinical records to census data for the areas served by the institutions providing the records.

In 1939, Faris and Dunham related diagnoses in public hospitals in Chicago to the characteristics of the residential areas from which the patients came. Levy and Rowitz (1973) repeated the study in Chicago years later, as Dunham himself did in Detroit (1965). Hollingshead and Redlich (1953) achieved a virtually complete count of treated cases by diagnosis in New Haven to study the relation between social class and the prevalence of specific diagnoses. Malzberg (1963) used records of the state hospitals of New York to study ethnic differences by disorder. These records have also served to link diagnosis to economic changes (Brenner, 1967).

Another boost to diagnostic epidemiology came with the development of psychiatric case registers. These registers made available area-wide diagnostic information for clinic outpatients and private patients both in and out of hospitals, as well as for patients of public hospitals, providing a count of all cases treated in the mental health specialty sector. In the United States, register-based research flourished (Bahn et al, 1966) until registers were discontinued because they were too expensive to maintain and the 1974 Privacy Law limited their research use. A great tradition of register-based research in Scotland and England suffered a similar loss of support.

The problems with epidemiologic studies based only on psychiatric record data from psychiatric facilities are fourfold: First, they omit cases treated by nonspecialists. Second, they tell us nothing about the frequency of untreated cases in the community. Third, the quality of the diagnoses may be below research standards. When Dunham repeated his study in Detroit, he returned to the records to satisfy himself that the cases diagnosed as schizophrenia actually deserved that diagnosis, and found many to reject. Thus, even the landmark study by Hollingshead and Redlich still leaves us uncertain as to whether the high rate of schizophrenia found in their lowest social class is a correct observation. Alternative explanations are that psychiatrists' diagnoses are class-biased, or that the findings are an artifact of differences in training backgrounds of those psychiatrists who serve the poor in public hospitals and those who treat the well-to-do in private offices. The fourth difficulty stems from the fact that the demographic information available in psychiatric records describes the patient as of the time of admission, but not the patient's characteristics before he or she became sick. This limits the items that can be treated as risk factors for a disorder rather than as its consequences to those that cannot change, such as sex and race. Socioeconomic status and place of residence cannot be interpreted since, for example, schizophrenics may cluster in the lower classes and live in the inner city, not because they began there, but only because their disorder made them unfit for well paid occupations (Goldberg and Morrison, 1963). Interviews can solve this problem by seeking historical information about place of rearing and father's occupation when the respondent was a child.

EVALUATING A DIAGNOSTIC INTERVIEW

Now that the onetime personal diagnostic interview has emerged as a feasible method for ascertaining symptoms and history of course of disorder in the general population, and a method in many ways superior to the use of routinely collected clinical records, we need to know how to assess and compare the usefulness of available interviews for various purposes. In the remainder of this chapter I will discuss how to evaluate their design, interviewer preparation, how to assess their reliability and validity, for which disorders they are inappropriate, populations in which they can be used, and, finally, their possible utility in clinical rather than epidemiological settings.

The ideal diagnostic interview produces accurate information reliably. To do so, it must not require unusual skills on the part of the interviewer, and it must not be unduly influenced by transitory states in the respondent. The data it produces must denote symptoms clearly enough so that a definite decision can be made as to whether the criteria of the diagnostic system in use have been met.

Question Design

Techniques developed by survey researchers for writing questions that are easily understood, inoffensive, and that elicit unambiguous responses can contribute a great deal to the accuracy and reliability of diagnostic interviews. These rules include keeping the language simple and nonjudgmental, covering only a single idea in a single question, and seeing that possible responses fall into predictable fixed alternatives (for example, "yes," "three"). Questions must specify the time span to be considered, and must avoid words that can be legitimately defined differently by different respondents or by the same respondent at different times. Common offenders are words such as "frequently" and "often." Preferable are phrases such as "more than once a week."

Many psychological tests reverse questions so that some yes responses signify health and others signify pathology to avoid response set or "nay-saying." This seldom works well for diagnostic interviews, and is likely to cause more confusion than remedy. These interviews transparently ask about problems, and it is easy for a respondent to deny them. Fortunately, most respondents in the general population are willing to answer accurately *so long as no adverse consequences can ensue.* To maximize valid answers, the respondent must understand that answers are confidential, and the interview must be conducted in private, where family and friends cannot listen in.

Interviewer Training

Interviewer training aims to prepare the interviewer for all possible responses to the questions through training manuals and supervised practice interviews, using prepared scripts covering examples of the range of responses that can be encountered. After training, careful and timely editing of interviews and occasional retesting against a criterion interview keep interviewers from drifting away from the practices learned in training.

Even when epidemiologic interviews spell out questions and follow-up probes to positive responses, they are not reliably and validly answered unless the interviewer listens carefully to answers to be certain that the question was understood and appropriately answered. Respondents eager to tell their stories often fail to listen to the whole question, but instead associate to it the problem on their mind. Teaching interviewers tactful ways of asking the respondent to pay attention to the question in full is a vital part of interviewer training. The fact that psychiatric interviews can be written for which *clinical* training is not a prerequisite does not mean that interviewers become automatons.

Measuring Reliability

There are two common methods for assessing reliability—an observer sitting in on an interview and scoring it independently, and a test-retest strategy with independent interviewers, both with skill levels and training characteristic of interviewers to be used in future studies, and both asking questions and recording responses, with the second interviewer blind to what happened in the first interview.

It has been widely agreed that the second strategy is the more rigorous, because it allows responses to vary as well as their scoring, and prevents the falsely high concordance in scoring that can arise because the observer guesses from the interviewer's behavior how he has scored a response. However, the test-retest design turns out to have its own problems.

A number of studies have now shown that second interviews produce fewer positive responses (Robins, 1985). This happens because there is no way to make a test-retest design *double* blind. The second interviewer can be blind to what was said in the first interview, but the respondent recalls the previous interview, and this seems to affect the second interview. A number of hypotheses have been offered as to why this might be so—the respondent is bored and unmotivated the second time; he or she has learned that positive answers lead to follow-up questions, and denies symptoms to keep the interview short; the respondent misunderstands the goal of the study and thinks it unnecessary to repeat what he or she remembers already having reported; the first interview was therapeutic, and the respondent's improved mental state makes his or her history of symptoms look less severe and not worth reporting; the first interview taught the respondent all the symptoms it is possible to have that he or she does *not* have, and the respondent's own burden now appears smaller; the respondent overreported in the first interview because he or she thought the interviewer would be disappointed with a long succession of negative responses; the respondent was caught off guard by the first interview and admitted to symptoms he or she now regrets having reported. Whatever the reasons for the negative bias in the second interview, the test-retest design cannot be a good measure of the reliability of the first interview, since the assumption that the two interviews are equivalent is clearly not met.

An additional problem with the test-retest design is that new symptoms can emerge in the interval between interviews which could not have been reported in the first interview. Unfortunately, reducing this problem by keeping the interval between interviews brief only increases the distortion caused by the respondent's recall during the second interview of what was said in the first.

No methods have yet been suggested to overcome these problems in assessing reliability. Although the development of the DIS can be faulted because rigorous tests for reliability have not been carried out, with these design problems, it is not clear how valuable such tests would be.

Assessing Validity

Testing the validity of a standardized personal diagnostic interview is equally problematic, because there are no laboratory tests for psychiatric disorders that can function as independent yardsticks to show whether it produces correct diagnoses. The external yardsticks that are available, such as the histories in hospital records, are generally themselves interview-based and therefore possibly biased by the same factors that have biased the standardized interview being tested.

CONTENT VALIDITY. The clarity with which symptoms are denoted can be determined in large part by examining the interview protocol itself along with its computer programs and comparing them to the diagnostic manual to be served. This assesses "content validity." The interview questions must match the sense of the criteria despite the constraint of having to be easily understood and answerable by fixed alternative responses. The decision rules specified by the diagnostic system must be clearly reflected in the computer algorithms.

EMPIRICAL TESTS OF VALIDITY. Other measures of validity require empirical tests of the interview's function. However, designing empirical studies to assess the validity of a psychiatric diagnostic instrument has turned out to be a difficult problem, for which our current tools seem not entirely adequate (Robins, 1985).

The options that have been considered for measuring validity are 1) comparing the diagnostic results of the standardized interview with diagnoses selected by an experienced clinician following a single interview—what Spitzer (1980) has called a test for "procedural" validity; 2) comparing the diagnostic results with a clinician's diagnosis using a set of data such as might be amassed in treating a patient, including not only the clinician's interview with the patient, but also a review of any existing records of treatment, an interview with an informed family member, and a physical examination (called a "best estimate" criterion) (Leckman et al, 1982); 3) assessment of the ability of the diagnostic interview to predict past and future functioning and past and future treatment seeking, positive response to treatments thought specific to the disorder, or the same diagnoses in family members. This latter set of tests constitute "predictive validity," which is generally thought to be the strongest test. However, even this test has its problems because a) the same disorder can have varying outcomes, and b) many disorders may share a similar outcome, such as disability. The value of predictive tests depends on how specific the outcome criterion is to the disorder of interest. Thus, a positive response to lithium is stronger evidence for affective disorder than is a response to psychotherapy or hospitalization; and a close relative's hospitalization for affective disorder is stronger evidence than is "mental disorder in the family."

Obviously, these alternative ways of assessing validity have very different costs and also differ greatly in how rapidly an answer is obtained. The comparison with an interview by a clinician is the cheapest and quickest, but probably the least satisfactory. Clinicians are notoriously unreliable diagnosticians. And when they are faced with making diagnoses from a system such as *DSM-III*, which contains over 200 diagnostic categories (each of which has specific criteria that must be met) the chances are low that they will apply criteria rigorously unless they use some sort of structured decision tree, which itself constitutes a standardized interview of untested accuracy. If a clinician's structured interview is used as the yardstick, the outcome will be influenced by how much agreement in interpretation of the diagnostic criteria there is between the authors of the two instruments. Because all diagnostic systems are ambiguous in some areas, differences of interpretation are not necessarily evidence for error.

An effort at assessing the predictive validity of first interviews in the St. Louis ECA data looks at responses to a follow-up interview one year later for more than 300 respondents who had been interviewed by both a lay interviewer and a psychiatrist (Helzer, 1986). Diagnoses made by the clinician were no better or worse than the diagnoses constructed by computer from the lay-administered epidemiologic diagnostic interview, in predicting whether one year later they would report similar psychiatric disorders in relatives, or whether they had sought treatment in the subsequent year; both diagnoses did much better than chance. These results question whether a clinician's interview has sufficiently better predictive validity than a fully structured interview given by a lay interviewer to warrant its use as a validity criterion.

Rigorous studies have yet to be done to compare the various options for assessing the validity of a structured diagnostic interview. One study (Leckman et al, 1982) suggested that the "best estimate" method might not be as great an improvement over a test for procedural validity as one might hope, because histories given about family members are much less reliable than a history given about oneself.

No matter which standard is selected against which to evaluate a structured interview, there remains the problem that a test of validity can predict the future success of an instrument only in a population with the same prevalence of disorder as the population in which the test was carried out. Sensitivity and specificity, the statistics traditionally used to assess validity, have been shown to vary with the prevalence of the disorder in the population (Robins, 1985). This means that an instrument with good validity in a clinical setting may do poorly in the community and vice versa. It also means that published validity data for two different interviews tested in different populations cannot be compared to decide which is the more valid instrument.

Other Criteria for the Value of a Diagnostic Interview

Validity and reliability are not the only grounds on which a diagnostic interview should be judged. Additional issues are the breadth of populations in which it can be used, the variety of diagnoses covered, and the versatility of data provided for each diagnosis.

BREADTH OF POPULATION: CROSS-CULTURAL APPROPRIATE-NESS. Interviews in wide current use were developed in western cultures where the opinion survey was a well accepted tradition. Although diagnostic interviews ask about feelings and behavior instead of attitudes, cooperation with them may have been prompted by the same motivation to contribute to scientific research that has motivated cooperation with public opinion surveys. One might imagine that gaining cooperation with diagnostic interviewing would be more difficult in cultures that lack this tradition. Surprisingly, experience with the DIS in less industrialized cultures shows lower refusal rates than in more industrialized settings (Canino in Puerto Rico, Yu in Shanghai, Hwu in Taiwan, personal communications). This parallels the higher levels of cooperation in rural than in urban areas of industrialized countries. Perhaps citizens in less industrialized settings have not been oversurveyed, and treat the professional interviewer with greater respect.

The fact that people will answer a diagnostic interview in a variety of cultures is no guarantee that their responses are comparable. Arguments remain as to whether some of the words and phrases describing symptoms in western culture have equivalents in other languages and, if not, whether the same sense can be evoked by circumlocutions. Answers to questions can have different meanings in different cultures. The DIS used in China, for example, had high rates of agreement to a question asking if one's sex life had been unimportant, something "one could have gotten along as well without" (Yu, personal communication.) In America this question worked well to detect inhibited sexual desire. In China it seemed to be asking the respondent whether he or she was a serious person, dedicated to important social goals, rather than hedonism; agreement was associated with high self-esteem, not psychiatric disorder. Such problems in translation and communication need to be confronted and solved by persons who know both cultures well.

BREADTH OF POPULATION: DEMOGRAPHIC SUBGROUPS. Within a given culture, questions should apply as broadly as possible. Thus there should be questions about school and homemaking chores as alternatives to questions about work for young people not yet in the work force and for homemakers, and questions about sexual partners for the unmarried.

Attempts to include children and adolescents present special problems. The issues still under discussion include the minimum age at which an interview designed for adults can be used, whether interviews for children and adults can have similar formats, by what age one can do without collaborative data from parents and teachers, and whether a single interview can be written that serves the whole age range in which interviewing children is feasible. Diagnostic interviews for children that do not require clinician interviews currently include the Diagnostic Interview Schedule for Children (DISC), developed under the guidance of NIMH, and the Diagnostic Interview for Children and Adolescents (DICA) developed at Washington University.

Diagnostic Coverage

The ideal would be a diagnostic interview that is comprehensive so that every psychiatrically disordered person could be correctly diagnosed. However, some psychiatric disorders limit the affected person's ability to participate in a psychiatric interview. Although persons with severe mental retardation or dementia can be tested by the interviewer for current intellectual impairment, they cannot respond accurately to questions about their histories. This makes it impossible to assign them on the basis of a personal interview alone to a specific organic mental disorder, since assignment requires knowing the etiology. Clearly an informant or medical records are necessary once impairment is established.

It is also difficult to make a diagnosis of schizophrenia in those whose psychotic symptoms are controlled by medication. In clinical practice as well as epidemiologic studies, they may fail to recall their psychotic symptoms. Records and informants must be sought whenever there are psychiatric hospitalizations, or periods in sheltered workshops or sheltered living arrangements that the respondent cannot account for. To detect such clues, a diagnostic interview should be accompanied by at least a few questions about history of impairment.

Other disorders that may require informant interviews are the personality disorders. The respondent may be unaware that he or she has the diagnostic trait. For example, few respondents with paranoid personality would recognize in themselves *DSM-III* Criterion C, lack of a true sense of humor.

THE PRODUCTS OF DIAGNOSTIC INTERVIEWS

We have focused on the ability of diagnostic interviews to categorize a respondent according to an established diagnostic system. A diagnosis by computer is achieved by putting together a variety of intermediary categorizations of symptoms and dates of onset and offset. These building blocks can have considerable value in their own right. The computer can put these items into narrative form for use in an individual patient's chart or tabulate them to describe groups of respondents. The limits are set by the detail in which questions are asked, and how many of the responses obtained are entered discretely into the computer.

Table 1 illustrates the range of data available from the most recent version of the DIS, Version III-B (Robins and Helzer, 1986), given its current set of computer algorithms. This long list does not exhaust the analyses that could be performed. The DIS provides a broader range of information than other diagnostic interviews because almost all items that contribute to a diagnostic decision are directly entered into the computer, and intermediate results are saved by the computer program. This allows describing the course of disorder and showing how it met criteria. When multiple diagnoses occur in the same individual, the computer programs show which came first and whether the diagnoses overlapped in time. With or without a positive diagnosis, the computer programs provide the number of symptoms, the correlations among symptoms, and the order in which symptoms emerge and disappear.

USE OF STANDARDIZED INTERVIEWS
IN CLINICAL PRACTICE

We have shown how diagnostic interviews for epidemiological research developed from clinical interviews, and how far they have come in applicability to a broad variety of populations. It is time now to consider whether these interviews can be of use to the clinician.

Table 1 is based on much the same data the clinician typically collects in the course of making a diagnosis, but which he or she may not record systematically, and which the clinician certainly does not computerize to discover the patterning of symptoms. If a structured interview is used and entered into a computer, these data become available. In addition, following its protocol assures the clinician that no important area of inquiry will have been overlooked, and protects against premature closure in making a diagnostic decision. The computer diagnosis makes certain that *DSM-III* diagnostic rules have been followed.

A structured diagnostic interview provides the novice psychiatrist or the primary care physician with question wordings that have been tested and shown to be understood by a wide variety of respondents. More experienced clinicians are likely to prefer their own wording. However, even they might be willing to consider sacrificing their preferred phrases in order to have the opportunity to compare their patient populations with normal and clinical populations surveyed in the course of the large number of studies using standardized interviews.

Table 1. Information That Can Be Obtained by Computer from the Diagnostic Interview Schedule (DIS), Version 3B

For a Single Patient

I. For any specified symptom:
Did the symptom ever occur?
Was it clinically significant?
May it be a psychiatric symptom or was it always explained by physical causes?
How old was the respondent the first time it occurred?
If this year, did it begin within the
last two weeks?
last month?
last six months?
last year?
How old was the respondent the last time it occurred?
If this year, did it occur within the
last two weeks?
last month?
last six months?
last year?

II. Across symptoms:
How many symptoms have ever occurred?
At what age did the symptom occur? (If this year, within the last two weeks, month, six months, year?)
How recently was the symptom experienced? (If this year, within the last two weeks, month, six months, year?)
How many symptoms were present in the last two weeks, last month, last six months, last year?
How many symptoms had occurred before any specified age?

III. For each diagnosis:
Has the respondent ever had a symptom of this diagnosis?
Which symptoms has the respondent had?
In what order did the symptoms appear?
How old was the respondent at the first symptom of this diagnosis?
Has the respondent discussed any of these symptoms with a doctor?
Which *DSM-III* criteria for the diagnosis has the respondent met?
At what age was each criterion first met?
Which criteria were met within the last two weeks, last month, last six months, last year?
How long was it between the first symptom and the last?
Has the respondent ever met all the criteria for this diagnosis? If so:
At what age were criteria first met?
Did the respondent meet all criteria in the last two weeks, last month, last six months, last year?
How long did the disorder last from the first symptom till the last?

IV. Across diagnoses:
   What diagnoses has the patient met criteria for in his or her lifetime?
      Which began first?
      Which diagnoses overlapped in time?
      Did any disorder occur only when another diagnosis was present?
   Of how many diagnoses has the respondent had at least one, two, or
      more symptoms?
   From what diagnosis was the respondent's earliest symptom?
   For which diagnosis did the respondent first meet criteria?
   What diagnoses overlapped temporally?
   Did symptoms of one or more diagnosis occur only within the period
      that another diagnosis was also present?

For a Population or a Sub-group
   I. For any specified symptom:
      What is its prevalence in the population in last two weeks, last month,
         six months, or year?
      What is its average age of onset?
      At what age does it typically remit?
      What is its average duration?
      In what population groups is it common?

   II. Across symptoms:
      On average, how many symptoms has the population ever experi-
         enced? In which diagnostic groups?
      How many symptoms, on average, have been experienced in the last
         two weeks, last month, six months, year?
      Across pairs of symptoms, which typically appears first?

   III. For any specific diagnosis:
      What is its prevalence in the population in last two weeks, last month,
         six months, or year?
      What is the average age of persons who currently show symptoms?
      What is the average age at which its first symptom appears?
      What is the average age of remission?
      What is the average age at which criteria are first met?
      In what population groups is it common?

   IV. Across diagnoses:
      Which diagnoses commonly coexist?
      If any pair of diagnoses both appear, which typically appears first?
      If any pair of diagnoses both appear, which typically remits first?

Spitzer has, in part jokingly, asked whether psychiatrists are still necessary
after the DIS (1983). The new interview he is preparing, the Structured Clinical
Interview for *DSM-III-R* (SCID) will continue to require psychiatrists as interviewers. But, in fact, he has nothing to worry about. Even if an interview
developed primarily to be used by lay interviewers did as well or better than

---

the average clinician at diagnostic assessment, there would be no need to fear that it would displace psychiatrists, any more than internists or general practitioners have been displaced by laboratory technicians' collecting blood samples and submitting them for computerized testing.

Standardized interviews that can be administered by a well trained office assistant can save a psychiatrist's time; and even the time of the office assistant can be saved if the interview is adapted to computer administration, so that a patient can fill in all or large parts of the history alone, producing a document that covers many of the topics the doctor would like answers to, and which can be quickly scanned to signal areas that need further investigation. But no matter how helpful the clinician may find the standardized interview in indicating current and past diagnoses, it will not produce a treatment plan or give an adequate picture of disability level or complicating social and medical factors. Diagnosis is only one step in planning and carrying out treatment.

For nonspecialists, the structured interview may be particularly helpful because it offers tried and true ways of asking questions about topics they may find difficult; and by putting the answers together to produce a diagnosis according to the official nomenclature, the structured interview can guide their referral decisions.

CONCLUSION

Standardized diagnostic interviews have been designed for use in the general population, and computer algorithms written to combine responses to these interviews to test whether criteria specific to many of the diagnoses in the standard psychiatric nomenclature have been met. The surveys in which they have been administered by persons without clinical experience, trained over a reasonably brief period, have response and completion rates equal to or better than those of well run opinion surveys, showing that the interviews are acceptable in the general population both in the United States and in other countries.

Diagnostic information collected by surveying the general population has clear advantages over results from surveys that obtain only global assessments of mental health, and results from studies that estimate prevalences by linking treatment records; and the studies undertaken show that diagnostic surveys are feasible. Yet their accuracy has not yet been firmly established because the tests that can be done quickly are not good measures of either reliability or validity. Longer range studies that use the results to predict course and correlates of disorder may give more definitive answers.

While diagnostic survey instruments were written for large-scale epidemiologic studies, they may be useful to the clinician who wants to be certain that he or she has been exhaustive in considering diagnostic alternatives and has applied diagnostic criteria rigorously, as well as to the clinician who wants to save time by having new patients prescreened for diagnosis-relevant symptoms by a medical assistant prior to a more detailed and intensive assessment. The novice psychiatrist and the nonpsychiatrist may find that they provide useful ways of phrasing difficult questions.

Because standardized diagnostic interviews can be important to epidemiological research and to clinicians, further efforts to develop methods for assessing their accuracy and improving their reliability, for example, by computerizing their administration, will be valuable.

REFERENCES

American Psychiatric Association: Diagnostic and Statistical Manual of Mental Disorders, Third Edition (DSM-III). Washington, DC, American Psychiatric Association, 1980

Bahn AK, Gardner EA, Alltop L, et al: Admission and prevalence rates for psychiatric facilities in four register areas. Am J Public Health 56:2033-2051, 1966

Brenner MH: Economic change and mental hospitalization: New York State, 1910–1960. Social Psychiatry 2:180-188, 1967

Brodman K, Deutschberger J, Erdmann AJ, et al: Prediction of adequacy for military service. U.S. Armed Forces Medical Journal 5:1802-1808, 1954

Brown GW, Davidson S, Harris T, et al: Psychiatric disorder in London and North Ulster. Soc Sci Med 2:367-377, 1977

Clayton P, Desmarais L, Winokur G: A study of normal bereavement. Am J Psychiatry 125:168-178, 1968

Cohen ME, Robins E, Purtell JJ, et al: Excessive surgery in hysteria. JAMA 151:997-986, 1953

Dohrenwend BP, Dohrenwend BS: Social Status and Psychological Disorder. New York, Wiley-Interscience, 1969

Dohrenwend BP, Dohrenwend BS: Perspectives on the past and future of psychiatric epidemiology. Am J Public Health 72:1271-1279, 1982

Dunham HW: Community and Schizophrenia. Detroit, Wayne State University Press, 1965

Eastwood MR: The Relation between Physical and Mental Illness. Toronto, University of Toronto Press, 1975

Essen-Moller E: Individual traits and morbidity in a Swedish rural population. Acta Psychiatrica et Neurologica Scandinavica (Suppl.) 100:1-60, 1956

Faris REL, Dunham HW: Mental Disorders in Urban Areas. New York, Hafner, 1960

Feighner JP, Robins E, Guze SB, et al: Diagnostic criteria for use in psychiatric research. Arch Gen Psychiatry 26:57-63, 1972

Goldberg EM, Morrison SL: Schizophrenia and social class. Br J Psychiatry 109:785-802, 1963

Gurin G, Veroff J, Feld S: Americans View their Mental Health. New York, Basic Books, 1960

Helgason T: Epidemiology of Mental Disorders in Iceland. Copenhagen, Munksgaard, 1964

Helzer JE: Psychiatric case identification in the general population—the DIS, in Proceedings of the International Symposium on Psychiatric Epidemiology. Edited by Yeh E-K (in press)

Helzer JE, Robins LN, Croughan JL, et al: Renard Diagnostic Interview: its reliability and procedural validity with physicians and lay interviewers. Arch Gen Psychiatry 38:393-398, 1981

Hollingshead AB, Redlich FC: Social stratification and psychiatric disorders. American Sociological Review 18:163-169, 1953

Husaini BA, Neff JA, Stone RH: Psychiatric impairment in rural communities. Journal of Community Psychology 7:137-146, 1979

Langner TS, Greene EL, Herson JH, et al: Psychiatric impairment in welfare and non-welfare children. Welfare in Review 7:10-21, 1969

Lapouse R, Monk MA: Fears and worries in a representative sample of children. Am J Orthopsychiatry 29:803-818, 1959

Leckman JF, Sholomskas D, Thompson WD, et al: Best estimate of lifetime psychiatric diagnosis. Arch Gen Psychiatry 39:879-883, 1982

Leighton DC, Harding JS, Macklin MA, et al: Psychiatric findings of the Stirling County study. Am J Psychiatry 119:1021-1026, 1963

Levy L, Rowitz L: The Ecology of Mental Disorder. New York, Behavioral Publications, 1973

Lin T-y: A study of the incidence of mental disorder in Chinese and other cultures. Psychiatry 16:313-336. 1953

Malzberg B: The Mental Health of the Negro. Albany, Research Foundation for Mental Hygiene, 1963

Othmer E, Penick EC, Powell BJ: Psychiatric Diagnostic Interview (PDI). Los Angeles, Western Psychological Services, 1981

Radloff LS: The CES–D scale: A self-report depression scale for research in the general population. Applied Psychological Measurement 1:385-401, 1977

Robins E, Murphy GE, Wilkinson RH Jr, et al: Some clinical considerations in the prevention of suicide based on a study of 134 successful suicides. Am J Public Health 49:888-889, 1959

Robins LN: The reluctant respondent. Public Opinion Quarterly 27:276-286, 1963

Robins LN: Deviant Children Grown Up. Baltimore, Williams & Wilkins, 1966.

Robins LN: The Vietnam Drug User Returns. Special Action Office Monograph, Series A, No. 2. Washington, DC, U.S. Government Printing Office, 1974

Robins LN: Epidemiology: reflections on testing the validity of psychiatric interviews. Arch Gen Psychiatry 42:918-924, 1985

Robins LN, Helzer JE: The Diagnostic Interview Schedule, Version 3B 1986

Robins LN, Murphy GE, Woodruff RA Jr, et al: The adult psychiatric status of black school boys. Arch Gen Psychiatry 24:338-345, 1971

Robins LN, West PA, Murphy GE: The high rate of suicide in older white men: a study testing 10 hypotheses. Social Psychiatry 12:1-20, 1977

Robins LN, Helzer JE, Croughan JL, et al: The NIMH Diagnostic Interview Schedule (DIS). Bethesda, Maryland, National Institutes of Health, 1979

Robins LN, Helzer JE, Weissman M, et al: Lifetime prevalence of specific psychiatric disorders in three sites. Arch Gen Psychiatry 41:949-958, 1984

Robins LN, Wing J, Helzer J: The Composite International Diagnostic Interview (CIDI). Geneva, World Health Organization, 1985

Spitzer RL: Psychiatric diagnosis: are clinicians still necessary? Compr Psychiatry 24:399-411, 1983

Spitzer RL, Endicott J: DIAGNO: A computer program for psychiatric diagnosis utilizing the differential diagnostic procedure. Arch Gen Psychiatry 18:746-756, 1968

Spitzer RL, Endicott J: Schedule for Affective Disorders and Schizophrenia. New York, 1977

Spitzer RL, Williams JBW. Classification of mental disorders and DSM-III, in Comprehensive Textbook of Psychiatry, third edition. Edited by Kaplan H, Freedman A, Sadock B. Baltimore, Williams & Wilkins, 1980

Spitzer RL, Endicott J, Robins E: Research diagnostic criteria: rationale and reliability. Arch Gen Psychiatry 35:773-782, 1978

Srole L, Langner TS, Michael ST, et al: Mental Health in the Metropolis. New York, McGraw-Hill, 1962

Star SA: The screening of psychoneurotics in the army, in Measurement and Prediction, vol 4. Edited by Stouffer SA, Guttman L, Suchman EA, et al. Princeton, Princeton University Press, 1950.

Uhlenhuth EH, Lipman RS, Balter MB, et al: Symptom intensity and life stress in the city. Arch Gen Psychiatry 31:759-764, 1974

Weissman MM, Myers JK: Psychiatric disorders in a U.S. urban community. Arch Gen Psychiatry 35:1304-1311, 1978

Wheeler EO, White PD, Reed EW, et al: Neurocirculatory asthenia (anxiety neurosis, effort syndrome, neurasthenia). JAMA 142:878-888, 1950

Wing JK, Cooper JE, Sartorius N: Measurement and Classification of Psychiatric Symptoms. Cambridge, England, Cambridge University Press, 1974

World Health Organization: Report of the International Pilot Study of Schizophrenia. Geneva, World Health Organization, 1973

Chapter 27

Psychiatric Disorders in the Community: The Epidemiologic Catchment Area Study

by Darrel A. Regier, M.D., M.P.H., and
Jack D. Burke, Jr., M.D., M.P.H.

Mental disorder epidemiology has been defined as the quantitative study of the distribution and causes of mental disorders in human populations (Regier and Burke, 1985). Epidemiologic studies begin by identifying a population about which information on the distribution and characteristics of individuals with mental disorders is desired. Although small populations in clinical settings are often studied by epidemiologic methods, the focus of this chapter will be on community studies of psychiatric disorder and their importance to clinicians.

CLINICAL USES OF EPIDEMIOLOGY

Community Diagnosis

Epidemiologic surveys of a community population may be conceptualized in public health terms as providing a community diagnosis in contrast to diagnosis of an individual patient. Community diagnostic information of this type is important for determining when rates of any illness or its consequences are higher than expected, such as in "epidemics" of youth suicide. Baseline information may also be provided for determining the proportion of individuals with mental disorders receiving services, and where they are treated, in order to develop an optimal treatment and referral system or establish the need for additional service resources.

Completing the Clinical Picture

Community studies are useful not only for identifying base rates and treatment rates, but also for identifying subclinical or mild cases of disorders that normally

The Epidemiologic Catchment Area Program is a series of five epidemiologic research studies performed by independent research teams in collaboration with staff of the Division of Biometry and Epidemiology (DBE) of the National Institute of Mental Health (NIMH). The NIMH Principal Collaborators are Darrel A. Regier, Ben Z. Locke, and Jack D. Burke, Jr.; the NIMH Project Officer is Carl A. Taube. The Principal Investigators and Co-Investigators from the five sites are: Yale University, U01 MH–34224—Jerome K. Myers, Myrna M. Weissman, and Gary Tischler; The Johns Hopkins University, U01 MH–33870—Morton Kramer, and Sam Shapiro; Washington University, St. Louis, U01 MH–33883—Lee M. Robins and John Helzer; Duke University, U01 MH–35386—Dan Blazer and Linda George; University of California, Los Angeles, U01 MH–35865—Marvin Karno, Richard L. Hough, Javier Escobar, Audrey Burnam, and Diane Timbers.

---

do not appear in physicians' offices. The identification of such disorders is important for determining the natural clinical course and prognosis for disorders in a representative sample. The alternative is to assess clinical outcome from a biased sample of the most severe cases which are found disproportionately in specialists' offices.

An additional benefit in completing the clinical picture is to identify the familial occurrence of disorders by pursuing a population genetics research strategy (discussed in Chapter 28). Follow-up studies with relatives of individuals with and without specific mental disorders may be drawn from a total community population, to avoid the same type of sampling bias with relatives that was discussed previously with patients.

Assessing Individual Risks

Once the base rates of disorders (including the full range of severity) are determined, and longitudinal follow-up studies are done of such cases, community studies may also be used to identify population groups with unusually high rates of a mental disorder. The correlates of disorders assessed may be physical, biological, social, and temporal characteristics of individuals and their environments. Characteristics associated with groups having high disorder rates are identified in order ultimately to identify risk factors, which, if altered, will interrupt a causal network producing a disorder. However, community studies are often so demanding in accomplishing the first objectives that additional case control or prospective cohort studies are required for more focused studies of putative risk factors.

EXAMPLES OF PAST STUDIES

Although there have been a large number of studies worldwide attempting to identify rates of mental disorders in communities, we will briefly mention three which have particular significance for the United States. These include the Stirling County study (Leighton, et al, 1963), the Midtown Manhattan study (Srole, 1962), and the Baltimore Morbidity study (Commission on Chronic Illness, 1957). All three studies took place in the early to mid-1950s, and were sophisticated advances for this period in identifying base rates of psychopathology in community populations. However, there was considerable variation both in their definition or diagnostic criteria for psychopathology and in the case identification instruments used in assessing the diagnostic status of their study subjects. A fourth community based study was conducted in New Haven in the mid-1970s which, although conducted on a relatively small, nonrepresentative sample, demonstrated use of an advanced diagnostic assessment instrument (Weissman et al, 1978).

The Stirling County study identified 32 detailed symptom patterns and used the general diagnostic guidelines of the *DSM-I* (American Psychiatric Association, 1952). The Baltimore study used the international statistical classification of disorders, but the Midtown Manhattan study focused entirely on a graded scale of mental ill-health covering six different levels of severity from mild to severe. Based on these differences in diagnostic criteria, there was also considerable variation in case identification technique, which ranged from lay survey interviewers with psychiatrists reviewing the information for final assessments, to general practitioners providing screening and diagnostic information later scored by psychiatrists.

What all three surveys shared was a sophisticated sampling design that allowed generalization from the study sample to the entire population of the community of interest. However, significant limitations existed in the clinical meaningfulness of the diagnostic criteria and the application of those criteria in the diagnostic assessment instruments used. It was difficult to assess the base rates of specific types of mental disorders which were seen in clinicians' inpatient wards or outpatient offices. Very limited data were obtained on the proportion of individuals with such disorders who actually received diagnostic and treatment services for primary care or specialty mental health settings. Finally, the complexity and idiosyncratic nature of many of these studies precluded replication to determine the degree to which findings were limited to given geographic or sociodemographic characteristics of the population studied.

THE EPIDEMIOLOGIC CATCHMENT AREA STUDY

Historical Context

It is of historical interest to note that the previously mentioned community studies took place shortly after World War II when there was a high level of concern about the large number of Americans who were rejected from the Armed Services because of psychiatric disorder, and because of the high number of psychiatric casualties that occurred under the stressful conditions of war. Public pressure for a determination of the total scope of mental disorders helped launch the National Institute of Mental Health and generated support for conducting the three previously mentioned community studies, as well as the Hollingshead and Redlich study of treated populations in New Haven published as *Social Class and Mental Illness* (Hollingshead and Redlich, 1958).

A different confluence of historical events made possible the Epidemiological Catchment Area (ECA) study, which is the definitive community epidemiological study of this generation. The major scientific development had been the progressive refinements of diagnostic criteria beginning with the Feighner criteria (Feighner et al, 1972), the Research Diagnostic Criteria (RDC), and the *DSM-III* criteria (American Pyschiatric Association, 1980)—all of which were attempts to make more explicit and measurable the descriptions of clinical diagnoses. The research goal was to improve reliability of diagnosis in clinical practice and research studies. The development of such criteria has led to a new generation of diagnostic instruments used to elicit the presence or absence of required symptom duration and severity for the criteria. Such instruments included the Renard Diagnostic Interview (RDI) (Helzer et al, 1981) for the Feighner criteria, and the Schedule for Affective Disorders and Schizophrenia (SADS) instrument for the RDC criteria. A modification was made of the SADS (Endicott and Spitzer, 1978) instrument to obtain lifetime history (SADS–L) of psychopathology in epidemiological studies. The application of the SADS–L in a community survey was demonstrated in the late 1970s by Myers and Weissman in a follow-up survey of 511 community residents studied 11 years earlier in New Haven (Weissman and Myers, 1978).

From the public policy standpoint, the major event was the President's

Commission on Mental Health initiated by President and Mrs. Carter in 1977 (The President's Commission on Mental Health, 1978). Several reviews were conducted of the current information on the scope of mental disorders in the U.S. population and the availability of services to treat such individuals.

Scientific Context

These reviews showed that the basic descriptive data for the prevalence of mental disorders and the use of mental health services was inadequate for the needs of the President's Commission on Mental Health. Previous estimates based on available data indicated that 15 percent of the population could be determined as having some type of mental disorder, and that approximately three percent of the population used specialty mental health services in one year (Regier, et al, 1978). However, the potential advantages of epidemiologic approaches mentioned previously could not be realized without the ability to identify specific mental disorders and related service use rates in community populations.

Fortunately, developments in clinical research had advanced by the late 1970s to the point where diagnostic criteria were sufficiently explicit so that an epidemiologic study using these criteria was feasible. The New Haven study had demonstrated that close approximations to clinical diagnoses could be made in a community by using a structured psychiatric interview based on such explicit diagnostic criteria. Obtaining the clinical and public health benefits of epidemiological studies already mentioned (for example, community diagnosis, completing the clinical picture, and assessing individual risks) was now a scientific possibility because of the advances in clinical research and nosology.

The fact that no information was available on the prevalence of currently defined mental disorders according to the emerging *DSM-III* criteria, and that insufficient information was available on the patterns of treatment, laid the groundwork for the NIMH staff proposal to conduct a new study of mental disorder in the community.

Before any such study could be conducted, it was necessary to develop a new diagnostic interview that would incorporate the *DSM-III* criteria which were still under development in the late 1970s. Because the NIMH had been responsible for supporting development of the Research Diagnostic Criteria, the SADS instrument, the SADS–L application in the New Haven study, and conducting the field trials of the *DSM-III*, the NIMH staff had good evidence both that the *DSM-III* would be widely accepted, and that it would be feasible to develop a reliable instrument built around those diagnostic criteria. Hence, in late 1977, one of the authors (DAR) was appointed as Director of the Division of Biometry and Epidemiology and took responsibility for coordinating the development of the instrument which later became known as the Diagnostic Interview Schedule (DIS) (Robins et al, 1981a, 1981b). This instrument (discussed by Dr. Robins in Chapter 26) was developed around the model of the Renard Diagnostic Interview, with Drs. Robins and Helzer as the principal developers in consultation with Drs. Spitzer and Williams—the principal APA coordinators for development of the *DSM-III* criteria. As a result of the close collaboration of all of these scientists, it was possible to produce the DIS interview and make it available for field trials at the same time in 1980 that the *DSM-III* criteria were officially published.

Research Objectives

Once the instrument feasibility was established, the NIMH staff developed the research design for the epidemiologic catchment area program in order to issue a request for contracts that would eventually enable a multisite collaborative study using a common case identification and survey methodology. Six major objectives were developed for the study.

The first of these was the requirement that the study would assess the prevalence of specific mental disorders defined by *DSM-III* rather than some global measure of mental ill health or impairment. Second, the study would assess the utilization of mental health services in specialty mental health, general medical, and other human services which had previously been defined as the De Facto U.S. Mental Health Service System. Third, a longitudinal design was required that would enable determination of the course of illness over at least two points in time and one year apart as well as a determination of incidence rates and service utilization rates over time. The fourth objective was to obtain both community and institutionalized population prevalence, incidence, and service use rates. The fifth objective was to test the validity and reliability of the *DSM-III* diagnostic criteria themselves, since this would be the first large-scale study using the newly published criteria. Finally, it was planned that an automatic replication of findings would be built into the study by designing a multisite collaborative study rather than one large national survey by a single contractor. The latter design would both draw in the best available epidemiologic and health services research expertise through the competitive application process, and would facilitate the collection of both institutional and community data in each geographical location.

Over a period of three years, successful applications for carrying out this study were submitted by Yale University, Johns Hopkins University, Washington University (St. Louis), Duke University, and UCLA.

EPIDEMIOLOGIC CATCHMENT AREA METHODS

Sampling the Population

Epidemiologic surveys typically sample individuals drawn from the population residing within a designated geographic area. In the case of the ECA survey, the designated area was to be one or more "catchment areas" that had been created after the Mental Health Act of 1963 to identify communities of about 200,000 people to be served by community mental health programs jointly funded by the states and the federal government. In addition to this routine aspect of the study, several unusual features were incorporated into the ECA study design to increase the precision of estimating rates of mental disorders in American communities.

First, the ECA program was designed as a multisite study, with five teams of investigators chosen to study five different communities. Being able to test for replication of findings within the program, using the same assessment instruments and uniform sampling procedures, ensured that the basic findings on mental disorders would be tested for consistency and reproducibility. The multisite design also permitted several more intensive investigations of specific subgroups who may not have been well represented in any single study as, for example, elderly subjects.

Second, the ECA samples were selected from both community populations and institutionalized populations. One typical advantage of epidemiologic surveys is that they include subjects who may have disorders but who do not enter the medical system; as a result, epidemiologic surveys have the potential to provide a more complete picture of a clinical condition than studies using only patients identified in treatment settings. However, especially for psychiatric disorders, surveys limited only to the community may still be incomplete, for many chronic patients reside in state and county mental hospitals, nursing homes, and other settings such as prisons. In the past, the pioneering surveys of psychiatric conditions in the general population were more limited and did not include comprehensive assessments of residents in various institutional settings.

Third, the ECA samples were intended to be large enough in each site to allow statistically stable estimates to be made of prevalence rates for specific mental disorders. For each site, this feature required that at least 3,000 community subjects and 500 institutional subjects be interviewed. Although the strategies for drawing these samples are relatively straightforward for survey statisticians, they required complex methods to ensure that each respondent had a known probability of selection; with that information, it is possible to weight the sample results accurately to reflect the rates in the population from which the sample has been drawn. However, since these studies are complex survey designs, they have also required use of unusually sophisticated computer programs to calculate the weighted population rates and the variances to be used in testing the statistical significance of any differences in rates among groups.

Identifying Psychiatric Disorders

Formulation of explicit diagnostic criteria for psychiatric disorders, first for research and then for clinical practice, encouraged efforts to develop standardized interview schedules for assessing subjects and assigning diagnoses. However, it was impossible to hire sufficient numbers of clinicians to undertake surveys of the magnitude of the ECA program using interviews designed for clinical research. The NIMH Diagnostic Interview Schedule (DIS) was constructed as a series of fully specified questions to elicit information for identifying the disorders considered by a set of consultants to be most important and/or most common. Criteria used in three classification systems were used for constructing the set of questions for each category: *Diagnostic and Statistical Manual of Mental Disorders, Third Edition*; Research Diagnostic Criteria; and Feighner Research Criteria (St. Louis).

These questions were to be read verbatim, which meant they could be suitable for administration by survey interviewers without clinical training; they were coupled to a set of probes to be sure the phenomena reported by the respondent were clinically meaningful and likely to be attributable to a psychiatric disorder.

In the ECA, information collected by these nonclinician interviewers using the DIS was reviewed by specially trained editors to ensure the logic of the interview schedule had been maintained; then it was scored by computer to generate diagnoses according to the criteria established by *DSM-III*. Initially, questions on the DIS ask whether particular experiences have occurred at any time in the respondent's lifetime (for example, "Have you ever . . ."). These lifetime reports are scored to determine if they have occurred in sufficient number and/or clustered together appropriately to cross the *DSM-III* threshold for the disorder. If so, the respondent is assigned the diagnosis on a "lifetime" basis. Once that assignment has been made, the respondent is asked when the symptoms for the particular disorder have most recently been active; such information is used to determine "current" cases, in categories of the past one month, six months, one year, or longer than one year.

The application of an interview schedule with prespecified questions and probes, by nonclinician survey interviewers, scored by computer, was an extension of methods developed in prior psychiatric epidemiology studies. To test the suitability of this DIS approach, a series of studies was undertaken as part of the ECA program and by other investigators. These included studies using a "test-retest" design, which compared the results of a DIS administered by a nonclinician to those from a DIS administered by a psychiatrist; and a "clinical comparison" design, which compared the results from a DIS, usually administered by a nonclinician, to the diagnoses assigned by a psychiatrist who used some other method to examine the same subject (Helzer, 1985; Anthony, 1985; Wittchen, 1985; Klerman, 1985; Burke, 1986).

Studying Special Issues

Although the ECA was designed principally to estimate prevalence rates for specific mental disorders, it was also possible to build into the study design features that laid the groundwork for further advances in epidemiologic research beyond this descriptive level.

Prevalence rates measure the proportion of individuals in a population who have a given disorder at the time of interview, or within some specified time period around the interview. However, for chronic disorders, the accumulated burden of subjects with long lasting or recurrent conditions can make it difficult to distinguish the "risk factors" that make an individual likely to develop the disorder initially from those characteristics that may tend to cause the disorder to persist or recur. To estimate the importance of "risk factors," epidemiologists prefer to use incidence rates, which measure the proportion of individuals who develop a new case of illness within a specified time period, typically within one year. As a first step to measuring incidence rates for specific disorders, the ECA program incorporated a one-year follow-up period, with a second administration of the DIS, to identify those who had never experienced a disorder at the first interview but who had developed it subsequently.

The calculation of incidence rates was expected to be a problem, especially for rare disorders, so the alternative of examining characteristics of those with a disorder at the first interview has also been used. While this approach cannot differentiate true risk factors that may contribute to onset of the illness from correlates that may result from having it or that cause it to persist, for example, it may be useful in generating hypotheses about further research.

A second, more specific use of epidemiologic methods is to examine the relationship between having a disorder and using medical services. One advantage of using a series of multisite studies, rather than a single large study, is to be able to study the patterns of illness in comparison to the patterns of using health services. In the ECA, elaborate questionnaires asked respondents about their use of general medical facilities as well as specialty mental health facilities for health and mental health problems. Besides the examination of different patterns of service use for specific disorders, this information also provides an estimate about those with a disorder who never receive medical attention.

A third use of an epidemiologic survey is to refine the same diagnostic criteria for case identification that made it possible. In the ECA, the use of *DSM-III* criteria in a large, community based study clarifies not only the distribution of the major disorders, but allows some examination of the effects of particular elements of the criteria written for a disorder. Of special interest is the ability to examine interrelationships among disorders in the total population, to escape the potential bias of overestimating co-occurrence of disorders from clinical samples ("Berkson's fallacy").

EPIDEMIOLOGIC CATCHMENT AREA RESULTS

Prevalence of Specific Disorders

In Table 1, the lifetime rates of major *DSM-III* disorders as identified with the DIS are presented for the household samples from the first three sites in the ECA program. These lifetime rates reflect the proportion of individuals whose report of clinically meaningful phenomena satisfied the *DSM-III* threshold some time during their lifetime, without regard to whether the disorder had recently been active. In these three sites, from 28 percent to 38 percent of the populations studied are estimated to have had at least one of the disorders covered on the DIS some time during their lifetimes. The most common conditions were anxiety disorders (ranging from 10.4 to 25.1 percent), substance use disorders (from 15.0 to 18.1 percent), and affective disorders (from 6.1 to 9.5 percent). (One advantage of modern survey practice, using advanced computer packages, is the ability to calculate standard errors to indicate the sampling variation in such point estimates of prevalence rates; these standard errors, which are necessary for determining statistical significance of any observed differences, are shown in the Tables but are not repeated in the text.)

In general, few significant differences emerged between sites; in this case replication may tend to lend confidence in the overall estimates. Although there were few significant differences between sites, one notable discrepancy occurred in the rates of phobias. At Baltimore, the rates were quite high (23.3 percent); at New Haven and St. Louis, the rates were substantially lower (7.8 and 9.4 percent). Initially, concern arose about possible methodologic differences in training the DIS interviewers at Baltimore. However, preliminary findings from the fourth and fifth sites in Durham and Los Angeles suggest that the rates of phobias in Durham were almost as high (about 19.5 percent) as in Baltimore, but that rates in Los Angeles were in the same range as New Haven and St. Louis. As a result, interest has also been directed at identifying factors that may be associated with this apparently higher prevalence of phobic disorders. At present, this finding of higher rates of phobia in the two mid-Atlantic sites represents an epidemiologic clue not yet fully understood.

Some differences also emerged in examining group rates within the sites. Consistently across the sites, women were more likely to experience major depressive episode, agoraphobia, and simple phobia; men were more likely to experience antisocial personality, alcohol abuse and dependence, and drug abuse

Table 1. Lifetime Prevalence Rates, Per 100*

Disorder	New Haven	Baltimore	St. Louis
Any DIS disorder	28.8(0.9)	38.0(0.9)	31.0(1.2)
Schizophrenia	1.9(0.3)	1.6(0.2)	1.0(0.2)
Manic episode	1.1(0.2)	0.6(0.2)	1.1(0.3)
Major depressive episode	6.7(0.5)	3.7(0.3)	5.5(0.6)
Dysthymia	3.2(0.4)	2.1(0.2)	3.8(0.4)
Alcohol abuse and dependence	11.5(0.6)	13.7(0.7)	15.7(0.9)
Drug abuse and dependence	5.8(0.4)	5.6(0.5)	5.5(0.6)
Phobia	7.8(0.4)	23.3(0.8)	9.4(0.6)
Panic	1.4(0.2)	1.4(0.2)	1.5(0.3)
Obsessive–compulsive disorder	2.6(0.3)	3.0(0.3)	1.9(0.3)
Somatization	0.1(0.1)	0.1(0.1)	0.1(0.1)
Antisocial personality	2.1(0.3)	2.6(0.3)	3.3(0.5)

*Numbers in parentheses are standard errors.

Reprinted from Robins LN, Helzer JE, Weissman MM, et al: Lifetime prevalence of specific psychiatric disorders in three sites. Arch Gen Psychiatry 41:959-967, 1984.

and dependence (Table 2). Overall, the findings by sex indicated that men and women have roughly equal rates of lifetime mental disorders, but that the pattern of disorders they have is different. In reporting these data, Robins and colleagues suggested that this finding tends to correct the impression that may be derived from treatment settings, where women may be more likely to attend than men, and from earlier epidemiologic studies, which concentrated on the depressive and anxiety disorders that seem more likely to affect women.

Several important findings emerged in terms of age differences. Not unexpectedly, the youngest age groups, 18–24 years old, had high rates of drug and alcohol dependence and abuse. A potentially important finding for affective disorders is that this same group also had substantial rates of major depressive episode, although the highest rates occurred in adults 25–44 years old.

But one surprising finding in age patterns occurred with most disorders studied. In considering lifetime illness, it would be reasonable to expect the highest rates to occur in the oldest age groups, since those who had the most years of adult life could be expected to have accumulated the highest rates of lifetime

Table 2. Selected Lifetime Prevalence Rates by Sex, Per 100*

	New Haven		Baltimore		St. Louis	
	Male	Female	Male	Female	Male	Female
Major depressive episode	4.4(0.6)	8.7(0.8)	2.3(0.4)	4.9(0.5)	2.5(0.5)	8.1(0.9)
Agoraphobia	1.5(0.4)	5.3(0.5)	5.2(0.6)	12.5(1.0)	1.5(0.3)	6.4(0.8)
Alcohol abuse and dependence	19.1(1.1)	4.8(0.5)	24.9(1.4)	4.2(0.4)	28.9(1.8)	4.3(0.6)
Antisocial personality	3.9(0.6)	0.5(0.2)	4.9(0.7)	0.7(0.2)	4.9(0.7)	1.2(0.3)

*Numbers in parentheses are standard errors.

Reprinted from Robins LN, Helzer JE, Weissman MM, et al: Lifetime prevalence of specific psychiatric disorders in three sites. Arch Gen Psychiatry 41:959-967, 1984.

Table 3. Selected Lifetime Prevalence Rates by Age, Per 100

	18–24 Years	25–44 Years	45–64 Years	65+ Years
Major depressive episode				
New Haven	7.5	10.4	4.2	1.8
Baltimore	4.1	7.5	4.2	1.4
St. Louis	4.5	8.0	5.2	0.8
Drug abuse and dependence				
New Haven	17.5	7.2	0.6	0.1
Baltimore	12.0	9.0	0.6	0.0
St. Louis	11.0	8.3	0.6	0.1

Reprinted from Robins LN, Helzer JE, Weissman MM, et al: Lifetime prevalence of specific psychiatric disorders in three sites. Arch Gen Psychiatry 41:959-967, 1984.

illness. However, in almost every category of illness and uniformly across sites, the older subjects reported the lowest rates of illness. Several explanations have been considered for such findings.

The first consideration is the adequacy of the assessment method being used. For older subjects trying to recall experiences from much earlier in their lives, it may be more difficult to report symptoms accurately. This difficulty in reporting lifetime symptoms is a potential methodologic problem with the "lifetime" framework of any diagnostic instrument.

A second possibility is that differential mortality for those with psychiatric illnesses may produce a cohort of older subjects who have experienced fewer psychiatric illnesses than others of their birth cohort who have already died by the time of the survey.

A third possibility that has intrigued some investigators is that some disorders, notably depression, may have been increasing in incidence among younger generations since mid-century, so that there are truly increased rates of illness in younger subjects; Klerman suggested this possible trend may produce an "age of melancholy." However, a cross-sectional study design like the ECA cannot offer definitive proof of such temporal changes in the occurrence of disease.

Any problems in recalling or reporting lifetime symptoms may be less serious with currently ill subjects. Six-month rates of mental disorders have also been reported from the ECA sites. Overall, it can be estimated from the findings of the first three sites that roughly 16.8–23.4 percent (average 18.9 percent) of adult Americans have a DIS/DSM-III diagnosable condition in the six months prior to interview. In general, phobia continued to be the most common disorder reported as being currently active (New Haven, 5.9 percent; Baltimore, 13.4 percent; St. Louis, 5.4 percent). Affective disorders were found with rates of 4.6 percent to 6.5 percent in the populations, with major depressive episode being the most common of the affective disorders studied. Currently active schizophrenia and schizophreniform disorder together were found in 0.6 to 1.2 percent of the population. Rates for these serious psychotic disorders are higher than had been anticipated with the strict criteria of *DSM-III*, and with the potential difficulty in detecting psychosis using a fully specified interview schedule administered by nonclinicians.

Although an approximation to clinical diagnosis of dementia could not be obtained with the DIS method, the instrument does incorporate the Mini-Mental Status Exam as a screening tool for "cognitive impairment." Using this MMSE, from 4.6 to 6.3 percent of men over age 65, and 3.6 to 4.8 percent of women over age 65, were determined to have severe cognitive impairment.

Use of Mental Health Services

Results from the health services questionnaire indicated that 57.7 to 59.8 percent of the populations in the three communities had made an outpatient visit for health or mental health reasons in the six months prior to the interview. This figure was somewhat higher for those subjects who had a DIS/*DSM-III* mental disorder in the previous six months; among those with a six-month diagnosis, from 65.7 to 69.1 percent had an ambulatory health visit.

The proportion visiting specifically for mental health reasons was much smaller, however. Of all those with a DIS/*DSM-III* disorder in the past six months, less than one in five (15.6 to 19.5 percent in the three sites) reported visiting either a general physician or a mental health specialist in the last six months for a mental health reason. Considering only mental health specialists, without counting visits to general physicians, only 8.1 to 12.4 percent reported a visit in the past six months.

For specific disorders, there was a substantial range in the proportion with the disorder who reported a mental health visit. Of those with a current diagnosis of schizophrenia or schizophreniform disorder, nearly one-half (from 38.6 to 53.2 percent) reported a mental health visit; of those with affective disorders, about one in three (31.2 to 31.7 percent) had a mental health visit; of those with cognitive impairment, fewer than one in 10 (3.6 to 7.6 percent) were known (by self-report or from information supplied by an informant) to have had a mental health visit.

Case-Finding in the Community

Studies that compared a DIS administered by a nonclinician to a DIS administered by a psychiatrist generally have demonstrated adequate agreement between the two versions. For example, for alcohol disorder, the range of kappa values used to measure the agreement found in several studies has been from 0.68 to 0.86. By contrast, the agreements for panic disorder have generally been about the lowest found, from 0.28 to 0.47.

Studies that compared the DIS to a psychiatrist's diagnoses made by some other procedure have been generally acceptable for most disorders but somewhat lower than the agreement using two examinations by the DIS (for example, kappa values for panic disorder of 0.30 to 0.32). The most relevant studies, but the hardest to interpret, are those which have used this "clinical comparison" strategy using community residents from the ECA. Both the study by Helzer and colleagues in St. Louis, and the one by Anthony and colleagues in Baltimore, have shown that agreement measured by the kappa statistic has been very low for the nonclinician's DIS and a psychiatrist's own diagnosis on the same subjects. However, two problems have been recognized in the effort to understand this finding.

Several investigators from the ECA and other studies have discussed the difficulty interpreting low values of kappa, which is attenuated in studies where the disorder occurs at low prevalence rates, for example, below five percent. Helzer and Spitznagel have demonstrated that other approaches to measuring agreement that are not affected by the prevalence rate yield acceptable values of agreement from the ECA studies of the DIS in St. Louis and Baltimore (Spitznagel and Helzer, 1985). However, this proposal to use other statistics besides kappa is controversial, and some interested investigators have argued that the "attenuation" of kappa in studying populations with low prevalence rates is unavoidable and appropriate.

A second problem in interpreting these studies has been the lack of a "gold standard" for psychiatric diagnosis. None of the alternative methods for assessing subjects and assigning diagnoses has been shown to be reliable or necessarily valid. For that reason, Spitzer has proposed that the best approach for evaluating the validity of diagnostic interviews is to use a "LEAD" approach: Longitudinal assessment by Experts of All the Data (Spitzer, 1983).

Nosologic Studies

Several types of studies have been conducted to examine the specific criteria used in *DSM-III* itself. Boyd and colleagues (1984) tested the assumptions built into the exclusion criteria for many disorders, and demonstrated a relative lack of specificity in the way pairs of disorders occur in the same individual. Concentrating on the relationship that *DSM-III* assumes between a specific pair of disorders, Boyd (personal communication) has also begun examining the pattern of co-occurrence between agoraphobia and panic disorder. Such empirical studies of the *DSM-III* criteria set will help improve future revisions of the classification system.

DISCUSSION

Early findings from the ECA program demonstrate the importance and common occurrence of mental disorders in the general population; nearly one in five adults in the three sites have had a diagnosable condition in the six months prior to interview. More intriguing than this overall finding are some specific results that may improve our understanding of specific clinical conditions.

Anxiety disorders, especially phobic disorders, have high prevalence in the community, and may be more significant than earlier believed. Although the need for treatment and degree of functional impairment associated with these disorders is not clear from the ECA, their common occurrence does reinforce the interest they have been receiving clinically and in the treatment research field over the past several years.

For younger adults especially, the reports of high rates of depression, and of alcohol and drug abuse, indicate that information about the age of onset and course of these conditions may need revision. In view of the possible "cohort effect" noticed by other investigators, the findings suggest that etiologic and pathogenic mechanisms need much clearer elucidation and that adolescent depression, for example, needs to be studied much more intensively. Together with evidence that individuals with these disorders are not commonly receiving treatment, the high prevalence suggests that a pressing public health need is to improve the detection, recognition, and treatment of these conditions.

For all disorders, and across all ages, the low proportion who reported a visit for mental health reasons is striking. While there may be some inaccuracy in the respondents' report of services use, the magnitude of such error will be estimated from a special study underway in Durham. Additional questions about the degree of functional impairment associated with these untreated conditions and about the reasons for lack of treatment need clarification; even for those who did report a visit, the effectiveness of any treatment received is unknown. Uncertainty about the proper role of general physicians in providing effective treatment for these disorders, and the apparently limited capacity of the mental health specialty sector to absorb a huge additional flow of patients, also indicate that there are major unresolved questions about the adequacy of treatment resources for those with mental disorders.

In other fields of medicine, epidemiologic research has led to great scientific and public health advances. The demonstration of associations linking cigarette smoking to lung cancer, and linking diet and lack of exercise to cardiovascular disease, is based on epidemiologic studies. Although psychiatric epidemiology is just at the edge of its promise to elucidate risk factors linked in a causal chain for specific disorders, it has already begun to make significant contributions to understanding the working of health services in the community and to completing the clinical picture of mental disorders. Future efforts to assess individual risks and understand causal mechanisms may now advance on the strength of this descriptive survey and the demonstration that new technology can be applied for approximating clinical diagnoses in large scale community surveys.

REFERENCES

American Psychiatric Association, Committee on Nomenclature and Statistics: Diagnostic and Statistical Manual of Mental Disorders. Washington, DC, American Psychiatric Association Mental Hospital Service, 1952

American Psychiatric Association, Committee on Nomenclature and Statistics: Diagnostic and Statistical Manual of Mental Disorders, Third Edition (DSM-III). Washington, DC, American Psychiatric Association, 1980

Anthony JC, Folstein M, Romanoski AJ, et al: Comparison of long DIS and a standardized psychiatric diagnosis: experience in eastern Baltimore. Arch Gen Psychiatry 42:665-667, 1985

Boyd JH, Burke JD, Gruenberg E, et al: Exclusion criteria of DSM-III: a study of co-occurrence of hierarchy-free syndromes. Arch Gen Psychiatry 41:983-989, 1984

Burke JD: Diagnostic categorization by the Diagnostic Interview Schedule: a comparison with other methods of assessment, in Mental Disorders in the Community. Edited by Barrett J, Rose R. New York, Guilford Press, 1986

Commission on Chronic Illness: Chronic Illness in the United States: Chronic Illness in a Large City, vol 4. Cambridge, Harvard University Press, 1957

Endicott J, Spitzer RL: A diagnostic interview: the Schedule for Affective Disorders and Schizophrenia. Arch Gen Psychiatry 35:837-844, 1978

Feighner JP, Robins E, Guze SB, et al: Diagnostic criteria for use in psychiatric research. Arch Gen Psychiatry 26:57-63, 1972

Helzer JE, Robins LN, Croughan JL, et al: Renard Diagnostic Interview. Arch Gen Psychiatry 38:393-398, 1981

Helzer JE, McEvoy LT, Robins LN, et al: Results of the St. Louis ECA physician reexamination study of the DIS Interview. Arch Gen Psychiatry 42:657-666, 1985

Hollingshead AB, Redlich FC: Social Class and Mental Illness. New York, John Wiley & Sons, 1958

Klerman GL: Diagnosis of psychiatric disorders in epidemiologic field studies. Arch Gen Psychiatry 42:723-724, 1985

Leighton DC, Harding JS, Macklin DB, et al: The Character of Danger. New York, Basic Books, 1963

Myers JK, Weissman MM, Tischler GL, et al: Six-month prevalence of psychiatric disorders in three communities: 1980-1982. Arch Gen Psychiatry 41:9471-978, 1984

President's Commission on Mental Health: Report to the President from the President's Commission on Mental Health. Washington, DC, stock No. 040–000–00390–8, vol. 1, 1978

Regier DA, Burke J: Epidemiology, in Kaplin HI, Sadock BJ (eds): Comprehensive Textbook of Psychiatry, fourth edition. Baltimore, Williams & Wilkins, 1985

Regier DA, Goldberg ID, Taube CA: The de facto U.S. mental health services system: a public health perspective. Arch Gen Psychiatry 35:685-693, 1978

Regier DA, Myers JK, Kramer M, et al: The NIMH Epidemiologic Catchment Area Program. Arch Gen Psychiatry 41:934-941, 1984

Robins LN, Helzer JE, Croughan J, et al: National Institute of Mental Health diagnostic interview schedule: its history, characteristics, and validity. Arch Gen Psychiatry 38:381-389, 1981a

Robins LN, Helzer JE, Croughan J, et al: NIMH Diagnostic Interview Schedule: Version III (May 1981). Rockville, Maryland, NIMH mimeo, 1981b

Robins LN, Helzer JE, Weissman MM, et al: Lifetime prevalence of specific psychiatric disorders in three sites. Arch Gen Psychiatry 41:959-967, 1984

Shapiro S, Skinner EA, Kessler LG, et al: Utilization of health and mental health services: three Epidemiologic Catchment Area sites. Arch Gen Psychiatry 41:971-978, 1984

Spitzer RL: Are clinicians still necessary? Compr Psychiatry 24:399-411, 1983

Spitznagel EL, Helzer JE: A proposed solution to the base rate problem in the kappa statistic. Arch Gen Psychiatry 42:725-728, 1985

Srole L: Mental Health in the Metropolis: The Midtown Manhattan Study. New York, McGraw-Hill Book Co, 1962

Weissman MM, Myers JK: Affective disorders in a U.S. urban community: the use of research diagnostic criteria in an epidemiological survey. Arch Gen Psychiatry 35:1304-1311, 1978

Weissman MM, Myers JK, Harding PS: Psychiatric disorders in a U.S. urban community: 1975–1976. Am J Psychiatry 135:459-462, 1978

Wittchen HU, Semler G, von Zerssen D: Comparing ICD diagnoses with DSM-III and RDC using the Diagnostic Interview Schedule (version II). Arch Gen Psychiatry 42:677-684, 1985

Chapter 28

Genetic Epidemiology of Psychiatric Disorders

by Kathleen R. Merikangas, Ph.D.

The importance of studying the role of genetic factors in the pathogenesis of psychiatric illness has long been recognized. In his book *Heredity and the Aetiology of the Neuroses*, Freud wrote, "Our opinion as to the aetiological role of heredity in nervous disease must assuredly be the result of an impartial statistical study . . ." (1896, p. 139).

The observation that genetic factors are involved in the etiology of numerous psychiatric disorders, including schizophrenia, alcoholism, and affective disorder, has been well established by twin, family, and cross-fostering studies. However, the degree of heritability and mode of genetic transmission of the major psychiatric disorders is unknown.

Genetic epidemiology, a science that deals with the etiology, distribution, and control of disease in groups of relatives and with the inherited (cultural or genetic) causes of disease in populations, is a relatively new discipline that has emerged from an integration of methods from the fields of population and clinical genetics, and chronic disease epidemiology (Neel and Schull, 1954; Morton and Chung, 1978). During the past three years, the discipline has introduced its own journal, *Genetic Epidemiology*, and published several textbooks describing a wide variety of applications and methods in genetic epidemiology.

This chapter will first describe the methods, applications, and contributions of each of the two derivative disciplines to psychiatry. The methods and advantages of the genetic epidemiologic approach to study the psychiatric disorders will then be discussed.

BACKGROUND: EPIDEMIOLOGY

Epidemiology may be defined as the study of the distribution and determinants of diseases in human populations. Epidemiologic studies are concerned with the *extent* and types of illnesses in *groups* of people and with the *factors* that influence their distribution (Mausner and Bahn, 1974).

Epidemiologists are concerned with the role of both intrinsic and extrinsic factors, consisting of interactions that may occur between the host, agent, and environment (the classic triangle of epidemiology) to produce a disease state. The ultimate aim of epidemiologic studies is to identify the *etiology* of a disease and thereby prevent or intervene in the progression of the disorder. In order to achieve this goal, epidemiologic studies generally proceed from descriptive

This work was supported in part by Research Scientist Development Award MH00499 from the National Institute of Mental Health. The suggestions of Drs. Neil J. Risch and Myrna M. Weissman are gratefully acknowledged.

studies which specify the amount and distribution of a disease within a population by person, place, and time (that is, descriptive epidemiology), to more focused studies of the *determinants* of disease in specific groups (that is, analytic epidemiology) (Mausner and Bahn, 1974). The three basic study designs in epidemiology are the cross-sectional study, the cohort study, and the case-control study. Whereas the former two designs may be descriptive or etiologic, the latter study type is usually etiologic (Kleinbaum et al, 1982).

The identification of risk factors for a disease comprises an intermediate step in the process of identifying a discrete and valid disorder, studying its distribution in the population, and conducting analytic studies that attempt to identify etiologic factors. There are several criteria for assessing the extent to which a risk factor is causally involved in a trait or disease within a particular study. These include the strength of the association, a dose-response effect, and a lack of temporal ambiguity. Broader criteria that can be applied to a set of studies on a putative etiologic risk factor include: consistency of the findings; biologic plausibility of the hypothesis; and specificity of the association (Kleinbaum et al, 1982).

The ultimate goal of epidemiology, the identification of the etiology of a disease, has often become lost in recent epidemiologic studies, in which the elucidation of population distribution and concomitant risk factors for psychiatric disorders have been viewed as final products of the application of epidemiologic methods. Furthermore, the term "risk factor" has often been applied inappropriately to descriptive factors that may be associated with, but do not cause, increased risk of the disorder.

The first formal use of the term "epidemiology" with respect to psychiatric disorders can be traced to a conference of the Milbank Memorial Fund in 1949, in which there was a consensus regarding the value of the application of the epidemiologic approach to causal research and its implications for administrative policy (Shepherd, 1984; Milbank Memorial Fund, 1950). However, prior to 1949 there were many classic descriptive epidemiologic studies of psychiatric disorders throughout the world (see Schwab and Schwab, 1978, for a complete description, and Chapter 25 in this volume).

Summaries of the post-World War II history of psychiatric epidemiology in the United States are presented by Weissman and Klerman, 1978; Robins, 1978; and Schwab and Schwab, 1983. The major methodologic contributions and recommendations for the application of epidemiology to psychiatric research are as follows:

1. development of *methods of assessment* of psychiatric illness such as structured diagnostic instruments
2. identification of the importance and development of assessments of *environmental factors* in the pathogenesis of psychiatric illness
3. development of *optimal sample designs* for studying population prevalence and identification of etiologic and precipitating risk factors
4. recognition of the importance of the *integration of several disciplines* including genetics, neurobiology, psychopharmacology, sociology, and anthropology in designing descriptive and analytic epidemiologic studies
5. identification of the *crucial role of the psychiatric clinician* in the development of diagnostic classification and assessments in epidemiologic studies

To date, however, these recommendations have not been simultaneously implemented in studies of psychiatric disorders. Jablensky (1984) recently noted that cross-fertilization between psychiatric epidemiology and the new wave of biological research in psychiatry has been a very rare phenomenon during the last decade. This is particularly striking if one considers the spectacular success of the application of epidemiologic methods in identifying the causes of pellagra and kuru.

Several characteristics of the psychiatric disorders have impeded etiological epidemiologic research: 1) classification of the major psychiatric disorders lacks adequate evidence of validity and reliability of measurement, despite the recent attention to this problem; 2) the probable heterogeneity of the major psychiatric disorders, which are likely to be comprised of etiologically distinct subtypes; 3) the lack of statistical power to detect differences (if such differences exist) among groups of subjects in most recent studies of risk factors for psychiatric disorders; and 4) the state of our basic knowledge about the structure and function of the brain remains primitive, thereby precluding major discoveries concerning the etiology and pathogenesis of specific mental disorders (Jablensky, 1984).

The recent integration of epidemiology and genetics is a major advance in the search for the ultimate causes, mechanisms, and treatment of psychiatric disease, as will be described below.

BACKGROUND: HUMAN GENETICS

Human genetics, the scientific study of heredity, began in the early 1900s after the rediscovery of Mendelian theory by Archibald Garrod and William Bateson (McKusick, 1969). Hardy and Weinberg, in 1908, and Castle (1903) laid the foundation of population genetics in describing the distribution of Mendelian traits in human populations. Since that time, the major subdivisions of human genetics that have evolved include: biochemical genetics, population genetics, cytogenetics, molecular genetics, and immunogenetics. Genetic epidemiology is primarily derived from the division of population genetics. Before reviewing the background and methods of population genetic studies, a brief review of basic genetic mechanisms will be presented.

Each normal human being has 23 pairs of chromosomes—the cellular components that are bearers of heredity—which are exclusively found in the nucleus of all living cells. There are 22 pairs of autosomes and one pair of sex chromosomes in humans, with one member of each pair respectively deriving from maternal and paternal lines. There are two components of chromosomes: *deoxyribonucleic acid* (DNA), and a class of small, positively charged proteins called *histones*. DNA is comprised of two complementary strands of *nucleotides*; there are four nucleotides, adenine and thymine, guanine and cytosine, each of which pairs exclusively with only one of the other three. Various combinations of three of these nucleotides code for amino acids, which are then joined sequentially to form specific proteins. The two intermediate steps in this process involve *transcription* of one of the DNA strands to its complement or messenger ribonucleic acid (mRNA) (which is identical to DNA except that the nucleotide uracil replaces thymine, and the sugar is ribose rather than deoxyribose) in the nucleus;

and *translation* of the mRNA into a sequence of amino acids with the assistance of transfer-RNA (tRNA) on the ribosomes in the cytoplasm of the cell.

All sequences of DNA are not active coding regions. Within genes, active coding sequences, or *exons*, are interspersed among *introns*, noncoding sequences and intervening sequences. Enhancers, promoters, and control sequences are located at one end of a gene (Gurling, 1985). Control of gene activity, or protein synthesis, is a complex process that can occur at several different levels. The signals that turn genes on and off are mediated by or generated within the cytoplasm of the cell by the presence of activating or inhibiting molecules, such as hormones (Watson et al, 1983; Wolpert, 1984).

However, even after a protein has been manufactured, there still remains a complex pathway to its final expression in the phenotype, which may depend upon the presence or absence of a variety of other genetic and environmental factors; for example, the disease phenylketonuria, a homozygous recessive condition results from a mutation in the gene coding for the enzyme phenylalanine hydroxylase, which converts the amino acid phenylalamine to tyrosine, resulting in permanent brain damage *only* if the vulnerable individual is exposed to typical levels of phenylalanine in the diet. One-to-one correspondence between genotype and disease is often absent, even for traits that are produced by known genetic loci (Cavalli-Sforza and Bodmer, 1971). Examples of this phenomenon include: *epistasis*, the interaction between distinct genes; *variable expressivity*, variation in the effects of a particular gene; *genotype–environment interaction*, genotypes that produce different phenotypes depending upon the environment in which they are expressed; and *reduced penetrance*, the situation in which persons with the relevant genotype express the phenotype mildly (formes fruste) or not at all. Conversely, a single gene can have multiple effects, or *pleitropy*. Because the complexity of the genotype is expected to exceed that of the phenotype which only has a limited repetoire of expression, Cloninger and colleagues (1983) recommend that investigations should begin with studies at a phenotypic level and proceed backwards toward the level of the genotype. However, Gurling (1985) and Kidd et al (1984) argue that genetic heterogeneity, together with the other factors that are related to a lack of one-to-one correspondence between the genotype and the phenotype, strongly limit the ability of phenotype studies to identify the underlying gene mechanisms. Instead, they suggest that molecular genetics studies of single large pedigrees are more likely to yield information on the genetic factors involved in a complex disorder.

There are four types of evidence that genetic factors contribute to a disease of unknown etiology:

1. significant aggregation of the illness within families
2. a higher concordance among monozygotic (MZ) twins than among dizygotic (DZ) twins
3. a higher incidence of the trait, irrespective of home environment, among biological offspring of affected individuals than among biological offspring of unaffected individuals; that is "positive" adoption study
4. genetic linkage of the illness with an identifiable allele at a marker locus

The types of studies that have been conducted to assess the role of genetic factors in the etiology of illnesses include: *family studies*, which can demonstrate significant degrees of aggregation of the trait among relatives of affected probands compared to expected rates from the population; *twin studies*, which compare concordance rates for monozygotic twins, who have identical genotypes, with those among dizygotic twins, who share an average of half of their genes in common; *adoption studies*, which compare the degree of similarity of an adoptee to his or her biologic parents from whom he or she was separated, to that with his or her adoptive parents, in order to determine the relative contribution of environmental and genetic effects; and *genetic linkage studies*, which examine the association between a known genetic trait and affectional status within pedigrees (but not necessarily *across* pedigrees).

A major advantage of studying diseases *within* families is that the assumption of homotypy of the underlying factors eliminates the effects of heterogeneity which are present in comparisons that are made *between* families. However, all individuals within a particular sibship are not expected to share equal genetic risk because of independent segregation of genes. However, if two members are affected, similar etiologic factors can be assumed, and variable forms of expression can be identified.

There are specific analytic techniques that are applicable to each of these types of studies. These include comparison of morbid risk or correlations among relatives of a proband to that in the population-at-large; path analysis, which partitions the total variance of the pairwise correlations between different types of relatives into genetic, cultural, and random environmental components; computation of pairwise or probandwise concordance for monozygotic versus dizygotic twins; comparison of correlations of adoptees with their biologic siblings or parents and those of their adoptive siblings or parents; and the sib pair and lod score methods of linkage analysis (as described below).

After the involvement of a genetic component in a disease has been established, there are numerous analytic methods for the detection and identification of the role of major genes, such as segregation analysis, disease-marker association studies, and linkage analysis. More extensive details of the application of each of these methods in psychiatry are given by Gershon et al (1977), Kidd (1981a), Gottesman and Carey (1983), Cloninger et al (1985), Suarez and Cox (1985), and Gurling (1985).

A summary of studies of the involvement of genetic factors in the major psychiatric disorders is presented in Table 1. Family studies have been conducted for nearly all of the major psychiatric disorders, with the exception of general anxiety disorder. A strong degree of familial aggregation has been reported for schizophrenia and bipolar affective disorder, with relative risks exceeding 10 for first degree relatives of patients compared to those of controls. Similarly, panic disorder, phobias, and alcoholism are strongly familial, with a range of relative risks from 3.0 to 5.5. The lowest degrees of familial aggregation has been observed for unipolar affective disorder and obsessive-compulsive disorder.

Numerous family studies of personality and its components have also demonstrated that although the heritability for personality is small, variation in heritability estimates among studies can be attributed to differences in the measurement scales, types of family members, degree of mate similarity, and the methods of analysis (Ahern et al, 1982). With the exception of antisocial personality, the heritability of the Axis II personality dimensions has not been widely studied.

Studies of concordance rates among twins have been conducted for all of the

Table 1. Summary of Genetic Studies of Psychiatric Disorders

	Twin	Family	Adoption	Marker		Review
				Association	Linkage	
Affective Disorders, All	+	+	+	−	?	Gershon (1983b)
bipolar	+	+	+	−	?	Gershon (1983a)
unipolar	+	+	−	−	?	Gershon (1983b)
Alcoholism	+	+	+	?	?	Goodwin (1979)
						Goodwin (1984)
Antisocial Personality	+	+	+	−	0	Hutchings & Mednick (1975)
						Cadoret (1982)
Anxiety Disorders, All	+	+	0	0	0	Carey & Gottesman (1984)
						Torgerson (1983)
general anxiety	−	0	0	0	0	Torgerson (1983)
obsessive-compulsive	+	?	0	−	0	Carey & Gottesman (1981)
						Insel et al. (1984)
panic	+	+	0	0	0	Crowe (1985)
phobia	+	+	0	0	0	Crowe (1985)
Schizophrenia	+	+	+	−	−	Kessler (1980)
						Goldin & Gershon (1983)
						Kendler (1985)

+ Majority Positive
? Discrepant Results
− Majority Negative
0 No Studies

major disorders. The results of these studies are nearly uniform in reporting significantly greater concordance rates for monozygotic compared to dizygotic twins. Large scale adoption studies of psychiatric disorders have been conducted for alcoholism (for example, Goodwin et al, 1973; Cadoret and Gath, 1978), antisocial personality (criminality) (for example, Schulsinger, 1975; Hutchings and Mednick, 1977), and schizophrenia (Heston, 1966; Kety et al, 1968; Gottesman and Shields, 1972). Similarity between adoptees and their biologic parents has been consistently greater than that between adoptees and their adoptive parents. However, this may vary according to diagnostic subtype and sex. For example, Cloninger and colleagues (1981) discriminated between two forms of alcoholism: "male-limited," in which biologic/genetic factors appear to predominate; and "milieu-limited," which was more strongly related to environmental factors in the adoptive families.

Recent twin and adoptive studies of unipolar affective disorders (Cadoret et al, 1985; Torgerson, 1983) and general anxiety disorder (Torgerson, 1983) have not indicated that genetic factors play an important role in these disorders. Cadoret and colleagues (1985) found that major depression among adoptees was positively, but not significantly, correlated with a biologic background of major depression. Instead, several environmental factors in the adoptive home, such as death of an adoptive parent before the age of 19, or the presence of a behavior disturbance in a member of the adoptive family, seemed to be related to a predisposition to depression in the adoptee. The two most recent twin studies of obsessive-compulsive disorder reported contradictory results. Whereas Carey and Gottesman (1981) found 87 percent concordance for obsessive-compulsive disorder in monozygotic twins as compared to 47 percent for dizygotic twins, Torgerson (1983) found no concordance among 12 pairs of twins in which one member was affected with obsessive-compulsive disorder.

There have been numerous studies of associations between biologic markers and psychiatric disorders. The general approach has been to study the relationship between a known genetic factor at a particular locus and disease status among probands, their relatives, and the general population. The most commonly studied genetic traits have been the human erythrocyte blood groups (ABO) and the human leukocyte antigens (HLA). The results of association studies in schizophrenia and the affective disorders have been inconsistent. There are no markers for which significant associations have been found in more than a single study (Goldin and Gershon, 1983).

The association between the enzyme monoamine oxidase (MAO) and all of the major psychiatric disorders has been widely studied. Two major forms of MAO have been studied in human populations: MAO–A, in plasma, and MAO–B, in platelets, with varying proportions in most tissues. Low levels of plasma MAO have been reported for alcoholism (for example, Major and Murphy, 1978), unipolar and bipolar depression (for example, Nies et al, 1974); schizophrenia (for example, Wyatt et al, 1979), and suicide (for example, Gottfries et al, 1974). However, a segregation analysis of MAO among pedigrees of schizophrenic subjects suggested that there was a rare allele that coded for *high* activity and was unrelated to disease status (Baron et al, 1985).

The lack of specificity for a particular disorder suggests that this enzyme cannot be used to identify susceptibility to a specific illness. Rather, it may be a nonspecific response to dysregulation of another neurochemical system.

Furthermore, there may be little or no relationship between the activity of MAO in brain and the periphery of humans, because of the possibility of the involvement of different genes, or differential regulation in the central nervous system (CNS) than in the periphery. This principle may also apply to other neurotransmitters, neuromodulators, hormones, and enzymes as well. This underscores the importance of including subjects with other psychiatric illnesses as controls, in addition to unaffected controls, when studying associations between markers and a particular psychiatric disorder. An extensive discussion of research strategies for studying genetic factors in psychiatry is presented by Rieder and Gershon (1978).

If a disease susceptibility locus is located close to a marker locus, they will tend to co-segregate within a pedigree. However, during the formation of gametes at meiosis, there is sometimes an exchange of genetic material, or recombination, between pairs of homologous chromosomes. The farther apart that the two loci are situated on the chromosome, the greater the tendency for recombination to occur between them. Conversely, two closely situated loci are unlikely to undergo recombination. This information is used to quantify genetic linkage. Linkage between a marker locus and disease does *not* imply that the marker is an etiologic factor in the disease; it only implies that the marker and disease locus are in close proximity on the chromosome.

Two major methods of genetic linkage analysis are: the *lod score method* (Morton, 1955), in which the log odds of the likelihood of a linkage between two loci within a pedigree is compared to that of the likelihood of independent segregation of the two loci, or a recombination frequency of 1/2; and the affected *sib-pair method*, derived from Penrose (1935), in which the sharing of marker alleles at a locus among affected sib pairs is examined. The null hypothesis of no linkage specifies probabilities of 1/4, 1/2, and 1/4 for sharing 2, 1, and 0 marker alleles among affected sibs. Excess sharing of 2 haplotypes (or conversely, diminished sharing of haplotypes) provides evidence for linkage.

Linkage studies of affective disorder and schizophrenia have been reviewed by Goldin and Gershon (1983), who conclude that the data do not consistently support linkage between either schizophrenia or affective disorders and any genetic marker. A possible exception is the observation of linkage between bipolar illness and loci on the long arm of the x chromosome. Although this, too, has been controversial, Risch and Baron (1982), reanalyzed the published studies on x-linkage in bipolar illness and confirmed that there was a subset of pedigrees in which there was co-segregation for the color-blindness and G6PD loci on the x chromosome and bipolar illness.

Despite the lack of conclusive data in favor of linkage for the psychiatric disorders, this situation is likely to change dramatically during the next decade. Although previous linkage studies were hampered by the limited number of known polymorphic markers, recent advances in molecular genetics have resulted in the identification of markers across the human genome. These markers, restriction fragment length polymorphisms (RFLPs), have enabled geneticists to identify disease loci for several major diseases, with Huntington's Disease and cystic fibrosis being dramatic examples (Gusella et al, 1983).

There are numerous disorders with psychiatric ramifications in which a specific gene defect has been identified (McKusick, 1985). These include the syndromes that lead to mental retardation such as Lesch Nyhan (Xq) (that is, chromosome;

Table 2. Known Genetic Loci of Relevance to Psychiatry

	Location
Alcohol dehydrogenase (ADH), Class I	4_q
Alcohol dehydrogenase (ADHE) (? Control of Expression)	1_p
Alcohol dehydrogenase (ADHX) Class III	4_q
Beta adrenergic receptor	5_q
Dopamine–beta–hydroxylase	?9
Manic-depressive illness	?6
Beta–adrenergic stimulation, response to	21_q
Monoamine oxidase A	X_q

Reprinted from McKusick VA: Human Gene Map. International Workshops on Human Gene Mapping, 1985.

p = short arm, q = long arm) and Prader-Willi (15q), and neurologic disorders that may present with psychiatric symptoms such as Huntington's disease (4p), acute intermittent porphyria (11q), and Wilson's disease (13q).

In addition, the loci for several biochemical parameters that are suspected to be involved in either etiology or outcome of the psychiatric disorders have been identified. Some of these relevant loci are shown in Table 2. It is important to note that many of these assignments are based upon a single study, and replication is clearly necessary. Identification of new loci is occurring at such a rapid rate that it is necessary to update the human map monthly. It is estimated that more than 10,000 gene loci will have been assigned to particular sites on chromosomes by the year 2000 (Suarez and Cox, 1985).

Application of this methodology to psychiatric disorders may be particularly fruitful in identifying major genes that are segregating in informative families. In a recent review of linkage analysis in psychiatry, Kidd and colleagues (1984) predicted that linkage analysis is likely to become the preferred tool for demonstrating unequivocally major genetic factors in complex disorders such as the psychiatric illnesses.

Table 3 summarizes the major models of disease transmission and the expected patterns of illness within pedigrees according to each model. However, adequate fit of these models to the observed data does *not* provide positive evidence regarding the mode of transmission of a disorder. Rather, those models that do not provide an adequate fit to the data can be excluded as explanations of the mode of transmission of a particular disorder, if the assumptions of the model are not violated.

The traditional single major locus Mendelian models have been rarely found to fit family data for the major psychiatric disorders (with the exception of some bipolar pedigrees as described above). However, these models may still provide a good fit to subtypes of the psychiatric disorders. Despite the recent progress in diagnostic nomenclature, definitions of psychiatric disorders still suffer from

Table 3. Observed Patterns of Transmission for the Major Genetic Models

Model		Observed Patterns
Single major locus (SML)	Autosomal dominant	• Every generation, no skipping • Unilineal transmission • Affected persons transmit to 1/2 (on average) of the offspring • Males = females
	Autosomal recessive	• Horizontal transmission • 1/4 of sibs of affected persons are affected • Males = females • Consanguinity may be increased in parents
	x-linked recessive	• Males >>> females • Absence of male-to-male transmission • 1/2 sons of carrier female are affected • All daughters of affected males are carriers
	x-linked dominant	• Females > males • Affected females transmit trait to 1/2 sons and 1/2 daughters • Affected males transmit to all daughters and not sons
Multifactorial	> 1 gene (polygenic) and/or > 1 nongenetic factor (cultural)	• Risk among relatives increased according to severity of the proband • Bilineal transmission common • Mean for offspring midway between parents and population values (continuous traits) • Recurrence risk (dichotomous traits) or correlation (continuous traits) among relatives is proportional to the degree of the genetic relationship
Mixed model	SML and multifactorial	• 3 distributions within a single skewed distribution

a lack of established reliability and validity, thereby casting doubt on assignment of affection status in probands and their families, and complicating genetic analyses. Furthermore, genetic heterogeneity, or different genetic factors resulting in similar phenotypic expression, is likely to be operating in the major psychiatric disorders, given the complexity of the underlying neural and developmental mechanisms.

The multifactorial model of disease transmission has been commonly found to adequately explain the observed patterns of transmission of some psychiatric disorders (for example, schizophrenia) (McGue et al, 1985). This model, first proposed by Falconer (1965), specifies that there are numerous genes and transmissible and nontransmissible cultural factors that are additively and independently (that is, without *epistasis*) involved in producing a phenotype. There is assumed to be a continuous underlying distribution, or liability, which is defined as the propensity for expressing a disease. The total liability includes a genetic (or transmitted) component and a nontransmitted component of the variance. The liability is assumed to be normally distributed with mean = 0 and a variance = 1. When a sufficient number of these factors is present, the individual will fall beyond the threshold, or the point on the distribution beyond which the disorder becomes manifest (see Figure 1).

Morton and MacLean (1974) have described a model which consists of both an autosomal major locus and a multifactorial component. According to this

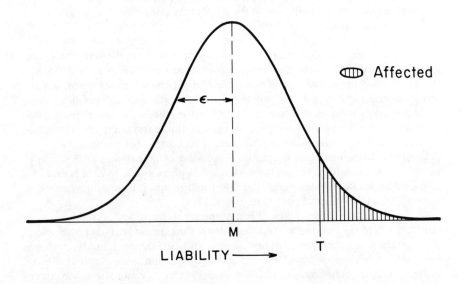

Figure 1. Polygenic thresholds model of disease transmission.

model, there are three major genotypes with heritable variation about the distribution for each genotype. The multifactorial background is comprised of both polygenic and environmental variation. This model is particularly useful when tested against a purely multifactorial model to determine whether the SML component significantly contributes to the fit of the model.

The analytic technique that has been frequently applied to resolve the polygenic and cultural components under multifactorial transmission is path analysis (Rao et al, 1981; Cloninger et al, 1985). The basic parameters are paths, co-paths, and correlations between pairs of relatives throughout an extended pedigree. Allowance is made for assortative mating, correlated environments between pairs of individuals, and unique environments of individuals. The observed and expected values of the correlations are compared and tested for statistical significance. Resolution of cultural and biological inheritance requires either extended familial relationships (that is, monozygotic twins, half sibs), or the identification of a relevant index of inherited environment.

More detailed descriptions of the assumptions, derivations, and computation of each of these models in psychiatry are discussed by Kidd (1981b); Reich et al (1980); and Cloninger et al (1985).

GENETIC EPIDEMIOLOGY OF PSYCHIATRIC DISORDERS

... our genes cannot make bricks without straw. The individual differences which men and women display are partly due to the fact that they receive different genes from their parents and partly due to the fact that the same genes live in different houses ... (Hogben, 1983, p. 1399)

There has been much progress during the past century in defining the epidemiology of psychiatric disorders since Jarvis' census of "lunatics" and "idiots" in 1850 (Jarvis, 1855). Through a rich interchange between sociologists, psychiatrists, psychologists, and epidemiologists, classification systems of psychiatric disorders have been established, standardized methods for ascertaining such classifications have been developed, and population parameters for psychiatric illnesses have been identified in both treated and untreated populations.

Similarly, there has been a dramatic explosion of knowledge in the field of genetics, with nearly 3,765 loci with Mendelian phenotypes having been identified, and with knowledge regarding the structure and function of genes incrementing at a monumental pace (McKusick, 1984).

There has been a general lack of communication, however, between individuals in the fields of genetics and epidemiology. Despite the goal of epidemiology to study the interaction between host, agent, and environment, epidemiologists have tended to neglect "host" characteristics other than demographics (Kuller, 1979). Similarly, geneticists have often neglected to consider the environment as a potential etiologic agent, either randomizing or controlling for it in their analyses. Geneticists consider the environment as noise and heredity the signal, whereas epidemiologists consider the opposite (Morton, 1982).

Despite their history of independence, the two fields share much common ground. Both are interested in determining the etiology of complex human disorders and predicting familial recurrence risks for such disorders. The advent of the new field of genetic epidemiology, defined as a science that deals with the etiology, distribution, and control of disease in groups of relatives, and with inherited (biological or cultural) causes of disease in populations, has served to bridge the gap between the two fields (Morton, 1982). As Morton notes, "synthesis of genetics and epidemiology is necessary before diseases of complex etiology can be understood and ultimately controlled" (p. 4).

The application of the techniques of the new field of genetic epidemiology, which is without either environmentalist or hereditarian bias, should result in substantial contributions to the understanding of psychiatric disorders. As in the study of other human disorders, genetic and epidemiologic methodologies have generally been applied independently to the study of psychiatric disorders.

The importance of the integration of epidemiologic methods in genetic studies is also underscored by the results of twin studies of numerous complex human disorders which suggest that 100 percent concordance rates for monozygotic twins are rarely observed. A recent panel of the Foundations' Fund for Research in Psychiatry studied the current state of research in identifying the role of gene–environment interactions in psychiatric disorders. They note how remarkable it is that despite the uniform agreement regarding the importance of environmental factors in psychiatric illness, nothing is known about what they are or how they act. Numerous experts from the fields of genetics and psychiatry concluded that an understanding of the genetic and environmental contributions to the etiology of psychiatric disorders will only occur through multidisciplinary studies which employ the best statistical–genetic methodology (Kidd and Matthysse, 1978).

The discipline of genetic epidemiology has directly built on the methods and analytic techniques of the field of population genetics by incorporating several methodologic techniques from the field of epidemiology. In general, genetic–epidemiologic studies differ from traditional genetic study paradigms by including control groups; assessing factors involved in sampling bias among treated populations; incorporating measurement of the environment such as diet, stress, and the social environment; studying the effects of cohabitation; examining time–space clustering; and employing analytic techniques such as methods of age correction that simultaneously control for confounding variables. Genetic epidemiology can also be distinguished from its two derivative fields in genetics. Whereas the emphasis of population genetics is on distributions of *traits*, both normal and aberrant, in *populations*, and focus of clinical genetics is on *individuals* who have genetic diseases, the major focus of genetic epidemiology is on *disease* in *populations*, or population subgroups.

The most common misconception regarding the role of genetic factors in the manifestation of a particular trait or disease is that the term "genetic" implies determinism by innate factors with a subsequently unalterable course. Nothing has impeded progress in knowledge of the development of human traits and disorders more than the nature *versus* nurture controversy. The concept was originally introduced by Galton (1894) as nature *and* nurture. The majority of known genetic traits are not fully expressed, or *totally* independent from the environment in which they are expressed. An illustrative example of gene–environment interaction is glucose–6–phosphate dehydrogenase (G6PD) deficiency, an x-linked disorder caused by a mutation on the long arm of the x chromosome. The expression of this disorder becomes manifest as hemolytic anemia only when the susceptible individual is exposed to certain drugs or fava beans. Genes may also be involved in the response or resistance to purely environmental agents such as diet, stress, exercise, drugs, and nutritional deficiencies, through the activity of immunogenetic factors of the major histocompatibility complex (Antel and Arnason, 1983).

Not only is the expression of genes modified by the environment, but there is now substantial evidence to indicate that numerous environmental factors may actually alter the genotype. For example, environmental agents may induce chromosomal mutations that lead to carcinoma, such as the role of Epstein–Barr virus in Burkitt's lymphoma, or tobacco smoking in small cell carcinoma of the lung.

Paradigms for the Analysis of Genetic Epidemiologic Studies

Descriptive epidemiologic studies are important in specifying the rates and distribution of disorders in the general population. These data can be applied to identify biases that may exist in treated populations and case registries from which persons who serve as probands in family, twin, and adoption studies are selected. Such individuals often constitute the "tip of the iceberg" of the disease and are not representative of the general population of similarly affected individuals with respect to demographic, social, or clinical characteristics (Reich et al, 1980).

The case-control study has been employed to study familial aggregation of disease in two ways: one in which the frequency of a positive family history among the cases is compared with that among the controls; and the other involves a retrospective cohort study (or combination case-control/cohort study), in which the retrospectively assessed course of relatives of the cases is compared to that of the controls.

After familial transmission of a trait has been established, the immediate goal of genetic epidemiologic studies is to identify the relative degree of phenotypic variance that can be attributed to genetic factors and transmissible and nontransmissible environmental factors. The ultimate purpose of such studies is to identify the specific agents that play an etiologic or contributing role to the development of the trait.

The two chief study paradigms for studying gene–environment interactions involve holding either the genetic background or the environment constant and evaluating systematic changes in the other (MacMahon, 1968; Susser, 1985). Examples of studies that hold genetic background constant while observing differential environmental exposures include: studies of discordant twins, migrant population studies, relatives exposed to a particular agent such as a virus, twins reared separately, or the family set design, in which comparisons are made among families of similar structure living in distinct environments.

Examples of paradigms in which the environment is held constant and genetic factors are allowed to vary include: monozygotic twins of affected individuals compared to dizygotic twins and nontwin siblings; offspring of consanguineous matings, compared to those of nonconsanguineous matings; half siblings compared to full siblings living in the same home; and first degree relatives of affected individuals.

In both types of studies, observations can be made regarding time–space clustering of disease, which can provide information regarding environmental agents, or a characteristic age of onset and course, which may provide information on genetic factors.

Ward (1980) suggests the following general steps in conducting genetic–epidemiologic studies:

1. construction of a biologically plausible definition of the problem
2. development of quasi-experimental studies
3. appropriate selection of controls
4. maximum use of phenotypic information
5. development of a hierarchy of hypothesis testing, in which one study builds upon another in a sequential manner

The basic analytic methods of genetic–epidemiologic studies entail a combination of the epidemiologic and genetic models described above. The general multifactorial model has been extended in numerous ways to allow for more refined estimates of familial and cultural transmission. Most recently, Kendler and Eaves (in press) have developed models for the joint effect of genes and environment on the liability to psychiatric illnesses; an additive effect of genotype and environment; genetic control of sensitivity to the environment; and genetic control of environmental exposure.

Application of the genetic–epidemiologic approach has yielded information on risk and etiologic factors for a number of disorders such as diabetes, hyperlipidemia, and coronary heart disease (King et al, 1984). An exemplary study of monozygotic twins who were concordant for heart disease but *discordant* for cigarette smoking demonstrated that smoking was not a risk factor for coronary heart disease. However, the twin pairs were found to be discordant for lung disease, which was found to be strongly related to cigarette exposure (Hauge et al, 1970). King and colleagues (1984) provide an excellent review of the genetic epidemiology of the major complex human disorders.

It is often difficult to distinguish between transmitted and genetic factors, because environmental factors are often confounded with genetic susceptibility to those factors. The effects of putative exogenous factors such as drugs, dietary factors, and physical factors such as stress, fever, and exercise, may be modified by immunogenetic factors, or genetic variation in enzymes, hormones, fatty acids, or neurochemicals (Antel and Arnason, 1983). In addition, factors that may appear to be purely environmental may actually be a result of transmissible factors. For example, the occurrence of parental divorce is generally considered to be an extrinsic risk factor to the development of drug abuse or alcoholism among the offspring. Yet the adoption study of Cadoret and Gath (1978) has demonstrated that divorce is "transmitted" among female offspring of alcoholics who neither reside with their biologic alcoholic parent nor develop alcoholism themselves. Although divorce is clearly not a transmissible phenomenon, the underlying factors that may lead to divorce, such as irritability or antisocial traits, may be transmissible and explain the tendency for divorce to run in families.

CLINICAL IMPLICATIONS OF GENETIC–EPIDEMIOLOGIC STUDIES IN PSYCHIATRY

In addition to the aforementioned contributions of genetic epidemiology, one major application of genetic–epidemiologic studies in psychiatry would be genetic counseling of affected persons and/or their spouses regarding the risk of transmission of the disorder to their offspring. Genetic counseling is defined as "the provision of information bearing upon the problems related to the occurrence, or risk of occurrence, of a genetic disorder in a family. The process is concerned with the risk and burden of the disorder and the options available for dealing with it" (Thompson and Thompson, 1980, p. 337). Genetic counseling is typically sought by couples with an affected child, or with a positive family history, who plan to conceive or have conceived another child. When the mode of transmission of the disorder is known, it is possible to estimate the recurrence risk in subsequent offspring. The presence of some disorders can be detected in utero by biochemical means if the defect is known, or through linked markers (with a certain confidence level) if the precise defect is not yet known. If the ongoing molecular genetics studies of the psychiatric disorders succeed in identifying disease markers, such markers could ultimately be used to detect a disease-predisposing genotype.

Because the mode of transmission of the major psychiatric disorders is not known, genetic counseling of couples-at-risk now involves specification of the empirical recurrence risks that have been derived from previous studies of the familial transmission of the disorder. The empirical recurrence risk should be refined according to the family's or individual's sociodemographic characteristics such as age, sex, socioeconomic status, and ethnicity, and the consultand's clinical characteristics including age at onset, co-morbidity, severity of illness, illness in the co-parent, and other factors which may be related to transmission of the disorder. It is also important to consider patterns of transmission in previous generations of the pedigree in estimating recurrence risks. For example, the range of recurrence risks for bipolar illness is three to seven percent but, as described above, there is also ample evidence that there may be certain pedigrees that manifest an x-linked mode of transmission. Investigation of transmission patterns in other lines of the pedigree may yield information regarding the presence of x-linked transmission in a particular family.

Approximate empirical recurrence risks for offspring of probands with the other major psychiatric disorders may be summarized as follows: schizophrenia: 10 percent (Kessler, 1980); agoraphobia/panic disorder: 30 percent (Crowe, 1985); antisocial personality: 16 percent (Robins, 1985); unipolar affective disorder: 12 percent (Gershon, 1983b); obsessive-compulsive disorder: 4 percent (Carey and Gottesman, 1981); and alcoholism: 25 percent males; 5 percent females (Goodwin, 1984). These estimates have been derived from reviews of controlled family studies that specify the recurrence risk in offspring of one psychiatrically ill parent. When both parents are affected, these estimates may double or triple.

Another major application of genetics to clinical psychiatry concerns the use of pharmacogenetics in formulating treatment decisions. For example, Pare and Mack (1971) found that relatives of probands with affective disorders shared the pattern of drug response or nonresponse with the proband. In eliciting a family history of a psychiatric disorder, clinicians should also examine the efficacy of specific pharmacologic agents among other family members with similar psychiatric syndromes to the patient who is being evaluated. The application of such information may conserve considerable time and effort in treatment decisions.

It is clear that most of the psychiatric disorders are related to major disruption in familial functioning. It has been difficult to identify whether the disruption in social functioning is causal, contributory, or residual to the illness. Nevertheless, such detrimental environments tend to be transmitted through families, and such combinations of vulnerable genotypes and negative environments are likely to interact in increasing the likelihood that offspring will be affected. The results of recent studies of populations at high risk for these disorders may yield information on premorbid indicators that may permit prediction of persons who are likely to develop a particular disorder. To date, there are no consistent premorbid biologic trait markers that would allow clinicians to identify vulnerable individuals for any of the major psychiatric disorders. However, recent studies of subjects at high risk for alcoholism have yielded some of the most promising results regarding neurophysiologic parameters as potential markers for subjects for alcoholism (Schuckit, 1985).

Finally, clinicians are often called upon by family members or prospective spouses to provide data on the course of a particular psychiatric illness. Again, a summary of empirical data relevant to that person's combination of demographic, social, and clinical characteristics should be carefully prepared. Unfortunately, the course of psychiatric disorders and their subtypes have been too often neglected in recent systems of diagnostic nomenclature. This is in direct contrast to the diagnostic approach prescribed by Kraepelin (1921), in which the course of illness was considered to be an essential element of diagnostic definitions.

FUTURE DIRECTIONS

There is a need for greater interchange between clinicians (who have extensive experience in attending to the diagnosis, treatment, course, and outcome of persons with psychiatric disorders) and genetic epidemiologists (who are designing and analyzing studies of such disorders). Problems of definition of who is affected, and to what degree, continue to plague the field and impede progress in identifying risk factors and modes of transmission of the psychiatric disorders. In particular, observations by clinicians regarding milder forms of manifestations of particular disorders, and diagnostic subtypes that are responsive to particular pharmacologic agents, may provide clues regarding etiologically distinct groups, the validity of which may be tested in genetic–epidemiologic studies. Although genetic–epidemiologic studies are useful in solving such problems regarding the validity of diagnostic categories, they are still dependent upon clinicians' definitions and identification of probands for inclusion.

Now that there has been an integration of the fields of genetics and epidemiology within psychiatry, it is necessary to merge the ongoing work in the fields of psychopharmacology and neurobiology to provide an even broader scope of investigation of the factors related to the pathogenesis of the major psychiatric disorders. Studies of familial aggregation should also include biologic trait measures, in which co-segregation of the marker with the disease may provide information on possible etiologic mechanisms, as well as milder manifestations and alternate forms of expression of particular disorders. Such studies will enhance our ability to specify mechanisms through which genes and their products interact with other factors within a particular genetic and environmental background, to produce the ultimate phenotype that comes to the attention of the clinician. Furthermore, knowledge of the research in biologic psychiatry will enable genetic epidemiologists to determine whether the theories that emerge from their studies make biologic sense.

Collaboration between genetic epidemiologists and immunologists and endocrinologists should be undertaken in order to examine how such systems modify host susceptibility and expression of transmitted psychiatric disorders. For example, it has been demonstrated that the female preponderance of depression and anxiety disorders cannot be attributed to the transmission of these disorders (Merikangas et al, 1985). Endocrine factors appear to play a major role in the enhanced expression of depression in women (Fischette et al, 1983; Halbreich and Rose, 1985). Similar findings have emerged for alcoholism, in which males outnumber females by four to one; and the sex difference is also not related to transmission (Reich et al, 1975).

Genetic linkage studies of psychiatric disorders need to be conducted to resolve the discrepant results obtained thus far, particularly for traits with known loci. The linkage studies that employ RFLPs or polymorphic markers with no known function should also be conducted on selected large pedigrees with clear segregation patterns.

Hybrid and novel designs should be applied, such as twin/offspring studies, combinations of family/high risk paradigms, half-sib/extended pedigree studies that are not limited to estimating the heritability of particular disorders, but also include identification of specific environmental factors that may be involved in the pathogenesis of these diseases.

In summary, the major psychiatric disorders consist of disorders for which the validity of definitions has yet to be established, the etiology is unknown, and the pathway from genotype to the phenotype is complex and probably heterogeneous. The new field of genetic epidemiology, with an integration of knowledge from clinical psychiatry, neurobiology, immunology, and endocrinology, provides hope of unraveling some of the complexity that continues to obscure the etiology and pathogenesis of the psychiatric conditions. Many of these disorders are among the most prevalent and distressing of all chronic human diseases. Specification of the role of genetic factors for a disease may also lead to the identification of critical environments for its expression. In fact, knowledge of the role of genetic factors may lead to prevention and amelioration of these diseases by purely environmental methods (Harris, 1977). Even without accomplishing the ultimate aim of specification of etiology, a considerable degree of optimism is warranted that the current generation of genetic–epidemiologic studies may yield information that will enable prevention and intervention efforts to minimize the effects of these disorders.

REFERENCES

Ahern FM, Johnson RC, Wilson JR, et al: Family resemblances in personality. Behav Genet 12:261-280, 1982

Antel JR, Arnason BGW: Genetic predisposition to environmental factors, in Genetics of Neurological and Psychiatric Disorders. Edited by Kety S, Rowland L, Sidman R, et al. New York, Raven Press, 1983

Baron M, Risch N, Levitt M, et al: Genetic analysis of platelet monoamine oxidase activity in families of schizophrenic patients. J Psychiatr Res 19:9-22, 1985

Cadoret R: Genotype–environment interaction in antisocial behavior. Psychol Med 12:235-239, 1982

Cadoret RJ, Gath A: Inheritance of alcoholism in adoptees. Br J Psychiatry 132:252-258, 1978

Cadoret RJ, O'Gorman TW, Heywood E, et al: Genetic and environmental factors in major depression. J Affect Dis 9:155-164, 1985

Carey G, Gottesman II: Twin and family studies of anxiety, phobic, and obsessive disorders, in Anxiety: New Research and Changing Concepts. Edited by Klein D, Rabkin J. New York, Raven Press, 1981

Carter CO: Polygenic inheritance and common diseases. Lancet 1:1252-1256, 1969

Castle WE: The laws of heredity of Galton and Mendel and some laws governing race and improvement by selection. Proceedings of the American Academy of Arts and Sciences 39:223-242, 1903

Cavalli-Sforza LL, Bodmer WF: The Genetics of Human Populations. San Francisco, WH Freeman, 1971

Cloninger CR, Reich T, Wetzel R: Alcoholism and affective disorders: familial associations and genetic models, in DW Goodwin, CK Erikson (eds): Alcoholism and Affective Disorders: Clinical, Genetic, and Biochemical Studies. Edited by Goodwin DW, Erikson CK. New York, SP Scientific Books, 1979

Cloninger CR, Bohman M. Sigvardsson S: Inheritance of alcohol abuse: cross-fostering analysis of adopted men. Arch Gen Psychiatry 38:861-868, 1981

Cloninger CR, Reich T, Yokoyama S: Genetic diversity, genome organization, and investigation of the etiology of psychiatric diseases. Psychiatr Dev 3:225-246, 1983

Cloninger CR, Reich T, Suarez BK, et al: The principles of genetics in relation to psychiatry, in Handbook of Psychiatry, vol. 5: The Scientific Foundations of Psychiatry. Edited by Shepherd M. Cambridge, Cambridge University Press, 1985

Crowe RR: The genetics of panic disorder and agoraphobia. Psychiatr Dev 2:171-186, 1985

Falconer DS: The inheritance of liability to certain diseases, estimated from the incidence among relatives. Ann Hum Genet 29:51-76, 1965

Fischette CT, Biegon A. McEwen BS: Sex differences in serotonin 1 receptor binding in rat brain. Science 222:333-335, 1983

Freud S: Collected Papers, vol 1. London, Hogarth Press, 1953

Galton F: Natural Inheritance. New York, MacMillan, 1894

Gershon ES: Genetics of major psychoses, in Genetics of Neurological and Psychiatric Disorders. Edited by Kety S, Rowland LP, Sidman RL, et al. New York, Raven, 1983a

Gershon ES. The genetics of affective disorders. Psychiatry Update: The American Psychiatric Association Annual Review, Vol. II. Edited by Grinspoon L. Washington, DC, American Psychiatric Press, Inc., 1983b

Gershon ES, Targum SD, Kessler LR, et al: Genetic Studies and Biologic Strategies in the Affective Disorders. Philadelphia, WB Saunders, 1977

Goldin LR, Gershon ES: Association and linkage studies of genetic marker loci in major psychiatric disorders, in Psychiatric Developments: Advances and Prospects in Research and Clinical Practice. Edited by Guze SB, Roth M. Oxford, Oxford University Press, 1983

Goodwin DW: Alcoholism and heredity: a review and hypothesis. Arch Gen Psychiatry 36:57-61, 1979

Goodwin DW: Studies of familial alcoholism: a review. J Clin Psychiatry 45:14-17, 1984

Goodwin DW, Schulsinger F, Hermansen L, et al: Alcohol problems in adoptees raised apart from biological parents. Arch Gen Psychiatry 28:238-243, 1973

Gottesman II, Carey G: Extracting meaning and direction from twin data. Psychiatr Dev 1:35-50, 1983

Gottesman II, Shields J: A critical review of recent adoption, twin, and family studies of schizophrenia: behavioral genetics perspectives. Schizophrenia Bull 2:360-401, 1976

Gottfries CG, Oreland L, Wiberg A, et al: Brain levels of monoamine oxidase in depression. Lancet 2:360-361, 1974

Gurling H. Application of molecular biology to mental illness: analysis of genomic DNA and brain RNA. Psychiatr Dev 3:257-273, 1985

Gusella JF, Wexler NS, Conneally PM, et al. A polymorphic DNA marker genetically linked to Huntington's Disease. Nature 306:234-238, 1983

Halbreich V, Rose R: Hormones and depression-conceptual transitioners. Pharmacol Bull 21:568-572, 1985

Harris H: Nature and Nurture. N Engl J Med 297:1399-1400, 1977

Hauge M, Horvald B, Reid D: A twin study of the influence of smoking on morbidity and mortality. Acta Genet Med Gemellol 19:335-336, 1970

Heston L: Psychiatric disorders in foster home reared children of schizophrenic mothers. Br J Psychiatry 112:819-825, 1966

Hogben LT: Nature and Nurture. London, Allen & Unwin, 1933

Hutchings B, Mednick SA: Criminality in adoptees and their adoptive and biological parents: a pilot study, in Biosocial Basis of Criminal Behavior. Edited by Mednick SA, Christiansen KO. New York, Gardner Press, 1977

Insel TR, Mueller EA III, Gillin JC, et al: Biological markers in obsessive-compulsive and affective disorders. J Psychiatr Res 18:407-424, 1984

Jablensky A: Epidemiological and clinical research as a guide in the search for risk factors and biological markers. J Psychiatr Res 18:541-554, 1984

Jarvis E: Insanity and idiocy in Massachusetts. Report of the Commission on Lunacy, 1855

Kendler K: Genetics of schizophrenia, in Psychiatry Update: The American Psychiatric Association Annual Review, Vol. 5. Edited by Frances AJ, Hales RE. Washington, DC, American Psychiatric Press, Inc., 1986

Kendler KK, Eaves LJ: Models for the joint effect of genotype and environment on liability to psychiatric illness. Am J Psychiatry 143:279-289, 1986

Kessler S: The genetics of schizophrenia: a review. Schizophrenia Bull 6:404-416, 1980

Kety SS, Rosenthal D, Wender PH: The types and prevalence of mental illness in the biological and adoptive families of adopted schizophrenics, in The Transmission of Schizophrenia. Edited by Rosenthal D, Kety S. London, Pergamon, 1968

Kidd KK: Genetic linkage markers in the psychiatric disorders, in E. Usdin and I. Hanin (eds): Biological Markers in Neurology and Psychiatry. Edited by Usdin E, Hanin I. Oxford, Pergamon, 1981a

Kidd KK: Genetic models for psychiatric disorders, in Genetic Research Strategies for Psychobiology and Psychiatry. Edited by Gershon ES, Matthysse S, Breakefield XP, et al. Pacific Grove, California, Boxwood Press, 1981b

Kidd KK, Matthysse S: Research designs for the study of gene–environment interactions in psychiatric disorders. Arch Gen Psychiatry 35:925-932, 1978

Kidd KK, Gerhard DS, Kidd JR, et al: Recombinant DNA methods in genetic studies of affective disorders, in Proceedings, 14th Collegium International of Neuropsychopharmacology Congress, Florence, Italy, 1984

King MC, Lee GM, Spinner NB, et al: Genetic epidemiology. Annu Rev Public Health 5:1-52, 1984

Kleinbaum DG, Kupper LL, Morgenstern H: Epidemiologic Research: Principles and Quantitative Methods. Belmont, California, Wadsworth, 1982

Kraepelin E: Manic-Depressive Insanity and Paranoia. Edited by Roberson G. Edinburgh, E & S Livingston, 1921

Kreitman N: Epidemiology in relation to psychiatry, in Handbook of Psychiatry, vol. 5: The Scientific Foundations of Psychiatry. Edited by Shepherd M. Cambridge, Cambridge University Press, 1985

Kuller LH: The role of population genetics in the study of the epidemiology of cardiovascular risk factors, in Genetic Analysis of Common Diseases: Applications to Predictive Factors in Coronary Disease. New York, Liss, 1979

MacMahon B: Gene–environment interaction in human disease. J Psychiatr Res 6 (Suppl 1):393-402, 1968

Major LF, Murphy DL: Platelet and plasma monoamine oxidase activity in alcoholic individuals. Br J Psychiatry 132:548-554, 1978

Mausner JS, Bahn AK: Epidemiology: An Introductory Text. Philadelphia, WB Saunders, 1974

McGue M. Gottesman II, Rao DC: Resolving genetic models for the transmission of schizophrenia. Genet Epidemiol 2:99-110, 1985

McGuffin P, Farmer AE, Gottesmann II, et al: Twin concordance for operationally defined schizophrenia: confirmation of familiality and heritability. Arch Gen Psychiatry 41:541-545, 1984

McKusick VE: Human gene map. Paper presented at Short Course on Human and Experimental Genetics. Bar Harbor, Maine, Jackson Laboratory, July 1985

McKusick VE: Human Genetics. Englewood Cliffs, New Jersey, Prentice-Hall, 1969

McKusick VE: Mendelian Inheritance in Man. Baltimore, Johns Hopkins University Press, 1984

Mednick SA, Finello KM. Biological factors and crime: implications for forensic psychiatry. Int J Law Psychiatry 6:1-15, 1983

Merikangas KR, Weissman MM, Pauls DL: Genetic factors in the sex ratio of major depression. Psychol Med 15:63-69, 1985

Milbank Memorial Fund: Epidemiology of Mental Disorder. New York, Milbank Memorial Fund, 1950

Morton NE: Sequential tests for the detection of linkage. Am J Hum Genet 7:277-318, 1955

Morton NE: Outline of Genetic Epidemiology. Basel, Karger, 1982

Morton NE, Chung CS (Eds): Genetic Epidemiology. New York, Academic Press, 1978

Morton NE, MacLean CJ: Analysis of familial resemblance, III: complex resemblance of quantitative traits. Am J Hum Genet 26:489-503, 1974

Murray RM, Clifford C, Gurling HMD: Current genetic and biological approaches to alcoholism. Psychiatr Dev 2:179-192, 1983

Neel JV, Shull WJ: Human Heredity. Chicago, University of Chicago Press, 1954

Nies A, Robinson DS, Harris LS, et al: Comparison of monoamine oxidase substrate activities in twins, schizophrenics, depressives, and controls. Adv Biochem Psychopharmacol 12:59-70, 1974

Pare CMB, Mack JW: Differentiation of two genetically specific types of depression by the response to antidepressant drug. J Med Genet 8:306-309, 1971

Penrose LS: The detection of autosomal linkage in data which consists of pairs of brothers and sisters of unspecified parentage. Annals of Eugenics 6:133-138, 1935

Rao DC, Morton NE, Gottesman II, et al: Path analysis of qualitative data on pairs of relatives: application to schizophrenia. Hum Hered 31:325-333, 1981

Regier DA, Myers JK, Kramer M, et al: The NIMH epidemiologic catchment area program: historical context, major objectives, and study population characteristics. Arch Gen Psychiatry 41:934-941, 1984

Reich T, Winokur G, Mullaney J. The transmission of alcoholism, in Genetic Research in Psychiatry. Edited by Fieve R, Rosenthal P, Britt H. Baltimore, Johns Hopkins University Press, 1975

Reich T, Suarez B, Rice J, et al: Current directions in genetic epidemiology, in Current Developments in Anthropological Genetics. Edited by Mielke J, Crawford M. New York, Plenum Press, 1980

Rieder RO, Gershon ES: Genetic strategies in biological psychiatry. Arch Gen Psychiatry 35:866-873, 1978

Risch N, Baron M: x-linkage and genetic heterogeneity in bipolar-related major affective illness: re-analysis of linkage data. Ann Hum Genet 46:153-166, 1982

Robins LN: Psychiatric epidemiology. Arch Gen Psychiatry 35:697-702, 1978

Robins LN: Epidemiology of antisocial personality, in Psychiatry, vol. 3. Edited by Cavenar JO. Philadelphia, JB Lippincott, 1985

Rosenthal D: Genetic Theory and Abnormal Behavior. New York, McGraw-Hill, 1970

Schwab JJ, Schwab ME: Sociocultural Roots of Mental Illness: An Epidemiologic Survey. New York, Plenum, 1978

Schwab JJ, Schwab ME: Psychiatric epidemiology: some clinical implications. Psychosomatics 24:95-103, 1983

Schuckit M: Studies of populations at high risk for alcoholism. Psychiatr Dev 3:31-64, 1985

Schulsinger F: Psychopathy: heredity and environment. International Journal of Mental Health 1:190-206, 1975

Shepherd M: The contribution of epidemiology to clinical psychiatry. Am J Psychiatry 141:1574-1576, 1984

Suarez BK, Cox NJ: Linkage analysis for psychiatric disorders, I: basic concepts. Psychiatr Dev 3:219-243, 1985

Susser M: Separating heredity and environment. American Journal of Preventive Medicine 1:5-23, 1985

Thompson JS, Thompson MW: Genetics in Medicine. Philadelphia, WB Saunders, 1980

Torgerson S: Genetic factors in anxiety disorders. Arch Gen Psychiatry 40:1085-1089, 1983

Ward RH: Genetic epidemiology. Soc Biol 27:85-99, 1980

Watson JD, Tooze J, Kurt DT: Recombinant DNA: A Short Course. New York, WH Freeman, 1983

Weissman MM, Klerman GL: Epidemiology of mental disorders. Arch Gen Psychiatry 35:705-712, 1978

Wolpert L: DNA and its message. Lancet 2:853-856, 1984

Wyatt RJ, Potkin SG, Murphy DL: Platelet monoamine oxidase activity in schizophrenia: a review of the data. Arch Gen Psychiatry 136:377-385, 1979

Chapter 29

Parental Mental Disorder as a Psychiatric Risk Factor

by Michael Rutter, C.B.E., M.D., F.R.C.P., F.R.C.Psych

STATISTICAL ASSOCIATIONS

More than 60 years have gone by since Janet drew attention to the importance of parental mental disorder as a psychiatric risk factor for children, and outlined the possible mechanisms that might be involved. Subsequent research has amply documented the reality of risk, as demonstrated by the consistent statistical associations between psychiatric disorder in parents and in their children (Rutter, 1966; Rutter and Quinton, 1984). Such associations have been demonstrated in numerous epidemiological studies of the general population; in case control comparisons of the parents of children with a psychiatric disorder; and in case control comparisons of the children of parents with a mental disorder. Moreover, the main risk is for persistent psychiatric disorders in the children rather than transient situational stress responses (Rutter and Quinton, 1984).

Of course, correlations do not prove causation and it could be that the problems of rearing a mentally disturbed child led to emotional disorder in the parent rather than the other way around. Doubtless that occurs; certainly there is evidence that the rearing of biologically handicapped children is associated with an increased rate of parental distress and disturbances (Breslau et al, 1982; Cooke et al, 1982) and there is some tentative evidence that maternal depression may be more likely to persist if one or more of the children has an emotional/behavioral disorder (Cox and Mills, 1983). Nevertheless, this does not seem to be the usual explanation if only because in many, if not most, cases the parental disorder antedates that in the child. Moreover, Richman and colleagues' (1982) prospective epidemiological/longitudinal study, showed that maternal depression when the children were aged three years (and free of psychiatric disorder) predicted the development of childhood disorder during the subsequent five years. It may be concluded that the risks to the children associated with parental psychiatric disorders are real.

Nevertheless, that conclusion does not necessarily mean that the risk derives from the parental illness per se. After all, childhood psychiatric disorder is also associated with chronic physical illness in the parents (Rutter, 1966), with parental death (Garmezy, 1983), with parental criminality (Rutter and Giller, 1983), as well as with family adversities of various kinds (Rutter and Madge, 1976). It could be that the risks stem from the psychosocial stressors associated with parental illness rather than from the illness as such. Also, insofar as the risks are a function of parental illness, they may be genetically or environmentally determined. Moreover, the environmental risks may stem from physical damage to the fetus (as from drugs or perinatal complications) or to the child (as from head injuries or other accidents deriving from lack of adequate parental supervision), as well as from psychosocial factors. If effective prevention or intervention is to follow identification of the risk factor, it is important that the relevant risk *mechanisms* or processes be identified. These constitute the main focus of this review. Obviously, the mechanisms involved may vary according to the type of parental illness that constitutes the risk variable or the type of child disorder that ensues; that possibility will be borne in mind in considering the relevant empirical findings.

GENETIC MECHANISMS

Much of the research on the risks to the children of parental mental disorders has been based on the premise that the risk is likely to be genetically determined. That premise derives from the empirical demonstration that genetic factors play a significant role in the determination of schizophrenia (Gottesman and Shields, 1976); of major affective disorders (Gershon et al, 1982; Weissman et al, 1984a); of antisocial personality disorders and criminality (Crowe, 1983); and of some varieties of alcoholism (Bohman et al, 1981; Cloninger et al, 1981). However, although there is an important heritable component to many types of major mental illness, genetic factors seem much less important in the broad run of emotional disorders that make up most of adult psychiatric outpatient practice (Torgersen, 1983).

Yet these disorders, when they occur in patients, are associated with a substantially increased psychiatric risk for the children (Rutter, 1966; Rutter and Quinton, 1984). But even when the parental condition is genetically determined in part, it does not follow that the risk to the children is genetically mediated. This is because: a) with all of the adult mental disorders there is a major *non-*genetic component; b) the continuity between mental disorders in children and adult life is far from complete (Rutter, 1985a) and, even when there is continuity, the genetic component may be greater for disorders that persist into adulthood than for those confined to the childhood years (Rutter and Giller, 1983); and c) parental mental disorder is frequently accompanied by major environmental disturbance. Thus, parental symptoms may directly impinge on or involve the children in some way (Rutter, 1966); the parental illness may interfere with parenting functions (Rodnick and Goldstein, 1974; Weissman and Paykel, 1974) or impair parent-child interactions (Cox, in press; Davenport et al, 1984); it may result in family disruption, with the children having to go into foster care (Rice et al, 1971); or the parental illness may be accompanied by marked marital discord and disharmony (Birtchnell and Kennard, 1983a, 1983b; Rutter and Quinton, 1984). This is associated with increased conflict over child-rearing, greater segregation in decision making, reduced affection, and altered patterns of dominance (Kreitman et al, 1971; Hinchcliffe et al, 1975).

Specificity of Effects

It is necessary, therefore, to consider how to test the hypothesis that the risk to the children is genetically mediated. A genetic transmission would be suggested if the risk to the children were relatively confined to certain specific types of parental disorder. However, the evidence is clear cut that this is *not* the case. Raised rates of psychiatric disorder in the children have been found, for example, for parental schizophrenia (Watt et al, 1985), depression (Beardslee et al, 1983; Keller et al, in press; Cytryn et al, 1986; Weissman et al, 1984b), alcoholism (Rydelius, 1981), and personality disorder (Rutter and Quinton, 1984).

Alternatively, the genetic hypothesis would receive some support if the disorders in the children tended to be of the same type as those in the parents or, at least, showed a degree of specificity in relation to the parental diagnosis. But even that does not seem to be generally the case. On the whole, there are only rather weak associations between the form of disorders in parents and children. However, there may be some limited specificity. Thus, although the children of schizophrenic parents may show a variety of psychiatric problems, there are some that are both particularly associated with this parental diagnosis and which appear to constitute the childhood precursors of adult schizophrenia (Rutter, 1985a). The key features comprise: 1) abnormalities in interpersonal relationships, shown by odd, unpredictable behavior, social isolation and rejection by peers, and (in males) solitary antisocial behavior in the home; 2) neurodevelopmental inactivities in the form of clumsiness, visuospatial difficulties, and verbal impairment; and 3) attention deficits characterized by poor signal-noise discrimination.

Second, there is some tendency for parental personality disorder to be associated with conduct disturbance in the sons (Stewart et al, 1980; Rutter and Quinton, 1984) and for parental alcoholism to be linked with both alcoholism and delinquency in the male offspring (Rydelius, 1981).

Third, and less certainly, major depression in the parents may be particularly likely to lead to depression in the children (Keller et al, in press; Cytryn et al, 1986; Weissman et al, 1984b). That about one-half of the psychiatric disorders in the children of seriously depressed parents are depressive in form has been shown through the use of standardized psychiatric assessments. The uncertainty stems from: a) the observation that half the disorders in the children are *not* depressive in type; b) the lack of evidence on whether the rate of childhood depression is higher than that found with *other* forms of parental mental disorder (mostly the comparisons have been with normal controls); and c) the limited knowledge on the extent to which childhood depression is synonymous with the major depressive disorders of adult life (Rutter et al, 1986). Nevertheless, there is some suggestion that depressive disorders in the children may be particularly linked with serious parental depression (Rutter and Quinton, 1984).

Environmental Effects

A third test of the genetic hypothesis is provided by studies that determine whether the association between disorders in parents and in their children can be accounted for by environmental variables. Rutter and Quinton (1984), in their study of a heterogeneous group of mentally ill parents, used a range of well tested discriminating measures of the family environment. Their results showed that the risk to the children was largely a function of the family discord and hostility associated with the parental mental disorder. Indeed, the risk to the children of mentally ill parents showed no significant increase over the level in the general population once the family adversity variables had been taken into account. It seems that the risk was largely nongenetic. However, there appear to be some important exceptions to the general finding. Emery et al (1982) found that whereas discord constituted the main factor involved in the conduct disturbances seen in the children of parents with depression or personality disorder, it did not account for the increased rate of disorders in the children of schizophrenics. Discord did account for conduct disturbances in the children of parents with Huntington's disease, but not for depression (Folstein et al, 1983).

Keller et al (in press) found that parental discord increased the risk of disorder in the children of depressed parents, but that the severity and chronicity of maternal depression also did so (it is not clear whether this was so after controlling for discord; also, the risk to the children was not significantly affected by depression in the father). Rutter and Quinton's (1984) findings are also compatible with some risk for childhood depression that is additional to that associated with discord.

Radke-Yarrow and colleagues (1985) found insecure attachment to be more frequent in the children of severely depressed mothers than controls; however, what was most characteristic was a type of insecurity associated with both resistance and avoidance, together with abnormal affect or stereotyped maladaptive behavior. As this is the pattern that may also be associated with child abuse, it seems unlikely that it is specific to parental depression. Nevertheless, it may represent a more pathological variety of insecure attachment. Radke-Yarrow and colleagues found that the problem was significantly associated with the severity and chronicity of mental depression; it was unaffected by whether or not the father was depressed, but it was associated with maternal negative expressed emotion to the child and with the absence of a father in the household. The lack of effect in this study and in that by Keller and colleagues (in press) of paternal depression, together with the effect of discord and of negative expressed emotions, suggests that genetic factors do not constitute a sufficient explanation.

Rutter and Quinton (1984) found that parental personality disorder (of antisocial and other types) was powerfully associated with disorder in the children. However, multivariate analyses showed that this was more a consequence of the children's exposure to hostile/aggressive behavior than of the parental diagnosis per se. Nevertheless, although the effect fell short of statistical significance, there was some suggestion that personality disorder put the children at an additional psychiatric risk beyond that accounted for by exposure to hostile behavior.

Away-Adopted Children

Probably the strongest test of the genetic hypothesis is provided by determination of rates of disorder in the children of mentally ill parents who are adopted in infancy and brought up by non-ill parents to whom they are not biologically related. This strategy has been employed with schizophrenia, in which several studies from Heston (1966) to Tienari et al (1985) have found an increased rate of schizophrenia in the away-adopted children. It has also been shown that the attention deficits found in the fostered children of schizophrenics who have been brought up away from the ill parents are similar to those found in remitted adult schizophrenics (see Rutter, 1985a).

The results of these studies provide strong evidence of a genetic mode of transmission. Tienari and colleagues (1985) are the only investigators to have made direct study of adopting parents. The data from analyses on the first 91 cases (one-half of the sample) showed that the psychiatric risk was increased when the adoptive family environment was disturbed, suggesting a gene–

environment interaction. However, this effect was evident for borderline and character disorders rather than for schizophrenic psychoses. Similar studies of the rearing environment of away-adopted children have not been undertaken for other types of parental mental disorder. However, Stewart and de Blois (1983) found that the associations between antisocial behavior in fathers and sons was greater when the fathers were in the home, although some association was found when fathers were absent.

Clinical Implications

The clearest conclusions apply to parental schizophrenia, where it is apparent that there is a definite genetically mediated increased risk of schizophrenia in the children; the increased risk for a broader range of "schizophrenia spectrum" disorders may also include a genetic component, but the criteria for such disorders remain quite uncertain and the genetic link with schizophrenia is as yet unestablished (Torgersen, 1984); in addition, there is an increased risk for other types of psychiatric disorders that probably is not genetically mediated. The clinical picture of social oddity, neurodevelopmental abnormalities, and attention deficits is most likely to represent a precursor of schizophrenic psychosis, but the criteria are not sufficiently clear-cut to warrant a definite diagnosis at that stage. Moreover, there is no advantage in creating an expectation of genetic predestination when there is such good evidence that environmental factors also play an important role in etiology.

Brown and colleagues (1962) showed that overinvolvement with relatives who express high levels of criticism (high EE) is associated with an increased risk of relapse in adult schizophrenia; Leff and colleagues found that this effect was additional to that obtained by appropriate medication; and a controlled therapeutic trial (Leff et al, 1982) demonstrated that social intervention with high EE families that resulted in a fall in EE significantly reduced the relapse rate. Doane and colleagues (1981) found that high EE and poor communication in the families of disturbed adolescents predicted a worse outcome (including the development of schizophrenic spectrum disorders). It may be inferred that when the children of schizophrenic parents develop psychiatric disorder, they are most likely to be helped by therapeutic interventions that reduce highly critical parental overinvolvement and that lead to harmonious parent–child communication.

It seems probable that genetic factors play some contributory role (although possibly a minor one) in the development of conduct disorders in the children of parents with personality disorders and of depression in the children of depressed parents. However, the genetic evidence is inconclusive and it provides no pointers to any particular mode of prevention or intervention. Alcoholism arising in the offspring of alcoholic parents probably does so for both genetic and environmental reasons. The treatment would be similar to that required for alcoholism generally. However, the reality of the risk means that clinicians treating alcoholic parents need to be alerted to the dangers for the offspring, and to the desirability of taking seriously the risks associated with heavy drinking or with drinking to relieve stress.

EFFECTS ON THE FETUS

Alcohol

It is known that high doses of alcohol in the first trimester of pregnancy act as a teratogen, causing mental retardation and a characteristic cranio-facial malformation that has come to be known as the fetal alcoholic syndrome (Porter et al, 1984). It seems that in the first 10 weeks alcohol is cytotoxic, causing a deficiency in brain growth; in mid-pregnancy there is a transient disorganization and delay of neural cell migration and development and interference with central nervous system (CNS) neurotransmitter production, leading to neuroendocrine abnormalities. It remains uncertain whether there is a threshold for this alcohol effect on the fetus, or whether there is a continuum of effects with subclinical damage at alcohol levels too low to cause the full syndrome; the balance of evidence suggests a continuum effect. Also, it is unclear whether the effect is specific to alcohol; some evidence suggests that marihuana may act in a similar way (Hinson et al, 1982).

Because parental alcoholism tends to be associated with so many postnatal environmental disturbances, it has proved difficult to separate fetal from postnatal effects when examining psychiatric disturbances in the children. Spohr and Steinhausen (see Porter et al, 1984), in a study of a small incomplete sample, found that the behavior of children with fetal alcohol effects tended to improve somewhat during the preschool years, provided there was not severe mental retardation; but hyperactivity tended to persist. The psychiatric outcome at 8½ years was not significantly associated with the extent of morphological damage as clinically assessed. Much the best data are provided by Streissguth and colleagues' (see Porter et al, 1984) detailed and systematic follow-up of some 500 infants, one-half of whom were born to heavy drinkers, and one-half to light and infrequent drinkers. Alcohol related behavior effects were still evident at four years of age after statistical adjustment for possible confounding variables. The effect was most evident for reaction time, response tendency, and attention, suggesting some impairment in the central processing of information. The findings suggested a dose-response rather than a threshold effect, but clinical abnormalities were found only at the heaviest drinking levels (more than 59g of absolute alcohol per day).

We lack knowledge on how best to treat these alcohol related attention deficits and associated behavioral disturbances. However, clearly, the most crucial need is to prevent the initial fetal damage (although some of the behavioral sequelae are likely to be related to postnatal influences). Public education on the damage from heavy drinking is a priority. It should be noted, however, that a reduction in drinking, or even abstinence from alcohol, once a woman realizes that she is pregnant, will not constitute effective prevention because the most serious damage occurs during the weeks before and just after the first missed menstrual period. People need to appreciate that the consumption of alcohol should be kept low whenever pregnancy is planned or considered likely.

Opioids

It is known that opioids pass the placental barrier and that offspring of heroin or morphine addicts will be born opioid dependent (Jeremy and Bernstein, 1984). Withdrawal after birth leads to an abstinence syndrome with marked irritability and rejection of overtures of comfort. Because this is likely to constitute difficult behavior for parents, there have been fears that it would lead to impaired parent–infant relationships. Very little evidence is available on the extent of that risk. Jeremy and Bernstein (1984) found little difference at four months between methadone-exposed and comparison infants in their patterns of interaction (in both, poor maternal communication was associated with greater infant tension and worse coordination). The mothers who abused drugs showed worse interaction and communication with their infants than controls, but poor maternal functioning was related more to lack of current emotional resources than to drug use per se. The findings, as far as they go, are consistent with a risk to the children of being reared by a mother who is addicted to opioids, but they suggest that the main risk does not stem from the infants' drug withdrawal syndrome in the neonatal period.

Pregnancy Complications

There has been much discussion of the possible role of pregnancy complications in the etiology of schizophrenia (Walker and Emory, 1983). The interest derives from the findings that schizophrenia is associated with a history of slightly raised incidence of obstetric complications; that such complications are more likely in schizophrenic twins than in their discordant monozygotic co-twins; and that pregnancy complications may lead to neurodevelopmental disabilities if the complications cause neural damage, such as by intraventricular hemorrhage (Stewart, 1983).

It was thought that if schizophrenic women were more likely to have abnormal pregnancies, this might constitute part of the reason for the psychiatric risk for the offspring. It is now clear that they are *not* more likely to have abnormal pregnancies, but it seems that the children born to schizophrenic mothers may be more *vulnerable* to damage from obstetric complications (Walker and Emory, 1983). There is some suggestion that the increased ventricular size found in some cases of schizophrenia may be associated with obstetric complications (Schulsinger et al, 1984), as well as being more common in schizophrenic individuals without a positive family history (Murray et al, 1985). Nevertheless, it remains quite uncertain whether pregnancy complications play other than a minor contributory role in the transmission of schizophrenia from parent to child.

FAMILY ENVIRONMENTAL EFFECTS

Exposure to Specific Parental Symptoms

Rutter's (1966) early study of child psychiatric disorders associated with parental mental illness suggested that the risk to the children was greater when parental symptoms directly impinged on or involved the children. Direct symptom impact occurred when parental delusions incorporated the children in some way; when children were forced to participate in parental rituals and compulsions; or when the parental illness led to marked restrictions in the children's social activities.

Many of these examples concerned severe and somewhat unusual types of parental disorders. Rutter and Quinton's (1984) four-year prospective study of a representative sample of the families of newly placed psychiatric patients, who were parents of children under 15 years of age, showed that such direct involvement in parental symptoms was *not* common and did not account for much of the risk to the children. Neither the children's exposure to psychiatric symptoms nor their exposure to parental affective symptoms was significantly associated with psychiatric disorder in the children once other factors had been taken into account. However, their exposure to hostile or aggressive behavior by the parent was very strongly associated with an increased risk of psychiatric disorder, irrespective of the parental diagnosis.

Family Discord

Marital discord constituted one important source of hostile behavior in the Rutter and Quinton study, and it showed a strong association with an increased psychiatric risk for the children. Sons tended to develop disturbances earlier than daughters in the presence of family discord, but if the discord persisted, the girls suffered in the long run, although not to quite the same extent as the boys (Rutter and Quinton, 1984). Similar findings derive from all other studies that have included systematic discriminating measures of parent–child and marital relationships (Keller et al, in press; Richman et al, 1982; Cox, in press; Radke-Yarrow et al, 1985). Most of the research has concerned the effects of parental depression, but the major psychiatric risks to the children associated with family discord and parental hostility or critical overinvolvement have been found with personality disorder (Rutter and Quinton, 1984) and Huntington's disease (Folstein et al, 1983), as well as with general population samples of parents who do not suffer from any mental illness (Emery, 1982; Rutter, 1982; Rutter and Giller, 1983). The effect is greater when discord is associated with other family adversities, but it is not necessary that such adversities include parental mental disorder.

The consistency and pervasiveness of the risk associated with serious persistent family discord that is found in quite disparate populations testifies to its importance as a psychiatric risk factor. Probably the risks are greatest when the discord results in parental criticism or hostility that is directly focused on one or more of the children, but the risk is still evident when the tension and quarrelling are mainly between the two parents. The crucial role of discord as a mediator of the psychiatric risks associated with parental mental disorder is a consequence both of the strength of the discord effect, and of the frequency with which mental disorder is associated with marital discord. The nature of the connections between mental disorder and marital discord are complex; there is evidence of causal influences in both directions and, in addition, both may be determined in part by family stresses and adversities outside the marriage. Nevertheless, however the discord arises, it serves as an important risk mechanism for the children.

Family Breakup

Parental mental disorder, especially when it is associated with other psychosocial hazards, not infrequently leads to temporary or permanent family breakup (Rice et al, 1971). Thus, a high proportion of children admitted to Children's Homes or to family foster care because of parenting difficulties or child neglect or abuse have mentally ill parents (Quinton and Rutter, in press). Even short admissions to residential care are associated with a substantially increased psychiatric risk for the children (Wolkind and Rutter, 1973). We lack studies in which there has been systematic psychiatric assessment of the parents whose children go into foster or institutional care. Nevertheless, such evidence as there is shows that in terms of psychiatric sequelae, both in childhood (Roy, 1983) and in early adulthood (Quinton and Rutter, in press), the main risks derive from the adverse experiences rather than from the parental mental illness per se. Probably the main adversity is not the child's separation from parents as such, but rather the multiple stresses with which it is associated, and the family discord that preceded and succeeded the child's admission into foster care (Wolkind and Rutter, 1985).

Brown and colleagues (1986) showed that with respect to effects on vulnerability to adult depression, parental loss created a risk factor only if it led to poor quality parental care that was lacking in warmth and affection. Nevertheless, the insecurities associated with going in and out of foster care may well add to the risks. This finding, however, poses real dilemmas for the clinician; children who return to their biological parents do poorly in adolescence (Hodges and Tizard, submitted for publication), but so do those who remain in Children's Homes (Quinton and Rutter, in press). The consequences are better if there is either stable family fostering (Roy, 1983) or harmony is restored in the biological family (Rutter, 1971); but fostering breakdown is all too common and the restoration of good relationships in the family is not easily brought about.

Physical Risks

A few studies have noted an increased rate of accidents in the children of depressed mothers (Brown and Davidson, 1978), and it is known that severe head injuries create a significant and substantial psychiatric risk (Rutter et al, 1983). While this mechanism (that is, brain damage stemming from head injuries resulting from inadequate parental supervision) may be important in individual children, the infrequency of severe head injury means that it is not a relevant factor in other than a minority of cases.

Parenting

Although it has been appreciated for some time that mental disorders, including schizophrenia (Rodnick and Goldstein, 1974) and depression (Weissman and Paykel, 1974) may significantly disorganize, distort, and impair parenting, it is only very recently that there have been systematic observational studies of the parenting of mentally ill mothers (fathers have yet to be studied). Radke-Yarrow and colleagues (1985) found that severe (but not minor) maternal depression, especially of the bipolar variety, was associated with a marked increase in an unusual (and presumably psychopathological) variety of resistant/avoidant insecure attachments. Depressed mothers were rated as more disorganized, unhappy, tense, inconsistent, and ineffective with their children than nondepressed mothers (Davenport et al, 1984). Cox (in press) and colleagues found that depressed mothers in the community differed from controls in being less likely to respond to their two-year-old children's overtures, less facilitative of social interactions, less adept in responding to their children's cues, and more likely to respond with control when their children were distressed. Stein and colleagues (in a paper submitted for publication) report similar findings from their longitudinal study of 49 women with postpartum depression and 49 individually matched nondepressed controls.

Observations of mother–child interaction when the children were aged 19 months showed that, compared with controls, the depressed women interacted less with their children and were less facilitating; their children showed less affective sharing, were much more likely to show marked distress during a planned brief departure from their parents' rooms, and were less likely to show initial sociability with a stranger. Similar, but reduced, effects were seen in the subgroup of families in which the mothers had been depressed postnatally but were no longer depressed. The findings suggest that the altered parenting quality is not a direct consequence of current depression.

The evidence is consistent in showing significant impairments in parenting associated with maternal depression, but all the studies have noted marked individual differences, with some depressed women parenting well. Also, they have been consistent in showing that the parenting differences tended to remain (albeit at a somewhat reduced level) after remission of the depression.

Less is known about parenting differences associated with other forms of parental mental disorder. Sameroff et al (1982) found that, compared with neurotic depression, maternal schizophrenia tended to be associated with less impairment in parenting and fewer emotional disturbances in infants. Naslund and colleagues (1984a, 1984b) found that the one-year-old offspring of women with schizophrenia or a cycloid psychosis differed from controls in showing a lack of fear of strangers. They also noted an increase of anxious attachment in the offspring of schizophrenics, but not in the children of mothers with other types of mental illness. As already noted, Radke-Yarrow and colleagues (1985) showed a marked increase in insecure attachment in the children of depressed mothers. While the evidence is contradictory as to whether there are effects on parenting that are specific to parental diagnosis, it seems probable that there are not. Most, if not all, forms of serious mental disorder may be associated with difficulties in or distortions of parenting. They are in turn associated with abnormalities in the dyadic relationship between mother and child, and probably this plays a role in leading to an increased psychiatric link (although direct evidence on this issue is lacking).

Clinical Implications

There is much evidence that parental mental disorder is frequently associated with widespread disturbances in many aspects of family interaction and of parenting; moreover, it is clear that these family disturbances constitute one of the main risk mechanisms by which parental mental disorder leads to psychiatric problems in the children. These associated psychosocial disturbances often continue well after acute parental symptoms abate (Bothwell and Weissman, 1977) and, hence, it is no surprise that there are no close connections between the ebb and flow of parental symptoms and the course of disorder in the children (Hobbs, 1982; Rutter and Quinton, 1984), or that the psychiatric risk to the children continues well after remission of the parental disorder (although the risk is greater if it persists) (Rutter and Quinton, 1984).

The most obvious implication is that clinicians treating parents with a mental disorder need to assess the extent to which the disorder is associated with family discord, with negative feelings to any of the children, and with impairments of parenting. The main risk to the children occurs when these family features are affected; the risk is much lower if they are not. Clearly, it is highly desirable to intervene therapeutically to improve patterns of family relationships, but this has not proved easy to accomplish in practice. Rounsaville and colleagues (1979) found that depressed women with serious marital difficulties had a poor outcome compared with those who were single or in supportive relationships, and that psychotherapy effected little improvement in the marriage although it was effective in enhancing other aspects of social functioning. Conjoint marital therapy might well be more effective, but not all husbands are willing to be engaged in treatment; nevertheless, this seems likely to be the preferred approach.

Equal attention needs to be paid to the difficulties in parenting associated with mental disorder. Most of the parenting differences involve quite subtle aspects of parent–child interaction (rather than gross neglect or abuse, although occasionally this occurs) (Hawton et al, 1985); nevertheless, the findings on insecurity of attachment indicate that there are significant consequences for the children. Of course, insecure attachments occur quite commonly in the general population; nevertheless, they are associated with later difficulties in peer relationships (Wolkind and Rutter, 1985). Radke-Yarrow and colleagues' (1985) findings suggest that the pattern of insecurity includes abnormal features not ordinarily seen in the absence of parental pathology. Sometimes there is a tendency to assume that very young children are not aware of family tensions and disputes, and hence are relatively protected from family discord. The evidence firmly contradicts this sanguine view. Not only does discord frequently interfere with parenting, but also it is clear that toddlers are quick to pick up negative feelings. Cummings and colleagues (1985) showed that two-year-olds typically responded with distress to angry verbal exchanges between adults, followed by subsequent increases in aggression with peers.

Parents who are depressed or suffering from some other form of mental disorder need to be helped to reduce intrafamilial conflicts, to avoid such conflicts' impinging on the children, and to improve their functioning as parents. In addition to direct efforts to bring about improved parenting, there are likely to be benefits from improving the parents' availability and use of emotional supports. For example, often it may be helpful to encourage the non-ill parent to take a greater role in looking after the children.

One specific issue that arises with puerperal psychosis is whether or not the mentally ill women should be encouraged to continue to look after their newborn infants or whether separation might be safer. We lack data on the factors that should be taken into account in making that decision. Mother and baby units in psychiatric hospitals have been available for many years (Rutter, 1966); often the results for both mothers and babies seem satisfactory, and there may be advantages in babies remaining with mothers while they are hospitalized (Grunebaum et al, 1975). Yet it is unclear that babies do not suffer from exposure to their severely ill mothers. The matter urgently needs further study. In the meantime it is necessary to seek to ensure that the care of infants is as good as it can be when mothers are mentally ill, whether the neonates are jointly admitted with the mother or remain at home with the father or other family members.

INDIVIDUAL DIFFERENCES IN CHILDREN'S RESPONSES

Finally, it is necessary to pay attention to the important universal observation that children differ markedly in their responses to parental mental illness. Ordinarily less than one-half succumb with any form of psychiatric disorder, many come through the experience without psychological damage, and often even seem to gain strength from having coped successfully with stress and adversity (El-Guebaly and Offord, 1980; Rutter 1985b). As already discussed, to some extent this individual variation is a function of the characteristics and context of the parental mental illness. The children are less likely to be affected adversely if the parental disorder is mild; if it is of short duration; if it is unassociated with family discord, conflict, and disorganization; if it is unaccompanied by impaired parenting; and if it does not result in family breakup. However, there are also other features that are associated with resilience or vulnerability.

Sex of Child

It has been found in many studies that boys tend to be more susceptible to ill-effects following exposure to family discord or disruption (Rutter, 1982); this sex difference is likely to influence children's responses to parental mental disorder (although we lack adequate data on whether boys do indeed differ from girls in this respect). Rutter and Quinton (1984) found little difference between boys and girls in their overall likelihood of developing disorder in association with parental mental disorder. However, boys tended to develop disorders earlier following family discord, and girls were somewhat more likely to develop disorder in the absence of discord. In children, there was some suggestion that children of the same sex as the ill parent were most at risk.

It is probable that several different mechanisms are involved in sex differences in response to discord. There may be a tendency for parents to be more likely to quarrel in front of their sons than their daughters (Hetherington et al, 1982). Also, boys are more liable to respond to conflict with aggression and girls with distress (Cummings et al, 1985). The boys' mode of response may lead to parents being less tolerant of their difficulties, and hence more likely to respond negatively with scapegoating or other forms of focused criticism.

Temperamental Factors

Children's temperamental features have been shown to be associated with differences in their response to a variety of stress situations. Rutter and Quinton (1984) showed that children of mentally ill parents with high risk temperamental attributes (defined in terms of the constellation of negative mood, low regularity, low malleability, and low fastidiousness) were twice as likely as temperamentally easy children to develop an emotional or behavioral disturbance. More detailed analyses suggested that the children's characteristics put them at increased risk because they elicited different parental behavior. Children with temperamental risk factors were only slightly more likely to come from discordant homes but, within such homes, they were more than twice as likely as other children to be the target of parental hostility and criticism. The implication is that the children's temperamental features in part determined the likelihood that they would be drawn into a maladaptive pattern of parental interaction, a pattern that in turn predisposed to the development of psychiatric disturbance in the child.

Protective Features

As with other stress situations, a good relationship with one or both parents has been found to be a protective factor (Rutter, 1971). The presence in the home of an emotionally supportive, mentally healthy other parent seems generally beneficial for both the children and the ill parent. Little is known about whether good relationships outside the home can serve a similar protective function. Presumably much depends on their closeness and intimacy, and hence on the extent to which they can be used supportively by the children. Schreiber (1985) found that the quality (but not quantity) of peer relationships was associated with levels of disorder in 9- to 12-year-old boys in both divorced and nondivorced families; it remains to be determined whether or not this protective effect applies with parental mental disorder.

Although good relationships are only one of several possible mitigating factors (El-Guebaly and Offord, 1980; Rutter, 1985b), others have been little studied in relation to the effects of mental illness in mothers or fathers. Bleuler (1978), discussing his study of the children of schizophrenic patients, commented that the stresses could be health-enhancing if they were both manageable and of a kind that gave rise to rewarding tasks that proved fulfilling. The suggestion is in keeping with the evidence from other situations that resilience is characterized by some sort of action to deal with the stress situation (Rutter, 1985b). Such self-efficacy is associated with a sense of self-esteem, a belief in one's own ability to cope with life's challenges, and a repertoire of social problem solving approaches. This positive cognitive set seems likely to be fostered by secure, stable affectional relationships, and prior experiences of success and achievement.

Clinical Implications

Three main implications stem from the findings on individual differences in children's responses to parental mental disorders. First, it is important to appreciate that such differences exist, and to focus clinically on how children in the families of adult patients are *actually* responding, rather than to assume that they are generally at risk. Second, resilience or vulnerability resides in patterns of patient–child interaction and transaction, and not just in some inherent constitutional qualities of children (although doubtless they play a role). Children put themselves at increased or reduced risk by the ways in which they react, ways which in turn influence parents' responses to them. There is a need to help children develop successful coping strategies, recognizing that there is a range of good strategies, and that what works best with one child may not work so well with another. Third, there needs to be a concern with the family as a whole (together with its kin and peer group links) and not just with the patient as an individual. As Kuipers and Bebbington (1985) note, the families of psychiatric patients should be seen as a positive and irreplaceable resource; their problems are real and need to be considered as a central concern of clinicians; and their positive qualities can make a significant difference in the course of the patient's disorder, as well as to its impact on the children.

SUMMARY

The children of mentally ill parents have an increased risk of developing psychiatric disorder themselves during their growing years; the risk is associated with a wide range of parental illnesses, and a variety of different mechanisms are involved. Genetic factors are involved in the clinical picture of social oddity, neurodevelopmental abnormalities, and attention deficits seen in some of the offspring of schizophrenics; however, it is possible that a nonintrusive, noncritical family environment may protect to some extent. It is probable that genetic factors play a contributory role in the development of conduct disorders in the children of parents with personality disorders, and of depression in the children of parents with a serious (especially a bipolar) affective disorder.

High doses of alcohol in the first trimester of pregnancy impair brain growth and may result in mental retardation (the fetal alcohol syndrome). Children born to heavy drinking mothers show an increased rate of attention deficits and behavior disturbances; this, too, may stem in part from fetal damage.

Marital discord and family disruption are frequent concomitants of many types of parental mental disorder; they also play a crucial role in the mediation of psychiatric risks for the children (especially when discord results in scapegoating of one of the children). Mental illness is often associated with impaired parenting and with a distorted dyadic relationship with some of the children. Even young infants are responsive to these adverse changes in the family environment, and the children of seriously depressed mothers show an increased rate of a maladaptive form of insecure attachment.

Children differ markedly in their responses to parental mental illness; less than one-half succumb with any form of psychiatric disorder, and some may even gain strength from having coped successfully with adversity. To an important extent, children's resilience or vulnerability resides in patterns of parent–child interaction and transaction, and not just in inherent constitutional qualities.

REFERENCES

Beardslee WR, Bemporad J, Keller MB, et al: Children of parents with major affective disorder: a review. Am J Psychiatry 140:832-852, 1983

Birtchnell J, Kennard J: Does marital maladjustment lead to mental health? Social Psychiatry 18:79-88, 1983a

Birtchnell J, Kennard J: Marriage and mental illness. Br J Psychiatry 142:193-198, 1983b

Bleuler M: The Schizophrenic Disorders: Long-Term Patient and Family Studies. New Haven, Yale University Press, 1978

Bohman M, Sigvardsson S, Cloninger R: Maternal inheritance of alcohol abuse: cross-fostering analysis of adopted women. Arch Gen Psychiatry 38:965-969, 1981

Bothwell S, Weissman MM: Social impairments four years after an acute depressive episode. Am J Orthopsychiatry 47:231-237, 1977

Breslau N, Staruch KS, Mortimer EA: Psychological distress in mothers of disabled children. Am J Dis Child 136:682-686, 1982

Brown GW, Davidson S: Social class, psychiatric disorder of mother, and accidents to children. Lancet 1:378-381, 1978

Brown GW, Monck EM, Carstairs GM, et al: Influence of family life on the course of schizophrenic illness. British Journal of Preventive Social Medicine 16:55-68, 1962

Brown GW, Harris TO, Bifulco A: Long-term effects of early loss of parent, in Depression in Young People: Developmental and Clinical Perspectives. Edited by Rutter M, Izard C, Read P. New York, Guilford Press, 1986

Cloninger CR, Bohman M, Sigvardsson S: Inheritance of alcohol abuse: cross-fostering analysis of adopted men. Arch Gen Psychiatry 38:861-868, 1981

Cooke K, Bradshaw J, Glendinning C, et al: 1970 cohort: 10-year follow-up study: interim report. Working paper of the Social Policy Unit, University of York. York, England, University of York, 1982

Cox AD: The impact of maternal depression on young children. J Child Psychol Psychiatry (in press)

Cox AD, Mills M: Paper presented to the British Psychological Society, Developmental Section, Annual Conference, Oxford, 1983

Crowe RR: Antisocial personality disorder, in The Child at Psychiatric Risk. Edited by Tarter RE. New York, Oxford University Press, 1983

Cummings EM, Lanott RJ, Zahn-Waxler C: Influence of conflict between adults on the emotions and aggression of young children. Developmental Psychology 21:495-507, 1985

Cytryn L, McKnew DW, Zahn-Waxler C, et al: Developmental issues in risk research: the offspring of affectively ill parents, in Depression in Young People: Developmental and Clinical Perspectives. Edited by Rutter M, Izard C, Read P. New York, Guilford Press, 1986

Davenport YB, Zahn-Waxler C, Adland MC, et al: Early child-rearing practices in families with a manic-depressive parent. Am J Psychiatry 141:230-235, 1984

Doane JA, Goldstein MJ, Rodnick EH: Parental patterns of affective style and the development of schizophrenia spectrum disorders. Fam Process 20:337-349, 1981

El-Guebaly N, Offord DR: The competent offspring of psychiatrically ill parents, I: a literature review. Can J Psychiatry 25:457-463, 1980

Emery RE: Interparental conflict and the children of discord and divorce. Psychol Bull 92:310-330, 1982

Emery RE, Weintraub S, Neale JM: Effects of marital discord on the school behavior of children with schizophrenic affective disorders and normal parents. J Abnorm Psychol 10:215-228, 1982

Folstein SE, Franz ML, Jensen BA, et al: Conduct disorder and affective disorder among the offspring of patients with Huntington's disease. Psychol Med 13:45-52, 1983

Garmezy N: Stressors of childhood, in Stress, Coping and Development in Children. Edited by Garmezy N, Rutter M, New York, McGraw-Hill, 1983

Gershon ES, Hamovit J, Guroff J, et al: A family study of schizoaffective, bipolar I, bipolar II, unipolar and normal controls. Arch Gen Psychiatry 39:1157-1167, 1982

Gottesman II, Shields J: A critical review of recent adoption, twin and family studies of schizophrenia: behavioral genetics perspective. Schizophr Bull 2:360-400, 1976

Grunebaum H, Weiss JL, Cohler BJ, et al: Mentally Ill Mothers and Their Children. Chicago, University of Chicago Press, 1975

Hawton K, Roberts J and Goodwin G: The risk of child abuse among mothers who attempt suicide. Brit J Psychiat 146:486-489, 1985

Heston LL: Psychiatric disorders in foster home reared children of schizophrenic mothers. Br J Psychiatry 112:819-825, 1966

Hetherington EM, Cox M, Cox R: Effects of divorce on parents and children, in Nontraditional families. Edited by Lamb ME. Hillside, New Jersey, Lawrence Erlbaum, 1982

Hinchcliffe M, Hooper D, Roberts FJ, et al: A study of the interaction between depressed patients and their spouses. Br J Psychiatry 126:164-172, 1975

Hingson R, Alpert JJ, Day N, et al: Effects of maternal drinking and marijuana use on fetal growth and development. Pediatrics 70:559-596, 1982

Hobbs P: The relative timing of psychiatric disorder in parents and children. Br J Psychiatry 140:37-43, 1982

Jeremy RJ, Bernstein VJ: Dyads at risk: methadone maintained women and their four-month-old infants. Child Dev 55:1141-1154, 1984

Keller MB, Beardslee WR, Dorer DJ, et al: Impact of severity and chronicity of parental affective illness on adaptive functioning and psychopathology in the children. Arch Gen Psychiatry (in press)

Kreitman N, Collins C, Nelson B, et al: Neurosis and marital interaction, IV: manifest psychological interaction. Br J Psychiatry 119:243-252, 1971

Kuipers L, Bebbington P: Relatives as a resource in the management of functional illness. Br J Psychiatry 147:465-470, 1985

Leff JP, Kuipers L, Berkowitz R, et al: A controlled trial of social intervention in the families of schizophrenic patients. Br J Psychiatry 141:121-134, 1982

Murray RM, Lewis SW, Reveley AM: Towards an aetiological classification of schizophrenia. Lancet 1:1023-1026, 1985

Naslund B, Persson-Blennow I, McNeil T, et al: Offspring of women with nonorganic psychosis: infant attachment to the mother at one year of age. Acta Psychiatr Scand 69:231-241, 1984a

Naslund B, Persson-Blennow I, McNeil T, et al: Offspring of women with nonorganic psychosis: fear of strangers during the first year of life. Acta Psychiatr Scand 69:435-444, 1984b

Porter R, O'Conner M, Whelan J (Eds): Mechanisms of Alcohol Damage in utero. Ciba Symposium 105. London, Pitman, 1984

Quinton D, Rutter M: Parenting Breakdown: Making and Breaking Inter-Generational Cycles. Aldershot, England, Gower (in press)

Radke-Yarrow M, Cummings ES, Kuczynski L, et al: Patterns of attachment in two- and three-year-olds in normal families and families with parental depression. Child Dev 56:884-893, 1985

Rice EP, Ekdahl MC, Miller L: Children of Mentally Ill Parents: Problems in Child Care. New York, Behavioral Publications, 1971

Richman N, Stevenson J, Graham PJ: Preschool to School: A Behavioural Study. London, Academic Press, 1982

Rodnick EH, Goldstein MJ: Premorbid adjustment and the recovery of mothering function in acute schizophrenic women. J Abnorm Psychol 83:632-628, 1974

Rounsaville BJ, Weissman MM, Prusoff BA, et al: Marital disputes and treatment outcome in depressed women. Compr Psychiatry 20:483-490, 1979

Roy P: Is continuity enough? Substitute care and socialization. Paper presented at Spring Scientific Meeting, Child and Adolescent Psychiatry Section, Royal College of Psychiatrists, London, March, 1983

Rutter M: Children of Sick Parents: An Environmental and Psychiatric Study. Institute of Psychiatry, Maudsley Monographs No. 16. London, Oxford University Press, 1966

Rutter M: Parent–child separation: psychological effects on the children. J Child Psychol Psychiatry 12:233-260, 1971

Rutter M: Epidemiological-longitudinal approaches to the study of development, in The Concept of Development. The Minnesota Symposia on Child Psychology, vol. 15. Edited by Collins WA. Hillsdale, New Jersey, Lawrence Erlbaum, 1982

Rutter M: Psychopathology and development: links between childhood and adult life, in Child and Adolescent Psychiatry: Modern Approaches, second edition. Edited by Rutter M, Hersov L. Oxford, Blackwell Scientific, 1985a

Rutter M: Resilience in the face of adversity: protective factors and resistance to psychiatric disorder. Br J Psychiatry 147:598-611, 1985b

Rutter M, Giller H: Juvenile Delinquency: Trends and Perspectives. Harmondsworth, Middlesex, Penguin, 1983

Rutter M, Madge N: Cycles of Disadvantage: A Review of Research. London, Heinemann Educational, 1976

Rutter M, Quinton D: Parental psychiatric disorder: effects on children. Psychol Med 14:853-880, 1984

Rutter M, Chadwick O, Shaffer D: Head Injury, in Developmental Neuropsychiatry. Edited by Rutter M. New York, Guilford Press, 1983

Rutter M, Izard C, Read P (Eds): Depression in Young People: Developmental and Clinical Perspectives. New York, Guilford Press, 1986

Rydelius PA: Children of alcoholic fathers. Acta Pediatrica Scandinavica Suppl 286: 1981

Sameroff AJ, Seifer R, Zax M: Early development of children at risk for emotional disorder. Monograph, Social Research in Child Development 47:199, 1982

Schreiber MD: Peer social support and coping in children of divorced and nondivorced families. Paper presented at the Annual Meeting of the American Psychological Association, Los Angeles, August 1985

Schulsinger F, Parnas J, Peterson ET, et al: Cerebral ventricular size in the offspring of schizophrenic mothers. Arch Gen Psychiatry 41:602-606, 1984

Stewart A: Severe perinatal hazards, in Developmental Neuropsychiatry. Edited by Rutter M. New York, Guilford Press, 1983

Stewart MA, De Blois S: Father–son resemblances in aggressive and antisocial behaviour. Br J Psychiatry 142:78-84; 143:310-311, 1983

Stewart MA, De Blois CS, Cummings C: Psychiatric disorder in parents of hyperactive boys and those with conduct disorder. J Child Psychol Psychiatry 21:283-292, 1980

Tienari P, Sorri A, Naarala M, et al: Interaction of genetic and psychosocial factors in schizophrenia. Acta Psychiatr Scand 71:19-30, 1985

Torgerson S: Genetics of neurosis: the effects of sampling variation upon the twin concordance ratio. Br J Psychiatry 142:126-132, 1983

Torgerson S: Genetic and neurological aspects of schizotypal and borderline personality disorders. Arch Gen Psychiatry 41:546-554, 1984

Walker E, Emory E: Infants at risk for psychopathology: offspring of schizophrenic parents. Child Dev 54:1269-1285, 1983

Watt N, Anthony EJ, Wynne LC, et al (Eds): Children at Risk for Schizophrenia: A Longitudinal Perspective. Cambridge, Cambridge University Press, 1985

Weissman MM, Paykel ES: The Depressed Woman: A Study of Social Relationships. Chicago, University of Chicago Press, 1974

Weissman MM, Gershon ES, Kidd KK, et al: Psychiatric disorders in the relatives of probands with affective disorders. Arch Gen Psychiatry 41:13-21, 1984a

Weissman MM, Prusoff BA, Gammon GD, et al: Psychopathology of the children (ages 6–18) of depressed and normal parents. J Am Acad Child Psychiatry 23:78-84, 1984b

Wolkind S, Rutter M: Children who have been "in-care": an epidemiological study. J Child Psychol Psychiatry 14:97-105, 1973

Wolkind S, Rutter M: Separation, loss and family relationships, in Child and Adolescent Psychiatry: Modern Approaches, second edition. Edited by Rutter M, Hersov L. Oxford, Blackwell Scientific, 1985

Chapter 30

Toward the Prevention of Psychiatric Disorders

by Felton Earls, M.D.

OVERVIEW

Prevention is the goal of all medical sciences. The conventional wisdom is that to prevent a disease it is first necessary to understand its causes. Once causal factors are isolated, the mechanism through which these factors operate to bring about the disease must be unraveled. With this accomplished, an experiment can then be conducted in an attempt to alter the disease mechanism. A successful experiment achieves a breakthrough in that it has shown that a disease can be prevented. The discovery of the immune response and the development of vaccines to protect children against common infectious illnesses such as polio, pertussis, diphtheria, and measles represent the most dramatic and important examples of prevention in modern medicine that have followed this scientific strategy.

To categorically predicate prevention on knowledge of the causal mechanism of a disease would be misleading, however. In tracing the cause of cholera to a geographically delimited water supply in London in the 1850s, John Snow had only a vague idea that a microorganism was involved (Snow, 1965). He was able to identify aspects of the microorganism's existence (that is, that it was strictly water-borne and not air-borne, as was the popular conception of his day) without being able to identify it as a bacterium. In fact, Vichow did not isolate the vibrio cholera until several decades later. In this century such examples have continued to occur. Goldberger proved that pellagra was not an infectious disease (the prevailing belief in the early part of this century) by tracing its cause to an absence of milk and eggs in the diets of institutional inmates (Goldberger et al, 1923). Yet he had no idea that the nutritional deficiency involved a vitamin. Indeed, vitamins had not yet been discovered.

Another example involves the link between cigarette smoking and lung cancer. For several decades epidemiologists carried out descriptive studies showing that the association was a replicable one (Doll and Hill, 1954; Dorn, 1959). Although the mechanism through which specific ingredients in cigarettes alter the biology of cells to produce a carcinoma was not understood, the association was so strong and plausibility of the argument so compelling that it led the Surgeon General in 1964 to conclude that a causal connection had been established, even in the absence of experimental evidence.

This research was supported by the John D. and Catherine T. MacArthur Foundation Mental Health Research Network on Risk and Protective Factors in the Major Mental Disorders, and by NIMH Grant No. MH–17104 for Training in Psychiatric Epidemiology and Biostatistics.

During the past 20 years a rather dramatic decline in mortality from cardio-vascular disease has occurred (Stamler, 1981). Risk factors, including a positive family history, hypertension, cigarette smoking, diets high in saturated fats, and a sedentary lifestyle have been identified, but the mechanism remains unclear despite the fact that a vast research empire has been established for this purpose. The decrease in mortality appears to be due to changes in lifestyle, this time not involving the Surgeon General's admonition. In fact, a decline of 30 to 40 percent in mortality from coronary and cerebrovascular disease has been paralleled by similar declines in per capita consumption of cigarettes, selected dairy products, and animal fats and oils (Walker, 1977).

An impressive example of this observation is found in a large preventive trial known as the Multiple Risk Factor Intervention Trial (MRFIT) (1982). In this project, healthy middle-aged males were assigned either to a preventive intervention consisting of regular exercise, cessation of smoking, and a controlled diet, or to a control group. Over several years of follow-up a similar decline in coronary heart disease was observed in both the experimental and control groups. It became clear as the study proceeded that men in the control group had become as aware of the identified risk factors as those in the experimental group. Participation in the trial had heightened their awareness of being at high risk for heart disease. Their awareness led them to adopt changes in lifestyle and habits which were similar to those that had been prescribed for the experimental group (Walker, 1983).

These contributions of epidemiology reflect an important and distinct perspective in modern medicine. As important as the discoveries were that led to the development of vaccines in conquering certain infectious diseases, changes in lifestyle customs and behavior are now known to serve as a basis for the prevention of heart disease and at least some types of cancer. The important point to be made from this brief overview is that clues to prevention can be obtained from observations on the way people behave and the conditions to which they are exposed. Interventions that are aimed at creating changes in these behaviors or exposures may lead to a reduction in disease rates, with little or no knowledge on how the disease was actually produced.

The science of observing how disease rates are influenced by the behaviors of human populations and their exposure to potential causal agents is epidemiology. Aside from certain administrative functions that involve epidemiological strategies, the primary purpose of this science is to detect causes and to prevent disease. The detection of possible causes is based on descriptive and observational approaches in carefully defined population groups, while the preventive function is discharged through the randomized controlled experiment, or preventive trial. Just as prevention is the aim of medical science generally, the preventive trial is the ultimate step in epidemiological research.

If changes in lifestyle can reduce the incidence of cardiovascular disease, is it not reasonable to ask what analogies there are in the field of mental health? Indeed, an impressive array of ideas exist: improvements in the social network to prevent depression, parent training and improvements in foster care to prevent conduct disorder, drug education to prevent substance abuse, and gun control to prevent suicide, among others. But, as yet, none of these ideas has been subjected to rigorous experimentation to evaluate their reasonableness. To evaluate the current status of prevention research, this chapter will first review a few of the solid achievements in psychiatry, then describe the requirements for a preventive trial, and conclude with a consideration of the feasibility of conducting such trials based on what we currently know about specific psychiatric disorders.

EXAMPLES OF SUCCESSFUL PREVENTION IN MENTAL HEALTH

Aside from Goldberger's detailed, systematic observations and experiment in instituting nutritional changes in the diets of inmates and patients in public institutions who either had pellagra or were at high risk of acquiring it, there are no examples of an equivalent success in dealing with the major mental disorders, with the exception of mental retardation. The recognition that inborn errors of metabolism are responsible for certain dietary induced forms of encephalopathy led to the discovery that phenylketonuria was a cause of mental retardation. A screening test to detect the disorder in neonates was devised and is now widely in use. The result is that a cause of moderate to profound mental retardation has been practically eliminated in the United States. Since the introduction of a vaccine in 1969, there has been a dramatic decline in the incidence of measles and, concomitantly, measles encephalitis (Bloch et al, 1985). This disease, once responsible for a high rate of mental retardation and behavior problems in children, including a particularly malignant sequelae—subacute sclerosing panencephalitis (SSPE)—has now nearly disappeared.

In addition to eliminating specific biological causes of mental retardation, progress has also been made in preventing milder, culturally influenced forms of mental retardation. The most carefully documented experiment, designed as a randomized control trial, is being conducted at the Frank Porter Graham Child Development Center at the University of North Carolina (Ramey et al, 1984). In this project, investigators assigned infants who were at risk of mild to borderline mental retardation either to an intervention employing a program of cognitive stimulation based in a day care center, or to a control group. The children were involved in the program for several years until they entered elementary school. Differences in intelligence first appeared in the second year of life, with children in the experimental group receiving higher scores. Their improved performance persisted until school entry. Benefits of this program were not only directed to the children, but to their mothers, as well. Notably, the mothers of infants in the experimental group achieved higher rates of job training and employment. As a properly conducted randomized controlled trial, the achievements of this experiment deserve particular attention. Based on the success of this project, a similar experiment, sponsored by the Robert Wood Johnson Foundation, is now underway in which the at-risk population of infants is defined by premature birth (less than 37 weeks gestational age).

The type of intervention employed in the Frank Porter Graham experiment was also employed in Project Head Start, a federally funded program aimed at achieving school readiness among indigent children at high risk of educational underachievement. A particularly well documented example of this project was the High Scope program based in Ypsilanti, Michigan. One hundred twenty-four children who were enrolled in the program at age three were followed into their late teens (Berrueta-Clement et al, 1984). Their test scores, academic performance, rates of school absenteeism, school drop-out, arrests, and delinquency were compared to a matched control group. The results were remarkable. Despite no significant differences in intelligence between groups, adolescents who participated in the program as preschoolers were better on every measure of educational achievement and social adjustment.

These social experiments are important because they constitute true efforts at prevention, rather than remediation (sometimes referred to as secondary or tertiary prevention). They also demonstrate that interventions that are specifically targeted to stimulate cognitive development have a general impact that not only enhances several aspects of functioning in the child, but the welfare of parents, as well.

After waiting two decades for the results of such time-consuming experiments, the results have encouraged a renewed interest in prevention research. A sense of optimism has been struck that is reminiscent of the mental hygiene movement at the beginning of this century. This enthusiasm is reflected in the National Institute of Mental Health's recent initiative to establish Preventive Intervention Research Centers. Several centers have been established with the objective of placing prevention strategies on a solid scientific foundation. It will be several years before the efforts of these projects can be thoroughly evaluated, however.

STRATEGIES INVOLVED IN PLANNING A PREVENTIVE TRIAL

A series of basic requirements must go into the planning of a preventive trial. First, it is necessary to have a clear concept of the condition to be prevented. This is a crucial point for psychiatry. For several years progress has been made in developing nosological systems to more objectively define psychiatric disorders and to distinguish specific disorders from more general and nonspecific mental health indicators. This is an important development because many experiments in prevention have defined psychiatric disorder in global or unitary terms. In some cases prevention experiments have been conducted in the absence of a specified outcome. For example, an effort to improve the social support of recently widowed women, conducted by the Laboratory of Social Psychiatry at Harvard in the 1960s, provided no specific outcome (Silverman, 1970), although it is presumed that the investigators had depressive disorders in mind.

Deciding upon a condition to prevent is predicated on knowledge of the natural history of that disorder and known risk factors that antedate its onset. Obviously, the more information available on these matters, the more likely it is that the intervention will be well timed and targeted on factors that have a good chance of reducing incidence. Because many psychiatric disorders, including alcoholism, affective disorders, personality disorders, and schizophrenia have a peak age of onset in young adulthood, it is reasonable to aim preventive experiments toward child and adolescent populations. However, only for the linkage between conduct disorder and antisocial personality disorder is a child–adult association established on the basis of longitudinal studies (Mellsop, 1972; Robins, 1978). For other disorders (with the exception, of course, of disorders with a childhood onset and chronic course, such as autism, Tourette's disorder, and obsessive-compulsive disorder) there are a variety of clues about childhood risk factors, but none that have been examined in longitudinal studies from the age of risk to the onset of the disorder to estimate the actual magnitude of risk. Although retrospective studies provide one means to accomplish this, prospective studies are much better for this purpose.

Information on the nature of the disorder should permit the design of a specific intervention, a decision on what age and under what circumstance to apply the intervention, and a satisfactory outcome measure. Once these aspects of an experiment are developed, what remains is the selection of an at-risk population, random assignment to intervention and control groups, and consistent application of the intervention over a planned period of time. During the course of the study the investigator will want to check at regular intervals to make certain that the intervention is proceeding as anticipated and that the control group is not being inadvertently influenced to behave as the experimental group. Finally, there must be a "blind" assessment of the outcome.

It is also wise for the investigator to keep an account of the various costs involved in carrying out the experiment, since a cost-effectiveness study will serve as an important aid to others who may be interested in replicating the results or in translating the results into public policy.

POSSIBLE EXAMPLES OF PREVENTION IN PSYCHIATRY

With these principles and characteristics of a preventive trial understood, it is now possible to consider some examples of the reasoning that must go into the planning of such an experiment in psychiatry. It is best to consider these examples in the context of present knowledge and current public health concerns regarding the desirability of prevention, since the history of preventive trials in psychiatry is spotty.

Consider alcoholism, the most prevalent of all psychiatric disorders and one of the costliest to society (Robins et al, 1985). Two leads exist. First, based on the retrospective reports of adult alcoholics, hyperactivity in childhood appears to be a precursor condition (Goodwin et al, 1975; Tarter, 1977). A number of prospective studies provide supporting evidence for this proposition, especially when symptoms of attention deficit, impulsivity, distractibility, and motor restlessness are examined together (Gittelman et al, 1985; Weiss et al, 1985). Family studies, family history studies, and adoption studies provide a different set of leads and suggest that the familial clustering of alcoholism in adult relatives and hyperactivity and conduct disorder in children may be genetically determined (Stewart et al, 1980; Stabenau, 1984; Cloninger, et al, 1981). This, in turn, has stimulated an intensive search for biological markers.

Putting together these two types of leads, hyperactive children of alcoholic parents may be at the highest risk for adult alcoholism. At least two possible mechanisms exist to explain how their high risk status leads to alcoholism. Behavior problems in high risk children and deviant peer influences may lead them to more readily abuse alcohol than others. Or, they may possess a biological vulnerability to metabolize alcohol less efficiently, which serves to deteriorate an already compromised state of behavioral and emotional control. But, we must ask, to what extent do these leads constitute a sure enough body of facts to warrant a preventive trial? A series of questions might help clarify what position to take:

1. Does successful treatment of childhood hyperactivity reduce the incidence of alcoholism?
2. Is it necessary to prevent hyperactivity in order to prevent alcoholism?
3. Do subtypes of hyperactivity exist that represent particularly high risk conditions for developing alcoholism?

The first question addresses the possibility that characteristics associated with hyperactivity are similar to those that place one at risk of developing alcoholism, with the implication that treatment of the prior condition should diminish the chances of acquiring the subsequent disorder. The answer to this question, unfortunately, is not known. Brain mechanisms responsible for hyperactivity may have nothing to do with hepatic enzymatic mechanisms responsible for the degradation of alcohol and its metabolites. Thus, effective treatment of the behavior symptoms with stimulant medications may have no appreciable effect on lowering the risk of alcoholism. On the other hand, a combination of psychological and pharmacological therapies may have their most pronounced effects on improving self-esteem and academic achievement, and reducing family tensions, rather than on the enhancement of brain function. In the context of knowing little about the effects of specific therapeutic interventions, such a multimodal treatment has its virtues and might be worth a preventive trial. But it would have to begin, at least, in middle childhood, and an answer to the success or failure of the trial would require 10 to 20 years' follow-up. Furthermore, the morbid risk of acquiring alcoholism in the presence of hyperactivity is not well established, making it difficult to determine the exact size of sample required for the trial.

If hyperactivity is a necessary precursor of adult alcoholism, then the treatment of hyperactivity represents a form of secondary prevention, according to the customary distinction between primary, secondary, and tertiary prevention. The question might be asked, "Why not prevent alcoholism by first preventing hyperactivity?" Of course, this gets back to the question of whether there is a common mechanism associated with both disorders. Such a study would also extend the period between the start of an intervention and reporting results. Of course, it could be argued that the double premium of preventing both a highly prevalent childhood disorder and an adult disorder of great cost to society easily makes up for the additional years of funding required in the primary prevention effort.

To answer the third question, regarding subtypes of hyperactivity at the highest risk for alcoholism, it is useful to begin with adoption studies. An adoption study of offspring of alcoholic parents has shown that two distinct forms of alcoholism appear to be heritable (Cloninger et al, 1981). One type, termed male-limited because it does not transmit to females, is associated with an early onset and antisocial behavior. The second type has a later onset and runs a milder course in terms of associated social problems. Hyperactivity in childhood exists in forms that suggest a similarity to this adult picture. This distinction is between pure hyperactivity on the one hand, and the co-existence of hyperactivity and conduct disorder on the other. When examining a clinical population of hyperactive boys, roughly one-half to two-thirds will characteristically be diagnosed to have both conditions (Stewart et al, 1981). Family studies indicate that boys with hyperactivity and conduct disorder are more likely to have alcoholic parents than are boys without alcoholic parents (Stewart et al, 1980). Therefore, it is currently reasonable to believe that children with hyperactivity and conduct disorder are at a higher risk for alcoholism than children with hyperactivity only, although we cannot firmly state that the mechanism subserving the behavior disorder has much to do with the mechanisms that specifically elevate the risk for alcoholism.

Given the public health concerns over alcoholism and strong interests in examining all possibilities for prevention, one might propose a simpler trial than the one briefly outlined above. Consider the following. A sample of hyperactive boys with alcoholic parents are randomly assigned during early adolescence either to a prevention program designed to provide education about alcohol use, or to a control group. Both groups would receive the conventional treatment for hyperactivity and in other ways would be appropriately matched. Thus, the only difference between the groups would be the educational intervention.

What is the likelihood that such an intervention would be successful? It represents a strategy similar to offering courses in sex education for schoolgirls at high risk for early pregnancy. The moral and medical imperatives to carry out efforts to prevent teenage pregnancy represent an immediate and compelling national concern, but there is little knowledge about what causes this condition that would serve as a basis for a preventive trial. While there are a few examples of demonstration projects that have reduced fertility among adolescents (Dryfoos, 1983), there are no published research reports of an experiment that adheres to a preventive trial in this area, despite its public health importance. But how compelling is an idea of this sort for the prevention of alcoholism? If the intervention proved successful, it almost certainly could be shown to be highly cost effective. However, the existence of a cost effective approach to prevention is no substitute for a scientifically based strategy. This illustrates the paradox of prevention researchers. Many more ideas seem justifiable, even reasonable, for a try at prevention than have a substantial scientific basis.

Next to alcoholism, it is desirable to consider the prevention of affective disorder based on its frequency in the population and the suffering associated with it (Robins et al, 1985). Again, we are dealing with a disorder that clusters in families, suggesting a genetic contribution (Weissman et al, 1984a). The adoption data are less clear than for alcoholism, leaving open the possibility that cultural transmission is more important for this disorder than genetic transmission (von Knorring et al, 1983). Moreover, the evidence linking a childhood behavior disorder to the adult depression is missing. Only recently has it been established that unipolar depression occurs in children and adolescents in much the same form as in adults (Kovacs et al, 1984). Family studies also indicate that while other disorders not clearly related to adult depression exist in the children of depressed parents, childhood depression exists almost exclusively in these families (Beardslee et al, 1983).

It is not clear whether depression with an onset in childhood runs the same course as depression with an onset in adulthood. A secular trend has been described in which the overall onset is shifting toward younger ages (Klerman et al, 1985). At the same time, there is evidence suggesting that early onset depression is more familial than the later onset disorder (Weissman et al, 1984b). If these findings are substantiated, it may be feasible to target families for an intervention in which the parents and adult relatives have an early onset depression.

But what should be done? Could a program to prevent depression be devised from what we know of the risks and natural history of the adult disorders? Perhaps the findings of a British study are most compelling, though still controversial (Brown and Harris, 1978). This study, conducted at the University of London, found that early loss of parent, low social class, an unsupportive marriage, and having more than one preschool child in the family were risk factors for depression in women. Since little can be done to prevent death of parents or to influence social class standing, one is left with attempts to provide psychological support for bereaved children, marital counseling, and family planning advice. Again, we have to ask, how compelling is this for a preventive trial? The answer seems to be based on even less of a data base than it was for alcoholism.

The Institute of Medicine (1984) recently concluded a study on the health consequences of bereavement, with the following conclusion relevant to preventive interventions:

> Because of this lack of evidence on the efficacy of the many intervention strategies, the committee cannot recommend that as a matter of public policy any particular approach be more widely adopted at this time. However, the efforts to devise conceptually sound programs to assist the bereaved are to be commended and certainly should not be discontinued. In fact . . . the committee believes it is time to subject various intervention strategies to rigorous study so as to determine their benefit to particular groups of bereaved individuals. (p. 286)

In many ways this commentary is applicable to other areas in which prevention is desirable, but not feasible.

This exercise in examining the possibilities for prevention in psychiatry could be extended to include other psychiatric morbidities such as: phobias, schizophrenia, obsessive-compulsive disorder, and anorexia nervosa. But as the list grows it becomes easy to recognize that the evidence for prevention becomes negligible. Even less is known about these conditions, which, though less prevalent than alcoholism and depression, still constitute handicapping conditions for large numbers of people. For schizophrenia in particular, given the heterogeneous nature of the condition, it might be best to envision its prevention using the combination of strategies that worked in mental retardation. Infectious, genetic, metabolic, and psychosocial mechanisms may be primarily responsible for different varieties of the disorder. By necessity, then, there must first be continued efforts to improve the capacity to recognize specific types of the disorder, and to describe the unique characteristics that distinguish each subtype. A similar condition prevailed at the turn of this century when mental retardation was first recognized as a medical disorder.

DESIGN OF A PREVENTIVE TRIAL TO DECREASE THE INCIDENCE OF CONDUCT DISORDER AND ANTISOCIAL PERSONALITY DISORDER

To conclude this chapter which has been directed more toward charting possibilities for a preventive psychiatry than on reviewing what has been done, a research design to prevent conduct disorder will be briefly outlined. In doing this, the objective is to illustrate that there is at least one condition in psychiatry in which we currently know enough to conduct a trial: conduct disorder and antisocial personality disorder. Ironically, it is the same condition at which one of the most remarkable preventive experiments in psychiatry was aimed 40 years ago and failed: the Cambridge–Somerville study (Powers and Witmer, 1951).

The prevention of conduct disorder and antisocial personality disorder is based on a long history of accumulating data describing its familial nature, early onset, and persisting course. It is possible to select a group of children who carry approximately a 50 percent morbid risk of conduct disorder on the basis of an existing antisocial personality disorder in the parent (usually the father) (Robins, 1978). If the selection were based on the presence of antisocial personality disorder in the mother, the morbid risk might be even higher, since assortative mating for antisocial characteristics may be higher when the proband is female rather than male.

With the availability of a representative sample of high risk children, a design can be constructed to select an intervention strategy, a proper time to intervene, and an outcome measure. Since conduct disorder may well have its earliest manifestations in the preschool period, it would be necessary to plan the intervention as early as possible. In fact, the variety of risk factors would include: 1) prenatal exposure to neurotoxins, perinatal distress, postnatal trauma and illnesses, and parental deprivation. Thus, the ideal sample would be selected from a group of pregnant women with antisocial disorder.

The intervention should be designed to offset the known risks. It would include adequate prenatal care and pediatric care following the delivery. Beginning in infancy high risk children would be assigned to a developmental center that would provide an experimental curriculum, the ingredients of which would include a component to increase language and social skills in the children, and a component directed toward providing support and training of parents. The educational skills would be directed primarily toward language and prereading skills, while the enhancement of prosocial development would involve teaching skills in interpersonal problem-solving, positive reinforcement for patience, warmth, and showing concern for others (Robins and Earls, 1986).

Following a random allocation procedure, children in the experimental and control groups would be followed periodically with blind developmental and behavioral assessments. If the intervention was successful, it would be assumed that differences would arise fairly quickly and would be detectable by the age of three. If significant differences were sustained to age 10, it could then be confidently concluded that the incidence of conduct disorder had been reduced and, by definition, the risk of antisocial personality disorder concomitantly diminished since this disorder seldom arises in adulthood in the absence of childhood conduct disorder. On the other hand, if differences were not detectable by the end of the preschool period, the project could be considered a failure, and this would necessitate a revision of causal thinking about the disorder.

There are several merits to this idea. First, antisocial personality lays a heavy burden on society through its association with criminality, violence, alcohol and substance abuse, and premature death from accidents, homicide, and suicide. A successful prevention would lead to substantial savings for the public and a reduction in unnecessary deaths. Second, conduct disorder represents one of the most common and treatment-resistant problems in child psychiatry. Primary prevention represents a logical alternative. Third, experience in the early intervention trials aimed at reducing the incidence of child abuse and school failure have provided experience and curricula that can be readily extrapolated to a preventive trial on conduct disorder. Fourth, given the heavy costs of antisocial personality to persons with the disorder, their families, and other victims, an intervention with even a modest effect should easily prove cost effective. Fifth, given the prolonged risk periods associated with most psychiatric disorders, the fact that an answer to an experiment to prevent conduct disorder could be obtained within a relatively short interval means that the duration of such a project is well within the productive life span of a single investigative team. Because the prevalence of antisocial personality affects approximately four to six percent of males and one to two percent of women, a successful intervention would help a very large number of persons. For example, it would benefit many more persons than would the successful prevention of schizophrenia, and it would help a larger proportion of persons with the disorder, since antisocial personality is a less heterogeneous disorder than schizophrenia. As in many prevention experiments, the results might also lead to wider social implications such as improvements in the quality of daycare, new insights into early emotional development, and unexpected benefits to parents.

CONCLUSION

By dismissing the customary distinction between primary, secondary, and tertiary prevention, the field of prevention research is severely restricted. In viewing prevention as a direct assault on reducing the incidence of specific disorders, accomplishments have been limited to a few disorders in this century, notably pellagra psychoses, general paresis, and several varieties of mental retardation. Given the difficulties of preventing any disease, these are not small achievements.

The new challenges for prevention are in areas such as alcoholism and substance abuse, depression, suicide, antisocial personality disorder, and, possibly, schizophrenia. Significant efforts have been made just in the past decade in recognizing these disorders as distinct conditions with different natural histories and causes. A variety of descriptive studies are currently underway which will soon add to our knowledge of risk factors and causal mechanisms. At some point in this progression experimental studies will become feasible. When they do, the possibility for a "leap forward" in understanding the nature of the disorder and how to prevent it will become possible. The essential lesson of epidemiology is that an experimental attitude, based on observation of patterns of the disease in carefully defined population groups and studies aimed at changing one or more putative causal factors, can lead to effective prevention even in the absence of detailed knowledge of the causal agents and causal mechanisms.

REFERENCES

Beardslee WR, Bemporad J, Keller MB, et al: Children of parents with major affective disorder: a review. Am J Psychiatry 140:825-832, 1983

Berrueta-Clement JR, Schweinhart LJ, Barnett WS, et al: Changed Lives: The Effects of the Perry Preschool Program on Youths Through Age 19. Monographs of the High/Scope Educational Research Foundation, No. 8. Ypsilanti, Michigan, The High/Scope Press, 1984

Bloch AB, Orenstein WA, Stetler HC, et al: Health impact of measles vaccination in the United States. Pediatrics 76:524-532, 1985

Brown GW, Harris T: Social Origins of Depression, London, Tavistock Press, 1978

Cloninger CR, Bohman M, Sigvardsson S: Inheritance of alcohol abuse: cross-fostering analysis of adopted men. Arch Gen Psychiatry 38:861-868, 1981

Doll R, Hill AB: The mortality of doctors in relation to their smoking habits: a preliminary report. Br Med J 1:1451-1455, 1954

Dorn H: Tobacco consumption and mortality from cancer and other diseases. Public Health Rep 74:581-593, 1959

Dryfoos J: Review of interventions in the field of prevention of adolescent pregnancy: preliminary report to the Rockefeller Foundation, October, 1983

Gittelman R, Mannuzza S, Shenker R, et al: Hyperactive boys almost grown up, I: psychiatric status. Arch Gen Psychiatry 42:937-947, 1985

Goldberger J, Waring CH, Tanner WF: Pellagra prevention by diet among institutional inmates. Public Health Rep 38:2361-2368, 1923

Goodwin D. Schulsinger F, Hermansen L, et al: Alcoholism and the hyperactive child syndrome. J Nerv Ment Dis 160:349-353, 1975

Institute of Medicine, Committee for the Study of Health Consequences of the Stress of Bereavement: Bereavement: Reactions, Consequences and Care. Washington, DC, National Academy Press, 1984

Klerman GL, Lavori PW, Rice J, et al: Birth-cohort trends in rates of major depressive disorder among relatives of patients with affective disorder. Arch Gen Psychiatry 42:689-695, 1985

Kovacs M, Feinberg M, Crouse-Novak SL, et al: Depressive disorders in childhood. Arch Gen Psychiatry 41:643-649, 1984

Mellsop GW: Psychiatric patients seen as children and adults: childhood predictors of adult illness. J Child Psychol Psychiatry 13:91-101, 1972

Multiple Risk Factor Intervention Trial Research Group: Multiple risk factor intervention trial: risk factor changes and mortality results: JAMA 248:1465-1477, 1982

Powers E, Witmer H: An Experiment in the Prevention of Delinquency: The Cambridge–Somerville Youth Study. New York, Columbia University Press, 1951

Ramey CT, Yeates KO, Short EJ: The plasticity of intellectual development: insights from preventive intervention. Child Dev 55:1913-1925, 1984

Robins LN: Sturdy childhood predictors of adult antisocial behavior: replication from longitudinal studies. Psychol Med 8:611-622, 1978

Robins LN, Earls F: A program for preventing antisocial behavior for high-risk infants and preschoolers: a research prospectus, in Psychiatric Epidemiology and Primary Prevention: The Possibilities. Edited by Hough R, Gongla P, Brown V, et al. Los Angeles, Neuropsychiatric Institute, University of California, 1986

Robins LN, Helzer JE, Weissman MM, et al: Prevalence of specific psychiatric disorders in three sites. Arch Gen Psychiatry 41:949-958, 1985

Silverman PR: The widow as caregiver in a program of prevention intervention with other widows. Mental Hygiene 54:540-547, 1970

Snow J: On the mode of communication of children, in: Snow on Cholera. A Reprint of Two Papers. Edited by Richardson BW. New York, Harper and Row, 1965

Stabenau JR: Implications of family history of alcoholism, antisocial personality, and sex differences in alcohol dependence. Am J Psychiatry 141:1178-1182, 1984

Stamler J: Primary prevention of coronary heart disease. Am J Cardiol 47:722-735, 1981

Stewart M, De Blois LS, Cummings C: Psychiatric disorder in the parents of hyperactive boys and those with conduct disorder. J Child Psychol Psychiatry 21:283-292, 1980

Stewart MA, Cummings C, Singer S, et al: The overlap between hyperactive and unso-cialized aggressive children. J Child Psychol Psychiatry 22:35-45, 1981

Tartar RE: Differentiation of alcoholics: childhood history of minimal brain dysfunction, family history and drinking pattern. Arch Gen Psychiatry 34:761-768, 1977

von Knorring AL, Cloninger, CR, Bohman M, et al: An adoption study of depressive disorders and substance abuse. Arch Gen Psychiatry 40:943-950, 1983

Walker WJ: Changing U.S. life-style and declining vascular mortality: cause or coinci-dence? N Engl J Med 297:163-165, 1977

Walker WJ: Changing U.S. life-style and declining vascular mortality: a retrospective. N Engl J Med 308:649-651, 1983

Weiss G, Hechtman L, Nulroy T, et al: Psychiatric status of hyperactives as adults: a controlled prospective 15-year followup of 63 hyperactive children. J Am Acad Child Psychiatry 24:211-220, 1985

Weissman MM, Gershon ES, Kidd K, et al: Psychiatric disorders in the relatives of probands with affective disorder. Arch Gen Psychiatry 41:13-21, 1984a

Weissman MM, Wickramaratne P, Merikangas KR, et al: Onset of depression in early adulthood. Arch Gen Psychiatry 41:1136-1143, 1984b

Chapter 31

Epidemiologic Findings from Disaster Research

Evelyn J. Bromet, Ph.D., and Herbert C. Schulberg, Ph.D.

Research on the mental health effects of disasters has both practical and theoretical value. From a practical viewpoint, results of such studies can be used for designing interventions tailored to different types of communities. For example, the National Institute of Mental Health's manual on crisis intervention programs for disaster victims in small communities (Tierney and Baisden, 1979) draws to a significant degree upon earlier empirical findings about stress reactions and coping mechanisms. From a theoretical perspective, disaster studies provide a unique opportunity to evaluate the immediate and long-term consequences of a major external stressor. Unlike studies of other stressful life events and psychiatric disorders in which the causal sequence is difficult to disentangle, research on disasters provides a natural experiment for understanding adaptation to externally induced stressful conditions, and for testing conceptual frameworks that include personal as well as situational variables.

Given the important uses to which disaster research can be put, we will review in this chapter the types of psychiatric conditions studied, the relevance of epidemiologic methods for evaluating the mental health effects of disasters, the prevalence of disorder occurring in both adults and children exposed to various disaster conditions and identified risk factors, and the preventive implications of this body of research. We will selectively review the published literature from the perspective of epidemiologists. Readers interested in the broader body of work not covered here are referred to the annotated bibliography on disaster and mental health compiled by Cohen and Ahearn (1980).

TYPES OF PSYCHIATRIC CONDITIONS

The mental health effects of a wide variety of disasters have been studied, including floods (Bennet, 1970; Gleser et al, 1981; Logue et al, 1979; Titchener and Kapp, 1976); tornadoes (Penick et al, 1976; Moore, 1958; Moore and Friedsam, 1959); fires or explosions (Adler, 1943; Leopold and Dillon, 1963; Green et al, 1985); cyclones (Parker, 1977); and volcanoes (Shore et al, 1986). The effects of the Three Mile Island accident, a man-made disaster, received intensive attention from several groups of investigators (Bromet et al, 1982; Collins et al, 1983; Houts and Goldhaber, 1981; Dohrenwend et al, 1981). In a review of psychiatric effects of natural disasters, Edwards (1976) identified a wide variety of signs and symptoms among individuals interviewed after such a traumatic experience. With respect to immediate effects, these included anger, guilt, defensive reactions, and, less frequently, panic. Prolonged disasters, such as the Belfast riots

This research was supported in part by funds from NIMH Grants MH–35425 and MH–15169.

(Lyons, 1971) and the Three Mile Island accident (Bromet et al, 1982) have led to elevations in affective conditions, such as reactive depression and anxiety states. The *Diagnostic and Statistical Manual of Mental Disorders, Third Edition (DSM-III)* (1980) also lists psychiatric impairment from disasters as a contributory element in post-traumatic stress disorder.

A significant influence upon the nature of reaction to a disaster is the severity and totality of the stress experience. Thus, following the Buffalo Creek flood of 1972, in which entire communities were destroyed, Titchener and Kapp (1976) described some of the survivors as evidencing psychic numbing—that is, being withdrawn from interpersonal relationships and preoccupied with somatic concerns—and likened their behavior to that of concentration camp survivors. Two years later, a flood in Australia affecting 6,700 households similarly produced not only widespread depression, irritability, and nervousness but also an increased use of sleeping medications (Abrahams et al, 1976).

A wide range of symptom responses has also been observed in children exposed to natural and man-made disasters, such as cyclones and tornadoes (Bloch et al, 1956; Milne, 1977); a group kidnapping (Terr, 1981); floods (Gleser et al, 1981; Burke et al, 1982; Ollendick and Hoffmann, 1982); war (Milgram and Milgram, 1976; Ziv and Israeli, 1973; Carey-Trefzer, 1949; Bodman, 1941); and the Three Mile Island accident (Bromet et al, 1984; Cornely and Bromet, 1986). The types of symptoms observed include aggressive behavior, anxiety, depressive symptoms, belligerence, fearful reactions, sleep disturbance, regressive behavior, and crying.

From the analysis above, it is clear that researchers have not found a singular pattern of psychiatric consequences to natural and man-made disasters. While this may be the result of their study methodologies, it more likely reflects the fact that disasters vary in intensity and duration and thus are capable of producing diverse psychological reactions among persons exposed to them. Moreover, Cassel (1976) emphasized the unlikelihood that different types of stressors would induce disease-specific consequences. Perry and Lindell (1978) have argued that some disaster victims display positive mental health effects as well. However, as Green (1982) concluded, the majority of the published evidence suggests adverse short- and long-term mental health consequences, particularly following disasters causing severe and pervasive damage.

In contemplating the nature of findings to date (Table 1), it also should be noted that there is growing concern about distinguishing effects resulting from natural as opposed to man-made disaster situations (Melick et al, 1982). Baum and colleagues (1983) have suggested that man-made situations are often more chronic, and the victims may view these types of events as preventable and hence more stressful. Thus, the ensuing psychological responses may be more severe than those resulting from acute, time-limited natural disasters. With regard to conceptual distinctions between acute and chronic stressors, Cohen and colleagues (1982) have used the dimension of "duration" to distinguish the following four types: 1) acute, time-limited; 2) sequential; 3) chronic intermittent; and 4) chronic. Since most stress research has been concerned primarily with the first two types, we still have relatively little understanding of the operative mechanisms, adaptive processes, and mental health consequences of the latter two types; disaster epidemiology can make major contributions to our understanding of chronic stress effects.

Table 1. Characteristics of Natural and Man-Made Disasters

Types of Disasters Studied in Psychiatric Research

Floods	Explosions	Nuclear accident
Tornadoes	Cyclones	Train wrecks
Fires	Volcanoes	Riots

*Common Phases of Disasters**
Threat
Warning
Impact
Recoil
Post-impact

Types of Psychological Symptoms Reported

Depression	Anxiety	Somatic complaints
Anger	Guilt	Psychic numbing

Etiologic Factors Affecting Outcome
Level of involvement (bereavement; injury)
Severity (catastrophic nature) of event
Prior psychiatric status

---

*Based on Kinston and Rosser, 1974

Fried (1982) noted the continuing uncertainty as to whether endemic stress is directly causal in the development of diagnosable illness, or whether its consequences emerge in a more indirect manner. Regardless of which causal pattern is truly operative, Fried suggested that the subclinical manifestations of long-term stress may be detected in such affective and behavioral indices as apathy, alienation, withdrawal, affective denial, decreased productivity, and resignation, symptoms which indeed have been reported in disaster victims. Of equal theoretic pertinence to a study of disaster's long-term consequences is Fried's speculation that clinical pathology most likely results when acute stressors are superimposed upon chronic ones, since previously marginal defenses are then overwhelmed. Since a disaster is best conceptualized as a series of events rather than a single occurrence, Fried's model is particularly appropriate.

There is also growing concern about distinguishing psychiatric sequelae that manifest themselves as transient symptoms from those achieving the severity of a clinically diagnosable condition. The former type are more prevalent than the latter, but there may well be vulnerable population subgroups who react to a disaster with a clinical episode of major depression, generalized anxiety, or even post-traumatic stress disorder. We, therefore, expect future disaster research increasingly to assess stress reactions with measures of both symptomatology per se and diagnosable pathology. Precedents for this methodology are seen in the present authors' study of the Three Mile Island nuclear accident (Bromet et al, 1982) and Shore and colleagues' study of the Mt. St. Helens volcano eruption (1986).

APPLICATION OF EPIDEMIOLOGIC METHODS

Despite the theoretical and clinical significance of how persons adapt to ongoing stressful circumstances and the value of empirical data, the mental health consequences of disasters have rarely been studied from a well-designed, epidemiologic perspective. Thus, the majority of earlier reports were case studies or research using volunteer or unrepresentative samples, and unstandardized clinical interviewing procedures; they failed to include control groups; and no specification was provided of moderating variables. As Perry and Lindell (1978) noted, these studies were typically atheoretical in nature. Moreover, the data collection occurred at varying points after the event, producing considerable confusion in attempts at estimating post-disaster prevalance rates (Chamberlin, 1980).

In the face of these earlier methodologic shortcomings, we would emphasize that epidemiologic research can be conducted on three levels: descriptive, analytic, and experimental. Descriptive studies are needed to provide information on numbers of individuals who can be expected to exhibit mental health problems following disaster situations. Such studies provide important information for disaster planners, as they may pinpoint vulnerable populations as well as geographic areas with relatively higher proportions of individuals in need of psychiatric intervention. Analytic research can demonstrate what the personal and environmental risk factors are that determine response to disaster. Such studies can provide data important to understanding the dynamics of the stress process per se, as well as suggest what factors might reduce the risk of impairment following a disaster. Finally, experimental intervention research can be used to firmly establish how best to intervene and prevent serious mental health problems in the short and long term. Given the frequency with which disasters occur (an average of 36 presidentially declared disasters affecting some 200,000 families annually), coupled with the limited number of epidemiologic studies (Kinston and Rosser, 1974), knowledge from all three levels of research is needed.

It is heartening to note that a growing number of investigations in the field of disaster research are indeed applying such epidemiologic strategies to their work. This is evidenced by a concern with drawing representative samples, including comparison groups, using standardized diagnostic instruments, and specifying potential moderating variables. Two large-scale investigations of disaster are described here to illustrate how epidemiologic methodology of the analytic type may be applied in such field studies (see Table 2).

The initial major epidemiological investigation of disaster was organized in response to the accident and subsequent stresses at the Three Mile Island nuclear power plant. Early reports about potentially adverse health consequences had suggested that morbidity would be manifested in psychological rather than physical difficulties. Thus Bromet and colleagues at the University of Pittsburgh (1986) designed a study that for the first time incorporated basic epidemiologic research principles. Their methodology was quasi-experimental and longitudinal. Representative samples of mothers of young children living near the plant, workers employed at the plant, and psychiatric outpatients living near the plant were administered the SADS–L (Endicott and Spitzer, 1978), a social support questionnaire, a symptom inventory (Derogatis, 1977), and other sociodemographic and health questionnaires on four occasions between 1979 (when the

Table 2. Comparison of Two Epidemiologic Studies of Disasters

	Three Mile Island Accident	Mount St. Helens Volcano
Source:	Bromet et al, 1982; Bromet and Schulberg, 1986	Shore et al, 1986
Severity:	Evacuation advisory for pregnant women and preschoolers residing within 5 miles of plant; no property damage or loss of life	Evacuation ordered; extensive property damage; 50 deaths due to volcano; continued threat of flooding
Samples:	Mothers of children born in 15 months prior to accident and living within 10 miles of plant; psychiatric outpatients living within 10 miles; nuclear workers employed at TMI; comparison groups drawn from an area with a nuclear plant and an area with a coal-fired plant	Randomly selected adult in each household suffering property damage or loss of life; random sample of adults in nondamaged but exposed households and in unexposed community
Timing:	Interviews conducted 9, 12, 30, and 42 months post-TMI	38-42 months post-eruption
Assessment:	RDC major depression and generalized anxiety (SADS-L); current symptomatology (SCL-90)	DSM-III depression, anxiety, post-traumatic stress disorder (DIS)
Results:	Twofold increase in rate of clinical disorder in TMI mothers; risk associated with proximity to plant and clinical history; no effects for outpatients or workers	Tenfold difference in onset rates in high-exposure group

accident occurred) and 1982. The mental health of each of these exposed populations was compared with that of similarly selected residents from western Pennsylvania. Thus, in the first two data waves occurring in 1979 and 1980 (9–10 months after the accident and at its first anniversary), comparison groups living near or working at another nuclear plant were interviewed. For the third and fourth data waves in 1981 and 1982, comparison groups living near or working at a fossil-fuel facility were also interviewed.

To briefly summarize the results, which are detailed elsewhere (Bromet et al, 1982), the study group most strikingly affected by the nuclear accident were the mothers of young children. They exhibited a twofold increase in their rate of major depression and/or generalized anxiety during the year after the accident; high levels of symptomatology were experienced throughout the study period as well. The three most important vulnerability factors were living closer to the plant, having a history of psychiatric problems prior to the accident, and having less adequate social support from friends, relatives, and/or spouse. The psychiatric status of the nuclear workers and community mental health center outpatients was similar to that of their respective controls. However, perceptions of Three Mile Island's danger were related to adverse mental health reactions among workers and patients, an association not found for the sample of mothers of young children.

The second major epidemiologic study of disaster sought to assess psychiatric reactions to the eruption of Mt. St. Helens on May 18, 1980. More than 50 people died and extensive property damage occurred as a result of the eruption and subsequent flooding; moreover, the threat of subsequent flooding and eruptions continued long after the initial explosion. Shore and colleagues (1986) focused on a community exposed to the eruption and severely affected by it (Castle Rock, Washington), and a demographically similar, nonexposed community (Estacada, Oregon). All property-damaged households and a random sample of nondamaged households were included in the exposed community study group. The prevalence of psychiatric disorder was determined by administering the Diagnostic Interview Schedule (DIS). The three most common psychiatric conditions were found to be depression, generalized anxiety disorder, and posttraumatic stress disorder. Onset rates for all disorders combined during the first year after the eruption were 21 percent among high-exposure females (that is, those experiencing extensive property damage and/or death of a relative), 6 percent among low-exposure females, and 2 percent among control females; among males, the rates were 11 percent in the high-exposure group, 2.5 percent in the low-exposure group, and 1 percent in the control group. This marked mental health effect (tenfold difference between high exposure and control group) still was observed after controlling for education, income, and employment history.

Taken together, the epidemiologic studies of Three Mile Island and Mt. St. Helens confirm the significant increase in psychiatric morbidity that ensues after major catastrophic events. Moreover, the studies demonstrate that the effects can linger far beyond the catastrophe itself. It should be noted, however, that not all epidemiologic studies have demonstrated such clear-cut effects (Robins et al, 1985; Smith et al, 1985; Logue et al, 1981). Thus, carefully designed, longitudinal research is needed to identify populations at risk for experiencing deleterious effects, and to provide information that might be used to design interventions to reduce potential long-term effects of major disasters.

ETIOLOGIC FACTORS AFFECTING RESPONSE TO DISASTER

Disaster induced stress is often transitory, with most people quickly reestablishing normal life patterns. For at least some groups, however, adaptation is a slower, if not an impossible, process. In adversely affected individuals, functioning at work and at home may be critically curtailed, and the ability to resume social relationships seriously impaired. Given our growing awareness of disaster's potentially long-term sequelae, increased efforts are being made to design follow-up studies that will validly determine which persons are affected in what ways over what time period by the trauma of natural or man-made upheavals.

The rates of psychiatric disorder following a disaster vary as greatly as the number of disasters studied, although it has been suggested that, on the average, 25 percent of an affected population can be expected to display disturbed responses (Melick et al, 1982). For example, in evaluating adult litigants in a class action suit following the Buffalo Creek flood, Gleser and colleagues (1981) administered a semistructured diagnostic interview and reported that more than 80 percent were significantly impaired two years later. Leopold and Dillon (1963) evaluated 36 survivors of a marine explosion, and found that a similarly high rate of 72 percent received psychiatric intervention over the subsequent four-year period. By contrast, the epidemiologic research of Shore and colleagues and Bromet and associates described above identified much lower pathology rates. In considering female samples, who can be expected to evidence higher prevalence rates than males, the epidemiologic findings for the one-year period following each event ranged from 26 percent in women with high exposure to Mt. St. Helens (Shore et al, 1986), to 14 percent in Three Mile Island mothers (Bromet et al, 1982), to 6 percent in women living near Mt. St. Helens but not experiencing any direct damage or loss of life. Wide variation in pathology has been found in studies of children as well. The reported symptom rates ranged from 4 percent following air raid attacks in England (Dunsdon, 1941) to 100 percent following a mass kidnapping and live burial of children on a school bus in California (Terr, 1981). As previously stated, these variations stem from several sources, including the multifaceted nature of disasters themselves, differences in types of coping responses evaluated, and the discrepant assessment techniques used to establish prevalence rates.

Regardless of the present ambiguity about the precise rate of disaster induced pathology, its magnitude undoubtedly is high enough to warrant concern about the accuracy with which we can identify risk factors affecting response to natural or man-made disasters. Again, however, the methodological variations across studies make it extremely difficult to identify consistent predictors of psychiatric disorder following disasters. Moreover, the disasters themselves were quite different in severity and long-term threat, and the timing of assessment interviews varied from a few weeks post-disaster to several months and, sometimes, even years later. The manner in which design variations have generated inconsistent findings regarding personal risk factors is evident in studies of children's distress levels. Although the majority of such investigations provided gender-

and age-specific findings, in one-third of these investigations no gender associations were found; one-third found that girls were more adversely affected; and the remaining one-third found that boys were more affected. Similarly, one-third of the studies found age unrelated to distress level; one-third of them found older children to be more distressed; and one-third found younger children to be more distressed (Bromet et al, 1984). Interestingly enough, the only risk factor consistently found to affect response to disaster is having a psychiatric diagnosis prior to its occurrence (Bennet, 1970; Bromet et al, 1982; Ahearn, 1981).

In contrast to the ambiguous findings about personal risk factors, most studies determined that one situational factor consistently predicted response to disaster, namely, the person's degree of direct involvement with the event. In fact, Chamberlin (1980) concluded from her review of disaster studies that the severity and totality of a disaster were more important determinants of subsequent distress level than an individual's intrapsychic predisposition. That is, individuals who were hospitalized as a result of a nightclub fire (Adler, 1943), who lived nearer to Three Mile Island (Bromet et al, 1982), who were directly affected by the Mount St. Helens volcano (Shore et al, 1986), who were directly affected by the floods caused by Hurricane Agnes (Logue et al, 1979), or who were directly affected by the flooding in Bristol, England (Bennet, 1970), and children whose parents were more upset by the disaster (Bloch et al, 1956; Lacey, 1972), were more distressed than individuals exposed to these events but not directly suffering loss of life or property.

It is important to note that while the affective responses are experienced more intensely by individuals more directly involved in a disaster, indications of cognitive distress are often more pronounced among persons threatened by but not actually experiencing a hazardous event. For example, Shippee and colleagues (1982) surveyed residents of two apartment complexes after a gangland-style slaying in which an automobile was bombed. Residents of the apartment dwelling more geographically distant from the bombing site were more likely to believe that another, similar event could occur in their area. These results are consistent with our own finding that mothers of young children living 5–10 miles from Three Mile Island were more likely than mothers within the immediate 5-mile radius to believe that Three Mile Island was dangerous (Dew et al, 1985). Shippee and colleagues concluded from their study that persons overtly unaffected by a disaster may be as fearful and in need of service as persons who clearly suffered physical and psychiatric distress.

CLINICAL AND PREVENTION IMPLICATIONS

The preceding review of the consequences of disaster has made it clear that psychiatric sequelae are to be expected among significant proportions of the affected populations, and that these clinical manifestations endure for varying periods of time. Indeed, the U.S. military established four cardinal principles in the treatment of psychiatric casualties: *immediacy* (that is, early intervention); *expectancy* (the attitude that the patient will soon return to duty); *simplicity* (simple forms of treatment that emphasize normality and anticipated recovery); and *centrality* (of facilities for treatment) (Jones and Johnson, 1975).

It is not surprising, then, that the need to provide crisis intervention services, and possibly long-term care, to disaster victims is now generally acknowledged.

Indeed, research findings have raised both the conceptual framework and the technology for such efforts to a sufficiently high level of sophistication that the federal government urges every community's health center to include a psychiatric team skilled in relevant crisis techniques (Institute for the Studies of Destructive Behavior, 1978). The specific scope and structure of a community's disaster intervention strategy undoubtedly will vary, in keeping with its unique characteristics. However, all communities are likely to include such program elements as an active outreach service and consultation–education initiatives, given our present awareness about the complex processes through which persons exposed to disaster cope with its immediate and long-term effects.

A key premise in the organization of disaster relief is that the human service systems' finite resources are most efficiently utilized when directed to high risk cohorts rather than to all residents of the affected locale. Within this planning framework, Cohen and Ahearn (1980) emphasized the value of a needs assessment that surveys affected groups to determine the extent of their problems. They also noted, however, that adequate time seldom exists during post-disaster field interviews for complete psychiatric history taking. Thus, it is vital for administrators and clinicians to have previously identified a community's psychiatrically vulnerable population, so that limited resources are deployed in the most expeditious and effective manner possible (Schulberg, 1974).

While the planning principles presented in Table 3 are easily espoused, their implementation creates various dilemmas for epidemiologists as well as service providers. First, the concept of vulnerability must be recognized as an essentially relative one. Which population is to be used as the yardstick in assessing degree of risk? Is it groups who have never experienced a psychiatric illness, groups who readily break down in the face of stressful life events, groups who lack a social support system to buffer the effects of stress, or others? A second dilemma in identifying vulnerable populations is the choice of a pathology index for assessing maladjustment. Should the index be that of symptomatology level alone, or is meeting criteria for psychiatric caseness the more useful measure for purposes of crisis intervention? Employing symptom ratings could be inefficient because of the significant number of "false positives" who then would be targeted for the service; conversely, by selecting for the intervention only those persons immediately meeting caseness criteria, clinicians could lose the opportunity to prevent later morbidity among high risk individuals.

A third and even more profound dilemma in the identification of populations potentially vulnerable to the effects of disaster is our present uncertainty about the relationship between short- and long-term adjustment processes (see Table 3, element 4). Do persons susceptible to stress in the immediate aftermath of disaster successfully adjust to its persisting sequelae, or do they exhibit prolonged maladjustment as well? Alternatively, does chronic stress develop only among those manifesting an initial vulnerability, or are differing individuals at risk in each distinctive phase of the readjustment cycle? Additional dilemmas confront those responsible for devising a community's disaster plan, but this last issue of how to identify long-term vulnerability is the one for which epidemiologic investigators may be particularly valuable. As an illustration of how such methodology can abet the design of post-disaster clinical interventions, we will discuss the long-term stress reactions of young mothers exposed to the Three Mile Island nuclear accident. By considering the prevalence rate for short- and long-term

Table 3. Critical Elements of a Disaster Plan*

1. Designation of Community Mental Health Center personnel as disaster workers

2. Designation of responsibilities of disaster workers, and training them to provide crisis intervention or emotional support, as well as practical assistance in helping victims utilize resources available through disaster relief agencies

3. Development of interagency agreements with disaster agencies, such as the Red Cross, Civil Defense, area hospitials, etc.

4. Responsiveness to changing needs of disaster victims over time:

   first phase (immediate impact): alleviate immediate cognitive disorganization and/or psychophysiologic reactions of the victims (goal—lessen stress)

   second phase (recoil): assess level of need and implement crisis counseling and therapy as needed (goal—crisis resolution)

   third phase (post-impact): assist those with social and legal problems, as well as those with vulnerable defenses who are unable to cope with new stressors, or those who are exhausted (goal—shore up dwindling post-disaster support systems)

*Adapted from Hartsough (1982), and Cohen and Ahearn (1980).

stress and the factors associated with each outcome in this potentially vulnerable population, we hope to clarify how epidemiologic data can focus intervention efforts in the successive phases of the post-disaster period.

We had mentioned previously that psychiatric adjustment to the Three Mile Island nuclear accident was assessed in terms of clinically diagnosable conditions as well as severity of symptomatology. We found that a high level of pathology on either index in the accident's immediate aftermath was significantly related to poor long-term outcome. When taken at face value, our data suggest that for case-finding purposes, those young mothers who react to a disaster with acute maladjustment patterns be carefully monitored for the development of chronic pathology as well.

While this strategy begins to target vulnerable individuals, it contains ineffi-ciencies by way of identifying numerous false positives; that is, women who are defined to be at high risk because of initial distress but who subsequently show little pathology. Thus, even among young mothers reporting significant pathology in the first 12 months after the Three Mile Island accident, two-thirds of the SADS-diagnosable women and one-third of those classified in the top quintile with respect to symptomatology did not continue in these categories over time. It therefore is necessary to define more precisely the characteristics of vulnerable persons who warrant long-term observation. Interestingly enough, in the Three Mile Island study no psychosocial or perceptual variables contributed to the prediction of continued affective disorder among those so diagnosed initially by the SADS–L. On the other hand, these variables did predict persisting high distress levels as measured by the SCL–90.

The differing rates of chronic distress uncovered by the outcome indices utilized in the Three Mile Island study, and the fact that we could better identify predictors of long-term pathology among highly symptomatic rather than clinically diagnosable women, raises the basic question of which type of assessment instrument is most valid and useful for case-finding purposes. It is clear that differing dimensions of psychopathology are measured by symptom scales and diagnostic schedules; for example, we found a correlation of only .13 between the SCL–90 and SADS–L for reports of affective distress during the first year following the Three Mile Island accident. Furthermore, if one conceives of the SCL–90 as a screening instrument to be used in detecting later diagnosable affective illness, it displayed a sensitivity of only .45 and a specificity of .75 in the Three Mile Island data set.

We suggest that a case-finding instrument be selected in terms of whether a disaster intervention program chooses to emphasize primary or secondary prevention in its clinical/consultation activities. When the former is the focus, symptom scales such as the SCL–90 should be utilized for their ability to identify a specifiable subcohort whose initial high level of distress is likely to be maintained over the long term. While a proportion of this subcohort will not become true psychiatric cases, intense distress levels nevertheless warrant clinical intervention to minimize possible later physical illnesses and adverse consequences for family members. Conversely, when it is determined that the community's limited caregiving resources should be used to intervene only with persons manifesting diagnosable pathology, then the SADS or DIS should be selected for case-finding purposes. Its key limitation for even this strategic purpose, however, stems from the fact that only a minority of persons meeting criteria for affective disorders immediately after a disaster are likely to maintain this severity level over time.

Regardless of which assessment instrument is chosen for case-finding purposes, questions remain about the psychiatric sector's role in disaster intervention. The ECA study of how health and mental health services are utilized by persons reporting recent *DSM-III* disorders found that only 16 to 19 percent of persons with affective disorders visited a mental health specialist; the remainder visited a general medical or other type of human service provider (Shapiro et al, 1984). Similar patterns of service utilization can be expected among disaster victims as well. This suggests that the mental health specialist's major, if not optimal, contribution may well be in the training of other human service workers in case identification techniques, and consulting with them about clinical intervention and referral procedures.

SUMMARY

During the past decade, increasingly rigorous methodologies have been used to investigate the psychiatric sequelae of natural and man-made disasters. State-of-the-art research includes the use of standardized assessment techniques and conceptual models specifying factors that might mediate the impact of stresses ensuing from the disaster. Most studies have used either descriptive or analytic epidemiologic approaches. We would suggest that it is timely to undertake experimental epidemiologic studies with identified high risk groups, particularly in situations in which direct or indirect predisaster mental health data are available. Such studies would serve the dual purpose of rigorously testing causal models of acute and chronic distress patterns, as well as evaluating the effectiveness of different types of intervention processes. This research can further examine the short- and long-term mental health consequences of various types of natural and man-made disasters whose severity and duration of threat differ. Recent research being undertaken by Baum and associates, in which investigators have identified geographic areas in the United States at high risk for disaster (1983), represents just such a state-of-the-art undertaking. Within this framework, epidemiologic studies of disasters can focus on the dynamics and consequences of long-term stress, and contribute on both a practical and theoretical level to our knowledge of the stress process.

REFERENCES

Abrahams MJ, Price J, Whitlock FA, et al: The Brisbane floods, January 1974: their impact on health. Med J Aust 2:936-939, 1976

Adler A: Neuropsychiatric complications in victims of Boston's Cocoanut Grove disaster. JAMA 123:1098-1101, 1943

Ahearn F: Disaster mental health: a pre- and post-earthquake comparison of psychiatric admission rates. The Urban and Social Change Review 14:22-28, 1981

American Psychiatric Association: Diagnostic and Statistical Manual of Mental Disorders, Third Edition (DSM-III). Washington,DC, American Psychiatric Association, 1980

Baum A, Fleming R, Davidson L: Natural disaster and technological catastrophe. Environment and Behavior 15:333-354, 1983

Bennet G: Bristol floods 1968: controlled survey of effects on health of local community disaster. Br Med J 3:454-458, 1970

Bloch D, Silber E, Perry S: Some factors in the emotional reaction of children to disaster. Am J Psychiatry 113:416-422, 1956

Bodman F: War conditions and the mental health of the child. Br Med J 2:486-488, 1941

Bromet E, Schulberg HC: The TMI disaster: a search for high risk groups, in Disaster Stress Studies: New Methods and Findings. Edited by Shore J. Washington, DC, American Psychiatric Press, 1986

Bromet E, Parkinson D, Schulberg H, et al: Mental health of residents near the Three Mile Island reactor: a comparative study of selected groups. Journal of Preventive Psychiatry 1:225-276, 1982

Bromet E, Hough L, Connell M: Mental health of children near the Three Mile Island reactor. Journal of Preventive Psychiatry 2:275-301, 1984

Burke J, Borus J, Burns B, et al: Changes in children's behavior after a natural disaster. Am J Psychiatry 139:1010-1014, 1982

Carey-Trefzer C: The results of a clinical study of war-damaged children who attended the Child Guidance Clinic, the Hospital for Sick Children, Great Ormond Street, London. Journal of Mental Science 95:535-559, 1949

Cassel J: The contribution of the social environment to host resistance. Am J Epidemiol 104:107-123, 1976

Chamberlin B: MAYO seminars in psychiatry: the psychological aftermath of disaster. J Clin Psychiatry 41:238-244, 1980

Cohen F, Horowitz H, Lazarus R, et al: Panel report on psychosocial assets and modifiers of stress, in Stress and Human Health. Edited by Elliott G. Eisdorfer C. New York, Springer, 1982

Cohen R, Ahearn F: Handbook for Mental Health Care of Disaster Victims. Baltimore, The Johns Hopkins University Press, 1980

Collins D, Baum A, Singer J: Coping with chronic stress at Three Mile Island: Psychological and biochemical evidence. Health Psychol 2:149-166, 1983

Cornely P, Bromet E: Prevalence of behavior problems in three-year-old children living near Three Mile Island: a comparative analysis. J Child Psychol Psychiatry 27:489-498, 1986

Derogatis L: The SCL–90 Manual I: Scoring, Administration and Procedures for the SCL–90. Baltimore, The Johns Hopkins University School of Medicine, Clinical Psychometrics Unit, 1977

Dew MA, Bromet E, Schulberg H: A comparative analysis of two community stressors' long-term mental health effects. Presented at the Annual Meeting of the American Psychological Association, Los Angeles, August, 1985

Dohrenwend BP, Dohrenwend BS, Warheit G, et al: Stress in the community: a report to the President's Commission on the accident at Three Mile Island. Ann NY Acad Sci 365:159-174, 1981

Dunsdon MI: A psychologist's contribution to air raid problems. Mental Health 2:37-41, 1941

Edwards JG: Psychiatric aspects of civilian disasters. Br Med J 1:944-947, 1976

Endicott J, Spitzer R: A diagnostic interview: the Schedule for Affective Disorders and Schizophrenia. Arch Gen Psychiatry 33:766-771, 1978

Fried M: Endemic stress: the psychology of resignation and the politics of scarcity. Am J Orthopsychiatry 52:4-19, 1982

Gleser G, Green B, Winget C: Prolonged Psychosocial Effects of Disaster: A Study of Buffalo Creek. New York, Academic Press, 1981

Green B: Assessing levels of psychological impairment following disaster: consideration of actual and methodological dimensions. J Nerv Ment Dis 170:544-552, 1982

Green B, Grace M, Gleser G: Identifying survivors at risk: long-term impairment following the Beverly Hills Supper Club Fire. J Consult Clin Psychol 53:672-678, 1985

Hartsough D: Planning for disaster: a new community outreach program for mental health centers. Journal of Community Psychology 10:255-264, 1982

Houts P, Goldhaber M: Psychological and social effects on the population surrounding Three Mile Island after the nuclear accident on March 28, 1979, in Energy, Environment and the Economy. Edited by Majumdar S. Easton, Pennsylvania, Pennsylvania Academy of Sciences, 1981

Institute for the Studies of Destructive Behaviors and the Los Angeles Suicide Prevention Center: Training Manual for Human Service Workers in Major Disasters. Washington, DC, U.S. HEW, 1978

Jones FD, Johnson AW: Medical and psychiatric treatment policy and practice in Vietnam. Journal of Social Issues 31:49-65, 1975

Kinston W, Rosser R: Disaster: effects on mental and physical state. J Psychosom Res 18:437-456, 1974

Lacey G: Observations on Aberfan. J Psychosom Res 16:257-260, 1972

Leopold RL, Dillon H: Psycho-anatomy of a disaster: a long term study of post-traumatic neuroses in survivors of a marine explosion. Am J Psychiatry 119:913-921, 1963

Logue J, Hansen H, Struening E: Emotional and physical distress following Hurricane Agnes in Wyoming Valley of Pennsylvania. Public Health Rep 94:495-502, 1979

Logue J, Melick M, Struening E: A study of health and mental health status following a major natural disaster, in Research in Community and Mental Health, vol. 2. Edited by Simmons R. Greenwich, JAI Press, 1981

Lyons HA: Psychiatric sequelae of the Belfast riots. Br J Psychiatry 118:265-273, 1971

Melick M, Logue J, Frederick C: Stress and disaster, in Handbook of Stress. Edited by Goldberger L, Breznitz S. New York, The Free Press, 1982

Milgram R, Milgram N: The effect of the Yom Kippur War on anxiety level in Israeli children. J Psychol 94:107-113, 1976

Milne G: Cyclone Tracy, II: the effects on Darwin children. Australian Psychologist 12:55-62, 1977

Moore HE: Some emotional concomitants of disaster. Mental Hygiene 42:45-50, 1958

Moore HE, Friedsam JH: Reported emotional stress following a disaster. Social Forces 38:135-139, 1959

Ollendick D, Hoffmann G: Assessment of psychological reactions in disaster victims. Journal of Community Psychology 10:157-167, 1982

Parker G: Cyclone Tracy and Darwin evacuees: On the restoration of the species. Br J Psychiatry 130:548-555, 1977

Penick E, Powell B, Sieck W: Mental health problems and natural disaster: tornado victims. Journal of Community Psychology 4:64-67, 1976

Perry R, Lindell M: The psychological consequences of natural disaster: a review of research on American communities. Mass Emergencies 3:105-115, 1978

Robins L, Smith E, Cottler L, et al: Impacts of disaster on mental health. Paper presented at the 138th Annual Meeting of the American Psychiatric Association, Dallas, Texas, May 18–24, 1985

Schulberg H: Disaster, crisis theory, and intervention strategies. Omega 5:77-87, 1974

Shapiro S, Skinner E, Kessler L, et al: Utilization of health and mental health services: three epidemiologic catchment area sites. Arch Gen Psychiatry 41:971-978, 1984

Shippee G, Bradford R, Gregory W: Community perceptions of natural disasters and post-disaster mental health services. Journal of Community Psychology 10:23-28, 1982

Shore J, Tatum E, Vollmer W: Evaluation of mental effects of disaster, Mount St. Helens eruption. Am J Public Health 76 (Suppl):76-83, 1986

Smith E, Robins L, Cottler L, et al: Psychosocial impact of a double disaster. Paper presented at the 138th Annual Meeting of the American Psychiatric Association, Dallas, Texas, May 18–24, 1985

Terr L: Psychic trauma in children: observations following the Chowchilla school-bus kidnapping. Am J Psychiatry 138:14-19, 1981

Tierney K, Baisden B: Crisis Intervention Programs for Disaster Victims: A Source Book and Manual for Smaller Communities. Washington, DC, U.S. Government Printing Office, 1979

Titchener JL, Kapp PT: Disaster at Buffalo Creek: family and character change at Buffalo Creek. Am J Psychiatry 133:295-299, 1976

Ziv A, Israeli R: Effects of bombardment on the manifest anxiety level of children living in Kibbutzim. J Consult Clin Psychol 40:287-291, 1973

Afterword

by Myrna M. Weissman, Ph.D.

The section has been organized around epidemiologic approaches rather than disorder-specific findings, since many of the findings based on these approaches have been routinely incorporated into reviews of specific psychiatric disorders. For example, most reviews of current knowledge on the affective disorders will routinely incorporate findings on rates and populations at increased risk, based on ECA studies described in Chapter 27, and/or from high risk studies described in Chapters 28 and 30. These reviews may include discussion of treatment based on findings from approaches discussed in Chapter 29, or may use diagnostic methods discussed in Chapter 26.

The merging of clinical thinking with epidemiology (Feinstein, 1985) is firmly a part of clinical psychiatry and of psychiatric research. The following developments are in their early stages in psychiatric epidemiology, are of relevance to clinicians, and are likely to have an impact in the next decade.

The ECA data, which will become available from all five sites and across all interview waves in 1986, will yield a rich source of information on the range, risks, and patterns of illness in different ethnic, age, and geographical groups, as well as insight into the diagnostic categories themselves. The risk factors included for assessment in the ECA study, however, are limited; no biological or familial assessments have been included, and only one-year longitudinal data are available. The ECA population-derived samples will be seen as a rich resource for testing specific risk factor hypotheses, and will be used in case-control family studies to determine familial patterns of psychiatric disorders, or in longitudinal studies of persons at risk for a disorder but without evidence of psychopathology, or, finally, to study the normal process of aging or of mild symptoms.

An epidemiologic assessment for children and adolescents is currently being developed under the aegis of the NIMH and in several university-based research groups. One major obstacle in these studies is the finding of a discrepancy between the parents' and children's reports of the child's psychopathology. The diagnostic dilemma will be resolved and the epidemiologic methods for assessing children will be ready to be included in community surveys comparable to the ECA. For the first time, studies on the magnitude and risks and patterns of specific psychiatric disorders in children will become possible.

Diagnostic methods that are compatible with a variety of international diagnostic systems are under development. When completed and tested they will open the way for cross-cultural studies never before undertaken. Diverse cultural contexts will provide natural experiments to observe and understand variations in rates. There will be opportunity to study the diagnostic differences in rates among countries, and to determine how much of the difference is real and how much is an artifact of semantics. The use of different diagnostic systems among the European countries and the U.S. will be resolved with the increasing interest in the *DSM-III* throughout the world, and the increasing communication among countries about these issues fostered conjointly by the ADAMHA and the World Health Organization.

There will be a merging of psychiatric epidemiology with what has been called "neuroepidemiology" (Kurtzke, 1984), due to the increasing interest in neuropsychiatric disorders, such as Tourette's, Huntington's, and Alzheimer's disease, as well as with the realization that children who later develop psychiatric disorders often have early soft sign abnormalities (Shaffer et al, 1985).

None of the epidemiologic diagnostic interviews adequately assess neurological or physical disorders that may be confused with psychiatric disorders. While there are some useful screening scales, such as the Mini-Mental Examination included in the ECA, further attention will be given to this problem beyond the screening phase.

Becasue of the promising results about familial factors in some of the psychiatric disorders, a family–genetic approach will be integrated into epidemiologic studies. This will be accomplished by: 1) studies of large pedigrees of biologically related individuals; 2) further studies of adoptees separated at birth from their biologically ill parents; 3) studies of individuals at high risk for a disorder by virtue of family history; or 4) studies of twins. There is increasing realization that genetics and epidemiology have much in common. Both disciplines are interested in familial resemblance, and there is an overlap in methodology. Both methods depend on collection of data dealing with disease frequency and both draw heavily on the application of mathematics to understand the patterns of disease distribution. Since few diseases are determined solely by either genes or environment, and since it frequently cannot be determined *a priori* whether a disease should best be studied by an epidemiologist or a geneticist, genetic epidemiology will increasingly emerge as a discipline.

Recent development of the first possible genetic tests for detecting Huntington's disease prenatally and in as yet unaffected individuals provides a potential model for the future collaboration between psychiatric epidemiologists and geneticists for primary prevention. Using the new molecular genetic techniques of gene splicing and searching for genetic markers in large and informative families with Huntington's disease, case identification is now possible. While most of the psychiatric disorders are more heterogenous and multifactorial in etiology than Huntington's disease, these new techniques will be seen as increasingly useful for subgroups of some psychiatric disorcers. The success of these techniques will demand careful diagnostic assessment of the phenotypes and careful collection and assessment of pedigrees. Thus, the collaboration between geneticists and clinical epidemiologists who have an astute appreciation and familarity with both the clinical phenomena and the appropriate methodology will be required.

In the future it may be difficult to present a separate section on psychiatric epidemiology because the approaches described here, including designs, sampling, and assessments, will be synonymous with well designed and well conducted psychiatric research.

REFERENCES

Feinstein AR: Clinical Epidemiology: The Architecture of Clinical Research. Philadelphia, W.B. Saunders, 1985

Kurtzke JF: Neuroepidemiology. Ann Neurol 16:265-277, 1984

Shaffer D, Schonfeld I, O'Connor PA, et al: Neurological soft signs. Arch Gen Psychiatry 42:342-353, 1985

VI

Psychopharmacology: Drug Side Effects and Interactions

Section

VI

Psycho-
pharmacology:
Drug Side
Effects and
Interactions

Contents

Section VI

Psychopharmacology: Drug Side Effects and Interactions

Foreword

by Leo E. Hollister, M.D., Section Editor

All drugs exact a price. No drug has a single pharmacologic action. Thus, for every wanted effect of a drug, we may have to accept one (or usually many more) unwanted effects. This fact of life has led to estimations of the cost–benefit ratios of drugs: Are the dangers or inconveniences of the unwanted effects acceptable in return for the wanted effects? With most psychotherapeutic drugs in use today, the balance is clearly in favor of the wanted effects. The unwanted effects of drugs may be avoided or mitigated in a number of ways. In this case, to be forewarned is truly to be forearmed.

Most side effects of drugs are extensions of their known pharmacological actions. The nonspecificity of effects of many psychotherapeutic drugs makes them especially prone to produce many unwanted effects. Most antipsychotics, as well as many tricyclic or heterocyclic antidepressants, affect a number of different receptor systems. As a result, many of the unwanted effects, such as excessive sedation, anticholinergic effects (dry mouth, blurred vision, constipation, urinary hesitancy, delirium), orthostatic hypotension, sexual dysfunction, and others are attributable to this nonspecificity of pharmacological actions. Carbamazepine has a similar multiplicity of actions. Lithium, working as it does primarily through cell membranes, also can affect many systems. Only the benzodiazepines seem to be relatively specific, affecting principally the central nervous system with relatively few effects on other systems.

Allergic and idiosyncratic reactions are far less common and are generally unpredictable. Thus, although little can be done to avoid these reactions the first time they occur, knowledge of their prior occurrence allows us to avoid repeating them.

I have had a long-standing interest in the side effects and complications of psychotherapeutic drugs. Early on in the history of modern psychotherapeutic drugs, I wrote the first comprehensive review of these effects (Hollister, 1957b). From this perspective, I shall provide a highly personal view of the major problems in current use of psychotherapeutic drugs. Most of these topics will be covered in greater depth in the succeeding chapters.

ANTIPSYCHOTICS

Initial concerns about antipsychotic drugs focused on two unwanted effects of chlorpromazine, agranulocytosis and cholestatic jaundice. Agranulocytosis was a potentially fatal complication that usually occurred early in the course of treatment. A directly toxic effect of the drug on maturing granulocytes in bone marrow was almost universal early in treatment. All but a rare patient, usually one who was old and frail and with complicating medical illnesses, was able to compensate for the initial toxicity. The exact prevalence of this complication was difficult to assess, but was believed to be on the order of 1:3,000 persons exposed. However, determining prevalence can be terribly tricky. We had four cases of agranulocytosis due to thioridazine at my hospital in a period of 18 months. We had used the drug for seven years previously without a single case, nor have we had another one during the subsequent 20 years. With the shift toward the high-potency, low-dose antipsychotics, concern about agranulocytosis has virtually disappeared as cases associated with newer drugs are exceedingly rare.

Cholestatic jaundice is another unwanted effect that is no longer of much concern. Initially, its prevalence from chlorpromazine was estimated to be three percent. My study of 17 cases, which was the largest series yet reported, clearly established it as an allergic reaction (Hollister, 1957a). I have often wondered what internal clock led me to consider 17 cases enough; had I chosen to accumulate 25, the paper would still be unpublished. For reasons that are not certain, the prevalence of this adverse reaction declined almost to the vanishing point.

So much for the good news. The bad news is that other complications of antipsychotics were not immediately recognized. The first of these was sudden death. Having officiated at several of these cases, I became greatly interested in why patients treated with antipsychotics, who were young and in perfectly good health, should drop dead. My first conclusion, which was wrong, was that they died of asphyxia. Only later did it become apparent that the deaths were cardiac, almost inevitably due to ventricular fibrillation (Hollister and Kosek, 1965). However, sudden death is by no means uncommon, and the recognition of a rare new event on a background of fairly frequent events is difficult to establish with certainty. Thus, this issue remains somewhat controversial, even though sudden death (unexpected and unexplained) is more common a cause of death than an obvious complication, such as agranulocytosis.

Many of us were slow to recognize tardive dyskinesia. George Crane was the gadfly who did most to bring it to the consciousness of American psychiatrists. This complication seems to be a prime example of how the body's homeostatic mechanisms may undo the effects of drugs which perturb the system. If a drug induced dopamine receptor supersensitivity is the mechanism for this motor complication, then prevention may require a minimal degree of drug exposure. Thus, this complication has led to the current interest in trying to minimize exposure to antipsychotics during maintenance treatment. As first suggested by Ungerstedt, the same homeostatic mechanism might also occur in the mesolimbic dopamine system and lead to tolerance to the antipsychotic effects of drugs. Evidence for such "tardive" or "supersensitivity" psychosis is still mostly anecdotal; fortunately it seems to be far less common than tardive dyskinesia. Yet these two long-term complications of treatment have had a major impact on current thinking about the therapeutic use of antipsychotic drugs.

The neuroleptic malignant syndrome is a potentially lethal side effect that was also slow to come into prominence. The number of case reports of this complication probably represents only a fraction of those that have occurred. Yet the largest series in the literature to date, reported from several clinics in Japan, is 14 cases (Itoh et al, 1977). Thus, it must be fairly uncommon. Rather than being due to homeostatic adjustments due to long-term exposure to a drug, it is most likely a manifestation of an abrupt change in homeostasis brought on by treatment with antipsychotics.

These examples were chosen to illustrate several points: 1) some side effects of treatment are mitigated by technical progress in developing new drugs; 2) some side effects remain uncertain and controversial; 3) and some may be due to homeostatic adjustments to the long-term presence of the drug or to too rapid disturbance by the drug of existing homeostasis. It is highly likely that drugs less valuable than antipsychotics would have long since been withdrawn. Bad as they are, present antipsychotic drugs remain the mainstay of treatment for one of the most disabling illnesses of mankind.

ANTIDEPRESSANTS

More antidepressants have been removed from the market because of unanticipated adverse reactions than any other class of drug. Iproniazid, the first monoamine oxidase (MAO) inhibitor, was quickly withdrawn when it became apparent that some patients developed hepatocellular jaundice. Alpha-ethyl tryptamine was withdrawn due to the most unusual complication of red-green color-blindness. Most recently, three promising new antidepressants have been withdrawn after brief periods of marketing.

Zimelidine, a specific uptake inhibitor of serotonin, had been marketed in several European countries and was considered to be highly effective and safe. Drug fever, with associated headache, arthralgias, and increases in hepatic enzymes, occurred in about 1.4 percent of patients but was not considered to be serious. Only in April 1983 did two cases of Guillain-Barre syndrome appear, to be followed over the next few months by six others, making eight cases among an estimated 200,000 patients treated with the drug. The findings suggested an unusual immunological reaction (Guillain-Barre syndrome is a previously unknown consequence of drug therapy) and led to withdrawal of the drug from the market.

Nomifensine was introduced into the U.S. after several years of use in many countries. An estimated 20 million patients had been exposed to the drug. Some immunological reactions, such as drug fever (approximately one to two percent of cases) and rare instances of vasculitis, hemolytic anemia, and systemic lupus-like illnesses, were known. The prevalence of such serious disorders was thought to be miniscule, in the range of 1:200–300,000. However, a series of cases of hemolytic anemia with intravascular hemolysis occurred in Britain that led to withdrawal of this drug.

Buproprion was developed in the U.S., and experience with the drug was limited to relatively few cases. Seizures were known to be dose-related, presumably occurring at doses of 600 mg/day or more. However, soon after introduction of this drug, seizures were found to occur at lower doses. It has been removed from the market pending a reassessment of recommended doses.

Thus, antidepressants have had unusually bad luck in turning up with side effects previously unrecognized or thought to be rare prior to marketing. Even the newer antidepressants that have survived have been less than notable for having fewer side effects. Amoxapine not only has most of the side effects of tricyclic antidepressants but also has some of those usually associated with antipsychotics. Maprotiline has sedative and anticholinergic side effects comparable to desipramine but produces seizures more frequently than any tricyclic.

Only trazodone may have fewer side effects, excessive sedation being the most common. Priapism is a rare and unusual side effect of this drug. The major problem is that clinical responses to this drug seem to be highly unpredictable.

The good news is that MAO inhibitors are being used more often and more successfully with fewer fears about their interactions with foods and other drugs. The hypertensive crises that occurred due to interactions with tyramine-containing foods or sympathomimetic drugs markedly restricted use of these drugs for many years. The dangers may have been overstated, for even with more intensive and successful treatment with the drugs, such interactions are no longer feared. With proper precautions, they can be prevented.

LITHIUM, CARBAMAZEPINE

Although lithium has many side effects and a narrow therapeutic margin, most side effects can be managed. Monitoring of serum concentrations helps to avoid toxicity. The greatest concern arose when it was reported that lithium produced an interstitial nephropathy that might have long-term adverse consequences (Hestbech et al, 1977). Further studies have indicated some doubt about the specificity of the nephropathy and very little evidence of possible renal failure. Rare instances of nephrotic syndrome have been largely unexplained. Thus, clinicians continue to use lithium with little fear of serious or irreversible renal damage.

When carbamazepine was first introduced into medical practice, both as an anticonvulsant and for treating facial neuralgia, blood dyscrasias were a feared complication. Despite the fact that the drug has now become one of the most widely used anticonvulsants and shows increasing utility as a psychotherapeutic drug, blood dyscrasias seem actually to be less of a problem. The reason for this apparent paradox is not known, but is good news for those who wish to exploit this drug as an alternative to lithium.

ANTIANXIETY AGENTS

The benzodiazepines must be one of the most widely used classes of drugs in medical history. They have been remarkably safe, with virtually all the adverse effects affecting the central nervous system. Rare instances of allergic or idiosyncratic reactions have been reported.

It was predictable that abuse of these drugs might lead to a withdrawal syndrome similar to that from alcohol and barbiturates. What was not anticipated was that the withdrawal syndrome from the longer-lasting members of this group would be attenuated, as compared with alcohol and short-acting barbiturates (Hollister et al, 1961). From the time of their introduction into the marketplace, the consequences of abuse of these drugs were well documented.

During the past decade, a new phenomenon, that of "therapeutic-dose dependence" on benzodiazepines has been repeatedly confirmed. The doses of drug have been those used therapeutically, but usually the duration of exposure has been long (Covi et al, 1973). Symptoms are often difficult to distinguish from those which were originally the patients' complaints, but the time course may suggest a true withdrawal syndrome as well as atypical symptoms such as headache, perceptual disturbances, weight loss, and clouding of consciousness.

As several million persons may be at risk for such minor degrees of dependence on benzodiazepines, the potential public health effects are large. However, this complication of treatment can be avoided (by interrupting courses of treatment) or mitigated (by slow withdrawal from the drugs). At present, the predominant feeling is that the benefits of benzodiazepine treatment outweigh the risks of this type of dependence.

WITHDRAWAL REACTIONS FROM OTHER PSYCHOTHERAPEUTIC DRUGS

Virtually all drugs that act on the central nervous system, as well as many that do not, may produce withdrawal reactions when long-term treatment is suddenly terminated. Withdrawal syndromes were described in the late 1950s for phenothiazines, and more recently for tricyclic antidepressants and lithium. In general, these withdrawal reactions have been mild and of little clinical consequence. Still, the usual practice now is to avoid abrupt withdrawal of centrally active drugs that have been administered for protracted periods.

TOXICITY IN OVERDOSE

While not strictly an adverse drug effect, overdoses of drugs may have very adverse effects. In general, overdoses of psychotherapeutic drugs have been relatively safe. Fatalities from overdoses of antipsychotics have been rare; most have been in children or with thioridazine. The number of fatal overdoses of benzodiazepines is minimal, usually due to patients taking very large doses and not being discovered in time to receive appropriate treatment.

Major problems with overdoses have involved drugs used for mood disorders, so that, paradoxically, the drugs used for treating these disorders may be lethal weapons in the hands of those patients most at risk for committing suicide. Overdose of tricyclic antidepressants produce lifethreatening cardiac arrhythmias, but if discovered early enough, most patients will survive.

The chapters that follow will describe in great detail the various side effects and problems associated with the use of psychotherapeutic drugs. While some, such as neuroleptic malignant syndrome and sudden death, are idiosyncratic and unpredictable, many are dose-related and can be anticipated from known pharmacological actions of the drugs. Thus, one should read these chapters with the question always in mind, "What might be done to prevent the side effect being described?" Of course, we all hope for better drugs that will not only be more efficacious, but also less prone to side effects. Until that happy day arrives, we shall have to do our best to make the use of existing drugs as safe for our patients as possible.

REFERENCES

Covi L, Lipman RS, Pattison JH, et al: Length of treatment with anxiolytic sedatives and response to their sudden withdrawal. Acta Psychiatr Scand 49:51-64, 1973

Hestbech J, Hansen HE, Amdisen A, et al: Chronic renal lesions following long-term treatment with lithium. Kidney Int 12:205-213, 1977

Hollister LE: Allergy to chlorpromazine manifested by jaundice. Am J Med 23:870-879, 1957a

Hollister LE: Medical progress: complications from the use of tranquilizing drugs. N Engl J Med 257:170-177, 1957b

Hollister LE, Kosek J: Sudden death during treatment with phenothiazine derivatives. JAMA 192:1035-1038, 1965

Hollister LE, Motzenbecker FP, Degan RO: Withdrawal reactions from chlordiazepoxide ("Librium"). Psychopharmacologia 2:63-68, 1961

Itoh H, Ohtsuka N, Ogita K, et al: Malignant neuroleptic syndrome: its present status in Japan and clinical problems. Folia Psychiatrica et Neurologica Japonica 31:565-577, 1977

Chapter 32

Antipsychotic Drug Side Effects

by Douglas F. Levinson, M.D., and George M. Simpson, M.D.

This chapter will focus on a group of antipsychotic drug side effects that have been the subject of recent research or controversy, including 1) extrapyramidal symptoms (EPS) and particularly tardive dyskinesia (TD); 2) syndromes of EPS with associated fever (the so-called neuroleptic malignant syndrome); 3) agranulocytosis; 4) cardiovascular effects; and 5) the potential for causing sudden death. Anticholinergic effects, hepatotoxicity, drug interactions, and other adverse effects will be discussed more briefly.

EXTRAPYRAMIDAL SYMPTOMS AND TARDIVE DYSKINESIA

All antipsychotic drugs currently available in the United States share two unique characteristics: at equivalent doses, they all ameliorate psychosis; and they all have the potential for causing extrapyramidal symptoms (Ayd, 1961; Simpson et al, 1981). These adverse effects may be classified into four groups: acute dystonic reactions, akathisia, parkinsonism, and the late onset dyskinetic disorders (tardive dyskinesia and tardive dystonia). Apart from tardive dyskinesia, all are totally reversible by prescribing anticholinergic agents and/or lowering the dose of the neuroleptic. Here we provide an overview of these syndromes, with a focus on aspects that have been more fully studied in recent years.

Acute Dystonia

Acute dystonic reactions consist of intermittent or sustained spasms of the muscles of the head and neck, producing such signs as torticollis (neck spasm), opisthotonus (spasm of spinal muscles with arching) oculogyric crisis (spasm of ocular muscles), macroglossia, grimacing, dysarthria and dysphasia, and in rare cases, even jaw dislocation. Early reports suggested an incidence of approximately two percent (Ayd, 1961), but more recent studies have found an incidence as high as 50 percent. This increase may reflect the increasing use of drugs such as haloperidol, with higher per-milligram potency and lower anticholinergic effects (which mitigate EPS) than chlorpromazine. There is a consensus that young males are more prone to such reactions, although the reason is not known. Acute dystonia typically occurs early in treatment, with the majority of reactions during the first 24 hours of treatment, and 90 percent by the third day (Sramek et al, 1986). In some cases there are later recurrences when dosage is increased or, more rarely, even when it is not. Acute dystonia responds dramatically to the use of intramuscular antiparkinsonism or antihistaminic drugs. Many clinicians prescribe antiparkinsonism agents from the beginning of treatment to prevent acute dystonia if high dosages of high potency neuroleptics must be used in the young.

Akathisia

Akathisia, a variant of the restless legs syndrome, is a state of motor restlessness associated with anxiety, tension, inability to sit or stand still, or to tolerate inactivity. In mild cases, the observable effects may appear almost normal; that is, increased swinging of crossed legs, jiggling of the foot, and shifting of weight. In more severe cases, patients are totally unable to keep still, and either pace or vigorously move their legs continuously in a kind of stomping movement. There may be myoclonic jerks of the feet. Sometimes there is increased perspiration.

Many clinicians do not inquire systematically about akathisia, which can easily be mistaken for anxiety. These patients usually realize that at least a component of the restlessness is felt in the legs, "as if my muscles were jumping out of my skin," or "as if my legs just have to move by themselves." Van Putten and colleagues (1984) recommend asking, "Do you feel restless or jittery inside? Is it difficult to sit still?" They suggest that routine inquiry from the beginning of treatment can help both patient and clinician to differentiate akathisia from other problems. Braude and colleagues (1983) report that most affected patients find it more difficult to stand still than to sit still. In some patients, restlessness is accompanied by intense dysphoria and inner turmoil, while in others, subjective complaints are absent. Normal volunteers report akathisia as a major source of discomfort after administration of neuroleptics (Anderson et al, 1981).

Akathisia has received increased attention in recent years because of the growing realization that it is a major reason for patients' subjective discomfort and poor compliance with medication. Akathisia may be misdiagnosed as worsening of psychotic symptoms, leading to prescription of increased neuroleptic doses, worsening of the akathisia and other adverse effects, and general clinical deterioration. Braude and colleagues (1983) reported a 25 percent incidence in acute patients, usually by the first week, with some improvement later. Van Putten and associates (1984) reported that of patients treated with 10 mg daily of haloperidol, or about 20–40 mg daily of thiothixene, 75 percent of the former and 46 percent of the latter experienced akathisia by day 7, mostly in the mild to moderate range (thiothixene patients had more somnolence and akinesia, however), with 20–40 percent of patients experiencing akathisia (some of it severe) after the first dose.

Akathisia is frequently poorly responsive to standard anticholinergic or antihistaminic drugs. Braude and colleagues (1983) report that this is particularly true for akathisia in the absence of other significant parkinsonism (the two types of symptoms do not correlate), and they review animal evidence suggesting that when akathisia appears alone it may be due to dopaminergic blockade in the mesocortical pathway or spinal cord, rather than the nigrostriatal pathway. Other proposed treatments include diazepam, lorazepam, and, more recently, beta-blockers or clonidine (Levinson and Simpson, in press). Beta-blockers and clonidine have the advantage for long-term treatment of not being prone to abuse, but the disadvantage is that hypotension can then be a problem, and that self-initiated discontinuation may produce rebound hypertension. In severe akathisia, it may be necessary to discontinue the neuroleptic for days or even weeks while treating the akathisia. Clearly, akathisia deserves more intensive study.

Parkinsonism

The syndrome of neuroleptic induced parkinsonism is identical to the classical idiopathic disorder associated with degeneration of the substantia nigra, or the post-encephalitic variety. It includes akinesia, rigidity, tremor, increased salivation, and abnormalities of posture and gait. It begins days to weeks after the onset of treatment. Akinesia may be the earliest or even the only manifestation in some cases, and may be mistaken for depression (Van Putten and May, 1978). Early signs of akinesia include diminished arm swing or arm dropping and deadening of facial expression. If unrecognized or untreated, it will proceed to a full blown parkinsonian "shuffling" gait, with arms flexed and trunk bent. The majority (up to 75 percent) of cases appear within one month of starting treatment. High dosages, parenteral medication, and long-acting drugs may produce akinesia within the first one or two days, along with dystonic reactions and other extrapyramidal symptoms. Incidence varies from a small minority, up to 90 percent of cases depending on drug and dose. Extrapyramidal symptoms have been found to correlate with blood levels of antipsychotics (which can vary widely among patients on the same dose) in some studies, although at some level further increases in EPS are not seen (Kane, 1985). Few mental health clinicians are trained in the use of standardized examinations for EPS that include assessment of rigidity (in wrists, elbows, shoulders, neck, and legs), gait, tremor (of extremities and tongue), and salivation (Simpson and Angus, 1970), as well as akathisia.

Anticholinergic drugs are the mainstay of treatment for this syndrome. Amantadine (which increases release of dopamine) has also been reported to be helpful (Borison, 1983). Severe drug induced rigidity may lead to a "catatonic" appearance, reduced respiration (with resulting pulmonary embolus or pneumonia), inability to eat (with dehydration and electrolyte abnormalities), and muscle damage (with myoglobinuria and a risk of renal failure). These are discussed further in relation to syndromes of EPS with fever, below, but are related to rigidity and need not be preceded by fever. In such severe cases, vigorous antiparkinsonism medication should be instituted, with discontinuation of neuroleptics if medical and psychiatric complications are present or seem likely. If parenteral anticholinergic agents are not rapidly effective, dopamine agonist therapy such as bromocriptine should be used.

In some patients, parkinsonism or akathisia are major obstacles to effective antipsychotic therapy. It remains an individual clinical decision whether to give prophylactic anticholinergic therapy at the start of treatment. With low or moderate doses of neuroleptics, many patients need little or no antiparkinsonism treatment. For outpatients, Rifkin and colleagues (1978) found that 54 percent of patients on long-term neuroleptics with anticholinergics had recurrence of EPS when anticholinergics were discontinued, and they recommended continuous treatment to avoid akinesia and noncompliance. On the other hand, 50 percent did not have recurrence. With the lower doses of maintenance neuroleptics often used today (for example, 0.5 cc fluphenazine decanoate every 2–3 weeks), many patients do not require continuous anticholinergics. Another problematic situation may occur with elderly patients with mild to moderate idiopathic parkinsonism (sometimes not previously appreciated) that worsens dramatically when a neuroleptic is begun. These patients' persistent parkinsonism may then be mistakenly considered a severe form of the drug induced disorder. Cautious treatment with thioridazine alone, or with another low potency drug plus an anticholinergic, may be attempted, but concurrent use of gradually increasing doses of L–dopa/carbidopa may also be necessary. In these and other cases of severe predilection for EPS, electroconvulsive therapy (ECT) may be considered as an alternative treatment for psychosis.

A rare form of EPS that deserves mention is the rabbit syndrome, characterized by rapid tremor of the lips. This was initially thought to be part of TD but it is responsive to antiparkinson agents and is no longer considered related to tardive dyskinesia.

Tardive Dyskinesia

Tardive dyskinesia refers to the appearance of abnormal movements later in the course of treatment. While TD is often associated with the assumption of irreversibility, even the earliest reports described improvement or resolution over time in many patients, a point that we shall emphasize. The earliest signs of TD most commonly involve mild, writhing (vermicular) movements of the tongue (Pi and Simpson, 1981). It is therefore recommended that all neuroleptic-treated patients be examined frequently for such movements (with the mouth in an open, relaxed position, and with distracting instructions such as to tap the fingers). Early signs usually include chewing, licking, smacking movements of the tongue and lips with lateral movements of the tongue and mouth that may cause the tongue to press toward and against the cheeks, the so-called bon-bon sign (all parts of the so-called buccal-lingual masticatory syndrome). Later, there may be choreiform and athetotic movements of the hands, fingers, and sometimes arms. This is frequently best observed by watching the patient walk away from the examiner while movements of fingers and wrists are observed. There also may be involvement of the feet and legs, the respiratory muscles, hemiballistic movements, or truncal movements with postural abnormalities, movements of the head and back, and swaying or thrusting of the pelvis.

These movements tend to worsen with stress, disappear during sleep, and decrease with sedation. Many patients are unaware of these movements and some deny them. The variability of movements during the course of the day sometimes leads psychiatric staff to the conclusion that they are intentional or manipulative, producing added psychic stress for the patient. Such accusations can be diminished by encouraging their proponents to attempt to mimic the patient's movements for a half-hour, an exhausting and usually impossible task.

While most cases occur after one year of treatment, some may be seen earlier. Kane and Smith (1982) found that the reported incidence of TD has increased over a 20-year period, probably due to the use of standardized rating instruments rather than to dramatic change in incidence. There are also a number of reports of a significant incidence of dyskinesias in elderly people (who may therefore be misdiagnosed as having drug induced TD after minimal drug exposure) and in schizophrenics not treated with neuroleptics, with suggestions of a higher incidence in the latter. Kane and Smith report that studies of untreated individuals yield a total incidence of five percent, while studies of neuroleptic-treated patients, taken together, show an incidence of 20 percent, suggesting a "true" incidence of 15 percent related to neuroleptic use. This is the best current estimate, but some studies have suggested higher rates of up to 50 percent.

Longitudinally, approximately four percent of neuroleptic-treated patients may develop the disorder each year (Kane et al, 1984).

Early TD will be missed if structured examinations are not used (Simpson et al, 1979). Still, diagnosis is problematic due to the difficulty of setting criteria for early or mild forms, the necessity of establishing the history of neuroleptic treatment, and the exclusion of other conditions such as spontaneous dyskinesias, idiopathic torsion dystonia, Wilson's disease, Huntington's disease, and stereotyped movements of schizophrenia or mental retardation. Women have a higher incidence of TD (particularly more severe forms), as do older people (but this may be due to greater persistence of TD in the elderly once it develops); but current data do not show increased risk for any type of neuroleptic, use of anticholinergics, polypharmacy or ECT, organic mental disorders, or presence or absence of drug free intervals as risk factors (Kane and Smith, 1982). Anecdotal evidence suggests that patients with affective disorders are at greater risk, but there are as yet no good controlled data.

It is of great interest to determine whether dosage and cumulative neuroleptic exposure are related to incidence of TD, as these are factors that might be controlled as a means of prevention. Studies are mixed, but suggest that the greatest risk may occur early, perhaps during the first 6–12 months of treatment at low to moderate doses. Thus it is imperative to give careful consideration to alternative diagnoses before initiating maintenance neuroleptic therapy, to give trials of drugs for affective disorders initially whenever there is a reasonable indication, and to attempt discontinuation of neuroleptics during the first year of treatment whenever possible. Once patients have passed through this initial treatment period, dosage does not correlate well with emergence of TD in many studies, suggesting that to some extent patients have differing propensities for the disorder. But because some studies suggest higher dose as a risk factor, and because improvement may be more likely on lowered doses (see below), the lowest effective doses should be used.

The cause of TD is unknown. Jeste and colleagues (1986) have reviewed current hypotheses. It had been proposed that post-synaptic striatal dopamine receptors increase in number following chronic neuroleptic administration, so that excess dopaminergic effects might either break through despite neuroleptic treatment (or be blocked by increasing doses), or might appear after drug discontinuation and exposure of the underlying "supersensitivity." This theory is problematic because all tested animals develop dopamine supersensitivity after brief neuroleptic treatment, whereas only a minority of patients develop TD after a much longer time, and because measurable supersensivity in animals disappears soon after drug withdrawal. It is possible that receptors are altered in some abnormal way in susceptible patients, and/or that other neurotransmitter systems are involved.

The natural course of TD is difficult to study. Based on the supersensitivity theory and uncontrolled clinical observations, it had been assumed that TD develops during treatment in susceptible patients, that the underlying sensitivity continues to worsen as long as neuroleptics are given, and that continued neuroleptic treatment simply masks this condition, with at least temporary worsening after drug discontinuation. The early results from prospective studies partially contradict these assumptions. For example, Casey (1986) reported that over a period of 7 years, 15 patients showed a 68 percent improvement although 12 patients continued on neuroleptics. Relatively low doses were used, and doses were reduced after onset of TD; the one patient who worsened had required several dosage increases. Thus, TD is at least partially reversible in many patients, if neuroleptics can be stopped or the dosage decreased, and improvement continues for a long time. The incidence of complete reversibility is not yet known.

The management of TD begins with careful documentation of the movements using a standardized rating scale, which can then be used to evaluate future changes. Early signs of TD should prompt consideration of discontinuing the drug, followed by long-term observation for improvement. If the drug is necessary, TD should be discussed with the patient, in terms the patient can comprehend cognitively and tolerate emotionally. Most such patients elect to continue treatment (many are not subjectively bothered by the movements), or ask to resume it after relapsing. Dosage should then be tapered to the lowest possible level, again with regular evaluations. During the early phase of drug discontinuation or withdrawal, TD may temporarily become worse before (usually) beginning to improve. Benzodiazepines, while in no way useful as therapy for TD, may help to ameliorate discomfort and anxiety during this phase.

A plethora of more active treatments have been advocated or tested for TD. None has proven successful in controlled studies. Although there is a hope of developing drugs with antipsychotic but not extrapyramidal effects, no such drug is currently available. Clozapine, an antipsychotic marketed in a number of other countries, is said to cause less TD, and also to be effective for some otherwise treatment resistant patients. Its actions on dopamine receptors and dopaminergic functions partially resemble and partially differ from standard neuroleptics; its lack of propensity to cause EPS may be due to some fundamental difference, or to its very high anticholinergic potency (Jenner and Marsden, 1983). There are reports that TD improved both during clozapine administration and following its withdrawal (Gerbino et al, 1980), but others report that TD worsened during clozapine withdrawal in some patients (Simpson et al, 1978), similar to the pattern with more typical neuroleptics. Unfortunately, clozapine can cause agranulocytosis (see discussion below), so that marketing has not been permitted in the U.S. Further investigation of clozapine in the U.S. has recently been resumed, and similar drugs are being tested (although none are close to marketing).

Tardive Dystonia

Tardive dystonia is a rare disorder which mainly affects young adults. The incidence is not known but must be well below one percent. Tardive dystonia has recently received greater attention because of the severely disabling nature of the symptoms and their frequent persistence. Abnormal movements can begin after brief exposure to neuroleptics. Such subjects may have acute dystonia but later develop similar but prolonged muscle spasms, with torsion movements. The neck and face are almost always involved. Burke and colleagues (1982) reported that 30 of their 42 cases also had dystonic movements of the trunk, arms, and/or legs. The tongue movements may be absent initially, but they can develop later. The subject's head may be constantly pulled back or to the side. Movements may make walking or even eating difficult. While some early cases improve after drug discontinuation, the disorder tends to be chronic.

Treatment remains experimental, with no controlled studies having been done.

High doses of anticholinergics (increasing to as high as 60–80 mg/day of tri-hexyphenidyl) are said to be helpful in some cases. Dopamine depleting agents such as tetrabenzine or reserpine have been used, but on theoretical grounds it would be anticipated that dopaminergic reduction would not prove useful in the long run. Large doses of clonazepam, baclofen, or benzodiazepines have been unsuccessful. We have seen a single, extraordinarily severe case in which (after multiple unsuccessful drug trials) bilateral stereotactic lesions of the anterior thalamic nuclei completely eliminated the dystonic movements (Goldman et al, 1985). It must be stressed that no surgical procedure has been suggested for the common, nondystonic forms of tardive dyskinesia.

SYNDROMES OF EXTRAPYRAMIDAL SYMPTOMS WITH FEVER

Delay and Deniker (1968) first described a *"syndrome malin"* (neuroleptic malignant syndrome) of fever, rigidity, and other signs, which was said to occur in 0.5–1.0 percent of neuroleptic-treated cases. There has been a recent explosion of interest in this syndrome: Caroff (1980) identified "over 60" reported cases, Levenson (1985) reviewed 53 subsequent cases, and Lazarus (1985) found over 100 publications related to neuroleptic malignant syndrome since 1980. Reported cases had received a variety of oral, intramuscular, or depot form neuroleptic drugs, ranging from a single dose to recent initiation of large or increased doses. In almost all of these cases, there was subsequent onset of severe rigidity and fever, with most showing some alteration of consciousness, abnormal blood pressure (increased, decreased, and/or labile) and sweating (distinguishing the presentation from heat stroke) (Levenson, 1985). Serum creatine phosphokinase has often been increased, presumably due to the degree of muscle contraction. Caroff (1980) reported a mortality rate of 20 percent, while Levenson (1985) reported a rate of 15 percent, in the more recent cases. It has been widely assumed that neuroleptic malignant syndrome represents a well established syndrome due to drug induced mechanisms.

We recently critically reviewed 40 reports (in English) between 1972 and 1984, with a total of 67 cases (Levinson and Simpson, 1986). In reviewing the 48 neuroleptic related cases that were described in detail, we found that concurrent medical disorders and complications had received insufficient attention as likely causes of fever and morbidity. Nine patients were found to have clear medical disorders that adequately explained fever and morbidity, with little apparent relationship to the neuroleptic treatment. Of the remaining 39 cases, we concluded that concurrent medical disorders probably contributed to fever in 16, and possibly contributed in another 9. The most common disorders were dehydration, pulmonary embolus and infection, other infections, and myoglobinuria with renal failure. In many cases, these medical complications appeared to be the result of severe and/or prolonged EPS, leading to immobilization, reduced oral intake, reduced respiratory excursion, and/or rhabdomyolysis. There were only 14 cases (36 percent of the 39, 21 percent of the entire series of 67) in which apparently healthy individuals were shown to develop otherwise unexplained fever with a time course suggesting a possible relationship with neuroleptic treatment. Hypertension was found in 38 percent, and increased creatine phosphokinase in 54 percent of the 39 cases.

There were 3 deaths among the 39 cases (8 percent), all attributable to known medical complications: complications of respirator therapy, pneumonia in a tracheostomized patient whose initial fever had resolved months previously, and rhabdomyolysis with renal failure and sepsis. There were no deaths among patients who received prompt treatment for severe extrapyramidal symptoms.

On the basis of this review, we would suggest that the existence of a "malignant" syndrome related to neuroleptic treatment has been accepted too uncritically. To establish a clear relationship between neuroleptic effects and fever and associated symptoms, it would be prudent to focus on those cases without pre-existing medical factors. These appear to be rare. Nevertheless, the appearance of fever in these cases remains unexplained, and the rapid resolution of symptoms sometimes seen after antiparkinsonism or muscle relaxant therapy suggests that a drug related mechanism may have been present.

Hypothesized mechanisms have included: 1) disruption of central dopaminergic thermoregulatory mechanisms; 2) excess heat production and adrenergic discharge secondary to muscle contraction related to central dopaminergic blockade; 3) possible direct effects of neuroleptics on muscle contraction, similar to the effect of anesthetic agents in the malignant hyperthermia syndrome; and 4) mechanisms unrelated to neuroleptic treatment, perhaps due to the underlying psychiatric illness (Levinson and Simpson, 1986). It seems likely that one or both central dopaminergic mechanisms are involved in most cases. While most reported neuroleptic malignant syndrome patients tested for malignant hypothermia-like sensitivity to halothane or caffeine have been negative, Caroff and colleagues (1983) have reported a malignant hypothermia-like effect of neuroleptics in a neuroleptic malignant syndrome patient. More data are needed in this area. Carmen and Wyatt (1977) have reported a patient with periodic psychotic excitement and fever in the absence of drug treatment, with evidence that both symptoms may have been related to calcium metabolism abnormalities. They suggest that such patients may have been included in the older category of "lethal catatonia," although the literature suggests that most patients with this diagnosis had extreme manic excitement with anorexia and subsequent dehydration, hypernatremia and other complications (Levinson and Simpson, 1986). It is of interest that in the cases we reviewed, there was a higher incidence of agitation prior to fever (59 percent) than any single medical symptom other than EPS and fever.

We would suggest that in most reported cases, neuroleptic malignant syndrome is a severe extrapyramidal symptom with secondary medical complications. A smaller number of cases may represent one or more neuroleptic-associated syndromes that include fever, but which are not specifically "malignant." Labelling a patient as having a "malignant" syndrome can have potentially harmful effects: treatment for severe rigidity may be withheld while the unusual syndrome is contemplated; and the understandably frightened clinician may be afraid (or be advised) not to give further neuroleptics to a psychotic patient. We prefer the designation "EPS with fever" for those syndromes without clear medical etiologies, pending further clarification. Vigorous treatment of rigidity should be the primary immediate concern. Rechallenge with neuroleptics has been uneventful in most reported cases (with cautious dosing and prophylactic anticholinergics).

If drug induced rigidity underlies both the fever and the medical complications, then reversal of dopaminergic blockade should be the most effective treatment for such patients. Some patients have responded to anticholinergic agents, but most reported cases represent those who were unresponsive to this routine initial step. In the presence of severe rigidity, with or without fever and associated signs, the neuroleptic should be temporarily discontinued. A number of reported cases have responded promptly to vigorous treatment with the direct acting dopamine agonist bromocriptine (typically at oral doses of 25–30 mg/day, with 60 mg reported necessary in one case), or the indirect acting agonists carbidopa/L–dopa (up to 50/200 mg four times a day, orally) or amantadine (200–300 mg/day orally). These patients have not experienced increased psychosis during treatment, presumably because the agonist is only partially compensating for existing, intense dopaminergic blockade. Bromocriptine would probably represent the most rational of these therapies, because of the direct action. Some cases have been reported to respond to muscle relaxant therapy, including dantrolene (0.8–1.25 mg/kg intravenously; 50–200 mg orally) or lorazepam (1.5–2.0 mg intravenously to start).

Prevention of these syndromes is likely to rest with avoidance of excessive neuroleptic dosages and early identification and treatment of neuroleptic induced rigidity.

AGRANULOCYTOSIS

Phenothiazines are among the leading causes of agranulocytosis in adults (Pisciotta, 1969). The high doses of chlorpromazine commonly used after its introduction in 1954 produced some decline in white blood count in a substantial proportion of patients (Mandel and Gross, 1968), perhaps as high as one-third (Pisciotta, 1969). The incidence of clinical agranulocytosis was in the range of 1:1200 to 1:2000 (Pisciotta, 1969; Litvak and Kaelbing, 1971), but while there have been no recent surveys, incidence appears to have decreased along with commonly prescribed doses. It is possible that concurrent medical disorders (Mandel and Gross, 1968) or a significant incidence of leukopenia among drug free psychiatric inpatients (Litvak and Kaelbing, 1971) may inflate these estimates to some extent.

Most reported cases, and thus most research, have involved chlorpromazine, probably because it has been the most widely used drug and because low potency drugs are used in high dosages. Cases have been reported with many phenothiazines. Onset is usually 10–90 days after initiation of the drug (occasionally later), more commonly but not exclusively at higher doses. Recovery occurs with standard supportive and antibiotic treatment over one to three weeks, and deaths are infrequent. Most cases occur rather suddenly and thus are identified after the appearance of clinical signs of infection, so that frequent white blood count monitoring in the absence of symptoms has proven ineffective and unnecessary, but a baseline complete blood count with differential is advised routinely. Rechallenge generally reproduces leukopenia, so that a switch to a nonphenothiazine is generally recommended.

It has been shown that granulocytes from recovered chlorpromazine induced agranulocytosis patients, but not from other patients, have a defect in the final stage of DNA synthesis. Chlorpromazine apparently interacts with this defect over time to inhibit granulocyte production (Pisciotta, 1971). This mechanism has not been studied with other antipsychotics.

Agranulocytosis has also been reported during therapy with clozapine. There has been renewed interest in clozapine, as discussed above. An unusual epidemic of agranulocytosis occurred among Finnish patients treated with clozapine in 1975, with a 1:175 incidence of leukopenia, a 1:215 incidence of agranulocytosis, and a 1:350 incidence of lethal agranulocytosis (Amsler et al, 1977). Of 379 patients treated for at least 6 weeks in U.S. studies, 3 developed total white blood counts of <1500/mm³, although none died (G. Honigfeld, personal communication, 5/21/86). In such cases the drug is stopped and supportive medical care instituted. Because of the high rate of tardive dyskinesia with all neuroleptics in current use, and growing appreciation of the problem of neuroleptic-resistant schizophrenia, clozapine has recently been reintroduced in the U.S. as an investigational drug for patients who fail to respond to neuroleptics, with close monitoring of blood counts in these studies.

CARDIOVASCULAR EFFECTS

Hypotension

The most common, potentially serious cardiovascular effect of neuroleptics is hypotension due to alpha-adrenergic blockade. Either orthostatic or persistent hypotension may lead to falls with serious morbidity, although the incidence of such events is not known.

Receptor binding studies using radioactive labelling of relevant ligands have shed some light on the alpha-adrenergic blocking properties of various neuroleptics. Alpha$_1$ blocking effects have been assayed by measuring the concentration of drug needed to inhibit specific binding of ^{3}H–WB–4101 (an alpha$_1$ antagonist) to rat brain tissue by 50 percent in vitro. Inhibition of WB–4101 binding has been shown to correlate with potency in blocking norepinephrine and epinephrine toxicity in rats, and with hypotensive and sedative effects in man, but not with clinical antipsychotic effects in humans (Peroutka et al, 1977).

Hypotensive and sedative potential can be estimated by the ratio of alpha-adrenergic to dopamine blocking effects (κ_i [^{3}H]WB–4101/κ_i [^{3}–H]haloperidol), with the latter providing a correction for clinical dosage (Peroutka et al, 1977). Table 1 shows: a) the κ_i[^{3}H]WB–4101 (nM) for a number of widely used antipsychotic drugs (lower κ_i means greater alpha$_1$ blocking potency); b) the κ_i [^{3}H]WB–4101/κ_i [^{3}–H]haloperidol ratio (again, lower ratio means more alpha$_1$ effects); and c) estimated relative alpha$_1$ blocking potency relative to trifluoperazine, the least potent of these drugs, calculated directly from (b) (higher number means higher potency); d) for comparison, the κ_iWB–4101 of phenoxybenzamine, an alpha receptor blocker in clinical use, showing that alpha blocking effects of antipsychotics are in the same range; that is, substantial.

The low potency drugs, chlorpromazine and thioridazine, thus have notably high potential for hypotensive and sedative effects, while trifluoperazine has the lowest (pimozide is similar). Richelson (1984) recently examined receptor affinities of a larger number of neuroleptic drugs using human brain tissue from autopsies of nonpsychiatric patients. While there has been reasonable consistency across earlier binding studies using rat brain, Richelson's data show different potencies than might have been expected for some drugs at some receptors, so that further confirmation will be required. The drugs listed in Table 1 did

Table 1. Alpha–Adrenergic Blocking Properties of Antipsychotic Drugs

Drug	$\kappa_i WB^1$ (Nm)	$\kappa_i WB/\kappa_i HALO^1$ (Nm)	Relative a_1* Potency vs. Trifluoperazine**
Trifluoperazine	46	22	1
Fluphenazine	9.9	11	2
Haloperidol	12	8.4	2.6
Thiothixene	6.6	4.4	5
Chlorpromazine	5.2	0.5	44
Thioridazine	5.4	0.4	55
Phenoxybenzamine	4.0		

*From Peroutka et al (1977). $\kappa_i = IC_{50}/(1 + [[^3H]-ligand]/\kappa_D)$. Note that lower κ_i means lower potency.

**Calculated from $\kappa_i WB/\kappa_i HALO$. This is the ratio of alpha$_1$=adrenergic to dopamine blocking effects, and thus represents a value approximately corrected for differences in dosage necessary to achieve dopaminergic blocking effects clinically. The relative alpha$_1$ potency listed here has been calculated by arbitrarily setting the potency of trifluoperazine as 1, and then dividing the $\kappa_i WB/\kappa_i HALO$ of trifluoperazine by that of each other drug. This may not reflect exact in vivo differences.

have a similar rank order of alpha$_1$ potency, however, so that these data may serve as a rough guide to the effects of some additional drugs. For alpha$_1$ blocking potency, mesoridazine was more potent than thioridazine, perphenazine was similar to fluphenazine (but is used at higher doses), and loxapine was similar to trifluoperazine (but is used at higher doses). Molindone showed unexpectedly low binding for all tested receptor sites, results that may not reflect in vivo activity.

Even the high potency drugs can have significant hypotensive effects. For example, 27 percent of geriatric patients on haloperidol developed hypotension, as did 22 percent on loxapine (Petrie et al, 1982). Patients vulnerable to hypotensive or sedative effects should be treated cautiously, with high potency drugs.

Effects on Cardiac Conduction and Rhythm

In animal studies, neuroleptic drugs have shown potential to decrease cardiac contractility, disrupt enzyme activity in cardiac cells, decrease tissue levels and increase circulating levels of catecholamines, and prolong atrial and ventricular conduction time and refractory periods (Risch et al, 1982). A small number of case reports have suggested that such effects might have caused serious cardiac effects, including ventricular arrhythmia and death, in neuroleptic-treated patients. Thioridazine, in particular, frequently causes characteristic changes in the electrocardiogram (ECG). Therefore, questions have often arisen as to whether cardiac effects of neuroleptics may be life threatening to some patients.

In the most extensive study to date, Swett and Shader (1977) monitored the incidence of cardiac side effects in several thousand psychiatric inpatients over a six-year period. There were 18 neuroleptic-treated patients with a prior cardiac diagnosis, of whom 2 had cardiac effects considered drug related (premature ventricular contractions in a patient treated with chlorpromazine; tachycardia believed related to thioridazine). In addition, a hypertensive patient treated with 2 mg/day of haloperidol plus diuretics and potassium suffered a myocardial infarction during a period of poorly monitored fluctuations in hydration and serum potassium concentrations. A total of 1,854 patients with no previous cardiac diagnosis received antipsychotic drugs alone at some point (some patients are counted more than once in this total). Of these, 10 had cardiac effects, of which 8 were tachycardia (> 100 beats per minute). One patient on thioridazine experienced premature ventricular contractions and one patient on fluphenazine hydrochloride had S–T segment depression with dyspnea. The only sudden death among neuroleptic-treated patients occurred in a patient with a seizure disorder who was receiving four anticonvulsant medications plus haloperidol; no seizure occurred at the time of death and no cause was determined. Thus, serious adverse cardiac effects appear to be rare in neuroleptic-treated patients.

Thioridazine is the one neuroleptic that predictably alters the ECG, although similar effects may be seen less frequently with other drugs. Axelsson and Aspenstrom (1982) have reported the most detailed data. In a sample of 43 patients, 42 developed T-wave changes during thioridazine treatment. Serial ECGs and blood level measurements of thioridazine and its metabolites revealed that progression from abnormally rounded T-waves to flattened and then notched (diphasic) T-waves was significantly correlated with thioridazine (but not metabolite) serum concentration. In fact, these authors suggest that appearance of flattended T-waves might be used as an index of thioridazine level, as most ECGs with this effect were associated with drug levels in a range believed by these authors to be therapeutic (1–4 μM/L). Individual patients followed longitudinally showed progression through this sequence of changes as serum levels increased, but most patients reached a maximal degree of T-wave flattening at some point without further effects at higher serum levels. A second type of T-wave change, complete T-wave inversion or diphasic waves with a downward component, was observed in seven patients, all women, without correlation with drug levels, and usually disappeared after one to two months. U-waves (indicating hazardous repolarization abnormality) were not observed, although these had been reported in two patients who suffered fatal arrhythmias attributed to thioridazine therapy (Kelly et al, 1963). It is likely that the higher doses of thioridazine formerly used were more hazardous in this regard (Nasrallah, 1978).

A pretreatment ECG is therefore advisable when initiating thioridazine in a patient likely to require high doses or with medical risk factors. Serial ECGs can be recommended when abnormally high serum levels are suspected, or when patients are believed to be at some risk for the development of conduction disturbance. Patients with such cardiac disorders are probably best treated with other drugs. It has been shown that in the elderly, for example, fluphenazine is much less likely than thioridazine to cause ECG changes (Branchey et al, 1978). Nasrallah (1978) has reviewed studies of factors influencing neuroleptic induced T-wave changes, and has concluded that 1) hypokalemia may be a factor in most serious neuroleptic-associated arrythmias, and potassium therapy (or propranolol) may reverse drug induced T-wave changes in some patients; 2) T-wave changes may vary with food intake, with more normal ECGs associated with the fasting state; and 3) thioridazine, more than other phenothiazines, may decrease cardiac output and contractile force, making heavy exercise a risk factor for some vulnerable patients.

It should be noted that tachycardia is undoubtedly the most common rhythm disturbance caused by neuroleptic drugs, probably related to anticholinergic effects (see below) and the increase in circulating norepinephrine levels cited above. Patients in whom tachycardia would be dangerous should be treated with drugs with low potential for anticholinergic and hypotensive effects. Interactions between neuroleptics and cardiac drugs are considered below.

SUDDEN DEATH

Leetsma and Koenig (1968) reviewed a series of case reports of psychiatric patients who died suddenly and unexpectedly, and concluded that neuroleptic drugs might cause sudden death in some patients by contributing to aspiration, to ventricular arrhythmia, and to hypotension. Concern about the possibility of drug related sudden death among psychiatric patients has focused on cardiac rhythm and hypotensive effects, suppression of the gag reflex and aspiration related to laryngeal dystonia or dyskinesia, and heat stroke (Simpson et al, 1984).

If neuroleptics can contribute to sudden death, available evidence suggests that it is too rare an occurrence to be demonstrable in large studies. Zhang and Davis (reported in Simpson et al, manuscript submitted) could find only 35 reported cases of sudden death among psychiatric patients between 1957 and 1980 meeting the following criteria: death discovered less than 24 hours after symptom onset in a healthy patient without pre-existing illness; taking usual doses of psychotropics; with an autopsy unable to explain cause of death; and with adequate medical data available for analysis. Mortality among psychiatric inpatients appears to have remained the same (Brill and Patton, 1962) or decreased (Craig and Lin, 1981) since the advent of neuroleptic drugs, although schizophrenic patients have a higher mortality rate from all causes than the general population regardless of treatment (Craig and Lin, 1981; Tsuang and Simpson, 1985). Swett and Shader (1977) failed to find cases of sudden death related to neuroleptic drugs in a large study of inpatients, described above. This body of evidence is reviewed in greater detail elsewhere (Simpson et al, manuscript submitted).

It therefore seems unlikely that sudden death is measurably increased among neuroleptic-treated patients. It should also be stressed that neuroleptic treatment has undoubtedly saved many lives. Most serious morbidity and mortality related to neuroleptic use is neither sudden nor unexplained, but is related to the occurrence of severe drug induced rigidity, dyskinesia, or hypotension. Serious adverse effects are most likely when excessive doses are used and when adverse effects are not systematically monitored. However, it is likely that in rare cases neuroleptics contribute to sudden death through cardiovascular or other mechanisms. The best preventive measures are likely to be avoidance of excessive doses, particularly of thioridazine, careful monitoring when treatment with multiple drugs is necessary and in the presence of prior cardiac risk factors, and proper management of patients with adverse effects such as hypotension, anticholinergic, and particularly the parkinsonian symptoms.

ANTICHOLINERGIC EFFECTS

Many antipsychotic drugs significantly antagonize acteylcholinergic receptors both centrally and peripherally. This effect can lead to dry mouth, constipation, ileus, urinary retention, blurred vision, tachycardia, arrhythmias, exacerbation of narrow angle glaucoma, inhibition of sweating and temperature regulation, sexual dysfunction, and delirium. Withdrawal from anticholinergic drugs (such as neuroleptics plus antiparkinson drugs) may be associated with nausea and autonomic symptoms. The propensity to cause these effects is highly correlated with in vitro inhibition of binding of the muscarinic (cholinergic) antagonist 3–quinuclidinyl benzilate (QNB) to rat brain. Table 2 shows estimates of relative anticholinergic potencies of several antipsychotic drugs. These potencies have been calculated from the QNB ED–50 concentrations (concentration necessary to inhibit 50 percent of QNB binding) reported by Snyder et al (1974), correcting for the drug's potency in inhibiting haloperidol binding as shown in Table 1, and then calculating potency relative to haloperidol (arbitrarily set as 1). For comparison, benztropine is approximately 20 times more potent than thioridazine (Miller and Hiley, 1974). Richelson's (1984) data for human brain tissue binding ranked the drugs shown in Table 1 in similar order, and suggest that, for anticholinergic (muscarinic) potency, mesoridazine is similar to chlorpromazine, loxapine is similar to trifluoperazine (but is typically used at higher doses), perphenazine would be similar to trifluoperazine at clinically similar doses, and thiothixene would be similar to fluphenazine. Clozapine has greater anticholinergic effects than thioridazine. Molindone, again, showed unusual results for all receptors in this study.

Serious clinical anticholinergic effects are usually due either to high doses of the most anticholinergic antipsychotics or to combinations of antipsychotics and other anticholinergic drugs, such as antiparkinson agents and antidepressants. Patients considered at special risk for anticholinergic effects and those on combi-

Table 2. Anticholinergic Potency of Antipsychotic Drugs

Drug	Anticholinergic Potency Relative to Haloperidol[1]
Haloperidol	1
Fluphenazine	2.6
Trifluoperazine	5.5
Chlorpromazine	340
Thioridazine	3400

[1]Calculated from the ratio of ED–50 concentration or QNB binding to rat brain (Snyder et al, 1974) to the κ_i for haloperidol (Peroutka et al, 1977), setting haloperidol potency arbitrarily as 1. Higher value means higher anticholinergic blocking potency.

nations of such drugs should be treated cautiously with antipsychotics of low anticholinergic potency. Peripheral anticholinergic effects can be treated with drugs such as bethanecol and glycopyrrolate. Central effects including delirium, as well as associated cardiac arrhythmias, should be treated with physotigmine by i.m. or slow (1 mg/min) intravenous injection. The usual dose is 1 mg (range of 0.5–2.0 mg), repeated every 15–30 minutes until slowing of heart rate and cognitive improvement are seen. Physostigmine is rapidly metabolized, so that repeated doses may be needed every 30–120 minutes until the offending drugs have been cleared.

The use of physostigmine to treat anticholinergic delirium deserves some emphasis. The combination of delirium, autonomic changes, and sometimes fever due to anticholinergic drugs may be confused with the so-called neuroleptic malignant syndrome and with worsening of psychosis, leading to mismanagement. When pupillary dilation, tachycardia, and other autonomic effects are seen in association with confusion, a trial of physostigmine, with repeat doses until heart rate is affected, can rapidly improve cognition and prove an anticholinergic etiology.

HEPATOTOXICITY

All classes of phenothiazines appear to be associated with an increased risk of hepatitis (Ishak and Irey, 1972; Jones et al, 1983), with an incidence estimated at 1.2 percent from a group of large studies (Ishak and Irey, 1972). Psychotropics rank second to the anesthetic halothane in the propensity to cause hepatitis, with most cases due to phenothiazines (Dossing and Andreasen, 1982). While butyrophenone and thioxanthene derivatives appear to be associated with a lower risk, individual cases have been reported (Simpson et al, 1984). Most cases are of a cholestatic type, although a minority are primarily cytotoxic (Dossing and Andreasen, 1982). Most patients have a prodromal period of 2–14 days, with onset typically within several weeks of starting the offending drug, with recovery over eight weeks in most cases, but with abnormal lab values for over one year in some (Ishak and Irey, 1972). Chronic hepatitis develops in about 10 percent, with some fatalities (Ishak and Irey, 1972; Dossing and Andreasen, 1982). Liver transaminase values are typically in the range of 50–300 Karmen units. Liver biopsy generally shows cholestatic changes with some degree of inflammation and focal necrosis.

The time course, low incidence, and frequent associated eosinophilia all suggest an immunological mechanism, although the much higher incidence of liver enzyme abnormalities in closely monitored patients (22–50 percent, according to Ishak and Irey's review) and of subtle cholestatic changes in biopsies of clinically well patients treated with chlorpromazine (Hollister and Hall, 1966) suggest cytotoxic effects. It has been suggested that cytotoxic effects on membranes might lead to hypersensitivity reactions in some patients (Sherlock, 1979). In the individual case, however, it should be remembered that as many as half of psychiatric inpatients may show liver enzyme elevations prior to drug treatment (Hollister and Hall, 1966), and that changes from drugs of abuse or infectious hepatitis may be confused with neuroleptic induced hepatitis. Thus, careful investigation of the time course and nature of changes in the individual case, with liver biopsy for cases with clinical signs, may be necessary before antipsychotics can be clearly implicated. Unfortunately, patients with minor enzyme elevations are often denied neuroleptics that have proven particularly effective for them; most such patients tolerate reintroduction of the drug.

When neuroleptic induced hepatitis has been well documented, rechallenge with neuroleptics often, but not always, causes recurrence. Nonphenothiazines are therefore recommended, although recurrence remains a possibility here as well. Patients with noncholestatic liver diseases are probably at special risk only because of their slowed metabolism and increased levels of drug, but use of nonphenothiazines would be prudent unless clinical response dictates use of a phenothiazine. Patients with cholestatic disease should not receive phenothiazine drugs. Patients with liver disease should have liver enzymes monitored over the first two months of antipsychotic therapy.

OTHER ADVERSE EFFECTS

Seizures

Neuroleptics alter background electroencephalogram (EEG) rhythm and can also rarely induce epileptiform activity, probably most commonly but not exclusively associated with the low potency drugs (Simpson et al, 1984). Risk factors have been reviewed by Sriwatanakul (1982). Oliver and colleagues (1982) have described an in vitro technique utilizing induction of spike activity in hippocampal slices to assess epileptogenic potential of individual drugs, suggesting that molindone has the lowest such potential among marketed drugs (along with the nonmarketed butaclamol and pimozide). Clinically, seizures are seldom observed in patients treated with appropriate doses of neuroleptics, and patients with seizure disorders are frequently treated safely with these drugs, along with anticonvulsants.

Other Central Nervous System Effects

Antipsychotics routinely increase prolactin levels in men as well as women after a single dose and during acute treatment, presumably due to the blocking of dopamine's inhibitory effect on prolactin release. In some patients, galactorrhea and gynecomastia may result, but breast cancer is apparently not increased. Meltzer and Fang (1976) reported prolactin levels of 140–470 ng/ml in women, and 55–195 ng/ml in men, during acute neuroleptic treatment. There is some controversy over how often prolactin levels normalize during treatment, and whether this predicts earlier relapse (Brown and Laughren, 1981). Neuroleptics may cause sexual dysfunction, including impotence and retrograde ejaculation (the latter primarily with the highly anticholinergic drug thioridazine), with specific effects including reduction of testosterone levels (Mitchell and Popkin, 1982). Weight gain is common, particularly in children taking thioridazine. Inappropriate anti-diuretic hormone secretion occurs, as does water retention and water intoxication (which may be seen in psychosis in the absence of drug treatment). Withdrawal from neuroleptics may involve a combination of central and peripheral dopaminergic and cholinergic effects, leading in some cases to vomiting, nausea, diarrhea, abdominal pain, anxiety, and other symptoms (Mitchell, 1981). Gradual withdrawal of anticholinergic agents after stopping neuroleptics may be helpful.

Ophthalmalogic Effects

Phenothiazines may cause lenticular and corneal deposits, probably due to melanin or melanin-drug complex deposition, the discovery of which should prompt change to a nonphenothiazine (Gowdey et al, 1985). Pigmentary retinopathy may also occur, primarily with thioridazine at doses over 800 mg/day (which has therefore been established as the maximum safe dose of the drug) (Simpson et al, 1981). It has been suggested that cataracts may also occur. Ophthalmalogic exam should be carried out for patients with complaints of impaired vision, impaired vision in the dark, or discoloration of vision.

Dermatologic Effects

Phenothiazines and particularly chlorpromazine are prone to cause benign skin rashes, although virtually any type of allergic reaction can occur. Photosensitivity (excessive sunburn) is also common, again particularly with chlorpromazine, so that neuroleptic-treated patients should be advised to use sunscreen lotions for heavy exposure. Skin discoloration may also occur with phenothiazines, due to melanin-drug complexes that may cause simultaneous lenticular deposits.

Pregnancy, Lactation, and Fertility

Limb reduction has been reported following haloperidol therapy during pregnancy (Kopelman et al, 1975), although little teratogenicity has been reported with neuroleptics generally. Newborns may suffer hypotonia, acute dystonia, jaundice, or corneal-lenticular melanin deposits (O'Connor et al, 1981). There is concern that the use of any psychotropic drugs during pregnancy could cause "behavioral teratogenicity." Electroconvulsive therapy may be considered as a safer alternative for treatment of acute psychosis. When maintenance therapy is needed, the older phenothiazine drugs may be preferred because of the absence of any documented teratogenicity over many years of use. Gradual withdrawal of the drug early in the third trimester might be considered in some cases to prevent postnatal effects. Neuroleptics are found in breast milk, so that breast feeding cannot be recommended. Data have been reported suggesting a potential for reduction in male fertility (Blair and Simpson, 1966).

Drug Interactions

Neuroleptics may increase hypotensive effects through alpha-adrenergic blocking activity; increase the effects of quinidine; increase beta-adrenergic effects of mixed alpha- and beta-pressor agents (by blocking alpha effects); increase analgesic and depressant effects of narcotics; potentiate the effects of central nervous system depressants generally; and add to anticholinergic effects of other drugs. They may increase blood levels of tricyclic antidepressants, which may lead to potentially toxic levels of some drugs or raise blood levels of nortriptyline beyond the apparent therapeutic window. Anticoagulant effects may be increased by phenothiazines but decreased by haloperidol, presumably by opposite effects on relevant enzymes. Blood levels of digoxin may be increased via impaired gastrointestinal motility. Chlorpromazine and propranolol have each been reported to raise blood levels of the other (and, presumably, of some related drugs). Neuroleptic drugs and phenytoin have each been reported to lower blood levels of the other. Antacids reduce phenothiazine absorption. Reviews of drug interactions of antipsychotics have been presented by Simpson and colleagues (1984) and by Shader and associates (1978).

REFERENCES

Amsler HA, Teerenhovi L, Barth E, et al: Agranulocytosis in patients treated with clozapine: a study of the Finnish epidemic. Acta Psychiatr Scand 56:241-248, 1977

Anderson BG, Reker D, Volavka J, et al: Prolonged adverse effects from haloperidol in normals. N Engl J Med 305:643-644, 1981

Axelsson R, Aspenstrom G: Electrocardiographic changes and serum concentrations in thioridazine-treated patients. J Clin Psychiatry 43:332-335, 1982

Ayd FJ: A survey of drug-induced extrapyramidal reactions. JAMA 175:1054-1060, 1961

Barnes TR: Akathisia variants and tardive dyskinesia. Arch Gen Psychiatry 42:874-878, 1985

Blair JH, Simpson GM: Effect of antipsychotic drugs on reproductive functions. Diseases of the Nervous System 27:645-647, 1966

Borison RL: Amantadine in the management of extrapyramidal side effects. Clin Neuropharmacol 6:S57-S63, 1983

Branchey MH, Lee JH, Amin R, et al: High- and low-potency neuroleptics in elderly psychiatric patients. JAMA 239:1860-1862, 1978

Braude WM, Barnes TRE, Gore SM: Clinical characteristics of akathisia: a systematic investigation of acute psychiatric inpatient admissions. Br J Psychiatry 143:139-150, 1983

Brill H, Patton RE: Clinical–statistical analysis of population changes in New York state mental hospitals since introduction of psychotropic drugs. Am J Psychiatry 119:20-35, 1962

Brown WA, Laughren TP: Tolerance to the prolactin-elevating effect of neuroleptics. Psychiatry Res 5:317-322, 1981

Burke RE, Fahn S, Jankovic J, et al: Tardive dystonia: late-onset and persistent dystonia caused by antipsychotic drugs. Neurology 32:1135-1346, 1982

Carmen JS, Wyatt RJ: Calcium and malignant catatonia. Lancet 1:1124-1125, 1977

Caroff SN: The neuroleptic malignant syndrome. J Clin Psychiatry 41:79-83, 1980

Caroff S. Rosenberg H, Gerber JC: Neuroleptic malignant syndrome and malignant hyperthermia. Lancet 1:244, 1983

Casey DE: Tardive dyskinesia: what is the long-term outcome? in Tardive Dyskinesia: From Dogma to Reason. Edited by Casey DE, Gardos G. Washington, DC, American Psychiatric Press, Inc., 1986

Craig TJ, Lin SP: Mortality among psychiatric inpatients: age-adjusted comparison of populations before and after psychotropic drug era. Arch Gen Psychiatry 38:935-938, 1981

Delay K, Deniker P: Drug induced extrapyramidal syndromes, in Handbook of Clinical Neurology. Edited by Pinken D, Gruyn G. New York, Elsevier Science Publishers, 1968

Dossing M, Andreasen B: Drug-induced liver disease in Denmark: an analysis of 572 cases of hepatotoxicity reported to the Danish board of adverse reactions to drugs. Scand J Gastroenterol 17:205-211, 1982

Gerbino L, Shopsin B, Collora M: Clozapine in the treatment of tardive dyskinesia: an interim report, in Tardive Dyskinesia Research and Treatment. Edited by Fann WE, Smith RC, Davis JM, et al. New York, Spectrum Publications, 1980

Goldman HW, Cooper IS, Simpson GM, et al: Reversal of severe tardive dyskinesia and dystonia following bilateral CT-guided stereotactic thalatomy. Philadelphia, Fourth World Congress of Biological Psychiatry, Sept. 1985

Gowdey CW, Coleman LM, Crawford EM: Ocular changes and phenothiazine derivatives in long-term residents of a mental retardation center. Psychiatr J Univ Ottawa 10:248-253, 1985

Hollister LE, Hall RA: Phenothiazine derivatives and morphologic changes in the liver. Am J Psychiatry 123:211-212, 1966

Ishak KG, Irey NS: Hepatic injury associated with the phenothiazines. Archives of Pathology 93:283-304, 1972

Jenner P, Marsden DC: Neuroleptics, in Psychopharmacology, Part I: Preclinical Psychopharmacology. Edited by Grahame-Smith DG, Cowen PJ. Oxford, Excerpta Medica, 1983

Jeste DV, Lohr JB, Kaufmann CA, et al: Pathophysiology of tardive dyskinesia: evaluation of supersensitivity theory and alternative hypotheses, in Tardive Dyskinesia: From Dogma to Reason. Edited by Casey DE, Gardos G. Washington, DC, American Psychiatric Press, Inc., 1986

Jones JK, Van de Carr SW, Zimmerman H, et al: Hepatotoxicity associated with phenothiazines. Psychopharmacol Bull 19:24-27, 1983

Kane JM: Antipsychotic drug side effects: their relationship to dose. J Clin Psychiatry 46:16-21, 1985

Kane JM, Smith JM: Tardive dyskinesia: prevalence and risk factors. Arch Gen Psychiatry 39:473-481, 1982

Kane JM, Woerner M, Weinhold P, et al: Incidence of tardive dyskinesia: five-year data from a prospective study. Psychopharmacol Bull 20:387-389, 1984

Kelly HG, Fay JE, Laverty SG: Thioridazine hydrochloride (Mellaril): its effect on the electrocardiogram and a report of two fatalities with electrocardiographic abnormalities. Can Med Assoc J 89:546-554, 1963

Kopelman AE, McCullan FW, Heggerness L: Limb malformations following maternal use of haloperidol. JAMA 231:62-65, 1975

Lazarus A: Neuroleptic malignant syndrome: detection and management. Psychiatric Annals 15:706-712, 1985

Leestma JE, Koenig KL: Sudden death and phenothiazines: a current controversy. Arch Gen Psychiatry 18:137-148, 1968

Levenson JL: Neuroleptic malignant syndrome. Am J Psychiatry 142:1137-1145, 1985

Levinson DF, Simpson GS: EPS with fever: heterogeneity of the neuroleptic malignant syndrome. Arch of Gen Psychiatry 43:839-848, 1986

Litvak R, Kaelbling R: Agranulocytosis, leukopenia, and psychotropic drugs. Arch Gen Psychiatry 24:265-267, 1971

Mandel A, Gross M: Agranulocytosis and phenothiazines. Diseases of the Nervous System 29:32-36, 1968

Meltzer HY, Fang VS: The effect of neuroleptics on serum prolactin in schizophrenic patients. Arch Gen Psychiatry 33:279-286, 1976

Miller RJ, Hiley CR: Anti-muscarinic properties of neuroleptics and drug-induced parkinsonism. Nature 248:596-597, 1974

Mitchell JR: Discontinuation of antipsychotic drug therapy. Psychosomatics 22:241-247, 1981

Mitchell JE, Popkin MK: Antipsychotic drug therapy and sexual dysfunction in men. Am J Psychiatry 139:663-667, 1982

Nasrallah HA: Factors influencing phenothiazine-induced ECG changes. Am J Psychiatry 135:118-119, 1978

O'Connor M, Johnson GH, James DI: Interuterine effect of phenothiazines. Med J Aust 1:416-417, 1981

Oliver AP, Luchins DJ, Wyatt RJ: Neuroleptic-induced seizures: an in vitro technique for assessing relative risk. Arch Gen Psychiatry 39:206-209, 1982

Peroutka SJ, U'Prichard DC, Greenberg DA, et al: Neuroleptic drug interactions with norepinephrine alpha receptor binding sites in rat brain. Psychopharmacology 16:549-556, 1977

Petrie WM, Ban TA, Berney S, et al: Loxapine in psychogeriatrics: a placebo- and standard controlled clinical investigation. J Clin Psychopharmacol 2:122-126, 1982

Pi EH, Simpson GM: Tardive dyskinesia and abnormal tongue movements. Br J Psychiatry 139:526-528, 1981

Pisciotta AV: Agranulocytosis induced by certain phenothiazine derivatives. JAMA 208:1862-1868, 1969

Pisciotta AV: Studies on agranulocytosis, IX: a biochemical defect in chlorpromazine-sensitive marrow cells. J Lab Clin Med 78:435-448, 1971

Richelson E: Neuroleptic affinities for human brain receptors and their use in predicting adverse effects. J Clin Psychiatry 45:331-336, 1984

Rifkin A, Quitkin F, Kane J, et al: Are prophylactic antiparkinson drugs necessary? a controlled study of procyclidine withdrawal. Arch Gen Psychiatry 35:483-489, 1978

Risch SC, Groom GP, Janowsky DS: The effects of psychotropic drugs on the cardiovascular system. J Clin Psychiatry 43:16-31, 1982

Shader RI, Ciraulo DA, Greenblatt DJ: Drug interactions involving psychotropic drugs. Psychosomatics 19:667-681, 1978

Sherlock S: Hepatic reactions to drugs. Gut 20:634-648, 1979

Siever LJ: The effect of amantadine on prolactin levels and galactorrhea in neuroleptic-treated patients. J Clin Psychopharmacol 1:2-7, 1981

Simpson GM, Angus JWS: A rating scale for extrapyramidal side effects. Acta Psychiatr Scand 212:11-19, 1970

Simpson GM, Levinson DF: Can we increase the response to somatic therapies in schizophrenia? Br J Psychiatry (in press)

Simpson GM, Lee JH, Shrivastava RK: Clozapine in tardive dyskinesia. Psychopharmacology 56:75-80, 1978

Simpson GM, Lee JH, Zoubok B, et al: A rating scale for tardive dyskinesia. Psychopharmacology 64:171-179, 1979

Simpson GM, Pi EH, Sramek JJ Jr: Adverse effects of antipsychotic agents. Drugs 21:138-151, 1981

Simpson GM, Pi EH, Sramek JJ Jr: Neuroleptics and antipsychotics, in Meyler's Side Effects of Drugs, 10th edition. Edited by Blackwell B. New York, Elsevier Science Publishers, 1984

Snyder S, Greenberg D, Yamamura HI: Antischizophrenic drugs and brain cholinergic receptors: affinity for muscarinic sites predicts extrapyramidal effects. Arch Gen Psychiatry 31:58-61, 1974

Sramek JJ, Simpson GM, Morrison RL, et al: A prospective study of anticholinergic agents for prophylaxis of neuroleptic-induced dystonic reactions. J Clin Psychiatry 47:305-309, 1986

Sriwatanakul K: Clinical pharmacology reports: Minimizing the risk of antipsychotic-associated seizures. Drug Ther 12:207-211, 1982

Swett CP, Shader RI: Cardiac side effects and sudden death in hospitalized psychiatric patients. Diseases of the Nervous System 38:69-72, 1977

Tarsy D: Neuroleptic-induced extrapyramidal reactions: classification, description, and diagnosis. Clin Neuropharmacol 6:S9-S26, 1983

Tsuang MT, Simpson JC: Mortality studies in psychiatry: should they stop or proceed? Arch Gen Psychiatry 42:98-103, 1985

Van Putten T, May PRA: Akinetic depression in schizophrenia. Arch Gen Psychiatry 35:1101-1107, 1978

Van Putten T, May PRA, Marder SR: Akathisia with haloperidol and thiothixene. Arch Gen Psychiatry 41:1036-1039, 1984

Chapter 33

Side Effects of Antidepressant Drugs

by Barry Blackwell, M.D.

SIDE EFFECTS AND ANTIDEPRESSANT DRUG DEVELOPMENT

Side effects have played a significant role in the evolution of antidepressant drugs (Ayd and Blackwell, 1970). From 1935 on, the addictive properties and adverse effects of the amphetamines, coupled with fear of electroconvulsive therapy (ECT), created a climate of ready acceptance when it was discovered in 1956 that iproniazid possessed the joint properties of elevating mood and inhibiting monoamine oxidase (MAO) in patients with tuberculosis.

Early reports of liver damage with iproniazid led to synthesis of newer, structurally different inhibitors. Simultaneously the same adverse effect with chlorpromazine encouraged the development of safer analogs, among them imipramine, which benefited depressed schizophrenic patients.

Both the MAO inhibitors and tricyclic compounds were in equal use as antidepressants until 1963, when the former fell into relative disuse after the discovery of hypertensive interactions provoked by tyramine in foods. Attempts to find reversible and selective inhibitors (Type 'A' or 'B') that will avoid this side effect are still underway. Only three MAO inhibitors, tranylcypromine, phenelzine, and isocarboxazid are in use in the United States (Table 1).

Since 1963 tricyclic antidepressants have proliferated and there are now at least 23 compounds available, of which only eight are in use in the United States (Table 2). The basic tricyclic structure has been manipulated in three ways; modification of the aliphatic side chain, insertions into the central seven-membered amino ring, and deletions or additions to the two benzene side rings. These structural modifications and resultant biochemical differences have produced few meaningful clinical advantages, but they do translate into side effect profiles that have occasional significance in clinical management.

The dangers of the MAO inhibitors, the fact that the tricyclic configuration had been extensively modified to little effect, with growing concern over cardiotoxicity and fatalities due to overdose, led to a search for new and safer compounds. Because it is more than 20 years since the antidepressant prototypes were discovered, these newer drugs are referred to as "second generation" compounds (Table 3). Of the seven such compounds available world-wide, only two are currently in use in the United States (maprotiline and trazodone) but others are in regulatory review.

STRUCTURE, MECHANISM OF ACTION, AND SIDE EFFECTS

Explanatory models of antidepressant drug action invoke at least three mechanisms, including blockade of amine re-uptake, regulation of receptor density,

Table 1. Monoamine Oxidase (MAO) Inhibitors

Compound	Structure	Comments
Iproniazid	Hydrazine	The first 7 drugs are earlier
Isocarboxazid*	Hydrazine	compounds which produced liver
Pheniprazine	Hydrazine	damage: obsolete in many
Mebanazine	Hydrazine	countries
Pivhydrazine	Hydrazine	
Phenoxypropazine	Hydrazine	
Nialamid	Hydrazine	
Phenelzine*	Phenylethylamine	Probably in widest use today
Tranylcypromine*	Phenylethylamine	Most "amphetamine-like"
Pargyline*	Propinylbenzylamine	Indicated for hypertension
Furizolidone*	Nitrofuran	Antimicrobial agent (giardiasis)
Procarbazine*	Methylhydrazine	Antineoplastic agent
Clorgyline	Propylamine	Experimental Type A MAO inhibitor (serotonin)
Deprenyl	Propinylamine	Experimental Type B MAO inhibitor (phenylethylamine)

*compounds that are commercially available in the United States

and direct interaction with receptors. At least five different neurotransmitter systems are involved, including norepinephrine (both alpha- and beta-adrenergic receptors), serotonin, dopamine, histamine, and acetylcholine (muscarinic) receptors. The manner in which these actions explain side effects is highly complex or speculative and often based on animal research or single dose experiments in humans (Richelson 1982).

The clinical claims for new drugs usually reflect on the deficiencies and drawbacks of existing compounds and often invoke different structures or mechanisms of action as an explanation. It is hoped that the new drug will have fewer anticholinergic actions, be safer in overdosage, and relatively free of serious effects such as cardiotoxicity or reduction in seizure threshold. These benefits are anticipated without the penalty of any novel or unique side effects.

While there is an element of reality to *some* of these claims, they must be interpreted with caution. Few biological derangements are restored to normal by drugs in less than a week. Few chemically active compounds are so selective that they work at a single site or bind to only one receptor. Delayed responses, unwanted effects, and multiple actions are to be expected, especially when drugs are directed at a finely tuned and well protected organ such as the brain. New structures must almost inevitably incur new side effects.

The data available on new drugs are always incomplete. Final categorization of each compound awaits widespread clinical use beyond the artificial confines of clinical trials. This includes the experience that accumulates among the victims of overdose, a tragic natural experiment in man that cannot be anticipated in

Table 2. Tricyclic Antidepressant Compounds

Compound	Structure	Comments
Imipramine*	Dibenzazepine: tertiary amine	Prototype compound
Desipramine*	Secondary amine	First metabolite of imipramine
Amitriptyline*	Dibenzocycloheptene: tertiary amine	Most widely prescribed
Nortriptyline	Secondary amine	First metabolite of amitriptyline
Protriptyline*	Secondary amine	Most potent: least sedative
Doxepin*	Dibenzoxepine ring	Sedative: widely used
Clomipramine	Halogenated ring	Available intravenously: Specific for obsessive-compulsive disorder; potential increased prolactin output; withdrawal effects
Dimethacrin	Acridine ring	Less sedative; weight loss; abnormal liver function
Lofepramine	Propylamino side chain	Hand tremor increased
Noxipitiline	Oxyimino side chain	Increased delirium
Butriptyline	Isobutyl side chain	More potent dopamine effects; similar to amitriptyline
Pizotifen	Piperidine side chain	Developmental: resembles amitriptyline
Imipramine N-oxide	Oxygenated ring; metabolite of imipramine	Similar to imipramine
Amitriptyline N-oxide	Oxygenated ring; metabolite of imipramine	Possibly fewer ECG effects
Dibenzepin	Dibenzodiazepine ring	Similar to imipramine
Melitracen	Anthracene ring	Similar to amitriptyline; possibly more rapid onset
Amoxapine*	Dibenzoxazepine ring; piperazine side chain	Possibly more rapid; less potent; fewer ECG effects; related to loxapine; galactorrhea reported
Iprindole	6-5-8 ring structure; indole nucleus	Cholestatic jaundice (allergic); little action on catecholamines
Prothiaden	Dibenzothiepine ring	Similar to imipramine
Trimipramine*	Propyl side chain	Similar to amitriptyline
Amineptine	7-carbon side chain	Less sedative profile; excessive liver damage reported
Omipramol	Piperidine side chain	A case of total hepatic necrosis reported
Dothiepin	Thio substitution	Similar to amitriptyline

*compounds that are commercially available in the United States

Table 3. Second Generation Antidepressant Drugs

Compound	Structure	Comments
Buproprion	Amino-keto alkyl	Structurally related to amphetamine: recently withdrawn due to concern over convulsions
Maprotiline*	Tetracyclic	Skin rashes (3%): increased incidence of seizures; similar side effect profile to tricyclic compounds
Mianserin	Tetracyclic	Sedative profile; increased incidence of agranulocytosis; possibly safer in overdose; fewer cardiodepressant effects
Nomifensine	Tricyclic (tetrahydro-isoquinoline) reported	Less sedative profile; possibly fewer peripheral anticholinergic activities; may have fewer cardiodepressant effects; recently withdrawn due to immune hemolytic anemia
Trazodone*	Triazolopyridine	Serotonin inhibitor; possibly fewer peripheral anticholinergic properties
Viloxazine	Bicyclic	Fewer anticholinergic or sedative effects and weight gain; causes nausea and vomiting and weight loss; may precipitate migraine; safer in overdose (fewer ECG effects)
Zimelidine	Bicyclic	Serotonin inhibitor; possibly less cardiodepressant activity; recently withdrawn from clinical use due to immune allergic responses

*compounds that are available at present in the United States

animals before a new drug is released. The information presented in Table 4 on each compound is derived from annual reviews of the international literature (Blackwell, 1984, 1985a, 1986).

Table 4. Major Characteristics of Antidepressant Drugs Available in the United States

Compound	Mechanism	Clinical Profile	Side Effects	Overdose
Tricyclics	Mixed actions on uptake and receptors for several neurotransmitters	Range of sedative actions All may be given once daily	Range of anticholinergic effects: Hypotension (nortriptyline less) Cardiotoxicity Seizures (amoxapine more) Withdrawal effects	Fatalities (? amoxapine worse)
MAO Inhibitors	Irreversible nonselective inhibitors of 'A' + 'B' enzymes	Tranylcypromine more stimulant; 2–3 times daily dosing	Hypotension Multiple interactions (including tyramine) Withdrawal effects Sexual dysfunction	Fatalities Difficult to manage
Maprotiline	Norepinephrine reuptake inhibitor	Same as imipramine	Increased seizures Skin rashes	Similar to tricyclics but exaggerated
Trazodone	Weak serotonin reuptake inhibitor Mixed receptor activity	Sedative profile Half as potent as tricyclics May be given once daily Questionable efficacy in severe depression	Sedation Behavioral-cognitive changes Less anticholinergic Low seizure incidence Ventricular ectopic beats Priapism	Relatively safe

MONOAMINE OXIDASE INHIBITORS

Contemporary Overview

The last several years have seen a reappraisal of the risk-to-benefit ratios of the monoamine oxidase inhibitors (MAOI) that has coincided with recognition that the advantages of 'second generation' drugs over the tricyclic compounds have been fewer than anticipated.

The scientific underpinnings of this renaissance are discussed in a review by Murphy and colleagues (1984). Much of the earlier work was conducted using inadequate doses of phenelzine, and recent investigations using adequate drug levels (to produce 85 percent or more enzyme inhibition) have validated the efficacy of this MAOI. Consensus among experts is clearly in favor of continued use, with the recognition that even if a specific responder is difficult to define, there are individuals who respond when all other drugs have failed (White and Simpson, 1985).

It is doubtful if the older MAO inhibitors will ever again obtain a place as 'first choice' compounds because of the large number of other drugs and tyramine-containing foods they have the potential to interact with. This includes both the tricyclic compounds and the second generation drugs that are serotonin reuptake inhibitors (Marley and Wozniak, 1984a, 1984b). The fact that the older MAO inhibitors act by irreversible enzyme inhibition (which only recovers gradually after drug cessation) means that if they fail to produce a response, other antidepressants cannot be given safely without a delay.

In addition, a recent comparison of side effects among patients treated with an MAO inhibitor or a tricyclic drug (Rabkin et al, 1984, 1985) found a significantly higher number of severe side effects due to MAO inhibitors, which led to discontinuation of the drug in 45 percent of patients.

It does remain possible that the newer, more selective and reversible compounds may have a different and safer side effect profile (Murphy et al, 1984) but they have not yet been fully studied or available in the United States.

Organ Systems

The central nervous sytem (CNS) effects of the MAO inhibitors differ among individuals and drugs. As many as one-half of the patients may complain of insomnia, and somewhat fewer of daytime sedation. Tranylcypromine in particular has an amphetamine-like structure and should not be prescribed later than mid-afternoon. In a recent review, conversion to a manic episode was the second most frequent side effect of phenelzine and occurred in 10 percent of those treated (Rabkin et al, 1984). Nocturnal myoclonic jerks also occur in some individuals and are worsened by the addition of tryptophan as a hypnotic or by rapid cessation of drug. With regard to the autonomic nervous system, a carefully controlled comparison of phenelzine with imipramine (Evans et al, 1982) found a comparable incidence of dry mouth, blurred vision, constipation, and urinary difficulty.

An unusual side effect influencing the peripheral nervous system is the development of carpal tunnel syndrome (Stewart et al, 1984), which is due to pyridoxine deficiency and can be corrected by appropriate vitamin supplements. The early symptoms of numbness and tingling are especially prone to misdiagnosis as somatization.

The MAO inhibitors are devoid of any direct cardiotoxic effects and may be useful in some patients with heart conditions or the elderly in cases where tricyclic and second generation compounds are contraindicated. However, they cause quite profound and persistent hypotension in some individuals, unlike that caused by tricyclic drugs, because it is more delayed in onset and effects supine blood pressure and not simply postural change (Razani et al, 1983).

Some (but not all) patients treated may experience a weight gain of more than 15 pounds during a course of treatment with an MAO inhibitor. In addition, peripheral edema may occur due to inappropriate secretion of antidiuretic hormone. Diuretics are not helpful, but dose reduction and wearing support stockings are helpful in some cases (Blackwell, 1984).

There have been a number of case reports of leukopenia due to MAO inhibitors, but the problem does not appear to be as frequent or severe as that experienced with tricyclic compounds. Hepatotoxicity was an early side effect reported with iproniazid, which led to the synthesis of the nonhydrazine derivatives. It does not appear to be a problem with the compounds currently in use in the United States, although isocarboxazid (which is rarely prescribed) could pose a potential hazard.

Probably the most common side effect of these drugs is disturbance in sexual function. Anorgasmia in women and impotence in men may occur in up to 20 percent of patients (Rabkin et al, 1984). These effects appear to be dose related and they disappear with dose reduction, if this can be accomplished without loss of therapeutic benefit.

Skin rashes occasionally occur, and rare instances of mouth sores and a lupus-like syndrome have been reported with hydrazine derivatives.

Because of its ampehtamine-like structure and mild euphoriant properties, a few cases of abuse have been reported with tranylcypromine (Griffen et al, 1981).

Drug Withdrawal

Interest in prophylactic therapy occurred only after the MAO inhibitors fell into disuse, but a new generation of research is beginning to address the issue (Tyrer, 1984). Sudden drug withdrawal in patients on phenelzine and tricyclic antidepressants produced a significantly greater number of symptoms after phenelzine was stopped. One-third of the patients formerly on phenelzine relapsed, while one-fourth of the patients formerly on tricyclic antidepressants relapsed.

An attempt to distinguish between withdrawal and relapse on the basis of rapidity and severity of symptoms did not produce a differentiation; approximately one-third of patients in both groups developed new symptoms of adrenergic hyperactivity, including anxiety and perceptual disturbances. Acute psychotic symptoms may also occur following abrupt withdrawal (Blackwell, 1986).

Overdose

More than 20 deaths due to overdose have previously been reported (Blackwell, 1984). The outcome is preceded by a 12-hour delay to the onset of increased neuromuscular activity followed by hyperthermia, coma, cardiovascular collapse, renal failure, and disseminated intravascular coagulation. Pharmacologic management is difficult due to the large number of drugs with which MAO inhibitors interact.

Special Risk Situations

It is inadvisable to administer MAO inhibitors to schizophrenic patients, even when they seem to be in an anergic or depressive state, since MAO inhibitors may precipitate psychotic crises. In addition, it is difficult to ensure that such patients respect dietary restrictions. The fact that MAO levels increase with age supports the use of these drugs in the elderly; but their hypotensive effects and interactions with other drugs and foods suggest that they be used with caution in a population exposed to polypharmacy, whose comprehension and compliance with warnings may be impaired. Even in a normal adult population given meticulous warnings to avoid tyramine-containing foods, eight percent of patients may still forget to do so and may experience hypertensive crises (Rabkin et al, 1984).

TRICYCLIC COMPOUNDS

Contemporary Overview

The major side effects of concern have been cardiotoxicity (especially in overdose), hypotension (particularly in the elderly), reduction in seizure threshold, and anticholinergic actions. Earlier alarm about some of these side effects has been tempered by subsequent experience and the opinion that their risks and contraindications have at times been somewhat inflated, especially in patients with heart disease (Glassman, 1984) or the elderly (Wasylenki, 1980).

A number of studies have attempted to define the relationship between the plasma levels of tricyclic antidepressants and their side effects, with conflicting results. Sporadic reports of severe side effects, mostly of the anticholinergic type, have sometimes been associated with high plasma levels; but at this stage of our knowledge routine measurements have no place in management (Nelson et al, 1982).

All the tricyclic compounds share the advantage of long half-lives, and therefore the ability to be prescribed once daily (especially at night). Some side effects (such as dry mouth or blurred vision) are obviously less troublesome during sleep, when single doses are given at bedtime. Other side effects may be more marked, including an increased frequency of frightening dreams. Elderly patients given large single doses at bedtime may be at risk for dizziness, ataxia, and confusion caused by postural hypotension when they attempt to get out of bed in the dark.

Organ Systems

The different tricyclic compounds vary significantly in their degree of sedative action. They range from the most sedating, such as amitriptyline, to the mildly stimulating, such as protriptyline. Paradoxical outbursts of rage or aggression may occur as they do with all sedative drugs, and may be a threshold or dose related phenomenon.

All tricyclic compounds lower seizure threshold in animals and may produce epileptic seizures in patients. The exact incidence is difficult to estimate but it is low, and seizures are more likely to occur in individuals with a history of epilepsy, brain damage, exposure to alcohol or drugs, and at times when dosage is abruptly increased. The addition of lithium to the treatment regimen may add to the risk in rare instances (Solomon, 1979).

Confusional episodes may occur with the provocation of delirium, particularly in patients treated concurrently with other drugs that have anticholinergic properties. The elderly may be more vulnerable to these effects, although the incidence may be somewhat lower than clinical lore indicates (Meyers and Mei-Tal, 1983).

Tricyclic antidepressants are often listed among the many drugs capable of producing bucco-facio-lingual or choreoathetoid movements (Fann et al, 1976). A putative mechanism is the central anticholinergic action of the antidepressant upsetting the balance between dopaminergic and cholinergic systems. A more clear-cut cause-and-effect relationship seems to be present in the parkinsonian symptoms that occasionally occur on high-dosage tricyclic therapy in susceptible individuals (particularly elderly females). Because of its piperazine side chain and structural resemblance to phenothiazines, amoxapine has antidopaminergic properties that appear to produce the full range of extrapyramidal reactions (Blackwell, 1985a).

Rarer side effects within the nervous system include difficulty in articulation described variously as a stutter, speech blockage, or dysarthria (Blackwell, 1985b). The disturbance is a delay in thinking and speech, in which the patient has difficulty transfering the next logical thought into words. Finally there have been a few reports of bilateral footdrop with peroneal nerve involvement.

A number of behavioral effects have been attributed to the tricyclic compounds. The naturally occurring tendency for depressed patients to become manic may be exacerbated in approximately 10 percent of patients treated with tricyclic antidepressants. Patients at risk are often younger, have an earlier onset of illness, and a positive first degree family history (Nasrallah et al, 1982). Another behavioral change attributed to tricyclic antidepressants has been the exacerbation of existing psychotic delusions.

The cardiac actions of the tricyclic antidepressants are complex (Blackwell, 1985a). Tricyclic antidepressants are highly concentrated in the myocardium: this may account for the vulnerability of the heart as a target organ, as well as for the inconsistent relationships reported between plasma levels and manifestations of cardiac toxicity. The drugs interfere with the rate, rhythm, and contractility of the heart through actions on nerve and muscle that are mediated by at least four different mechanisms, including an anticholinergic action, interference with re-uptake of adrenergic amines, direct myocardial depression, and alterations in membrane permeability due to lipophilic and surfactant properties.

The most readily observable change in cardiac function is the sinus tachycardia, which occurs in a majority of patients. Its presence can serve as an indirect measure of compliance but is seldom a cause for concern, except in individuals who anxiously monitor their own physiological function.

The changes in conduction and repolarization are manifested as prolongation of the PR, QRS, and QT intervals and flattening or inversion of the T-waves on routine electrocardiograms, (ECGs); the conduction delay occurs distal to the atrioventricular node and is apparent as a prolonged H–V interval (time from activation of the bundle of His to contraction of ventricular muscle). This effect resembles that due to Type I cardiac arrhythmic drugs such as quinidine and procainamide. These conduction changes may result in atrioventricular or bundle-branch block and may predispose to re-entrant excitation currents with ventricular ectopic beats, tachycardia, or fibrillation.

The quinidine-like action of these drugs may even be beneficial in some patients with supraventricular arrhythmias. Nevertheless, caution should be exercised in patients who have had a recent myocardial infarction and who have evidence of impaired conduction (first degree heart block, bundle-branch block, or prolonged QT interval), since tricyclic antidepressants might theoretically add to the already increased risk of ventricular fibrillation. Routine plasma level monitoring does not seem indicated, since plasma levels account for only a small part of the variance in cardiac effects. If an individual patient shows significant changes clinically or on repeat ECG, then a spot measurement may reveal an elevated plasma level requiring dose reduction.

To date there have been no prospective studies that have clearly demonstrated increased mortality in cardiac patients following use of a tricyclic antidepressant. Even in patients who have chronic heart disease, the risks of effective treatment with a tricyclic appear minimal (Veith et al, 1982).

Among the tricyclic antidepressants, there has been conflicting evidence as to whether doxepin may have significantly less of a direct cardiotoxic effect. However, doxepin overdose may still cause lethal arrhythmias, probably by producing more marked respiratory depression.

The effect of tricyclic drugs on blood pressure is a much more common concern than the myocardial actions. As many as 20 percent of the patients treated with adequate doses of a tricyclic may experience marked postural hypotension; this effect does not appear to be consistently correlated with plasma level of drug, and tolerance does not develop during treatment. The mechanism for this effect remains uncertain; it has been attributed to a peripheral antiadrenergic action, to a myocardial depressant effect, and to an action mediated by alpha-adrenergic receptors in the CNS.

Postural hypotension can lead to significant problems in some patients, including severe falls and lacerations. Its occurrence may be predictable, since patients who have elevated systolic pressures and who show a pronounced postural drop before treatment are most likely to experience drug induced hypotension. Such patients should rise slowly from sedentary positions. Since the hypotensive effect is not directly related to plasma levels it may not improve with dose reduction, and the wisdom of using sympathomimetic drugs to counter this unwanted effect is questionable.

Recent studies conclude that there is less relative risk of hypotension in patients treated with nortriptyline compared with other tricyclic compounds (Blackwell, 1984).

A number of endocrine and metabolic changes may occur as a result of treatment with a tricyclic compound. Weight gain may be part of the improved mental state, or due to increased appetite or enhanced taste perception; but there also appears to be a physiological component with an increased craving for carbohydrates. No abnormalities have been found in fasting glucose and insulin levels or in intravenous insulin tolerance tests.

Inappropriate secretion of antidiuretic hormone may occur and contribute to edema and weight gain. It does not respond to diuretics and a change of drug may be necessary.

Galactorrhea has been reported with amoxapine (Gelenberg et al, 1979), accompanied by scanty menstruation and increased prolactin levels related to its dopamine-blocking activity.

Tricyclic drugs have rare but serious effects on the hemopoietic system. Twenty-one cases of agranulocytosis have been reported (Albertine and Penders, 1978). These usually occur within the first few weeks of treatment, presenting as a persistent febrile illness. A majority recover with aggressive management but eight deaths have occurred. Rare instances of purpura and thrombocytopenia have also been reported (Nixon, 1972).

Elevation of liver enzymes, especially transaminases and alkaline phosphatases, is quite common during treatment with tricyclic antidepressants. Such findings are usually benign. More serious and sometimes fatal liver necrosis has been reported with a number of different tricyclic structures, and probably represents an extreme form of allergic hypersensitivity (Schiff, 1982). A particular hazard appears to be posed by the drug amineptine.

A review of the literature by Mitchell and Poplin (1983) examines sexual dysfunction during treatment with antidepressants. Impotence due to loss of erectile function has been reported in at least 30 cases involving most of the commonly used tricyclic compounds in the low normal dose ranges.

Delayed and occasionally painful ejaculation appears to occur with a similar frequency. Both increased and decreased libido have been reported, and a small number of uncontrolled studies have reported therapeutic benefits due to antidepressant medication in patients with premature ejaculation or disturbed sexual function accompanied by clinical depression (Renshaw, 1975).

The mechanism of action mediating sexual dysfunction is controversial. One article (Quirk and Einarson, 1982) examines adrenergic mechanisms, while another invokes the anticholinergic system and suggests taking physostigmine 15 mg, one hour before intercourse, to reverse ejaculatory dysfunction (Kraupl-Taylor, 1972).

Several organ systems are targets for the anticholinergic (muscarinic) activity of tricyclic compounds. They constitute the most common adverse effects of the tricyclic antidepressants, but the peripheral anticholinergic actions may also be put to therapeutic use in such conditions as irritable bowel syndrome, premature ejaculation, and nocturnal enuresis.

Comparison of five compounds on human subjects revealed that amitriptyline and doxepin were the most potent and desipramine the least potent, with imipramine and nortriptyline being intermediate (Blackwell et al, 1980). Protriptyline is probably the most anticholinergic compound, while trimipramine is highly sedative but has little anticholinergic activity. It is valuable to know that anticholinergic effects occur immediately following the first dose of a tricyclic antidepressant, but it is difficult to predict which particular organ system will become the major target. Some patients complain bitterly of dry mouth, others report blurred vision, and some develop bowel or bladder symptoms. Careful history-taking and physical examination will often reveal a possible contributory cause based on the patient's previous response to similar drugs, existing disease (such as narrow-angle glaucoma, enlarged prostate, constipation), or advancing age.

Troublesome dry mouth can often be alleviated by instructing the patient to suck sugarless candy or chew gum. Although generally benign, prolonged dry mouth due to high dosage of tricyclic compounds can lead to severe dental caries. More serious complications that can arise include paralytic ileus which may be life-threatening, especially in the elderly. A less well known adverse effect is the potential for aggravating or even possibly inducing a hiatus hernia, presumably due to the anticholinergic action of these drugs on the cardiac sphincter (Tyber, 1975).

Clinical experiments have shown that the tricyclic antidepressants increase bladder sphincter tone and the volume of fluid necessary to trigger detrusor contraction. Such effects may account for the efficacy of tricyclic antidepressants in nocturnal enuresis, where the benefit occurs early and at a low dosage consistent with anticholinergic activity (Hendler, 1982). This pharmacological action may produce hesitancy, and more serious problems with urinary retention can occur, especially in predisposed males who have an enlarged prostate gland.

Loss of accommodation and blurred vision are common inconveniences that can usually be tolerated. Exacerbation of narrow angle glaucoma can occur, but is not an absolute contraindiction to treatment with a tricyclic antidepressant, since the anticholinergic effects can be balanced by judicious use of pilocarpine. Decreased lacrimation and accumulation of mucoid secretions may also promote potential damage to the corneal epithelium in patients who wear contact lenses (Litovitz, 1984).

Skin rashes are so common that it is difficult to determine a cause-and-effect relation to drug treatment. A choice must be made between waiting to see if the rash clears or switching to a different compound. Skin reactions to tricyclic antidepressants include cutaneous vasculitis, urticaria, and photosensitivity. The risk of allergic reactions is reported to be somewhat higher with amitriptyline than with imipramine. Cross-allergenicity does not necessarily occur, and a switch to another tricyclic compound may be worthy of a trial if the therapeutic response has been good.

Another example of an unwanted effect to appear after prolonged availability is the tinnitus reported to occur during treatment with tricyclic antidepressants. Symptoms usually decrease with dose reduction and are thought to be due to alterations in blood flow to the inner ear (Fleishhauer, 1982).

Drug Withdrawal

The evidence for a withdrawal syndrome due to abrupt discontinuation of tricyclic antidepressants is now compelling. Its significance is heightened by the increasing tendency to prescribe such drugs either as maintenance therapy or for prophylaxis against future episodes. Symptoms occur as early as the morning following a missed dose, but more often after 48 hours and up to 2 weeks following discontinuation. Symptoms include anxiety, restlessness, diaphoresis, diarrhea, hot or cold flashes, and piloerection. Delirium following discontinuation has been reported, as have instances of mania.

A review article (Dilsaver and Greden, 1984) summarizes the observations from 23 studies. The authors subscribe to the "cholinergic overdrive hypothesis" and speculate that withdrawal effects will not be observed in those second generation drugs that have few or no anticholinergic properties. The authors also recommend a management regimen. In most instances, reinstitution of the drug and tapered withdrawal are adequate. In instances in which rapid cessation is required (because of other toxicity or induction of mania) the use of atropine sulphate or other tertiary belladonna alkaloids is recommended, using an initial dose of 0.8 mg followed, if necessary, by further dosages every three to four hours.

Overdosage

The mean ingested overdose of a tricyclic antidepressant in adults is approximately 1,000 mg, but only about 3 percent of patients take a sufficient amount to cause fatal complications. Plasma levels in excess of 1,000 ng/ml are often associated with coma, convulsions, cardiac arrhythmias, and a need for supportive measures.

Symptoms often appear within four hours of ingestion, are usually maximal at 24 hours, and most patients regain consciousness within 36 hours. Manifestations include dry mouth, blurred vision, dilated pupils, tachycardia, neurological signs, and either excitement or depression. Epileptic seizures and cardiovascular complications also occur. Gastric aspiration may be helpful for up to 12 hours after ingestion because of pylorospasm induced by the anticholinergic effect of the drugs. Continuous aspiration and the use of activated charcoal have been advised to reduce the delayed toxic effects due to enterohepatic circulation and slow absorption of the drug.

Attempts to shorten coma by the use of physostigmine are based on the assumption that coma, delirium, and confusion are contributed to by the central anticholinergic action of tricyclic compounds. When used, physostigmine is given in dosages of 2 mg intravenously, but its rapid metabolism may necessitate repeating this dose every three to four hours. Results have been conflicting. The drug may produce unwanted cholinergic effects including bradycardia, hypersalivation, and aggravation of heart block. Physostigmine usually fails to control convulsions, which are best treated with intravenous diazepam and not with barbiturates, diphenylhydantoin, or paraldehyde.

Acidosis should be corrected and hypoxia treated with artificial ventilation. Hemodialysis is generally unhelpful, because the bulk of the tricyclic antidepressant is bound to plasma proteins.

A bleak picture of amoxapine is evolving with regard to its toxicity in overdose, with evidence for increased CNS effects as well as renal damage (Blackwell, 1985a).

Effects on Fetus and Neonate

In spite of reports negating a possible association between tricyclics and teratogenicity (Crombie et al, 1972), it might be advisable to avoid these drugs during pregnancy, especially in the first trimester, unless a compelling need exists.

Instances of distress in the newborn have been reported following treatment of the mothers with tricyclics prior to delivery. Clinical manifestations are thought to result from both the adrenergic and anticholinergic effects of the drug, which readily passes the placenta and should be avoided during the perinatal period.

Detectable levels of both imipramine and desipramine are present in breast milk and caution is advised because of the known hypersensitivity of young children to tricyclic antidepressants.

Special Risk Situations

A number of special risk situations in the use of tricyclic antidepressants have been alluded to in this chapter, including risks to children, the elderly, the physically impaired, and patients who are suicidal.

The elderly are often taking other drugs that may cause depression or interact with tricyclic antidepressant treatment. Safe practice dictates that treatment in the elderly be initiated at lower dosages (50 mg imipramine or equivalent daily) in divided amounts with smaller increments (50 mg imipramine per week) and reduced total dose range (75–150 mg daily, except in unusual circumstances). Close attention should be paid to the potential anticholinergic, neurological, or cardiovascular complications to which the elderly are vulnerable.

SECOND GENERATION COMPOUNDS

Much less is known about the second generation compounds than is known about the two other major categories of antidepressant drugs. To date, they have not been shown to have withdrawal effects or to produce effects on the fetus or neonate, although experience is still limited. These sections are therefore omitted and a brief summary has been added on the advantages and limitations of each compound as compared to the older drugs.

Buproprion

CONTEMPORARY OVERVIEW. Buproprion is a substituted chloropropiophenone with a structure reminiscent of stimulant and anoretic drugs such as diethylproprion.

Buproprion was synthesized and tested almost exclusively in the United States. Very little had been published until the appearance of a complete issue of the *Journal of Clinical Psychiatry* in May 1983 (Vol. 5, No. 2). Distribution of buproprion was abruptly halted in March 1986 due to the occurrence of seizures in 3 out of 55 patients receiving up to 400 mg daily in a 3-center study of buproprion for bulimia. The manufacturers are currently negotiating with the Food and Drug Administration (FDA) over the conduct of additional research to more accurately assess the risk of seizures.

Preclinical testing revealed a profile of mild stimulant properties and a specific but atypical antidepressant effect. The compound appears to have a relatively selective action on dopamine re-uptake, and in animal experiments the compound lacks any significant action on serotonergic, histaminic, or cholinergic mechanisms.

Buproprion is rapidly absorbed, with peak plasma concentrations within two hours (Lai and Schroeder, 1983), and a plasma half-life of 11 to 14 hours. It has been evaluated in dosages between 300 and 750 mgs daily, given three times a day for periods of up to six months (Shopsin, 1983). Plasma levels vary tenfold and appear unrelated to dosage or age.

ORGAN SYSTEMS. Buproprion has significantly fewer anticholinergic side effects than amitriptyline, but is not free of them. There is a noticeable absence of sedation, but there is the occurrence in some patients of stimulant effects including excitement, increased palpitations, tremor, agitation, increased motor activity, and an occasional toxic confusional state. Because of the lack of sedation and stimulant side effects, sedative-hypnotics may be required for insomnia or anxiety in depressed patients. Skin rashes and gastrointestinal disturbances (nausea and vomiting) are also reported.

One unusual side effect (reported by Becker and Dufresne, 1983) has been the occurrence of perceptual disturbances, including an alteration in time sense, sensitivity to sensory stimuli, and vivid dreaming. These actions may be related to buproprion's influence on dopamine metabolism and appear more likely to occur in patients with a schizophrenic diathesis.

Other side effects related to buproprion's chemical and stimulant profile include evidence of an average weight loss of one to two pounds during four weeks of treatment, as well as concern over the potential for amphetamine-like abuse. The compound is self-administered by primates, and tests at the Addiction Research Center clearly discriminated buproprion from amphetamines, but did suggest some dose dependent increases in lysergic acid diethylamide (LSD) and morphine-benzedrine scales (Blackwell, 1984).

Patients with prior sexual dysfunction on tricyclic compounds (impaired libido and partial erection) regained normal function after switching to buproprion, probably because of fewer anticholinergic and adrenergic actions (Gardner and Johnston, 1985).

Buproprion lowers the seizure threshold in animals, and at least 10 clinical cases of epilepsy are reported. As noted above, concern about this side effect has recently halted distribution of the compound.

There appear to be few, if any, cardiotoxic effects with buproprion in the clinical trials to date (Glassman, 1984). The compound has produced no significant ECG or conduction changes and no alterations in pulse or blood pressure, even in patients with previous postural hypotension on tricyclic drugs (Farid et al, 1983).

OVERDOSAGE. The substantial size of buproprion tablets (over 10 mm) may deter patients from large overdoses. Five patients are reported to have survived up to 3,000 mg (six times the therapeutic dose) without impaired consciousness, seizures, or cardiovascular complications (Preskorn and Othmer, 1984).

ADVANTAGES AND LIMITATIONS. Buproprion has a profile that may make it useful for selected segments of the population, particularly those sensitive to the sedative, anticholinergic, or cardiovascular complications of tricyclic drugs. Patients who are overweight may also benefit. The compound also has several limitations. It is not suitable for once-daily dosing, and patients may require adjunctive sedative or hypnotic drugs. The stimulant and dissociative tendencies will restrict its use in schizophrenic patients.

Maprotiline

CONTEMPORARY OVERVIEW. Maprotiline is a modification of the basic tricyclic configuration by the addition of an ethylene bridge to the middle ring. The compound was the first of the second generation drugs to become available. It has been marketed in other countries for more than 10 years, and in the United States since 1981.

The compound has a similar pharmacologic profile to tricyclic antidepressants in general and desipramine or nortriptyline in particular. In animals it is relatively selective in blocking norepinephrine uptake and inactive on serotonergic mechanisms (Lloyd, 1977), but it also has strong antihistaminic and anticholinergic properties.

Maprotiline is equipotent to imipramine and has a long elimination half-life of 43 hours, providing a steady state level toward the end of one week and permitting once-daily regimens. Plasma levels vary tenfold from one individual to another, but there are inadequate data to correlate outcome or side effects to blood level in a predictable manner.

ORGAN SYSTEMS. Although earlier reports claimed fewer side effects, there is no consistent evidence to support this (Robinson, 1984). The principal side effects are peripheral anticholinergic manifestations in up to 30 percent of patients, followed by drowsiness in over 15 percent.

In some animal models and at low dosage in humans (below 100 mgs), maprotiline has been reported to have fewer cardiac effects, but in usual therapeutic dosages and in overdose its effects are indistinguishable from those of the tricyclic compounds (Coccaro and Siever, 1985).

Maprotiline possesses two side effects present in higher frequency compared to tricyclic compounds. Approximately three percent of patients develop an exanthematous skin rash, usually within two weeks of treatment, which is probably allergic in nature and which disappears rapidly on drug cessation.

Of more serious concern is an increased ability to lower the seizure threshold, with an increased incidence of epileptic seizures during treatment and complicating overdose. It is usual to avoid treatment with maprotiline in patients with a personal or family history of epilepsy, and to reduce the risk of seizures by initiating treatment in low dosage and avoiding upward titration until steady state is reached.

OVERDOSAGE. In a study of a large series of overdoses on maprotiline (Knudsen and Heath, 1984), the outcome was similar to tricyclic complications, although prolonged coma (over 72 hours) and seizures (in 36 percent of patients) were troublesome. Seizures appeared more likely to occur in patients with cardiac conduction defects. Deaths due to overdose have also been recorded (Blackwell, 1984). Overall, the morbidity associated with overdose due to maprotiline may be worsened by its long half-life and delayed excretion.

ADVANTAGES AND LIMITATIONS. Maprotiline is similar to tricyclic compounds, with little evidence of any useful clinical distinctions. It has the additional disadvantages of an unusually long life and a higher incidence of seizures, skin rashes, and complications of overdose. It is possible that selected patients who fail to respond to a tricyclic compound may benefit from maprotiline but there is no documented evidence for this, and switching to a more clinically and structurally differentiated second generation drug would be a more rational choice.

Trazodone

CONTEMPORARY OVERVIEW. Trazodone is a triazolopyridine derivative related to oxypertine, a compound with antipsychotic and antianxiety properties (Hollister, 1981).

The compound was the first really novel nontricyclic compound to appear, and it was tested in Europe and in the United States. The first double blind studies were published in 1979, but the majority of clinical research appeared in a special supplement to the *Journal of Clinical Psychopharmacology* in November 1981, prior to FDA approval and marketing of the compound in the United States in 1982.

Trazodone is a relatively selective but weak inhibitor of serotonin re-uptake.

Its action on receptors is more complex. It does not bind to muscarinic receptors but is active at both serotonergic and alpha-adrenergic receptors (Richelson, 1981).

Trazodone is rapidly absorbed with peak plasma levels 0.5 to 2 hours after ingestion. It has a relatively short half-life of 6 to 11 hours for the parent compound, and 13 for the total drug and metabolites. Despite this short half-life, studies by the general practitioner group in Britain (Wheatley, 1980) found comparable efficacy with once, twice, and thrice daily dose regimens.

A study comparing therapeutic response to plasma levels (Mann et al, 1981) found an eightfold variation in plasma levels among individuals, with no significant relation to outcome.

ORGAN SYSTEMS. In studies on endogenous depression treated with trazodone or imipramine, the side effects differed markedly among active drugs (Brogden et al, 1981). Anticholinergic effects (dry mouth, blurred vision, and bowel and bladder disturbance) occurred in 20 percent of patients on trazodone, 15 percent on placebo, and 51 percent on imipramine. Other side effects were more common with trazodone. The most common was sedation, reported in 24 percent of patients on trazodone, 12 percent of those on imipramine, and 6 percent on placebo. Trazodone also produced a variety of behavioral changes (indecision, loss of interest, forgetfulness, hostility, and fuzzy feeling or confusion), which occurred in 22 percent of patients, compared to 11 percent on imipramine and 4 percent on placebo.

Although these results support the common belief (also based on animal pharmacology) that trazodone is relatively free of anticholinergic side effects, the data from controlled outpatient studies compared to amitriptyline found that dry mouth and visual disturbances occurred with almost equal frequency in both drugs and in excess of placebo. It is possible that some of the side effects normally attributed to peripheral antimuscarinic actions may be mediated by other mechanisms.

In one long-term study (Feigner et al, 1981), patients on trazodone who survived one year of treatment reported a much higher incidence of drowsiness (56 percent, compared to 19 percent on imipramine), but less dry mouth (16 percent, compared to 39 percent on imipramine).

Trazodone appears to possess some significant advantages with respect to the more serious side effects attributed to tricyclic compounds. Reports of seizures have occurred in 30 cases (Blackwell, 1986) but the overall incidence appears to be low and the majority of patients have had a seizure predisposition or concurrent contributing condition.

Based on animal experiments and the early clinical trials, trazodone appeared free from direct cardiac toxicity, although it does produce hypotension, a fact subsequently supported by reports of postural changes and syncope in a series of 27 patients (Robinson, 1984). This effect is reported to occur shortly after the drug is ingested, particularly on an empty stomach, and to disappear after four to six hours (Glassman, 1984). With the exception of one reported case of heart block (Rausch et al, 1984), it is fairly well established that trazodone has no action on the conduction system of the heart (Burgess, 1981). It does, however, appear to cause ventricular ectopic beats in some patients (Janowsky et al, 1983) and, in contrast to the tricyclic compounds, may increase cardiac irritability.

The only other severe side effect unique to trazodone reported to date has been priapism. Eleven cases have been described (Sher et al, 1983), of which five required corrective surgery and three suffered permanent loss of erectile function due to scarring and fibrosis of the corpora cavernosa. This rare occurrence had not been reported before as a side effect of antidepressants, but has occurred with a number of other psychoactive and antihypertensive drugs (phenothiazines, methaqualone, guanethidine, and hydralazine).

When first released, the side effect profile of trazodone appeared to differentiate it clearly from tricyclic compounds. As use has increased and experience has accumulated, this impression has lessened. Reports of toxic delirium, liver toxicity, skin rashes, conversion to mania, and inhibition of ejaculation have begun to appear (Blackwell, 1986).

OVERDOSAGE. Trazodone appears to be significantly safer than tricyclic compounds in overdose. A review (Faillace, 1983) documents 68 cases in amounts ranging up to 5g (12 times the maximum therapeutic dose). The predominant symptom is drowsiness and, in rare cases, coma. There have been no deaths in patients who took trazodone alone, and only two deaths in patients who took trazodone in combination with other potentially lethal drugs. Cardiovascular complications have not occurred.

ADVANTAGES AND LIMITATIONS. Trazodone was the first of the second generation drugs to possess a truly distinct structure and profile. Its major advantages are safety in overdose and a reduced frequency of anticholinergic side effects. Other claimed advantages are relative rather than absolute, and seem to lessen as experience accumulates.

The principal drawbacks to trazodone are its highly sedative profile and obtunding effect, as well as concerns about its efficacy in true melancholia. Priapism is a serious concern that may limit its use in males.

The present place of trazodone in therapy appears to be in patients who have marked anxiety, agitation, or insomnia without melancholic features, who may be sensitive to anticholinergic side effects or who have exhibited intolerance to the cardiovascular or other specific side effects of tricyclic compounds.

SIDE EFFECTS AND CLINICAL DECISIONS

In heterogeneous populations of depressed patients all of the available drugs are equally effective in short-term clinical trials. Choice among them is based neither on differences in efficacy, alleged biochemical mechanisms, or valid clinical subtypes of depression.

The possibility or presence of unwanted effects, however, has a powerful influence on decisions about which drug to prescribe, what to say to the patient, and how to deal with treatment emergent complaints.

Drug Choice

Selection from among the compounds listed in Table 4 is based on history of previous response to drug therapy, concurrent medications (to avoid interactions), and matching the patient's physical and psychological status with the side effect and sedative profile of the drug. This questioning will reveal any relative contraindications to a particular drug or category.

Because of their extent of use and knowledge about their side effects, tricyclic compounds are usually chosen first. Second generation drugs are preferred next for treatment refractory or side-effect sensitive individuals whose pre-existing physical condition or idiosyncratic responses make them susceptible to tricyclic compounds.

The monoamine oxidase inhibitors are reserved as a last choice because of their dangers and interactions, and because if given first their irreversible enzyme inhibition prevents the clinician from prescribing other drugs for two weeks should the patient fail to respond.

Within the three categories of antidepressants, choice of a particular drug is based on the need for sedative action (depending on insomnia, anxiety, or retardation) and the likely tolerance for potential adverse effects of the particular drug.

With the exception of maprotiline, which shares all the side effects of the tricyclic compounds, the second generation drugs possess some advantages, including freedom from anticholinergic and autonomic side effects and relative safety in overdose. They also have reduced cardiotoxicity, although trazodone has direct myocardial actions despite the lack of conduction effects. This means that there is no sedative second generation drug with a totally clean cardiac profile.

All of the second generation drugs may lower seizure threshold and, as shown in Table 4, each has potential disadvantages of its own.

Discussion with the Patient

Discussion with the patient should include explanation of the likely occurrence and rapid onset of common adverse effects. This can be done in a manner that encourages belief in efficacy, if unwanted effects are explained as evidence of drug availability and action. If fear is unnecessarily provoked, the patient's ability to understand explanations about treatment, as well as subsequent compliance, may be reduced. Comprehension of instructions and explanations should be checked at the end of the interview by asking patients to relate back what they have heard. During therapy, nonjudgmental and open-ended inquiries about problems with taking medication also serve as checks to compliance.

The expected duration of treatment can be predicted on the basis of the natural history of depressive disorders in general, as well as on the individual's experience during previous episodes. The decision to end treatment is aided by careful monitoring of the patient's capacity to cope and is accomplished by gradual dose reduction (¼ of the daily dose each week or two) to restore the patient's confidence in the ability to cope without medication, and to minimize the possibility of any withdrawal effects that might undermine this. If long-term maintenance therapy seems necessary, careful consideration should be given to its risks and benefits, and the dose used should be carefully titrated to the lowest possible level.

Treatment Emergent Effects

Accurate interpretation of side effects that occur during treatment is complicated by the fact that the biological features of depression such as dry mouth or constipation may mimic drug action, as well as by the tendency of depressed patients to somatization. Significant side effects may be overlooked as a result. Examples include the headaches due to hypertensive crises with MAO inhibitors and the flu-like symptoms that have masked allergic-immune responses to some of the second generation drugs.

An accurate pretreatment baseline, and a detailed history and careful clinical evaluation of any treatment-emergent condition is essential. Once the drug relatedness of the complaint is established, the clinician has the choice of reducing dosage, stopping treatment, or adding another drug designed to counteract the unwanted side effects.

Dose reduction carries the obvious hazard of losing benefit, but this is not necessarily inevitable, because therapeutic and unwanted effects are sometimes due to different pharmacologic actions with discrepant dose relationships. Stopping treatment also involves the risk of withdrawal effects, which may then be erroneously attributed to the next drug administered, further complicating management. This can be avoided by tapering the first drug while the second is cautiously introduced. The addition of a drug to suppress side effects carries its own risk of complicating the interpretation of outcome, but is occasionally indicated when therapeutic benefit is unequivocal or alternative drugs are unavailable.

The drug relatedness of a particular side effect can sometimes only be established with certainty by a carefully planned rechallenge, provided this can be justified on grounds of safety and because of the unavailability of alternative therapy.

REFERENCES

Albertini RS, Penders TM: Agranulocytosis associated with tricyclics J Clin Psychiatry 39:483-485, 1978

Ayd FJ, Blackwell B (Eds): Discoveries in Biological Psychiatry. Philadelphia, J.B. Lippincott, 1970

Becker RE, Dufresne RL: Perceptual changes with buprorion, a novel antidepressant. Am J Psychiatry 139:1200-1203, 1983

Blackwell B: Antidepressant drugs, in Meyler's Side Effects of Drugs, 10th edition. Edited by Dukes MNG. Amsterdam, Excerpta Medica, 1984

Blackwell B: Antidepressant drugs, in Meyler's Side Effects of Drugs Annual 9. Edited by Dukes MNG. Amsterdam, Excerpta Medica, 1985a

Blackwell B: In the pipeline. Psychopharmacol Bull 21:357-358, 1985b

Blackwell B: Antidepressant drugs, in Meyler's Side Effects of Drugs Annual 10. Edited by Dukes MNG. Amsterdam, Excerpta Medica, 1986

Blackwell B, Peterson GR, Kuzma RJ, et al: The effect of five tricyclic antidepressants on salivary flow and mood in healthy volunteers. Community Psychopharmacology 4:255-261, 1980

Brogden RN, Heel RC, Speight TM, et al: Nomifensine: a review of its pharmacological properties and therapeutic efficacy in depressive illness. Drugs 18:1-24, 1979

Burgess CD: Effects of antidepressants on cardiac function. Acta Psychiatr Scand 63:370-379, 1981

Burgess CD, Montgomery S, Wadsworth J, et al: Cardiovascular effects of amitriptyline, mianserin, zimelidine, and nomifensine in depressed patients. Postgrad Med J 55:704-708, 1979

Coccaro EF, Siever LJ: Second generation antidepressants: a comparative review. J Clin Pharmacol 25:241-260, 1985

Crombie DL, Pinsent RJ, Fleming D: Imipramine in pregnancy. Br Med J 1:745, 1972

Dilsaver SC, Greden JF: Antidepressant withdrawal phenomena. Biol Psychiatry 19:237-256, 1984

Evans DL, Davidson J, Raft D: Early and late side effects of phenelzine J Clin Psychopharmacol 2:208-210, 1982

Faillace LA: In antidepressant therapy: risks and alternatives. Emergency Medicine Special Supplement Jan. 20, 1983

Fann WE, Sullivan J, Richman BW: Dyskinesias associated with tricyclic antidepressants. Br J Psychiatry 128:490-493, 1976

Farid FF, Wenger TL, Tsai SY, et al: Use of buproprion in patients who exhibit orthostatic hypotension on tricyclic antidepressants. J Clin Psychiatry 44:170-173, 1983

Feighner JP, Merideth CH, Hendrickson G: Maintenance antidepressant therapy: a double-blind comparison of trazadone and imipramine. J Clin Psychopharmacol 1 (Suppl):45S-48S, 1981

Fleischhauer J: Acute hypacusis of the inner ear as a result of reduced blood pressure by amitriptyline: a rare complication of the therapy with amitriptyline. International Journal of Pharmacopsychiatry 17:123-128, 1982

Gardner EA, Johnston JA: Buproprion—an antidepressant without sexual pathophysiological action. J Clin Psychopharmacol 5:24-29, 1985

Gelenberg AJ, Cooper DS, Doller JC, et al: Galactorrhea and hyperprolactinemia associated with amoxapine therapy. JAMA 242:1900-1901, 1979

Glassman AH: Cardiovascular effects of tricyclic antidepressants. Annu Rev Med 35:503-511, 1984

Griffin N, Draper RJ, Webb MGT: Addiction to tranylcypromine. Br Med J 283:346, 1981

Hendler N: The anatomy and pharmacology of chronic pain. J Clin Psychiatry 43:15-20, 1982

Hollister LE: 'Second generation' antidepressant drugs. Psychosomatics 22:872-879, 1981

Janowsky D, Curtis G, Zisook S, et al: Trazodone aggravated ventricular arrhythmias. J Clin Psychopharmacol 3:372-376, 1983

Knudsen K, Heath A: Effects of self-poisoning with maprotiline. Br Med J 288:601-603, 1984

Kraupl-Taylor F: Loss of libido in depression. Br Med J 1:305, 1972

Lai AA, Schroeder DH: Clinical pharmacokinetics of buproprion: a review. J Clin Psychiatry 44:82-84, 1983

Litovitz GL: Amitriptyline and contact lenses. J Clin Psychiatry, 45:188, 1984

Lloyd AH: Practical consideration in the use of maprotiline (Ludiomil) in general practice. J Int Med Res 5 (Suppl 4):122-125, 1977

Mann JJ, Georgotas A, Newton R, et al: A controlled study of trazadone, imipramine and placebo in outpatients with endogenous depression. J Clin Psychopharmacol 1:75-80, 1981

Marley E, Wozniak KM: Interactions of a non-selective monoamine oxidase inhibitor, phenelzine, with inhibitors of 5–hydroxytryptamine, dopamine or noradrenaline re-uptake. J Psychiatr Res 18:173-189, 1984a

Marley E, Wozniak KM: Interactions of non-selective monamine oxidase inhibitors, tranylcypromine and nialamide, with inhibitors of 5–hydroxytryptamine, dopamine or noradrenaline re-uptake. J Psychiatric Res 18:191-203, 1984b

Meyers BS, Mei-Tal V: Psychiatric reactions during tricyclic treatment of the elderly reconsidered. J Clin Psychopharmacol 3:2-6, 1983

Mitchell JE, Popkin MK: Antidepressant drug therapy and sexual dysfunction in men: a review J Clin Psychopharmacol 3:76-79, 1983

Murphy DL, Sunderland T, Cohen RM: Monoamine oxidase-inhibiting antidepressants: a clinical update. Psychiatr Clin North Am 73:549-562, 1984

Nasrallah HA, Lyskowski J, Schroeder D: TCA-induced mania: differences between switchers and non-switchers. Biol Psychiatry 17:271-274, 1982

Nelson JC, Jatlow PI, Bock J, et al: Major adverse reactions during desipramine treatment. Arch Gen Psychiatry 39:1055-1061, 1982

Nixon DD: Thrombocytopenia following doxepin treatment. JAMA 220:418, 1972

Peck AW, Stern WC, Watkinson C: Incidence of seizures during treatment with tricyclic antidepressant drugs and buproprion. J Clin Psychiatry 44:197-201, 1983

Preskorn SH, Othmer SC: Evaluation of buproprion hydrochloride: the first of a new class of atypical antidepressants. Pharmacotherapy 4:20-34, 1984

Quirk KC, Einarson TR: Sexual dysfunction and clomipramine. Can J Psychiatry 27:228-231, 1982

Rabkin J, Quitkin F, Harrison W, et al: Adverse reactions to monoamine oxidase inhibitors, part 1: a comparative study. J Clin Psychopharmacol 4:270-278, 1984a

Rabkin J, Quitkin F, Harrison W, et al: Adverse reactions to monoamine oxidase inhibitors, part II: treatment correlates and clinical management. J Clin Psychopharmacol 5:2-9, 1984b

Rausch JL, Pavlinac DM, Newman PE: Complete heart block following a single dose of trazodone. Am J Psychiatry 141:1472-1473, 1984

Razani J, White KL, White J, et al: The safety and efficacy of combined amitriptyline and tranylcypromine antidepressant treatment: a controlled trial. Arch Gen Psychiatry, 40:657-661, 1983

Renshaw DC: Doxepin treatment of sexual dysfunction associated with depression, in Sinequan: A Monograph of Clinical Studies. Amsterdam, Excerpta Medica, 1975

Richelson E: Tricyclic antidepressants: interactions with histamine and muscarinic acetylcholine receptors, in Antidepressants: Neurochemical, Behavioral, and Clinical Perspectives. Edited by Enna SJ. New York, Raven Press, 1981

Richelson E. Pharmacology of antidepressants in the United States. J Clin Psychiatry 43:4-11, 1982

Robinson DS: Adverse reactions, toxicities, and drug interactions of newer antidepressants: anticholinergic, sedative, and other side effects. Psychopharmacol Bull 20:280-290, 1984

Schiff L (Ed): Diseases of the Liver. Philadelphia, JB Lippincott, 1982

Sher M, Krieger JN, Juergens S: Trazodone and priapism. Am J Psychiatry 140:1362-1364, 1983

Shopsin B: Buproprion: a new clinical profile in the psychobiology of depression. J Clin Psychiatry 44:140-142, 1983

Solomon JG: Seizures during lithium-amitriptyline therapy. Postgrad Med 66:1-6, 1979

Stewart JW, Harrison W, Quitkin F, et al: Phenelzine-induced pyridoxine deficiency. J Clin Psychopharmacol 4:225-226, 1984

Tyber MA: The relationship between hiatus hernia and tricyclic antidepressants: a report of five cases. Am J Psychiatry 132:652-653, 1975

Tyrer P: Clinical effects of abrupt withdrawal from tricyclic antidepressants and monoamine oxidase inhibitors after long-term treatment. J Affective Disorders 6:1-7, 1984

Veith RC, Raskind M, Caldwell JH, et al: Cardiovascular effects of tricyclic antidepressants in depressed patients with chronic heart disease. N Engl J Med 306:954-959, 1982

Wasylenki D: Depression in the elderly. Can Med Assoc J 122:525-532, 1980

Wheatley D: Trazadone in depression. International Journal of Pharmacopsychiatry 15:240-246, 1980

White K, Simpson G: Should the use of MAO inhibitors be abandoned? Integrative Psychiatry 3:34-45, 1985

Chapter 34

Lithium Carbonate and Carbamazepine Side Effects

by James W. Jefferson, M.D., and John H. Greist, M.D.

Lithium has a well established role in psychiatry while carbamazepine is a newer, promising, but relatively untested arrival. Food and Drug Administration (FDA) labelling approval of lithium for mania (1970) and bipolar maintenance (1974), while belated, is now a matter of history. Carbamazepine, on the other hand, is still seeking a firm psychiatric nitch, and, while a workhorse of neurology, tends to be viewed with hope, skepticism, and even fear by many psychiatrists.

Neither drug is benign in terms of side effects, yet in proper hands, both can be used with a margin of safety that should ensure their widespread clinical use and general acceptance.

Establishing an appropriate therapeutic indication for a drug is but one aspect of insuring its successful use. Equally important is the ability to recognize and deal with side effects, avoiding those of a serious nature and minimizing those that are milder but often unavoidable. A drug that is discontinued because of adverse reactions will never achieve its therapeutic promise. This sentiment has been captured in cartoon captions such as "I feel a lot better since I ran out of those pills you gave me" and "I stopped taking the medicine because I prefer the original disease to the side effects." In short, being able to anticipate, recognize, and effectively prevent or treat side effects is essential to the successful use of any drug.

Patients and their families as well as clinicians must be educated in these areas. A successful therapeutic outcome requires active collaboration between doctor and patient with education being a critical link. In recent years, requests to the Lithium Information Center have come in increasing numbers from nonprofessionals. Publications for lay persons (Bohn and Jefferson, 1982) have been widely accepted and play a vital role in assuring the knowledgeable and safe use of this drug. The growing use of carbamazepine in psychiatry has led to publication of a companion lay guide on carbamazepine (Medenwald et al, 1986).

This review has been weighted in the direction of lithium, which has had far greater use in psychiatry than carbamazepine. In addition, there is much more literature dealing with adverse reactions to lithium and far more investigational work done with this drug. The Lithium Information Center has been gathering, organizing, cross-referencing, and disseminating information for more than 10 years (over 15,000 articles are on file). Many articles have been written reviewing the side effects and toxicity of lithium. On the other hand, there is no "Carbamazepine Information Center" and, until now, little has been published in the way of a comprehensive review of its adverse effects.

Prior to discussing specific side effects and their treatment, several points should be made. Symptoms associated with the underlying disorder may be misconstrued as drug side effects unless a careful pre-drug history is taken. For example, Abou-Saleh and Coppen (1983) evaluated drug-free depressed inpatients, lithium-treated outpatients, and controls. Compared to controls, patients taking lithium complained more of "poor memory, trembling hands, excessive thirst, dry mouth and drowsiness" (but less often of headache). But when compared to drug-free depressed patients, those taking lithium had a *lower* incidence of diarrhea, metallic taste, trembling hands, and poor memory, suggesting that some symptoms associated with lithium therapy may actually reflect coexisting illness and personality characteristics.

Other studies of side effect rates can be faulted for failure to include controls or to define a control population matched closely enough in all characteristics except for presence of the drug. For example, in one study, Smith and Helms (1982) examined lithium side effects in "acutely ill elderly patients" (mean age 69.7 years) and used a control group that was not matched in terms of age (mean age 35.1 years), sex, psychiatric diagnosis, associated illnesses, or use of other drugs. The lithium-kidney controversy highlighted the need for proper controls when it was noted that patients with affective disorders *who had never taken lithium* had more morphological abnormalities than nonpsychiatric controls. Case reports can be an important tipoff to previously unrecognized side effects yet, at the same time, can cause mischief by placing unsubstantiated, inconclusive observations in the literature where they may be accepted as fact simply because of the power of the written word.

Finally, when evaluating side effects, the yield will be considerably higher if patients are specifically questioned rather than asked only global questions such as: "Are you having any problems with the drug?" or still worse, left to volunteer any difficulties they might be having. An organ system approach to side effect screening can be applied in a relatively brief time, yet be sufficiently thorough to ensure a comprehensive evaluation.

LITHIUM SIDE EFFECTS: OVERVIEW

Several studies have examined the frequency of lithium side effects. The data provided in Table 1 give a general "flavor" of the percentage of patients experiencing certain of these problems. Because of differences among these studies, direct comparisons cannot be made. The yield in such studies varies depending on factors such as 1) length of time on lithium, 2) serum lithium level, 3) diagnosis, 4) use of associated drugs, 5) age, 6) sex (for example, tremor is more common in men and hypothyroidism in women), 7) interview technique (questionnaire versus live interview; specific versus global questions), and 8) quantitative decisions as to when a symptom becomes a side effect. The side effects listed in Table 1 are representative but far from inclusive. Omitted are areas such as central nervous system (CNS) side effects (except for tremor) and gastrointestinal side effects (except for diarrhea).

One point bears stressing—*most* patients taking lithium have side effects. With the exception of findings by Johnston and colleagues (1979), a consistent finding was that less than 20 percent of patients had no complaints. Fortunately, the majority of patients classify side effects as mild. In their longitudinal one-year study of 67 patients, Lyskowski and colleagues (1982) found that only 30 percent complained of moderate to severe problems.

Table 1. Percentage of Patients with Lithium Side Effects

	Johnston et al (1979) n = 49	Bone et al (1980) n = 65	Vestergaard et al (1980) n = 237	Lyskowski et al (1982) n = 64	Duncavage et al (1983) n = 21
Tremor	31	25	45	10	14
Thirst	45[a]	23	70	19	48
Excessive urination	45[a]	38	—	22	57
Nocturia	—	—	17	—	62
Edema	—	—	10	1	—
Diarrhea	—	10	20	—	10
Weight gain	—	—	20	4	43
No complaints	37	18	10	7	19

[a] Thirst/polyuria was a combined symptom in this study.

Also, the true incidence of side effects must be underestimated, since studies tend to involve only patients in active treatment. Those with intolerable side effects discontinue lithium and are not available for inclusion.

Whether the frequency of side effects varies with length of time on lithium has not been fully resolved. Although it is accepted that tolerance develops as patients adjust to the drug, additional explanations for fewer side effects over time include 1) those with severe reactions stop taking lithium, 2) dosage reduction, 3) improvement in underlying illness, and 4) discontinuation of other drugs. Peselow and colleagues (1981) evaluated 49 patients over a six-month period for "ten well-known innocuous side effects of lithium therapy" (thirst, nausea, dizziness, fine tremor, diarrhea, excessive urination, abdominal pain, fatigue, lethargy, and muscle weakness). They found that these complaints were most prevalent during the first month of treatment, diminished over time, and were unrelated to plasma lithium level. On the other hand, when Duncavage and colleagues (1983) evaluated patients after one and five months on lithium, no difference was found in the frequency of tremor, weight gain, increased thirst, increased urination, and nocturia.

As with any drug, one must assume that *any* symptom can be a side effect of lithium. As will be discussed, some side effects are more common and can be considered characteristic of lithium. Others may be idiosyncratic reactions occurring rarely for unknown reasons. When doubt exists as to the relationship of lithium to a symptom, less or no medication for a few days may provide the answer. Any symptoms suggestive of lithium intoxication should be a reason for temporary drug discontinuation pending resolution of the issue.

NEUROLOGICAL EFFECTS

The neurological effects of lithium range from benign to lethal, with the most extreme being those associated with intoxication. It is generally accepted that factors such as extremes of age, debilitation, coexisting neurological and other medical disorders, and other central nervous system drugs will increase susceptibility to neurological side effects. As in other areas, studies of neurological function often suffer from methological problems such as failure to consider associated mood state, educational level, other illnesses (including lithium induced hypothyroidism), associated drugs, and failure to use fully matched controls.

Benign, Nontoxic

It is common, especially early in the course of lithium therapy, for patients to complain of symptoms such as lethargy, dysphoria, impaired memory, difficulty concentrating, intellectual inefficiency, reduced reactivity to stimuli, slowed response times, and a general lack of spontaneity.

Attempts to more formally study these subtle symptoms have produced mixed results. Clinical reports of memory impairment are common, with complaints such as "spotty memory loss for recent and remote events," inability to recall details to the point of interfering with daily functioning," and "gaps in recall of past information." On the other hand, a number of studies specifically designed to evaluate memory found no impairment that could be attributed to lithium.

In normal volunteers, one study found reversible performance decrements in three of five tasks measuring cognitive and/or motor functions (double blind), and another found delayed reaction time during stimulation. This latter finding was contrary to the normal reaction times in patients with Meniere's disease.

All in all, it is not surprising that lithium can exert subtle (and at times not so subtle) influences on cognitive function. Should patients taking lithium complain of impaired memory or other cognitive difficulties, the possibility of a mild depressive relapse or lithium induced hypothyroidism should be considered. When in doubt about the relationship of lithium to impaired memory, a trial at a lower serum level may resolve the issue.

Creativity

Both the qualitative and quantitative aspects of creativity can be influenced by lithium and the underlying mood state. Sustained hypomania may be associated with great creativity, while more severe mania can destroy the creative process. What constitutes creativity is also quite subjective, and opinions may differ between an individual and independent observers. In some, the flame of creativity may be stabilized by lithium while in others it may be extinguished. Schou found that depending on the individual, mood stabilization with lithium led to increased, decreased, or altered (qualitatively but not quantitatively different) creativity (Schou, 1979).

Patients who complain that lithium is having an adverse effect on creativity and productivity should be encouraged to give the drug an adequate chance, and to take it long enough to adjust to the stability it imparts. Those who complain of being "overcontrolled" by lithium may benefit favorably from dosage reduction (but also be at greater risk for relapse).

Tremor

Tremor is a common lithium side effect occurring in the majority of patients early in the course of therapy. Predisposing factors include high serum lithium levels, associated use of antidepressant drugs, increased age, male sex, anxiety, excessive caffeine use, and a personal or family history of essential tremor. The tremor has a frequency of 7–16 Hz (similar to physiologic and essential tremor) and is aggravated by movements requiring fine motor control (threading a needle, eating soup, drilling teeth). While Vestergaard and colleagues (1980) reported that 45 percent found tremor to be socially or professionally embarrassing, others (including ourselves) find this to be far less common.

Evaluation for tremor should be an integral part of every patient visit and should consist of observation of the outstretched hands and specific questioning regarding daily activities. Lithium tremor may also take on extrapyramidal characteristics. Tyrer and colleagues (1981) found a frequency shift into the parkinsonian range (4–7 Hz) in patients who had been on long-term lithium. While the fine tremor associated with lithium therapy is considered benign, a worsening of tremor in terms of quality (coarseness), severity, or generalization suggests impending lithium intoxication and should be investigated immediately.

Treatments for nontoxic lithium tremor include:

1. the passage of time
2. dosage reduction
3. use of a slow-release preparation
4. reduction or elimination of caffeine intake
5. anxiety reduction (psychotherapy and/or the short-term use of a benzodiazepine anxiolytic)
6. beta-adrenergic receptor blocking drugs: While propranolol has been best studied (20–120 mgs. or more daily in divided doses), oxprenolol, pindolol, nadolol, and metoprolol have also been used successfully

Given the wide variety of treatment approaches that can be utilized alone or in combination, it would be quite unusual for a patient to remain intolerant of lithium because of a benign, nontoxic tremor.

Extrapyramidal Effects

Extrapyramidal manifestations are common during lithium intoxication. They have also been reported in patients on long-term lithium therapy in the absence of elevated serum lithium levels and neuroleptic drugs. The true frequency is difficult to estimate since some patients in these reports were currently receiving or had recently received neuroleptics. Whether the long-term use of lithium increases susceptibility to Parkinson's disease has not been established (one author, JJ, has seen slowly progressive parkinsonism develop in two patients at ages 44 and 51).

Peripheral Neuropathy

Peripheral neuropathy has been described as a long-term sequelae of lithium intoxication, and a significant decrease in conduction velocity and amplitude noted in median, ulnar, perineal, and sural nerves during the course of lithium therapy. Also, abnormalities in nerve conduction velocities have been noted in both bipolar patients and normal volunteers taking lithium. The findings in the bipolar patients were inconclusive, however, since pre-lithium values were not obtained and confounding variables were not controlled. The changes in the volunteers were small and within normal limits, yet were consistently noted and reversible with lithium discontinuation.

Overall, it is unlikely that lithium in therapeutic amounts causes peripheral neuropathy. Should such a problem occur in a patient taking lithium, alternative causes should be sought. In the absence of an obvious etiology, a trial off lithium may be indicated.

Neuromuscular Effects (Myasthenia Gravis-like Syndrome)

Lithium may inhibit acetylcholine synthesis and release and alter depolarization and repolarization of the motor end plate. While being treated for manic-depression, one patient experienced four episodes of myasthenia gravis which resolved when lithium was reduced or stopped (Neil et al, 1976). Two additional cases have been described, one on therapeutic amounts, and one associated with intoxication. Based on these observations, myasthenia gravis should be a relative contraindication to the use of lithium.

Electroencephalogram (EEG)

Lithium can cause reversible EEG changes consisting of increased amplitude and generalized slowing, with increased theta and delta and decreased alpha activity. It has been suggested (and seems reasonable) that pre-existing EEG abnormalities may predispose patients to neurotoxic side effects.

Seizures

Seizures, including status epilepticus, may complicate lithium intoxication. Seizures have also been reported during the course of lithium therapy, although the incidence is quite low (case reports), and unless there are predisposing factors, the risk should be considered negligible. When used in the presence of epilepsy, lithium has been reported to both decrease and increase seizure frequency.

Overall, lithium is not contraindicated in the presence of epilepsy, although carbamazepine may have more appeal given its dual anticonvulsant and anti-manic activity.

Sleep

Disordered sleep is not a clinically important complication with lithium therapy unless it occurs for secondary reasons such as lithium induced polyuria with nocturia. The drug does appear to cause alterations in the sleep EEG, including increased slow-wave (delta) sleep, decreased REM duration, and increased REM latency without REM-rebound upon discontinuation. Sleep studies are difficult to evaluate since the number of subjects involved is small and underlying mood state has been a confounding variable.

Tardive Dyskinesia

Lithium has been used therapeutically with mixed results in the treatment of tardive dyskinesia (Jefferson et al, 1986). The likelihood that lithium can cause, activate, or aggravate tardive dyskinesia is difficult to assess. There have been occasional reports of tardive dyskinesia or a tardive dyskinesia-like syndrome occurring in association with lithium therapy. Given otherwise appropriate indications, tardive dyskinesia is not a contraindication to lithium therapy, although patients should be carefully observed for aggravation of their movement disorder.

Pseudotumor Cerebri (Benign Intracranial Hypertension)

Several cases of pseudotumor cerebri (increased intracranial pressure, normal or small ventricles, normal cerebrospinal fluid (CSF) constituents, papilledema, headache, and blurred vision) have been reported in patients taking lithium (Saul et al, 1985). Improvement was noted when lithium was stopped. If there is a causal association it is extremely rare, and routine periodic funduscopic evaluation of *asymptomatic* lithium patients does not seem necessary.

Intoxication

Neurotoxicity is the central feature of lithium intoxication. Severity depends on individual susceptibility combined with both the duration and magnitude of exposure to toxic amounts of lithium. While intoxication can occur at therapeutic levels, an elevated serum level is usually present. Despite similar or even higher serum lithium levels, patients with acute intoxication (for example, deliberate overdose) may have fewer symptoms than patients gradually intoxicated, since there has been less time for tissue saturation. Conversely, improvement in neurotoxic symptoms may lag considerably (many days) behind a fall in serum level in patients with prolonged exposure to toxic levels.

Early findings of intoxication include dysarthria, ataxia, lethargy, weakness, coarse tremor, and muscle twitches as well as nausea, vomiting, diarrhea, and abdominal cramps. In more severe cases these findings progress and, in addition, disorientation, confusion, muscular irritability, impaired consciousness, seizures, and incontinence may occur. Coma and death may follow. Other organ systems, including cardiovascular and renal, may also be involved. While recovery may be complete, some who survive suffer permanent neurological and renal damage.

Intoxication can be caused by a variety of factors including excessive intake of an accidental or deliberate nature, reduced excretion due to renal or prerenal causes (dehydration, congestive heart failure), a negative sodium balance, or drug interactions which reduce lithium clearance (such as thiazide diuretics and nonsteroidal anti-inflammatory drugs).

Preventing intoxication is an integral aspect of lithium treatment. Educating patients and significant others about causes and manifestations of toxicity is essential. When in doubt, patients should be instructed to discontinue the drug and seek immediate evaluation.

Treating intoxication involves minimizing absorption, maximizing excretion, and providing general support. Hemodialysis, the treatment of choice for severe intoxication, should be started promptly and be of sufficient frequency and duration to insure that the serum lithium levels *remain* below 1.0 mEq/1. This is best established by measuring serum lithium six to eight hours after completion of dialysis, since a rebound increase in serum level occurs for several hours as lithium continues to shift from tissues to blood. There are no absolute guidelines as to when to dialyze. This decision should be based on evaluation of both clinical condition and serum level. Given the potential lethality of lithium, one should err in the direction of early dialysis.

Less severe intoxication has been treated successfully with hydration and forced diuresis with osmotic diuretics and furosemide.

If large amounts of lithium have been ingested, absorption should be minimized by induced emesis or gastric lavage. Since lithium carbonate may form poorly soluble aggregates and be absorbed gradually over long periods of time, repeated lavage may be of value. Measures to increase gastrointestinal transit time may also be helpful.

All patients with lithium intoxication must receive supportive therapy and careful monitoring until serum levels remain below 1.0 mEq/1 and clinical condition has stabilized (Winchester, 1983; Hansen and Amdisen, 1978). Clinical improvement may lag *days* behind the fall in serum level, reflecting a slower decrease in tissue levels and, perhaps, other lithium effects at a cellular level.

OCULAR EFFECTS

Volunteers

Ocular side effects are not common but when carefully "looked" for may be more prevalent than expected. The short-term (10-day) administration of lithium to volunteers at serum levels between 0.5–1.0 mEq/1 caused no clinically or statistically significant changes in a variety of measurements including acuity, visual fields, tear secretion, accommodation, and intraocular pressure (Kaufman et al, 1985). At the same time, 10 of 13 subjects in this nonblind study had subjective visual or ocular complaints of a nonspecific nature such as dry eyes with inability to wear contact lenses, difficulty focusing on small print, blurred vision, slowed adaptation to darkness, tired and bloodshot eyes, and the sensation of objects being darker. In another study, lithium caused no ocular changes except an inhibitory effect on the electrooculogram (EOG), which was of questionable clinical significance.

Patients

When 73 patients on long-term lithium were evaluated, no long-term ocular lesions were found that could be attribued to lithium (Hiroz et al, 1981).

Rare reports have linked therapeutic lithium levels to a variety of ocular changes in ways that are difficult to substantiate. These include worsening of cataracts and reduced accommodation, senile macular degeneration, downbeat nystagmus, papilledema, eye irritation, and exophthalmos. Lithium also caused abnormal smooth-pursuit eye movements in patients and a reduction in visual perception when tested with backward masking.

All in all, lithium does not appear to have consistent adverse ocular effects. This does not exclude the possibility that such effects may occur in given individuals. In asymptomatic patients, we do not feel that routine periodic eye examinations are necessary (although some would disagree). Certainly, lithium patients with ocular complaints should be evaluated and, at times, a brief trial off lithium may prove diagnostic.

Reports of suspected or confirmed ocular side effects should be sent to both 1) the Lithium Information Center, and 2) National Registry of Drug-Induced

Ocular Side Effects, University of Oregon Health Science Center, 3181 S.W., Sam Jackson Park Road, Portland, Oregon 97701 [(503) 255–8456].

EAR, NOSE, AND THROAT EFFECTS

Other than the possibility of a tablet or capsule lodging in an oral or nasal orifice, the ears and the nose are not adversely affected by lithium.

Lithium has had a variety of effects on taste which range from causing a bad taste (metallic, salty) through either direct contact or salivary lithium secretion, to alterations in flavor perception. Also reported have been a spoiled taste from dairy products containing butterfat, an altered taste of celery, and a single case of complete loss of taste for salt. Patients, in general, prefer lithium capsules or coated tablets because of the unpleasant taste caused by regular tablets.

Dry mouth is a common complaint and has generally been felt to be secondary to lithium induced polyuria. There is some evidence that lithium may also cause xerostomia due to a reduction in salivary flow, although normal salivary flow has also been reported. It has also been suggested, but not confirmed, that dental caries occur more frequently in lithium patients, possibly due to 1) dry mouth from reduced salivary flow and fluid loss secondary to polyuria and 2) attempts to quench thirst with hard candies or sugar-containing beverages.

Case reports have described contact stomatitis from lithium carbonate tablets (a lichenoid stomatitis from lithium carbonate capsules, which resolved on discontinuation and recurred with rechallenge), and a nonspecific stomatitis.

ENDOCRINE EFFECTS

Thyroid

THYROID FUNCTION. Abnormalities in thyroid function are common during the course of lithium therapy but, fortunately, clinically meaningful alterations are not (Wilson and Jefferson, 1985). Through a number of mechanisms (Wolff, 1979), the most important of which is inhibiting the release of thyroid hormones, T3 uptake (T3U), T4 and protein-bound iodine (PBI) are reduced, thyroid-stimulating hormone (TSH) increased, and TSH response to thyrotropin-releasing hormone (TRH) infusion accentuated. Antithyroid antibody titers may also increase in some patients.

Over time, despite continued lithium use, many, if not most, of these laboratory alterations return to normal. For example, in a prospective study of 51 patients, Smigan and colleagues (1984) found a decrease in T4 and T3U and an increase in TSH at four months, with spontaneous improvement by 12 months with T4 and T3U at pretreatment levels, and TSH lower than at four months. Only 3 of 51 patients had significant antithyroid antibody titers and only 1 patient developed clinical hypothyroidism requiring treatment with L-thyroxine.

THYROID MORPHOLOGY. Whether lithium causes consistent and/or persistent abnormalities in thyroid morphology is unclear, but since lithium concentrations in the gland are 2½–5 times those in serum, the possibility must be considered.

HYPOTHYROIDISM. In certain individuals, lithium causes clinical hypothyroidism. While figures vary, it can be estimated that perhaps five percent of patients will experience this condition (versus 0.03–1.3 percent in the general population), with women nine times more likely than men, and those with a pre-lithium history of thyroid abnormalities, at higher risk.

When in the course of lithium therapy hypothyroidism develops is not predictable. Mannisto (1974) noted a wide variation in the interval between the start of lithium and the diagnosis of hypothyroidism (2 weeks to 6 years, with a mean of 18 months).

While clinical symptoms may be classic (cold intolerance, fatigue, dry, thickened edematous skin, hair loss, constipation, and so forth, atypical presentations must be considered. It is our practice to be quite liberal in testing thyroid function any time clinical conditions so dictate. For example, what at first glance may appear to be breakthrough depression might actually be a manifestation of hypothyroidism.

Clinical hypothyroidism should always be treated. Discontinuing lithium usually results in return to the euthyroid state, although there have been a few reports of persistent hypothyroidism (whether this is due to an unrelated cause or a persistent lithium induced change in a susceptible individual is open to question). If lithium must be continued, supplementary treatment with exogenous thyroid hormone will restore euthyroidism. The combined use of lithium and L–thyroxine has proven safe and well tolerated over substantial periods of time.

Whether subclinical (chemical) hypothyroidism should be treated is more controversial. Given Amdisen and Anderson's findings that all 10 patients with a serum TSH > 35 eventually became clinically hypothyroid (Amdisen and Andersen, 1982), it would appear that even asymptomatic patients should receive thyroid supplementation if TSH is substantially elevated.

Whether milder TSH elevations should be treated is less clear. In the same study, TSH levels returned to normal without treatment in 7/8 patients who had elevations between 10–34.9 (one patient became clinically hypothyroid). It has been suggested that only in the presence of latent autoimmune thyroiditis is lithium likely to cause clinical hypothyroidism, and that monitoring antithyroid antibody titers may be of value (Calabrese et al, 1985). We do not feel that patients whose only abnormality is a slight increase in TSH or an inappropriate TSH response to TRH infusion should be treated with thyroid hormone, although this is an area of active research interest.

Patients with rapid cycling bipolar disorder have a higher prevalence of both clinical hypothyroidism and abnormal thyroid function tests than do nonrapid cyclers (Cowdry et al, 1983). In such patients, the use of replacement thyroid hormone should follow the same guidelines as mentioned above, although in those in whom lithium is ineffective, a trial of supplemental thyroid should be considered regardless of laboratory values. Unfortunately, the response of rapid cycling to thyroid hormone supplementation has been inconsistent, even in the presence of overt hypothyroidism.

GOITER. Both euthyroid and hypothyroid goiter may occur in association with lithium therapy. In a literature review, Wolff (1979) found a 6.1 percent incidence of euthyroid goiter (n = 876) and a 3.7 percent incidence of hypothyroid goiter (n = 491). Only rarely will goiter become a cosmetic problem, and after several years of unrewarded effort, we discontinued routine thyroid gland palpation. With discontinuation of lithium or treatment with supplemental exogenous thyroid, goiters tend to regress in size, although there have been reports of persistence. Goiters have been reported in infants exposed to lithium prenatally.

HYPERTHYROIDISM. Hyperthyroidism has been described both during the course of lithium therapy and following dosage reduction or discontinuation. Lithium's antithyroid effect may explain why this phenomenon is quite uncommon and why withdrawal of lithium may allow a hyperthyroid "rebound" to occur in predisposed individuals. Lithium has been used on an experimental basis to treat hyperthyroidism.

EXOPHTHALMUS. Using special measurements, exophthalmus was found in 23 percent of euthyroid lithium patients (Lazarus et al, 1981). There have been case reports of exophthalmus both with and without associated hyperthyroidism. It is possible that lithium masks the development of hyperthyroidism but not the ocular changes. Despite these observations, clinically significant exophthalmus is so uncommon during lithium therapy that routine exophthalmometry is not indicated.

MONITORING. Both baseline and periodic assessment of thyroid function should be an integral part of lithium therapy. There is an unfortunate tendency to neglect clinical evaluation and depend entirely on laboratory testing. We found that patients were rarely so cooperative as to become hypothyroid at the time of their yearly testing and, consequently, we abandoned routine testing in favor of evaluating thyroid function whenever our clinical suspicion is aroused (there are others who prefer testing every 6–12 months on a routine basis). Measurement of serum T4 and T3 uptake is often adequate, although serum TSH is a more sensitive (and expensive) indicator of primary hypothyroidism and many clinicians prefer this latter test.

Parathyroid Hormone and Calcium Metabolism

A mild elevation of serum calcium, magnesium, and parathyroid hormone level is common during the course of lithium therapy. Both decreased and increased bone mineral content have been described. In general, lithium's effects on parathyroid function and calcium metabolism are not of clinical importance, and routine monitoring of serum calcium, magnesium, and parathyroid hormone is not considered necessary. There have been, however, at least nine cases of parathyroid adenoma developing during the course of lithium therapy (Graze, 1981) so that certain clinical situations may demand more extensive investigation.

Diabetes Mellitus, Insulin, Carbohydrate Metabolism

The effect of lithium on blood glucose levels and insulin responsiveness both in nondiabetics and diabetics is not predictable (Russell and Johnson, 1981). The drug can affect carbohydrate metabolism in a number of ways, and these changes have been postulated to be responsible for weight gain in susceptible individuals.

One study of 49 patients on lithium for 1–10 years found a higher incidence of abnormal glucose tolerance tests in patients over 40 years of age than would have been anticipated in the general population (Muller-Oerlinghausen et al, 1979). A number of studies in animals have shown that insulin secretion in response to glucose loading is inhibited by acute administration of lithium (Russell and Johnson, 1981).

While such reports suggest that lithium might regularly induce or aggravate diabetes mellitus, this seems to be the exception rather than the rule. There have been case reports of both first appearance and exacerbation of diabetes mellitus in association with lithium use and, in at least one patient, glucose tolerance returned to normal when lithium was discontinued and became abnormal again when the drug was restarted. On the other hand, this illness has also been reported to improve or be unaffected by lithium therapy.

Lithium use is not contraindicated in the presence of juvenile or adult-onset diabetes mellitus. It would be wise, however, to closely monitor blood glucose when lithium is started, early in the course of therapy, and when dosage is changed. Since glucosuria is a cause of increased urine volume, the coexistence of poorly controlled diabetes mellitus and lithium therapy may complicate the evaluation and treatment of polyuria, which could be due to either or both of these factors. It is also worth remembering that mood state may favorably or unfavorably alter glucose metabolism.

Should diabetes mellitus appear during the course of lithium therapy or should preexisting diabetes mellitus become more difficult to control, a decision to discontinue lithium must be weighed against the severity of the affective illness and the ability to effectively treat the diabetes with diet, exercise, and drugs.

Adrenal

While lithium has been shown experimentally to alter adrenal cortical function in terms of both cortisol and aldosterone secretion, these changes have not been shown to be of practical clinical importance.

Weight Gain

Weight gain while taking lithium is common. For example, Vendsborg and colleagues (1976) found that 64 percent of 70 patients gained an average of 10 kg during 2–6 years on lithium, and Vestergaard and colleagues (1980) noted a similar weight gain in 20 percent of 237 patients on lithium for an average of 5.2 years.

A number of factors may contribute to the weight gain occurring during lithium therapy. Lithium may work indirectly through mood stabilization, allowing weight loss related to mania or depression to be corrected. A positive correlation was noted between beneficial response to lithium and weight gain. Although uncommon and not likely to be persistent, fluid retention secondary to lithium induced edema is another possibility. Increased thirst secondary to nephrogenic polyuria and, perhaps, a central mechanism may lead to increased caloric intake in the form of beverages used for fluid replacement. Hypothyroidism induced by lithium is another possible cause of weight gain. The associated use of neuroleptic and/or antidepressant medication may also play a contributory role. Finally, lithium does have a number of effects on carbohydrate and lipid metabolism, which also might play a role in weight gain. It is conceivable, although not proven, that lithium alters "set-point" in a way that directs calories away from thermogenesis. Given these possibilities it is, perhaps, more surprising that all patients on long-term lithium therapy do not gain weight rather than that a smaller percentage do.

In addition to the health hazards of obesity, weight gain also adversely affects body image and increases the risk of lithium noncompliance. Treatment of this side effect should begin with preventive education, good dietary habits, regular exercise, and monitoring of weight (we weigh our patients each time we see them).

Should undesired weight gain occur, the following should be considered:

1. rule out hypothyroidism
2. instruct patient in the use of low or no calorie beverages to quench thirst
3. treat lithium induced polyuria
4. instruct patient in a sensible weight reduction diet
5. encourage participation in a program such as Weight Watchers
6. encourage regular exercise

Grof (1983) suggests that a lithium holiday of a minimum of four weeks may result in gratifying weight reduction and a greater ease of dietary control of weight once lithium is restarted. How practical such an approach is remains open to question.

Edema

While generally considered uncommon during the course of lithium therapy, Vestergaard and colleagues (1980) found complaints of intermittent edema in 10 percent of 237 patients. Before concluding that edema is lithium induced, other possible causes such as heart failure, liver disease, and thyroid dysfunction must be excluded. Edema associated with lithium tends to occur in the absence of cardiovascular or renal disease or electrolyte imbalance and may be due to altered aldosterone metabolism. It often regresses spontaneously but should treatment be necessary, spironolactone may be beneficial (the possibility of increased serum lithium level must be considered when diuretics are used).

HEMATOLOGIC EFFECTS

White Cells

Lithium often causes a mild, benign leukocytosis that may persist throughout the course of therapy but remit upon discontinuation of the drug. This increase in granulocyte numbers may be relative (not exceeding the upper range of normal) or absolute (total counts are usually less than 15,000). While higher white counts have been reported, extreme values should be suspect and alternative etiologies sought. The cells produced appear to be mature granulocytes with intact phagocytic ability, possibly produced by lithium induced enhancement of colony stimulating factor. While neutrophils are increased, other granulocytes may be increased or unchanged, with an associated decrease in the absolute or relative number of lymphocytes.

Given this ability to stimulate granulocyte production, concern has been expressed that lithium might have carcinogenic potential, perhaps by enhancing proliferation of silent leukemic clones. While there have been case reports of leukemia occurring during the course of lithium therapy, a causal relationship has not been established. Recently Norton and Whalley (1984) found no increase in deaths from cancer or leukemia in 791 patients who had been treated with lithium for 2 months to 10 years. In a controlled study of lithium to treat granulocytopenia associated with chemotherapy of acute myelogenous leukemia, no adverse effect was noted on duration or number of remissions (Stein et al, 1980). In addition, lithium has not been listed as an actual or potential carcinogen or co-carcinogen by the U.S. Environmental Protection Agency (or any other government agency).

Red Blood Cells

Lithium has no clinically important effects on red blood cells. While one case of fatal aplastic anemia was reported, it occurred in the presence of other drugs and a week after lithium had been discontinued. There are actually several case reports of lithium having been used beneficially to treat aplastic anemia.

Platelets and Coagulation

Platelet counts may be slightly increased or remain unchanged in the presence of lithium. The drug has been noted to increase the rate and extent of platelet aggregation, which could conceivably have cardiovascular implications. Overall, lithium does not appear to cause problems with blood coagulation.

Conclusion

Routine monitoring of the hemogram is not an essential aspect of lithium therapy. In the absence of clinical findings to the contrary, a mild leukocytosis is almost certain to be benign and does not require more invasive investigation.

CARDIOVASCULAR EFFECTS

Fetal Malformation

The risk of major cardiovascular malformations (especially Ebstein's malformation of the tricuspid valve) appears to be increased in babies exposed to lithium during the first trimester (see section on teratogenesis for details).

Arrhythmias and the Electrocardiogram

Benign, reversible T-wave lowering, flattening, or inversion occur commonly during the course of lithium therapy. These changes often develop early in the course of treatment and may persist, wax and wane, or disappear spontaneously. Displacement of intracellular potassium by lithium may be an explanation for these changes.

A variety of arrhythmias has been reported in association with lithium therapy. These 1) include abnormalities of sinus node impulse generation, atrioventricular (AV) blocks, and ventricular ectopy; 2) are mostly case reports; and 3) often lack substantiation as to cause and effect (summarized in Jefferson and Greist, 1979; Mitchell and Mackenzie, 1982).

Middelhoff and Paschen (1974) found a high incidence of supraventricular and ventricular extrasystoles (24 percent) and conduction abnormalities (40 percent)—mainly first degree AV block—in a series of 31 patients; and Martin and Piascik (1985) noted first degree AV block in 5 of 18 patients. These findings are unusual and have not been found in other studies. It would seem that arrhythmias induced by therapeutic levels of lithium are uncommon and are more likely to occur in patients with coexisting cardiovascular disease.

Lithium may have some predilection for the sinus node as evidenced by a number of arrhythmias indicative of sinus node dysfunction. These include sinus arrest, sinoatrial block, and brady-tachy arrhythmias such as might be seen in the "sick sinus syndrome." At present, there have been at least 37 case reports occurring at both therapeutic and toxic lithium levels, in both symptomatic and asymptomatic individuals (usually elderly). If such an arrhythmia appears, lithium should be discontinued. Pre-existing sick sinus syndrome is a relative contraindication to lithium therapy and a condition for which a pacemaker might be considered if lithium must be used.

In the presence of lithium intoxication, cardiac rhythm and conduction disturbances are more common and careful monitoring is indicated. Even under overdose conditions, lithium does not appear to have the malignant cardiovascular profile of the tricyclic antidepressants.

Heart Failure and Myocardiopathy

While there have been isolated reports of heart failure and myocardiopathy associated with lithium use, they are quite rare and have usually occurred in the presence of other drugs or conditions which were likely to cause or contribute to the cardiac pathology.

Blood Pressure

Lithium does not affect blood pressure in any way that would be of clinical concern. Even with intoxication, the blood pressure tends to remain stable unless secondary complications occur (an exception being a patient with a serum level of 2.2 mEq/1 whose pressure rose to 230/150 mm Hg).

Sudden Death

In a study of the effect of lithium on chemotherapy induced leukopenia in patients with lung cancer, lithium significantly increased the risk of sudden death in those with pre-existing cardiovascular disease, especially if they were also receiving theophylline derivatives (Lyman et al, 1984).

Shopsin and colleagues (1979) also described a higher than expected rate of sudden cardiac death in their male lithium patients (a similar rate was found in relatives who were not taking lithium), leading them to speculate that "lithium may contribute to and uncover an underlying cardiac defect in highly susceptible individuals. . . ."

Whether generalizations can be made from these two reports is questionable. While lithium has not been shown to increase the risk of sudden death in other populations and clinical experience suggests that lithium patients are not dropping dead at unusually high rates, no study has conclusively resolved the issue.

Conclusion

Overall, lithium is well tolerated by the cardiovascular system. Its use is not absolutely contraindicated in patients with coexisting cardiovascular disease but, if used, appropriate cautions must be taken (Jefferson and Greist, 1979).

GASTROINTESTINAL EFFECTS

Lithium is one of many exogenous substances that can upset the gastrointestinal tract, through local initiation and central mechanisms. Side effects include appetite loss, nausea, vomiting, loose stools, and abdominal pain. Mild symptoms are common early in the course of therapy. In general, such symptoms are mild and transient, may be associated with large doses or rapidly rising serum levels, and generally improve 1) with time, 2) by reducing the number of pills taken in a single dose, 3) by taking doses on a full stomach, or 4) by the use of a different lithium preparation. In a report of three patients with abdominal distress from lithium carbonate, relief was obtained by switching to lithium citrate syrup (Vasile and Shelton, 1982). Improvement may have been due to differences between carbonate and citrate in absorption, gastric pH, or gastrin release.

Since there are many other causes of common gastrointestinal symptoms, it is often difficult to decide whether lithium is causing, aggravating, or merely coexisting as an "innocent bystander." When in doubt, temporarily stopping the drug is a safe, conservative approach. We feel that, more often than not, a bout of vomiting and/or diarrhea during the course of lithium therapy is of viral etiology. Nonetheless, even a viral gastorenteritis may be worsened by lithium, and dehydration associated with such an illness could lead to lithium intoxication.

Gastrointestinal symptoms are not always benign. More severe and persistent symptoms may indicate the prodromal stages of lithium intoxication. In a fashion similar to digitalis, anorexia in a patient on lithium can be a tipoff to impending toxicity. When in doubt, the drug should be discontinued, serum level measured, and appropriate corrective measures taken.

Lithium is not known to be a hepatotoxin. Occasionally hepatitis has occurred in patients taking lithium (unpublished reports to the Lithium Information Center) but the association is more likely casual than causal, and there is no evidence suggesting anything more than a chance association. A single case of ascites developing during the course of lithium therapy in association with normal hepatic and renal function is difficult to interpret.

RENAL EFFECTS

No adverse aspect of lithium therapy has generated as much interest, attention, and concern as has the effects of the drug on the kidney. Is it a potent nephrotoxin or does it merely cause benign, sometimes annoying alterations in renal function? Extensive investigations in recent years have been more supportive of the latter position. While generalizations cannot be made from a single case, it is reassuring to know that after 30 years of treatment, one of Cade's first lithium patients had a normal serum creatinine and more than adequate glomerular function, despite some morphological abnormalities and a marked concentrating defect (Chiu et al, 1983).

Kidney Morphology

There is little question that lithium can cause morphological abnormalities in the kidney. The most common finding is a nonspecific intersitital fibrosis which, in turn, has been associated with impaired renal concentrating ability. An additional lesion, felt to be distinctive to lithium, has been described in the distal tubules and collecting ducts by Walker and colleagues (1983) and awaits confirmation by other investigators.

The extent of the morphological alterations attributable to lithium appears to be less significant than originally thought. Patients with affective disorders who have never been on lithium fall somewhere between lithium patients and healthy controls in terms of renal anatomical abnormalities. In his review, Bendz concluded that "irreversibly reduced tubular function due to a tubulo-interstitial nephropathy is sometimes a consequence of long-term (> 2 years) lithium treatment even in the absence of intoxication" (Bendz, 1983). Two studies found that approximately 15 percent of patients had major histological abnormalities, and approximately 30–35 percent showed more moderate changes.

Glomerular Filtration Rate (GFR)

Glomerular filtration rate does not deteriorate in a relentless and ultimately fatal fashion during the course of long-term lithium therapy. Long-term therapy may, however, cause some decrease in GFR, although changes appear small and of little or no clinical consequence. For example, Amsterdam and colleagues (1985), in a prospective two–three-year study, found a slight but statistically significant increase in serum creatinine (still within the range of normal) and a nonsignificant trend toward a decrease in creatinine clearance. Jensen and Rickers (1984) found no overall decrease in GFR in 13 patients followed prospectively for a mean of 16.5 months, but a significant although not dramatic, fall did occur in two patients. Lokkegaard and colleagues (1985) measured GFR (51 Cr–EDTA clearance) in 153 patients who had been on lithium for a mean of 10 years (range 5–17 years). Results were corrected for age and surface area, and a significant decrease in GFR was found across the 5–17-year treatment. Nonetheless, changes were mild with the regression line intersecting the lower limits of normal after approximately 17 years of treatment. Only a few patients showed more marked changes.

In his review, Bendz (1983) also concluded that lithium has the potential for causing irreversible reduction in glomerular function but that changes develop very slowly. Whether patients on "ultra" long-term lithium therapy (20–50 exposure years) will be at risk for more serious changes cannot be answered. Overall, Bendz concluded that no greater than 10 percent of patients on lithium had a decrease in GFR that could not be explained by factors other than lithium.

In evaluating GFR, a number of points should be made:

1. A distinction must be made between reversible and irreversible reduction in GFR. In the presence of volume contraction due to lithium-induced polyuria, a *reversible*, pre-renal reduction in GFR may occur.
2. When creatinine clearance is used as an index of glomerular filtration, an incomplete 24-hour urine collection will result in an artifactual reduction in clearance.
3. Serum creatinine levels may be increased by exercise and diet, and analytic errors among different measurement techniques can be as great as 10–40 percent. Hence, a pre-exercise, fasting sample processed in the same laboratory by the same technique is most likely to produce useful information.
4. A reduction in GFR cannot be automatically assumed to be caused by lithium. The possibility of unrelated renal disease must always be considered.
5. Age, alone, has adverse effects on renal function, with GFR decreasing by 30 percent between the ages of 30 and 80 years. In addition, due to the

decreased muscle mass associated with aging, less creatinine is produced and a greater reduction in GFR is necessary before it is reflected in a serum creatinine increase above normal.

6. The trend in recent years toward effective maintenance therapy at lower serum lithium levels may further reduce the risk of nephrotoxicity.
7. Despite these confounding factors, most patients on lithium can have adequate monitoring of GFR merely by properly measuring serum creatinine two to three times yearly. We feel (and some may disagree) that *routine* measurement of 24-hour creatinine clearance is not an essential part of routine monitoring.

Renal Concentrating Ability

There is no disagreement about the effect of lithium on the concentrating ability of the kidney. It is impaired in the majority of patients taking lithium in a fashion that appears related to dose and duration of treatment. Bendz (1983), in his review, found a concentrating defect in 30–96 percent of patients. In patients on lithium for a mean duration of six years, Vestergaard and Amdisen (1981) found a progressive decrease in concentrating capacity with duration of treatment. Lokkegaard and colleagues (1985) found a significantly reduced concentrating capacity in their group of patients studied 5–17 years (mean 10 years) after the start of treatment, the severity of which correlated with total lithium dose but not with duration of treatment. The authors concluded that "the change in renal concentrating capacity mainly takes place during the first 5–6 years and thereafter the concentrating capacity remains relatively constant" (p. 353).

These abnormalities in concentrating capacity appear to be lithium induced even when several potentially confounding factors are considered: 1) studies vary greatly in the methods used to measure concentrating capacity; 2) studies are usually not controlled for the gradual, progressive decrease in concentrating capacity that occurs with normal aging; and 3) studies often fail to consider that affectively ill patients who have never been on lithium have lower concentrating capacity than normal controls.

While the irreversibility of these changes has not been firmly established, they may persist in less severe form after discontinuation of lithium. Since *long-term* post-lithium studies have not been done, the full extent of impairment remains to be determined. Since some correlation has been found between the extent of chronic morphological tubular changes and impaired concentrating capacity, it is reasonable to anticipate some irreversibility in some patients.

Polyuria and Diabetes Insipidus

One of the more troublesome lithium side effects is polyuria (arbitrarily defined as a urine volume of greater than 3,000 cc per day), which affects up to 35–40 percent of patients (reviewed in Bendz, 1983). It usually, but not always, occurs in association with a renal concentrating defect, and may be related to cumulative lithium exposure. Symptoms of frequent urination and thirst may appear early or develop after months or years of treatment. While excessive thirst is generally felt to be secondary to lithium's effect on the kidney, in some studies complaints of thirst exceed those of polyuria (Vestergaard et al, 1980). There is evidence that lithium can also have a direct effect on central control of thirst regulation.

While a slight increase in urine output is a well tolerated side effect, large urine volumes can be quite troublesome. Consequences of polyuria include 1) dehydration with the risk of lithium intoxication, especially in patients attempting to control output by reducing intake; 2) social and occupational inconvenience and embarrassment; 3) insomnia secondary to nocturia; 4) weight gain, improper diet, and dental caries secondary to high caloric fluid replacement; and 5) noncompliance with lithium therapy. In the process of evaluating lithium induced polyuria, consideration must be given to other diagnostic possibilities such as 1) psychogenic polydipsia, 2) urinary tract infection, 3) renal medullary disease, 4) osmotic diuresis (such as glucosuria from diabetes mellitus), and 5) other drugs (diuretics, nephrotoxins). Recently described was a syndrome of urinary urgency and incontinence in the absence of large urine volumes.

Treatment of polyuria begins with the preventive measure of using the lowest effective maintenance dose of lithium. The trend in recent years toward keeping serum levels between 0.6–0.8 mEq/1 instead of 0.8–1.0 has resulted in lower urine volumes. The type of lithium preparation used and dosage schedule may also influence urine volume, although the initial promising findings with single daily dose, standard lithium carbonate having lower 24-hour urine volumes than divided dose, slow-release lithium have not been firmly substantiated (Bendz, 1983).

Patients must be cautioned not to attempt to reduce polyuria by reducing fluid intake. This can lead to dehydration and an increased risk of lithium intoxication.

Both thiazide and potassium-sparing diuretics alone and in combination have been useful for treating lithium induced nephrogenic diabetes insipidus. Thiazides decrease urine volume by reducing extracellular volume and cause an associated reduction in lithium clearance and increase in serum lithium level. Thus, when thiazides are started (for example, hydrochlorothiazide 25 mg twice a day), lithium dosage usually must be reduced to maintain a stable serum level. The potassium-sparing diuretic, amiloride, in a dose of 5–10 mg twice a day, may work through a different mechanism by blunting the inhibitory effect of lithium on the collecting ducts, and in some patients, urine volume decreases without an associated increase in serum lithium level (Batlle et al, 1985).

Thiazides alone have the disadvantage of causing hypokalemia which, in turn, can cause medical problems, including aggravation of polyuria. Evidence in rats shows that dietary potassium supplementation has a protective effect against lithium induced polyuria. While supplemental dietary potassium in the absence of hypokalemia is not advised in man, the use of potassium-sparing diuretics such as amiloride, or a combination diuretic such as Dyazide (hydrochlorothiazide and triamterine) or Moduretic (hydrochlorothiazide and amiloride), may be preferable.

Nephrotic Syndrome

There have been at least 10 cases of nephrotic syndrome (proteinuria, hypoalbuminemia, edema, and hyperlipidemia) reported in patients on lithium (Kalina and Burnett, 1984). In three, a possible causal relationship was established when the syndrome improved when lithium was stopped, and worsened when it was restarted. While lithium appears to induce nephrotic syndrome in a few individuals, what determines this idiosyncratic susceptibility is not known.

Renal Tubular Acidosis

Lithium can interfere with distal tubular hydrogen secretion and produce an incomplete distal renal tubular acidosis. This defect does not appear to be of clinical significance, although patients could be more susceptible to metabolic acidosis if their acid excretory systems were stressed by acid loads. The measurement of blood pH, CO_2, and bicarbonate levels is not a necessary part of routine lithium monitoring.

Monitoring Renal Function

Distinction must be made between patient care (safety) and research with regard to the extent of renal function monitoring during the course of lithium therapy. Experts differ in their recommendations, with some suggesting baseline and periodic testing of 24-hour creatinine clearance, urinalysis, and renal concentrating capacity, while others feel that for routine purposes baseline and periodic (2–4 per year) serum creatinine levels are adequate with urine volume estimated by questioning about nocturia and daytime frequency. While our basic laboratory evaluation is restricted to serum creatinine, we are not reluctant to expand testing as dictated by the clinical state of our patients.

REPRODUCTIVE EFFECTS

Teratogenesis

Although results have been somewhat conflicting, it is generally accepted that lithium, in sufficient amounts, is a teratogen in premammalian species. While less firm, evidence in humans suggests that maternal exposure to therapeutic amounts of lithium during the first trimester increases the risk of fetal malformation. As of 1980, the Register of Lithium Babies found an 11 percent incidence of malformation in 225 births versus a rate of about 3 percent in the general population (Weinstein, 1980). This figure may be artifactually high since normal births are less likely to be reported. The proportion of major cardiovascular abnormalities to total malformations is considerably higher in lithium babies than in the general population, suggesting that lithium may be a cardiovascular teratogen. Ebstein's malformation of the tricuspid valve is especially overrepresented. For example, information from the Swedish Medical Birth Registry showed a seven times greater incidence of cardiovascular malformations in lithium babies compared to babies of manic-depressive women who had not taken lithium during pregnancy (Kallen and Tandberg, 1983).

In view of these findings, if at all possible, lithium should be avoided at conception and during at least the first trimester. It should be noted, however, that the vast majority of "lithium" babies are normal and first trimester exposure to lithium is usually not considered grounds for therapeutic abortion. Since fetal echocardiography can detect major abnormalities at a time when abortion is still possible, this procedure may be a useful screening technique.

Concern has been expressed that fetal exposure to lithium may cause less obvious changes in the developing nervous system (behavioral teratology). In the only study to date, lithium babies who were normal at birth grew and developed normally (Schou, 1976). It is possible that more sophisticated evaluation methods could detect subtle abnormalities, but this remains conjecture.

Pregnancy and Delivery

The physiologic changes occurring during pregnancy are complex. For example, GFR and effective renal plasma flow increase by 30–50 percent, plasma volume by 50 percent, and filtered sodium load by 5,000–10,000 mEq/day. Additional factors that might complicate lithium therapy include edema and hypertension, sodium restriction, and the use of diuretics. In view of these changes, and because little work has been done with lithium under these circumstances, monitoring must be especially thorough. While it has been suggested that serum lithium level may decrease during pregnancy (due to increased lithium clearance) and abruptly return to pre-pregnancy levels following delivery (Weinstein, 1980), the opposite has also been reported.

The fetus is exposed to lithium concentrations at least as high as those found in maternal blood. To minimize risk to the newborn, maternal lithium should be temporarily discontinued just prior to delivery. There have been reports of neonatal lithium toxicity and thyroid abnormalities.

Postpartum and Breast Feeding

The risk of affective relapses increases in the postpartum period, which may necessitate the reinstitution of lithium maintenance. It has been estimated that 40 percent of bipolar women will experience a postpartum affective episode.

Whether breast-feeding poses a substantial risk to the infant has not been determined. Lithium is present in breast milk and the serum lithium concentration in breast-fed babies ranges from 10–50 percent of that of the mother (Weinstein, 1980). There have been two reports of lithium toxicity in breast-fed infants. Because the effects of lithium in young children are unknown and because infants may be at higher risk for lithium intoxication during episodes of dehydration and febrile illness, breast-feeding is generally discouraged. There may be times, however, when the psychological and immunological advantages of breast-feeding outweigh the potential risks.

Sexual Dysfunction

While quite rare, there have been reports of both reduced libido and erectile dysfunction in men on lithium that have been confirmed under single and double blind conditions. There have also been reports of lithium altering sperm viability and motility, but it is not known if fertility is affected.

Mutagenesis

Few studies have examined the effect of lithium on chromosomes, and most of these found no mutagenic effect. Those that did have been faulted for failure to control for factors such as affective illness and other drugs.

DERMATOLOGIC EFFECTS

Hair

Hair loss is an uncommon but reasonably well documented side effect of lithium. In a review of 24 published cases, Mortimer and Dawber (1984) noted that all but two were women, three were hypothyroid, seven had diffuse loss, three had increased shedding rates, and one had alopecia areata. In some, regrowth occurred despite continued use of lithium, while in others discontinuation of the drug was necessary and rechallenge led to recurrence of the problem. A more recent survey found that 42 percent of patients noted hair changes while on lithium (thinning in 19 percent and loss of curl or wave in 23 percent) (McCreadie and Morrison, 1985). The Lithium Information Center has had reports of increased curliness associated with lithium use.

Should hair loss occur during the course of lithium therapy, we suggest: 1) evaluation for nonlithium related causes; 2) rule out lithium induced hypothyroidism; 3) if mild, follow for spontaneous regrowth; and 4) if necessary, reduce or discontinue lithium. Hair samples (at least two teaspoons from the nape of the neck) are being sought by the Lithium Information Center for future research considerations.

Skin

The most common dermatologic problems associated with lithium have been acne and psoriasis, which may appear for the first time or be exacerbated during treatment. Acneiform eruptions may spontaneously clear or improve during the course of lithium therapy but, should treatment be necessary, standard dermatological approaches are usually effective. Since body image is often quite important, especially to younger patients, acne as a cause of lithium noncompliance should not be underestimated. Since acne is a common condition, its appearance in some lithium patients may be nothing more than coincidence.

Lithium appears especially troublesome with regard to psoriasis in that it may exacerbate the condition, and prevent otherwise effective treatment from working (Skott et al, 1977).

Other skin changes reported with lithium use include folliculitis, maculopapular rash, and other less well specified eruptions. A lupus-like syndrome with butterfly rash and positive antinuclear antibodies was described in one patient shortly after starting lithium. The issue of lithium "allergy" is periodically raised, and while it is unlikely that an element (atomic number 3) would be an allergen, the same cannot be said for some of the fillers and dyes that go into the makeup of capsules and tablets.

Nails

A single report of lithium-associated golden discoloration of the toenails has not yet been confirmed.

MUSCULOSKELETAL EFFECTS

While myalgia and arthritis have been attributed to lithium by a number of patients, a causal relationship has not been established. Studies of the effect of lithium on bone have produced conflicting results. Some found evidence of bone mineral loss during the course of lithium therapy, while another found an increase in bone mineral content. While there is no evidence that lithium poses a clinical risk in this area, there is insufficient evidence to know if there would be subtle long-term osteopathic effects. Further studies are indicated, especially in groups which might be at high risk such as children and post-menopausal women.

CARBAMAZEPINE SIDE EFFECTS: OVERVIEW

Immediately after the words "Tegretol" and "carbamazepine," the Physicians' Desk Reference (1986) contains the following warning:

> Warning: Serious and sometimes fatal abnormalities of blood cells (aplastic anemia, agranulocytosis, thrombocytopenia, and leukopenia) have been reported following treatment with Tegretol, carbamazepine. Early detection of hematologic change is important, since, in some patients, aplastic anemia is reversible.
>
> Complete pretreatment blood counts, including platelet and possibly reticulocyte and serum iron, should be obtained. Any significant abnormality should rule out use of the drug. These same tests should be repeated at frequent intervals, possibly weekly during the first three months of therapy and monthly thereafter for at least two to three years. The drug should be stopped if any evidence of bone marrow depression develops.
>
> Patients should be made aware of the early toxic signs and symptoms of a potential hematologic problem, such as fever, sore throat, ulcers in the mouth, easy bruising, petechial or purpuric hemorrhage, and should be advised to discontinue the drug and to report to the physician immediately if any such signs or symptoms appear.

Carbamazepine (CBZ), chemically similar to imipramine, was introduced into neurologic practice in 1959 and has come to play an important role in the treatment of partial, tonic, clonic, and tonic-clonic seizure disorders, as well as trigeminal and glossopharyngeal neuralgias. Carbamazepine is generally well tolerated and less than five percent of patients have such severe side effects that treatment must be discontinued. Nevertheless, CBZ has caused deaths because of hematologic and hepatic side effects, and also can adversely affect the skin, electrolytes, and neurologic, endocrinologic, reproductive, cardiovascular, and renal systems. Some adverse effects are dose related while others appear to be idiosyncratic.

Neurologists soon observed that CBZ had generally beneficial effects on the behavioral and psychological functioning of adult epileptic patients. Characteristic slowness, perseverations and apathy found in many patients with severe and long-lasting epilepsy diminished, in contrast to little if any improvement with phenobarbital and phenytoin. Reduction or abolition of irritability, impulsivity, aggressivity, dysphoria, depression, and other adverse affective states often occurred. It was perhaps inevitable that CBZ would be tried in patients with primary affective disorders, and there is growing evidence that CBZ has a role to play in the treatment of bipolar patients unresponsive to lithium, and may be especially helpful in patients with rapid cycling (more than four episodes per year). There is also preliminary evidence that CBZ may have antidepressant effects in patients with primary unipolar depressive disorders. There have also been case reports of benefit in schizophrenia and episodic dyscontrol. As psychiatrists increase their use of CBZ, awareness of CBZ side effects becomes more important. The following review is based primarily on the larger literature regarding the use of CBZ in patients with epilepsy. There is no indication, at present, that patients with affective disorders differ significantly in their reactions to CBZ from patients with epilepsy.

As with lithium, plasma CBZ levels are helpful in determining a minimum dose likely to be therapeutic and avoiding doses with a high potential for adverse effects. The usual therapeutic range of plasma CBZ levels for epilepsy is 4–12 micrograms per milliliter and the same range is being used for psychiatric disorders, although clear dose/response relations have not been established. Rate of rise of plasma level also affects the frequency and severity of side effects so that gradual increases in dose are preferable when the patient's clinical condition permits such an approach.

NEUROLOGICAL EFFECTS

Although less life-threatening than some hematologic and hepatic side effects, adverse neurological effects are more common and more likely to lead to modification or discontinuation of carbamazepine treatment. Table 2 lists common side effects reported in a study of 255 epileptic patients (Livingston et al, 1974) and from a separate report of neurotoxic reactions in 510 patients with trigeminal neuralgia (Gayford and Redpath, 1969). Other side effects mentioned in several studies were: asterixis, dystonia, memory impairment, nystamus, tremor, neuritis, and psychosis.

Neurological side effects account for about 50 percent of all reported CBZ side effects and are positively correlated with plasma level, rate of dosage increase and, possibly, age. Most neurotoxic effects occur in the first few weeks of treatment and frequently disappear without dosage reduction. While a few cases of

Table 2. Neurotoxicity of Carbamazepine

	Livingston et al (1974) N = 255 %	Gayford and Redpath (1969) N = 510 %
Central nervous system effects		
Drowsiness	11	12
Vertigo		11
Ataxia		9
Dizziness	3	
Paresthesias	3	0.2
Headache		0.8
Depression		0.2
Tinnitis		0.2
Confusion		0.6
Peripheral nervous system effects		
Diplopia	16	0.2
Blurred vision	6	

psychosis have been reported, this outcome is uncommon and the mood normalizing effects of CBZ far outweigh the occasional reports of patients becoming depressed or manic.

Cognitive and memory function appear little affected and sometimes improve in individuals receiving CBZ at therapeutic plasma levels. Normal volunteers exhibited some decrease in motor but not in mental speed, as well as reductions in memory for new information. New epileptics well controlled on CBZ alone performed better on memory tasks and a tracking task than patients controlled on phenytoin alone.

While neurotoxic effects are as common as all other side effects combined, they substantially affect less than five percent of patients receiving CBZ and may be minimized by increasing dose gradually and keeping plasma levels as low as consistent with therapeutic effect. Most neurotoxic symptoms abate within a few weeks even if dose is not reduced. Neither long-term nor irreversible neurotoxic effects have been identified, but recent awareness of insidious late effects of hydantoins and barbiturates indicate the need for continued monitoring for neurotoxic effects in patients receiving CBZ.

HEMATOLOGIC EFFECTS

Physicians must be aware of carbamazepine's several hematologic effects to avoid either an over-cautious or cavalier approach to its use. By 1985, aplastic anemia had been reported in 22 patients receiving CBZ, all but 3 of whom were also receiving other medications. Fifteen died. This reported lethality often raises concerns in physicians, especially those who are prescribing CBZ for the first time. Aplastic anemia appears idiosyncratic and unrelated to dose, and may appear between three weeks and two years after initiation of CBZ treatment. The incidence and prevalence of aplastic anemia in patients treated with CBZ is estimated to be quite low (see Table 3). Nevertheless, new cases continue to appear and at least one was a psychiatric patient receiving CBZ for treatment of an atypical psychotic illness.

Transient leukopenia (primarily reduction of granulocytes) occurs in about 10 percent of CBZ treated patients and persistent leukopenia in approximately 2 percent, with average white blood cell decreases from 0 to 1000 per mm3 in different studies. Transient leukopenia is associated with greater age but not with dose of CBZ. Leukopenia usually abates despite continued CBZ treatment and does not appear to progress to aplastic anemia, suggesting that these hematologic disorders are unrelated. Persistent leukopenia of significant proportions usually appears in the first few weeks of treatment and remits with discontinuation of CBZ. Interestingly, CBZ induced leukocytosis has also been reported in one patient.

A series of 43 psychiatric patients treated with CBZ exhibited a statistically significant, but clinically insignificant, decrease in white blood cell and erythrocyte counts, which tended to return toward normal over a four-week period (Joffe et al, 1985). Agranulocytosis is rare but a fatal case was reported in a psychiatric patient treated with CBZ and antipsychotics. Transient eosinophilia is not uncommon in the first weeks of treatment.

Thrombocytopenia has also been reported in patients with epilepsy as well

Table 3. Hematological Toxicity of Carbamazepine

Aplastic anemia
  Estimated prevalence: < 1/50,000
  Estimated incidence: 0.5/100,000/yr

Leukopenia (neutropenia)
  Prevalence
    Transient: 10% (range, 2–60%)
    Persistent: 2% (range, 0–8%)
  Average change: 0 to 1,000 mm^3

Thrombocytopenia
  Prevalence: 2%
  Average change: 0 to 20,000 per mm^3

Anemia
  Prevalence: < 5% (range, 0–10%)
  Average change: 0 to 0.5 gm Hb/dl

Adapted from Hart and Easton, 1982

as in psychiatric patients. Most reported falls in platelet counts have been small and occur in the first month of CBZ therapy.

Mild anemia (decreases of 0 to 0.5 grams of hemoglobin) occurs in less than five percent of patients receiving CBZ for extended periods. Anemia disappears with discontinuation of CBZ, but this is seldom necessary. A single case of CBZ induced hemolytic anemia has been reported. A single case of CBZ induced reticulocytosis in a woman with bipolar disorder was reported in the absence of usual explanations for reticulocytosis.

The incidence of aplastic anemia in chloramphenicol treated patients has been calculated to be between 1 in 20,000 and 1 in 40,000, leading to the conclusion that "the extreme rarity of aplastic anemia precludes its identification by routine blood counts" (Pisciotta, 1975). Estimates of the incidence of aplastic anemia with CBZ are even lower, leading to questions about the necessity of following the PDR hematologic monitoring guidelines (Hart and Easton, 1982). Five years ago, the yearly cost of administering 1,000 mg of CBZ per day was estimated at $978 of which $730 was for laboratory tests and only $248 for the medication itself (Goldberg, 1981).

If the manufacturer's full recommendations were followed, the first year cost would be over $2,000 and, projected across the approximately 200,000 patients receiving CBZ in the United States, laboratory costs would exceed $300,000,000 each year! Hart and Easton offer the following modified recommendations for laboratory monitoring:

1. Reports of serious hematological complications of CBZ must be submitted to the manufacturer to establish the incidence and benefit of laboratory monitoring as well as other characteristics of these complications.
2. Blood and platelet counts should be performed before the initiation of CBZ therapy. Patients with abnormalities on these tests and those taking other

myelotoxic drugs should be considered at special risk. CBZ therapy in these groups should be monitored closely or avoided.

3. Complete blood counts should be made every two weeks for the first two months. If no abnormalities appear, counts should be obtained quarterly or with the appearance of symptoms or signs of bone marrow suppression. Patients should be instructed to contact their physicians immediately if petechiae, pallor, undue weakness, fever, or infection occurs.

4. If leukopenia develops, it should be monitored at two-week intervals seeking the expected return to baseline. The drug dose should be reduced if possible, and the presence of infection or severe leukopenia ($<3,000$ WBC/mm^3 or $<1,500$ neutrophils/mm^3) calls for immediate cessation of CBZ use (p. 311).

While it is not uncommon for patients to experience a small and transient leukopenia, persistent leukopenia of clinical significance is uncommon. Leukopenia often abates spontaneously without discontinuation of CBZ and does so consistently when CBZ is discontinued (as do the less common thrombocytopenia and anemia). Aplastic anemia is rare, idiosyncratic, and unlikely to be detected by regular laboratory monitoring. On the other hand, patients with low pretreatment white blood cell, erythrocyte, or platelet counts and patients receiving other myelotoxic agents are at special risk, and should be monitored more closely or not treated at all with CBZ.

The manufacturer's recommendations on hematologic monitoring are observed infrequently by neurologists, and those offered above probably reflect current thinking and practice.

GASTROINTESTINAL EFFECTS

The most common gastrointestinal side effects are nausea and occasional vomiting, which appear to be dose related and may be minimized by gradual increase in dose. Also common are elevations in liver function tests. Alkaline phosphatase was elevated in 22 percent of one adult patient population without concomitant elevations in transaminase levels (Livingston et al, 1974). These patients had no other evidence of liver disease or progression of abnormal laboratory values despite continued CBZ treatment. Four percent of adult patients in another series experienced elevation in SGOT levels (Ramsay, 1967), while a group of 61 children followed for at least one year showed neither clinical nor laboratory evidence of hepatic dysfunction (Marotta, 1967).

Most alarming are very rare (20 reported cases as of 1985), idiosyncratic, nondose related hypersensitivity reactions usually occurring in the first month of CBZ treatment. Patients present with fever, rash, hepatic tenderness, and, sometimes, eosinophilia. Biopsies revealed variable amounts of hepatocellular degeneration and necrosis, canalicular cholestasis, bile duct proliferation, and granulomas (some containing eosinophiles). Fatality rates approaching 25 percent have been reported. A few patients have been rechallenged with CBZ and promptly developed symptoms of recurrence of this cholestatic hepatitis.

At least one case of more direct hepatocellular injury in the absence of cholestasis has been reported. Symptoms, signs, and laboratory evidence of hepatitis appeared four months after CBZ therapy was initiated, and may have been related to an accumulation of a metabolite of CBZ (CBZ-epoxide), perhaps appearing in greater concentration because of the concomitant administration of phenytoin, which is known to induce enzymes involved in CBZ metabolism.

While nausea and vomiting may appear as early and transient dose related gastrointestinal side effects, and about 20 percent and 5 percent of adult patients may exhibit small and nonprogressive increases in alkaline phosphatase and transaminase levels, respectively, the only dangerous gastrointestinal side effects recognized are a rare idiosyncratic cholestatic granulomatous hepatitis, and an even more rare heptocellular hepatitis probably occurring as a result of accumulation of CBZ metabolites. The relatively great frequency of inconsequential elevations of liver function tests and the exceedingly small frequency of dangerous hepatitis suggests that slight elevations of routine liver function tests may alert clinicians to the possibility of mild hepatic dysfunction, but should not raise undue alarm about drug induced hepatitis. Careful evaluation of any symptoms suggestive of hepatitis (fever, rash, and right upper quadrant tenderness), including liver function studies, is essential.

CARDIOVASCULAR EFFECTS

While "congestive heart failure, edema, aggravation of hypertension, hypotension, syncopy and collapse, aggravation of coronary artery disease, arrhythmias and A-V block, primary thrombophlebitis, recurrence of thrombophlebitis and adenopathy or lymphadenopathy" (Physicians Desk Reference, 1986) have been associated with CBZ treatment and "some of these cardiovascular complications have resulted in fatalities," most reported cardiovascular problems are described in elderly patients with probable underlying arteriosclerotic cardiovascular disease, which apparently predisposes them to cardiotoxicity. This suggests that these patients are either predisposed to CBZ cardiotoxicity or that the association may be casual rather than causal.

Both sinus bradycadia and varying degrees of A-V block have been reported, as well as a probable decrease in ventricular automaticity. The average age of eight patients experiencing sinus node dysfunction or A-V block was 77, and several of these patients experienced remission with a 200 mg reduction in CBZ dose and return of blockade with re-elevation of dose (after implacement of a cardiac pacemaker). Heart block can produce syncope and myocardial ischemia, particularly in patients with already compromised coronary arteries. Patients with, or at risk for, significant arteriosclerotic disease should have careful cardiovascular evaluation including an electrocardiogram before treatment with CBZ, and ongoing monitoring of pulse for rhythm disturbances and electrocardiographic evaluation, as indicated. The dose related nature of the rhythm disturbances argues strongly for use of the minimum effective dose.

DERMATOLOGIC EFFECTS

The 1986 Physicians Desk Reference lists dermatologic side effects of "pruritic and erythematous rashes, urticaria, Stevens-Johnson syndrome, photosensitivity reactions, alteration of skin pigmentation, exfoliative dermatitis, erythema multiforme and nodosum, purpura, aggravation of disseminated lupus erythematosus, alopecia and diaphoresis." Approximately three percent of patients taking CBZ develop rashes, and some dermatologic reactions are severe enough that treatment must be discontinued. Rarely, as with patients who develop Stevens-Johnson syndrome (erythema multiforme skin lesions and bulbous or vesicular lesions of two or more mucous membranes), exfoliative dermatitis, toxic epidermal necrolysis, and a systemic lupus erythematosus (LE-like reaction), skin disorders may be life-threatening. Common in vitro tests for CBZ hypersensitivity have produced unpredictable results, which lead to the unfortunate necessity of rechallenging patients if one is to confirm or refute the diagnosis of drug hypersensitivity. In the case of severe reactions, rechallenge is a last resort, to be tried only when other effective treatments are not available.

ELECTROLYTES

Mild hyponatremia (serum sodium <135 mEq/1) is a well recognized side effect of CBZ treatment in epileptic patients, occurring in 15 and 23 percent of single serum sodium determinations in two separate studies (Henry et al, 1977; Perucca et al, 1978). Serum sodium seldom declines below 130 mEq/1 but, even at levels slightly above 130 mEq/1, symptoms of dysphoria may occur. Rarely, patients develop severe hyponatremia, even on doses as low as 300 mg CBZ per day. Increasing dose and serum level (CBZ levels >6 micrograms/mL increased risk 3.5 times) and greater age (four times greater risk for those over age 30) were associated with increased risk of hyponatremia (Lahr, 1985). Further emphasizing the effect of increased age was a failure to find any cases of hyponatremia in 28 CBZ treated epileptic children (Helin et al, 1977). In one study, vasopressin (ADH) was decreased in 7 of 12 hyponatremic subjects while cyclic AMP was normal, suggesting that CBZ may have direct vasopressin-like properties.

A group of 12 patients receiving CBZ treatment for affective disorders exhibited statistically significant decreases in serum sodium from 141.3 mEq/1 to 139.0 mEq/1 ($p < 0.01$) (Uhde and Post, 1983). One-third of these patients had values below 135 mEq/1. These small decreases in serum sodium were dose related, and patients with lowest initial serum sodium values had the greatest fall in sodium levels. There was a nonsignificant trend for CBZ responsive patients to exhibit greater sodium decreases than nonresponders. Statistically but not clinically significant reductions in calcium and chloride levels were also observed and attributed to hemodilution. No changes were found in potassium or magnesium levels.

Interestingly, the antidiuretic effect of CBZ was found to be of no benefit in reducing urine production in lithium treated patients experiencing polyuria.

Carbamazepine commonly produces small and clinically insignificant decreases in serum sodium but may infrequently cause clinically significant hyponatremia. Increasing age, low initial serum sodium levels, and higher CBZ doses are associated with greatest decreases in sodium levels. Routine monitoring of serum electrolytes does not appear necessary. Electrolytes may help explain dysphoria and are essential in evaluating possible signs of severe hyponatremia such as edema, clouding of consciousness, coma, or seizures.

ENDOCRINE EFFECTS

Epileptics treated with CBZ have been shown to have reductions of total serum T4 and T3, which usually remain in the normal range. This effect correlates positively with dose and a few patients have hormone levels that fall below the normal range. Thyroid-stimulating hormone and TRH stimulation tests were normal and none of these patients became clinically hypothyroid.

Fifty affectively ill patients (40 bipolar and 10 unipolar) treated with CBZ exhibited statistically significant decreases in peripheral thyroid hormone levels (30 percent decrease in free T4 ($p < 0.001$); 17 percent decrease in T3 ($p < 0.001$) and a smaller but still significant decrease in TSH (10 percent) ($p < 0.01$) (Roy-Byrne et al, 1984). Somewhat greater decreases were observed in responders than in nonresponders, and levels returned to normal two weeks after CBZ treatment was discontinued. A thyrotropin stimulation test employing TRH in six depressed patients demonstrated a reduction in TSH response to TRH, suggesting that CBZ's effect on thyroid function in depressed patients may occur primarily at the level of the pituitary (Joffe et al, 1984).

Carbamazepine is far less likely than lithium to produce clinically significant hypothyroidism. Thyroid function tests are not necessary routinely but should be obtained if there are concerns about hypothyroidism.

REPRODUCTIVE EFFECTS

Carbamazepine rapidly crosses the placenta, and fetal blood concentrations are approximately 60 percent of those found in the mother. The same relative concentration is found in breast milk.

It is estimated that most of the 11,550 infants born to epileptic mothers each year will have been exposed to anticonvulsant medications and some of them to CBZ. However, a review of the literature did not specifically mention teratogenicity of CBZ in humans and reported that, among teratogenic studies of anticonvulsants in animals, "the highest teratogenicity is due to diphenylhydantoin, *least with CBZ*, minimal with clonazepam and ethosuximide, and modest with phenobarbital and primidone" (Kelly, 1984, p. 428). A prospective study conducted by the same author's group followed 468 women enrolled in their epilepsy clinic who gave birth to 171 children during a five-year period. Only two children were exposed to CBZ alone, and neither exhibited congenital defects. One major conclusion of the study was that multicenter collaborative protocols would be necessary to collect enough subjects so that meaningful results could be obtained.

Based on animal data and the absence of congenital abnormalities in humans, CBZ appears to be comparatively safe if it must be taken during pregnancy. As with all medications where insufficient information is available, avoidance during pregnancy is prudent, and when avoidance is not possible, minimum doses that are effective should be used.

RESPIRATORY EFFECTS

Except for uncommon pulmonary eosinophilia and pneumonitis associated with uncommon hypersensitivity to CBZ, pulmonary effects appear to be clinically insignificant.

GENITOURINARY EFFECTS

The Physicians Desk Reference (1986) lists "urinary frequency, acute urinary retention, oliguria with elevated blood pressure, azotemia, renal failure and impotence" as well as "albuminuria, glycosuria, elevated BUN and microscopic deposits in the urine." The literature describing renal side effects is remarkably limited. An apparent CBZ induced acute tubulo-interstitial hypersensitivity nephritis was reported in one patient, as well as a single case of overflow urinary incontinence.

FEVER

Fever in patients taking CBZ may be a sign of hypersensitivity reaction or infection secondary to neutropenia. Twice daily fever has also been attributed to CBZ in a single patient. Fever in patients taking CBZ requires consideration of hypersensitivity and neutropenic complications.

OVERDOSE

Carbamazepine has a similar overdose profile to imipramine. Major problems arise from cardiovascular toxicity primarily in the form of prolonged conduction times and A-V nodal blocks, and associated hypotension and hypoxia. Neurologic complications range from mild ataxia to stage IV coma with respiratory failure. Neurologic changes are dose related, with stupor or coma, as well as myoclonic or convulsive activity commonly being found at plasma levels greater than 30 to 40 micrograms/mL. Depression or absence of doll's head phenomenon (conjugate deviation away from the side to which the head is turned), gag reflex, and response to caloric stimulation may occur, as well as acute respiratory failure, suggesting both central and peripheral nervous system dysfunction (May, 1984). As plasma levels fall to between 15 and 30 micrograms/mL, combative and stereotypic behaviors may appear. At drug levels of 10 to 20 micrograms/mL, responsiveness to verbal stimuli and deep tendon reflexes commonly return in the presence of residual cerebellar dysfunction. Three deaths associated with CBZ overdose have been reported, two of which involved aspiration pneumonitis. Nausea and vomiting may be associated with gastrointestinal irritation, hypotension on a cardiovascular basis or seizures. The lethality of CBZ seems lower than from tricyclic antidepressants.

Overdose management initially involves emptying the stomach with syrup of ipecac in alert patients, or by gastric lavage after endotracheal intubation for patients who have a depressed gag reflex. Repeated administration (every four hours) of activated charcoal has been found to increase CBZ clearance by 50 percent. Rebound rises in serum levels suggest the development of a gastric coagulum or concretion of CBZ which is gradually released and absorbed. Whether large doses can overload the enzymatic pathways for metabolism is an issue of debate, although a patient who had a serum CBZ level of 65.9 micrograms/mL (the highest reported level found in our review) exhibited no metabolic pathway saturation.

Since most CBZ is protein-bound (65 to 92 percent, average 73 percent), hemodialysis has not been found to substantially accelerate the removal of toxic levels of drug. Charcoal hemoperfusion, which passes blood over an absorbing surface, has been advocated to increase the removal of protein- and lipid-bound drugs but requires heparinization to prevent the absorption of platelets. In one patient treated this way, slightly less than 200 micrograms of CBZ per hour could be removed. The importance of this increased rate of removal is uncertain.

Most CBZ overdoses respond well to conservative measures aimed at gastrointestinal elimination of unabsorbed drug, accompanied by monitoring and general supportive measures until metabolism and excretion of CBZ have occurred. There appears to be little role for hemodialysis, and experience with hemoperfusion is limited.

SUMMARY

Based on more than 25 years of use of CBZ in neurology and early experience in psychiatry, it seems clear that most side effects are dose related, relatively benign, well tolerated, and likely to decrease as patients adjust to the medication or with dose reduction. Rare, idiosyncratic hypersensitivity reactions involving hematological or hepatic systems may be fatal, but are so infrequent that routine repetitive monitoring with laboratory tests is unlikely to detect these serious reactions before clear clinical clues to their presence emerge. Pretreatment hematologic screening for all patients, and EKGs of patients likely to have cardiac disease are appropriate, as are repeat hematologic indices over the first few months of treatment.

Most patients can be treated with minimal side effects. In the end, considerations of risk–benefit ratio and informed patient consent, as well as prudent monitoring of clinical and laboratory indices, are cornerstones of good treatment. The proper role of CBZ in the treatment of affective and other psychiatric disorders remains to be defined, but adverse effects are unlikely to be a major factor limiting its use.

CONCLUSION

While most patients taking lithium or carbamazepine experience some side effects, only 5–10 percent find them intolerable. The most common side effects are usually benign, and if they do not decrease with time they can be modified by reducing dose or alternating dosage schedule. Both drugs can be fatal if consumed in toxic amounts, and even at therapeutic levels certain adverse reactions are potentially dangerous (for example, nephrogenic diabetes insipidus from lithium and aplastic anemia from carbamazepine). Careful clinical and laboratory monitoring coupled with patient education will do much to minimize the risks from these drugs and allow them to maximize their therapeutic potential.

Due to space limitations, comprehensive referencing has not been possible. Additional references are available on request.

REFERENCES

Abou-Saleh MT, Coppen A: Subjective side-effects of amitriptyline and lithium in affective disorders. Br J Psychiatry 142:391-397, 1983

Amdisen A, Andersen CJ: Lithium treatment and thyroid function: A survey of 237 patients in long term lithium treatment. Pharmacopsychiatria 15:149-155, 1982

Amsterdam JD, Jorkasky D, Potter L, et al: A prospective study of lithium-induced nephropathy: preliminary results. Psychopharmacol Bull 21:81-84, 1985

Batlle DC, Von Riotte AB, Gaviria M, et al: Amelioration of polyuria by amiloride in patients receiving long-term lithium therapy. N Engl J Med 312:408-414, 1985

Bendz H: Kidney function in lithium-treated patients: A literature survey. Acta Psychiatr Scand 68:303-324, 1983

Bohn J, Jefferson JW: Lithium and Manic Depression: A Guide. First edition, 1982; revised editions, 1982, 1983, 1984. Board of Regents of the University of Wisconsin System (Lithium Information Center): Madison, Wisconsin, 1982

Bone S, Roose SP, Dunner DL, et al: Incidence of side effects in patients on long-term lithium therapy. Am J Psychiatry 137:103-104, 1980

Calabrese JR, Gulledge AD, Hahn K, et al: Autoimmune thyroiditis in manic-depressive patients treated with lithium. Am J Psychiatry 142:1318-1321, 1985

Chiu E, Davies B, Walker R, et al: Renal findings after 30 years on lithium. Br J Psychiatry 143:424-425, 1983

Cowdry RW, Wehr TA, Zis AP, et al: Thyroid abnormalities associated with rapid-cycling bipolar illness. Arch Gen Psychiatry 40:414-420, 1983

Duncavage MB, Nasr SJ, Altman EG: Subjective side effects of lithium carbonate: A longitudinal study. J Clin Psychopharmacol 3:100-102, 1983

Gayford JJ, Redpath TH: The side-effects of carbamazepine. Proceedings of the Royal Society of Medicine, 62:615-616, 1969

Goldberg MA: Costs of anticonvulsant therapy. Ann Neurol 9:95, 1981

Graze KK: Hyperparathyroidism in association with lithium therapy. J Clin Psychiatry 42:38-39, 1981

Grof P: Lithium update: selected issues, in Affective Disorders Reassessed: 1983. Edited by Ayd FJ, Taylor IJ, Taylor BT. Baltimore, Ayd Medical Communications, 1983

Hansen HE, Amdisen A: Lithium intoxication (report of 23 cases and review of 100 cases from the literature). Q J Med 47:123-144, 1978

Hart RG, Easton JD: Carbamazepine and hematological monitoring. Ann Neurol 11:309-312, 1982

Helin I, Nilsson KO, Bjerre I, et al: Serum sodium and osmolality during carbamazepine treatment in children. Br Med J 2:558, 1977

Henry DA, Lawson DH, Reavey P, et al: Hyponatraemia during carbamazepine treatment. Br Med J 1:83-84, 1977

Hiroz CA, Assimacopoulos T, Cuendet JF, et al: Ophthalmological side effects of lithium (in French, English abstract). Encephale 7:123-128, 1981

Jefferson JW, Greist JH: The Cardiovascular Effects and Toxicity of Lithium, in Psychopharmacology Update: New and Neglected Areas. Edited by Davis JM, Greenblatt, D. New York, Grune & Stratton, 1979

Jefferson JW, Greist JH, Ackerman DL, et al: Lithium Encyclopedia for Clinical Practice (2nd edition). Washington, DC, American Psychiatric Press, 1987

Jensen SB, Rickers H: Glomerular filtration rate during lithium therapy: A longitudinal study. Acta Psychiatr Scand 70:235-238, 1984

Joffe RT, Gold PW, Uhde TW, et al: The effects of carbamazepine on the thyrotropin response to thyrotropin-releasing hormone. Psychiatry Res 12:161-166, 1984

Joffe RT, Post RM, Roy-Byrne PP, et al: Hematological effects of carbamazepine in patients with affective illness. Am J Psychiatry 142:1196-1199, 1985

Johnston BB, Dick EG, Naylor GJ, et al: Lithium side effects in a routine lithium clinic. Br J Psychiatry 134:482-487, 1979

Kalina KM, Burnett GB: Lithium and the nephrotic syndrome. J Clin Psychopharmacol 4:148-150, 1984

Kallen B, Tandberg A: Lithium and pregnancy: A cohort study on manic depressive women. Acta Psychiatr Scand 68:134-139, 1983

Kaufman PL, Jefferson JW, Ackerman D, et al: Ocular effects of oral lithium in humans. Acta Ophthalmol (Copenhagen) 63:327-332, 1985

Kelly TE: Teratogenicity of anticonvulsant drugs, I: review of the literature. Am J Med Genet 19:413-434, 1984

Lahr MB: Hyponatremia during carbamazepine therapy. Clin Pharmacol Ther 37:693-696, 1985

Lazarus JH, John R, Bennie EH, et al: Lithium therapy and thyroid function: a long-term study. Psychol Med 11:85-92, 1981

Livingston S, Pauli LL, Berman W: Carbamazepine (Tegretol) in epilepsy: nine year follow-up study with special emphasis on untoward reactions. Diseases of the Nervous System 35:103-107, 1974

Lokkegaard H, Andersen NF, Henriksen E, et al: Renal function in 153 manic-depressive patients treated with lithium for more than five years. Acta Psychiatr Scand 71:347-355, 1985

Lyman GH, Williams CC, Dinwoodi WR, et al: Sudden death in cancer patients receiving lithium. Journal of Clinical Oncology 2:1270-1276, 1984

Lyskowski J, Nasrallah HA, Dunner FJ, et al: A Longitudinal survey of side effects in a lithium clinic. J Clin Psychiatry 43:284-286, 1982

Mannisto PT: Hypothyroidism during lithium treatment: A review of 49 cases. Psychiatria Fennica 299-305, 1974

Marotta JT: A long-term study of trigeminal neuralgia. Headache 9:83-87, 1967

Martin CA, Piascik MT: First degree A-V block in patients on lithium carbonate. Can J Psychiatry 30:114-116, 1985

May DC: Acute carbamazepine intoxication: Clinical spectrum and management. South Med J 77:24-26, 1984

McCreadie RG, Morrison DP: The impact of lithium in south-west Scotland, I: demographic and clinical findings. Br J Psychiatry 146:70-74, 1985

Medenwald J, Greist JH, Jefferson JW, et al: Carbamazepine and Manic-Depressive Illness: A Patient Guide. Madison, Wisconsin, Board of Regents of the University of Wisconsin System (Lithium Information Center), 1986

Middelhoff HD, Paschen K: Effects of Lithium on the EKG (in German; English abstract). Pharmakopsychiatr Neuropsychopharmakol 7:254-264, 1974

Mitchell JE, Mackenzie TB: Cardiac effects of lithium therapy in man: a review. J Clin Psychiatry 43:47-51, 1982

Mortimer PS, Dawber RPR: Hair loss and lithium. Int J Dermatol 23:603-604, 1984

Muller-Oerlinghausen B, Passoth P-M, Poser W, et al: Impaired glucose tolerance in long-term lithium-treated patients. International Journal of Pharmacopsychiatry 14:350-362, 1979

Neil JF, Himmelhoch JM, Licata SM: Emergence of myasthenia gravis during treatment with lithium carbonate. Arch Gen Psychiatry 33:1090-1092, 1976

Norton B, Whalley LJ: Mortality of a lithium-treated population. Br J Psychiatry 145:277-282, 1984

Perucca E, Garratt A, Hebdige S, et al: Water intoxication in epileptic patients receiving carbamazepine. J Neurol Neurosurg Psychiatry 41:713-718, 1978

Peselow ED, Dunner DL, Fieve RR, et al: Course and relationship of lithium side effects to plasma lithium levels. Psychiatr Clin (Basel) 14:178-183, 1981

Physicians' Desk Reference: PDR (40th edition). Oradell, NJ, Medical Economics Company, 1986

Pisciotta AV: Hematologic toxicity of carbamazepine. Adv Neurol 11:355-368, 1975

Ramsay ID: Carbamazepine-induced jaundice. Br Med J 4:155, 1967

Roy-Byrne PP, Joffe RT, Uhde TW, et al: Carbamazepine in thyroid function in affectively ill patients. Arch Gen Psychiatry 41:1150-1153, 1984

Russell JD, Johnson GFS: Affective disorders, diabetes mellitus and lithium. Aust NZ J Psychiatry 15:349-353, 1981

Saul RF, Hamburger HA, Selhorst JB: Pseudotumor cerebri secondary to lithium carbonate. JAMA 253:2869-2870, 1985

Schou M: What happened later to the lithium babies? A follow-up study of children born without malformations. Acta Psychiatr Scand 54:193-197, 1976

Schou M: Artistic productivity and lithium prophylaxis in manic-depressive illness. Br J Psychiatry 135:97-103, 1979

Shopsin B, Temple H, Ingwer M, et al: Sudden death during lithium carbonate maintenance, in Lithium: Controversies and Unresolved Issues. Edited by Cooper TB, Gershon S, Kline NS, et al. Amsterdam, Excerpta Medica, 1979

Skott A, Mobacken H, Starmark JE: Exacerbation of psoriasis during lithium treatment. Br J Dermatol 96:445-448, 1977

Smigan L, Wahlin A, Jacobsson L, et al: Lithium therapy and thyroid function tests: A prospective study. Neuropsychobiology 11:39-43, 1984

Smith RE, Helms PM: Adverse effects of lithium therapy in the acutely ill elderly patient. J Clin Psychiatry 43:94-99, 1982

Stein RS, Flexner JH, Graber SE: Lithium and granulocytopenia during induction therapy of acute myelogenous leukemia: update of an ongoing trial. Adv Exp Med Biol 127:187-198, 1980

Tyrer P, Lee I, Trotter C: Physiological characteristics of tremor after chronic lithium therapy. Br J Psychiatry 139:59-61, 1981

Uhde TW, Post RM: Effects of carbamazepine on serum electrolytes: clinical and theoretical implications. J Clin Psychopharmacol 3:103-106, 1983

Vasile RG, Shelton RP: Alleviating gastrointestinal side effects of lithium carbonate by substituting lithium citrate. J Clin Psychopharmacol 2:420-423, 1982

Vendsborg PB, Bech P, Rafaelsen OJ: Lithium treatment and weight gain. Acta Psychiatr Scand 53:139-147, 1976

Vestergaard P, Amdisen A: Lithium treatment and kidney function: A follow-up study of 237 patients in long-term treatment. Acta Psychiatr Scand 63:333-345, 1981

Vestergaard P, Amdisen A, Schou M: Clinically significant side effects of lithium treatment: A survey of 237 patients in long-term treatment. Acta Psychiatr Scand 62:193-200, 1980

Walker RG, Dowling JP, Alcorn D, et al: Renal pathology associated with lithium therapy. Pathology 15:403-411, 1983

Weinstein MR: Lithium treatment of women during pregnancy and in the post-delivery period, in Handbook of Lithium Therapy. Edited by Johnson FN. Lancaster, England, MTP Press, 1980

Wilson WH, Jefferson JW: Thyroid disease, behavior, and psychopharmacology. Psychosomatics 26:481-492, 1985

Winchester JF: Lithium, in Clinical Management of Poisoning and Drug Overdose. Edited by Haddad LM, Winchester JF. Philadelphia, WB Saunders, 1983

Wolff J: Lithium interactions with the thyroid gland, in Lithium: Controversies and Unresolved Issues. Edited by Cooper TB, Gershon S, Kline NS, et al. Amsterdam, Excerpta Medica, 1979

Chapter 35

Benzodiazepine Side Effects

by Karl Rickels, M.D., Edward Schweizer, M.D., and Irwin Lucki, Ph.D.

Benzodiazepines constitute one of the most widely prescribed classes of drugs, and are by far the most widely used of the anxiolytics and hypnotics. The first benzodiazepine, chlordiazepoxide, was introduced in 1960. Since then, 12 benzodiazepines have been marketed in the United States, and double that number are available worldwide. Remarkably, no benzodiazepine has ever had to be withdrawn from the world market. After a quarter of a century of use and misuse, low dose, high dose, and overdose, in all manner of clinically appropriate and inappropriate settings, benzodiazepines have emerged, perhaps not unscathed, but with a record of safety almost unparalleled among prescription drugs. Few drugs could have withstood the trials that benzodiazepines have undergone in the past generation. It has required a vocal media effort in the last few years (Gordon, 1979) to remind the public and the physician alike that benzodiazepines are controlled substances with potential risks, which should be reserved for specific diagnoses and should be used only under medical supervision. All of this must be kept in mind as we undertake in this chapter to review the side effects and risks of benzodiazepine treatment. Considerations of space, and the desire to produce a more thorough review, have led us to exclude barbiturates and beta blockers from the present discussion. Reviews of their side effects are available elsewhere (Harvey, 1980; Davies, 1977).

The most comprehensive clinical review of the full range of benzodiazepine side effects and risks still is *Benzodiazepines in Clinical Practice* (Greenblatt and Shader, 1974). *Benzodiazepines: From Molecular Biology to Clinical Practice* (Costa, 1983) provides a useful update with an extensive preclinical introduction to the behavioral and neuropharmacological effects of the benzodiazepines. Since the publication 12 years ago of Greenblatt and Shader's book, nothing has emerged to seriously shake our confidence in the essential safety of benzodiazepines. Several clinical issues, however, have been the focus of recent research. Prominent among them are the phenomena of benzodiazepine dependence (especially at low dose) and the associated withdrawal syndrome. Increased knowledge of the twin issues of dependence and withdrawal is already having a significant impact on how benzodiazepines are utilized.

The cognitive and behavioral effects of benzodiazepines have also been the focus of considerable investigation. Adverse cognitive and behavioral effects can be subtle, but may have important clinical consequences. This is an area in which experimental and preclinical research can illuminate clinical practice. For example, memory effects from benzodiazepines were not mentioned in a recent summary of side effects obtained by self-report from 45 controlled clinical trials on a total of 3,634 patients (Greenblatt et al, 1984). Yet experimental assessments of amnestic effects (Lister, 1985) suggests that they are characteristic of all benzodiazepines, and specific inquiry about benzodiazepine memory effects in clinically anxious populations yields, in our experience, a notably higher rate than that generated by self-report. Any discussion of benzodiazepine side effects must broaden its scope beyond sole reliance on self-report and epidemiology to include more experimental assessments of the impact of benzodiazepines on physiological, behavioral, and cognitive parameters.

This principle will be evident as we first review central nervous system (CNS) effects of benzodiazepines, including effects on cognitive function, memory, behavior, and performance. We will then review systemic effects of benzodiazepines, concluding with a discussion of benzodiazepines in pregnancy. Finally we will review benzodiazepine overdosage, dependence, and withdrawal.

BEHAVIORAL AND COGNITIVE EFFECTS OF BENZODIAZEPINES

The behavioral and cognitive effects of benzodiazepines can be discussed, for the sake of convenience, under four different headings: First, the effect of benzodiazepines on alertness and arousal; second, their effect on general behavioral activity; third, the effect of benzodiazepines on psychomotor performance, with special attention to their impact on operating automobiles or other machinery; and fourth, their effect on cognitive function and memory. Consideration will be given to the effect of chronic benzodiazepine use on these parameters, and to the effect of benzodiazepines when used as hypnotics.

Effects on Alertness and Arousal

The primary pharmacologic action of benzodiazepines in the central nervous system is their facilitation of GABAergic neurotransmission (Haefely et al, 1983). GABA is considered to be the most extensive inhibitory neurotransmitter in the CNS (Haefely et al, 1983), with 30–50 percent of all synapses estimated to be GABAergic. In light of this, it is not surprising that CNS depression is the most commonly observed unwanted effect of benzodiazepine treatment. It is perhaps more accurately characterized as an extension of the therapeutic effect of the benzodiazepines than as a side effect, and in general terms is merely a function of too large a dose for a specific person. Central nervous system depression is reflected in typical electroencephalogram (EEG) changes (Greenblatt and Shader, 1974). Clinically, CNS depression due to benzodiazepine use is reported as feelings of drowsiness, lethargy, fatigue, lightheadedness or dizziness, and mental or physical slowing. Blunting of initiative or motivational drive can be observed. There also appears to be a neuromuscular component, with complaints of ataxia, uncoordination, and dysarthria. Pooled data from controlled studies of benzodiazepines (Greenblatt et al, 1984) finds the CNS depressant effects to be the only adverse reaction consistently and significantly in excess of that seen with placebo.

Intensity of anxiety and dose of benzodiazepine are two obvious factors influencing the development of CNS depression. Factors that alter rates of absorption or excretion of benzodiazepines also can influence development of sedative side effects. Geriatric patients are well known to have an increased susceptibility to sedation. It is unclear whether this differential sensitivity can be attributed to alterations in the CNS substrate, or to peripheral metabolic considerations, or both.

The sedative effect of benzodiazepines can be rapid in onset. Even with oral doses it can occur, in some cases, in less than 30 minutes. Diazepam, the most lipophilic benzodiazepine, has the fastest onset of action in this regard. Maximal sedation after an acute dose occurs in the first one to two hours after ingestion, and often begins to subside before benzodiazepine plasma levels have significantly dropped. Pharmacodynamic effects involving both systemic drug distribution and local benzodiazepine receptor binding and dissociation (Jack et al, 1983) may account for this seeming anomaly. Certain benzodiazepines, in equipotent doses, appear to have somewhat different sedating properties, possibly due to similar mechanisms (Ellinwood et al, 1985).

Unwanted benzodiazepine sedation not infrequently can limit the therapeutic effectiveness of the drug, especially in conditions of severe anxiety such as panic disorder, which often require relatively high doses for treatment. Tolerance to the sedative effects occurs with time. Caution should of course be exercised in combined use of other sedating substances such as antihistamines or alcohol. Flexible dosing, taking benzodiazepines with meals, and sparing use of caffeinated beverages all facilitate accommodation to the sedative effect of benzodiazepines. The use of caffeine is an effective adjunct that often produces surprisingly little anxiogenesis in the face of adequate benzodiazepine plasma levels (Downing and Rickels, 1981). Heavy cigarette smoking has also been shown to militate against benzodiazepine sedative effects, but overcoming sedation by this means may be a Pyrrhic victory (Downing and Rickels, 1981). Finally, nonspecific personality factors and premorbid psychopathology also affect intensity of reported sedation (Downing et al, 1979).

General Behavioral Reactions

The development of verbal or behavioral irritability, hostility, or aggression due to benzodiazepines has long been noted (Greenblatt and Shader, 1974; Hall and Zisook, 1981) and occasionally has been contested (Rickels and Downing, 1974). The latter view is largely supported by multiple clinical trials that have found a low rate of marked behavioral reactions to benzodiazepines. When notable hostility does occur, it is usually characterized as a "paradoxical" reaction, since the therapeutic effect of benzodiazepines is most often conceived of as a general tranquilizing or calming effect. This perhaps oversimplified perception can be traced back to early experiments in which vicious macaque monkeys were "tamed" by benzodiazepines (Randall et al, 1960).

However, in quite a few preclinical studies, as reviewed by Greenblatt and Shader (1974) and Thiébot and Soubrié (1983), benzodiazepines either have no effect on aggressive behavior, or actually facilitate it. This may be part of a more general "releasing" effect of benzodiazepines behaviorally: in experimental paradigms one of the most reliable effects of benzodiazepines is their *disinhibition* of behavior normally suppressed by anticipated negative or aversive consequences (Gray et al, 1983). These findings for benzodiazepines suggest that clinically observed hostile and irritable reactions may be a manifestation of this disinhibition, rather than a paradoxical side effect. Benzodiazepines appear, in fact, to facilitate not only aggressiveness, but a variety of other, more socially acceptable behaviors (Rickels and Clyde, 1967).

It has been suggested (Greenblatt and Shader, 1974; Rosenbaum et al, 1984) that premorbid personality features such as poor impulse control, chronic resentment, or passive-aggressive tendencies may combine with benzodiazepine influence in social situations marked by interpersonal tension, to yield overt expressions of irritability, even rage. These latter reactions appear to be unusual, and are much less frequent than intense behavioral reactions reported for alcohol. Other studies, however (Greenblatt and Shader, 1974; Kochansky et al, 1975) suggest that a milder disinhibition of irritability/aggression may be a frequent concomitant of benzodiazepine treatment.

There is some suggestion (Kochansky et al, 1975; Kroef, 1979; Rosenbaum et al, 1984) that certain benzodiazepines (such as the triazolo-benzodiazepines) might possess a greater potential for precipitating extreme disinhibition of behavioral control, though still less than that observed for alcohol. This may be due as much to their high potency as to some unique property of the triazolo ring. The effect of benzodiazepines on behavioral dyscontrol usually occurs in the first week of treatment, often after one or two doses. It is unknown whether tolerance develops to these behavioral effects.

Benzodiazepines have also been reported (France and Krishnan, 1984; Strahan et al, 1985) to cause manic-like excited states in depressed-anxious patients. They also are thought, not uncommonly, to induce depression, especially in high doses when administered chronically (Hall and Zisook, 1981). This effect, however, is difficult to disentangle from the depression which complicates the history of anxiety disorders in well over 50 percent of patients. Finally, there are isolated case reports of miscellaneous other behavioral disturbances due to benzodiazepines: confusional states (attributed to triazolam), hallucinations, paranoid reactions, vivid dreams, and nightmares (Hall and Zisook, 1981).

Psychomotor Performance

Many experimental studies employing objective measures of human performance have been conducted with benzodiazepine medications in order to characterize the nature of any behavioral deficits that patients are likely to experience. Objective measures are apt to be more reliable and precise indicators of behavioral impairment than subjective reports, because subjects frequently misjudge their own performance abilities. The behavioral measures most sensitive to impairment by benzodiazepines include critical flicker fusion (CFF) thresholds, reaction time, and the repetition of simple motor acts such as finger tapping, motor manipulations, card sorting, and letter cancellation (Vogel, 1979). In addition, many studies have reported benzodiazepines to disturb performance on vigilance and coding tasks such as symbol copying and the digit-symbol substitution test (DSST). Thus, a variety of psychomotor skills are significantly disturbed by the acute administration of benzodiazepine medications.

The sensitivity of tasks measuring vigilance or the speed of motor performance to benzodiazepines may reflect merely general CNS depression. In contrast, tasks involving accuracy or judgment as measures of performance may be more variable in showing impairment with benzodiazepines, especially if subjects are allowed to compensate on a difficult task by performing it more slowly.

In general, all currently marketed benzodiazepines produce dose dependent behavioral impairments when administered acutely to normal volunteers, though doses at the moderate to high end of the therapeutic range are often required. In the case of diazepam, for example, 10 mg and 20 mg doses reliably impair behavioral performance when administered acutely, whereas 5 mg doses produce inconsistent or weak effects on psychomotor functions (Ghoneim et al, 1984c). Most studies evaluating psychomotor performance have examined the effects of benzodiazepines administered to normal volunteers. Performance-impairing effects of benzodiazepines have been demonstrated in some anxious subjects (Ghoneim et al, 1984a), but not in all (Oblowitz and Robins, 1983), possibly because reduction of intense anxiety can itself improve performance.

Another problem in extrapolating easily from experimental paradigm to clinical setting is the divergence of conditions and motivational contexts between the former and the latter. This is of some public health interest in light of the possible impact of benzodiazepines in situations such as driving, which require some degree of psychomotor skill. There has been great concern that the increased use of benzodiazepine medications may contribute to a larger number of traffic accidents or accidents in the workplace (Skegg et al, 1979). Many of the skills evaluated by psychomotor tests—that is, reaction time, visuo-motor coordination, and vigilance—are skills used in driving; the impairment of these behaviors by benzodiazepines in laboratory tests suggests that caution should be exercised by patients while driving. The acute administration of benzodiazepine medications at moderate doses has been shown to impair driving performance judged by trained evaluators or with automated driving simulators (de Gier, 1984). However, since tolerance develops to the psychomotor-impairing effects of benzodiazepines with their continued administration, and because patients with anxiety neurosis will become less tense and nervous from the therapeutic effects of benzodiazepines over time, it is important to evaluate these skills in patients that have taken benzodiazepine medications for some time. In addition, since alcohol is known to contribute to traffic accidents, many problems with driving may arise from the potentiation of alcohol's effects when benzodiazepines are taken simultaneously.

Effects on Memory

The initial reports of the ability of benzodiazepines to inhibit memory emerged from the inability of patients to recall events that occurred prior to surgery when benzodiazepines were used as preanesthetic medicants. Oral administration of benzodiazepines at therapeutic doses, however, also causes impairment of the recall ability in normal volunteers (Ghoneim et al, 1984b) and in anxious subjects (Angus and Romney, 1984). The memory impairment does not appear to be merely a manifestation of the drug's sedative effects. Most experimenters agree that benzodiazepines reduce the acquisition of new information presented subsequent to drug intake, and that such information is not consolidated adequately into long-term memory storage. The effects are relatively specific, since recall tests show that immediate memory or short-term memory are not severely affected by benzodiazepines (for review, see Lister, 1985). Neither do benzodiazepines impair the recall of information received prior to drug intake. It is unlikely that state-dependent learning explanations account for the disruptions of memory. Although some tolerance may develop to the memory-impairing effects of diazepam in normal volunteers, anxious subjects who were long-term users of benzodiazepine medications still demonstrate memory-impairing effects shortly after taking their benzodiazepine medications (Lucki et al, 1985; 1986).

The clinical significance of the disruptions in memory detected with laboratory tests remain to be determined. As with experimentally determined psychomotor deficits, lack of realistic motivation may be a confounding variable. In addition, since only acquisition of new information presented shortly after drug intake appears altered, it is not clear to what extent anxious subjects actually experience clinically relevant memory impairments as a result of therapy with benzodiazepines. Although memory problems are rarely cited spontaneously by patients when self-report is relied on, evidence for memory impairments might require more specific questions.

Benzodiazepine effects on memory no doubt vary depending on drug, dose, and frequency of administration. In addition, certain patient populations, such as cardiac-impaired patients or the elderly, may have a special susceptibility to these effects on memory (Pomara et al, 1984).

Pharmacokinetic/Pharmacodynamic Considerations

The benzodiazepine medications commonly used to treat anxiety disorders in the United States have differing rates of absorption, distribution, and elimination (for review, see Greenblatt and Shader, 1974). Other differences among potential medications involve the recommended dose or potency of these compounds, ranging from very potent (for example, alprazolam or lorazepam) to less potent (for example, diazepam, clorazepate, or chlordiazepoxide), although such differences are adjusted by the doses recommended for treatment. The prospective mechanism of action may involve only direct actions of the parent compound, or could include several active metabolites.

Recently, it has become increasingly clear that aspects of pharmacodynamic interactions with active receptor sites in the CNS play a critical role in determining the behavioral effects of benzodiazepine medications. The recovery from impaired visual tracking ability produced by diazepam was relatively rapid (less than two hours), while the plasma half-life of diazepam and its active metabolites was 33 hours (Ellinwood et al, 1983). This pattern of rapid behavioral recovery preceding the fall of plasma levels of benzodiazepines or other sedatives has been called acute tolerance. The implication of this finding is that behavioral impairment associated with a particular plasma level during a drug's absorptive phase will not correlate with plasma levels measured during a drug's elimination phase or at steady state. Ellinwood and colleagues (1985) compared the time course of behavioral effects produced by the acute administration of clinically equivalent doses of diazepam, alprazolam, and lorazepam. The behavioral impairment caused by diazepam showed the most rapid recovery despite the longest half-life. The recovery from impairment with alprazolam was still more rapid than that from lorazepam, even though both drugs had similar elimination half-lives that were much shorter than diazepam. Clearly, drug distribution, not elimination, terminates the action of a single benzodiazepine dose. The peak behavioral impairment obtained after acute administration of lorazepam occurred at two to four hours, and may correspond better with declining plasma concentrations (Seppala et al, 1976). Since lorazepam is lower in lipid solubility than diazepam, its time course may reflect difficulty in transport to active sites in the CNS. Importantly, however, diazepam dissociates from receptors in the brain more rapidly than does lorazepam, and this might allow the duration of its CNS-impairing effects to be shorter in duration (Jack et al, 1983). Such pharmacodynamic differences among benzodiazepine medications could also contribute to differences in their therapeutic effects or to their propensities for causing other side effects.

Effects with Long-Term Use

Benzodiazepines are, on occasion, administered chronically. In general, tolerance rapidly develops to the subjective sedative effects of benzodiazepines in anxious subjects (Rickels et al, 1983). Tolerance has also been shown to develop to the peformance-impairing effects of benzodiazepines after their administration to normal volunteers for just a few weeks (Aranko et al, 1983). Improvement of performance may be evident even after a single administration. Thus, chronic benzodiazepine use will significantly reduce the disruptions to behavior caused by these drugs.

On the other hand, there has been growing concern about deleterious psychological effects that may be produced when benzodiazepine medications have been taken for years. Petursson and Lader (1984) have reported impaired performance by long-term benzodiazepine users on the DSST and symbol copying test, although reaction time and letter cancellation were not altered. In a subsequent study, however, Lucki and colleagues (1985; 1986) found that the DSST and symbol copying ability of long-term benzodiazepine users did not differ from a matched group of drug free anxious subjects. In those studies, the acute effects of benzodiazepines were examined in long-term users shortly after having taken an acute dose of medication. In this setting, benzodiazepines increased feelings of tranquilization and reduced critical flicker fusion (CFF) thresholds, but did not cause sedation or alter DSST, symbol copying, or letter cancellation performance in the chronic benzodiazepine users. The effects of benzodiazepines at impairing motor performance and producing sedation were reduced following their chronic administration, probably due to the development of tolerance. However, acute administration of benzodiazepine medications caused memory-impairing effects even in the chronic users, similar to acute effects caused in drug-naive subjects. Thus, certain behavioral effects of benzodiazepine medications, such as their tranquilizing ability, reduced CFF threshold, and short-term memory impairments, do not show significant tolerance after chronic use.

Sedative-Hypnotics and Behavioral Performance

Benzodiazepines are often prescribed to be taken at night to improve the quality of sleep for patients with insomnia. The rationale for medical treatment of insomnia often assumes that increased or improved sleep for insomniacs should lead to better performance during the day. Yet many studies in sleep laboratories have shown that benzodiazepine or barbiturate sedative-hypnotics often lead to impairments in behavioral performance the day following their administration.

Johnson and Chernik (1982) reviewed 52 studies examining the residual effects of bedtime ingestion of hypnotics on behavioral performance measured during the following day. There is convincing evidence that such bedtime use may impair psychological functioning the following day, and that the risk of such "hangover" effects or residual behavioral effects ought to be considered when making the decision to prescribe these medications for patients. The behavioral tests found to be most affected were card sorting, DSST and symbol copying performance, and tapping rate. Tests of vigilance, reaction time, visuo-motor coordination, and arithmetic ability also demonstrated decrements (Johnson and Chernik, 1982). In general, tasks that involved the measurement of speed or motor components were the most sensitive to impairment by hypnotics. Benzodiazepine hypnotics also exert anterograde amnesic effects, so that patients may not recall events that woke them during the night (Roth et al, 1984).

In general, all of the benzodiazepine hypnotics studied demonstrated the pattern of producing increased decrements as higher doses were used. There is a distinct trend for those benzodiazepine hypnotics with long half-lives or with active metabolites that are not readily eliminated (such as flurazepam and nitrazepam) to produce greater residual impairment of performance than benzodiazepine hypnotics with shorter elimination half-lives (such as triazolam or temazepam). Although elimination half-life may play an important role in producing residual behavioral decrements, this factor does not alone appear to be a sufficient criterion for evaluating the probability of "hangover effects" for different medications. For example, the night-time ingestion of diazepam (5–10 mg) did not appear to cause similar morning residual effects, although it has a relatively long half-life (14–90 hours), and, in consequence, substantial plasma levels of the parent compound and active metabolite would be present the next day (Clarke and Nicholson, 1978). The residual impairment caused by hypnotics might also be tolerated better after multiple nights of drug administration (Church and Johnson, 1979), even if plasma levels of active benzodiazepines would be increasing in subjects over time.

Pharmacokinetic effects (cited above) undoubtedly influence behavioral effects. In addition, certain populations may be especially susceptible to daytime behavioral impairments by benzodiazepines used as hypnotics. These include the elderly (Castleden et al, 1977), heavy snorers (see Respiratory section), or patients with other medical problems.

The decision to prescribe a hypnotic for a patient with sleeping problems involves a weighing of benefits and risks. The benefits from a good night's sleep may consist more in the psychological relief from worrying about insomnia than in any demonstrable improvement in behavioral efficiency the next day. If sleeplessness has continued for some time, such benefits may be an overriding consideration. However, physicians should be cautioned against prescribing hypnotics for an extended period of time without evaluating the cause of the insomnia, since this practice may merely cover more serious psychopathology. The choice of a hypnotic drug should be influenced by the expected duration of behavioral effects, and the dosage should be adjusted to minimize reductions in behavioral efficiency during the day following treatment.

SYSTEMIC EFFECTS OF BENZODIAZEPINES

Respiratory Effects of Benzodiazepines

Benzodiazepines may produce mild respiratory depression in therapeutic doses (Rudolf et al, 1978). Discernible effects are largely, but not solely, limited to patients with pulmonary disease, and are mostly seen with parenteral or higher oral doses. Respiratory impairment appears to stem from several causes, including direct effects on upper airway neuromusculature (Leiter et al, 1985), and decreased central respiratory drive as assessed by reduced ventilatory response to CO_2 (Rudolf et al, 1978). These effects are most pronounced in patients diagnosed with chronic obstructive lung disease, and can become clinically significant, even to the point of respiratory failure (Model and Berry, 1974). In contrast, pilot data (Mitchell-Heggs et al, 1980) suggest that benzodiazepines might safely reduce dyspnea (due to anxiety reduction) in nonhypercapneic emphysematous "pink puffers." Benzodiazepines also appear to have no deleterious effects on airway resistance in asthmatics (Heinonen and Muittari, 1972).

An underrecognized concern is the effect of benzodiazepines on respiration during sleep. It is estimated that at least one percent of the general population has sleep apnea, strictly defined (Lavie, 1983). Habitual snoring occurs in another 5–10 percent of the population (Partinen, 1985), and may represent a forme fruste of the sleep apnea syndrome. Benzodiazepines, like alcohol, can cause a significant worsening of nocturnal respiration in these patient groups (Issa and Sullivan, 1982). In fact, 30 mg of flurazepam has been shown (Dolly and Block, 1982) to significantly increase sleep-disordered breathing and oxygen desaturation, even in asymptomatic subjects. It has been suggested (Mendelson et al, 1981) that the "hangover" effect observed when using bedtime benzodiazepines may be attributable, in part, to their effects on nocturnal respiration and oxygenation.

In summary, the respiratory depressive effects of benzodiazepines are mild but occasionally of clinical significance. They should perhaps be used circumspectly in patients with chronic lung disease, or in habitual snorers or other patients with sleep disordered breathing.

Cardiovascular Effects of Benzodiazepines

Benzodiazepines appear to lack significant cardiovascular toxicity. This has allowed benzodiazepines to assume a central role in the induction of anesthesia, and as a premedicant for a variety of other procedures ranging from cardioversion to endoscopy. This lack of untoward cardiovascular effects has been borne out by the benign anecdotal evidence of (often massive) benzodiazepine overdosage (Greenblatt and Shader, 1974).

This is not to suggest that benzodiazepines are totally without cardiovascular effects, even at doses in the therapeutic range. For example, intravenous benzodiazepines have been demonstrated to cause coronary artery vasodilation in animals and in humans (Ikram et al, 1973), both with and without coronary artery disease. The mechanism is unknown, but there is experimental evidence that benzodiazepines have a direct relaxing effect on vascular smooth muscle and that this effect may be due, in part, to calcium channel blocking effects (Ishii et al, 1983). Although there have been reports of antihypertensive effects from benzodiazepines, they are not generally felt to possess clinically significant effects on blood pressure (Medical Letter, 1974), except transiently in parenteral doses.

Benzodiazepines have also demonstrated intrinsic antiarrhythmic properties experimentally (Wang and James, 1979), and may potentiate the antiarrhythmic effects of other agents such as lidocaine. Anecdotal confirmation in humans of an antiarrhythmic benefit from benzodiazepines has also been provided (Spracklen et al, 1970).

Parenteral administration of benzodiazepines tends to be irritating and can cause burning, stinging, and erythema at the injection site in up to one-quarter of patients (Ameer and Greenblatt, 1981). In 5–10 percent of patients, thrombolphlebitis is a complication. Dilution of the drug, and injection into larger antecubital veins, may serve to reduce the incidence of local complications (Ameer and Greenblatt, 1981).

In general, benzodiazepines have established a remarkable track record of cardiovascular safety.

Gastrointestinal and Hepatic Effects

Gastrointestinal (GI) complaints such as nausea, diarrhea, or constipation are not infrequently reported by patients during the course of treatment with benzodiazepines. Gastrointestinal side effects, however, appear with comparable frequency in placebo-treated populations, and as often as not are attributable to the underlying anxiety disorder that initially led to treatment. Still, rare but incontrovertible GI side effects do occasionally crop up.

Hepatotoxicity from benzodiazepines is very low, but there are rare and isolated case reports (Cobden et al, 1981; Reynolds et al, 1981) in which benzodiazepine induced cholestatic jaundice seems likely. In general, benzodiazepines have no effect on liver function tests (Donlon and Singer, 1979), although isolated cases of benzodiazepine induced hepatitis have been reported (Roy-Byrne et al, 1983). They also do not appear to cause significant induction to hepatic microsomal enzymes (Greenblatt and Shader, 1974).

Since their introduction, benzodiazepines have been anecdotally reported to cause increased appetite and weight gain in selected patients. It is surprising that this effect is so rare, given the well documented appetite enhancing effects of benzodiazepines in a variety of mammalian species (Cooper, 1980). In fact, there have been reports of slight but significant weight loss when benzodiazepines are used as hypnotics (Oswald and Adam, 1980).

Neuromuscular Effects

Along with anticonvulsant activity and anticonflict effects, muscle relaxation represents one of the defining features of benzodiazepines preclinically. Increased GABAergic inhibition of pathways controlling skeletal muscle tone appears to account for these muscle relaxant effects (Haefely et al, 1983). Inhibition occurs at both a spinal and supraspinal level, including the cerebellum. Feelings of weakness and ataxia are the most frequently reported side effects attributable to these mechanisms, but are seldom serious at therapeutic doses.

Cutaneous and Allergic Reactions

Benzodiazepines, like almost all known drugs, can cause allergic or hypersensitivity reactions that are idiosyncratic and not dose related. Dermatologic reactions to benzodiazepines, reviewed by Greenblatt and Shader (1974), include urticaria, exanthematous reactions, vesicular/bulbous eruptions, erythema multiforme, and purpura. Very few cases have been verified by rechallenge (Copperman, 1967), therefore erroneous associations have, no doubt, been asserted. In extremely rare instances benzodiazepines, like most other drugs, can cause anaphylaxis (Jerram, 1984).

Hematologic and Immunologic Effects

As with cutaneous and allergic reactions, benzodiazepines have been reported in rare and usually unsubstantiated cases to cause hematologic reactions ranging from leukopenia and thrombocytopenia to aplastic anemia or leukocytosis (Greenblatt and Shader, 1974; deGruchy, 1975). Benzodiazepines have not, to our knowledge, been generally demonstrated to have clinically significant effects on red blood cell indices or immune function.

Experimentally, various benzodiazepines have been shown to significantly inhibit platelet aggregation and prostaglandin synthesis (Romstedt and Juzour-Akbar, 1985). In fact, there are suggestions that prostaglandin A may be an endogenous ligand for the benzodiazepine receptor (Asano and Ogasawara, 1982). Triazolo-benzodiazepines are potent inhibitors of platelet-activating factor (Kornecki et al, 1984), a phospholipid which serves as a mediator of such diverse physiologic functions as platelet aggregation, bronchoconstriction, and inflammation. The clinical significance of these experimental findings is not readily evident as side effects, and requires further investigation. For the time being, benzodiazepines appear to be extremely safe hematologically.

Ophthalmic and Ear, Nose, and Throat Effects

The effect of benzodiazepines on various aspects of ocular functioning has not, to our knowledge, been systematically investigated. Relaxation of ocular muscles would appear to underlie problems in accommodation that are occasionally noted as blurring of vision. There have also been rare reports of conjunctivitis due to benzodiazepines (Lutz, 1975).

Benzodiazepines occasionally cause dry mouth, despite minimal anticholinergic effect. A bad or metallic taste in the mouth is also sometimes complained of. This is more common for flurazepam than for other benzodiazepines (Greenblatt et al, 1984).

Endocrine Effects

In contrast to other psychotropics, such as lithium or the neuroleptics, the benzodiazepines are remarkably free of endocrine effects. The changes that are observed are generally not physiologically relevant at therapeutic doses.

Diazepam has been demonstrated to stimulate growth hormone release, an effect which may become blunted with chronic administration (Shur et al, 1984). This growth hormone response occurs only in a subset of challenged patients, and it has been suggested that it may be secondary to benzodiazepine sleep induction (Levin et al, 1984).

Benzodiazepines appear to have minor or no effect on the thyroid axis (Greenblatt and Shader, 1974). Conflicting reports have suggested that benzodiazepine use may result in a rise (Beary et al, 1983) or no change (Wilson et al, 1979) in plasma prolactin and cortisol. There have been several case reports of gynecomastia in males on diazepam, which was associated with lowered testosterone, raised estradiol, and normal prolactin levels (Bergman et al, 1981). The frequency of these, and other, benzodiazepine related endocrine changes appears to be quite rare.

USE IN PREGNANCY, LABOR, AND LACTATION

The effects of benzodiazepine use in pregnancy is a complex issue of special public health concern, especially in light of the preponderance of women of childbearing potential who are diagnosed as having anxiety disorder. Assess-

---

ment of risk from maternal benzodiazepine ingestion must focus on at least four separate areas: organ teratogenesis, direct fetal and neonatal drug effects, postnatal CNS/behavioral toxicity, and effects from lactation.

Organ Teratogenesis

Concern over congenital malformations due to prenatal benzodiazepine use has focused almost exclusively on diazepam and its possible etiologic role in cleft lip, with or without associated cleft palate. This correctable anomaly has a natural incidence of about 1 per 1,000 live births. Three case-control studies (Saxen and Saxen, 1975; Safra and Oakley, 1975; Aarskog, 1975) suggest that diazepam may confer a three- to fourfold increased relative risk for cleft lip. These findings are contradicted by two subsequent case-control studies (Rosenberg et al, 1983; Creizel, 1976) and other post-hoc analyses (Shiono and Mills, 1984).

Embryologically, in humans, the palatal shelf forms at about the sixth week of gestation. A report of a craniofacial cleft after a one-time maternal ingestion of high-dose diazepam (580 mg) at about the 43rd day of gestation is very etiopathologically suggestive (Rivas et al, 1984). In addition, experimental research in mice (Zimmerman, 1985) suggests that palatal shelf orientation is profoundly influenced by GABAergic mechanisms.

Though definitive evidence is lacking to link maternal benzodiazepine treatment to oral clefts, its use in the first trimester should be sparing and circumspect, especially since use of benzodiazepines is rarely a matter of clinical urgency. Teratogenic effects of benzodiazepines other than diazepam have been much less well studied, but should probably be considered to pose at least a comparable risk. There have been mixed reports (Milkovich and van der Berg, 1974; Hartz et al, 1975) of chlordiazepoxide possibly being associated with a slightly increased incidence of various congenital anomalies and fetal death.

Direct Fetal and Neonatal Drug Effects

All marketed benzodiazepines appear to cross the placenta readily and, since fetal metabolism and excretion are slower, they tend to accumulate on the fetal side with repeated dosing (Kanto, 1982). Significant neonatal effects have been reported (Kanto, 1982) for acute dosages of benzodiazepines during labor (≥ 30 mg of diazepam or its equivalent), or more chronic administration of benzodiazepines during the last weeks of pregnancy. The latter have been demonstrated even at doses as low as 10–15 mg of diazepam daily (Speight, 1977). In these situations CNS depression is not infrequently observed, characterized as the "floppy infant syndrome," and manifesting as general flaccidity, poor feeding, apneic episodes, and hypothermia. In addition, in rare instances, infants may undergo a benzodiazepine withdrawal syndrome in the first week after birth (Rementeria and Bhatt, 1977).

Postnatal CNS/Behavioral Toxicity

Long-lasting neurochemical, cognitive, and behavioral sequellae to early developmental exposure to centrally acting drugs is one of the most neglected areas of research on human drug effects (Kellog, 1985). There is substantial evidence that pre- and early postnatal exposure to benzodiazepines in animals can result in subsequent emergence of significant alterations in behavioral, cognitive, and neurochemical function (Frieder et al, 1984; Simmons et al, 1984). At present there is no evidence of comparable effects in humans, nor are we aware of any research that addresses the issue.

Lactation

All benzodiazepines studied have been shown to be excreted in breast milk (Kanto, 1982). Passage from maternal blood to milk is limited to the nonprotein bound fraction of the drug. Therapeutic doses of benzodiazepines generally are insufficient to produce discernible effects on nursing infants, though there have been case reports of significant passive tranquilization from nursing mothers treated with diazepam at 30 mg per day (Ananth, 1978).

OVERDOSAGE

In the past 15 years benzodiazepines have been implicated in one-fourth to one-half of all overdoses that reach medical attention (and probably a higher percent that do not) (Prescott, 1983). In most documented overdoses involving benzodiazepines other drugs are also involved, and in overdosage resulting in death this almost invariably is the case. A survey (Finkle et al, 1979) of 1,239 diazepam-related fatalities yielded only two that might be attributable to diazepam alone. A similar result was found for 8,000 benzodiazepine overdoses, in which only one death (apparent respiratory arrest) was attributable to benzodiazepines alone (Prescott, 1983).

The clinical features of benzodiazepine overdosage reflect a CNS depression that progresses from drowsiness, dysarthria, and ataxia to stuporous sedation. Marked coma with associated hypotension and hypothermia are rare, except where there are extenuating circumstances. These include concomitant use of other drugs or alcohol, intercurrent medical conditions, or old age. Recovery tends to occur over a 12–24 hour period, and patients often become notably more alert despite benzodiazepine plasma levels that are still quite elevated (Greenblatt et al, 1978). Since benzodiazepines tend to be highly protein bound, dialysis generally offers little, and is rarely required anyway.

The general lack of life-threatening coma due to benzodiazepine overdosage stands in sharp contrast to this not infrequent outcome for comparable barbiturate overdosage. The development of some form of acute tolerance has been invoked to explain why patients "wake up" from benzodiazepine overdosage so much more readily than they do from barbiturate overdosage. The mechanism may also be rooted in the self-limiting role of the GABAergic system in the CNS. The GABAergic system forms recurrent inhibitory pathways almost exclusively. As Haefely and colleagues have suggested (1983), as activity in the principal neuronal system becomes depressed, feedback inhibition by GABA necessarily decreases, no matter how much benzodiazepine facilitation is occurring. As far as we know, benzodiazepines act only through these GABA receptor mechanisms, and have no direct membrane depressant effects. Judicious use of newer benzodiazepine antagonists would be of interest in cases of massive overdose. To our knowledge this has never been attempted.

DEPENDENCE AND WITHDRAWAL

The development of physical dependence on benzodiazepines, and symptoms of withdrawal upon discontinuation, have been issues of intense public concern.

Yet, they have been remarkably elusive phenomena to adequately document. Initial reports of benzodiazepine withdrawal syndromes began to appear soon after their first introduction 25 years ago, but they were generally anecdotal and reported on excessive dosages given for prolonged periods of time which were abruptly stopped. Prior to 1980 there were no systematic, controlled studies of dependence or withdrawal from benzodiazepines at therapeutic doses—what has been called low dose dependence.

Benzodiazepine dependence and withdrawal responses can be usefully viewed from several perspectives. From a neurochemical standpoint, there is increasing evidence that benzodiazepines produce their pharmacological effects, as mentioned above, by enhancing GABA transmission. During long-term exposure to benzodiazepines, GABA receptors show evidence of adaptive changes which would tend to reduce the effect of benzodiazepine. Abrupt cessation of benzodiazepine treatment might therefore lead to an acute reduction in inhibitory GABA function. There has been speculation (Cowen and Nutt, 1982) that such adaptive changes (often termed down-regulation) might underlie the symptoms associated with benzodiazepine withdrawal. Such withdrawal responses to abrupt drug discontinuation are not unique to benzodiazepines. They have also been reported for propranolol, clonidine, and the tricyclic antidepressants, and here also are thought to reflect receptor related rebound phenomena.

From an epidemiologic standpoint, the degree of physical dependence liability incurred by benzodiazepine treatment does not appear to be great. Marks (1978) was able to confirm only 28 cases of benzodiazepine dependence for 17 years and 150 million "patient-months" of benzodiazepine use in the United Kingdom. More recent surveys (Mellinger and Balter, 1981; Uhlenhuth et al, 1983) suggest that this low incidence may, in part, be due to the fact that patients actually consume benzodiazepines much less frequently, and at lower doses, than they are prescribed.

From the standpoint of behavioral pharmacology, benzodiazepines appear to have very weak self-reinforcing properties in animals and humans (DeWitt et al, 1984). This is not the profile seen with highly addictive substances. The preconditions leading to benzodiazepine dependence, therefore, appear to be weak when compared to other substances that produce physical dependence.

Withdrawal reactions, physical dependence on benzodiazepines, and withdrawal after abrupt discontinuation (even at low or therapeutic doses), indisputably occur, as has now been carefully documented (Winokur et al, 1980). The syndrome of withdrawal includes symptoms of adrenergic overactivity such as diaphoresis, tremor, restlessness, and tachycardia. It is a mistake, however, to conceive of benzodiazepine withdrawal as solely a hyper-adrenergic state, and indeed pilot and anecdotal evidence suggests that beta-blockers and clonidine only partially reduce benzodiazepine withdrawal symptoms. Other aspects of withdrawal encompass a diverse range of symptoms, including insomnia; gastrointestinal complaints (nausea, diarrhea, constipation, anorexia, and weight loss); neuromuscular complaints (head and muscle aches, fasciculations, and cramps); sensory complaints (including increased acuity, increased startle, perceptual distortions, blurred vision, tinnitus, sore eyes, metallic taste, and paresthesias); and cognitive complaints (such as impaired memory or concentration, impaired organization and expression of thoughts, and depersonalization feelings). Psychosis, paranoia, delirium, or convulsions are largely reserved for patients undergoing abrupt discontinuation of ≥40 mg diazepam or its equivalent (DeBard, 1979).

The time course of withdrawal symptoms is often distinctive and provides one of the best clues for discriminating withdrawal from return of original symptoms. Withdrawal symptoms usually begin 24–72 hours after discontinuing the benzodiazepine, though these symptoms may have an even earlier onset in drugs with a shorter half-life. Withdrawal reactions generally peak within seven days and, if untreated, gradually decrease with time (Rickels, 1981). Definite withdrawal usually produces a great degree of psychic distress, often much more than the original symptoms ever did, and it usually includes symptoms not previously reported. Not infrequently a patient experiences both a return of original symptoms as well as withdrawal symptoms, and only a prolonged observation of such a patient off medication will provide a better answer as to whether the patient suffers from a mixture of both or only from a return of original symptoms.

More research is needed to characterize what factors predispose to or predict the occurrence, intensity, and duration of benzodiazepine withdrawal responses. Preliminary work suggests that dosage level, duration of treatment, drug half-life, how the drug is discontinued, and premorbid psychopathology are all significant influences. Though the subtleties of how these various factors interact remains to be elucidated, several tentative comments can be made. As to drug dosage, in our NIMH Benzodiazepine Discontinuation Program (Rickels et al, 1986) we have observed withdrawal to occur after abrupt discontinuation of as low as one milligram of lorazepam (roughly equivalent to 5 mg diazepam). Prior slow taper was a confounding variable in some cases, and all patients had had protracted benzodiazepine treatment.

While some rebound anxiety may already occur in selected patients after only four to six weeks of benzodiazepine therapy (Fontaine et al, 1984), incidence of withdrawal reactions to the abrupt discontinuation of benzodiazepine therapy in therapeutic doses is rather small after short-term (one to three months) treatment. This incidence rate increases to 5–10 percent in patients treated from 4–12 months' (Rickels et al, 1983). Thereafter, the incidence rises steeply and may reach substantial levels (Petursson and Lader, 1984). In the only prospective study known to the authors (Rickels et al, 1983) and restricted to *DSM-III* diagnosed generalized anxiety disorder (GAD) patients, 43 percent clear-cut and 14 percent transient withdrawal responses were observed when patients were taking benzodiazepine for more than one year. These percentages were reduced to five percent and four percent respectively for patients treated for shorter periods of time.

Withdrawal from benzodiazepine therapy should be most cautiously conducted for those patients who are treated with excessive daily dosages of benzodiazepines for prolonged periods of time as, for example, patients treated for severe panic and agoraphobia with 4–8 mg per day of alprazolam, the equivalent of 40–80 mg of diazepam. In our own research program, abrupt discontinuation produced withdrawal symptoms in 82 percent of patients, regardless of benzodiazepine half-life. Severity of withdrawal, however, was clearly related to benzodiazepine half-life, with short half-life benzodiazepines causing a more severe withdrawal reaction during the first week of abrupt placebo substitution than long half-life benzodiazepines.

For most patients who received only low therapeutic dosages for a short period of time, or if given chronically only on an intermittent basis, discontinuation usually causes only minor problems. Benzodiazepine discontinuation can in most instances be effectively managed by tapering drug intake slowly (Winokur et al, 1980; Smith, 1979). And while many patients may experience few or no symptoms at all when gradually withdrawn, this certainly is not true for all patients. Some of the latter patients actually prefer the option of a more intense withdrawal response lasting for a shorter period of time.

In our experience (Rickels et al, 1986), chronically benzodiazepine-dependent patients tend to have significant and often inadequately treated psychiatric symptoms and illness. In many instances the use of benzodiazepines was not the best treatment available. More than 90 percent had *DSM-III* diagnoses by structured interview, and almost all were in need of a great deal of support and reassurance. A follow-up of 62 patients 12 months after participation in our discontinuation program indicated that 24 percent of them were off medication, 37 percent had been treated with antidepressants, and 38 percent were still taking benzodiazepines, frequently on an occasional or low daily dosage.

It was of interest to note that there was a subset of 10 patients who had no *DSM-III* psychiatric diagnosis and had normal Hamilton Anxiety scores prior to discontinuation. These 10 patients experienced notably milder withdrawal symptoms, and (despite comparable benzodiazepine doses) all were able to successfully withdraw. None required further psychiatric medication at follow-up. This raises the intriguing possibility that the intensity of benzodiazepine withdrawal may be only partially a function of the chemistry of declining blood levels. Instead, the intensity of the benzodiazepine withdrawal syndrome appears also to be a function of the degree of the patient's psychopathology, including his premorbid personality characteristics. This parallels the experience of Nelson and colleagues (1984), who found antidepressant side effects to be more closely correlated with premorbid psychopathology than with actual antidepressant blood levels.

Optimal management of withdrawal from chronic benzodiazepine use would appear to involve monitored dosage reductions of ¼ to ⅛ every one to two weeks, a switch to a long half-life benzodiazepine when necessary, the judicious use of adjunctive medication such as beta-blockers, antihistamines, and chloral hydrate as needed, and plenty of moral support. Last, but far from least, adequate diagnosis and treatment of underlying psychiatric problems is imperative if withdrawal from benzodiazepines is to be tolerated and maintained.

SUMMARY

Benzodiazepines have been in clinical use for a quarter of a century, and their effectiveness has been shown to be matched by their safety. In reviewing the side effects of benzodiazepines we have attempted to go beyond a mere list of reported adverse reactions. It is our belief that enlightened psychopharmacology should incorporate an understanding of the nuances of a drug's behavioral, physiological, and psychological effects, and an inkling about mechanism of action where possible. This is especially important for benzodiazepines, in which blatant side effects are rare, but more subtle side effects may have important consequences.

Research is currently in progress to further investigate the cognitive, memory, and performance effects of benzodiazepines and to clarify the nature and extent of dependence and withdrawal syndromes. Out of these studies should emerge a clearer picture of the benefits and risks of benzodiazepine treatment, and what constitutes judicious and appropriate use.

REFERENCES

Aarskog D: Association between maternal intake of diazepam and oral clefts. Lancet 2:921, 1975

Ameer B, Greenblatt DJ: Lorazepam: a review of its clinical pharmacologic properties and therapeutic uses. Drugs 21:161-200, 1981

Ananth J: Side effects in the neonate from psychotropic agents excreted through breast-feeding. Am J Psychiatry 135:801-805, 1978

Angus WR, Romney DM: The effect of diazepam on patient's memory. J Clin Psychopharmacol 4:203-206, 1984

Aranko K, Mattila MJ, Seppala T: Development of tolerance and cross-tolerance to the psychomotor actions of lorazepam and diazepam in man. Br J Clin Pharmacol 15:545-552, 1983

Asano T, Ogasawara N: Prostaglandins A as possible endogenous ligands of benzodiazepine receptor. Eur J Pharmacol 80:271-274, 1982

Beary MD, Lacey JH, Bhat AV: The neuroendocrine impact of 3–hydroxy-diazepam (temazepam) in women. Psychopharmacology (Berlin) 79:295-297, 1983

Bergman D, Futterweit W, Segal R, et al: Increased oestradiol in diazepam related gynecomastia. Lancet 1:1225-1226, 1981

Castleden CM, George CF, Marcer D, et al: Increased sensitivity to nitrazepam in old age. Br Med J 1:10-12, 1977

Church MW, Johnson LC: Mood and performance of poor sleepers during repeated use of flurazepam. Psychopharmacology 61:309-316, 1979

Clarke CH, Nicholson AN: Immediate and residual effects in man of the metabolites of diazepam. Br J Clin Pharmacol 6:325-331, 1978

Cobden I, Record CO, White RWB: Fatal intrahepatic cholestasis associated with triazolam. Postgrad Med J 57:730-731, 1981

Cooper SJ: Benzodiazepines as appetite enhancing compounds. Appetite 1:7-19, 1980

Copperman IJ: Purpura in a patient taking chlordiazepoxide. Br Med J 4:485-486, 1967

Costa E (Ed): Benzodiazepines: From Molecular Biology to Clinical Practice. New York, Raven Press, 1983

Cowen PJ, Nutt DJ: Abstinence symptoms after withdrawal of tranquilizing drugs: is there a common neurochemical mechanism? Lancet 1:360-362, 1982

Creizel A: Diazepam, phenytoin, and etiology of cleft lip or cleft palate. Lancet 1:810, 1976

Davies DM: Textbook of Adverse Drug Reactions. Oxford, Oxford University Press, 1977

DeBard ML: Diazepam withdrawal syndrome: a case with psychosis, seizure and coma. Am J Psychiatry 136:104-105, 1979

de Gier JJ: Driving tests with patients. Br J Clin Pharmacol 18:1035-1085, 1984

deGruchy GC: Drug-induced blood disorders. London, Blackwell, 1975

Dewitt H, Johanson CE, Uhlenhuth EH: The dependence potential of benzodiazepines. Curr Med Res Opin 8(suppl 4):48-52, 1984

Dolly FR, Block AJ: Effect of flurazepam on sleep-disordered breathing and nocturnal oxygen saturation in asymptomatic subjects. Am J Med 73:239-243, 1982

Donlon PT, Singer JM: Clobazam versus placebo for anxiety and tension in psychoneurotic outpatients. J Clin Pharmacol 19:297-301, 1979

Downing RW, Rickels K: Coffee consumption, cigarette smoking and the reporting of drowsiness in anxious patients treated with benzodiazepines or placebo. Acta Psychiatr Scand 64:398-408, 1981

Downing RW, Rickels K, Rickels LA, et al: Nonspecific factors and side effects complaints. Acta Psychiatr Scand 60:438-448, 1979

Ellinwood EH Jr, Linnoila M, Easler ME, et al: Profile of acute tolerance to three sedative anxiolytics. Psychopharmacology 79:137-141, 1983

Ellinwood EH Jr, Heatherly DG, Nikaido AM, et al: Comparative pharmacokinetics and pharmacodynamics of lorazepam, alprazolam and diazepam. Psychopharmacology 86:392-399, 1985

Finkle BS, McCloskey KL, Goodman LS: Diazepam and drug-associated deaths. A survey in the United States and Canada. JAMA 242:429-434, 1979

Fontaine R, Chouinard G, Annable L: Rebound anxiety in anxious patients after abrupt withdrawal of benzodiazepine treatment. Am J Psychiatry 141:848-852, 1984

France RD, Krishnan KRR: Alprazolam-induced manic reaction. Am J Psychiatry 141:1127-1128, 1984

Frieder B, Epstein S, Grimm VE: The effects of exposure to diazepam during various stages of gestation or during lactation on the development and behavior of rat pups. Psychopharmacology (Berlin) 83:51-55, 1984

Ghoneim MM, Hinrichs JV, Noyes R, et al: Behavioral effects of diazepam and propranolol in patients with panic disorder and agoraphobia. Neuropsychobiology 11:229-235, 1984a

Ghoneim MM, Hinrichs JV, Mewaldt SP: Dose-response analysis of the behavioral effects of diazepam, I: learning and memory. Psychopharmacology 82:291-295, 1984b

Ghoneim MM, Mewaldt SP, Hinrichs JV: Dose-response analysis of the behavioral effects of diazepam, II: psychomotor performance, cognition and mood. Psychopharmacology 82:296-300, 1984c

Gordon B: I'm Dancing as Fast as I Can. New York, Harper & Row, 1979

Graham CW, Pagano RR, Katz RL: Thrombophlebitis after IV diazepam—can it be prevented? Anesthesia and Analgesis 56:409-413, 1977

Gray JA, Holt L, McNaughton N: Clinical implications of the experimental pharmacology of the benzodiazepines, in The Benzodiazepines: From Molecular Biology to Clinical Practice. Edited by Costa E. New York, Raven Press, 1983

Greenblatt DJ. Shader RI: Benzodiazepines in Clinical Practice. New York Raven Press, 1974

Greenblatt DJ, Woo E, Allen MD, et al: Rapid recovery from massive diazepam overdose. JAMA 240:1872-1874, 1978

Greenblatt DJ, Shader RI, Divoll M, et al: Adverse reactions to triazolam, flurazepam and placebo in controlled clinical trials. J Clin Psychiatry 45:192-195, 1984

Haefely W, Pole P, Pieri L, et al: Neuropharmacology of benzodiazepines: synaptic mechanisms and neural basis of action, in The Benzodiazepines: From Molecular Biology to Clinical Practice. Edited by Costa E. New York, Raven Press, 1983

Hall RCW, Zisook S: Paradoxical reactions to benzodiazepines. Br J Clin Pharmacol 11:995-1045, 1981

Hartz SC, Heinonen OP, Shapiro S, et al: Antenatal exposure to meprobamate and chlordiazepoxide in relation to malformations, mental development and childhood mortality. N Engl J Med 292:726-728, 1975

Harvey SC: Hypnotics and sedatives, in The Pharmacologic Basis of Therapeutics, sixth edition. Edited by Goodman, Gilman. New York, Macmillan, 1980

Heinonen J, Muittari A: The effect of diazepam on airway resistance in asthmatics. Anesthesia 27:37-40, 1972

Ikram H, Rubin AP, Jewkes RF: Effect of diazepam on myocardial blood flow of patients with and without coronary artery disease. Br Heart J 35:626-630, 1973

Ishii K, Kano T, Ando J: Pharmacological effects of flurazepam and diazepam on isolated canine arteries. Japan Journal of Pharmacology 33:65-71, 1983

Issa FG, Sullivan CE: Alcohol, snoring and sleep apnea. J Neurol Neurosurg Psychiatry 45:353-359, 1982

Jack ML, Corborn WA, Spirit NM, et al: A pharmacokinetic/pharmacodynamic receptor binding model to predict the onset and duration of pharmacological activity of the benzodiazepines. Prog Neuropsychopharmacol Biol Psychiatry 7:5-6, 1983

Jerram T: Hypnotics and sedatives, in Meyler's Side Effects of Drugs, 10th edition. Edited by Dukes MNG. New York, Elsevier, 1984

Johnson LC, Chernik DA: Sedative-hypnotics and human performance. Psychopharmacology 76:101-113, 1982

Kanto JH: Use of benzodiazepines during pregnancy, labor and lactation, with particular reference to pharmacokinetic considerations. Drugs 23:354-380, 1982

Kellog CK: Drugs and chemicals that act on the central nervous system: interpretation of experimental evidence. Prog Clin Biol Res 163c:147-153, 1985

Kochansky GE, Salzman C, Shader RI, et al: The differential effects of chlordiazepoxide and oxazepam on hostility in a small group setting. Am J Psychiatry 132:861-863, 1975

Kornecki E, Ehrlich YH, Lenox RH: Platelet-activating factor induced aggregation of human platelets specifically inhibited by triazolobenzodiazepines. Science 226:1454-1456, 1984

Kroef C: Reactions to triazolam. Lancet 2:526, 1979

Lavie P: Incidence of sleep apnea in a presumably healthy working population: a significant relationship with excessive daytime sleepiness. Sleep 6:312-318, 1983

Leiter JC, Knuth SL, Krol RC, et al: The effect of diazepam on genioglossal muscle activity in normal human subjects. Am Rev Respir Dis 132:216-219, 1985

Levin ER, Sharp B, Carlson HE: Failure to confirm consistent stimulation of growth hormone by diazepam. Horm Res 19:86-90, 1984

Lister RG: The amnesic action of benzodiazepine in man. Neurosci Biobehav Rev 9:87-94, 1985

Lucki I, Rickels R, Geller AM: Psychomotor performance following the long-term use of benzodiazepines. Psychopharmacol Bull 21:93-96, 1985

Lucki I, Rickels R, Geller AM: Chronic use of benzodiazepines and psychomotor and cognitive test performance. Psychopharmacology 88:426-433, 1986

Lutz EG: Allergic conjunctivitis due to diazepam. Am J Psychiatry 132:548, 1975

Marks J: The Benzodiazepines: Use, Overuse, Misuse, Abuse. Lancaster, England, MTP Press, 1978

Medical Letter: Diazepam (Valium) in hypertension. Medical Letter Drug Therapy 16:96, 1974

Mellinger GD, Balter MB: Prevalence and patterns of use of psychotherapeutic drugs: results from a 1979 national survey of American adults, in Epidemiological Impact of Psychotropic Drugs. Edited by Tognoni G, Bellantuono C, Lader M. New York, Elsevier/North Holland Biomedical Press, 1981

Mendelson WB, Garnett D, Gillin JC: Flurazepam-induced sleep apnea syndrome in a patient with insomnia and mild sleep-related respiratory changes. J Nerv Ment Dis 169:261-264, 1981

Milkovich L, van der Berg BJ: Effects of prenatal meprobamate and chlordiazepoxide hydrochloride on human embryonic and fetal development. N Engl J Med 291:1268-1271, 1974

Mitchell-Heggs P, Murphy K, Minty K, et al: Diazepam in the treatment of dyspnea in the "pink puffer" syndrome. J Med 49:9-20, 1980

Model DG, Berry DJ: Effects of chlordiazepoxide in respiratory failure due to chronic bronchitis. Lancet 2:869-870, 1974

Nelson JC, Jatlow PI, Quinlan DM: Subjective complaints during desipramine treatment. Arch Gen Psychiatry 41:55-59, 1984

Oblowitz H, Robins AH: The effect of clobazam and lorazepam on the psychomotor performance of anxious patients. Br J Clin Pharmacol 16:95-99, 1983

Oswald I, Adam K: Benzodiazepines cause small loss of body weight. Br Med J 281:1039-1040, 1980

Partinen M, Palomäli H: Snoring and cerebral infarction. Lancet 2:1325-1326, 1985

Petursson H, Lader M: Dependence on Tranquilizers. New York, Oxford University Press, 1984

Petursson H, Gudjonsson GH, Lader MH: Psychometric performance during withdrawal from long-term benzodiazepine treatment. Psychopharmacology 81:345-349, 1983

Pomara N, Stanley B, Block R, et al: Adverse effects of single therapeutic doses of diazepam on performance in normal geriatric subjects: relationship to plasma concentrations. Psychopharmacology 84:342-346, 1984

Prescott LF: Safety of the benzodiazepines, in The Benzodiazepines: From Molecular Biology to Clinical Practice. Edited by Costa E. New York, Raven Press, 1983

Randall LO, Schalle KW, Helse GA, et al: The psychosedative properties of methamino-diazepoxide. J Pharmacol Exp Ther 129:163-171, 1960

Rementeria JC, Bhatt K: Withdrawal syndrome in neonates from intrauterine exposure to diazepam. J Pediatrics 90:123-126, 1977

Reynolds R, Lloyd DA, Slinger RP: Cholestatic jaundice induced by flurazepam hydrochloride. Can Med Assoc J 124:893-894, 1981

Rickels K: Are benzodiazepines overused and abused? Br J Clin Pharmacol 11:715-835, 1981

Rickels K, Clyde DJ: Clyde mood scale changes in anxious outpatients produced by chlordiazepoxide therapy. J Nerv Ment Dis 145:154-157, 1967

Rickels K, Downing RW: Chlordiazepoxide and hostility in anxious outpatients. Am J Psychiatry 131:442-444, 1974

Rickels K, Case WG, Downing RW, et al: Long-term diazepam therapy and clinical outcome. JAMA 250:767-771, 1983

Rickels K, Case WG, Schweizer E, et al: Low dose dependence in chronic benzodiazepine users: a preliminary report on 119 patients. Psychopharmacol Bull 22:407-415, 1986

Rivas F, Hernandez A, Cantu JM: Acentric craniofacial cleft in a newborn female prenatally exposed to a high dose of diazepam. Teratology 30:179-180, 1984

Romstedt K, Juzour-Akbar A: Benzodiazepines inhibit human platelet activation: comparison of the mechanism of antiplatelet actions of flurazepam and diazepam. Thromb Res 38:361-374, 1985

Rosenbaum JF, Woods SW, Groues JE, et al: Emergence of hostility during alprazolam treatment. Am J Psychiatry 141:792-793, 1984

Rosenberg L, Mitchell AA, Parsells JL, et al: Lack of relation of oral clefts to diazepam use during pregnancy. N Engl J Med 309:1282-1285, 1983

Roth T, Roehrs T, Wittig R, et al: Benzodiazepines and memory. Br J Clin Pharmacol 18:455-515, 1984

Roy-Byrne P, Vittore BJ, Uhde TW: Alprazolam-related hepatotoxicity. Lancet 2:786-787, 1983

Rudolf M, Geddes DM, Turner JAM, et al: Depression of central respiratory drive by nitrazepam. Thorax 33:97-100, 1978

Safra MJ, Oakley GP: Association between cleft lip with or without cleft palate and prenatal exposure to diazepam. Lancet 2:478-480, 1975

Saxen I, Saxen L: Association between maternal use of diazepam and oral clefts. Lancet 2:498, 1975

Seppala T, Kortilla K, Hakkinen S: Residual effects and skills related to driving after a single oral administration of diazepam, medazepam, or lorazepam. Br J Clin Pharmacol 3:831-841, 1976

Shiono PH, Mills JL: Oral clefts and diazepam use during pregnancy. N Engl J Med 311:919-920, 1984

Shur E, Petursson H, Checkley S, et al: Long-term benzodiazepine administration blunts growth hormone response to diazepam. Arch Gen Psychiatry 40:1105-1108, 1984

Simmons RD, Kellog CK, Miller RK: Prenatal diazepam exposure in rats: long-lasting receptor-mediated effects on hypothalamic norepinephrine-containing neurons. Brain Res 293:73-83, 1984

Skegg DCG, Richards SM, Doll R: Minor tranquilizers and road accidents. Br Med J 1:917-919, 1979

Smith DE: Importance of gradual dosage reduction following low dose benzodiazepine therapy. Newsletter, California Society for the Treatment of Alcohol and Drug Dependence 6:1-3, 1979

Speight ANP: Floppy infant syndrome and maternal diazepam and/or nitrazepam. Lancet 2:878, 1977

Spracklen FHW, Chambers RJ, Schrire V: Value of diazepam in treatment of cardiac arrhythmias. Br Heart J 32:827-832, 1970

Strahan A, Rosenthal J, Kaswan M, et al: Three case reports of acute paroxysmal excitement associated with alprazolam treatment. Am J Psychiatry 142:859-861, 1985

Thiébot MH, Soubrié P: Behavioral pharmacology of the benzodiazepines, in The Benzodiazepines: From Molecular Biology to Clinical Practice, Edited by Costa E. New York, Raven Press, 1983

Uhlenhuth EH, Balter MB, Mellinger GD, et al: Symptom checklist syndromes in the general population. Arch Gen Psychiatry 40:1167-1173, 1983

Vogel JR: Objective measurement of human performance changes produced by antianxiety drugs, in Anxiolytics. Edited by Fielding S, Lal H. New York, Futura Publishing Company, 1979

Wang CM, James CA: An analysis of the direct effect of chlordiazepoxide on mammalian cardiac tissues and crayfish and squid giant axons: possible basis of antiarrhythmic activity. Life Sci 24:1357-1366, 1979

Wilson JD, King DJ, Sheridan B: Tranquilizers and plasma prolactin. Br Med J 1:123-124, 1979

Winokur A, Rickels K, Greenblatt DJ, et al: Withdrawal reaction from long-term low-dosage administration of diazepam—a double-blind, placebo-controlled case study. Arch Gen Psychiatry 37:101-105, 1980

Zimmerman EF: Role of neurotransmitters in palate development and teratologic implications. Prog Clin Biol Res 171:283-294, 1985

Chapter 36

Clinically Significant Psychoactive Drug Interactions

by John G. Csernansky, M.D., and Harvey A. Whiteford, M.B., B.S., M.R.A.N.Z.C.P.

Because of the wide use of psychoactive and other drugs, the recognition and understanding of drug interactions has become essential for the clinician. Sometimes drug interactions can be used to enhance therapy as, for example, when anticholinergics are given to ameliorate the dystonic or parkinsonian effects produced by antipsychotics. At other times they decrease efficacy or produce unwanted side effects. Two major varieties of drug interactions may occur: pharmacokinetic or pharmacodynamic.

Pharmacokinetic drug interactions occur when one drug alters the absorption, distribution, metabolism, or elimination of another. In some but not all cases, altered pharmacokinetics of the first drug can be demonstrated by measuring plasma drug levels, cerebrospinal drug levels, and so forth. A well known example of such an interaction is cimetidines's ability to raise plasma levels of some benzodiazepines by inhibiting their dealkylation and oxidation.

Pharmacodynamic drug interactions occur when one drug alters the action of another at an effector site (for example, neurotransmitter receptor). No change in the plasma levels of the first drug occurs. For example, since phenothiazine antipsychotics and tricyclic antidepressants are both capable of blocking muscarinic acetylcholine receptors, their combined use may produce additive anticholinergic effects. Also, the action of any drug occurs within a physiological milieu. Thus, pharmacodynamic drug interactions may occur when one drug alters some parameter of that milieu (for example, pH, lipid mobility, and so on), thereby affecting the action of another.

ANTIANXIETY AND SEDATIVE-HYPNOTIC DRUGS

Benzodiazepines

Despite their recent decline in popularity the benzodiazepines continue to be among the most widely prescribed classes of drugs. This high level of use increases the chance that these compounds may be involved in significant drug interactions. Despite this, benzodiazepines display a wide margin of safety, and the clinician has a relatively small number of interactions for which to be alert.

There are few significant pharmacokinetic interactions involving the absorption, protein binding, or elimination of benzodiazepines. Antacids and anticholinergics may delay their oral absorption but this is rarely of clinical importance. Pharmacokinetic interactions are mainly attributable to interference with the hepatic metabolism of benzodiazepines.

A wide variety of benzodiazepines are currently marketed worldwide. Some of these (such as oxazepam, temazepam, and lorazepam) are predominantly metabolized by glucuronide conjugation to inactive metabolites. Conjugation is minimally affected by the coadministration of other drugs. Most benzodiazepines, however, are metabolized by N–dealkylation or aliphatic hydroxylation prior to conjugation, and these steps can be associated with significant interactions (Table 1) (Blackwell and Schmidt 1984, Greenblatt et al, 1983).

Microsomal enzyme inhibition has been reported with cimetidine, disulfiram, alcohol, and isoniazid. Of these, the most significant seems to be the interaction with cimetidine. Increases of up to 50 percent in plasma levels of diazepam have been noted (Klotz and Reimann, 1981). Microsomal enzyme induction is seen with a variety of agents but these are seldom of clinical significance.

Interactions with drugs possessing central sedative effects are probably the most important of the pharmacodynamic interactions. Alcohol is of major concern here (Sellers and Busto, 1982), as are other hypnosedative compounds (Table 1). Antagonism of the therapeutic effects of the benzodiazepines may occur with stimulant drugs (for example, appetite suppressants).

Table 1. Drug Interactions Involving Benzodiazepines (bz)

Interacting Compound	Mechanism of Interaction	Clinical Outcome
Cimetidine	Inhibit hepatic enzymes	Increase plasma bz levels
Disulfiram	Inhibit hepatic enzymes	Increase plasma bz levels
Alcohol (acute effect)	Inhibit hepatic enzymes	Increase plasma bz levels
Isoniazid	Inhibit hepatic enzymes	Increase plasma bz levels
Estrogens	Inhibit metabolism bz	Increase plasma bz levels
Cigarette smoking	Induce hepatic enzymes	Decrease plasma bz levels
Rifampin	Induce hepatic enzymes	Decrease plasma bz levels
Alcohol (chronic effect)	Induce hepatic enzymes	Decrease plasma bz levels
Levodopa	Unknown	Reduced antiparkinson effect of L dopa
Digoxin	Unknown	Increased half life digoxin
CNS depressants (alcohol, hypnosedatives, antihistamines, narcotics)	Additive CNS depression	Increased sedation
CNS stimulants (amphetamines, appetite suppressants, caffeine)	Antagonism of anxiolytic effect	Loss of bz efficacy

Barbiturates

Barbiturates have a well known ability to induce hepatic microsomal enzymes. This is most pronounced for the longer acting compounds (such as phenobarbital) and forms the basis for many of their significant interactions. The end result of this enzyme induction is a decrease in the plasma levels (and therefore the efficacy) of drugs metabolized by this system. In addition, the cessation of barbiturate intake can lead to a rapid increase in the plasma levels of these drugs, sometimes with potentially serious consequences (such as bleeding due to increased levels of warfarin). The other major interaction involving the barbiturates is central nervous system (CNS) depression. This occurs when barbiturates are combined with agents possessing central sedative properties.

Overall, barbiturates are of potential concern in a wide range of drug interactions. The interactions of greatest concern are found in Table 2. A more extensive list is available in pharmacology reference texts (Goodman-Gilman et al, 1980; Shinn and Shrewsbury, 1985; Hansten 1985).

Others

CHLORAL HYDRATE. The relative safety of this hypnosedative is well established. One interaction of concern takes place with anticoagulants. The major metabolite of chloral hydrate, trichloroacetic acid, displaces warfarin from albumin binding sites. This causes prolonged prothrombin times and increased metabolism of warfarin. This response is relatively short lived and with continuous coadministration, prothrombin times return to pre-chloral hydrate values. It should also be remembered that chloral hydrate is a CNS depressant and this effect is potentiated in combination with alcohol.

HYDROXYZINE. This histamine H1 antagonist is a relatively safe hypnosedative. It displays antihistaminic and antiemetic properties and may potentiate the actions of other CNS depressants.

BUSPIRONE. This nonbenzodiazepine anxiolytic has recently become available in the United States. It is from the azaspirodecanedione class of compounds and lacks anticonvulsant activity. It interacts minimally with CNS depressants such as alcohol, and does not seem to cause muscle relaxation. The drug is reported to cause minimal sedation and no impairment of psychomotor coordination (Dommisse and DeVane 1985). However, as with all new drugs, significant clinical exposure will be required to assemble an adequate safety profile.

ANTIDEPRESSANT DRUGS

Tricyclic Compounds

The tricyclic antidepressants (TCAs) have a wide range of pharmacologic actions. These include blockade of the neuronal uptake of biogenic amines (especially norepinephrine and serotonin), blockade of histamine (H1) receptors, blockade of muscarinic cholinergic receptors, and blockade of alpha-adrenergic receptors. This wide pharmacologic spectrum increases the potential for drug interactions. Potentially significant interactions involving the TCAs are listed in Table 3.

Until the recent introduction of the second generation antidepressants, the

Table 2. Major Drug Interactions Involving Barbiturates

Interacting Compound	Mechanism of Interaction	Clinical Outcome
Cholestyramine resin	Decreased absorption of barbiturates	Decrease plasma levels barbiturates
Oral anticoagulants	Induction hepatic enzymes	Decrease plasma levels anticoagulants
Tricyclic antidepressants	Induction hepatic enzymes	Decrease plasma levels TCAs
Beta-blockers	Induction hepatic enzymes	Decrease plasma beta-blockers
Chloramphenicol	Induction hepatic enzymes	Decrease plasma levels chloramphenicol (increase plasma levels barbiturates)
Oral contraceptives	Induction hepatic enzymes	Decrease plasma levels oral contraceptives
Corticosteroids	Induction hepatic enzymes	Decrease plasma levels corticosteroids
Phenothiazines	Induction hepatic enzymes	Decrease plasma levels phenothiazines
Phenytoin	Induction hepatic enzymes (normal doses of barbiturates)	Decrease plasma levels phenytoin
	Competitive inhibition of metabolism (high doses of barbiturates)	Increase plasma levels phenytoin
Propoxyphene	Inhibition barbiturate metabolism	Decrease plasma levels barbiturates
Quinidine	Induction hepatic enzymes	Decrease plasma levels quinidine
Tetracyclines	Induction hepatic enzymes	Decrease plasma levels tetracyclines
All CNS depressants (alcohol, sedatives, narcotics, antihistamines, etc.)	Additive central CNS depression	Increased sedation
MAOIs	Additive central CNS depression (can be counteracted by decreased barbiturate metabolism; see Table 4)	Increased sedation

Table 3. Drug Interactions Involving Tricyclic Antidepressants (TCAs)

Interacting Compound	Mechanism of Interaction	Clinical Outcome
Antipsychotics (especially chlorpromazine)	Inhibit hepatic enzymes	Increase plasma levels of TCA (especially imipramine and nortriptyline)
Disulfiram	Inhibit hepatic enzymes	Increase plasma levels of TCA
Cimetidine	Inhibit hepatic enzymes	Increase plasma levels of TCA
Methylphenidate	Inhibit hepatic enzymes	Increase plasma levels of TCA
Estrogens	Inhibit hepatic enzymes	Increase plasma levels of TCA
Cigarette smoking	Induce hepatic enzymes	Decrease plasma levels of TCA
Barbiturates	Induce hepatic enzymes	Decrease plasma levels of TCA
Phenytoin	Inhibit metabolism phenytoin	Increase plasma level of phenytoin
Guanethidine	Decrease neuronal uptake of guanethidine	Antagonism of antihypertensive action
Clonidine (also methyldopa)	TCAs down regulate alpha$_2$ presynaptic noradrenergic receptors	Antagonism of antihypertensive action of clonidine
MAOIs	Increase amount of amine available in synapse	Excitation, tremor, sweating, confusion, convulsions, coma
Sympathomimetic agents	Increase amount of amine available in synapse	Hypertension, hyperpyrexia
Alcohol, hypnosedatives and other CNS depressants	Additive central CNS depression	Increased sedation
Anticholinergics (including aliphatic and piperidine phenothiazines)	Additive anticholinergic effects	Blurred vision, dry mouth, urinary retention, paralytic ileus, confusion

TCAs and monoamine oxidase inhibitors (MAOIs) have been the major pharmacological treatments available for depressive illness. The temptation to combine these agents in refractory patients is often resisted because of well documented dangers (Table 3). However, recent reports suggest that this combination can be used safely if adequate precautions are taken (White and Simpson, 1981; Feighner et al, 1985; Pare, 1985). The wisest course of action is to take the patient off either drug for at least a week and then commence the two together. A TCA should not be added to the regimen of a patient taking an MAOI without ceasing the latter for at least seven days. Low doses of both agents are advisable at first. The recommended tricyclics for this combination therapy are amitriptyline, trimipramine, and doxepin. Imipramine is best avoided. Phenelzine is the MAOI preferred over tranylcypromine.

The treatment of psychotic depression or depressive illness occurring in a schizophrenic may lead to the combined use of a TCA and a phenothiazine. As both of these psychotropics use the hepatic cytochrome P–450 system, concurrent administration may increase TCA plasma levels by up to 70 percent (Blackwell and Schmidt, 1984). This exposes the individual to increased risk from TCA side effects. In addition, additive side effects of the phenothiazines (especially thioridazine) and the TCAs is a potentially serious problem. Reports of seizures and cardiotoxicity have occurred.

Depression and cardiovascular disease are two of the most common disorders afflicting Western society. Not infrequently, clinicians are required to treat both conditions coexisting in an individual patient. Several of the drugs used in the treatment of hypertension interact with TCAs (Table 3) and the clinician needs to be highly vigilant in the therapy of these persons.

Heterocyclics

It takes many years to accrue a complete safety profile for any new drug. To identify a rare (though serious) adverse reaction occurring in 1 in 40–50,000 patients will probably require 700,000 to 1 million patient exposures (Robinson, 1984). Similarly, to detect a clinically significant drug interaction often requires widespread use of the compound. This is particularly the case if the interaction cannot be predicted from the known pharmacology of the two drugs. As the heterocyclics (the so-called second generation antidepressants) have only become available worldwide in the last decade, information concerning drug interaction is still being accumulated.

Maprotiline is structurally similar to the existing TCAs and is a potent noradrenergic reuptake blocker. It also has strong antihistaminic and moderate anticholinergic effects. It is as sedating as the standard tricyclic compounds. On theoretical grounds, many of the interactions listed in Table 3 could occur with maprotiline (Shinn and Shrewsbury, 1985). Antagonism of the antihypertensive action of guanethidine and related drugs has been reported (Briant and George, 1974). Of particular concern with this drug has been a lowering of the seizure threshold. It should therefore be used with caution in epileptic patients, and in combination with drugs also known to lower the seizure threshold (Coccaro and Siever, 1985).

The antidepressant amoxapine is a derivative of the neuroleptic drug loxapine. It has been associated with extrapyramidal symptoms, akathisia, and tardive dyskinesia (Robinson, 1984). Therefore, it should be avoided in patients who are using dopamine blocking drugs (such as phenothiazines). In addition, amoxapine has the potential to be associated with many of the interactions listed in Table 3 (Shinn and Shrewsbury, 1985).

A triazolopyridine derivative, trazodone has a safety profile differing in significant ways from existing antidepressants. It has a low incidence of anticholinergic effects and would therefore not be expected to potentiate other compounds with anticholinergic properties (such as thioridazine). However, it does have significant sedative properties which would be of concern when used in combination with other CNS depressants. In addition, trazodone has been reported to increase serum digoxin and phenytoin levels (Robinson, 1984).

The tetrahydroisoquinoline antidepressant nomifensine displays both noradrenergic and dopaminergic reuptake blocking properties. It has few anticholinergic effects and is one of the least sedative of the available antidepressants (Coccaro and Siever, 1985). In fact, it may be stimulating in some patients, producing insomnia if taken at bedtime. From a theoretical perspective it should not significantly potentiate other drugs with anticholinergic or CNS depressive effects. There is some preliminary evidence that nomifensine does not potentiate the impairment in psychomotor function produced by alcohol (Taeuber, 1974). It is best avoided in patients taking antipsychotics, as its dopamine reuptake blocking properties may produce a decrease in efficacy of the antipsychotic.

Buproprion is a trimethylated monocyclic phenylaminoketone that has been shown to possess antidepressant properties equivalent to the standard TCAs. It has minimal sedative, anticholinergic, and cardiotoxic effects. Buproprion does not appear to enhance ethanol or benzodiazepine impairment of psychomotor function (Robinson, 1984). Its exact mechanism of action remains unclear, but buproprion has been shown to block norepinephrine and dopamine reuptake. The major area of concern at this time is an increased seizure risk when taking the drug (Dufresne et al, 1984). Reports suggest that this risk may be associated with the concurrent administration of lithium or antipsychotics (Robinson, 1984).

Monoamine Oxidase Inhibitors (MAOIs)

All of the available MAOIs act by irreversible competitive inhibition of mitochondrial MAO. This inhibition is only overcome by the synthesis of new enzyme. Monoamine oxidase inhibitors can be divided into two classes: the hydrazines (iproniazid, phenelzine, isocarboxazid) and the nonhydrazines (tranylcypromine). Some of the significant interactions with MAOIs are outlined in Table 4. A complete list is found in standard pharmacologic reference texts (Goodman-Gilman et al, 1980; Shinn and Shrewsbury, 1985; Hansten, 1985). These interactions occur by way of two mechanisms (Blackwell, 1984). The first is an exacerbation or prolongation of the normal actions of a drug resulting from hepatic enzyme inhibition by the MAOI (for example, CNS depression caused by narcotics). The second is the well known hypertensive crisis due to the release and potentiation of catecholamines following the intake of tyramine-containing foods or sympathomimetic drugs.

ANTIPSYCHOTIC DRUGS

The significant drug interactions involving antipsychotics are outlined in Table 5. Those of special importance to the clinician are discussed in more detail below.

Table 4. Examples of Drug Interactions Involving Monoamine Oxidase Inhibitors (MAOIs)

Hepatic enzyme inhibition by MAOI causing increased drug plasma levels of the following agents:

  barbiturates
  chloral hydrate
  oral anticoagulants
  phenothiazines
  narcotics (meperidine)
  anticholinergics

Sympathomimetics (direct, indirect, mixed) and similar compounds predisposing to a potential hypertensive crisis in combination with MAOI:

  amphetamine and congeners
  methylphenidate
  ephedrine, pseudoephedrine and congeners
  reserpine
  phenylpropranolamine
  L–dopa

Tyramine-containing foods and beverages predisposing to a potential hypertensive crisis in combination with MAOI:

  cheese
  yeast extracts
  pickled herring
  Bovril
  fava beans
  Chianti wine
  chicken livers

Other

  MAOI antagonizes the antihypertensive effects of guanethidine and methyldopa

  MAOI can enhance or prolong the hypoglycemic response to insulin and sulfonylurea hypoglycemics

  MAOI in combination with tryptophan can cause a behavioral or neurologic toxic state

---

The coadministration of phenothiazine antipsychotic drugs and antacids such as aluminum hydroxide should be avoided, since they may form adsorption complexes which limit the absorption of the antipsychotics (Forrest et al, 1970). Antipsychotics with substantial anticholinergic effects, such as chlorpromazine and thioridazine, may slow gastrointestinal motility, thereby increasing the absorption of various other drugs.

The administration of anticholinergic medications, such as benztropine mesyl-

Table 5. Drug Interactions Involving Antipsychotic Drugs

Interacting Compound	Mechanism of Interaction	Clinical Outcome
Aluminum hydroxide (and other antacids)	Decreased gastrointestinal absorption	Decreased antipsychotic efficacy
Oral anticoagulants	Antipsychotic may inhibit hepatic microsomal enzymes	Increased anticoagulent activity
Tricyclic antidepressants (TCAs)	Antipsychotic may inhibit hepatic microsomal enzymes	Increased plasma levels TCA
Benztropine mesylate (and other anticholinergics)	Unknown	Decreased antipsychotic plasma levels, efficacy and side effects
Barbiturates	Induction of hepatic microsomal enzymes	Decreased plasma levels of antipsychotics
Alcohol (and other CNS depressants)	Additive CNS depressant effect	Increased sedation
Amphetamine (also levodopa)	Antagonize dopamine blockade	Decreased efficacy of antipsychotics
Benztropine mesylate (and other anticholinergics)	Anticholinergic interaction	Reverse parkinsonism, increased anticholinergic and sedative side effects (e.g., dry mouth, blurred vision)
Lithium carbonate	CNS irritant	Enhancement of neurotoxic effects, (e.g., dyskinesia, ataxia)
Phenytoin (and other anticonvulsants)	Antipsychotic may lower seizure threshold	Decreased efficacy of anticonvulsant
Propranolol (and other beta-blockers)	Additive antihypertensive interaction	Exaggerated antihypertensive effects
Chlorothiazide (and other diuretics)	Additive antihypertensive interaction	Exaggerated antihypertensive effects
Methyldopa	False transmitter for dopamine	Increase in antipsychotic effect and side effects

ate, has been shown to decrease antipsychotic plasma levels (Gautier et al, 1977). In fact, this interaction has been postulated to account for some of the ability of anticholinergics to reverse antipsychotic drug induced parkinsonism. Phenobarbital and other barbiturates may decrease antipsychotic drug plasma levels by induction of hepatic microsomal enzymes.

Since antipsychotic drugs have some sedative properties, other sedative-hypnotics must be coadministered with caution in order to avoid an adverse pharmacodynamic interaction. Amphetamine and levodopa have pharmacologic effects on dopamine function that are opposite to those of antipsychotics. Therefore, administration of such drugs may decrease antipsychotic efficacy.

In the extrapyramidal motor pathway, dopamine, and acetylcholine function to create a neurochemical balance (Hollister, 1983). Because of this, anticholinergic drugs are used to reverse antipsychotic drug-involved parkinsonism due to the antidopaminergic properties of antipsychotics. However, since some antipsychotics have considerable anticholinergic effects themselves, coadministration of these agents can sometimes cause serious atropinism (that is, delirium, blurred vision, hyperthermia, and so on).

In 1974, Cohen and Cohen reported four cases of irreversible neurotoxicity due to combined treatment with haloperidol and lithium. However, it now appears that when lithium is combined with various antipsychotics, enhanced neurotoxicity of both drugs can be observed (Spring and Frankel, 1981). This interaction need not prohibit the coadministration of antipsychotics and lithium. In fact, combination treatment of this kind is often indicated for patients with schizoaffective disorder (Lipinski and Pope 1978; Biederman et al, 1979). Moderate doses of both drugs should be employed when utilizing this combination.

Since antipsychotics lower the seizure threshold, they may diminish the efficacy of administered anticonvulsants. On the other hand, thioridazine has been shown to inhibit the metabolism of phenytoin, leading to phenytoin toxicity (Vincent, 1980). Several antipsychotics, such as chlorpromazine, have significant anti-alpha adrenergic effects and produce hypotension. Therefore, they should be used cautiously in combination with antihypertensives. In addition, one antihypertensive, alpha-methyldopa, acts as a false transmitter for dopamine, and may enhance the side effects of antipsychotics.

LITHIUM CARBONATE AND CARBAMAZEPINE

Lithium

Lithium is used widely for the treatment of various affective disorders. Its efficacy remains best proven in bipolar affective disorder.

Several drugs alter the renal clearance of lithium. Acetazolamide increases lithium excretion and may lead to decreased serum lithium levels. Conversely, chlorothiazide and other thiazide-type diuretics decrease lithium clearance, and may lead to increased serum lithium levels and toxicity. Other drugs are known to alter serum lithium levels through poorly understood mechanisms. Tetracycline and indomethacin increase serum lithium levels, and may also lead to toxicity. Theophylline decreases serum lithium levels and may produce inadequate control of affective symptoms (see Table 6).

One of the more serious pharmacodynamic interactions involves the coad-

Table 6. Drug Interactions Involving Lithium

Interacting Compound	Mechanism of Interaction	Clinical Outcome
Acetazolomide	Increased urinary excretion of lithium	Decreased plasma lithium levels
Chlorothiazide	Decreased urinary clearance of lithium	Increased plasma lithium levels; possible toxicity
Tetracycline	Unknown	Increased lithium levels; possible toxicity
Theophlylline	Unknown	Decreased lithium levels
Indomethacin (and other nonsteroidal anti-inflammatory drugs)	Unknown (?inhibition of renal prostaglandins)	Increased lithium levels; possible toxicity
Neuroleptics	CNS irritant	Enhancement of neurotoxic effects
Carbamazepine	Unknown	Increased possibility of neurotoxicity
Potassium iodide (and other iodine-containing compounds)	Decreased T_4 release	Potentiate lithium-induced hypothyroidism and goiter

ministration of lithium and antipsychotic drugs, discussed in the previous section. In addition, phenytoin has been shown to precipitate lithium toxicity without apparently altering serum lithium levels (MacCallum, 1980). Carbamazepine has also been reported to enhance lithium's neurotoxic effects (Ghose, 1980). Despite these reports, combined use of lithium and carbamazepine has been found to be safe and particularly beneficial for some patients with schizoaffective and bipolar affective disorder (Lipinski and Pope, 1978).

Lithium is known to decrease release of thyroid hormone, sometimes leading to goiter or hypothyroidism. Lithium should therefore be cautiously coadministered with various iodide-containing compounds which also decrease thyroid hormone release.

Carbamazepine

Carbamazepine is being increasingly used to treat affective disorder, sometimes as an alternative to lithium. Because carbamazepine is chemically similar to the tricyclic antidepressants, one might hypothesize that using it in conjunction with monoamine oxidase inhibitor antidepressants is dangerous. However, no adverse interaction between these two drugs has been reported. Cimetidine has been reported to raise plasma carbamazepine levels by decreasing hepatic metabolism (Telerman-Toppet et al, 1981). Erythromycin, isoniazid, and propoxyphene have also been reported to increase plasma carbamazepine levels (Wong et al, 1983; Valsalan et al, 1982; Dam et al, 1977). Conversely, phenobarbital has been reported to decrease plasma carbamazepine levels, probably by enhancing its metabolism to an epoxide (Rane et al, 1976).

CONCLUSION

If severe and deleterious interactions are known to occur regularly when two drugs are given concurrently, then prevention is a matter of education and surveillance. However, most interactions are infrequent, vary in severity, and are tolerated differently by individual patients. Patient characteristics such as age, sex, physical health, and other variables can be important factors in drug interactions. Often, value judgments must be made when weighing the potential benefits and possible risks of a course of therapy.

There are some general guidelines that can enable the physician to minimize the risk of clinically significant drug interactions:

1. A detailed drug history is mandatory (Stewart et al, 1983). This should include past drug reactions as well as a family history of unusual responses to medication. It is important to include "over the counter" drugs and illicit drugs, as well as prescribed ones. Alcohol should not be forgotten. If possible, independent confirmation of the history obtained should be sought.
2. Patient education is highly desirable, and if necessary written advice and/or instructions should be given.
3. Identification of "at risk" groups is important. The age of the patient is a critical factor. Older patients and infants are overrepresented in serious drug interactions. Several disease states predispose to adverse reactions in general. These include glaucoma, hypertension, peptic ulcer, renal or hepatic disease, and diabetes. Duration of therapy is also important. Enzyme induction requires several days to occur, whereas inhibition of metabolism usually occurs more rapidly. An increase in half-life may not be immediately apparent until a new steady state is achieved. This requires four to six drug half-lives.

   In addition to these factors, psychiatric patients may be "at risk" for erratic compliance or increased coadministration of drugs because of a range of mental state factors. These should be fully assessed and regularly monitored by the treating physician. Somatic complaints by psychiatric patients should not be automatically dismissed without adequate assessment and investigation.
4. It is advisable to have available a detailed updated reference source to assess potential drug interactions. Excellent reference texts are available (Goodman-Gilman et al, 1980; Shinn and Shrewsbury, 1985; Hansten, 1985).
5. Finally, the physician should avoid unnecessary polypharmacy. Ineffective drugs should be withdrawn before new ones are added unless there are sound reasons for doing otherwise.

REFERENCES

Biederman J, Lerner Y, Belmaker RH: Combination of lithium carbonate and haloperidol in schizo-affective disorder. Arch Gen Psychiatry 36:327-333, 1979

Blackwell B: Antidepressant Drugs, in Meylers' Side Effects of Drugs, vol. 8. 10th edition. Edited by Dukes MNG. Amsterdam, Elsevier, 1984

Blackwell B, Schmidt GL: Drug interactions in psychopharmacology. Psychiatr Clin North Am 7:625-637, 1984

Briant RH, George CF: The assessment of potential drug interactions with a new antidepressant drug. Br J Clin Pharmacol 3 (suppl. 2):113-118, 1974

Coccaro EF, Siever LJ: Second generation antidepressants: a comparative review. J Clin Pharmacol 25:241-260, 1985

Cohen WJ, Cohen NH: Lithium carbonate, haloperidol and irreversible brain damage. JAMA 230:1283-1287, 1974

Dam M, Kristensen CB, Hansen BS, et al: Interaction between carbamazepine and propoxyphene in man. Acta Neurol Scand 56:603-607, 1977

Dommisse CS, DeVane CL: Buspirone: a new type of anxiolytic. Drug Intell Clin Pharm 19:624-628, 1985

Dufresne RL, Weber SS, Becker RE: Buproprion hydrochloride. Drug Intell Clin Pharm 18:957-964, 1984

Feighner JP, Herbstein J, Damlouji N: Combined MAOI, TCA and direct stimulant therapy of treatment-resistant depression. J Clin Psychiatry 46:206-209, 1985

Forrest FM, Forrest IS, Serra MT: Modification of chlorpromazine metabolism by some other drugs frequently administered to psychiatric patients. Biol Psychiatry 2:53-58, 1970

Gautier J, Jus A, Villeneuve A, et al: Influence of the antiparkinsonian drugs on the plasma level of neuroleptics. Biol Psychiatry 12:389-399, 1977

Ghose K: Interaction between lithium and carbamazepine. Br Med J 280:1122, 1980

Goodman-Gilman A, Goodman LS, Gilman A (Eds): The Pharmacological Basis of Therapeutics. New York, Macmillan, 1980

Greenblatt DJ, Shader RI, Abernathy DR: Current status of benzodiazepines. N Engl J Med 309:354-358, 1983

Hansten PD: Drug Interactions. Philadelphia, Lea and Febiger, 1985

Hollister LE: Clinical Pharmacology of Psychotherapeutic Drugs, 2nd edition. New York, Churchill Livingstone, 1983

Klotz V, Reimann I: Evaluation of steady state diazepam levels by cimetidine. Clin Pharmacol Ther 30:513-517, 1981

Lawson DH, Lowe-Gordon DO: Drug therapy reviews: clinical use of anticoagulant drugs. Am J Hosp Pharm 34:1225-1234, 1977

Lipinski JF, Pope HG: Diagnosis in schizophrenia and manic-depressive illness. Arch Gen Psychiatry 35:811-28, 1978

MacCallum W: Interaction of lithium and phenytoin. Br Med J 280:610-611, 1980

Pare CMB: The present status of monoamine oxidase inhibitors. Br J Psychiatry 146:576-584, 1985

Rane A, Hojer B, Wilson JT: Kinetic of carbamazepine and its 10, 11–epoxide metabolite in children. Clin Pharmacol Ther 19:276-283, 1976

Reynolds JEF (Ed): The Extra Pharmacopoeia. London, The Pharmaceutical Press, 1982

Rivera-Calimlim L, Castaneda L, Lasagna L: Effects of mode of management on plasma chlorpromazine in psychiatric patients. Clin Pharmacol Ther 14:978-986, 1973

Robinson DS: Adverse reactions, toxicities and drug interactions of newer antidepressants: anticholinergic, sedative and other side effects. Psychopharmacol Bull 20:280-290, 1984

Sellers EM, Busto U: Benzodiazepines and ethanol: assessment of the effects and consequences of psychotropic drug interaction. J Clin Psychopharmacol 2:249-262, 1982

Shinn AF, Shrewsbury RP: Evaluations of Drug Interactions. St. Louis, C.V. Mosby, 1985

Spring G, Frankel M: New data on lithium and haloperidol incompatibility. Am J Psychiatry 138:818-821, 1981

Stewart RB, Springer PK, Moskovitz RA: The value of expanded medication histories for psychiatric inpatients. Hosp Community Psychiatry 34:722-743, 1983

Taeuber K: Relevance of screening tests in human psychopharmacology: the psychological point of view [Human screening tests for the clinical investigation of nomifensine]. Symposia Medica Hoechst 10. Stuttgart, Schattauer Verlag, 1974

Telerman-Toppet N, Duret M, Coers C: Cimetidine interaction with carbamazepine. Ann Intern Med 94:544, 1981

Valsalan V, Cooper G: Carbamazepine intoxication caused by interaction with isoniazid. Br Med J 285:261-262, 1982

Vincent FM: Phenothiazine-induced phenytoin intoxication. Ann Intern Med 93:56-57, 1980

White K, Simpson G: Combined MAOI-tricyclic antidepressant treatment: a reevaluation. J Clin Psychopharmacol 5:264-282, 1981

Wong Y, Ludden T, Bell R: Effect of erythromycin on carbamazepine kinetics. Clin Pharmacol Ther 33:460-464, 1983

Afterword

by Philip A. Berger, M.D., Section Editor

Discussions of the side effects of medications can often paint a bleak and dismal picture. Drug side effects range from troublesome to fatal, and can create problems with patient compliance and with drug approval by government agencies. The chapters in this section are a comprehensive summary of the unwanted and sometimes dangerous pharmacological actions of the major psychotropic drug classes. The information presented is essential for good patient care, yet the summary necessarily concentrates on the negative rather than the positive aspects of psychopharmacology. The medications discussed in these chapters are responsible for a revolution in the care of patients suffering from anxiety, depression, mania, and schizophrenia. The studies that scientifically established the therapeutic efficacy of these medications are among the largest and most carefully conducted investigations in the history of pharmacology. These studies are responsible for the introduction of quantitative methods for the assessment of symptom patterns and severity in psychiatric patients. Finally, the study of these medications has led to enormous advances in human understanding of the mechanisms of the brain in both sickness and health (Berger, 1978).

This Afterword will briefly present one aspect of the future of psychopharmacology. It is a selected summary of recent case reports that propose pharmacological treatments that may ameliorate psychotropic drug side effects. Each of these treatments has yet to be confirmed with the type of systematic investigation necessary for establishing therapeutic efficacy. Nevertheless, in the course of clinical treatment, these proposed drug treatments for drug side effects may prove valuable for a particular patient.

One of the major problems with monoamine oxidase inhibitors (MAOIs) and tricyclic antidepressants (TCAs) is their tendency to cause sexual dysfunction. Several recent anecdotal reports suggest that the antihistamine and serotonin-blocking drug cyproheptadine may be a pharmacological remedy for some individuals with sexual dysfunction caused by antidepressants. In these case reports, cyproheptadine is described as restoring orgasmic function in both male and female patients with anorgasmia secondary to MAOI or TCA treatment (Sovner, 1985; DeCastro, 1985). Another report describes the reversal of anorgasmia by cyproheptadine in a woman treated with the MAOI phenelzine. This woman had the return of orgasmic function 48 hours after treatment with 2mg/day cyproheptadine at bedtime, but side effects of drowsiness, nasal congestion, and dry mouth and nose led to a reduction to 1mg/day. There is at least one other report that suggests that cyproheptadine may be a safe and effective antidote for sexual dysfunction with antidepressant drugs. While these reports are anecdotal, cyproheptadine might be tried in patients for whom anorgasmia is a problem complicating MAOI or TCA treatment.

Many patients taking MAOIs experience dizziness because of orthostatic hypotension. As pointed out by Blackwell in Chapter 33, this is a common complaint. It may affect as many as 11 percent of patients taking phenelzine, and 14 percent of patients taking tranylcypromine. The orthostatic hypotension usually appears during the first two months of treatment and can be less of a problem on maintenance therapy. Patients with MAOI-related orthostatic hypotension should have a thorough work-up to search for additional contributing factors, such as low calorie or low salt diet, dehydration, concomitant use of diuretics or antihypertensive drugs, hypothyroidism, or hypoadrenalism. Sometimes orthostatic hypotension can be treated by switching the time of the dose; that is, either dividing the dose or giving the entire dose at bedtime, depending on the pattern of the hypotension. Dose reduction can sometimes be helpful. Some patients benefit from the use of support stockings, while others find them inconvenient and uncomfortable. Pharmacological treatments that have been suggested for the orthostatic hypotension caused by MAOIs include salt tablets or fludrocortisone. The salt tablets and fludrocortisone expand the intravascular volume and can be quite effective for orthostatic hypotension in some patients who could not otherwise continue on the MAOI. However, both salt tablets and fludrocortisone can cause problems for elderly patients or for patients with kidney or heart disease (Evans et al, 1982; Rabkin et al, 1984).

Another troublesome side effect with MAOIs, again mentioned by Blackwell in Chapter 33, is the carpal tunnel syndrome (CTS). It has recently been suggested that the MAOI phenelzine may share pharmacological characteristics with other hydrazine drugs (isoniazid (INH), hydralazine) and may occasionally cause pyridoxine (vitamin B_6) deficiency. Pyridoxine deficiency can cause neuropsychiatric complications such as peripheral neuropathy, CTS, hyperacusis, irritability, depression and, in rare cases, convulsions, coma, and death. Recently, one group of investigators described CTS in several patients being treated with a nonhydrazine MAOI, tranylcypromine, which suggests that these patients may also develop pyridoxine deficiency (Harrison et al, 1983).

A number of patients have reported numbness, edema of the hands, and electric shock-like sensations (usually in the head and neck, but sometimes in the arms), which begin anywhere from six weeks to six months after the initiation of treatment with phenelzine. Several of the patients with these symptoms and with low plasma pyridoxine levels have been reported to be improved by the introduction of pyridoxine (Stewart et al, 1984). Interestingly, other patients with similar syndromes but without lowered pyridoxine levels did not respond to pyridoxine. There are no systematic studies of pyridoxine treatment of these troublesome neurological symptoms in patients taking MAOIs. However, an empirical trial of pyridoxine supplementation might be worthwhile in patients who develop symptoms that are similar to those described with pyridoxine deficiency.

Dry mouth is perhaps the most common complaint of patients taking TCAs, and is also a common complaint of patients taking neuroleptics and antiparkinsonism drugs. Many of these patients get into difficulties by self-treating this syndrome with sugar-containing hard candies and soft drinks. These treatments can lead to dental caries (Bassuk et al, 1978). Healthier ways to treat the dry mouth caused by TCAs, antiparkinsonism drugs, and neuroleptics include switching to medication with less anticholinergic activity, increasing hydration while avoiding sugar-containing beverages, and using saliva substitutes approved by the American Dental Association. Pharmacological approaches include administering bethanechol hydrochloride. Bethanechol has been reported to help some patients with dry mouth due to anticholinergic medications, and also to help some patients who have urinary retention or constipation. However, not all patients have benefited from this treatment (Everett, 1975).

Lithium carbonate and tricyclic antidepressants produce hand tremors that can be a problem for patients whose activities require fine hand muscle coordination. As described by Blackwell in Chapter 33, and by Jefferson and Griest in Chapter 34, hand tremors produced by tricyclic antidepressants or lithium carbonate can be diminished by dose reduction. In addition, propranolol, a beta-adrenergic blocking drug, may alleviate both tricyclic and lithium induced tremor (Kronfol et al, 1983).

Polydipsia and polyuria are common complaints of patients treated with lithium salts. As described by Jefferson and Griest in Chapter 34, this pharmacological action can be troublesome, annoying, or at times dangerous, causing dehydration and possibly leading to lithium toxicity. When dietary strategies do not work, treatment with amiloride, a potassium-sparing diuretic that acts on the cortical collecting tubule, has been reported to increase renal concentrating capacity in patients with lithium induced polyuria. Thiazide diuretics have the same effect but can lead to elevated serum concentrations of lithium, sometimes causing lithium toxicity. In addition, thiazide diuretics can ultimately produce hypokalemia. Thus, amiloride may be a superior pharmacological treatment for lithium induced nephrogenic diabetes insipidus (NDI), since it will not raise plasma concentrations of lithium or lower plasma concentrations of potassium in most patients (Battle et al, 1985).

Neuroleptic induced akathisia is an extremely dysphoric symptom. The inability to sit still, leading to agitation, restlessness, and extreme subjective discomfort, can cause severe suffering. As described by Levinson and Simpson in Chapter 32, akathisia sometimes responds to anticholinergic antiparkinsonism drugs, or to antihistamines; however, akathisia does not respond as well as other extrapyramidal syndromes. One recent case report suggests that the beta-blocker propranolol may be useful as a treatment for akathisia. Another patient with akathisia was treated with clonidine by the same group of investigators and also responded (Lipinski et al, 1983; Zubenko et al, 1985). Empirical trials of propranolol or clonidine for akathisia that does not respond to standard treatments may be useful.

The neuroleptic malignant syndrome (NMS) may be overdiagnosed, as suggested by Levinson and Simpson. However, a small minority of patients do develop a toxic syndrome including rigidity, fever, tachycardia, hypertension, and other medical complications. The most important treatment for these patients is careful symptomatic medical management. However, in the literature in case reports, a number of pharmacological agents have been reported to be effective. Dantrolene, bromocriptine, amantadine, pancuronium and, recently, the antihypertensive agent sodium nitroprusside have been reported to help in the management of this toxic syndrome (Blue et al, 1986; Coons et al, 1982; Khan et al, 1985; Lazarus, 1985; Sangal and Dimitrijevic, 1985; and Zubenko and Pope, 1983).

Drug treatments for anxiety, depression, mania, and schizophrenia that are free of troublesome and dangerous side effects are certainly a goal of new psychotropic drug development. Another goal of psychopharmacology research is to develop new categories of psychotropic drugs to treat disorders and illnesses that are not currently treated pharmacologically, or are only minimally affected

---

by available medications. Interestingly, the side effects of current psychotropic drugs give us clues to some of these new pharmacological categories.

The search for the mechanism of action of the benzodiazepines uncovered the endogenous benzodiazepine receptor in mammalian brain (Paul et al, 1986). Studies of ligands for this receptor have nearly succeeded in separating four major pharmacological actions of the benzodiazepines: sedation, anxiolytic activity, muscle relaxation, and anticonvulsant activity. Benzodiazepine antagonists can inhibit these actions of classical benzodiazepines, while recently synthesized inverse agonists have pharmacological activity that is opposite from classical benzodiazepine agonists. Animal studies suggest that a benzodiazepine counteragonist to the sedative actions may produce wakefulness or alertness (Paul et al, 1986). Amphetamines and cocaine also produce alertness but eventually cause paranoid psychosis (Berger and Dunn, 1986). Caffeine and other alkylxanthines produce alertness by inhibiting the inhibitory neurotransmitter adenosine, but also seem to produce anxiety (Daly et al, 1981). Will it be possible to separate the production of alertness from anxiety and paranoia with a benzodiazepine inverse agonist?

A major troublesome side effect of neuroleptic antipsychotics, antidepressants, and lithium salts is weight gain and carbohydrate craving. At least four antidepressants, none of which is currently in clinical use, may produce appetite suppression. This suggests that an effective appetite suppressant might be developed that does not produce the rapid tolerance seen when amphetamine and other psychostimulants are used in weight reduction regimens. Zimelidine, fluoxetine, nomifensine, and buproprion were all reported to produce an antidepressant effect while suppressing appetite. Zimelidine and nomifensine have been removed from worldwide clinical use because of other side effects, while fluoxetine and buproprion await approval by the FDA.

Neuroleptic antipsychotics often decrease aggressive behavior in patients with psychosis by reducing psychotic symptoms. Both lithium carbonate and carbamazepine have been suggested to reduce aggression in a more general way in populations of aggressive individuals. More carefully controlled prospective studies are needed, but these preliminary reports suggest that a medication to reduce aggression is possible (Eichelman, 1986).

The anticholinergic activity of psychotropic medications frequently mentioned in these chapters can lead to the side effect of cognitive disturbance, including memory problems in psychiatric patients. One human model for the memory disturbances found in Alzheimer's disease is based on the administration of the anticholinergic agent scopolamine to normal human subjects (Drachman and Leavitt, 1974). This and other considerations have led to numerous animal and human demonstrations that cholinomimetics can enhance memory in some subjects and under some circumstances (Berger et al, 1979). Benzodiazepines are reported to cause anterograde amnesia (Mac et al, 1985). The existence of the benzodiazepine receptor and the production of benzodiazepine inverse agonists may offer another approach to the search for a memory-enhancing medication.

The use of tricyclic antidepressants has recently increased in multidisciplinary clinics organized to care for patients with chronic pain syndromes who do not respond to conventional therapy. Tricyclic antidepressants, for example, are sometimes useful in the treatment of migraine headaches and painful diabetic neuropathies (Bonica and Chapman, 1986). Since the antidepressants used in this way do not produce morphine-like tolerance or withdrawal syndromes, a nonaddicting analgesic may be possible for certain pain syndromes.

REFERENCES

Bassuk E, Schoonover S: Rampant dental caries in the treatment of depression. J Clin Psychiatry 39:163-165, 1978

Battle DC, von Riott AB, Gaviria M, et al: Amelioration of polyuria by amiloride in patients receiving long-term lithium therapy. N Engl J Med 12:408-414, 1985

Berger PA: Medical treatment of mental illness. Science 200:974-981, 1978

Berger PA, Dunn MJ: The biology and treatment of substance abuse, in The American Handbook of Psychiatry, vol VIII. Edited by Berger PA, Brodie HKH. New York, Basic Books, 1986

Berger PA, Davis KL, Hollister LE: Cholinomimetics in mania, schizophrenia and memory disorders, in Nutrition and the Brain. Edited by A. Barbeau A, Growdon J, Wurtman R. New York, Raven Press, 1979

Blue MG, Schneider SM, Noro S, et al: Successful treatment of neuroleptic malignant syndrome with sodium nitroprusside. Ann Intern Med 104:56-57, 1986

Bonica JJ, Chapman CR: Biology, pathophysiology, and therapy of chronic pain, in: The American Handbook of Psychiatry, vol. VIII. Edited by Berger PA, Brodie HKH. New York, Basic Books, 1986

Coons DJ, Hillman FJ, Marshall RW: Treatment of neuroleptic malignant syndrome with dantrolene sodium: a case report. Am J Psychiatry 139:944-945, 1982

Daly JW, Bruns RF, Snyder S: Adenosine receptors in the central nervous system: relationship to central actions of methylxanthines. Life Sci 28:2083-2097, 1981

DeCastro R: Reversal of MAOI-induced anorgasmia with cyproheptadine (letter). Am J Psychiatry 142:783, 1985

Drachman DA, Leavitt J: Human memory and the cholinergic system. Arch Neurol 30:113, 1974

Eichelman B: The biology and somatic experimental treatment of aggressive disorders, in The American Handbook of Psychiatry, vol. VIII. Edited by Berger PA, Brodie HKH. New York, Basic Books, 1986

Evans DL, Davidson J, Raft D: Early and late side effects of phenelzine. J Clin Psychopharmacol 2:208-210, 1982

Everett HC: The use of bethanechol hydrochloride with tricyclic antidepressants. Am J Psychiatry 132:1202-1204, 1975

Harrison W, Stewart JW, Lovelace R, et al: A case report of carpal tunnel syndrome with tranylcypromine. Am J Psychiatry 140:1229-1230, 1983

Khan A, Jaffe JH, Nelson WH, et al: Resolution of neuroleptic malignant syndrome with dantrolene sodium: case report. J Clin Psychiatry 46:244-246, 1985

Kronfol Z, Greden JF, Zis AP: Imipramine-induced tremor: effects of a beta-adrenergic blocking agent. J Clin Psychiatry 44:225-226, 1983

Lazarus A: Neuroleptic malignant syndrome: detection and management. Psychiatric Annals 15:706-712, 1985

Lipinski JF, Zubenko GS, Cohen BM, et al: Propranolol in the treatment of neuroleptic-induced akathisia (letter). Lancet 1:685-686, 1983

Mac DS, Kumar R, Goodwin DW: Anterograde amnesia with oral lorazepam. J Clin Psychiatry 46:137-138, 1985

Paul SM, Crawley JN, Skolnick P: The neurobiology of anxiety: the role of the GABA/benzodiazepine receptor complex, in: The American Handbook of Psychiatry, vol. VIII. Edited by Berger PA, Brodie HKH. New York, Basic Books, 1986

Rabkin J, Quitkin F, Harrison W, et al: Adverse reactions to MAOIs: part I: a comparative study. J Clin Psychopharmacol 4:270-278, 1984

Sangal R, Dimitrijevic R: Neuroleptic malignant syndrome; successful treatment with pancuronium. JAMA 254:2795-2796, 1985

Sovner R: Treatment of tricyclic antidepressant-induced orgasmic inhibition with cyproheptadine (letter). J Clin Psychopharmacol 4:169, 1985

Stewart JW, Harrison W, Quitkin FM, et al: Phenelzine-induced pyridoxine deficiency. J Clin Psychopharmacol 4:225-226, 1984

Zubenko G, Pope HG Jr: Management of a case of neuroleptic malignant syndrome with bromocriptine. Am J Psychiatry 140:1619-1620, 1983

Zubenko GS, Cohen BM, Lipinski JF, et al: Use of clonidine in treating neuroleptic-induced akathisia. Psychiatry Res 13:253-259, 1985

Afterword

Afterword

by Robert E. Hales, M.D., and Allen J. Frances, M.D.

Volume 6 of the *Annual Review* has been both a great pleasure and a difficult challenge for us. We imagine that the exhausted, but, we hope, enlightened reader must by now share many of our own feelings toward the book. The rapid progress in psychiatry that is presented is a wonder and a delight, but it also places a heavy burden of responsibility upon all of us to stay current in the face of an almost exponentially growing literature.

In this spirit we are now already hard at work on Volume 7. Perhaps because this will be our last effort together as Co-Editors of the *Annual Review* series, we are hopeful that Volume 7 will be especially memorable. Certainly the choice of topics, section editors, and contributors gives us reason to expect a fine swan song. Section editors and topics include Drs. Katherine Shear and David Barlow on "Panic Disorder"; Dr. Martin Keller on "Unipolar Depression"; Drs. J. John Mann and Michael Stanley on "Suicide"; Drs. Robert Rose and Harold Pincus on "Electroconvulsive Therapy"; and Drs. A. John Rush and Aaron Beck on "Cognitive Therapy." Each of these areas has been enriched recently by important research findings, with direct clinical implications influencing the way in which all of us practice. We are learning a great deal in preparing Volume 7 and believe that you will find it helpful.

Until then.

Index

Alprazolam:
  alcohol and, 422
  antidepressant effects, 141
  beta-adrenergic receptor down-
    regulation, 170
  disinhibition of self- and other-directed
    violence, 516
Alzheimer, 260
Alzheimer's disease:
  CNS effects, 500
  immunity in, 227
  sleep disturbances in, 236-237
Amenorrhea, anorexia nervosa and, 193-
  195
American Psychiatric Association Task
  Force on Restraint and Seclusion, 522,
  554, 566
  principles for monitoring, 530-531
Amphetamines, 496
  schizophrenia, and dopamine, 179
  violent behavior and, 457
Amitriptyline, metabolization to
  nortriptyline, 160-161
Anaphylaxis, 210
  avoidance learning and, 219
  leukotrienes, 211, 212
  studies of, and hypothalamus, 214-215
Androgens, violence and, 453-454
Anemia, pernicious, 497, 500
Anergia, SAD and, 72-74
Anesthesia, general, and lithium, 94
Anger, recognition in self, by violent
  patient, 539
Anhedonia, 361, 503
Anorexia nervosa, 289
  DST and, 190
  endocrine abnormalities, 193-194
  general atrophy on CT scan, 267
Anorgasmia, MAOIs and, 421, 422
Antianxiety agents:
  side effects and interactions, 701-702,
    781
  violent patient, 515-516, 521
Antibodies, 211
  antinuclear, 224
  autoimmune, in schizophrenia, 226-227
  HTLV-III, 497
  suppression, by distressing
    environmental stimuli, 219
Anticholinergic system, antipsychotic side
  effects on, 717-718
Anticholinergics, neuroleptic-aggravated
  delirium, 518
Anticonvulsants, 27
  for treatment-refractory bipolar
    disorders, 127-143
  violent patient, 542
Antidepressants:
  bipolar III and, 13

buproprion, 737-738
development of, and side effects, 724
distinctly noradrenergic or
  serotonergically mediated, 166
dose–response relationship, 180-182
induction of rapid cycling by, 70-71
major characteristics of, 728
MAOIs, 725, 729-731
maprotiline, 738-739
noncompliance, 418
plasma levels, 171
second-generation, 727, 737-741
side effects and interactions, 700-701,
  724-743
structure and mechanism of action, 724-
  728
trazodone, 739-741
tricyclics, see Tricyclics
Antigens, specific, target, 211, 212
Antipsychotics:
  alpha-adrenergic-blocking properties,
    714
  anticholinergic effects, 717-718
  biological mechanism of action, 178-180
  cardiovascular effects, 713-716
  CNS effects, 719-721
  hepatotoxicity, 718-719
  plasma levels, 180-182
  pregnancy, lactation, fertility effects,
    720
  seizures, 719
  side effects and interactions, 698-700,
    704-721
  sudden death from, 716-717
Antisocial behavior, group treatments for,
  356
Antisocial personality disorder, 502-503
  hypoglycemia and, 454
Anxiety disorders:
  psychopharmacologic treatments, 419-
    423
  therapeutic techniques, 383-384
Anxiety management strategies, 382
Apathy, 280, 282
Apneas, sleep, 242-244, 251
  and alcohol, 244
Appendix, noradrenergic innervation, 217
Arousal, reticular formation and, 236
  See also Sleep–wake cycle
Arrhythmias, lithium-induced, 759-760
Arson, 447, 465
  frequency, 469
Assassination, 448, 465, 481-482
Assaults, 467-472
  aggravated, 469
  frequency of, 469, 470
  mental health settings, 510
  sexual, 447, 453, 458-459, 465, 469, 566
  simple, 466

Asthma, 212
  hypothalamus and, 214
  nocturnal, 247
ATP, see Adenotriphosphatase
Attention, impairment in, 280, 282
Attention deficit disorder (ADD), 503
  bipolar disorder and, 25-26
Authority, resistance to, 391, 392, 505
Autism:
  cell-mediated immune function, against
    myelin protein in, 227
  reversed brain asymmetry in, 273
Autoimmune disorders, 212
  of CNS, schizophrenia as, 226-227
Autoimmune processes, depression and,
  224
Avolition, 282

B cells, 211-213, 224
  changes, in schizophrenia, 226
Bacteria:
  humoral immunity against, 211-212
  intracellular, 212
BDH, see Buss–Durkee Hostility Inventory
BEAM, see Brain electrical activity
  mapping
Bedwetting, 247, 253
Behavior, organization and continuity of,
  318
Behavior therapy:
  applied to various diagnoses, 382-386
  brief, 406
  for depression, 383
Benzodiazepines:
  elective, oral, for agitated nonpsychotic,
    515
  endocrine effects, 200
  short-acting, 420
  side effects and interactions, 701-702,
    781-797
  withdrawal symptoms, 420
Bereavement:
  conjugal, and lymphocyte function, 220-
    221
  morbidity and mortality following, 221
  treatment format, 367
Biofeedback, 385-386
Biogenic amine theory, of depression,
  159, 188
Bion, W., 357
Bipolar disorders, 5-151
  age of onset, 92
  biological findings in, 32-56
  bipolar I, 10-12, 14-15, 20-21
  bipolar II, 10, 11, 14-15, 21
  bipolar III, 10
  chronobiology and, 245
  classification of, 10-16
  communication of information, in
    treatment, 108-110, 122

cyclothymia, 10, 13-14
diagnostic distinction, from unipolar, 6-
  7, 10, 13, 32-33, 53, 56, 62
disease model, 5
drug treatment, and therapeutic
  alliance, 108-111
follow-up care, 110-111
history of violence, 537
hydrogen proton behavior
  abnormalities, in, 286
hypothalamic effects of light, 65
lithium side effects, 746-768
lithium toxicity symptoms, 96
long-term course, effects of drugs on,
  38-40
maintenance (prophylactic) treatment
  of, 91-101
medication monitoring, 81, 93-96, 100,
  110
natural course of, 10, 20-21
personality and, 22-23
psychotherapeutic issues, 108-113
schizoaffective disorder and, 15-16
seasonality of, 72-75
sleep, and biological rhythms, 61-76
strengths and assets ameliorating, 115-
  117
subclassification of, 7
suicide prevention, 113-123
switch periods, 6, 63, 66, 68-69, 75-76
treatment of, 81-103, 108-111
treatment-resistant, 9, 81, 125-145
unipolar mania, 10, 13
valproic acid in, 138-140
ventricular enlargement in, 270
  See also Depression; Mania
Bipolarity, definition of, 10
Birth, complications of, 267, 283, 292-293
Body size, interpretation of biologic data
  and, 40
Bombings, 448, 465, 485-486
Bone marrow:
  lymphocytes in, 211
  noradrenergic innervation, 217
Borderline personality disorder, 409
  manic depression and, 26
  unstable, 503
Bowlby, John, 355
Box-score method, of research review, 358
Brain:
  atrophy of structures forming lateral
    ventricle boundaries, 291-292
  corpus callosum abnormalities, 284-285
  evoked potential mapping, 300, 308-312
  frontal lobes, and schizophrenia, 279-
    282
  functional imaging techniques, 158, 300-
    319
  gender differences, 282, 285
  hemispheres of, 273, 284

imaging techniques, 260-319
impaired capacity to grow, 282-283, 292-293
interhemispheric communication, 284-285
noninvasive approaches to, 287
schizophrenia as autoimmune disorder of, 226-227
septal region high-affinity globulin, 226
sleep-promoting areas, 239
structural imaging techniques, 158, 260-293
structure of, changes in schizophrenia, 262-274
theta activity, and sleep, 241
Brain electrical activity mapping (BEAM), 280
diagnosis of violent patient, 497
Breathing:
control systems, 243
sleep and, 242-244, 251
Bruxism, sleep-related, 253
Bulimia, DST and, 190
Bullying, 458
Buproprion:
norepinephrine down-regulation, 170
overdose, 738
side effects and interactions, 737-738
Buss–Durkee Hostility Inventory (BDH), 453
Bystanders, effect on violence, 459-460

Calcitonin, 42
Calcium:
abnormality, in depression and/or (hypo)mania, 41
hypercalcemia, 204
hypocalcemia, 42
metabolism, lithium effects, 756
Calcium-channel blockers, 42, 142-143
Carbamazepine:
acute antidepressant effects, 130
antikindling properties, 38
antimanic effects, 127-130
compliance, 136
cycle-frequency reduction, 39
hepatitis from, 136, 138
interactions and side effects, 135-138, 700, 768-777
phenytoin versus, 140-141
predictors of antdepressant response to, 131
prophylaxis, 130-132
side effects, 135-138
supplemental thyroid and, 137
for treatment-refractory bipolar disorders, 127-138
violent patient, 542-543
Carbohydrates:
craving for, and SAD, 72-74

metabolism, lithium effects, 756-757
Castration, hormonal, for sex offenders, 453
CAT, see Computerized axial tomography
Catatonia, prolonged, 289
Catecholamines, increased excretion from peripheral ANS, 168
Cells:
B, 211-213, 224
mast, 211
natural killer (NK), 212-216
T, 211-213, 224
white, lithium and, 758-759
Central nervous system (CNS):
antipsychotic side effects on, 719-721
disorders of, 499, 500
feedback with immune system, 210, 223-224
MAOI side effects, 729-730
modulation of immunity by, 210, 214-219
norepinephrine, as signal modulator, 53-54
Cerebellum, changes, on CT, 272-273
Cerebrospinal fluid (CSF), neurotransmitter/depression studies, 47-53
Cerebrum:
asymmetries of, 273, 284
size, in schizophrenia, 282
Change:
adaptation to, 318
defining markers of, 391, 392
family- and lifestyle-related, 366
intensity and, 403
levels of, 387
process of, 387
Character change:
and brief therapies, 407
and therapist's gender, 430, 440
Children:
abuse of, 447, 457-458, 505, 565, 566
adopted-away, of mentally disordered parent, 650
of alcoholics, 364
autistic, 227, 273
bipolar disorders in, 25-26
cruelty in, 458
of depressed mothers, 655
depressive-equivalent assaultiveness in, 502
DST in, 189
family therapy with, 355
gender of, 658
homicide and, 481
individual differences in response, 658-659
lithium in, 541-542
of mentally disordered, 647-660
treatment format, 467-468

disinhibition, 68
hypercortisolism, 188, 201
levels, and recirculating lymphocyte
    traffic, 222
as marker of CNS serotonergic function,
    46
rhythms of, 244
Costs:
    chronic care, 346
    deinstitutionalization and institutional
        care, 348
    hospitalization, 336, 343
    third-party payers, 332, 333, 336, 342,
        398, 401, 406
Counterconditioning, 387
Countertransference:
    with bipolar patients, 111-112, 122-123
    violent patient, 449, 507, 513, 539, 543-
        544
Couples therapy, 362
    for agoraphobia, 363-364
    treatment length, 406
Creativity, lithium effects on, 749
CRF, see Corticotropin-releasing factor
Crime:
    expressive, 448
    instrumental, 448
    organized, 485
    racial inequality and stress, 459
    social control of, 459-460
Crime in the United States, F.B.I., 468
Crime Watch, 460
Criminal Victimization in the United States,
    468
Crisis home, 341
Crisis intervention, 339-342
    character changes, 407
    defined, 34
    length of treatment, 406
    setting, 438
Crisis management strategies, 363
Criticism:
    in families of schizophrenics, 349, 360-
        361
    inability to tolerate, 505
Cruelty:
    childhood, 458
    violent offenders, 456
CSF, see Cerebrospinal fluid
Cucalon v. State, 550
Cushing's syndrome, 188, 189, 203-204
    CNS effects, 500
    DST and, 191
    pseudo-, 201
    violence associated with, 453
Cyclicity:
    of mania and depression, 6-7, 61
    in violent feelings, 115
Cycling, rapid, 46, 62-63, 67-71, 416
    doses of thyroid and, 46

kindling, 38
sleep and, 62-63
sleep deprivation and, 67
Cytotoxicity reactions, T cells in, 212

Dangerousness, prediction of, 506-507
Davis v. Hubbard, 551, 553, 554, 555
Death:
    of spouse, 220-221
    sudden, as antipsychotic side effect,
        716-717
Deinstitutionalization, 347, 348
    limits of, 438-439
Delirium, violence and, 500
Delusional depression,
    psychopharmacology of, 415-416
Delusions, violence and, 457
Dementia, violence and, 500
Demographic characteristics, therapist–
    patient, 381
Dependency, patient–therapist, 381
Depression:
    acute, 87-91, 130
    alcohol and, 110
    animal models of, 54
    antidepressant effects of light, 245
    antidepressant effects of sleep
        deprivation, 64, 66-68
    bereavement and, 221
    bipolar, acute, 87-91
    body rhythms and, 61
    breakthrough, 87, 98-100
    circadian phase-advance hypothesis, 63-
        66, 73-74, 245
    cognitive modification therapies for, 383
    delusional, 415-416
    dopamine in, 159, 167-168
    drug decision-tree approach, 88-89
    EEG abnormalities, 62-63
    fall–winter, 72
    family treatments for, 362
    hospitalization for, 90
    inborn need, extra interpersonal
        support and encouragement, 369
    increased peripheral ANS
        catecholamine excretion, 168
    late spring attacks, 72
    low brain norepinephrine/serotonin,
        159, 160, 166, 169-171
    maternal, 368, 655
    neurobiology of sleep disturbances in,
        249, 254
    neuroendocrine abnormalities in, 44-46,
        188-195
    norepinephrine theory of, 159, 160, 169-
        170
    polarity change, to mania, 13
    pretreatment evaluation, importance of,
        81-82, 88, 93, 94
    pseudounipolar, 56

clinical decisions and side effects, 741-743
concurrent, 415
differential therapeutics, 415-425
endocrine effects, 198-200
hyperprolactinemia-inducing, 196
interactions, 96-97, 415
interpreting biologic data, 40
lithium, and other, 96-97
pharmacological bridge, 35-40
psychotropics, 334
side effects, *see* Side effects, drug
systems vulnerable to, 81
with three classes of action on bipolar illness, 38-39
violent behavior and, 457, 472, 475-476, 566
violent patient, 515-522
See also Psychopharmacology
DSM-II, *see Diagnostic and Statistical Manual of Mental Disorders, Second Edition*
DSM-III, *see Diagnostic and Statistical Manual of Mental Disorders, Third Edition*
DST, *see* Dexamethasone suppression test
Duration, of treatment, 332, 334, 398-412
conclusions and recommendations concerning, 411-412, 439-440
covariables, and factors increasing or decreasing, 399
research on, 400-401
Dysarthria, intoxication and, 495
Dyslexia, reversed brain asymmetry in, 273
Dysphoria:
acting out, 505
versus true depression, 418
Dysregulation, of biologic systems, in bipolar disorders, 33

Eating disorders, therapeutic techniques, 384
ECA, *see* Epidemiological Catchment Area study
Eclecticism:
meaning of term, 389
systematic therapeutic, 387-388
technical, 386, 387
Edema:
lithium-induced, 758
MAOIs and, 421, 422
PMS and, 455
Education:
for diagnostic interviewer, 598-599
violence and, 458, 459
EE, *see* Emotion, high expressed
Ego, strengths and motivation, low, 409
Egocentricity, violence and, 505
Ejaculation, premature, 385
Electroencephalogram (EEG),

computerized, 300, 308-312
Electrolytes:
and bipolar disorders, 41-42
imbalances in, and lithium or carbamazepine, 84
Emergency care, violent patient, 510-532
assessment, 512-514
choice of intervention, 511-512
medication intervention, 515-522
physical intervention, 522-532
seclusion versus restraint, 531-532
technique, 514-515
Emotion:
high expressed, and schizophrenia, 349
lability of, 505
overcontrolled, 491, 497
Endocrine system:
abnormalities in schizophrenia, 195-198
affective disorder abnormalities, 188-195
diseases of, psychiatric abnormalities in, 202-204
effect on immune processes, 221
effects of psychiatric medications on, 198-200
endocrinopathies, 500
endogenous-hormone allergy, and PMS, 455
hypothalamus and, 214
lithium effects on, 754-758
rhythms during sleep, 246
Endocrinology:
of aging, 201-202
See also Psychoendocrinology
Endorphins:
in bipolar disorders, 41, 43-45
schizophrenia and, 197
Enuresis, sleep-related, 247, 253
Environment:
adopted-away children, 650-651
parental mental disorder and, 649-657
Epidemiologic Catchment Area (ECA) study, 610-623
historical context, 611-613
methods, 614-617
prevalence of specific disorders, 617-621
research objectives, 614
results, 617-622
scientific context, 613
Epidemiology, psychiatric
basic concepts, 575-576, 625-627
bipolar disorders, 10, 23-24, 72
clinical research and, 584-585
clinical uses, 610-611
defined, 574, 625
genetic, 625-642
history of, 580-584
method and scope, 574-575
overview of, 574-585, 625-627
prevention, overview, 664-666
seasonal trends, in mania and

specific psychiatric disorders and, 224-227

stimulatory effect of lithium, 101

stress and, 219-223

Immunity:
cell-mediated, 211, 212, 219
humoral, 211-212, 214-215, 219, 226

Immunization, as experimental paradigm, 213

Immunoglobulin (Ig):
abnormal, in schizophrenics, 226-227

Impulse control, 491, 503, 505

Incidence, defined, 23

Indifference, 280

Infanticides, 481

Informed consent, 553
with manic patients, 87

Initiative, lack of, 317

Insight:
poor, 317
regarding dynamics of violence, 539-540, 545

Insomnias, 246-247, 250-251
light therapy for, 249
mania and, 62

Institutionalization, see Hospitalization

Insulin:
lithium and, 756-757
resistance, in depression, 192-193

Integration, neurologic/immunologic, in biological adaptation, 210

Interactions, psychoactive drug, clinically significant, 802-813
antipsychotics, 720-721

Interferon:
feedback between immune system and CNS, 223
T cell release of, 212

Interleukin-1 (IL-1), lymphocyte-activating factor, 212, 213

Intermittent explosive disorder, 499
ego-dystonic violence, 503

Interpersonal therapy
applied to various diagnoses, 382-386
treatment manual, 380

Intervention programs, violence, 565

Interviews, clinical, 589-606
modification for epidemiologic use, 596
See also Diagnostic interviews

Intoxication
idiosyncratic, 500, 502
lithium, 752-753
obvious signs of, 495

Iprindole, norepinephrine down-regulation, 170

Jamison v. Farabee, 553

Jealousy, abnormal, 363-364

Jet lag, 64, 247, 249
chronobiology and, 245

Judgment, poor, 317

Kidnapping, 465

Killers:
mercy, 485
serial, 465, 484-485
set-and-run, 483-484
See also Murder

Kindling:
amygdala, paradigm, 143
MAOI or TCA, 38

Kinins, 211

Korsakoff's syndrome, CNS effects, 500

Kraepelin, Emil, 5, 10
department of psychiatry, 260

La Cosa Nostra, 485

Lactation, antipsychotic side effects on, 720

Language:
increase in verbal ability, 449
lateralization of, in brain, 261, 273

Lateralization, in cognitive task performance, 261, 273, 284-285

Latitude, seasonality of suicide and, 72

LC, see Locus coeruleus

Lectins, plant, 213
of violence by psychiatric patients, 549-562

Legal considerations:
mechanical restraint or seclusion, 523, 523, 528, 530
Tarasoff, 447, 543, 545, 546, 557-558

Lethargy, 361

Leukocytes:
abnormal, in peripheral blood of disordered, 224
abnormal, in schizophrenics and their relatives, 226
depression and, 169
See also Immune system

Lewin, Kurt, 356

LH, see Luteinizing hormone

LHRH, see Luteinizing-hormone-releasing hormone

Libido:
diminished, and neuroleptics, 199
loss of, 202

Librium rage, 516

Life chart:
retrospective, 125-127, 144
in pretreatment evaluation of bipolar disorders, 81

Life narrative, psychodynamic, 408

Light, phototherapy, 249
for breakthrough depressions, 99-100
brightness and duration of, and depression, 72
hypothalamic effects, in manic-depressives, 65
natural, timing and/or duration of, 73

phase response curve, 245
for SAD patients, 72-75
sleep deprivation and, 75
treatment-resistant bipolar patients and,
81
utility in clinical disorders, 245
Light–dark cycle:
affective illness and, 61
chronobiology and, 244-245
Lithium:
breakthrough depressions and, 87, 96,
98-100
cardiovascular effects, 759-760
combined with a MAOI, 88, 89
compliance, 96, 108, 112-113, 118, 136,
363
creativity, effect on, 749
cycle-frequency reduction, 39
diabetes, insulin, and carbohydrate
effects, 756-757
dry mouth from, 754
edema from, 757, 758
effects on norepinephrine, 54-55
endocrine effects, 199, 754-758
general anesthesia and, 94
genetic factors, in response to, 88
goiter, 755-756
hematologic effects, 758-759
holidays, 100-101
interactions and side effects, 95-98, 112,
136, 700, 746-768
intoxication, 752-753
intracranial hypertension, 752
maintenance (prophylactic) treatment
with, 91-101
management of mania with, 82-86
monitoring, maintenance, 93-96, 100
neuroleptics with, 86
neurological effects, 749-753
ocular effects, 753-754
other effects, 97-98
during pregnancy, 138
rapid-cycling patients on, 70
renal tubular function, 81, 83
side effects, management of, 95-96, 112
sodium and, membrane processes, 42-
43
stimulatory effect, on immune system,
101
studies on effects of, 6
T1 relaxation time and, 286-287
tardive dyskinesia and, 751-752
taste, effects on, 754
thirst induced by, 96, 754
thyroid effects, 96, 112, 754-756
timing of the dose, 100
toxicity, treatment of, 96
tremor, 750
valproate with, 138
violent patient, 541-542

weight gain from, 96, 112, 757-758
Liver, mania and, 84
Locus coeruleus (LC):
age-related degenerative changes, 189-
190
inhibition of antigravity musculature,
240
signal-to-noise ratio, and
norepinephrine, 53
Luteinizing hormone (LH):
effects of substance abuse, 200
sleep-related secretion pattern, 246
Luteinizing-hormone-releasing hormone
(LHRH), 200
in hypothalamus of postmenopausal
women, 202
Lymph nodes, noradrenergic innervation,
217
Lymphocytes:
age-related changes in function, 225
bereavement and, 220-221
cytotoxic, 212
function, in depression, 224
hormone and neurotransmitter
receptors on, 210
peripheral blood, in schizophrenia, 226
recirculating traffic, 221-222
stimulation, in vitro technique, 213
types of, 211
See also Immune system

Macrophages, 211, 212
Magnesium, abnormality, in depression
and/or (hypo)mania, 41-42
Magnesium pemoline, paranoid psychosis
from, 179
Magnetic resonance imaging (MRI), in
psychiatry, 260-261, 275-293
approaches to research using, 279-287
principles of, 275-279
Malformation, fetal, lithium-induced, 759,
765-766
Mania:
acute, 82-87, 127-130
body rhythms and, 61
breakthrough, management of, 87, 96,
98-100
delirious, 11
diagnostic features, 12
differentiation from nonorganic
psychiatric syndromes, 18
first bipolar disorder episode, 92
high brain norepinephrine/serotonin
theory, 159, 160, 169-171
hospitalization for, 87
hyperactivity of, and pregnancy, 84
hypomania and, 10, 16-19
nature and severity of symptoms, 82
norepinephrine/dopamine agonist
precipitation of, 37-38, 50

organic causes, 16-18
plasma and CSF norepinephrine in, 50
premorbid cyclothymic personality, 14
sleep deprivation and, 67
sleep reduction in, 62
spring-summer, 72
treatment and prevention of, 67, 82-87
unipolar, 10, 13
Manuals, treatment, 364, 380
MAOIs, *see* Monoamine oxidase inhibitors
Maprotiline, side effects and interactions, 738-739
Marathon sessions, 398, 402
Markers, change, in psychotherapy, 391, 392
Marriage:
  bereavement, 220-221, 367,
  couples therapy, 354, 362-364, 406
  disruption of, 458-459
  marital conflict, 369
  spouse abuse, 447, 458, 565, 566
  See also Family
Martial arts, 466
Masochism, 409
Mass media, violence and, 458, 565
Mass murder, 483-484
Mast cells, 211
Maternal depression, accidents to children and, 655
Maternal intoxication or addiction, effects on fetus, 652-653
Maturation, stress and, 407-408
Media, mass, violence and, 458, 565
Medical problems, 408
  dysphoria attending, 418
  psychotherapeutic techniques for, 385-386
Medication strategies, violent patient, 515-522
Melatonin:
  circadian rhythm, 65
  light–dark cycle and, 245
  nocturnal pineal secretion, and phototherapy, 74
  in SAD patients, 73
Membrane transport, bipolar disorders and, 41-43
Men, *see* Gender
Menstrual cycle, 97
  amenorrhea, 193-195
  associated psychoses, 141
  LHRH in hypothalamus of postmenopausal women, 202
  lithium mood change intensification, 97
  neuroleptic effects, 199
  phases of, and affective symptoms, 61
  PMS, 195, 454-455
  prolactin and, 196
  rapid manic-depressive cycling and, 69
  violent feelings and, 115, 454-455

Mental health:
  successful prevention in, 666-667
  See also Epidemiology
Mental health services:
  intervention programs, 565
  use of (ECA), 621
Meta-analysis:
  of low MHPG and imipramine response, 165
  of MHPG levels in depression, 161-165
  research review by, 358
  of results, various therapy forms, for depression, 383
Methyldopa, precipitation of depression, 35
Mianserin, norepinephrine synthesis, 170
Migraine, 267
Mills v. Rogers, 553
Minnesota Multiphasic Personality Inventory, Overcontrolled Hostility Scale, 497
Mitogens, 213
MMPI, *see* Minnesota Multiphasic Personality Inventory
Modeling procedures, 382
Monoamine oxidase inhibitors (MAOIs), 725, 729-731
  in depression, 88-90
  effects on norepinephrine, 54-55
  genetic factors, 88
  and kindling, 38
  organ effects, 729-730
  overdose, 730
  withdrawal from, 730
Monocytes, 211
Mood:
  diurnal rhythms in, 61, 244
  fluctuations, calendar for assessing, 126
  multiple sclerosis and, 83
  sleep and, 66
  stress effects of, and lithium, 101
Morbid risk, defined, 23
Motivation, of violent patient, in psychotherapy, 538
Mouth, dry, from lithium, 754
MRI, *see* Magnetic resonance imaging
Multiple sclerosis, 267
  associated mood lability, and lithium, 83
  CNS effects, 500
  mania and, 16, 17
  NMRI and, 290, 291
Murder, 477-481
  mass, 448, 465, 483-484
  serial, 465, 484-485, 565
Murder–suicide, 483, 502
Myasthenia gravis:
  lithium neuromuscular effects, 751
  mania and, 83

Organic brain syndrome (OBS), substance-induced, 495
Organization, and continuity, of behavior, 318
Orgasm, dysfunction, 385
   anorgasmia, 421
   and neuroleptics, 199
Outpatients, committed, 561-562
Overcontrolled Hostility Scale, of MMPI, 497
Overdose:
   buproprion, 738
   MAOI, 730
   maprotiline, 739
   toxicity in, 702
   trazodone, 741
Overinvolvement, families of schizophrenics, 349, 360-361

Pacemaker, circadian rhythm, 64-65
   mammalian, 245
Panic disorder, psychopharmacologic treatments, 420-423
Panic management procedures, 364
Paradoxical injunctions, 382
Paradoxical sleep, 235
Paranoia, mass murders and, 483
Parasomnias, 247, 252
Parsons, Talcott, 356
Parathyroid gland:
   hyperfunction, and hypercalcemia, 204
   lithium effects on, 756
Parental mental disorder:
   clinical implications, 651, 656-657, 659
   effects on adopted-away children, 650-651
   environmental effects, 649-657
   exposure to specific symptoms of parents, 652-657
   fetal effects, 652
   genetic mechanisms, 648-651
   individual differences in children's responses, 658-659
   protective features against, 658-659
   as psychiatric risk factor, 647-660
   statistical association, 647-648
Parkinson's disease, as dopamine-deficiency state, 178
Parkinsonism, mania and, 83
Patient:
   belief system of, 381, 392
   likelihood of spontaneous improvement, 410
   oppositional, 410
   patient's role, 391, 392
   personal characteristics of, 380-382, 384, 386
   personality match, with therapist, 430, 431

at risk for no, or negative, response, 409
   role induction, 392
   suicidal, 108, 113-123
   technique choice, and patient variables, 379, 386
   treatment preference of, 371, 392
   variables, and treatment duration, 399
   violent, 447-562
Pavor nocturnus, 247, 253
Payne Whitney Clinic, differential therapeutics course, 431-432
PCP, see Phencyclidine
PEG, see Pneumoencephalography
Pellagra, 500
Penis:
   erectile and ejaculatory dysfunction, and neuroleptics, 199
   nocturnal tumescence, 236, 253
Peptides, bipolar disorders and, 41, 43-45-47
Personality:
   bipolar disorders and, 22-23
   value of specific therapies and, 381, 390, 391
Personality disorders:
   overcontrolled types of, 457
   treatment format, 365
   violence and, 457, 537-538
PET, see Positron emission tomography
PHA, see Phytohemagglutinin
Pharmacodynamics, defined, 160
Pharmacokinetics, defined, 160
Pharmacological bridge, between neurotransmitters and depression, 35-40
Pharmacology, see Psychopharmacology
Pharmacotherapy, mania and depression, 81
Phase advance, circadian-oscillator, 63-66, 73-74, 245, 249, 254
Phase-delay syndrome:
   chronobiology and, 245
   in night owls, 245, 247-249
Phencyclidine (PCP), 495
   toxic screen for, 496
Phenelzine, side effects, 421
Phenytoin:
   antimanic action, and carbamazepine, 140-141
   episodic dyscontrol syndrome, 542
Phobias:
   exposure treatments, 382, 389
   therapeutic techniques, 382
Phototherapy, 65, 72, 245, 249
   for breakthrough depressions, 99-100
   for SAD, 72-75
   sleep deprivation and, 75
   treatment-resistant bipolar patients and, 81

Physostigmine, 179-180
  influence on affective states, 171
Phytohemagglutinin (PHA), 213, 215, 220,
  222, 224, 225
Placebo, response to, in depression, 178
PMS, *see* Premenstrual tension syndrome
Pneumoencephalography (PEG), 261
Pokeweed mitogen (PWM), 213, 224, 225
Polypharmacy, 415
Polyuria, lithium-induced, 95, 136
Ponto–geniculo–occipital (PGO) waves,
  REM sleep and, 241-242
Positron emission tomography (PET), 261,
  280, 300-308
  psychiatric research employing, 302-308
Posttraumatic stress disorder, 503
  assault victims, 472
Potassium, in manic-depressive illness,
  41-42
Poverty, violence and, 458-459, 475, 565
Power, struggles over, with bipolar
  patients, 111
Pratt, Joseph, 355-356
Prediction, of violent behavior, 494, 504,
  565
Pregnancy:
  antipsychotic side effects on, 720
  complications of, 652-653
  developmental abnormalities,
    schizophrenia and, 282-283, 292-293
  DST and, 189, 191
  lithium effects on fetus, 84, 138, 759,
    765-766
  prolactin in, 196
Premenstrual tension syndrome (PMS),
  195
  violence and, 454-455
President, and other public figures,
  threats to, 467
Prevalence:
  point, definition of, 23
  specific disorders (ECA), 617-621
Prevention:
  psychiatric disorders, 664-673
  of violence, 459, 512, 514-515, 565
Problem-solving therapy, brief, 406
Process S, sleep-inducing, homeostatic,
  245
Progabide, antidepressant properties, 141-
  142
Progesterone, deficiency, 455
Prolactin:
  depression and, 45, 46
  hyperprolactinemia, 196
  inhibition, 68
  neuroleptics and, 198-199
  PMS and, 195
  in SAD patients, 73
  schizophrenia and, 195-197
  sleep and, 246

Prophylaxis:
  in bipolar disorders, 91-101
  carbamazepine, 130-132
  pharmacoprophylaxis and affective
    illness course, 143
Propranolol:
  precipitation of depression, 35
  violent patient, 543
Protection, child of mentally disordered,
  651, 655-657, 659
Proteins, abnormal, in schizophrenia, 226-
  227
Pseudocommandos, 483
Psychiatric disorders:
  assessment of diagnosis, 589-607
  disaster research findings, 676-687
  ECA study, 610-623
  epidemiology of, 572-691
  genetic epidemiology, 625-642
  measures of, 567, 576-577
  parental, as risk factor, 647-660
  preventing, 664-673
Psychodynamic life narrative, 408
Psychodynamic therapy:
  applied to various diagnoses, 382-386
  brief, 407-408
  treatment manual, 380
Psychoeducation, 341, 349, 362-363
Psychoendocrinology, in clinical
  psychiatry, 188-205
  See also Endocrine system
Psychoimmunology, in clinical psychiatry,
  210-228
Psychopathology, violent crime expressive
  of, 448
Psychopharmacology:
  in clinical psychiatry, 159-183
  differential therapeutics, 415-425
  mania and depression, 81
  research in, 331
  side effects and interactions, 698-821
Psychosis:
  premenstrual, 195
  postpartum or perimenstrually related,
    141
  supposed, and murder, 485
Psychosomatic disorders, 356
Psychotherapy:
  for bipolar disorders, 108, 111-112
  brief, 406-408
  categories of, 382
  continuous or intermittent, 401, 403-404
  in-depth, contraindicated for the
    suicidal, 121
  indicators for, 390-391
  long-term, 401, 404-405
  patients at risk for no or negative
    response, 409
  prescriptive methods, 380-389
  open-ended, 404

supportive, 403-404, 411
treatment holidays, 405
PWM, *see* Pokeweed mitogen

Question design, diagnostic interviews, 598

Race, violence and, 458-459, 471, 475-476, 480
Rape, 447, 453, 465, 566
frequency, 469
Rapid-cycling affective disorder:
and biological rhythms, 68-71
treatment of, 71
Rapid-eye-movement (REM) sleep, 61-62
acetylcholine and, 240-242
arousal during, 235
cholinergic systems and, 240-242
density, 62, 73, 235-236, 249
deprivation, 68
duration of, 98
latency, 62-64, 73, 98, 235, 244, 245, 249, 254
narcolepsy and, 254
neurobiology of, 236-242
peripheral muscle atonia, 235, 240-241
timing and amount of, 61-64
Regional cerebral blood flow (RCBF), 261, 280, 300, 313-316
diagnosis of violent patient by, 497
Regression:
iatrogenic, 403
need for, 407
Rehabilitation:
clinical considerations, 343-344
inpatient, 342-343
interrupting the sick role, 343
partial hospital, 343
research data, 344-346
settings, 337, 342-346
Relapse/recurrence:
among bipolar patients, 20
prevention, in depression, 90-91
schizophrenic, predicting, 424
Relatives:
mentally disordered, 647-660
See also Heredity
Relaxation training, 383, 385-386
Remission:
psychomotor stimulants and, 179
spontaneous, 410
Research:
approaches to, using MRI, 279
bipolar illness, 5-6
design, in biologic psychiatry, 577-580, 584
on differential therapeutics, 433-435
disaster, epidemiologic findings, 676-687
genetic epidemiology, future, 641-642

limitations of, 333
psychiatric preventive trial, 667-668, 671-673
psychotherapy design, 331-332
sleep, 235-236, 247-248, 250-254
on treatment formats, 372
on violence, 565
See also Studies
Reserpine, depression and, 35, 159
Restraint, of violent patient, 522-532
incidence of, 524
legal regulation of, 554-555
precipitants to, 526-527
technique, 528-530
versus seclusion, risks and benefits, 531-532
Reticular formation:
arousal and, 236
REM sleep and, 241-242
Rhythms, biological, 97-98
bipolar disorders and, 6, 7, 61-76
circadian, *see* Circadian rhythms
light and, 73
menstrual cycle, 61, 69, 97, 115,141, 193-196, 199, 202, 454-455
violence and, 469-470
See also Sleep–wake cycle
Risk:
factor, psychiatric, parental disorder as, 647-660
individual psychiatric, assessing, 611
morbid, defined, 23
physical, to children of mentally disordered, 655
rapid neuroleptization, 518-522
suicide, 113-115, 117-118
of violence, 504-506
Robbery, 472-476
career criminals' work, 465, 472
frequency, 469, 470
Rogers v. Commissioner, 553, 554
Romeo, Nicholas, 550-551
Rules, animal ability to develop, and change, 318

SAD, *see* Seasonal affective disorder
Sadists, psychopathic sexual, 484-485
Sadness, versus true depression, 418
Safety:
of potential victims, 511, 545-546
therapist's, 447, 495, 510, 511, 539, 544-545, 566
Sampling, population, ECA, 614-615
Schizoaffective disorder:
bipolar disorder and, 15-16
ventricular enlargement in, 270
Schizophrenia:
aggravation of, by dopaminergic activity increase, 179
altered immunity and, 226-227

Theories:
of differential therapeutics, 386
See also Hypotheses
Therapeutic alliance, 392
countertransference, 111-112, 122-123,
449, 507, 513, 539, 543-544
in drug treatment of bipolar disorders,
108-111
as predictor of outcome, 430
transference, 356, 407, 430, 440, 513,
539, 545
Therapist:
belief system of, 381, 392
co-variables, and treatment duration,
399
flexibility in, 438
gender of, 430, 440
inappropriate reactions, to violent
patient, 543
personal characteristics of, 380-382, 384,
386
personality match, with patient, 430
potential liability, for violent patient,
549-551
relative lack of skill in, 409
role, 391, 392
safety of, 447, 510, 539, 544-545, 566
for suicidal bipolar patient, 111-112,
119, 121-123
variables, and technique choice, 379
violent patient's, 492-493, 495, 507
Therapy:
brief, 398, 401, 406-408
couples, 354, 362, 406
directive and nondirective procedures,
392
dosage of, 334, 398-412
family, 349, 354-355, 360, 406
group, 349, 355-357
individual, 354, 359-360
maintenance, 337
mode of delivery, 353-372
occupational, 349
See also Treatment
Theta activity, sleep and, 241
Thirst, lithium-induced, 136
Threats, of violence, to public figures, 467
Thymus:
lymphocytes from, 211
noradrenergic innervation to, 217
Thyroid extract, endocrine effects, 199-200
Thyroid gland:
diseases of, 69, 203
lithium effects on, 754-756
maintaining optimal function in bipolar
patients, 143
and rapid cycling, 69
Thyroid-stimulating hormone (TSH), 45,
46
disinhibition, 68

rhythms of, 244
test, diagnosing thyroid, nonthyroid,
and depressive diseases, 190-192
Time, psychotherapy and, 398-412
Timing, of violence, 469-470
Toxic screen:
indications for, 500
for violent patient, 496
Training in Community Living (TCL), 341
Tranquilization, rapid, with neuroleptics,
516-522
paradoxical effect, 519
Tranquilizers–sedatives, violent behavior
and abuse of, 457
Transference, 407, 440
in group therapy, 356
mutual, difficulties with, 430
therapist's gender and, 430
violent patient, 513, 539, 545
Transplantation reactions, cell-mediated
immune response, 212
Trazodone, side effects and interactions,
739-741
Treatment, 331-440
administrative issues, 435-436
of bipolar disorders, 81-103
clinical issues, 335, 428-431
differential therapeutics, 331-440
duration, 332, 334, 398-412
educational issues, 335, 431-433
format, 332, 334, 353-372
frequency, 334, 402-403
global orientations, and diagnosis, 382-
386
goals of, 336, 359, 392, 399, 430
holidays from, 405
involuntary, 560-562
long-term, violent patient, 537-546
medication, 334, 415-425
none, 334, 401, 408-410
phase of, and course of illness, 361, 371
plan, 391-393
premature standardization of, 333
preparing patient for, 392-393
psychiatric, specificity of, 332
reliability, lack of, 379-380
research issues, 433-435
resistance to differential therapeutics,
332-333
setting, 332, 334, 336-350
social systems needed in, 369-371
somatic, recommendations concerning,
440
spontaneous improvement, 410
techniques, 334, 378-393
time-limited, 406
violent patient, 447
weekly planning conference, 432
See also Therapy

medications for, 515-522, 540-543
outpatient characteristics, 537
personnel participating in evaluation, 492-493
potential victims, protecting, 545-546
social interventions, 540
techniques to avoid provoking, 514-515, 565
therapist's safety, 544-545
toxic screen, 496
weakness as key dynamic in, 540, 546
Violent patient–victim therapy, 545
Viruses, immunity against, 211, 212
cell-mediated, 212
Vitamins:
B_6, myoclonic jerks, MAOIs and, 421, 422
B_{12}, serum, 496, 497
deficiencies, 455, 500
folate, 496, 497
Volition, decreased, 280

Wakefulness, duration of, and slow-wave sleep, 62
War neurosis, group treatment for, 356
Weakness, as key dynamic in violent patient, 540, 546

Weight:
cranial, cerebral, and frontal lobe size by, 282
gain, lithium-induced, 96, 112, 136, 757-758
and SAD, gain in, 73
Wilson's disease, 497
CNS effects, 500
Wisconsin Card Sort test, cognitive activation state, 314-316
Withdrawal, pychotherapeutic drug reactions, 702
from benzodiazepines, 420
MAOIs, 730
opioid, 495
tricyclic antidepressants, 735-736
Women, postmenopausal, LHRH in hypothalamus of, 202
See also Gender
Wyatt v. Stickney, 551, 554, 555

X-ray computed tomography, in psychiatry, 260-275, 287-293

Youngberg v. Romeo, 550-551, 554, 555

Zemelidine, norepinephrine-uptake inhibition, 170